Pathologies

SIXTH EDITION

A Massage Therapist's Guide to Pathology

Ruth Werner, LMP, NCTMB

Wolters Kluwer

Philadelphia • Baltimore • New York • London
Buenos Aires • Hong Kong • Sydney • Tokyo

Acquisitions Editor: Jay Campbell
Product Development Editor: Linda G. Francis
Marketing Manager: Leah Thomson
Editorial Assistant: Tish Rogers
Design Coordinator: Stephen Druding
Manufacturing Coordinator: Margie Orzech
Prepress Vendor: SPi Global

Sixth edition

Two Commerce Square
2001 Market Street
Philadelphia, PA 19103 USA
LWW.com

Printed in China

Library of Congress Cataloging-in-Publication Data
Werner, Ruth (Ruth A.), author.
A massage therapist's guide to pathology / Ruth Werner. — Sixth edition.
p. ; cm.
Includes bibliographical references and index.
ISBN 978-1-4963-1082-8 (alk. paper)
I. Title.
[DNLM: 1. Massage. 2. Diagnosis, Differential. WB 537]
RM721
615.8'22—dc23

2015005686

Care has been taken to confirm the accuracy of the information presented and to describe generally accepted practices. However, the authors, editors, and publisher are not responsible for errors or omissions or for any consequences from application of the information in this book and make no warranty, expressed or implied, with respect to the currency, completeness, or accuracy of the contents of the publication. Application of the information in a particular situation remains the professional responsibility of the practitioner.

The authors, editors, and publisher have exerted every effort to ensure that drug selection and dosage set forth in this text are in accordance with current recommendations and practice at the time of publication. However, in view of ongoing research, changes in government regulations, and the constant flow of information relating to drug therapy and drug reactions, the reader is urged to check the package insert for each drug for any change in indications and dosage and for added warnings and precautions. This is particularly important when the recommended agent is a new or infrequently employed drug.

Some drugs and medical devices presented in the publication have Food and Drug Administration (FDA) clearance for limited use in restricted research settings. It is the responsibility of the health care provider to ascertain the FDA status of each drug or device planned for use in their clinical practice.

To purchase additional copies of this book, call our customer service department at (800) 638-3030 or fax orders to (301) 223-2320. International customers should call (301) 223-2300.

Visit Lippincott Williams & Wilkins on the Internet: at LWW.com. Lippincott Williams & Wilkins customer service representatives are available from 8:30 am to 6 pm, EST.

10 9 8 7 6 5 4 3 2 1

This book is and will forever be dedicated to
the memory of my grandmother, Dora Charak Beckhard,
who probably never got a massage in her life—
but she sure could have used one.

I think of you every day, Dodie.

Reviewers

Steven N. Blair, PED
Departments of Exercise Science and Epidemiology & Biostatistics
Arnold School of Public Health
University of South Carolina

Fran Candelaria, MPH, BA, LMT
Kaplan College

Che Chinn, BS, LMT
International School of Skin, Nailcare & Massage Therapy

Amanda Hooten, LMT, CHT
Cumberland Institute of Holistic Therapies

Dave MacDougall, MA, LMT
North Country Community College

Niki Munk, PhD, LMT
Department of Health Sciences
School of Health and Rehabilitation Sciences
Indiana University

Susan Prasch, MEd, LMT
River Valley Community College

Tracy Walton, MS, LMT
Tracy Walton & Associates, LLC

Lisa B.S. Weaver, PTA, LMT, NCTMB
Northeast Wisconsin Technical College

About the Author

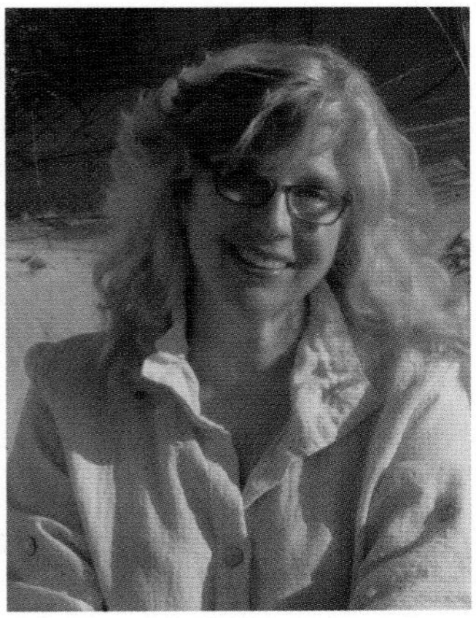

Ruth Werner is a retired massage therapist and lifelong educator with a passionate interest in the role of massage and bodywork for people who struggle with illness. She began teaching while she was still a student of massage and discovered she has a gift for taking complex topics and breaking them down to easily assimilated pieces so that learners can rebuild those ideas in their own framework. Her love of teaching has been a center point of her career, and in 2005, Ruth was honored to win the Jerome Perlinski AMTA Council of Schools Teacher of the Year award.

The first edition of *A Massage Therapist's Guide to Pathology* was published in 1998. Her second book, *Disease Handbook for Massage Therapists*, was published in 2010.

In addition to keeping *A Massage Therapist's Guide to Pathology* up to date, Ruth is a columnist for *Massage and Bodywork magazine* and is a frequent contributor to other trade journals.

Her success as a writer and educator allows her to devote time and energy to many volunteer efforts. Ruth has served on committees for the American Massage Therapy Association, the National Committee for Therapeutic Massage and Bodywork, the Federation of State Massage Therapy Boards, the Alliance for Massage Therapy Education, and the Fascia Research Society. It has been her privilege to serve as President and Trustee for the Massage Therapy Foundation..

Ruth lives on the Oregon Coast, within sight and sound of the Pacific Ocean. When she is not writing, she paints, quilts, gardens, and walks her dogs on the beach.

Acknowledgments

The thought of acknowledging all the people who have helped to shape MTGP 6e is almost paralyzing. It might be easier just to say, "Everybody I know helped me with this. Except maybe the tree trimmer. No, wait, him too."

But here is the short list anyway:

- As always, my first massage teacher, mentor, boss, model for aiming for excellence in all things, Brian Utting, and with him my first contraindications instructor, Suzanne Carlson: the two of you began a Big Thing, whether you knew it or not.
- Students, workshop participants, Facebook correspondents, and all the people I talk to about pathology: your kindness feeds everything that I do, and the users of this text will benefit from your generosity.
- The editorial staff at *Massage & Bodywork Magazine* (Leslie A. Young, PhD, and Darren Buford): your support has helped me hone my writing skills and your influence touches these pages.
- Trustees and staff at the Massage Therapy Foundation: you inspire me to be always learning.
- Friends and colleagues at Wolters Kluwer, especially Linda Francis: you are the writers' North Star. If we know where you are—and as long as you are happy—then we are safe and homeward bound. We are lucky to have you.
- The Hatters: You let me rage and boast and vent and exult on a regular basis. That's a rare privilege. Thank you.
- Special helpers: Katherine Mayerovitch, my invaluable assistant throughout, and Nathan Martin, my short-term but essential extern: this would not have happened on the timeline it did without your help. Kat, your gentle good humor and imaginative problem solving did much to keep me sane and moving forward.
- Reviewers: we worked hard on getting a wide range of eyes on this edition. A lot of the reviewers were unknown to me, so thank you in advance for your wise input. And a couple of them are very well known to me, and they both helped improve the final product in tangible, crucial ways. So, to Tracy Walton and Niki Munk: my very great gratitude.

And of course, my ever-evolving family:

Curtis, Nathan, and Lily Anne Rose, my heroes. Words fail, love triumphs. All the time, every minute, no matter what.

Preface

Thank you for picking up *A Massage Therapist's Guide to Pathology*, sixth edition, referred to here as MTGP 6e. This textbook is the culmination of over 20 years' worth of learning about massage therapy, learning about diseases and conditions, and learning about what we can observe or predict when the two meet. As the practice of massage therapy continues its journey toward being part of conventional health care, it is increasingly important for massage therapists to be able to make knowledgeable decisions as part of evidence-informed practice, and my goal is for this book to be helpful in the process.

Pathology can be a daunting subject. It can feel scary, too personal, or needlessly technical. I—to my complete surprise—turn out to love this topic, and I love writing and teaching about it. I can understand how the body breaks down, but I get really excited about how it rebuilds itself; to me this is practically miraculous. I invite readers into a learning environment that is friendly without being trivial; clear without being simplistic; and sensitive, not only to the struggles that we and our clients may live with but also to the complexities of the decisions that we must make in that context.

MTGP 6e has come a long, long way from its first edition. Williams & Wilkins took a big risk with this project in 1998, but a combination of factors that included excellent editorial support and unsurpassed book design, along with some hard work, good luck, and evolution in the massage therapy field, all combined so the book entered the market at exactly the right moment. MTGP 1e became one of the first widely adopted professionally published textbooks specifically for massage therapy in the country.

W&W is now LWW (Lippincott Williams & Wilkins), and they continue to take risks to bring the best to massage therapy education. MTGP 6e is the first project in its department to be available as a fully functioning interactive electronic textbook. All of the resources that are built into the eBook are also available to traditional hard copy users, but of course the interface is less integrated. It is a thrill to be on the leading edge of massage therapy educational systems. I had the privilege of being in that position with 1e, and years later, here we are again.

It is my hope that as massage therapy education continues to evolve, resources like this one will help our field make the transition into integrative health care easier. Massage therapy has much to offer, but only if massage therapists are critical thinkers—that is, able to balance many evaluated sources of information to come to a highly informed conclusion. Among those pieces of information …

- How does the human body work when it is healthy?
- How does a disease or condition change that process?
- Where does massage or bodywork best enter that dance?

And in the choices about massage therapy …

- What are the best possible benefits massage can offer this person?
- What are the possible risks?
- *How can I create a session that achieves the best possible benefits and avoids the risks?*

This text will help to answer all those questions except the last: that one is up to you. Your skills are yours alone, and no one will ever give a massage exactly like yours, with your unique perspective and expertise. So you alone can answer this question, using what you know about how massage works, and how your clients' challenges might be addressed by your one-of-a-kind approach.

Reader, you are doing important work. The world needs you to do it well.

Finally, my traditional closing words: I invite you to read this with joy. Do more research in what interests you. Share your findings with others. Remember that some of the questions dealt with here will probably never be completely answered. And what we think we know today may be revised or proved wrong tomorrow. Isn't that terrific?

Many thanks and many blessings,

Ruth Werner
Waldport, OR
Winter, 2015

Key Features of *A Massage Therapist's Guide to Pathology, Sixth Edition*

The Text

Conditions List

A full list of all the conditions with their subtypes and page numbers can be found on the Pathologies pages that start just after the inside front cover.

Introduction to Concepts

Chapter 1 is dedicated to introducing the language and basic concepts that frame our discussion of pathology. Here you will find Greek and Latin word roots, basic vocabulary, a discussion of adverse effects and evidence-informed practice, a discussion of pathogens and their mechanisms, hygiene for massage settings, and an overview of the inflammatory process.

The Systems and Conditions

Chapters 2 to 11 provide information organized by body systems. Each chapter begins with an overview of how the system works when it is healthy, to provide a context for what happens when disease or injury occurs. Then each condition is discussed with a definition, etiology, signs and symptoms, treatment options, medications that are likely to be in use, and a brief discussion of massage risks and benefits.

- *Chapter Objectives and Review Questions*: Chapter Objectives appear at the beginning of each chapter (with a link to expanded objectives housed on thePoint®); Chapter Review Questions appear at the end of each chapter. Each of these features has been thoroughly revised to place additional emphasis on critical thinking and practical application of the concepts discussed here.
- *Key terms*: New to the sixth edition, brief definitions of key terms are included within the chapter text: no more shuffling back and forth to the glossary.
- *Sidebars*: These contain information that is interesting, but perhaps not central to a discussion. Sidebars also contain the cancer staging protocols for all the types of cancer discussed.
- *Research boxes*: If current research is available that addresses massage or bodywork in the context of a specific condition, a brief synopsis of findings, along with links to abstracts or full articles, is included along with the risk/benefit discussion.
- *Other features*: Look for *Case Histories*, in which a person shares a personal experience of living with a specific condition; *Compare and Contrast* charts, which line up similar conditions for a side-by-side comparison; and *Notable Cases* provide examples of well-known public figures affected by a specific condition.

Cancer

Although various types of cancer are covered in the appropriate chapters, Chapter 12 is dedicated solely to a discussion of massage therapy in the context of cancer in general. This chapter contains a look at the process of metastasis, what treatment options are available, and a thorough description of when and how massage therapy applications must be adapted for the special challenges of these diseases and their treatments.

Appendices

Appendix A, **Medications** is a fully revised and updated, with a new piece on the most commonly prescribed medications in the United States; each of those drugs is described in the appendix, along with many others.

Appendix B, **Evidence-Informed Practice** picks up on themes introduced in Chapter 1, with guidance about how to become a research literate professional, and how to use that skill to achieve the best possible client outcomes.

Appendix C, **Extra Conditions—At a Glance**: this feature provides a thumbnail sketch of about 100 conditions and subtypes that are not often seen in everyday practice but that have some important relevance for massage therapists.

Bibliography

A textbook is only as good as its sources. A full bibliography is provided so that readers who want to learn more about any given topic can pursue it through resources that have already been shown to be useful. Do you have a client with a particular condition, and you want to get more information? Look for that topic in the bibliography, and start with those resources.

Online Resources for Learners

- *Audio glossary*: if you can't say a word, you don't own it. Have you found a difficult-to-pronounce term? Check the audio glossary.
- *Video extras*: taken from LWW's extensive library, we offer short animations, patient interviews, cadaver videos, and extra commentary from the author to create a more full and rich understanding of given topics.
- *Quick Reference Guide*: This is a very brief look at every condition in the text, providing a definition, signs and symptoms, and proposed massage risks and benefits. This is also formatted as an electronic flash card for self-quizzing.
- *Interactive art*: Most chapters have at least one illustration that has been made available as a student activity to label.
- *Full Chapter Objectives:* Each chapter in the text begins with Chapter Objectives. In Chapters 2 to 11, these apply to the introduction only. Expanded Chapter Objectives for each condition can be found at thePoint®. Your instructor can pick and choose which ones to share with you, depending on which conditions are included in your syllabus.
- *Chapter Review Question answers:* Check your understanding with these answers.
- *Chapter Practice Quizzes:* These are a great way to practice your multiple-choice skills, as well as preparing for school and credentialing exams.
- *Chapter Games:* Learning games have become a popular feature of MTGP. The sixth edition offers specially created versions of …
    - **Robot Man** (Like Hangman, only less violent)
    - **Crossword puzzles** (Self-evident)
    - **Quiz Show** (Answer questions! Imagine winning big prizes!)
    - And new with this edition…
        - **Vocabulary Game**: specific to Chapter 1, solidify your foundation in pathology by making sure you understand the key terms.
        - **Design a Session**: intake forms filled out by fictional characters will provide information on which you must design what to include, what to omit, and what especially to emphasize in session design.
        - **Sequence the Sequelae**: steps in the disease process are all mixed up; you must put them in the correct order.

Resources for Educators

MTGP 6e and its support materials have been configured to make teaching pathology as exciting and rich as possible. The text can carry students from basic vocabulary up through complex decision making, with your help to identify the key decision-making points along the way.

Curriculum Guide and Entry Level Analysis Program (ELAP)

For educators who are hoping for some guidance in building a curriculum and creating a usable syllabus, a document offering some suggestions is available.

All of the teaching ancillaries have been designed to coordinate with ELAP recommendations for curriculum development and assessment. Questions in the text and the Test Bank address the cognitive domain and are formulated on two levels of understanding: Level 1 ("Receive and Respond") and Level 2 ("Apply").

Other student activities, especially the *Design a Session* game and the *What Would You Do?* questions address Level 3 cognitive processes ("Choose and Plan"). This scaffolding of information from building blocks to complex decision making is the basis of effective learning, and we have worked to create a resource that supports this process in the classroom and in independent study.

Lecture Notes, Handouts

Lecture notes using the outline structure of the text are available by chapter or by topic, so you can select the items you want for a specific lecture. These can also be adapted to be used as student handouts.

Power Point Slides

Power point slides are also organized by chapter or by topic, so you can customize your own slide deck for each class. Slides and lecture notes contain essentially the same text, but the slides also have embedded illustrations and links to supporting video.

Chapter Objectives

Each chapter in the text begins with Chapter Objectives. In Chapters 2 to 11, these apply to the introduction only. Expanded Chapter Objectives for each condition can be found in the educator ancillaries, and you can pick and choose which ones to share with students when you select conditions to be included in your syllabus.

Chapter Review Questions

The Chapter Review Questions help to reinforce key concepts in multiple choice, matching, and short-answer formats. These can be used as student assignments, study recommendations, or small group activities.

Student Activities

Suggested Student Activities and games range from labeling unmarked illustrations to role-playing complex and nuanced client-therapist interactions. These can be used during class time or as supplementary work.

Test Bank

The Test Bank is thoroughly revised and updated, and each item is coded to match specific Chapter Objectives at either Level 1 or Level 2. You can pull a selection of questions for a quiz or test that apply to a given objective. You can also use items from the Test Bank as independent study assignments, to help cover material that is not addressed during lectures.

User's Guide

A *Massage Therapist's Guide* to Pathology gives you the tools to make informed decisions about bodywork for clients who live with a wide variety of diseases and conditions. This user's guide shows how to put the book's features to work for you.

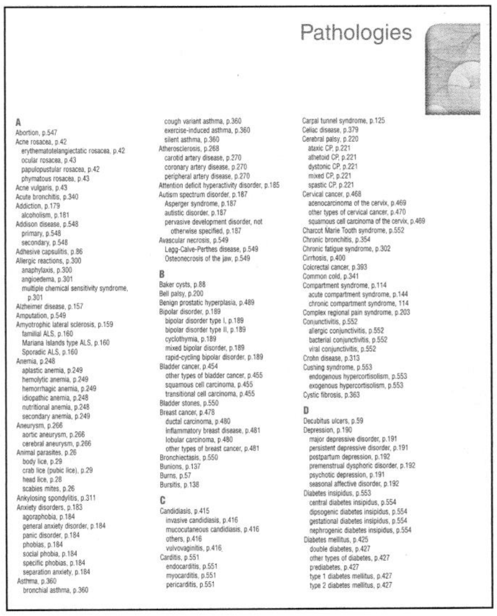

Pathologies

A
Abortion, p.547
Acne rosacea, p.42
erythematotelangiectatic rosacea, p.42
ocular rosacea, p.43
papulopustular rosacea, p.42
phymatous rosacea, p.43
Acne vulgaris, p.43
Acute bronchitis, p.340
Addiction, p.179
alcoholism, p.181
Addison disease, p.548
primary, p.548
secondary, p.548
Adhesive capsulitis, p.86
Allergic reactions, p.300
anaphylaxis, p.300
angioedema, p.301
multiple chemical sensitivity syndrome, p.301
Alzheimer disease, p.157
Amputation, p.549
Amyotrophic lateral sclerosis, p.159
familial ALS, p.160
Mariana Islands type ALS, p.160
Sporadic ALS, p.160
Anemia, p.248
aplastic anemia, p.249
hemolytic anemia, p.249
hemorrhagic anemia, p.249
idiopathic anemia, p.248
nutritional anemia, p.248
secondary anemia, p.249
Aneurysm, p.266
aortic aneurysm, p.266
cerebral aneurysm, p.266
Animal parasites, p.26
body lice, p.29
crab lice (pubic lice), p.29
head lice, p.28
scabies mites, p.26
Ankylosing spondylitis, p.311
Anxiety disorders, p.183
agoraphobia, p.184
general anxiety disorder, p.184
panic disorder, p.184
phobias, p.184
social phobia, p.184
specific phobias, p.184
separation anxiety, p.184
Asthma, p.360
bronchial asthma, p.360
cough variant asthma, p.360
exercise-induced asthma, p.360
silent asthma, p.360
Atherosclerosis, p.268
carotid artery disease, p.270
coronary artery disease, p.270
peripheral artery disease, p.270
Attention deficit hyperactivity disorder, p.185
Autism spectrum disorder, p.187
Asperger syndrome, p.187
autistic disorder, p.187
pervasive development disorder, not otherwise specified, p.187
Avascular necrosis, p.549
Legg-Calve-Perthes disease, p.549
Osteonecrosis of the jaw, p.549

B
Baker cysts, p.88
Bell palsy, p.200
Benign prostatic hyperplasia, p.489
Bipolar disorder, p.189
bipolar disorder type I, p.189
bipolar disorder type II, p.189
cyclothymia, p.189
mixed bipolar disorder, p.189
rapid-cycling bipolar disorder, p.189
Bladder cancer, p.454
other types of bladder cancer, p.455
squamous cell carcinoma, p.455
transitional cell carcinoma, p.455
Bladder stones, p.550
Breast cancer, p.478
ductal carcinoma, p.480
inflammatory breast disease, p.481
lobular carcinoma, p.480
other types of breast cancer, p.481
Bronchiectasis, p.550
Bunions, p.137
Burns, p.57
Bursitis, p.138

C
Candidiasis, p.415
invasive candidiasis, p.416
mucocutaneous candidiasis, p.416
others, p.416
vulvovaginitis, p.416
Carditis, p.551
endocarditis, p.551
myocarditis, p.551
pericarditis, p.551
Carpal tunnel syndrome, p.125
Celiac disease, p.379
Cerebral palsy, p.220
ataxic CP, p.221
athetoid CP, p.221
dystonic CP, p.221
mixed CP, p.221
spastic CP, p.221
Cervical cancer, p.468
acenocarcinoma of the cervix, p.469
other types of cervical cancer, p.470
squamous cell carcinoma of the cervix, p.469
Charcot Marie Tooth syndrome, p.552
Chronic bronchitis, p.354
Chronic fatigue syndrome, p.302
Cirrhosis, p.400
Colcrectal cancer, p.393
Common cold, p.341
Compartment syndrome, p.114
acute compartment syndrome, p.144
chronic compartment syndrome, 114
Complex regional pain syndrome, p.203
Conjunctivitis, p.552
allergic conjunctivitis, p.552
bacterial conjunctivitis, p.552
viral conjunctivitis, p.552
Crohn disease, p.313
Cushing syndrome, p.553
endogenous hypercortisolism, p.553
exogenous hypercortisolism, p.553
Cystic fibrosis, p.363

D
Decubitus ulcers, p.59
Depression, p.190
major depressive disorder, p.191
persistent depressive disorder, p.191
postpartum depression, p.192
premenstrual dysphoric disorder, p.192
psychotic depression, p.191
seasonal affective disorder, p.192
Diabetes insipidus, p.553
central diabetes insipidus, p.554
dipsogenic diabetes insipidus, p.554
gestational diabetes insipidus, p.554
nephrogenic diabetes insipidus, p.554
Diabetes mellitus, p.425
double diabetes, p.427
other types of diabetes, p.427
prediabetes, p.427
type 1 diabetes mellitus, p.427
type 2 diabetes mellitus, p.427

The Pathologies

Every condition in the book and its subtypes are listed in alphabetical order with page numbers; this list is in the front matter of the text.

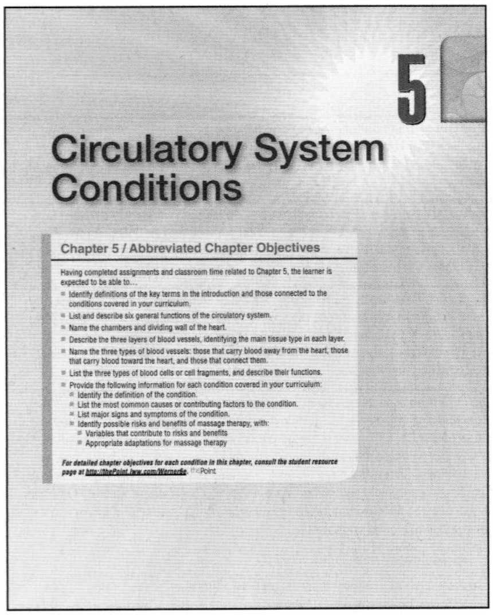

5

Circulatory System Conditions

Chapter 5 / Abbreviated Chapter Objectives

Having completed assignments and classroom time related to Chapter 5, the learner is expected to be able to...

- Identify definitions of the key terms in the introduction and those connected to the conditions covered in your curriculum.
- List and describe six general functions of the circulatory system.
- Name the chambers and dividing wall of the heart.
- Describe the three layers of blood vessels, identifying the main tissue type in each layer.
- Name the three types of blood vessels: those that carry blood away from the heart, those that carry blood toward the heart, and those that connect them.
- List the three types of blood cells or cell fragments, and describe their functions.
- Provide the following information for each condition covered in your curriculum:
  - Identify the definition of the condition.
  - List the most common causes or contributing factors to the condition.
  - List major signs and symptoms of the condition.
  - Identify possible risks and benefits of massage therapy, with:
    - Variables that contribute to risks and benefits
    - Appropriate adaptations for massage therapy

For detailed chapter objectives for each condition in this chapter, consult the student resource page at http://thePoint.lww.com/Werner6e. thePoint

Chapter Objectives

Newly revised Objectives begin every chapter, alerting the reader to important concepts and providing a framework for independent study. For a more targeted focus, chapter objectives specific to particular conditions appear online.

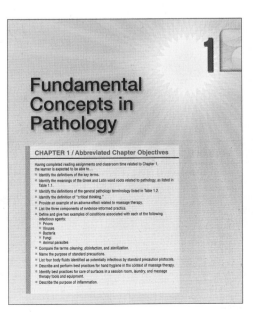

1

Fundamental Concepts in Pathology

CHAPTER 1 / Abbreviated Chapter Objectives

Having completed reading assignments and classroom time related to Chapter 1, the learner is expected to be able to...

- Identify the definitions of the key terms.
- Identify the meanings of the Greek and Latin word roots related to pathology, as listed in Table 1.1.
- Identify the definitions of the general pathology terminology listed in Table 1.2.
- Identify the definition of "critical thinking."
- Provide an example of an adverse effect related to massage therapy.
- List the three components of evidence-informed practice.
- Define and give two examples of conditions associated with each of the following infectious agents:
  - Prions
  - Viruses
  - Bacteria
  - Fungi
  - Animal parasites
- Compare the terms *cleaning, disinfection,* and *sterilization.*
- Name the purpose of standard precautions.
- List four body fluids identified as potentially infectious by standard precaution protocols.
- Describe and perform best practices for hand hygiene in the context of massage therapy.
- Identify best practices for care of surfaces in a session room, laundry, and massage therapy tools and equipment.
- Describe the purpose of inflammation.

Introductory Chapter

Chapter 1 introduces key concepts on which the study of pathology is built. Terminology, infectious agents, hygienic methods, and the inflammatory agents are discussed here. This chapter also covers adverse effects of massage, as well as the importance of evidence-informed practice.

Body System Overviews

Chapters 2 to 11 open with a brief review of the body system under discussion, with special emphasis on processes that may be interrupted by conditions that change the way we function.

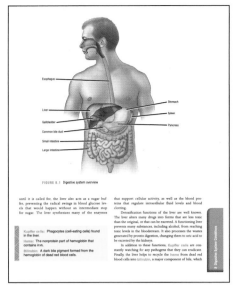

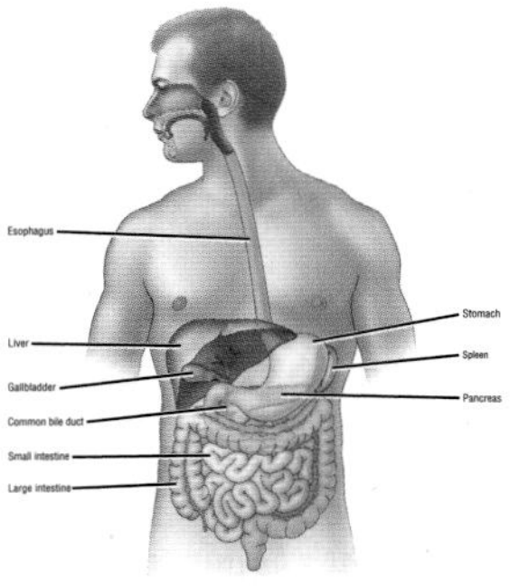

FIGURE 9.1 Digestive system overview

until it is called for, the liver also acts as a sugar buffer, preventing the radical swings in blood glucose levels that would happen without an intermediate stop for sugar. The liver synthesizes many of the enzymes that support cellular activity, as well as the blood proteins that regulate intracellular fluid levels and blood clotting.

Detoxification functions of the liver are well known. The liver alters many drugs into forms that are less toxic than the original, or that can be excreted. A functioning liver prevents many substances, including alcohol, from reaching toxic levels in the bloodstream. It also processes the wastes generated by protein digestion, changing them to uric acid to be excreted by the kidneys.

In addition to these functions, Kupffer cells are constantly watching for any pathogens that they can eradicate. Finally, the liver helps to recycle the heme from dead red blood cells into bilirubin, a major component of bile, which

Kupffer cells: Phagocytes (cell-eating cells) found in the liver.
Heme: The nonprotein part of hemoglobin that contains iron.
Bilirubin: A dark bile pigment formed from the hemoglobin of dead red blood cells.

9 Digestive System Conditions

HPA axis: The hypothalamic-pituitary-adrenal axis, consisting of the complex interactions between these three glands.
Neuroplasticity: The ability of the central nervous system to change functionally and structurally as a result of injury or damage.

Key Terms Boxes

For easy access while reading, key terms and their definitions appear on the page where they are first discussed. These terms also appear in the Glossary.

Massage Therapy Implications

With this edition, we've made our "Risks/Benefits/Options" tables even more useful by including a "Research" row in selected conditions. This reinforces the habit of looking to the latest evidence before determining the best approach to therapy.

Massage Therapy Implications

RISKS	A client with a history of drug or alcohol abuse is at higher-than-average risk for secondary health problems, including liver damage, bacterial infections, HIV/AIDS, hepatitis, and heart problems. All of these require adjustments in bodywork choices if they impact a client's general health and resilience.
BENEFITS	Some rehabilitation facilities employ massage therapists to help ameliorate withdrawal symptoms, speed detoxification, and reduce the need for tranquilizers and other drugs. Clients who are in long-term recovery and good health can enjoy the same benefits from bodywork as the rest of the population.
OPTIONS	Current alcohol or other drug use at the time of an appointment contraindicates massage, mainly because of the risk of overwhelming the system leading to nausea and vomiting. This guideline can be a judgment call, based on the level of intoxication (one glass of wine is different from a fifth of vodka), the setting of the massage session, the behavior of the client, and the boundaries set by the therapist.
RESEARCH	Massage therapy has been used as an alternative or in addition to tranquilizers to soften the process of withdrawal and detoxification for various types of substance abuse. One study found that compared with rest, a seated massage was connected to more positive withdrawal symptom scores for an alcohol rehabilitation program.[1] Another found that massage was an effective way to manage withdrawal-related anxiety for people transitioning off of psychoactive drugs, including alcohol, cocaine, and opiates.[2] An emphasis at the National Institutes of Health on finding ways to manage pain without the risk of addictive drugs may lead to increasing interest in massage therapy for this population. 1. Reader M, Young R, Connor JP. Massage therapy improves the management of alcohol withdrawal syndrome. *Journal of Alternative and Complementary Medicine* 2005;11(2):311–313. http://www.ncbi.nlm.nih.gov/pubmed/15865498 2. Black S, Jacques K, Webber A, et al. Chair massage for treating anxiety in patients withdrawing from psychoactive drugs. *Journal of Alternative and Complementary Medicine* 2010;16(9):979–987. http://www.ncbi.nlm.nih.gov/pubmed/20799900

SIDEBAR 9.2 Managing Diabetes: Blood Glucose Highs and Lows

Keeping blood glucose within a limited range of variation can be a complicated undertaking. Normal fasting blood sugar (a measurement that is taken before eating in the morning) is 110 mg/dL of blood or less. Diabetes is diagnosed when fasting levels rise over 126 mg/dL for 2 or more consecutive days.

Another test, called the hemoglobin A1c test, measures how much sugar sticks to the hemoglobin in circulating erythrocytes. This is often considered a better long-term test, since it reflects general blood sugar levels for 3 months or more, instead of in increments of several hours. A normal reading is 4% to 5.9%; diabetes is diagnosed when A1c tests show 8% or more glucose.

The opposite problem with blood sugar can also be a problem for people with diabetes. Hypoglycemia can develop quickly if the schedule of eating and medication is disrupted in such a way that insulin levels are high, but not enough sugar is entering the bloodstream from the intestines. Hypoglycemia is recognized when circulating levels of glucose dip below 70 mg/dL.

Signs and symptoms of hypoglycemia include confusion and dizziness, feeling shaky, alterations in vision and hearing, hunger, headache, and irritability. Pale skin, racing pulse, sweating and weakness are also possible. Hypoglycemia can be dangerous; it can lead to loss of consciousness and coma. More often it simply calls for some easily absorbable simple sugar, in a hurry. Many people with diabetes will have a favorite option for this: sugar tablets, a gel tube, fruit juice, or hard candies are common options.

Hypoglycemia can develop occasionally in people who don't have diabetes, but it is typically a serious, ongoing problem only for those with a history of liver, kidney or pancreatic diseases, who have been through stomach surgery, or who have other metabolic problems.

Because massage therapy has been seen to lead to lower blood sugar levels, it is important to inform clients who have diabetes of this phenomenon, and to have a plan ahead of time in case a diabetic client feels unsteady after a session.

Sidebars

These present information that is important but peripheral to the core discussion. Disease histories, some statistics, and specific cancer staging protocols are provided in the sidebars.

CASE HISTORY 8.1 Hepatitis C: "I feel totally worthless. It sucks."

I spent a lot of time in Southeast Asia—Vietnam and afterwards. I was probably infected with hepatitis C when I was in the military.

In the late 80s I felt healthy. I was a musician and a music producer. I was into playing, engineering, stage-managing. I was on the road a lot. And it was the culture—I indulged in drugs, especially cocaine.

Then I was told I had "hep non-A, non-B."

It was all a guessing game to figure out how it happened or what to do. Everyone contradicts everyone else.

RANDY, AGE 64

Eventually, you have to go by what you trust. I ended up using some herbal remedies and supplements. I stopped drinking, and reduced stress, and things seemed to be okay. I got married, had kids, and got away from big crowds. I had learned building as another way to earn a living.

But my energy levels just got worse and worse. That was my big indicator.

It can get to where I can only work 3 or 4 hours a day. My desire to do things—to go fishing, to play music—are gone. Some days nothing matters. It impacts my home, my relationships. I feel totally worthless. It sucks.

I never treated my hep C with interferon—it turns out that the type of virus coming out of Southeast Asia had a really poor response to that. I am hoping to start a new treatment protocol this year. I feel like hep C has taken more than my energy. It's taken my personality—my whole psyche. I hope I can get some of that back.

Case Histories

These provide an important voice to the people who live with a variety of diseases and conditions. They offer insight into how some disorders powerfully influence people's lives.

COMPARE & CONTRAST 4.1 Fibromyalgia versus Myofascial Pain Syndrome

Fibromyalgia and MPS are frequently confused. Because they call for quite different treatment options, it is important to be able to recognize both their similarities and their unique qualities.

CHARACTERISTICS	FIBROMYALGIA SYNDROME	MYOFASCIAL PAIN SYNDROME
Prevalence	Up to 3% of the US population	Unknown
Demographics	85%–90% of all diagnoses are in women.	Women and men are equally affected
Prognosis	Lifelong problem; can be managed	Can be a short-term problem that is permanently solved
Primary symptoms	Tender points: predictable areas; light touch elicits intense, diffuse pain at the site	Trigger points: predictable areas in muscles; may be nodular or appear as a taut band that generates a twitch response with pressure. Manual pressure elicits pain locally and at distant areas
Implications for massage	Careful massage can help, but patients are often hypersensitive and easy to overtreat.	Responds well to massage: rhythmic pressure and release can interrupt dysfunctional signals at trigger point sites

Compare And Contrast Boxes

These put key features of closely connected disorders side by side for a point-by-point comparison of similarities and differences.

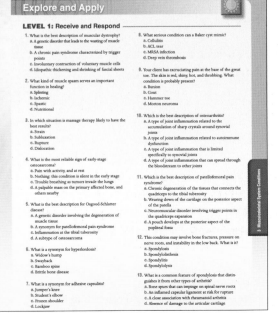

Explore and Apply

LEVEL 1: Receive and Respond

1. What is the best description of muscular dystrophy?
   a. A genetic disorder that leads to the wasting of muscle tissue
   b. A chronic pain syndrome characterized by trigger points
   c. Involuntary contraction of voluntary muscle cells
   d. Idiopathic thickening and shrinking of fascial sheets
2. What kind of muscle spasm serves an important function in healing?
   a. Splinting
   b. Ischemic
   c. Spastic
   d. Nutritional
3. In which situation is massage therapy likely to have the best results?
   a. Strain
   b. Subluxation
   c. Rupture
   d. Dislocation
4. What is the most reliable sign of early-stage osteosarcoma?
   a. Pain with activity, and at rest
   b. Nothing: this condition is silent in the early stage
   c. Trouble breathing as tumors invade the lungs
   d. A palpable mass on the primary affected bone, and others nearby
5. What is the best description for Osgood-Schlatter disease?
   a. A genetic disorder involving the degeneration of muscle tissue
   b. A synonym for patellofemoral pain syndrome
   c. Inflammation at the tibial tuberosity
   d. A subtype of osteosarcoma
6. What is a synonym for hyperlordosis?
   a. Widow's hump
   b. Swayback
   c. Bamboo spine
   d. Brittle bone disease
7. What is a synonym for adhesive capsulitis?
   a. Jumper's knee
   b. Student's elbow
   c. Frozen shoulder
   d. Lockjaw
8. What serious condition can a Baker cyst mimic?
   a. Cellulitis
   b. ACL tear
   c. MRSA infection
   d. Deep vein thrombosis
9. Your client has excruciating pain at the base of the great toe. The skin is red, shiny, hot, and throbbing. What condition is probably present?
   a. Bunion
   b. Gout
   c. Hammer toe
   d. Morton neuroma
10. Which is the best description of osteoarthritis?
    a. A type of joint inflammation related to the accumulation of sharp crystals around synovial joints
    b. A type of joint inflammation related to autoimmune dysfunction
    c. A type of joint inflammation that is limited specifically to synovial joints
    d. A type of joint inflammation that can spread through the bloodstream to other joints
11. Which is the best description of patellofemoral pain syndrome?
    a. Chronic degeneration of the tissues that connects the quadriceps to the tibial tuberosity
    b. Wearing down of the cartilage on the posterior aspect of the patella
    c. Neuromuscular disorder involving trigger points in the quadriceps expansion
    d. A pouch develops at the posterior aspect of the popliteal fossa
12. This condition may involve bone fractures, pressure on nerve roots, and instability in the low back. What is it?
    a. Spondylosis
    b. Spondylolisthesis
    c. Spondylitis
    d. Spondylolysis
13. What is a common feature of spondylosis that distinguishes it from other types of arthritis?
    a. Bone spurs that can impinge on spinal nerve roots
    b. An inflamed capsular ligament at risk for rupture
    c. A close association with rheumatoid arthritis
    d. Absence of damage to the articular cartilage

3 Musculoskeletal System Conditions

Explore and Apply

This expanded review section gives readers a variety of ways to test their knowledge, comprehension, and application of the concepts presented in the chapter. In addition to objective questions, "What Would You Do?" allows you to practice thinking like a therapist. Suggested Activities encourage more exploration to deepen your understanding even further.

Appendices

This text has three valuable appendices to take readers deeper into pathology studies.

- **Appendix A, Medications:** This appendix addresses the role of bodywork when clients use medications to treat or manage their conditions.
- **Appendix B, Research Literacy, Research Capacity:** This appendix introduces concepts in research literacy so that therapists may become familiar with the skills of reading, interpreting, and possibly even conducting research projects about massage therapy.
- **Appendix C, Extra Conditions at a Glance:** This is a collection of conditions that are interesting and pertinent, but that can be somewhat abbreviated because they are rare or seldom seen in an acute stage.

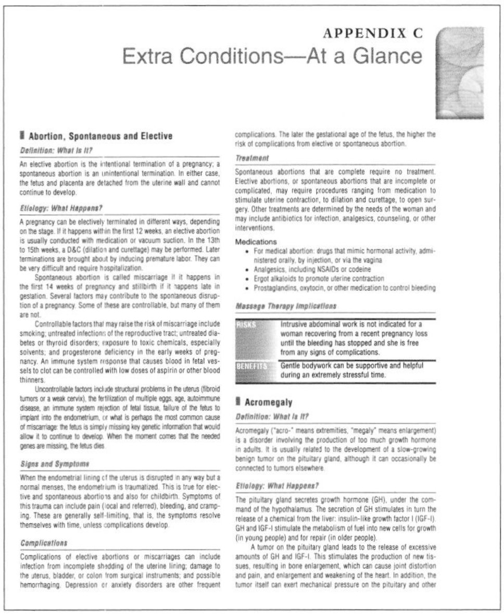
APPENDIX C

Extra Conditions—At a Glance

Abortion, Spontaneous and Elective

Definition: What Is It?

An elective abortion is the intentional termination of a pregnancy; a spontaneous abortion is an unintentional termination. In either case, the fetus and placenta are detached from the uterine wall and cannot continue to develop.

Etiology: What Happens?

A pregnancy can be electively terminated in different ways, depending on the stage. If it happens within the first 12 weeks, an elective abortion is usually conducted with medication or vacuum suction. In the 13th to 15th weeks, a D&C (dilation and curettage) may be performed. Later terminations are brought about by inducing premature labor. They can be very difficult and require hospitalization.

Spontaneous abortion is called miscarriage if it happens in the first 14 weeks of pregnancy and stillbirth if it happens late in gestation. Several factors may contribute to the spontaneous disruption of a pregnancy. Some of these are controllable, but many of them are not.

Controllable factors that may raise the risk of miscarriage include smoking; untreated infections of the reproductive tract; untreated diabetes or thyroid disorders; exposure to toxic chemicals, especially solvents; and progesterone deficiency in the early weeks of pregnancy. An immune system response that causes blood in fetal vessels to clot can be controlled with low doses of aspirin or other blood thinners.

Uncontrollable factors include structural problems in the uterus (fibroid tumors or a weak cervix), the fertilization of multiple eggs, age, autoimmune disease, an immune system rejection of fetal tissue, failure of the fetus to implant into the endometrium, or what is perhaps the most common cause of miscarriage: the fetus is simply missing key genetic information that would allow it to continue to develop. When the moment comes that the needed genes are missing, the fetus dies.

Signs and Symptoms

When the endometrial lining of the uterus is disrupted in any way but a normal menses, the endometrium is traumatized. This is true for elective and spontaneous abortions and also for childbirth. Symptoms of this trauma can include pain (local and referred), bleeding, and cramping. These are generally self-limiting, that is, the symptoms resolve themselves with time, unless complications develop.

Complications

Complications of elective abortions or miscarriages can include infection from incomplete shedding of the uterine lining; damage to the uterus, bladder, or colon from surgical instruments; and possible hemorrhaging. Depression or anxiety disorders are other frequent complications. The later the gestational age of the fetus, the higher the risk of complications from elective or spontaneous abortion.

Treatment

Spontaneous abortions that are complete require no treatment. Elective abortions, or spontaneous abortions that are incomplete or complicated, may require procedures ranging from medication to stimulate uterine contraction, to dilation and curettage, to open surgery. Other treatments are determined by the needs of the woman and may include antibiotics for infection, analgesics, counseling, or other interventions.

Medications

- For medical abortion: drugs that mimic hormonal activity, administered orally, by injection, or via the vagina
- Analgesics, including NSAIDs or codeine
- Ergot alkaloids to promote uterine contraction
- Prostaglandins, oxytocin, or other medication to control bleeding

Massage Therapy Implications

RISKS	Intrusive abdominal work is not indicated for a woman recovering from a recent pregnancy loss until the bleeding has stopped and she is free from any signs of complications.
BENEFITS	Gentle bodywork can be supportive and helpful during an extremely stressful time.

Acromegaly

Definition: What Is It?

Acromegaly ("acro-" means extremities, "megaly" means enlargement) is a disorder involving the production of too much growth hormone in adults. It is usually related to the development of a slow-growing benign tumor on the pituitary gland, although it can occasionally be connected to tumors elsewhere.

Etiology: What Happens?

The pituitary gland secretes growth hormone (GH), under the command of the hypothalamus. The secretion of GH stimulates in turn the release of a chemical from the liver: insulin-like growth factor I (IGF-I). GH and IGF-I stimulate the metabolism of fuel into new cells for growth (in young people) and for repair (in older people).

A tumor on the pituitary gland leads to the release of excessive amounts of GH and IGF-I. This stimulates the production of new tissues, resulting in bone enlargement, which can cause joint distortion and pain, and enlargement and weakening of the heart. In addition, the tumor itself can exert mechanical pressure on the pituitary and other

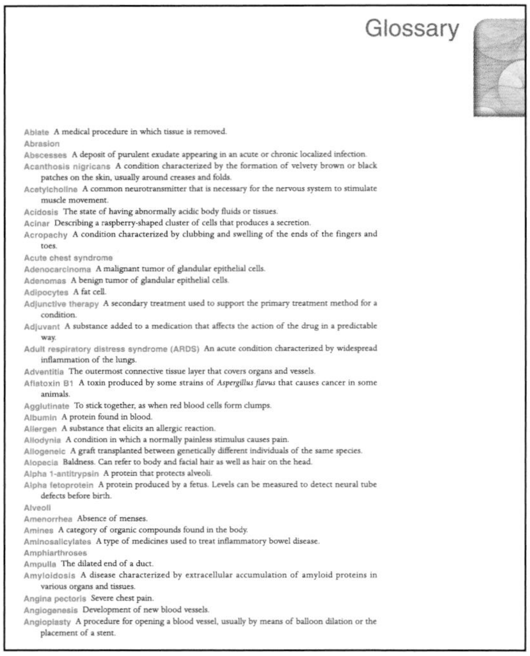
Glossary

Abiate A medical procedure in which tissue is removed.
Abrasion
Abscesses A deposit of purulent exudate appearing in an acute or chronic localized infection.
Acanthosis nigricans A condition characterized by the formation of velvety brown or black patches on the skin, usually around creases and folds.
Acetylcholine A common neurotransmitter that is necessary for the nervous system to stimulate muscle movement.
Acidosis The state of having abnormally acidic body fluids or tissues.
Acinar Describing a raspberry-shaped cluster of cells that produces a secretion.
Acropachy A condition characterized by clubbing and swelling of the ends of the fingers and toes.
Acute chest syndrome
Adenocarcinoma A malignant tumor of glandular epithelial cells.
Adenomas A benign tumor of glandular epithelial cells.
Adipocytes A fat cell.
Adjunctive therapy A secondary treatment used to support the primary treatment method for a condition.
Adjuvant A substance added to a medication that affects the action of the drug in a predictable way.
Adult respiratory distress syndrome (ARDS) An acute condition characterized by widespread inflammation of the lungs.
Adventitia The outermost connective tissue layer that covers organs and vessels.
Aflatoxin B1 A toxin produced by some strains of *Aspergillus flavus* that causes cancer in some animals.
Agglutinate To stick together, as when red blood cells form clumps.
Albumin A protein found in blood.
Allergen A substance that elicits an allergic reaction.
Allodynia A condition in which a normally painless stimulus causes pain.
Allogeneic A graft transplanted between genetically different individuals of the same species.
Alopecia Baldness. Can refer to body and facial hair as well as hair on the head.
Alpha 1-antitrypsin A protein that protects alveoli.
Alpha fetoprotein A protein produced by a fetus. Levels can be measured to detect neural tube defects before birth.
Alveoli
Amenorrhea Absence of menses.
Amines A category of organic compounds found in the body.
Aminosalicylates A type of medicines used to treat inflammatory bowel disease.
Amphiarthroses
Ampulla The dilated end of a duct.
Amyloidosis A disease characterized by extracellular accumulation of amyloid proteins in various organs and tissues.
Angina pectoris Severe chest pain.
Angiogenesis Development of new blood vessels.
Angioplasty A procedure for opening a blood vessel, usually by means of balloon dilation or the placement of a stent.

Glossary

A full glossary with definitions is provided in the text.

Online Resources

Student Resources

- Interactive quiz bank, arranged by chapter
- Animations and video clips to demonstrate several anatomical features or disease processes
- Answers to the Chapter Review questions
- Audio Glossary
- Flash cards of Greek and Latin roots and their English equivalents
- Games, including a sequencing game, crossword puzzles, robotman, and other activities
- Taking a Client History provides information on how to gather a full picture of each client's health history, with printable intake forms
- Full bibliography, including the print and electronic resources used to gather information for the text, is listed here to point the way for further research

Online Instructor's Resources

- **Pathology curriculum guidelines.** This document is based on many years of experience. It provides suggestions for how to customize a pathology course to individual needs, including how to choose content, how to use quizzes and examinations, examples of student projects, and much more
- **Syllabi.** These suggested syllabi for 40- and 60-hour pathology courses have schedules, grading guidelines, and suggested timing for quizzes and examinations
- **Lecture notes in printable form.** These outlines of the text can be used for teaching notes, student handouts, or both
- **Lecture notes as PowerPoint slides.** These can project content outlines with images embedded in the appropriate places. Condition-specific slide presentations allow instructors to easily select the tools they need for a given class
- **Images.** All of the art from the text is available in an easily downloadable format
- **Test bank.** More than 1,000 multiple-choice questions for the new edition have been compiled in a Brownstone test generator. These can be used for quizzes, tests, or homework assignments. They are coded for the Chapter Objectives as well as the ELAP recommendations.

Artwork and Photos

These are rendered in full color throughout the book to help illustrate key points. They provide a valuable resource to help readers recognize a wide range of skin conditions in various stages of severity, and explain how disease affects the body.

Contents

1

Fundamental Concepts in Pathology

CHAPTER 1 / Abbreviated Chapter Objectives

Having completed reading assignments and classroom time related to Chapter 1, the learner is expected to be able to…

- Identify the definitions of the key terms.
- Identify the meanings of the Greek and Latin word roots related to pathology, as listed in Table 1.1.
- Identify the definitions of the general pathology terminology listed in Table 1.2.
- Identify the definition of "critical thinking."
- Provide an example of an adverse effect related to massage therapy.
- List the three components of evidence-informed practice.
- Define and give two examples of conditions associated with each of the following infectious agents:
  - Prions
  - Viruses
  - Bacteria
  - Fungi
  - Animal parasites
- Compare the terms *cleaning*, *disinfection*, and *sterilization*.
- Name the purpose of standard precautions.
- List four body fluids identified as potentially infectious by standard precaution protocols.
- Describe and perform best practices for hand hygiene in the context of massage therapy.
- Identify best practices for care of surfaces in a session room, laundry, and massage therapy tools and equipment.
- Describe the purpose of inflammation.

- List four signs or symptoms of inflammation.
- Label and describe what happens during each of the three major stages of healing.
- Name three possible consequences of chronic inflammation.
- Describe three situations in which inflammation contraindicates massage.
- Describe a situation in which inflammation indicates massage.
- Identify how conventional treatment for inflammation might influence massage choices.

Introduction to Fundamental Concepts in Pathology

To undertake the study of diseases and disorders in the context of massage therapy can feel like an overwhelming task to students and practitioners. Some consider that the subject is irrelevant, either because they doubt massage has much impact on the health and disease process or because they plan to work only with healthy clients. Many massage therapists are intimidated by the thought of all the things that can go wrong with the human body. They may find medical writing confusing and obscure, or they may be squeamish about looking at pictures of sick people.

The wonderful thing about studying pathology, though, is the discovery that much of the time, even after a serious illness, *people get better*. The reparative capacity of the human body is awe-inspiring, and the study of pathology illuminates that process. And for people who don't recover—for those who live with chronic diseases that can be managed but not eradicated, or those whose condition marks the end of life—those people too have much to teach us about living in grace and finding power, pleasure, and fullness from every moment. It is a deep and important privilege for a massage therapist to be invited into that process.

This chapter lays out some of the starting principles for the study of pathology for massage therapists. Being familiar with key concepts will help the reader integrate and mentally organize the rest of the material in this text. We introduce ideas about critical thinking and evidence-informed practice, and terminology for pathology discussions, and then look at common infectious agents, hygienic practices, and principles of the inflammatory process.

Critical Thinking and Practical Application

A Massage Therapist's Guide to Pathology: Critical Thinking and Practical Application is dedicated to helping massage therapists achieve the best results with clients who have simple or complex health issues. We will emphasize how to use the information you find here to make choices that are informed by the many variables that lead to the best possible client outcomes.

Critical Thinking

The term "critical thinking" has a specific meaning in this context. It means taking information that you have acquired and evaluated, and using it to guide your actions. Every time we touch a client, we process a huge amount of information. Some of it isn't important, and lots of it flies under the radar of our consciousness. But the best massage therapists develop their ability to filter out unimportant noise and to process relevant input, using it help their clients. This can happen in real time with hands on the client, and in preparation time, as we get ready to offer our best work. Ultimately, this is what the study of pathology requires as well: the ability to hone in on what is important and to use that information to make the best choices for your client.

Practical Application

Some readers of this textbook will find it fascinating and exciting, and they will want to go on to learn more about the details of diseases and conditions that interest them. That's wonderful, but that is not the intended outcome for this book. The primary purposes of this text are twofold: they are to provide knowledge about important topics and to provide ideas for how to put that knowledge to use in your session room. For example, knowing that herpes simplex is a tough, resilient virus is one thing, but knowing how to manage infection risk in a massage practice is even more important.

One of the ways that this book emphasizes turning critical thinking into action is in the "Explore and Apply" section of each chapter. There you will find questions based on basic vocabulary and ideas ("Receive and Respond") and another set of questions based on how to put those ideas to use ("Practical Application").

Adverse Effects, and How to Avoid Them

Among the variables that we need to process with our clients is the possibility of an **adverse effect**. An "adverse effect" or "adverse event" is a harmful or undesired outcome from some intervention. Every health care intervention has the potential for a negative outcome. The more invasive the intervention is, the higher the risks are for a bad outcome: the possible adverse effects for orthopedic surgery, for instance, include forming a blood clot that goes to the lungs (**pulmonary embolism**) or developing a life-threatening secondary infection.

Massage therapy is not usually considered to be a high-risk intervention, as the adverse effect most often seen with our work is minor muscle soreness for a day or two. Massage therapy is not risk free, however, and one of the reasons for pathology courses is to help massage therapists to work safely.

Adverse effects relating to massage have been documented and published in the medical literature, usually by the medical doctors who treat the aftermath of sessions gone wrong. A 2012 systematic review of articles lists massage session–related injuries ranging from **spinal cord injury**, to rupture of the bladder, to rhabdomyolysis: an emergency situation that can lead **to renal failure**. Other publications include case reports on massage and a ruptured renal cyst, damage to the spinal accessory nerve, and the collapse and fragmenting of stents in the iliac arteries.

It is important to point out that adverse effects in massage are relatively rare. Further, not all of these events were related to work being done by a trained massage therapist; in many of the reports, the practitioner is not identified by a title, or the treatment was done with a tool or machine rather than by hand.

That doesn't let us off the hook, however. What is reported in the medical literature is only a tiny portion of the damage that happens in massage session rooms every day. And as more and more clients seek massage to help deal with stress and medical conditions, the process of making informed decisions on their behalf becomes increasingly complicated.

Pathologies cannot be "rubber-stamped" for the appropriateness of massage, because clients' needs change from day to day. A physician's permission does not guarantee that a massage therapist's work will be safe or that a client won't be harmed. The best way to move forward is to be able to identify the key variables in each client's situation that will provide the information to answer these questions:

- What is the best thing that massage can provide to this client?
- What is the worst thing that could happen if this client receives the wrong kind of bodywork?
- How can I design a session that eliminates the risks while maximizing those benefits?

Only you can answer that last question. Your best answers will be based on three things: your own training and expertise, the client's needs and priorities, and finally, what the research says about massage in that context: this is the essence of **evidence-informed practice**.

> **Adverse effect:** A harmful or undesired outcome from some intervention.
>
> **Evidence-informed practice:** The use of client goals and values, practitioner judgment, and research findings to inform therapeutic choices.

Evidence-Informed Practice

Evidence-based practice is a term developed in 1992 and described as "the conscientious, explicit, and judicious use of current best evidence in making decisions about the care of individual patients."[1]

Amazingly, the medical profession had no publicly stated expectation of, or commitment to, using the results of research in clinical decision making before then.

By 1996, the novel idea of using what the research says (as opposed to relying mainly on tradition and folklore) to inform decisions in medical practice was further developed to include three major points of focus: the expertise of the clinician, the desires and goals of the patient, and what the best research evidence reveals (Figure 1.1). Ideally, all three of these components should contribute to clinical decision making.

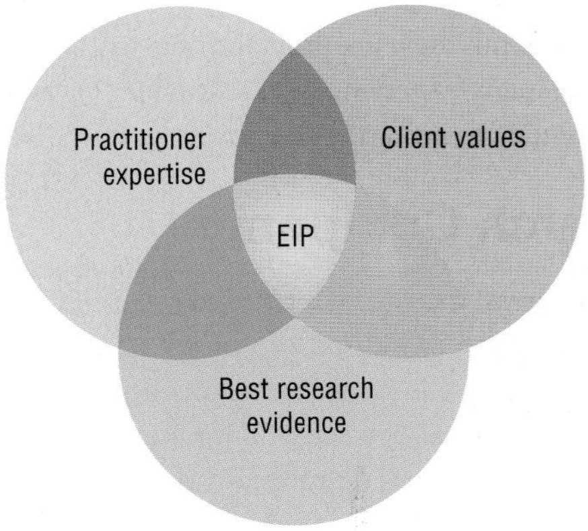

FIGURE 1.1 Evidence-informed practice encompasses practitioner expertise, client goals and values, and the best research evidence to create a treatment strategy

[1]Sackett DL, Rosenberg WM, Gray JAM, et al. Evidence based medicine: what it is and what it isn't. *British Medical Journal* 1996;312:71–72.

Clinical decision making must go through the same steps in the practice of massage therapy as it does in any health care profession. It involves considering a multitude of variables connected to these three components and then developing session strategies that address the client's goals, while maximizing benefits and minimizing any potential risks.

Client Component

A Massage Therapist's Guide to Pathology: Critical Thinking, Practical Application provides information that can help identify the variables connected to the client's place in evidence-informed practice. In the "client" circle, we find his or her values, along with goals, priorities, and current physical state. Too often, the client's goals give way to the massage therapist's goals. In these situations, someone with sore legs gets a long shoulder massage, or someone who wants to relax gets a massage that challenges her pain threshold. It is critical that every session begin with the question "what would you like to accomplish today?" whether it is a first-time massage or a hundredth-time massage.

In the context of pathology, this means the massage therapist must consider the general health, resilience, and adaptability of the client, along with any conditions that may be present, and in what stage they may be. Any treatment regimens, including exercise protocols, surgery, or medications, may also influence predictions about the possible risks and benefits of massage therapy.

Practitioner Component

The "practitioner" circle must be informed by your own knowledge, skills, and abilities. You alone can determine whether the work you do is within your client's capacity to adapt, regardless of whether you call your massage modality "deep tissue," "myofascial release," or "Pfrimmering." Some guidance about massage modalities is provided in the online Modality Recommendation Charts available at http://thePoint.lww.com. thePoint, but these are provided only to give some insight about what many experienced practitioners have found; they are not intended to prescribe or limit types of massage.

Research Component

To help address the "research" circle, a brief synopsis of current relevant research accompanies many of the items in this book, but this is by no means a comprehensive or exhaustively analyzed list; nor will it remain timely. Research findings about massage therapy are produced and updated frequently, and if we want to claim that we commit to evidence-informed practice, we need to incorporate those findings into our clinical decision making alongside our client's priorities and our own expertise. This requires a basic level of research literacy: the ability to find, read, evaluate, and apply research findings. More information on research literacy is provided in Appendix B.

In the absence of accessible research findings, other textbooks and reliable online sources are still valuable, but it is important to become an informed and discerning consumer of information.

It can be challenging to keep all these factors in mind as we strategize plans for our clients. We need to be able to analyze and synthesize information from multiple sources to help us make good decisions in the moment. This is the essence of critical thinking: turning carefully evaluated information into appropriate action on behalf of our clients. No book or single resource can do that for you; all we can do here is provide some of the information that will influence your choices. The rest is up to you.

Terminology

Critical thinking in pathology begins with breaking down the language barrier. Many people who are new to the field of massage are surprised to find that the study of anatomy, physiology, and pathology requires learning a new language. It doesn't take much, but a smattering of Greek and Latin not only can help to demystify anatomical terminology but can even make it fun. Knowing that *vermiform appendix* really means *hanging thing that looks like a worm* adds tremendous satisfaction to learning new ways to describe the body.

The list in Table 1.1 includes the Greek and Latin fragments that are most useful in the study of pathology. This is not a comprehensive or exhaustive list, and it omits many of the terms that turn up in beginning anatomy courses. It does include most of the roots for terms that are used in this book, however. Familiarity with these word fragments will make the study of pathology much more enjoyable.

In addition to Greek and Latin word roots that form the basis for much medical terminology, it is important to define some central ideas. Table 1.2 provides basic definitions for key terms used throughout this text. Finally, some vocabulary that may be new to you appears in each chapter. To help you with these words, you will find them in the margins, close to where they are first used (see p. 3 for example).

Infectious Agents

Disease-causing organisms are called pathogens. The many thousands of pathogens that can threaten human health have been categorized into five basic types: prions, viruses, bacteria, fungi, and animal parasites. These organisms are the causes of many diseases, some of which are communicable. However, any individual's ability to resist pathogenic invasion may be at least partly determined by other modifiable factors. That is to say, a person who exercises carefully and eats well, who gets plenty of good-quality sleep, and who has a generally positive

TABLE 1.1 Greek and Latin Word Parts

Word Parts	Meaning	Example
a-, an-	Without	Malignant melanoma lesions may show as **a**symmetrical discolorations on the skin.
acro-	Extremity	**Acral** lentiginous melanoma usually begins on the fingers or toes.
adeno-	Glandular	**Adeno**carcinoma is cancer that begins in glands.
-algia	Pain	An an**alge**sic is a painkiller.
angio-	Blood or lymph vessels	**Angio**genesis is the production of new blood vessels.
arthr-	Joint	**Arthro**plasty is surgical implantation of an artificial joint, often to treat osteo**arthr**itis.
brady-	Slow	**Brady**cardia means slow heartbeat.
carcin-	Crab (cancer)	A **carcin**ogen is a cancer-triggering agent.
cardio-	Heart	**Cardio**myopathy refers to damaged heart muscle.
cervi-, cervico-	Neck	**Cervi**cal cancer originates in cells found in the neck of the uterus.
-cele	Swelling, hernia	In spina bifida meningo**cele**, the dura mater and arachnoid protrude through an incompletely closed vertebral arch.
cep-, ceph-	Head, brain	En**ceph**alitis refers to inflammation of the brain.
chole	Bile	**Chole**cyst is another term for gallbladder.
com-, con-	With, together	A **con**centric muscle **con**traction brings the bony attachments closer together.
contra-	Against	A coup-**contre**coup head injury occurs when the brain hits the opposite side of the cranium from the direction of the original blow.
cyst	Hollow organ	Chole**cyst**itis is inflammation of the gallbladder.
demo-	People	**Demo**graphics is recorded information about a specific group of people.
derm-	Skin	**Derm**atophytosis is the condition of having plants (in this case fungi) growing on the skin.
dia-	Through	**Dia**betes mellitus means *sweetness flowing through*, referring to excessive production of urine that is high in sugar.
dys-	Difficulty	**Dys**phagia is difficulty with swallowing or eating.
ecto-, -ectomy	Outside, removal	An append**ectomy** is the removal of the appendix.
-emia	Blood	Septic**emia** is a type of infection of the blood.
endo-	Inside	An **endo**scopy is a test to examine the lining of the gastrointestinal tract.
epi-	Upon	An **epi**demic is a contagious disease that affects a lot of people. (Literally this word means *upon the people*.)
erythr-	Red	**Erythr**opoietin is a hormone that stimulates production of red blood cells.
ex-	Out of	**Ex**ophthalmos is a condition in which the eyes bulge out of their usual position.
-gen	Beginning, producing	An aller**gen** is an allergy-producing substance.

(table continues on page 6)

TABLE 1.1 Greek and Latin Word Parts (continued)

Word Parts	Meaning	Example
glyco-	Relating to sugar	Hypo**glyc**emia is another term for low blood sugar.
-graphy	Recording, writing	Veno**graphy** is a test to measure blood flow through veins.
hemi-	Half	**Hemi**plegic cerebral palsy affects half of the body.
hemo-	Blood	**Hemo**rrhage means *flowing blood.*
hepat-	Liver	**Hepat**itis is inflammation of the liver.
hydro-	Water	**Hydro**cephalus is a condition involving too much cerebrospinal fluid.
hyper-	Above, too much	**Hyper**uricemia describes having too much uric acid in the blood.
hypo-	Below, too little	**Hypo**tension is another term for low blood pressure.
-itis	Inflammation	Arthr**itis** is inflammation of a joint.
kine-	Movement	**Kinesiology** is the study of movement.
-lepsis	Seizure	Epi**lepsy** is a type of seizure disorder.
leuko-	White	**Leuk**emia is a cancer involving overproduction of white blood cells.
lipo-	Fat	Hyper**lip**idemia describes high levels of fat in the blood.
litho-	Rock	The presence of a kidney stone is nephro**lith**iasis.
-logy	Study	Patho**logy** is the study of disease.
-lysis, -lyso	Destruction	Para**lysis** is the loss of normal function.
mega-	Large	Spleno**mega**ly (enlarged spleen) is a potential complication of mononucleosis.
meno-	Month	**Men**struation is the monthly detachment and expulsion of the uterine lining.
metr-	Mother (uterus)	The endo**metr**ium is the inner lining of the uterus.
micro-	Small	**Micro**graphia (shrinking of handwriting) is a possible symptom of Parkinson disease.
myco-	Fungus	**Myco**sis is any disease caused by a yeast or a fungus.
mye-	Marrow or spinal cord	A **mye**locele is a protrusion of the spinal cord, seen with some types of spina bifida.
myo-	Muscle	Fibro**my**algia describes "fiber muscle pain."
narco-	Stupor	**Narco**lepsy means sleep seizure.
necro-	Death	**Necro**sis is the condition of tissue death.
neo-	New	A **neo**plasm is a new formation; it sometimes refers to a cancerous growth.
nephro-	Kidney	**Neph**ritis is the inflammation of a kidney.
neuro-	Nerve	Peripheral **neuro**pathy is a complication of untreated diabetes mellitus.
-oid	Resembles	The sigm**oid** colon looks like an **S**.
-oma	Tumor	A lip**oma** is a benign fatty tumor.
onco-	Tumor	An **onco**logist is a doctor who specializes in cancer.

Word Parts	Meaning	Example
onyx-	Nail	**Onych**olysis describes the destruction of the nail.
orchi-	Testes	**Orchi**tis is inflammation of the testicles.
-osis	Pathologic condition	Hyperkyph**osis** is the condition of having an accentuated kyphotic curve.
osteo-	Bone	**Osteo**porosis is the condition of developing porous bones.
para-	Alongside, near	The **para**spinal muscles run **para**llel to the spine.
-penia	Lack of, shortage	Leuko**penia** refers to an abnormally low number of white blood cells.
peri-	Around	The **peri**cardium wraps around the heart.
phagia-	Eating	Poly**phagia**, or constant hunger, is a symptom of diabetes mellitus.
-philia	Affinity	Hemo**philia** is a blood clotting disorder.
phleb-	Vein	Thrombo**phleb**itis is inflammation of a vein because of a clot.
phyto-	Plants	Dermato**phyto**sis is another term for fungal infection of the skin.
-plasia	Growth	Hyper**plasia** means too much growth.
-plasm, -plasma	Formed	A wart is a type of neo**plasm**.
patho-	Disease state	A **patho**gen is a disease-causing organism.
physio-	Nature	**Physio**logy is the study of normal life functions.
pseudo-	False	**Pseudo**gout involves different chemical deposits from those seen with acute gouty arthritis.
psych-	The mind, mental	**Psych**ogenic tremor develops in stressful situations.
Radix	Root	**Radic**ulopathy is a disorder of spinal nerve roots.
ren-	Kidney	The ad**ren**al glands are on top of the kidneys.
-rrhagia, -rrhea	Flowing	A hemo**rrhage** is uncontrolled bleeding.
rhino-	Nose	A **rhino**plasty is a nose job.
sarco-	Flesh	Kaposi s**arco**ma is a type of cancer.
sclero-	Hardness, scarring	**Sclero**derma is a disease involving the hardening of the skin.
spondy-	Spine	**Spondy**losis is osteoarthritis in the spine.
-stasis	Stagnation, standing still	**Stasis** dermatitis is related to poor circulation.
stoma-	An opening; mouth	**Stoma**titis is the development of inflamed lesions at the corners of the mouth.
syn-, sym-	With	The two pubic bones come together at the **sym**physis pubis.
thrombo-	Clot	Deep vein **thrombo**sis is a risk factor for pulmonary embolism.
therm-	Temperature	Hypo**therm**ia is the state of getting too cold.
-trophy, -trophic	Nutrition, growth	Muscular dys**trophy** is a condition in which muscles degenerate.
vaso-	Blood vessel	Raynaud syndrome involves severe **vaso**spasm in the extremities.

TABLE 1.2 Pathology Terms

Term	Definition
Acute	Rapid onset, brief, can be severe
Chronic	Prolonged, long-term, can be low intensity
Comorbid, comorbidity	Coexistence of two or more disease processes
Complication	A process or event that occurs during the course of a disease that is not an essential part of that disease
Contraindicated	Describing an intervention that may have a negative outcome in a given condition
Demographic	An identified group of people about which information is gathered
Diagnosis	The determination of the nature of a disease, injury, or defect
Endemic	A pattern of disease incidence that is limited to a particular population or area
Epidemic	Widespread outbreak of a contagious disease
Idiopathic	A disease of unknown origin
Incidence	The number of new cases of people falling ill with a specified disease during a specific period within a specific population
Indication	The basis for an intervention that is likely to have a positive outcome in a given condition
Lesion	A pathologic change in tissue
Local	Describing a limited area of the body
Morbidity	A diseased state; the ratio of sick to well people within a population
Mortality	Death rate from a specific disease
Pandemic	A contagious disease affecting the global population
Prevalence	The number of cases of a disease existing in a given population during a specific period or at a particular moment; the proportion of people affected
Prodrome	An early or predictive symptom of a disease
Prognosis	Expected outcome of a disease or disorder
Sequela/ae	A condition following the consequence of a disease
Sign	An objectively observable indication of a disease or disorder
Stenosis	Abnormal narrowing of any canal or orifice
Subacute	Between acute and chronic; a stage in healing or tissue repair
Symptom	A subjective experience relating to a disease or disorder
Syndrome	A collection of signs and symptoms associated with a specific disease process
Systemic	Describing a whole-body involvement
Trauma	Any physical or mental injury

attitude toward life is often better equipped to fight off the same pathogens that actively threaten someone who is sleep deprived and stressed out. In other words, while viruses cause colds, other factors may influence immune system activity, which can enhance or interfere with a person's ability to resist getting sick.

Prions

Prions are unique among pathogens: although they are composed of proteins, they contain neither DNA nor RNA. They begin as slightly malformed proteins in neurons that essentially get in the way of normal neuronal activity (Figure 1.2). In ways that aren't entirely clear, prions cause infected cells to produce more prions (similarly to the way viruses work). They spread among humans via contaminated blood or transplant tissue, contaminated surgical instruments, or consumption of infected meat products. Prion diseases can also be inherited or the result of spontaneous mutations.

Prions are the causative agents for bovine spongiform encephalopathy (also called mad cow disease), Creutzfeldt-Jakob disease, kuru (a disease that used to be seen among human cannibals), scrapie in sheep and goats, chronic wasting disease among deer and elk, and a few other rare diseases. All prion diseases affect the nervous system, and all are eventually fatal.

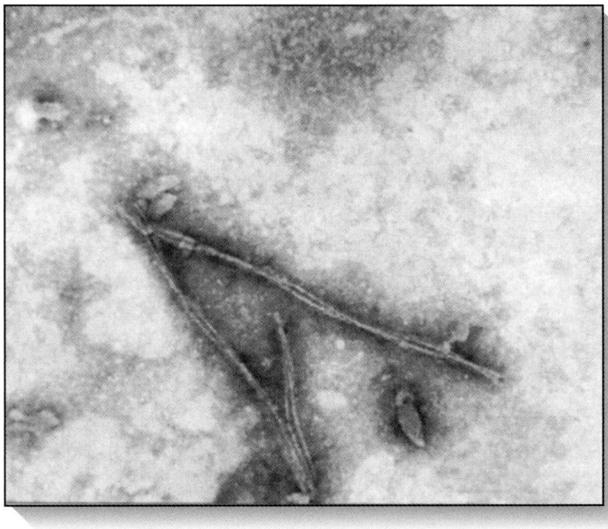

FIGURE 1.2 Fibrillar prion proteins accumulate in the brains of patients with BSE

Viruses

Viruses are packets of DNA or RNA wrapped in a protein coat called a capsid (Figure 1.3). They can't replicate outside of a host; instead, they use the machinery of the cells they

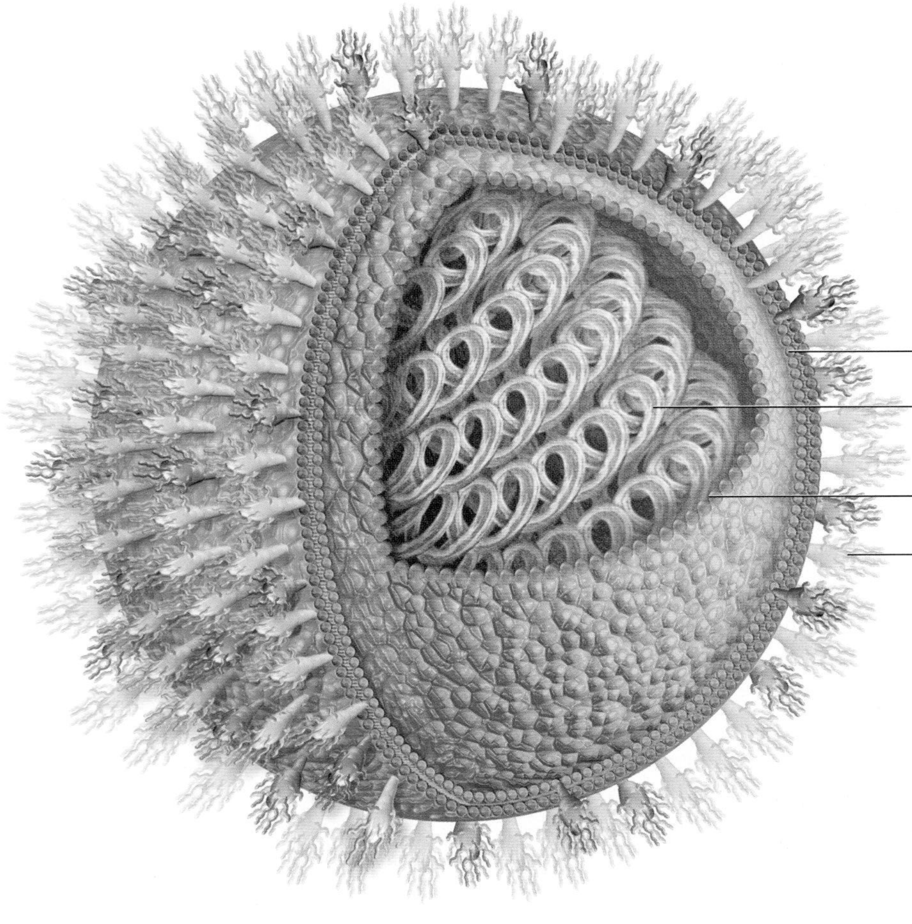

FIGURE 1.3 General structure of a virus

invade to make more viruses. The infected cell eventually releases many copies of the virus, or viral particles called virions, which may then invade other nearby cells. Every virus that affects humans has at least one specific target cell, although some viruses have multiple levels of infectious activity. Poliovirus, for example, first invades cells in the gastrointestinal tract and then migrates to motor neurons in the spinal cord.

Outside of a host, many viruses are fragile and disintegrate quickly. Some, however, are extremely stable and can retain infectious potential for weeks or longer. The most common stable viruses that massage therapists are likely to encounter include **herpes simplex, hepatitis B, and hepatitis C**. These infections are discussed in detail in Chapters 2 and 8, respectively.

Bacteria

Bacteria are single-celled microorganisms that can survive outside of a host. Not all bacteria are pathogenic; many are necessary for good health. But others can cause serious illnesses, either by invading healthy tissues or by releasing enzymes or toxins that destroy healthy cells.

Antibiotics are a group of drugs that either kill bacteria directly or interfere with bacterial replication. Aggressive bacterial infections with a high replication rate often respond to antibiotic therapy better than do slow-growing infections. Another feature that helps to determine the virulence of a bacterium is whether it develops a tough waxy coat that protects it from the environment. Coated bacteria, sometimes called spores, can survive for extended periods outside a host. **Tuberculosis**, tetanus, and anthrax are infections caused by spore-bearing bacteria.

Bacteria come in several basic forms, although some species show an ability to change their shape depending on environmental factors.

- *Cocci* are spherical bacteria that appear in predictable patterns.
  - *Diplococci* are paired cocci. These bacteria are associated with a type of pneumonia (Figure 1.4).
  - *Staphylococci* clump together in groups that resemble bunches of grapes (Figure 1.5). Staph infections of the skin are usually, but not always, localized to a specific area. Some varieties of staph have become resistant to common antibiotics and can be difficult to treat. One example is methicillin-resistant *Staphylococcus aureus,* or MRSA, which is discussed in the section on **staphylococcus infections** in Chapter 2.
  - *Streptococci* cling together in chains (Figure 1.6). They tend to cause systemic infections such as strep throat or rheumatic fever. **Necrotizing fasciitis**, or "flesh-eating bacteria," is often a strep infection, although some other agents have been seen with this condition as well.

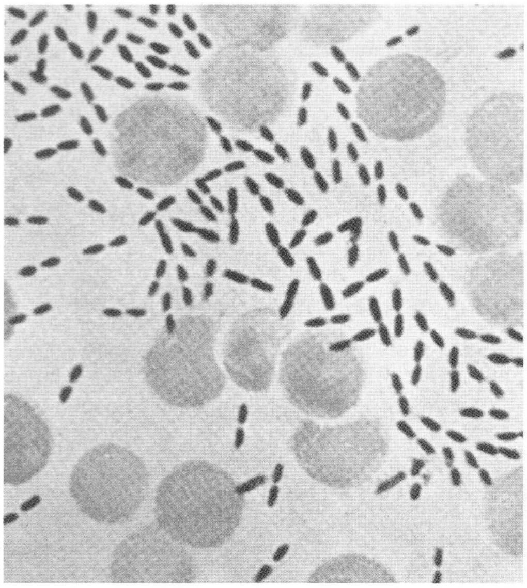

FIGURE 1.4 Diplococci, in pairs

- *Bacilli* are elongated, rod-shaped bacteria. These are the most capable of forming spores (Figure 1.7).
- *Spirochetes* are spiral bacteria. Technically, they are greatly elongated bacilli, with filaments that wind around the cell wall, pulling them into a spiral. Infections caused by spirochetes include **syphilis** (*Treponema pallidum*) and **Lyme disease** (*Borrelia burgdorferi*) (Figure 1.8.)
- *Mycoplasma* are very tiny microorganisms that lack a cell wall, which means they are resistant to some antibiotics. They cause some sexually transmitted infections and a common type of **pneumonia**.

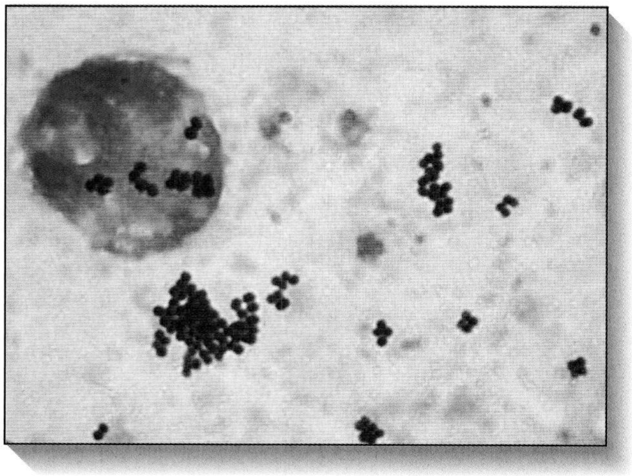

FIGURE 1.5 Staphylococci, in clumps like bunches of grapes

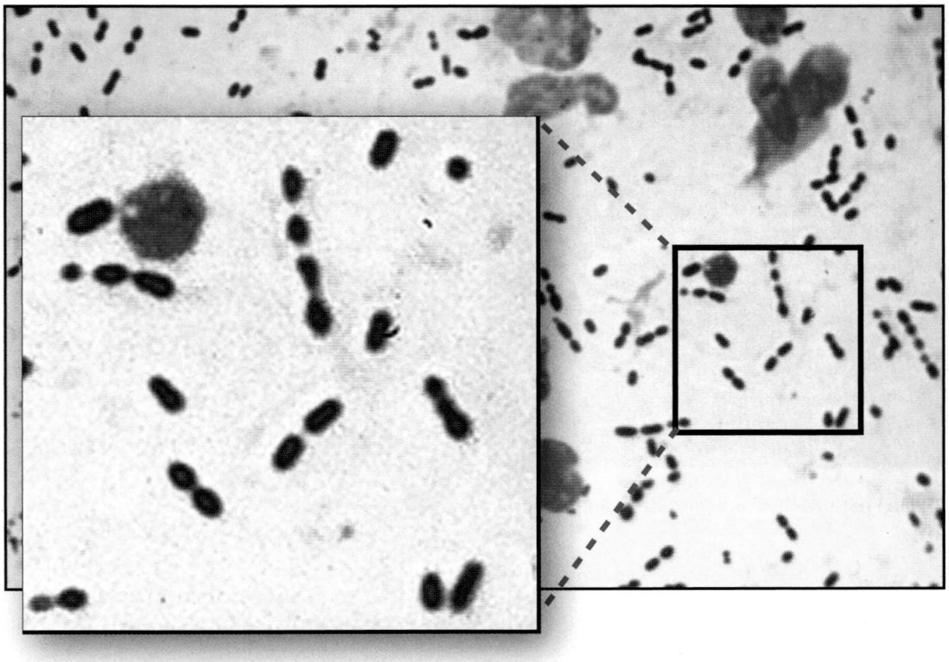

FIGURE 1.6 Streptococci, in chains like pearls

Fungi

Fungi are a group of organisms that includes both yeasts and molds. Most internal fungal infections are indications of imbalances that allow normal yeasts to replicate uncontrollably; **candidiasis**, discussed in Chapter 8, is an example. Other fungal infections are usually limited to the skin. **Ringworm, athlete's foot**, and **jock itch** are superficial fungal infections that are discussed in Chapter 2.

Animal Parasites

Animal parasites can be unicellular or multicellular. The parasites listed here are animals that live on or in a host rather than those that visit one host after another. Animal parasites are annoying in their own right, but they can also function as vectors for other contagious diseases.

- *Protozoa*. These single-celled organisms cause diseases that include giardiasis, malaria, and cryptosporidiosis. The protozoan associated with **malaria** is vector borne through mosquitoes, but giardiasis and cryptosporidiosis are transmitted through oral-fecal contamination (Figure 1.9).
- *Helminths and roundworms*. Parasitic worms colonize various places in the body, including the gastrointestinal tract, the liver, and the urinary bladder. Most helminths have been eradicated from the United States, but they are still a significant public health issue in developing countries. Roundworms are still common infestations in the United

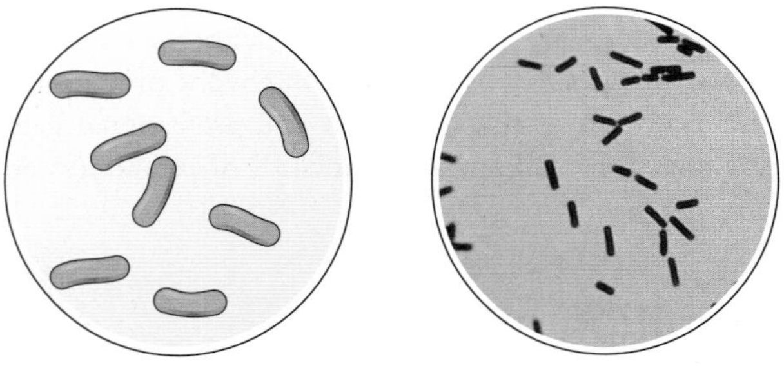

A Bacilli **B** Bacilli, photomicrograph

FIGURE 1.7 Bacillus: a rod-shaped bacterium

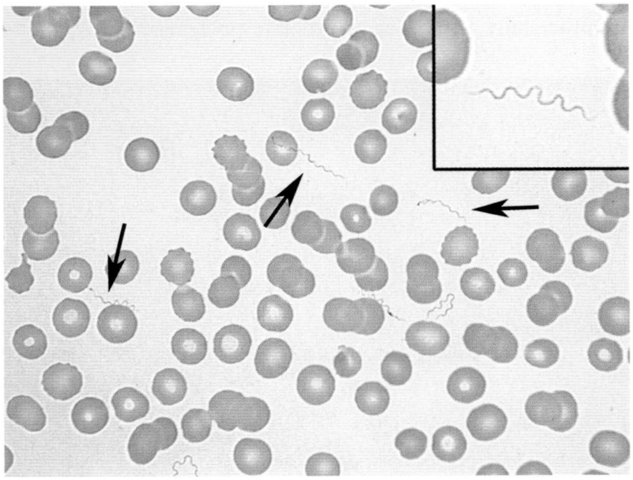

FIGURE 1.8 Spirochetes, like corkscrews (*arrows*)

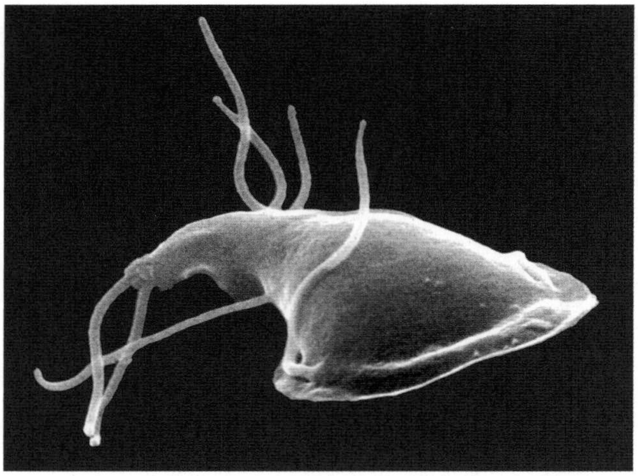

FIGURE 1.9 Giardia: a paramecium transferred through oral-fecal contamination

States and the rest of the world, although they tend to be most prevalent in warm climates. Schistosomiasis, which can cause bladder cancer, and trichinosis are worm-related diseases.

- *Arthropods.* **Head lice, crab lice**, and the mites that cause **scabies** are animal parasites that colonize human skin. They are discussed in detail in Chapter 2.
- *Others.* Other animal parasites don't necessarily live on or in a host, but they are worth mentioning because they can spread other pathogens. Mosquitoes (malaria, **West Nile virus**), ticks (**Lyme disease**, Rocky Mountain spotted fever), and fleas (bubonic plague) are common disease vectors (Figures 1.10 and 1.11).

Hygienic Practices for Massage Therapists

Massage therapists work with a physical intimacy unmatched by practically any other health care profession. How many

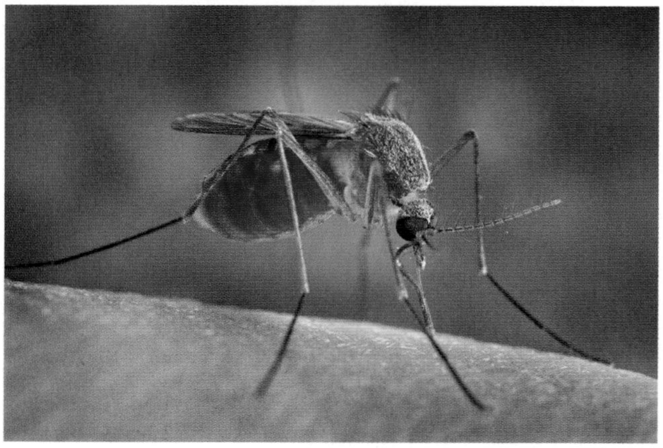

FIGURE 1.10 Mosquito: vector for West Nile virus

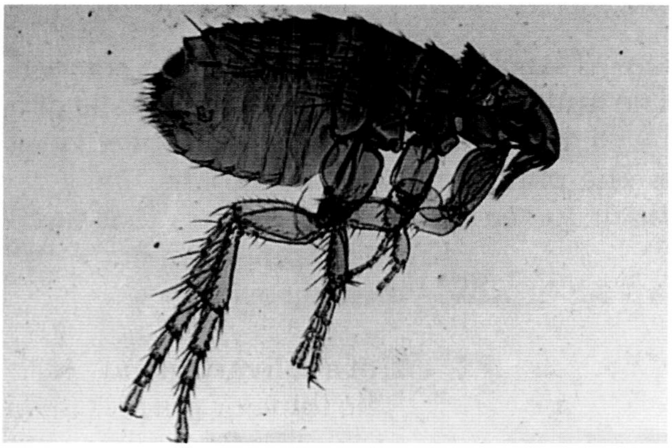

FIGURE 1.11 Flea: vector for bubonic plague

health professionals, outside of nurses, surgeons, dentists, and dental hygienists, spend an hour or more devoting the total of their concentration and focus, as well as their touch, to the well-being of their clients? This prolonged close contact puts both therapists and clients at risk for sharing pathogens.

The ways infectious agents jump the gap from one host to another have been exhaustively studied. The process essentially boils down to three issues: a reservoir or source of the infectious agent, a susceptible new host, and a mode of transport. Possible reservoirs can include other humans or animals, or environmental habitats like contaminated computer keyboards or food that harbors potentially dangerous bacteria. The susceptibility of a new host depends on a number of variables, from species to inborn immunity, to variable resistance. Finally, the mode of transport can be direct (like blood-to-blood exchange) or indirect through the air with respiratory secretions, or from an intermediate object like a doorknob or a light switch. These disease-relaying objects are sometimes called fomites.

The hygienic practice guidelines provided here are drawn from recommendations by the Centers for Disease Control, the World Health Organization, and other resources for health care professionals in hospital, dental, and home care settings. Individual states may also have specific guidelines for massage therapists. These recommendations are probably more elaborate than most massage therapists observe, but bodywork practitioners are conceivably at risk for illness and professional liability if they don't follow strict standards of cleanliness and professionalism.

Definition of Terms

- *Cleaning* is the removal of soil through manual or mechanical means, often in preparation for disinfection or sterilization.

- *Disinfection* is the destruction of pathogenic microorganisms or their toxins by direct exposure to chemical or physical agents. Disinfectants are described as low, intermediate, and high level. These interventions can kill most pathogens, but bacterial spores may be spared.
- *Sterilization* is the destruction of all microorganisms in a given field. It is accomplished with baking, steam under pressure, or chemicals under pressure.
- *Sanitation* is the use of measures designed to promote health and prevent disease; it usually refers to creating a clean environment but does not specify the level of cleanliness.
- *Plain soap* is any detergent that contains no antimicrobial products or only small amounts of antimicrobial products to act as preservatives.
- *Antimicrobial soap* is a detergent that contains antimicrobial substances.
- *Alcohol-based hand rub* contains 60% to 95% alcohol (usually ethanol, isopropanol, or both).
- *Standard precautions* are a set of protocols that create some uniformity in how medical professionals, especially dentists, should limit contact with body fluids in the working environment. Standard precautions include guidelines on how to avoid exposure to all potentially harmful body fluids. The following fluids are specifically mentioned in standard precautions as potentially infectious: semen, vaginal secretions, breast milk, cerebrospinal fluid, synovial fluid, pleural fluid, pericardial fluid, amniotic fluid, blood, blood-tinged saliva, and vomit (emesis). Sweat and tears are not described as infectious fluids.

Practical Applications for Massage Therapists

Hand Washing

Healthy skin is composed of several layers of cells that are manufactured deep in the epidermis. As they mature, new cells underneath push older cells toward the surface. By the time they reach the superficial layers of the skin, the cells are dead and they have been filled with keratin to create a tough, waterproof covering. A layer of intercellular lipid anchors the epidermis. This lipid layer, with the stratum corneum, forms an effective barrier between the inside and the outside of the body.

Various types of bacteria colonize the epidermis. Transient bacteria are found in the superficial layers of the skin; these microbes are easily removed with soap and water or other friction. Resident bacteria colonize deeper layers of the skin, and they are more difficult to remove. Fortunately, they also tend to be less aggressive and less likely to cause serious infections.

Hand washing with soap and running water removes new dirt and some transient bacteria, at least temporarily. Depending on the temperature of the water and the nature of the soap, frequent hand washing can also interfere with the function of the lipid layer: hot water and some detergents can reduce intercellular lipids and increase cell proliferation. This can interfere with the uptake of essential fatty acids that help to preserve the impermeability of the skin. In other words, too-frequent hand washing with hot water and harsh soap can actually make the skin more vulnerable to infection by compromising the shield.

After extensive research comparing the benefits and risks of frequent hand washing with plain soap and water, antimicrobial soap, and alcohol-based gels, well-accepted recommendations for normal use and for health care workers have been developed. Running warm water (not hot water, which raises the risk of skin irritation) plus plain soap for 30 seconds with all rings, bracelets, and watches removed is adequate for most everyday use. Special focus must be given to the fingernails and cuticles, where pathogens may not be removed without specific attention. Long sleeves are not recommended for health care providers, because they can carry pathogens that cannot be removed with hand washing (Figure 1.12).

Washing with warm running water and plain soap is always recommended to remove any visible or palpable dirt or fluids. It is preferable to dispense soap in liquid form, because bacteria can colonize bar soap. Rinsing so that water runs from the hands down the fingers and into the sink is preferable, so contaminated water does not run up toward the elbow.

Using alcohol-based gel or foam according to manufacturers' directions (which means using the amount prescribed and rubbing until the skin is dry) is often faster and more convenient than is washing with soap and water, and it is an effective antibacterial and antiviral mechanism, but it does not remove dirt, and it is not effective against spore-forming bacteria. Hand cleaning with alcohol gel or foam is often recommended in medical settings where a trip to the sink for a full soap-and-water treatment takes too long. Alcohol-soaked towelettes are specifically not recommended because their alcohol concentration isn't high enough to be effective.

To view an excellent demonstration, see the video "Hand Washing/Hand Antisepsis," available at http://thePoint.lww.com/Werner6e. thePoint

Washing hands with water and antimicrobial soap is effective but carries a higher risk for negative reactions in the form of allergies or contact dermatitis than does washing with plain soap. No evidence supports the theory that antibacterial soap provides significant benefits compared to plain soap, but scientists have found that some com-

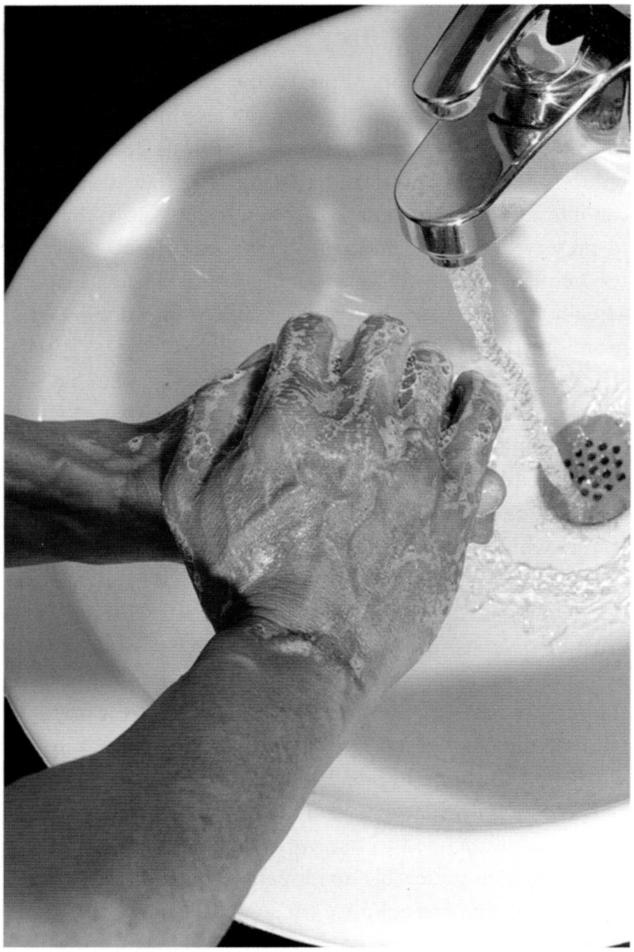

FIGURE 1.12 Hand washing

mon bacteria have developed resistance to triclosan, the substance used to limit bacterial activity in antimicrobial soaps.

For people whose skin is very sensitive, it is important to choose a soap with no or minimal dyes or perfumes. These substances raise the risk of developing allergic contact dermatitis, which can compromise the integrity of the skin. In addition, using an emollient that is likewise free of dye or perfume can help support a healthy epidermis and lipid layer while minimizing the risk of an allergic reaction. One benefit of alcohol gels is a relatively low risk of irritating skin reactions; this problem is often cited as a barrier to regular hand hygiene.

Other Hand Care

In addition to keeping hands and nails clean, massage therapists must be vigilant about the risk of open lesions. Hangnails that peel and fray can become portals of entry for serious infections. Hangnails must be kept short and controlled; a good pair of cuticle scissors and appropriate lotion can help with this.

Any other open lesions on the hands must be covered during a massage. This can be done with a simple bandage if it is in a place that doesn't come in direct contact with a client and is changed with each session; a liquid bandage (which can be washed with regular hand washing); or a finger cot, a small latex or nitrile sheath that must be replaced for every session.

Fingernails must be kept short, of course, and artificial nails should be avoided. Scrapings from the fingernails of health care workers have been cultured to reveal colonies of yeasts and gram-negative bacilli. Imagine getting a massage from someone with long nails, knowing what could be growing under there ... how relaxing could that be?

Care of Surfaces and Equipment

In a massage therapy workspace, it is a good goal to create an environment where nothing that one client touches directly or indirectly is touched by another client before it is cleaned. This means isolating table linens and other fabrics, and cleaning massage furniture, massage tools, lubricant dispensers, and any other items that might come into use during a session.

Fabrics

The fabrics that clients directly contact include linens on the massage table, face cradle covers, bolster and pillow covers, and the therapist's clothing. Any fabric item that a client contacts should be laundered before another client touches it. Similarly, any item that a massage therapist touches during a session with one client should be cleaned or re-covered before it is used again.

Therapists have some choices about their own clothing. Some wear aprons that can be changed with every appointment; this is appropriate as long as the client does not directly contact other articles of clothing. It is also possible to own several uniform shirts that can be changed between sessions. Aprons, uniform shirts, and other clothing items can be laundered with linens.

Guidelines for laundering are not universally agreed upon, but here are some important factors to bear in mind:

- Professional laundering services use water that is 160°F (71.1°C) or above, with a minimum of 25 minutes of agitation to reduce microbial populations.
- Good antimicrobial effect is found with temperatures from 71°F to 77°F (21.6°C to 25°C), if the detergent is strong and used according to manufacturers' directions.
- If bleach is added to the wash, it becomes most active at temperatures above 135°F (62.7°C). Most home hot water heaters heat water to 120°F to 140°F (48.4°C to 60°C), so bleach in the washing machine may not reach

its full potential. The recommended amount of bleach is a ratio of 50 to 150 ppm (parts per million).
- Bleached laundry must be thoroughly rinsed to minimize irritation to users.
- Laundry must not be left damp for any significant length of time.
- All laundry should be dried on high heat (160°F, 71.1°C). Ironing adds extra antimicrobial action, but this is probably not a practical suggestion for most massage therapists.
- Clean laundry must be packaged to keep it clean until its next use. It could be wrapped in plastic or stored in a closed, freshly disinfected container.

Therapists who use a professional laundry service will probably rent their sheets from the service. This means the therapist has no control over the quality, texture, color, or newness of the linens. Also, all items except sheets must be laundered by the therapist. This includes towels, face cradle covers, bolster covers, pillow cases, and clothing.

Therapists who do their own laundry should be aware that adding bleach will shorten the life of their fabrics, and of course it is impractical for colored sheets or clothing. Nonchlorine bleach does not have antimicrobial effect. Washing with strong detergent and drying on high heat are sufficient for most situations, however.

Other fabric items include mattress pads, bolsters, pillows, blankets, and heating pad covers. Any of these should be laundered if a client touched it directly, but if the contact was through some other covering (i.e., a mattress pad that is *always* covered by a sheet), then laundering for every session is unnecessary. The exception to this rule is when there are signs of contamination (i.e., bleeding or other fluid seepage) that may penetrate through the protective layer of fabric.

Other Equipment

Massage tables and chairs can be swabbed with disinfectant between clients. This is especially important for face cradles, of course. Therapists may choose which product they prefer, but it should be at least an intermediate-level disinfectant. The CDC recommends a 10% bleach solution for high-touch surfaces; this is inexpensive and easily available. It is important to mix fresh solution frequently however, as bleach solutions lose potency if they are not used promptly, and if they are stored in translucent bottles. Bleach-infused wipes can be useful in this application, but it is important to read the labels for best results: some of them require at least 10 minutes of exposure to be effective. Alcohol is specifically not recommended for cleaning surfaces because it evaporates too quickly; it works best with prolonged contact against targeted pathogens.

Massage lubricants must be kept free from the risk of cross-contamination. Lubricants that are solid at room temperature (e.g., beeswax, coconut oil) must be dispensed into individual containers and leftovers discarded so that double dipping never occurs. Liquid lubricants must be dispensed in bottles that are washed between every session. Bottles should be kept away from possibly contaminated surfaces, such as desktops or the floor.

Hot or cold rocks and crystals may be the only massage tools that lend themselves to full sterilization. Depending on their composition, these may be boiled or baked between uses to ensure removal of all pathogens. Items that are not disposable, such as massage tools, vibrators, and hot and cold packs, must have their contacting surfaces disinfected every time they are used.

The Massage Environment

Research indicates that fabrics such as curtains, carpeting, and upholstery are not significant sites of transmission for infectious agents, but they may harbor pet hair or dander that could cause an allergic reaction. For this reason, upholstery and carpets should be vacuumed frequently. Vinyl or leather upholstery can be swabbed with disinfectant. Any carpeting that gets wet can harbor bacteria and fungi; it should be replaced if it isn't completely dry within a few hours. Hard floors can be washed regularly with detergent, but no particular benefit has been found in washing frequently with high-level disinfectants.

Other surfaces that clients and therapists contact should also be cleaned frequently. These include doorknobs, bathroom fixtures, light switch plates, telephones, and coat rack or hooks. If a therapist uses a computer in the office, the keyboard may provide a rich growth medium for pathogens. This can be ameliorated with antiseptic-soaked towelettes or keyboard covers that can be washed in the sink. Also, cash is not called "filthy lucre" for nothing; it is typically handled by numerous dirty hands and is an excellent vector for communicable diseases.

The guidelines suggested here may seem unnecessarily alarmist. However, as more people seek massage, and as new and stronger forms of pathogens develop, it becomes increasingly important for massage therapists in any setting to create the most professional and safest environment possible.

The Inflammatory Process

What Is Inflammation?

Inflammation is a tissue response to damage or the threat of invasion by **antigens**: bits of nonself. It is typically caused by physical injury (trauma, chemical burn, hypothermia),

> **Antigen:** Any substance that elicits an immune response on contact with sensitive cells.

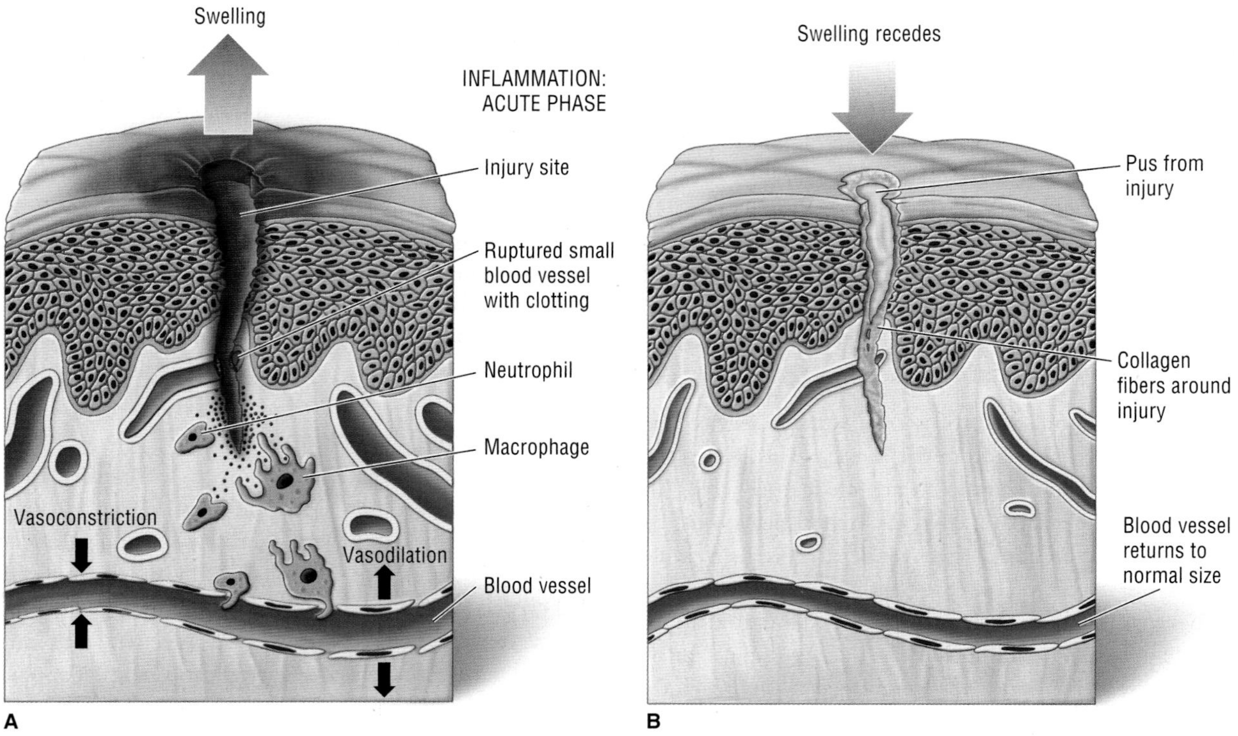

FIGURE 1.13 Many cellular changes happen with the inflammatory response **(A)** to protect the body from infection and prepare the area for healing **(B)**

invasion with foreign bodies (pathogens, splinters, shrapnel), hormonal changes, or autoimmune activity. The inflammatory response is expressed through cellular and vascular functions that are coordinated by chemical mediators.

The purpose of inflammation is to protect the body from pathogenic invasion, to limit the range of contamination, and to prepare damaged tissue for healing. Once an acute inflammatory response has begun, it has only a few possible courses: complete resolution with no significant tissue changes, accumulation of scar tissue, or chronic inflammation, possibly with the formation of cysts and **abscesses**.

Components of Inflammation: Vascular Activity

The vascular component of inflammation comes into play when tissue is damaged by trauma or other factors. For the sake of simplicity, consider a basic laceration or puncture wound as a model, although the same principles hold true for any kind of local injury (Figure 1.13A and B). In the first moments, **vasoconstriction** occurs. This is easily observable on scratching the skin: a white wheal is followed by a red mark within a few seconds. The vasoconstrictive stage is over within moments for a minor injury, and several minutes for a more serious one.

Vasodilation is the next step in vascular activity. Damaged endothelial cells and mast cells release a host of chemicals that increase the permeability of blood vessel walls, reinforce capillary dilation, attract platelets, and slow blood flow away from the area, limiting the risk of deeper penetration of pathogens.

Vasodilation is short lived with minor injuries, but it may last for several days with more severe injuries. In some situations, the vascular reaction to tissue damage is delayed for several hours; this is the case with sunburns, for instance.

> **Abscess:** A deposit of purulent exudate appearing in an acute or chronic localized infection.
>
> **Vasoconstriction:** Tightening of blood vessels, including capillaries.
>
> **Vasodilation:** Loosening of blood vessels, including capillaries.
>
> **Angiogenesis:** Development of new blood vessels.

Components of Inflammation: Cellular Activity

Many cells are recruited to manage tissue damage and contamination risk with injury:

- *Endothelial cells.* The endothelial cells of damaged blood vessels release chemicals that activate platelets and allow white blood cells to escape their boundaries. These cells are also sensitive to chemical signals to proliferate: in later stages of healing, endothelial cells build capillaries to supply new tissue growth: this is called **angiogenesis**.

- *Platelets*. When **platelets** are stimulated, they become jagged and sticky, and they release several chemicals that interact with plasma proteins to weave the net of fibrin that forms a blood clot and the scaffolding for future scar tissue.
- *White blood cells*. Several types of white blood cells participate in the inflammatory process. Which types depends on how long the injury has been present and what types of pathogens are involved.
  - *Neutrophils*. **Neutrophils** are the most common type of leukocyte to be involved in early stages of inflammation. These tiny white blood cells are associated with bacterial infection and musculoskeletal injury.
  - *Mast cells*. **Mast cells** are found in tissues most vulnerable to damage: skin, the respiratory tract, and gastrointestinal tract. When they are activated, they release histamine and other chemicals that reinforce and prolong the inflammatory response.
  - *Monocytes and macrophages*. **Monocytes** are large, mobile white blood cells. They are sensitive to chemical signals that call them to sites of injury or potential infection. Monocytes can become permanently fixed **macrophages**. They are typically involved in later stages of inflammation: they help clean up cellular debris to prepare the area for healing.
  - *Lymphocytes*. Some lymphocytes are involved in the resolution of inflammation. They work with macrophages to clean up dead and damaged cells and to help form scar tissue and new blood vessels.
- *Fibroblasts*. **Fibroblasts** produce collagen and other components of connective tissue **extracellular matrix**. They also respond to chemical signals that call them to the site of injury or invasion. They typically begin by migrating to local blood clots and may proliferate to create more scar tissue if necessary.

Platelet: An irregularly shaped fragment of a megakaryocyte that aids in blood clotting.

Neutrophil: A type of mature white blood cell formed in the bone marrow.

Mast cell: A white blood cell found in connective tissue that contains heparin and histamine.

Monocyte: A relatively large leukocyte that normally constitutes 3% to 7% of the leukocytes in circulating blood.

Macrophage: A type of phagocytic white blood cell.

Fibroblast: A cell capable of forming collagen fibers and other extracellular matrix.

Extracellular matrix: A collective term for connective tissue fibers and the liquid medium in which they are suspended.

Complement: A combination of many serum proteins that react with each other in various ways to disable antigens and assist immune system response.

Kinin: Any of a variety of chemicals with physiological effects on cell activity, including visceral muscle contraction along with vascular muscle relaxation, which leads to vasodilation.

Basophil: A phagocytic leukocyte.

Granulation tissue: Vascular connective tissue that forms on the surface of a healing wound.

Collagen: A major protein forming the white fibers of connective tissue.

Components of Inflammation: Chemical Mediators

All cells involved in inflammation are coordinated by chemical messages that tell them what to do. Some of these chemicals are suspended in plasma (clotting factors, **complement**, and a group of chemicals called **kinins** that increase pain sensation and the permeability of capillaries). Platelets, mast cells, and **basophils** release histamine and serotonin, which also promote vasodilation and capillary permeability. Injured cell membranes release chemicals that activate platelets to form clots, and other proinflammatory chemicals. The study of proinflammatory chemicals continues to reveal new secrets about this remarkable and intricate process.

For another view of the inflammatory process, view the animation "Acute Inflammation" available at http://thePoint.lww.com/Werner6e. thePoint

Stages of Healing

The process of healing from injury or infection is extremely complex. It requires the highly coordinated interaction of vascular, cellular, and chemical components to come to a successful resolution. Healing typically happens in three stages.

- *Acute stage*. In this initial inflammatory phase, damaged cells release their chemicals, causing vasoconstriction and vasodilation, the accumulation of fluid between cells (edema), and the attraction of platelets and fast-moving white blood cells. Tissue exudate begins to form: this can take the shape of the fluid that fills blisters, pus, or other material that indicates immune system activity and the possibility of infection. Depending on the severity of the injury, the acute stage may last 1 to 3 days or longer.
- *Subacute stage*. Also called the proliferative stage, this is the phase when specific cells accumulate and work to fill in damaged tissue. Endothelial cells grow into new capillaries to supply **granulation tissue**, the framework for new cells. If the damage affects deeper layers, fibroblasts spin new **collagen** fibers and other components of extracellular matrix. At the same time, slower moving white blood cells begin to clean up dead pathogens and

other cellular debris. The subacute stage may last for 2 to 3 weeks, depending on the severity and depth of the injury and the healing capacity of the person who has been injured.

- *Postacute stage.* Also called the maturation stage, this is when new collagen undergoes changes: it is remodeled and reshaped, and it becomes denser and aligns according to force. In other words, if a muscle, tendon, or ligament is injured and accumulates scar tissue, and if that structure is stretched and exercised carefully, those new collagen fibers eventually lie down in alignment with uninjured fibers.

Chronic or Unsuccessful Inflammation

Occasionally the inflammatory process is not wholly successful. Pathogens or irritants are not removed from the body, and the immune system continually attacks some type of tissue. When this happens, the result is called chronic inflammation. This is different from standard inflammation, involving different types of cells and holding a different prognosis.

When chronic inflammation is connected to an infection or an autoimmune process, several things can happen. Pus that is never reabsorbed is surrounded by a wall of connective tissue; this is a cyst or abscess: the body's attempt to remove this foreign material. Abscesses carry a risk of rupture and dangerous infection. Another form of chronic inflammation can cause persistent signals to fibroblasts, so that an accumulation of scar tissue interferes with organ function, as seen with **cirrhosis** of the liver. Scar tissue can also block the digestive tract or other passageways; this is called a **stricture**, which can cause stenosis: obstruction of an important passageway. When tubes are otherwise blocked, the body sometimes attempts to build new "exit routes" or drainage channels. When these release onto the skin, they are called **sinuses**; when they connect to other hollow organs, they are called **fistulae**. Sinuses and fistulae are possible complications of chronic inflammatory conditions such as **ulcerative colitis**, **Crohn disease** (both in Chapter 6), and others.

An unsuccessful inflammatory process can also cause problems in musculoskeletal tissues. Under normal circumstances when a fibrous structure like a muscle, tendon, or ligament is injured, it undergoes a typical inflammatory response. Neutrophils arrive to scout the area for potential invaders; monocytes and fibroblasts follow afterward to clean up the debris and lay down the framework for new collagen fibers. But sometimes, the quality of the new collagen is never well established, and the injured structure never satisfactorily heals. While inflammation subsides and no proinflammatory cells are present, pain, weakness, and limitation may continue. This situation, called tendinosis when it affects tendons, is discussed in the section on **tendinopathies** in Chapter 3.

To learn more about this condition and its impact, see the author's "Chronic Inflammation" available at http://thePoint.lww.com/Werner6e. thePoint

> **Stricture:** Narrowing of a tube, duct, or hollow structure.
>
> **Sinus:** A channel for the passage of material without the coats of an ordinary vessel.
>
> **Fistula, fistulae:** An abnormal passage from one epithelialized surface to another.

Signs and Symptoms of Inflammation

The Latin terms for the signs and symptoms of inflammation are still taught today: *dolor* (pain), *calor* (heat), *rubor* (redness), *tumor* (swelling). *Functio laesa* (loss of function) was added later. Pain, heat, redness, swelling, and loss of function make up a litany every massage therapist needs to know. In some cases, itching, clotting, and pus formation can be added to this list.

The sources of these symptoms are easy to identify. Vasodilation brings about the redness, heat, and swelling by drawing extra blood and interstitial fluid to an isolated area. Pain and itching can be the result of several factors: edematous pressure, damaged nerve endings, irritating pathogenic toxins, and inflammatory chemicals that increase pain sensation. If the inflammation limits movement, the injured or invaded area loses function. Clotting and pus formation have already been discussed. Not all of these symptoms are present in all cases of inflammation.

Treatment

The typical treatment for inflammation is no surprise; a wide variety of anti-inflammatory drugs have been developed to interfere with the production of proinflammatory chemicals, and decrease pain perception at various steps along the sensory pathways. Several of these medications are discussed in detail in Appendix A. Regardless of their chemical effect on the body, orally administered anti-inflammatories impact massage decisions, because they may hide the results of overtreatment, raising the risk that massage can cause injury. If a client takes anti-inflammatories for a condition that does not contraindicate massage, it is wise to schedule the session when the drug is at its lowest activity. In this way, it is possible to get the most accurate feedback from the client's tissues about the effects of the massage.

Isolated injuries without signs of infection may also be treated with the PRICE protocol: protection, rest, ice, compression, and elevation. This traditional approach is under scrutiny for whether it is the best way to treat common musculoskeletal injuries, where the early introduction of movement and careful weight-bearing stress (as opposed to rest) is an important strategy in the healing process.

Medications

- Over-the-counter anti-inflammatories
- Prescription nonsteroidal anti-inflammatories
- Prescription steroidal anti-inflammatories

Massage Therapy Implications

RISKS

Acute systemic infections like cold or flu contraindicate some types of bodywork because of the risk of communicability to the practitioner, and because the immune system may not keep up with the additional challenge of rigorous massage.

Acute local skin infections like boils or small lesions locally contraindicate massage because of the risk of communicability, and the possibility of overwhelming the body's ability to isolate the infectious agents.

Inflammation that is not related to infection may be appropriate for various types of bodywork, depending on the stage.

Clients who have used anti-inflammatory drugs prior to their massage session may be less sensitive to pressure and consequently vulnerable to overtreatment.

BENEFITS

Lymph drainage and other gentle techniques can be useful for acute inflammation when no infection is present. Postacute local inflammation may respond well to careful massage, which may help to improve sluggish and congested circulation in the postacute stages of infection and inflammation.

More information about using massage therapy to take advantage of specific stages of healing will be addressed with specific condition discussions.

RESEARCH

Only a few studies have examined the role of massage in the inflammatory process in the past several years. One article suggests that the mechanical action of massage on cells in the skin and superficial fascia leads to altered pathways in the production of proinflammatory and anti-inflammatory chemicals.[1] These researchers suggest that massage could decrease secondary injury, decrease nerve sensitization, and provide a number of other benefits. Two other studies[2,3] found that massage may accelerate the recovery of muscle function after exercise-induced injury; both studies hypothesized that this occurs through changes in the secretion of proinflammatory chemicals.

These findings can be perceived as a bit surprising, since massage appears to increase heat and redness, if only temporarily and only at the site of contact, but that is the nature of research: we must be open to surprising findings. These studies don't allow us to make any blanket statements about massage and inflammation, but as more information is generated we may see some stronger evidence on the anti-inflammatory aspects of massage therapy.

1. Waters-Banker C, Dupont-Versteegden EE, Kitzman PH, et al. Investigating the mechanisms of massage efficacy: the role of mechanical immunomodulation. *Journal of Athletic Training* 2014;49(2):266–273, http://www.ncbi.nlm.nih.gov/pubmed/24641083
2. Best TM, Gharaibeh B, Huard J. Stem cells, angiogenesis and muscle healing: a potential role in massage therapies? *Postgraduate Medical Journal* 2013;89(1057):666–670, http://www.ncbi.nlm.nih.gov/pubmed/24129034
3. Crane JD, Ogborn DI, Cupido C, et al. Massage therapy attenuates inflammatory signaling after exercise-induced muscle damage. *Science Translational Medicine* 2012;4(119):119ra113, http://www.ncbi.nlm.nih.gov/pubmed/24129034

Explore and Apply

LEVEL 1: Receive and Respond

1. Which of the following makes extracellular matrix?
   a. Fibroblasts
   b. Mast cells
   c. Basophils
   d. Monocytes

2. Define these words using Table 1.1:
   a. Hypodermic
   b. Orchiectomy
   c. Acromegaly
   d. Leukocyte

3. Your client has a runny nose and a headache. Which one of these is the symptom, and which one is the sign?

4. When a client is very sore the day following a massage, this is called a/an...
   a. Prognosis
   b. Expected outcome
   c. Morbidity
   d. Adverse effect

5. Evidence-informed practice means using ________ to make clinical decisions:
   a. Client income, therapist availability, doctor's permission
   b. Client willingness, therapist expertise, available equipment
   c. Client priorities, therapist expertise, current research
   d. Client availability, therapist strength, current research

6. Critical thinking means...
   a. Looking for the flaws in information so it can be improved
   b. Using evaluated information to make decisions and take action
   c. Weighing risks and benefits for every client
   d. Developing an algorithm to help make clinical decisions

7. Label the following conditions with the type of microorganisms that cause them (prions, bacteria, viruses, paramecia, or fungi):
   a. Creutzfeldt-Jakob disease
   b. Tuberculosis
   c. Hepatitis B
   d. Methicillin-resistant *Staphylococcus aureus*
   e. Giardia
   f. Ringworm
   g. Herpes simplex
   h. Mad cow disease
   i. Jock itch
   j. Malaria

8. Which is the most rigorous level of hygiene?
   a. Cleaning
   b. Sterilization
   c. Disinfection
   d. Antisepsis

9. "Standard precautions" refers to ...
   a. A group of guidelines designed to protect doctors from contracting HIV
   b. A book of rules that all health care providers are required by law to follow
   c. A set of protocols that guide hygienic practices in health care settings
   d. A list of concerns regarding infectious agents in public settings

10. Which body fluid is considered to be most potentially infectious?
    a. Saliva
    b. Semen
    c. Sweat
    d. Sebum

11. What is the best choice for soap in a massage clinic bathroom?
    a. Bar soap on a dish near the sink
    b. Antimicrobial liquid soap
    c. Plain liquid soap
    d. Liquid detergent that can also be used for surfaces

12. What is the best substance to use to clean a massage table?
    a. 10% bleach solution
    b. 80% ethanol
    c. Alcohol wipes
    d. Ammonia

13. Which is the best list of the purposes of acute inflammation?
    a. Put a wall around antigens; prevent future exposure; protect the injured area
    b. Prepare for healing; route blood to the area; kill pathogens
    c. Limit the range of contamination; repel new pathogens; build scar tissue
    d. Protect from invasion; limit the range of contamination; prepare for healing

14. Translate the following:
    a. Rubor
    b. Calor
    c. Dolor
    d. Tumor

15. Which of the following happens in the acute stage of healing?
    a. Collagen is remodeled and reshaped
    b. Vasoconstriction followed by vasodilation
    c. Pus is encapsulated by an abscess
    d. White blood cells clean up debris

16. Which of these happens in an unsuccessful inflammatory response?
    a. Collagen is remodeled and reshaped
    b. Vasoconstriction followed by vasodilation
    c. Pus is encapsulated by an abscess
    d. White blood cells clean up debris

17. Which medication will a client most likely use to manage mild inflammation related to a sore knee?
    a. NSAIDs
    b. Steroidal anti-inflammatories
    c. Immune-suppressant drugs
    d. Diuretics

LEVEL 2: Application of Concepts

1. Your client calls you the day after a session to complain about having a headache and muscle soreness where you worked on her neck. This is an example of a/an…
    a. Delayed reaction
    b. Acute inflammatory response
    c. Chronic inflammatory response
    d. Adverse effect

2. When you wipe your massage table with 10% bleach, you are…
    a. Disinfecting
    b. Sterilizing
    c. Lubricating
    d. Laundering

3. You are working at a busy outdoor venue, and the nearest sink or water facilities are several minutes away. What is your best option for fast hygiene?
    a. Use 10% bleach solution on your face cradle and alcohol gel on your hands
    b. Use alcohol wipes on your hands and face cradle
    c. Use 10% bleach solution on your hands and alcohol gel on your face cradle
    d. Use alcohol gel on your hands and face cradle

4. Your client was pruning her roses 3 days ago, and she has a painful laceration on her forearm. The 10-inch long wound is marked by a scab, and the edges are hot, red, and swollen. Close examination shows that the wound is beginning to seep, and pus is collecting in various places along the scab. What is happening?
    a. The lesion is in the proliferative stage of the inflammatory process
    b. The lesion is in the maturation stage of the inflammatory process
    c. The lesion is showing signs of infection
    d. The lesion is showing signs of chronic inflammation

5. One of the dangerous sequelae of chronic inflammation is…
    a. Accumulation of scar tissue that can interfere with organ function
    b. Hyperproduction of white blood cells that can lead to leukemia
    c. Suppressed immune system function
    d. Hypertrophic scar formation in injured tendons

Explore and Apply (continued)

6. Why might the PRICES protocol for acute inflammation of injured muscles and tendons be questioned?
   a. It is too expensive to use at home
   b. It places too much emphasis on icing
   c. It places too much emphasis on rest
   d. It is too easy to overtreat

7. A new client is on her way to your office. She has a condition you've never heard of, and it isn't in your pathology book. What is your best course of action?
   a. For her safety, refuse to see her
   b. Look up her condition in a medical text or on a trusted online resource and make decisions about her safety from that information
   c. Call her doctor for permission to work with her
   d. Deliver a standard relaxation massage regardless of her condition and resilience, because that is always a safe choice

Note to educators: Due to space considerations, these review questions skim over only the most important material from Chapter 1. The Test Bank provides a much more comprehensive selection of questions, all of which are keyed to the appropriate chapter objectives.

What Would *You* Do?

Use the list of Greek and Latin word fragments in Table 1.1 to suggest words for "runny nose," "headache," and "slow movement." Can you think of some other health-related compound words? Leaf through a textbook or medical dictionary, or read an article online about an illness, and find some words that you can now define based on their Greek and Latin roots.

Hand Washing

Research shows that health care workers are often inconsistent about hand washing. What would bar you from washing your hands frequently enough to be safe and healthy? What solutions do you see for this problem?

Hygiene Application

How often do you swab your table or chair? What about your face cradle? When was the last time you wiped your doorknobs and switch plates? Are you sure that the products you use are effective? How do you know?

Adverse Effects

What if you injured a client? What would you do about it to….

- Make it right with the client?
- Be sure it never happens again?
- Educate your colleagues so they can avoid making that mistake?

Standard Precautions

You have two clients, both of whom slid into second base and have large, half-healed abrasions on their thighs. You know that one of the clients is HIV positive. How do you manage the hygiene and infection control aspects of each session differently?

Suggested Activities

1. Write one multiple choice question for each of the following sections of Chapter 1. Share your questions with your classmates as you study together.
   a. Adverse effects
   b. Evidence-informed practice
   c. Terminology
   d. Infectious agents
   e. Hygienic practices
   f. Inflammatory process
2. Use the student resources on thePoint to find printable flash cards for the terms in Tables 1.1 and 1.2. Practice these cards until you are comfortable with this new vocabulary.
3. Use the student resources on thePoint to find practice quiz questions and games.

2

Integumentary System Conditions

CHAPTER 2 / Abbreviated Chapter Objectives

Having completed assignments and classroom time related to Chapter 2, the learner is expected to be able to...

- Identify definitions of the key terms in the introduction and those connected to the conditions covered in your curriculum.
- Name four functions of the skin.
- Describe the structure of the skin with three main layers.
- Explain why damaged skin contraindicates massage therapy.
- Provide the following information for each condition covered in your curriculum:
  - Identify the definition of the condition.
  - List the most common causes or contributing factors to the condition.
  - List major signs and symptoms of the condition.
  - Identify possible risks and benefits of massage therapy, with:
    - Variables that contribute to risks and benefits
    - Appropriate adaptations for massage therapy

For detailed chapter objectives for each condition in this chapter, consult the student resources page at http://thePoint.lww.com/Werner6e. thePoint®

Introduction: Function and Construction of the Skin

Massage practitioners speak in a language of touch. The messages we convey are invitations to a number of different possibilities: to enjoy a state of well-being, to heal and repair what is broken, and to reacquaint a client with his or her own body. All this happens through the skin, a medium equipped like no other tissue in the body to take in information and respond to it, largely on a subconscious level. The goal of massage practitioners is to anticipate these reactions and set the stage for them in a way that is most beneficial for their clients.

Functions of the Skin

A student once said that the purpose of skin is to keep our insides from falling out. That's true, but that's not all skin does; its many functions work to keep the body healthy and safe, and all wrapped up in a tidy 8- to 10-pound, 22–square foot package.

Protection

Intact skin keeps pathogens out of the body, and it discourages their growth on its surface by secreting the acidic substances that also keep hair shafts lubricated. Furthermore, by constantly sloughing off dead cells, it sloughs off potential invaders too.

The skin is the first line of defense against invasion; it is the physical barrier that defines our boundaries. Although it is made of relatively delicate tissue, skin cells are **labile**: they quickly and efficiently replace themselves. Think of scraping your knuckle on a cheese grater at night, and how the wound is well on its way to healing by the next morning. Lability can sometimes backfire, however, with dangerous results.

In addition to fast repair, the abundance of immune system cells located in superficial fascia offers protection from potential invasion. When these defense mechanisms become hyperactive, they can cause certain types of rashes and other skin problems.

Homeostasis

The skin protects us from fluid loss, a top homeostatic priority, and one of the most dangerous functions to lose when the skin is damaged. The skin also helps to maintain a stable internal temperature through three mechanisms: superficial capillaries dilate or constrict in response to external temperature; fat in the subcutaneous layer acts as insulation against cold; and the evaporation of sweat is a powerful cooling device when the ambient humidity is low.

> **Labile:** (Of cells) constantly multiplying.
>
> **Excretion:** Material that has been excreted (discharged) by the body, because it serves no further use.
>
> **Callus:** A thickening of the skin in response to repeated friction or pressure.

Sensory Envelope

With as many as 19,000 sensory receptors in every square inch of skin, it's obvious that this is the organ (or tissue, or membrane, or system—depending on context) that tells us the most about our environment. Massage therapists must develop the skill of becoming conscious of the subtle information their hands pick up when they touch their clients, and must understand that every sensation on a client's skin causes ripples of reactions all through that person's body.

Absorption and Excretion

The skin can be recruited as an organ of absorption and **excretion**, but only under certain circumstances. The skin does not typically absorb topical substances into the bloodstream unless they are of a particular molecular size, or administered with a chemical that allows for transcutaneous absorption; this is the mechanism behind nicotine patches, birth control patches, and some other medications.

The skin excretes limited metabolic wastes through sweat under normal circumstances, but when the liver, colon, or kidneys are so overwhelmed that they can't process waste products adequately, sweat can carry other noxious chemicals out of the body.

Construction of the Skin

Skin varies from being very thin (on the lips) to remarkably thick (on the heels). It remodels according to stresses put upon it. **Callus** is an example of this phenomenon: it is simply extra-thick, extra-hard epidermis on places that really take a beating.

The construction of the skin is important, because it has relevance for how disease occurs and how easily it can spread. Three basic layers of tissue define the skin, and within those layers are more layers. The deepest layer has three possible names: the subcutaneous layer, subdermis, or superficial fascia. It is composed of a loose collagen and elastin framework that holds fat cells and some other structures (Figure 2.1).

The middle layer is the dermis, or "true skin." This is the location of hair shafts, oil and sweat glands, and some nerve endings. The outermost layer of dermis, the basal layer, lies just deep to the epidermis and has the best

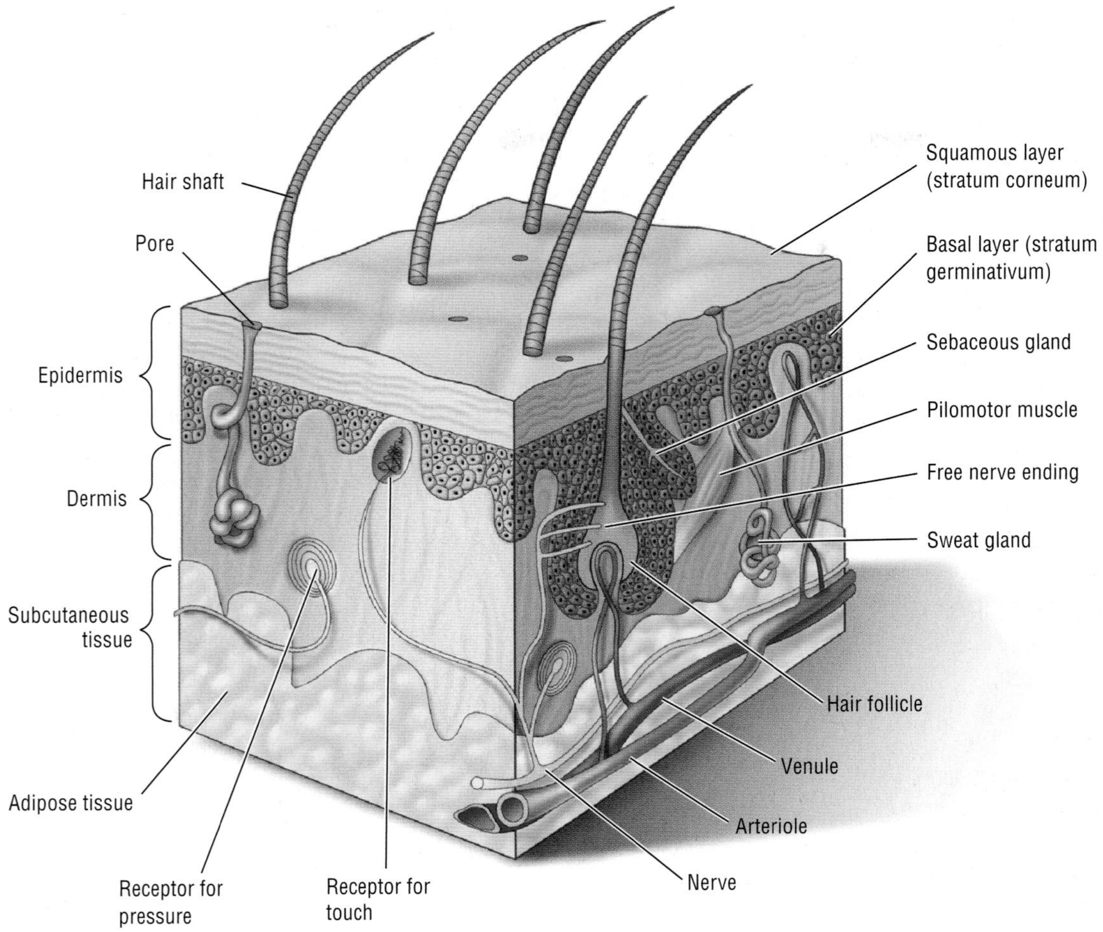

FIGURE 2.1 Layers of skin

capillary supply. This is where new skin cells arise. It is also the site of pigment cells or melanocytes, which produce melanin to protect people from harmful ultraviolet (UV) rays.

The epidermis is the most superficial layer of skin. It is composed of many layers of cells called keratinocytes that are produced in the basal layer of the dermis. As these cells are pushed toward the surface, they fill with keratin, becoming water resistant and scaly in the process. By the time they reach the surface, they are long dead and are eventually exfoliated to become the major ingredient of household dust. Bacteria colonize these layers of keratinocytes. Transient bacteria, which tend to be more aggressive, are found in the superficial layers. They are removed with friction and running water but are quickly replaced. Resident bacteria, which tend to be less aggressive, colonize deeper layers of the epidermis.

Implications for Massage

Skin conditions have a special relevance for massage therapists because we are in a position to notice lesions and blemishes that clients often don't know are present. This is why it is especially important to be able to recognize most common skin conditions, at least to recommend that clients investigate further with their own doctor. Many skin conditions contraindicate massage because they might be contagious, or they might spread further on the body. But beyond that danger, the one cardinal rule for skin conditions and massage is this: *if the skin in not intact, the client is a walking invitation to infection.* Open skin, broken skin, scabbed skin, oozing skin, or any skin that allows access to the blood vessels inside is a red flag for bodywork practitioners.

To hear more of the author's point of view about massage therapy and skin conditions, see "Skin Diseases," a video available at http://thePoint.lww.com/Werner6e. thePoint®

Integumentary System Conditions

Contagious Skin Disorders

- Animal parasites
  - Head lice
  - Crab lice (pubic lice)
  - Body lice
  - Scabies mites
- Fungal infections of the skin
  - Tinea capitis
  - Tinea corporis
  - Tinea cruris (jock itch)
  - Tinea pedis (athlete's foot)
  - Tinea manuum
  - Onychomycosis
  - Tinea versicolor
- Herpes simplex
  - Oral herpes
  - Genital herpes
  - Herpes whitlow
  - Herpes gladiatorum
  - Herpes sycosis
  - Eczema herpeticum
  - Ocular herpes
- Staphylococcal infections of the skin
  - Boils
  - Folliculitis
  - Methicillin-resistant *Staphylococcus aureus* (MRSA)
  - Hidradenitis suppurativa
  - Pilonidal cysts
- Streptococcal infections of the skin
  - Cellulitis
  - Erysipelas (St. Anthony's fire)
  - Necrotizing fasciitis
- Warts
  - Common warts
  - Plantar warts
  - Cystic warts
  - Plane warts
  - Filiform warts
  - Molluscum contagiosum
  - Genital warts
  - Butchers' warts
  - Focal epithelia hyperplasia
  - Epidermodysplasia verruciformis

Noncontagious Inflammatory Skin Disorders

- Acne rosacea
  - Erythrotelangecteal rosacea
  - Papulopustular rosacea
  - Phymatous rosacea
  - Ocular rosacea
- Acne vulgaris
- Eczema, dermatitis
  - Eczema
    - Atopic dermatitis
    - Seborrheic eczema
    - Dyshidrosis
    - Nummular eczema
  - Contact dermatitis
    - Irritant contact dermatitis
    - Allergic contact dermatitis
  - Other types of dermatitis
    - Stasis dermatitis
    - Neurodermatitis

Neoplastic Skin Disorders

- Seborrheic keratosis (SK)
- Skin cancer
  - Basal cell carcinoma (BCC)
    - Nodular BCC
    - Pigmented BCC
    - Superficial BCC
    - Micronodular BCC
    - Morpheaform BCC
  - Squamous cell carcinoma (SCC)
    - Actinic keratosis (AK)
    - Actinic cheilitis
    - Leukoplakia
    - Bowen disease
  - Malignant melanoma
    - Superficial spreading melanoma
    - Lentigo melanoma
    - Acral lentiginous melanoma
    - Uveal melanoma

Skin Injuries

- Burns
- Decubitus ulcers
- Scar tissue
  - Keloid scars
  - Hypertrophic scars
  - Contracture scars

Contagious Skin Disorders

Animal Parasites

Many massage therapists fear parasitic infestations, because we are so vulnerable to whatever is crawling around on our clients' skins. But here, as in all things fearful, the best defense is information. This discussion will be limited to animals that live in or on humans or their clothing.

Types of Animal Parasites

Mites

Definition: What Are They?

Mites (*Sarcoptes scabeii*) are microscopic arthropods that cause the skin lesions called scabies (Figure 2.2). The females burrow into the epidermis where they feed on damaged skin cells, defecate and urinate, and lay eggs so the next generation can carry on. The average life cycle of a female mite is

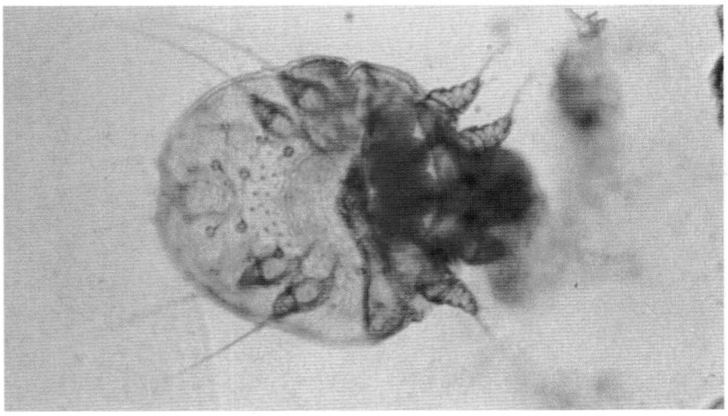

FIGURE 2.2 Scabies mite (microscopic)

30 to 60 days. As an adult, she lays approximately three eggs per day, although only a small percentage of them hatch. Newly hatched mites migrate to the surface of the skin, where it takes about 14 days for them to achieve maturity.

The mites' waste is highly irritating, causing a delayed itchy allergic reaction in most hosts. If scratching damages the skin, the risk of secondary infection is high.

One type of scabies, called crusting or Norwegian scabies, is particularly prevalent among immunocompromised people. It can involve thousands or even millions of mites, and it is highly contagious. The lesions cover large areas and develop dry, flaky scabs, but they tend not to itch as much as typical scabies lesions.

How Do They Spread?

Mites spread readily through skin-to-skin contact or through contact with something someone else has recently worn or lain on, including massage sheets. Depending on local conditions, mites can live up to 3 days in clothing or bedding. They can spread before they cause any symptoms, so if a person is diagnosed with them, all of the members of that household are counseled to be treated for an infestation. (Case History 2.1).

Signs and Symptoms

Scabies mites are too small to see with the naked eye, so a visual diagnosis is based on the trails they leave behind. Sometimes their burrows are visible; these look like reddish or grayish lines around the areas the mites favor: the groin, axilla,

CASE HISTORY 2.1 Scabies, Valerie

Valerie was a massage student. She worked with a variety of people, including fellow students, friends, her student internship group, and people with AIDS.

One day Valerie noted that she had some areas on the outsides of her elbows that were slightly but persistently itchy during the day. They gradually developed red bumps. Ironically, this occurred while Valerie was studying skin conditions in her massage course. "It's natural to convince yourself that you have symptoms of a lot of things. I knew something was going on, and it seemed like it *could* be scabies, but my symptoms were different from anything I'd seen described," she said. The itching was not particularly worse at night, and there were no tracks or typical signs of infestation. Even the site of the infestation was unusual: scabies mites usually seek out warm, moist, protected areas like skin folds on the *insides* of elbows but not the outsides.

Eventually, Valerie went to her general practitioner, who pronounced her condition a "mystery rash" and suggested a corticosteroid cream to limit the itchiness. In a way, Valerie was relieved by this diagnosis. "You never want to think you have scabies," she said. When her husband also developed symptoms, however, he went straight to a dermatologist, who immediately diagnosed scabies and prescribed enough pesticidal soap for both of them.

The cream was applied all over the body up to the chin; evidently scabies do not infest the head or face. "That night after I washed off the cream, I was really, really, *really* itchy, and then for 4 or 5 weeks my skin was raw and uncomfortable." The cream itself can cause symptoms that mimic a scabies infestation for weeks at a time. This can lead to scabiosis, in which a person is convinced of the need to medicate for scabies again and again, although the infestation is gone. Scabiosis can become a life-threatening condition, if the person repeatedly self-medicates.

Six to eight weeks passed between the onset of Valerie's symptoms and a final diagnosis. During this time, Valerie continued to work on friends and clients and to receive massage from other students. Two other classmates were infested and finally diagnosed. "The first few days (after we knew it was scabies) were full of panic and fear. Within a couple of days of people getting over their fear and paranoia, there was a lot of support. People had the attitude that this is just one of the things that can happen when you're a bodyworker."

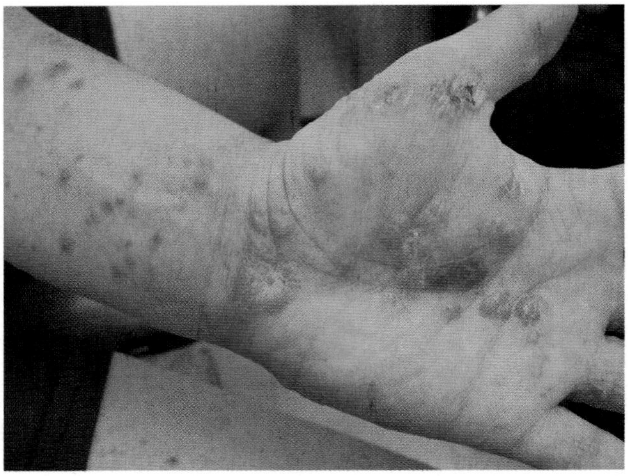

FIGURE 2.3 Scabies lesions

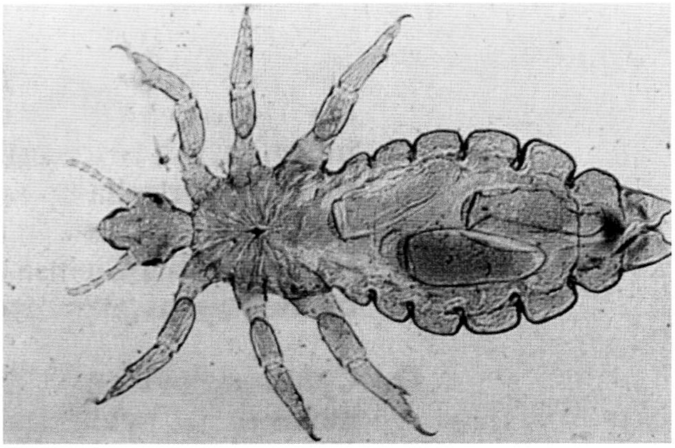

FIGURE 2.4 Head louse

elbows, belt line, or between fingers. Other signs of mite infestation are secondary bacterial infection and the irritated blisters and nodules that arise from allergic reactions to their waste (Figure 2.3). The itching caused by mites has a distinctive unrelenting quality. Where other itchy conditions like eczema or mosquito bites might itch intermittently and then subside, the itching with mites gets progressively worse.

Diagnosis

Scabies lesions can be tricky to diagnose if a parasite isn't isolated and identified. A typical test involves taking a skin scraping to look for mites or their wastes, but doctors can also test for mite DNA, elevated IgE antibodies, and a high number of eosinophils that indicate an infestation.

Scabies can resemble **psoriasis**, **eczema**, **chickenpox**, and several other conditions, so it is important to get an accurate diagnosis. Missing the correct diagnosis increases the risk of further spread and secondary infection; a false-positive diagnosis means a person may be unnecessarily exposed to potentially toxic medication.

Head Lice

Definition: What Are They?

Head lice are wingless insects (*Pediculus humanus capitis*) that live in head hair and suck blood from the scalp. Infestation with lice is sometimes called pediculosis. Lice are quite a bit larger than mites and can easily be seen without a microscope (Figure 2.4). Their saliva is very irritating, causing itching and creating the possibility of secondary infection. Lice gestate for 7 to 16 days depending on ambient temperature. When they hatch, they go through three molts and live an average of 2 to 3 weeks. Their life consists mainly of taking blood meals, mating, and laying eggs.

Historically, head lice and body lice (which can interbreed) have been vectors of diseases that include typhus, relapsing fever, and trench fever. While no longer considered a health threat in developed countries, these diseases are still spread by lice in refugee camps and other areas where people live in close contact and where good hygiene is difficult to maintain.

Demographics

Animal parasites are a common part of the human condition, especially where people live in close quarters with little access to hygiene. About 12 million people are diagnosed with head lice in the United States each year; most of them are school children.

How Do They Spread?

Head lice spread most easily through direct contact: human heat allows them to move quickly from scalp to scalp during sports, camping trips, and other close-contact events. When they are separated from a host, they tend to be more sluggish. While head lice don't jump or fly, they can be dislodged to find new hosts with hair dryers, removal of clothing, or rigorous towelling.

Lice can also use hats, scarves, and upholstery as fomites. They may live in batters' helmets that are shared by Little League teams, hairbrushes that are shared by best friends, and car seats that are shared by carpool buddies.

Signs and Symptoms

If a person has lice, the actual insects may or may not be obvious; when they are warm, they move fast and can hide. But they lay eggs called nits that are glued to hair shafts and look like tiny grains of rice (Figure 2.5). Newly laid nits are usually found at the base of the hair shaft, mostly behind the ears and along the back of the head. They hatch after about a week on a human host, but nits laid on hairbrushes or clothing may gestate up to a month. Dark nits may not yet have hatched, but light-colored nits are usually the empty shells. Nits are a definitive feature for pediculosis; anything else of that size and color (like dandruff or dried hairspray) brushes out easily.

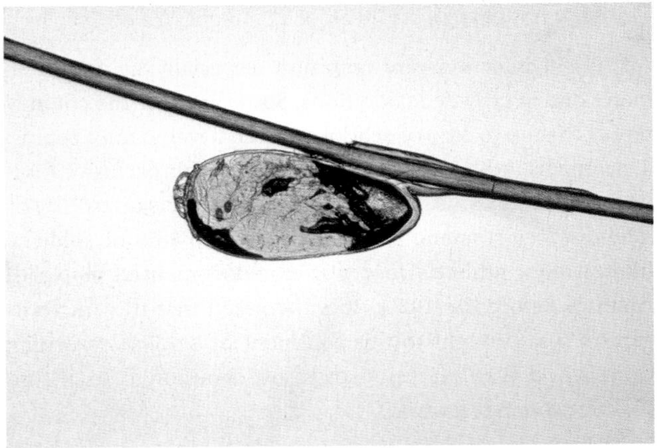

FIGURE 2.5 Nit attached to a hair shaft

A person with head lice experiences itchiness and the sensation of movement on the scalp. Rigorous scratching can damage the skin and open the door to secondary bacterial infection.

Body Lice

Definition: What Are They?

Body lice (*Pediculus humanus corporis*) are closely related to head lice, but they have different living and feeding patterns. Body lice tend not to live directly on their host but in the host's clothing, especially in the seams. They are a bit bigger than head lice, and they also take blood meals, causing an itchy reaction.

Body lice are fairly rare except among homeless and transient populations who have limited access to laundry facilities and so spend a lot of time in unwashed clothing. Like head lice, body lice are potential vectors of communicable diseases.

How Do They Spread?

Body lice live in clothing, so sharing unwashed clothing is the most efficient way for them to spread from one host to another. They may also crawl from infested clothing to other clothing in a laundry basket or other close proximity.

Signs and Symptoms

The primary sign of body lice is an itchy rash that gets worse. The insects seldom live directly on the skin, and they usually lay eggs in clothing, so unless the clothing is examined, a live body louse may not be found.

Pubic Lice

Definition: What Are They?

Pubic lice (*Pthirus pubis*) are tiny animals that look a lot like their nickname, crabs (Figure 2.6). Crabs often infest hair in the groin, but they also live in armpit hair and other coarse body hair (Figure 2.7). They may also be found in mustaches, beards, eyebrows, eyelashes, and on the margins of head hair.

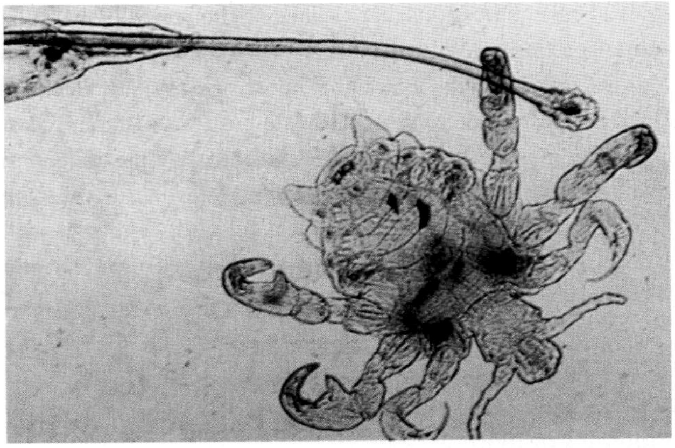

FIGURE 2.6 Crab louse

How Do They Spread?

Pubic lice are usually spread through sexual contact, but infested clothing, linens, or massage sheets can spread them too. They can survive only for a day off a host.

Signs and Symptoms

Pubic lice look like tiny crabs. Like all of the infestations being discussed, the primary symptom is itching that gets progressively worse without treatment.

Treatment for Animal Parasites

Parasitic infestations carry a powerful social stigma that is negatively (and inaccurately) associated with poverty and poor hygiene. Anybody can have this problem, and manual therapists are in a position to spread parasites to clients before any symptoms develop, so it is important to be compassionate, nonjudgmental, and well informed.

Of all the infestations discussed here, the easiest to eradicate is body lice: these animals are destroyed with good hygiene and clean clothes.

Mites, head lice, and crab lice are typically treated with pesticidal cream or shampoo. These substances can be toxic, especially to young children, so they must be used with great

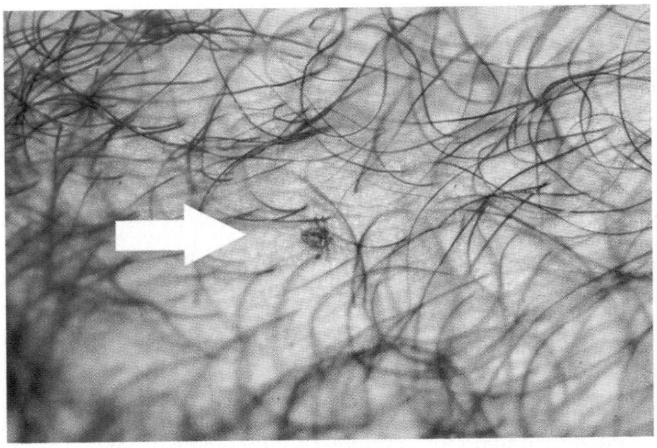

FIGURE 2.7 Crab louse in body hair

care. These medications don't kill eggs; they only kill hatched animals. Consequently, they must be used at least twice to remove any animals that hatch after the first application. Head lice resistance to typical topical pesticides is an increasing problem, so conscientious use is important. Head lice can also be treated with less toxic substances, but this must be followed by careful manual removal of adults and nits with a nit comb—this is the source of the terms "nitpicky" and "fine-toothed comb."

Washing or isolating bedding, clothing, upholstery, and soft toys for up to 2 weeks is also recommended. Head lice die when water temperatures reach 131°F, 55°C for 5 minutes or more.

Medications

- Topical pesticides include preparations of pyrethrum, malathion, and lindane
- Oral medications are sometimes prescribed
- Antihistamines to control itching
- Antibiotics for secondary infection

Massage Therapy Implications

RISKS	Animal parasites are communicable through direct contact. Even though the risk of transmission may be low, the safest choice is to delay massage for a client with an infestation for after treatment is complete.
BENEFITS	Any client who has completely treated his or her condition can enjoy the same benefits of bodywork as the rest of the population.

Fungal Infections

Definition: What Is It?

The nomenclature for superficial fungal infections is dizzying. Fungal infections of human skin, also called mycoses, can be caused by several different types of fungi (**dermatophytes**). Dermatophytosis, then, is another term for **mycosis**. The lesions the infections create are called **tinea**, a Latin word for "gnawing worm": this, and the fact that many lesions look like expanding circles on the skin, is the source for the common and misleading term for these fungal infections, "ringworm."

Dermatophyte: A fungus that causes superficial infections of the skin, hair, and nails.

Mycosis: Any disease caused by a fungus.

Tinea: A fungal infection of the skin, hair, or nails.

Kerion: A secondary bacterial infection of tinea capitis, leading to a raised, spongy lesion.

Demographics

All fungal infections are common, especially in warm climates and in crowded conditions. Some areas of the country report that up to 30% of school children develop tinea capitis. Tinea pedis (athlete's foot) is associated with occlusive footwear and community shower facilities. It affects up to 30% of long-distance runners, 73% of miners, and 58% of soldiers. Interestingly, athlete's foot was not documented in North America before the 1920s. It is theorized that this microorganism was brought to this continent by soldiers returning from World War I. It is now the most common form of fungal infection in the world.

Etiology: What Happens?

Fungal infections are transmitted via touch: either skin to skin, or skin to any possible vector or fomite, like pets, shower floors, garden soil, or the family hairbrush. It takes anywhere from 4 to 14 days for lesions to appear, and during that time the carrier can spread the fungus, which makes this condition very hard to control (Case History 2.2).

Dermatophytes on a new host secrete enzymes that dissolve keratin, which allows them to invade the stratum corneum of the epidermis. They thrive in warm, moist places like skin folds between toes or around the groin.

Several types of dermatophytes may create tinea lesions. Most cases of ringworm are related to colonies of *Trichophyton*, *Epidermophyton*, or *Microsporum* fungi.

Types of Fungal Infections

- ***Tinea capitis:***This is a fungal infection of the scalp. It is most common in children before the onset of puberty. It can cause hair loss, and a particularly extreme form can cause an inflammatory response leading to the formation of pus-filled sores called **kerions**. Some of the causative fungi for tinea capitis fluoresce under blacklight; this is a common diagnostic tool for this condition (Figure 2.8).
- ***Tinea corporis:*** This is "body ringworm" that typically develops on the trunk or extremities. It generally begins as one small round, red, scaly, itchy patch of skin on the trunk. Scratching spreads the fungus to other parts of the body, and other lesions appear. They heal from the center first, and they soon take on the appearance of red circles or rings with a scaly edge that may gradually increase in size as the fungus spreads out for new food sources (Figure 2.9).
- ***Tinea cruris:*** Also called "jock itch," this is a fungal infection of the groin area. It is much more common in males than females. It is typically associated with warm, damp conditions and tight clothing. Men who are obese or who have diabetes are more at risk for jock itch than are the general public. It usually spares the penis and scrotum, but may affect the skin around the groin, thighs, and low back (Figure 2.10).

CASE HISTORY 2.2 Ringworm, Delores G

In June 1994, I was working hard in massage school. I was living in a house where some stray kittens were close by. I wanted to pet them, so I brought them some food. They came out, and I got to pet them while they were eating.

I was sitting down next to them with my knees up. I had shorts on. I was petting them with my left hand, and then I held my legs with the same hand when I was done. I also folded my arms, so my left hand touched my right biceps.

About 9 days later, I found round red spots, the size of a half-dollar, on my left calf, and then on my right arm. It wasn't until I remembered petting the kittens that I realized where they came from. About a week after the spots appeared, they started really burning and keeping me awake.

Having ringworm was awful. It turns out that I had massaged only two people between being exposed and being diagnosed, so it didn't spread through the class, but I had to wait until I was cleared up before I could work again. I sat out of practices, which was really depressing, *plus* it was spreading all over me, from my right arm to my right breast, and on my other calf.

I treated it by showering and then putting tea tree oil and antifungal vaginal cream all over me. I did that for 2 or 3 weeks before it started clearing up. I was all cleared up in about 4 weeks. I waited an extra week just to be sure, so I missed a total of 3 weeks of massage.

When I got ringworm, I was extremely run down from school, which probably made me susceptible. My teacher said it was interesting that my body chose ringworm as the thing that would slow me down, but it worked!

- ***Tinea pedis*:** This is "athlete's foot," but it is not specific to athletes. It usually starts between the third and fourth digits (Figure 2.11). Athlete's foot burns and itches, and it carries the additional complication of weeping blisters, cracking, peeling skin, and the possibility of a dangerous secondary infection. One variety of athlete's foot fungus presents as dry, scaly, itchy lesions on the heel and sole of the foot. This is called a "moccasin distribution" (Figure 2.12).
- ***Tinea manuum*:** Many people who handle their athlete's foot develop secondary fungal infections on their hands; this is tinea manus. (Figure 2.13).
- ***Onychomycosis*:** Also called tinea unguium, this is the result when a fungal infection invades the skin under finger or toenails. It can lead to pitted, eroded, and discolored nails that may eventually detach from the nail bed (Figure 2.14). Destruction of the nail is called onycholysis.
- ***Tinea versicolor*:** This fungal infection is unique in that the vast majority of adults have colonies of the causative agent (usually *Malassezia globosa* or *Malassezia furfur*) as part of the normal flora of the skin. In some situations, these normally benign organisms become more aggressive, causing patches of hypo- or hyperpigmented skin that heal within a few months. Because the fungi associated with tinea versicolor are part of most people's naturally occurring skin colonies, this is not considered to be a contagious condition (Figure 2.15).

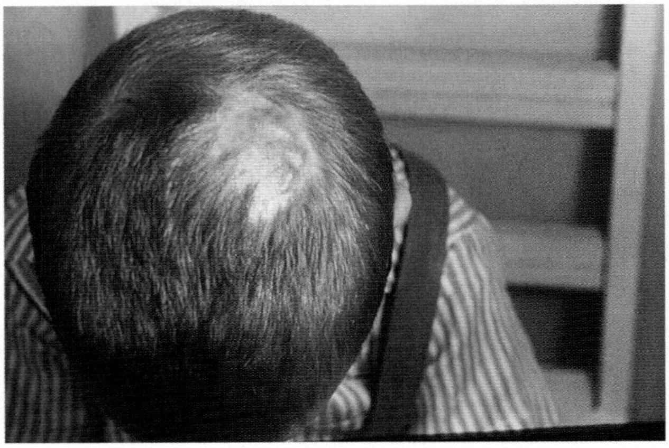

FIGURE 2.8 Tinea capitis: head ringworm

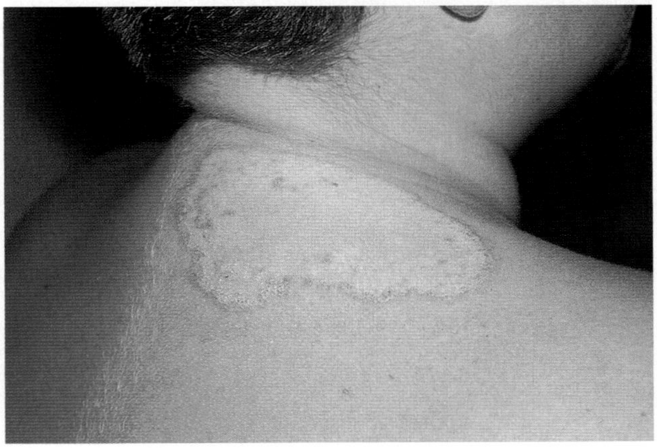

FIGURE 2.9 Tinea corporis: note the raised red edge, and the paler skin in the middle of the lesion

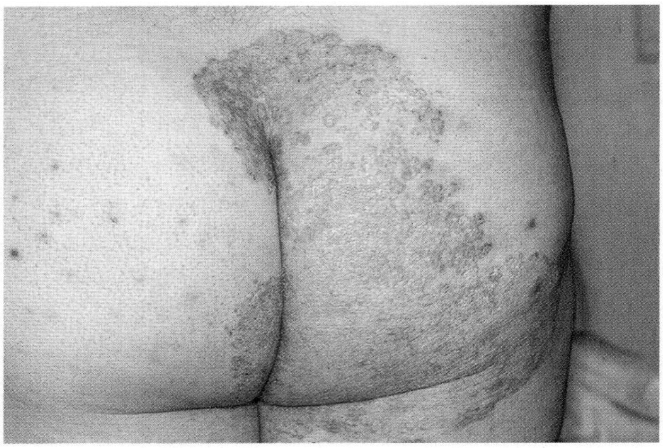

FIGURE 2.10 Tinea cruris: jock itch. Note that the lesions extend beyond the area that is usually covered by a drape.

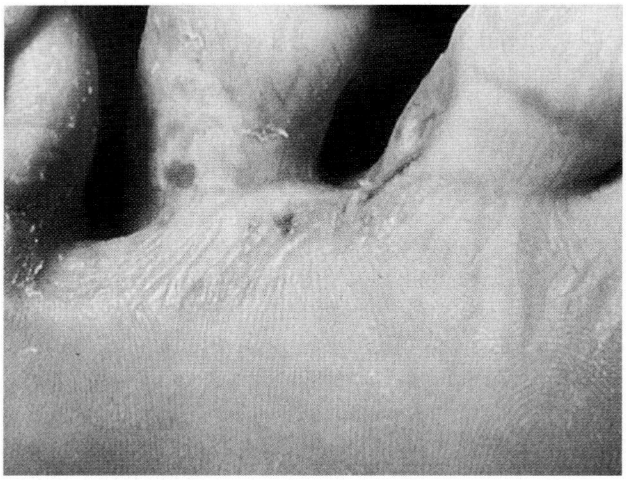

FIGURE 2.11 Tinea pedis: athlete's foot

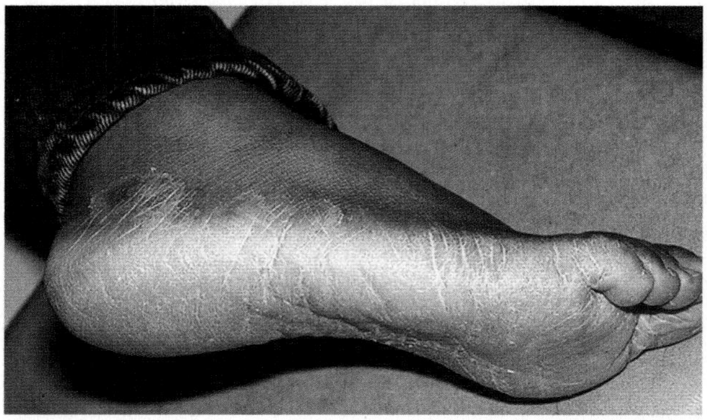

FIGURE 2.12 Tinea pedis: moccasin distribution

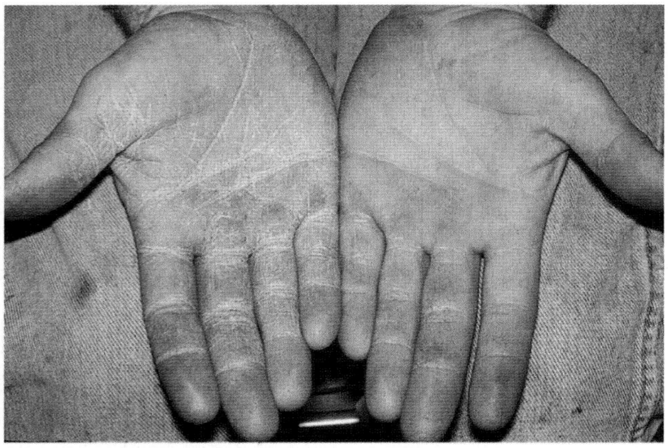

FIGURE 2.13 Tinea manuum: hand ringworm

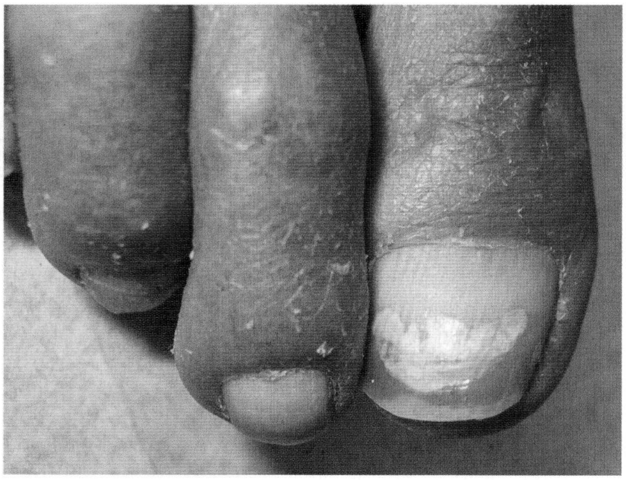

FIGURE 2.14 Onychomycosis: fungal infection of toenails

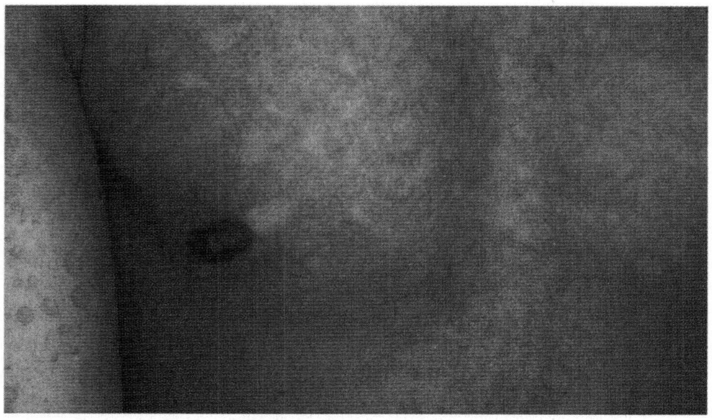

FIGURE 2.15 Tinea versicolor

Signs and Symptoms

Symptoms of tinea infections vary considerably depending on the causative agent and where they appear. The characteristic "ringworm" lesion is a slowly enlarging reddish scaly circle that is pale in the middle: this shows where the fungi have already taken advantage what nutrients are available. Interestingly, mushrooms grow in essentially the same pattern: an enlarging circle around an initial colony.

Subtypes of fungal infections may also involve fluid-filled blisters, ulcerations, or pus-filled sores. Individuals who are immune suppressed are more likely to experience atypical fungal infections with abscesses and deep scarring. It is important to remember that any compromise of the skin creates a risk for secondary bacterial infection.

Treatment

Tinea capitis tends not to respond to topical treatment, so a systemic medication is usually prescribed for diagnosed patients; it may also be recommended for other members of the household, along with caregivers and playmates. Treatment for other fungal infections typically begins with topical antifungal creams or powders. If these are insufficient, oral antifungal medication may be prescribed.

Nonpharmacological treatment for fungal infections includes laser treatment, photodynamic therapy, and surgical removal of the nail for onychomycosis.

Along with treatment, most fungal infections improve when the skin is kept dry. Many patients are advised to avoid tight clothing that may irritate the skin and exacerbate symptoms. Preventive measures (not sharing towels or clothing; using footwear in public showers, etc.) are important for anyone prone to fungal infections.

Medications

- Topical antifungal applications
- Oral antifungal medications

Massage Therapy Implications

RISKS	Tinea infections tend not to be aggressive, but it is important not to promote their spread. Consequently, they at least locally contraindicate bodywork.
BENEFITS	If a client has a localized fungal infection that is covered and well controlled, massage for the rest of the body is safe and appropriate.
OPTIONS	If a client has athlete's foot but has no open blisters, it may be safe to work on his or her feet through the sheet. This can minimize the risk of spreading the fungi any further on the foot, to the other foot, or from the client to the therapist.

Herpes Simplex

Definition: What Is It?

Among the several viruses in the herpes family that affect humans, herpes simplex viruses are especially common. Herpes simplex type 1 (HSV-1) is typically associated with lesions that appear around the mouth, while herpes simplex type 2 (HSV-2) is associated with genital herpes. Because the treatment options for type 1 and type 2 are identical, the distinction between them is less important than it used to be.

Etiology: What Happens?

Oral herpes is transmitted through oral or respiratory secretions. Genital herpes is transmitted through mucous membranes. In either case, the virus spreads most efficiently through direct contact. A person's first outbreak, which usually occurs 2 to 20 days after exposure, is called primary herpes. All subsequent outbreaks are called recurrent herpes.

A primary herpes outbreak may be very severe or almost unnoticeable. Most cases of oral herpes are picked up during early childhood, and the new carrier may never be aware of his or her infection. In extreme cases, the primary infection may be accompanied by fever, swollen glands, and many painful sores that may last 2 to 6 weeks.

One of the distinguishing features of all herpesviruses is that they are never fully expelled from the body. After the primary outbreak, the HSV goes into hiding in the dorsal root ganglia of the spine or the trigeminal nerve. There it waits for an appropriate trigger, which could be a fever, a systemic infection, a sunburn, stress, menstruation, or some other stimulus. When the virus reactivates, a recurrent outbreak occurs, usually at or near the site of the original infection.

Oral herpes lesions are sometimes referred to as "cold sores" or "fever blisters." This reflects the fact that blisters often erupt when the immune system is suppressed as a person deals with another infection; it is very common to have a herpes outbreak while recovering from a cold, for instance.

Herpes simplex carries some risk for complications. Secondary bacterial infection is a common problem at herpes lesions. People who are coinfected with HIV and genital herpes have a greater risk of communicating HIV to sexual partners, and people with active genital herpes lesions have an increased risk of contracting HIV from an infected partner. Vaginally delivered newborns of mothers with active genital herpes may develop blindness, pneumonia, or brain damage; this is why women with a history of this condition may be counseled to deliver their children by C-section.

Communicability

While herpes spreads most efficiently through direct skin-to-skin contact, the virus can persist on surfaces from several hours to several days. This means that the face pad used by

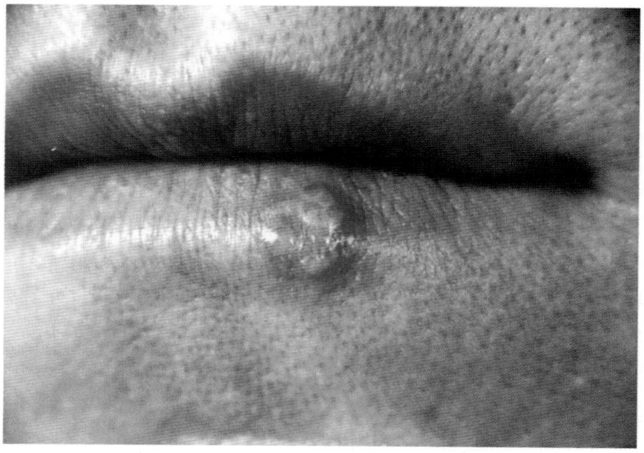

FIGURE 2.16 Oral herpes

an infected client can pass the virus to someone else, or the doorknob may now have some virus from when the client touched an itchy blister and then closed the door. Even leaving aside the possibility of spreading an infection to other people, herpes can also spread to other parts of the body; this is called autoinoculation. Touching a cold sore and then touching the eye, for instance, can result in a painful and harmful infection of the cornea or conjunctiva.

It is important to understand that herpes virus is highly concentrated in the fluid-filled blisters, but it can also be shed from skin that has no visible lesion; this is especially likely during the **prodrome** stage. In other words, the carrier doesn't need to have a visible lesion to spread the virus to other people.

While this sounds very alarming, herpes simplex can only cause a new infection in someone who has never been exposed. Because the vast majority of adults in the United States are positive for herpes simplex virus antibodies, the risk of establishing a new infection in a client or a therapist is relatively low.

Types of Herpes Simplex

- *Oral herpes* or herpes labialis tends to erupt when immunity is otherwise depressed; during hormonal changes, as in pregnancy or menstruation; after prolonged exposure to sunlight or extreme temperatures; or following any emotional stress. They appear most often on the lips and on the skin around the mouth (Figure 2.16). They may be a lifelong problem.
- *Genital herpes* outbreaks also correspond to depressed immunity and general stress levels, but they typically appear with decreasing frequency until finally they simply never come back. These blisters may appear on the genitals, but they can also be found on the thighs, buttocks, and on the skin over the sacrum (Figure 2.17). People who are immune suppressed tend to have outbreaks over larger areas of the body than do others. The lesions are usually quite painful, but if they are inside the vaginal canal, a woman may be unaware of them; this has important implications for communicability. Genital herpes outbreaks are sometimes accompanied by systemic symptoms: fever, muscular aches, swelling in the inguinal lymph nodes, and difficult or painful urination.
- *Herpes whitlow* is an outbreak of lesions around the nail beds of the hands. This condition has traditionally been associated with children who suck their thumbs, and before the days of consistent glove use, with health care workers, especially dental hygienists (Figure 2.18). Because massage therapists often work without gloves,

> **Prodrome:** An early symptom or warning of the onset of a disease.

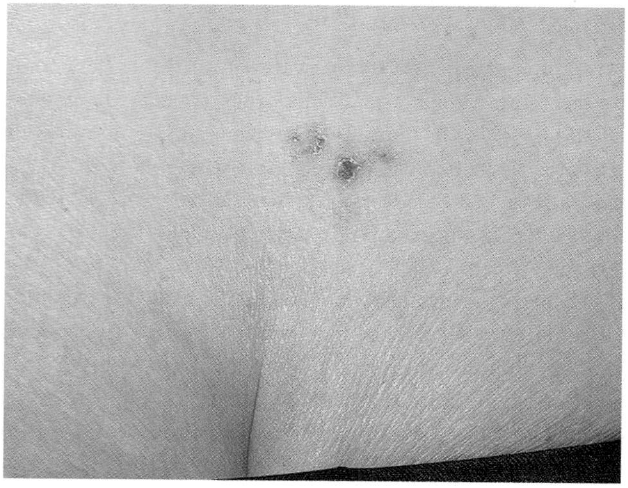

FIGURE 2.17 Genital herpes can appear on areas outside the genitalia, including where massage therapists may work

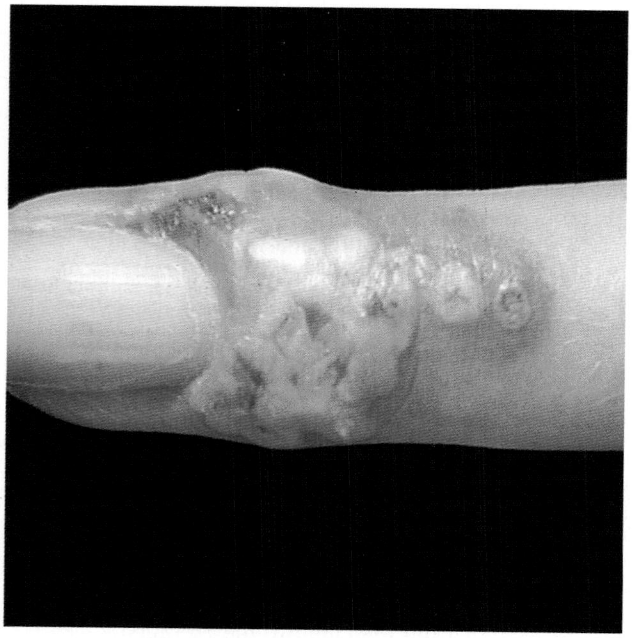

FIGURE 2.18 Herpes whitlow

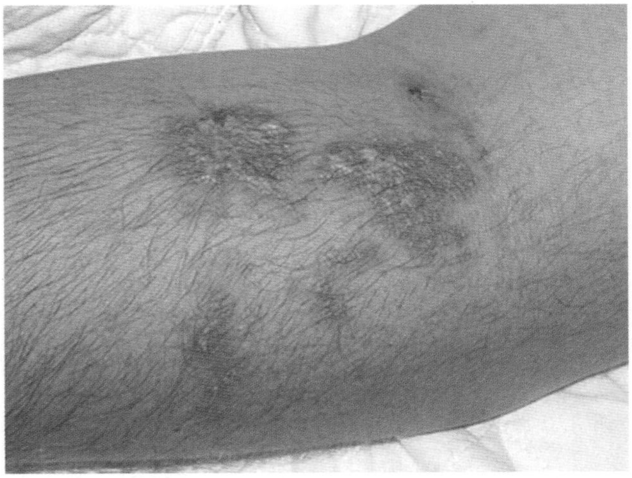

FIGURE 2.19 Herpes gladiatorum

we may be at risk for herpes whitlow if clients are shedding virus from any accessible herpes lesion.

- *Herpes gladiatorum* occurs on the trunk and extremities of wrestlers and other athletes who share skin-to-skin contact. In this situation, **vesicles** often rupture, so the lesions may look more like painful ulcers than blisters on a red base (Figure 2.19).
- *Herpetic sycosis* is a condition in which multiple herpes lesions develop over the beard area. It is the result of repeated shaving while a lesion is active; this allows the virus to spread into tiny cuts all over the face.
- *Eczema herpeticum* is a condition in which herpes simplex is associated with atopic dermatitis, a type of eczema. It is most common in children and produces a widespread outbreak of herpes lesions.
- *Ocular herpes* occurs when the virus affects the eyelid, conjunctiva, or cornea of the eye. One outbreak may not cause scarring, but repeated infections can lead to permanent damage.

Signs and Symptoms

Whether type 1 or type 2 herpes simplex usually presents in the same way: the affected area may have some pain or tingling a few days before an outbreak (the prodromic stage); then a blister or cluster of blisters appears on a red base. The blisters erupt and ooze virus-rich liquid all around the area. The blisters scab over after a week or 10 days, ending the most contagious phase of the disease. Altogether the outbreak lasts about 2 to 3 weeks.

Not all mouth sores are herpes. See Sidebar 2.1 for a description of other situations that can cause painful lesions in and around the mouth.

Vesicle: A blister.

SIDEBAR 2.1 When is a Mouth Sore Not Herpes?

Oral herpes causes the familiar lesions we call fever blisters or cold sores, but not all sores around the mouth are caused by herpesvirus.

Angular stomatitis is a condition involving painful irritated cracks around the corners of the mouth. This is often associated with denture wearers, who may drool while they sleep. The accumulation of saliva around the corners of the mouth provides a rich growth medium for the yeast that causes these lesions.

Aphthae, or "*canker sores,*" are lesions inside the mouth, often on the gums and cheeks. These are small, painful ulcers whose cause is unknown. Aphthae may be viral, but they do not appear to be contagious.

Treatment

No treatment fully eradicates herpes simplex from the body, so emphasis is placed on prevention and reducing the frequency of outbreaks by keeping as healthy as possible.

Medications

- Antiviral medications to shorten the duration of an outbreak
- Topical creams for oral herpes
- Prophylactic medications that reduce the frequency of genital herpes outbreaks

Massage Therapy Implications

RISKS	Active herpes locally contraindicates massage, and if a client knows he or she is developing a lesion, it is a courtesy to reschedule a massage appointment.
BENEFITS	Massage has no specific benefits for herpes outbreaks, but a client who has no current signs can enjoy the same benefits of bodywork as do the rest of the population. Conceivably, the stress management qualities of massage might reduce the frequency of herpes outbreaks for people who find that stress is a trigger.
OPTIONS	Because it is so difficult to resist touching the itchy, burning blisters of herpes simplex, some massage therapists choose not to work with their clients' hands (or to work on the hands through a sheet) while a client has an active outbreak.

Staphylococcus Infections of the Skin

Definition: What Are They?

Staphylococcus aureus (named *staphyle*, Greek for grapes, and *aureus* for its yellow color under a microscope) or staph, is a group of bacteria known for colonizing human skin and nasal passages. Staph infections have different names, depending on where they are found or what subtypes of bacteria are present. The lesions described in this section may involve pathogens other than *Staphylococcus*, but this is the most commonly found pathogen in these contexts.

Etiology: What Happens?

Staphylococcus bacteria use two mechanisms to cause damage: active invasion of healthy tissue, and the release of corrosive chemicals that can kill cells so that the bacterial colony can expand. When staph infections occur on the skin, they typically involve painful pus-filled vesicles, occasionally with signs of systemic infection (fever, headache, swollen lymph nodes, malaise).

Most people have colonies of staph bacteria on their skin or in their nasal passages. While these pathogens can be transmitted through person-to-person contact or via contaminated surfaces where the bacteria can survive for months in hostile environments, they can also be transferred from one area to another. In other words, if a person wipes his nose and then scratches his scabbed knee, the knee wound could develop a new staph infection. Further, once such an infection is established at a site where the skin is damaged, it is possible for the bacteria to travel through the bloodstream to set up infections elsewhere. Pneumonia, bone and joint infections, endocarditis, and varieties of toxic shock syndrome are all rare but possible complications of superficial staph infections. These are particular risks for people who are already immunocompromised. Staph infections often occur at sebaceous glands or hair shafts that are clogged by dirt, dead skin cells, or other debris, but they can begin wherever the skin has been compromised by a cut, scrape, or friction. An aggressive immune response to this pathogen leads to the classic redness, swelling, pain, and pus formation at the sites of these localized infections.

Types of Staphylococcus Infections

- ***Boils***: Boils, also called furuncles, are local infections of the skin. Boils typically occur one at a time (Figure 2.20). A group of boils connected by channels under the skin is called a carbuncle. Boils have much in common with acne, but *S. aureus* is a virulent, aggressive bacterium that actively attacks healthy tissue; this is not true of the pathogen associated with common **acne** (see Compare & Contrast 2.2, with the discussion of acne).

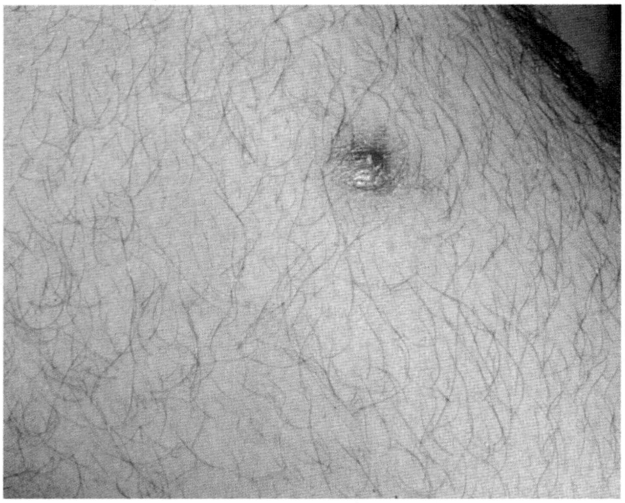

FIGURE 2.20 *Staphylococcus* infection: a single boil

- ***Methicillin-resistant Staphylococcus aureus (MRSA)*** MRSA are a group of infection-causing staph bacteria that have been recognized in hospital settings since the 1950s and are now common outside of health care facilities. About 73,000 MRSA infections are reported each year in this country in hospitals and in the community. Hospital-acquired MRSA usually takes the form of pneumonia, kidney infection, or an infected surgical wound. Community-acquired MRSA is often associated with athletic facilities and high-density, low-hygiene settings. These skin infections can be spread through indirect contact, like sharing towels or razors (Figure 2.21). MRSA occurs in several subtypes, but they are all resistant to several antibiotics, including penicillin, methicillin, amoxicillin, and others. The antibiotic resistance issue is so serious that many specialists recommend lancing or surgically excising cutaneous MRSA infections rather than trying to treat them with medication (Figure 2.22).

MRSA is a particular risk for massage therapists, who must be especially vigilant about hygienic practices because of this pathogen. To provide the best protection

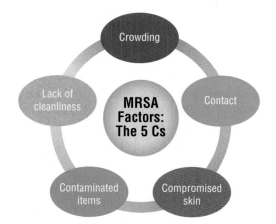

FIGURE 2.21 Five Cs of MRSA communicability, from the Centers for Disease Control and Prevention

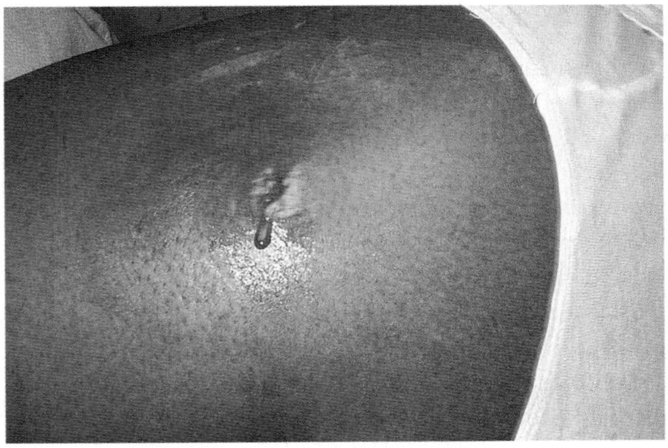

FIGURE 2.22 This MRSA infection is seeping bacteria-rich fluid

against being impacted by these bacteria, we can take extra steps (wiping down surfaces between clients and following good protocols with laundry) while making sure that any open lesions on our hands are covered.

Dangerous MRSA infections in health care settings are becoming less common, but community-acquired MRSA is pervasive. The risks of antibiotic resistance and communicability are so high that manual therapists are encouraged to view any pus-creating skin lesion, including the others listed in this article, as potential MRSA infections.

To learn more about massage in the context of this condition, see the author's video "MRSA" at http://thePoint.lww.com/Werner6e. thePoint®

- ***Folliculitis***: This condition refers to multiple boils in close proximity usually affecting hair follicles. This kind of outbreak occurs in a predictable diamond-shaped pattern (Figure 2.23). "Hot tub folliculitis" or "wetsuit folliculitis" describes a situation where **pustules** form several hours after exposure to contaminated water in the area contacted by a bathing suit or wetsuit. It can be a staph infection, or another pathogen called *Pseudomonas* can cause this. A "sty" is a version of folliculitis that affects the hair follicle of an eyelash.
- ***Pilonidal cysts***: Pilonidal cysts describe a large encysted infection at the sacrococcygeal region. They are most common among young men in their late teens to early 20s. These cysts frequently recur and may have to be surgically excised.
- ***Hidradenitis suppurativa***: This refers to deep boils that occur where hair follicles and apocrine sweat glands are numerous; the axillae and groin are the most typical locations. A defect in the epithelium of hair shafts among the apocrine glands makes a rich environment for bacterial infections here, and as the body encysts the infection, it also develops sinuses for drainage to the surface (Figure 2.24). The process can leave permanent **keloid scars.** About 1% to 2% of the population will experience this condition at some point, mostly between 11 and 50 years of age.

Pustule: A small bump in the skin containing pus. A pimple.

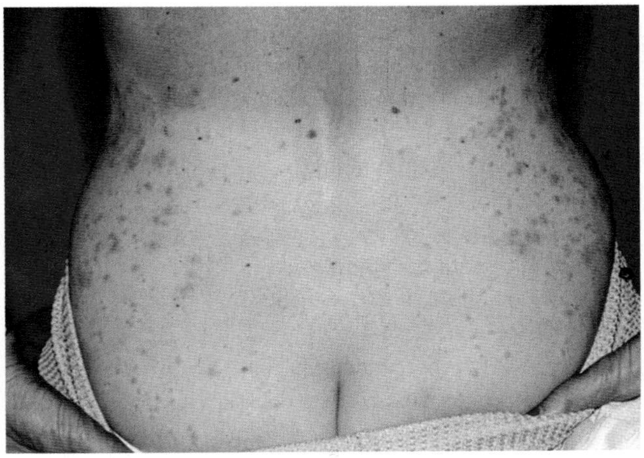

FIGURE 2.23 Folliculitis: this condition developed in the areas contacted by a bathing suit

Signs and Symptoms

A staph infection of the skin typically begins as a hard, painful, red or pinkish bump that develops over a day or two. For the next several days it increases in size, and the center of the abscess fills with pus: bacteria, dead leukocytes, and necrotic tissue. It may grow to the size of a golf ball during this time. Finally, unless it is surgically drained, the boil spontaneously ruptures and resolves. Large infections that penetrate into deep layers of the skin may leave permanent scars.

NOTABLE CASES It is rumored that the original draft of *Das Kapital* was spattered with bloodstains from Karl Marx's lanced boils.

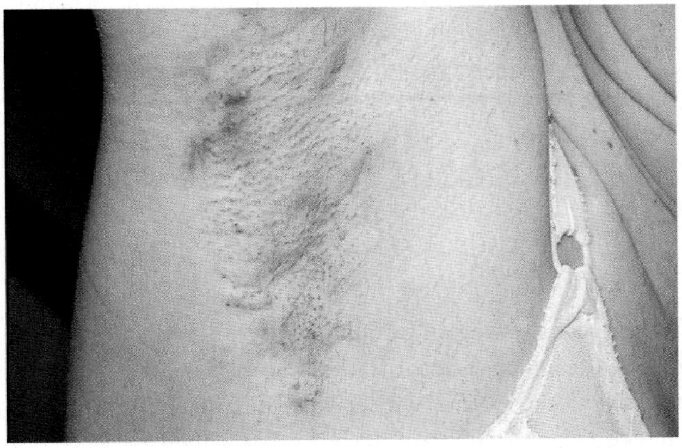

FIGURE 2.24 *Staphylococcus* infection: hidradenitis suppurativa

Treatment

People who are obese and who have poorly controlled diabetes are at increased risk for serious bacterial infections of the skin. Management of both these conditions is often a high priority to help prevent boils and other skin infections.

Conservative treatment for localized staph infections begins with warm compresses, loose clothing, and topical antibiotic ointment. If this is not sufficient, a physician may lance and drain or excise the lesion. Oral antibiotics are sometimes prescribed, but they tend to be slow acting and have the best effect for people who have a recurring problem. Untreated or incompletely treated staph infections may lead to life-threatening complications, so it is important to treat these infections aggressively and fully.

It is important never to try to squeeze or pop an infection. It could force the infection deeper into tissues, or spread the bacteria over the surface of the skin.

Medications

- Topical antibacterial ointment
- Oral or IV antibiotics, if necessary

Massage Therapy Implications

RISKS	A staph infection involves virulent, hardy bacteria that can spread deeper into the body, to another location on the body, or from one person to another. These qualities make staph infections at very least a local contraindication. If signs of systemic infection (fever, swelling at nearby lymph nodes, discomfort anywhere other than the site of the boil) are present, it is necessary to reschedule the massage.
BENEFITS	A client who has recovered from a *Staphylococcus* infection can enjoy the same benefits of massage and bodywork as the rest of the population.
OPTIONS	A client who has a well-controlled local staph infection with no systemic symptoms may receive massage, but not on or near the lesion.

Streptococcus Infections of the Skin

Definition: What Are They?

Streptococcal (strep) infections of the skin usually involve one of the group A class of *Streptococcus* bacteria. These bacteria are also associated with strep throat, **impetigo**, and toxic shock syndrome. Some of the lesions described in this section can involve multiple classes of bacteria, but *Streptococcus* is the most common pathogen found in these contexts.

Etiology: What Happens?

Bacteria, including streptococci, colonize both superficial and deep layers of the skin. Surface pathogens may be temporarily dislodged with washing, but they are quickly replaced. When they gain access through some breach in the defenses, the enzymes they produce can kill healthy cells, causing a very aggressive immune system response.

To cause an infection, streptococcal bacteria must cross the barrier of the skin through some portal of entry. This can be a cut or scratch, athlete's foot, an insect bite, surgery, or some other skin injury. People with stasis dermatitis or unresolved skin ulcers are particularly vulnerable.

A typical streptococcal infection of the skin begins at a skin wound, and may spread to affect a large area. These infections carry a high risk of becoming systemic, even complicating to blood poisoning, so it is important to treat them aggressively.

Types of *Streptococcus* Infections of the Skin

- ***Cellulitis***: This is a general streptococcal infection of deep layers of the skin and subcutaneous tissues. It is often a complication of simple injuries like a scraped knee or a contaminated blister from athlete's foot. Most cases of cellulitis begin on the lower leg; a smaller percentage begin on the face (Figure 2.25). Cellulitis is differentiated from boils and other staph infections by the absence of an abscess or draining wound. These infections are broader and less isolated than most staph infections.
- ***Necrotizing fasciitis***: This is "flesh-eating bacteria." In truth, necrotizing fasciitis isn't always a strep infection; it could also be clostridial (as seen with gas gangrene) or it could involve multiple pathogens. The most common cause, however, is group A beta-hemolytic *Streptococcus* bacteria, which excrete powerful toxins that can cause circulatory shock and death. Necrotizing fasciitis moves quickly along fascial planes, and can progress from a minor skin wound to a limb-threatening or life-threatening infection in a matter of hours.

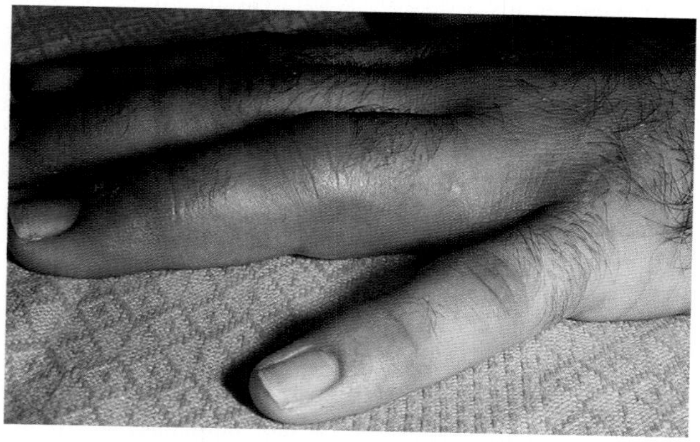

FIGURE 2.25 *Streptococcus* infection: cellulitis beginning from a minor hand wound

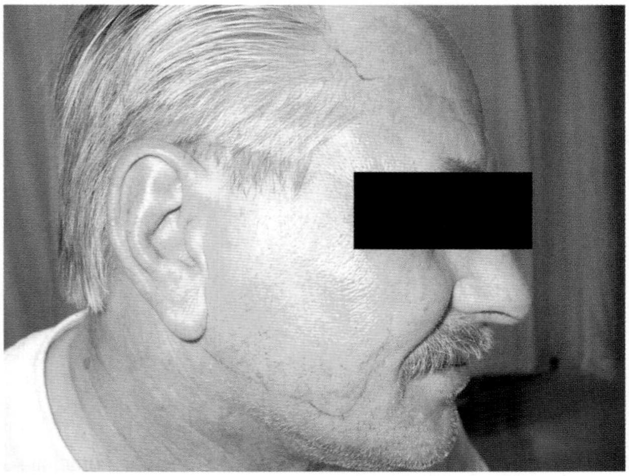

FIGURE 2.26 *Streptococcus* infection: erysipelas. Note the clear border at the edge of the redness.

- ***Erysipelas (St. Anthony's fire)***: This describes a streptococcal infection of superficial layers of the skin. Unlike other strep infections, erysipelas shows a sharp margin between involved and uninvolved skin; the red edges are usually very clear (Figure 2.26). The affected area becomes hard, shiny, and red. Blisters may develop, and superficial skin cells may shed. Erysipelas usually has a positive outcome, with no lasting damage unless the patient is especially vulnerable due to age or immune system compromise.

Signs and Symptoms

Sometimes indications of systemic infection (fever, swollen nodes, headache) precede an obvious skin injury, but signs often begin with a tender, red, swollen area. The wound may develop red streaks running toward the nearest set of lymph nodes. This is also an indicator of **lymphangitis**: infection of the lymphatic vessels. If the infection starts on the face, a raised, hot, tender, red area may spread across the bridge of the nose and forehead.

When the infection has thoroughly engaged the immune system, symptoms include fever, chills, and systemic discomfort. Facial infections are particularly dangerous because of the risk of intracranial spreading through lymphatic capillaries. If strep infections are left untreated, the bacteria may get past the lymph system and enter the circulatory system, leading quickly and perhaps fatally to septicemia, or blood poisoning.

Treatment

Most *Streptococcus* bacteria are sensitive to antibiotics. If the infection is well contained, oral antibiotics are generally recommended. If the infection has penetrated to the lymph or circulatory system, aggressive treatment with intravenous antibiotics is probably called for. Surgical removal of damaged tissue may be part of treatment for necrotizing fasciitis.

Medications

- Topical antibacterial ointment
- Oral or IV antibiotics, if necessary

Massage Therapy Implications

RISKS	Streptococcal infections of the skin involve tissue damage, a highly contagious bacterial infection, and a risk of blood poisoning. This situation systemically contraindicates massage until all signs of infection have passed.
BENEFITS	Clients who have fully recovered from strep infections and are good candidates for any kind of bodywork. Clients who have had surgery to deal with this infection may need extensive rehabilitative therapy afterwards; massage therapy can be an important part of that.

Warts

Definition: What Are They?

Warts are small, benign growths caused by varieties of human papillomavirus (HPV) that invade keratinocytes deep in the stratum basale of skin and some mucous membranes. Contrary to folklore, toads do not carry warts; HPV affects only humans.

Demographics

Children and teenagers have skin warts more often than does the rest of the population; it is estimated that 10% to 20% of all children have **verruca** vulgaris at some time. Among the rest of the population, the incidence is probably about 7% to 20%. People with suppressed immune systems are also more likely than is the general population to develop warts, and to have them in extreme forms. Because common skin warts are not reported, it is impossible to determine how many people are affected by this common condition.

Etiology: What Happens?

HPV is a group of over 100 pathogens that have been associated with several types of human warts. These pathogens are loosely categorized into three categories according to their genomic sequences: mucosal warts (cervical and anogenital warts are examples), epidermodysplasia verruciformis

Verruca: A wart.

(a genetic disease with wartlike lesions), and the subject of this section: nongenital cutaneous warts.

These varieties of HPV are spread when someone with compromised skin directly touches a wart, or through indirect contact, when a new host picks up the virus from a surface or contaminated item. They often develop on areas that are chronically irritated like hangnails, or that take a lot of friction, especially knuckles, knees, and feet. Most warts grow extremely slowly, sometimes taking months or years to fully develop.

When a person irritates a wart or damages skin nearby (like picking at hangnails or biting fingernails near a wart), the virus can spread and more warts may appear. The same caution exists for trying to clip or cut away warts: the blood from these injuries may carry the virus to cause new infections nearby.

HPV tends not to elicit an aggressive immune system response, so untreated warts can persist for months or years. Several treatment options work by irritating the site so that an inflammatory reaction recruits a more directed immune system response in the area.

Types of Warts

- *Common warts* or verruca vulgaris typically appear on the hands, knees, and elbows. They are hard, flesh-colored flaky nodules that vary in size (Figure 2.27). When a person has a wart on one finger, he or she is likely to develop another on the adjoining finger; these are called "kissing warts."
- *Plantar warts* grow on the soles of the feet (Figure 2.28). Plantar warts are easy to mistake for callus, but it is important not to try to clip or file them away (see Compare & Contrast 2.1). When several plantar warts grow in the same area, the resulting lesion is called mosaic warts. When warts on the sole of the foot grow in the deepest layers of the skin, they are called myrmecia.

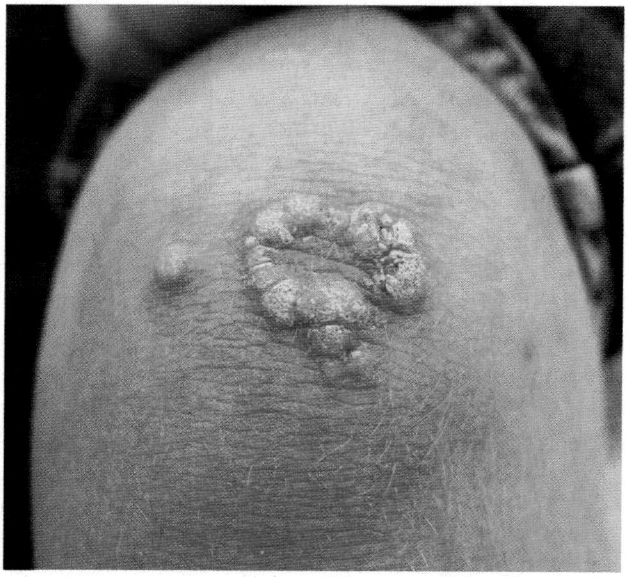

FIGURE 2.27 Common warts: verruca vulgaris on a knee

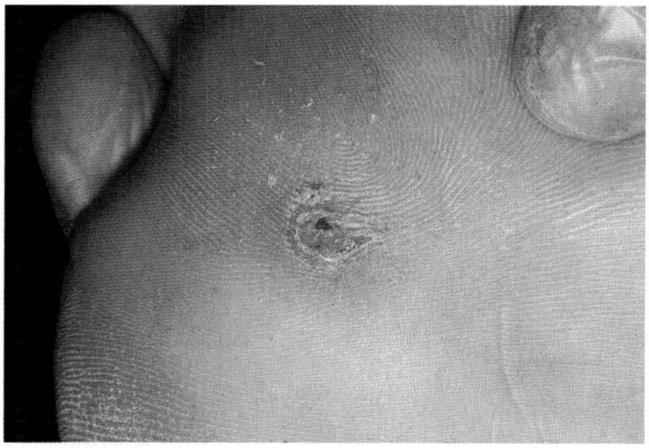

FIGURE 2.28 Plantar wart: note the dark spots and potential bleeding

- *Cystic warts* usually occur on the sole of the foot, but unlike plantar warts, they are smooth and soft. When they are excised, a cheesy substance can be squeezed out. Some experts suggest that they may involve blocked sweat glands or an attempt to encyst the original viral infection.
- *Plane or flat warts* are small, brown, smooth warts. They can grow a few at a time or with hundreds spread over a large area (Figure 2.29). Plane warts may spread during shaving, which is why they are often found on women's legs and on men's beard areas.
- *Filiform warts* are also called facial warts. They are fast-growing threadlike warts that appear on eyelids, lips, and the neck (Figure 2.30). They are painless unless irritated, and they spread readily to other areas.
- *Molluscum contagiosum* is usually a children's malady involving small white lumps, sometimes with accompanying **eczema**. The pathogen is not HPV; it is from the pox family of viruses. Molluscum contagiosum in adults can be related to immune suppression or a **sexually transmitted infection**.
- *Genital warts* are a sexually transmitted infection caused by several varieties of HPV. Most genital warts come and go with no symptoms, but others may trigger cellular activity leading to **cervical cancer**, which is discussed elsewhere.
- *Butchers' warts* are associated with meat handling. They look like common warts but are caused by a different variety of HPV.
- *Focal epithelial hyperplasia (Heck disease)* is a form of wart that forms in the mouth, on the lower lip, or on the tongue. It is most common in Native Americans and Aleuts.
- *Epidermodysplasia verruciformis* is a form of flat wart connected to a genetic disease that involves suppressed immunity and an increased risk of **squamous cell carcinoma**.

COMPARE & CONTRAST 2.1 Plantar Warts vs. Calluses

Plantar warts often look like simple calluses: the thick skin that grows on areas of the feet subject to a lot of wear and tear. The problem is that while people may file or snip off their calluses with no ill effects, to do the same with a plantar wart is to risk having that wart virus spread all over the foot, leading to more growths until it becomes impossible to walk without pain.

Massage therapists are in a unique position to observe their clients' feet and notice the subtle differences between plantar warts and callus. They may be able to give clients guidance about getting the right kind of care.

CHARACTERISTICS	PLANTAR WARTS	CALLUS
Location	Anywhere on plantar surface of foot. Usually *not* bilateral.	Appears in areas of wear and tear, especially back of heels and lateral aspect of feet. Callus usually grows in a similar pattern on both feet.
Appearance	May be white, but with darker speckling under thickened skin; this is the capillary supply.	Thick, white skin.
Sensation	Very hard and unyielding, like stepping on a pebble.	No particular sensation.

Signs and Symptoms

Warts come in several different presentations, depending on where they are found and the causative strain of HPV; descriptions are listed with the types of warts. Sometimes dark spots or "wart seeds" are seen near the base of warts: these are not in fact seeds; they are tiny thrombosed capillaries.

Treatment

Treatment options for warts vary from psychosomatic suggestion ("cut a potato into six pieces, then bury each piece in a different place and never tell anyone where you buried them") to low-tech applications of garlic juice or duct tape, to cryotherapy with liquid nitrogen or invasive electrocauterization, surgery, or lasers. At this point, no single intervention works permanently on all warts, but most people can find relief one way or another.

NOTABLE CASES Oliver Cromwell demanded that his portraitist protray him, "warts and all." His death mask has clearly discernable warts.

Wart treatment may be classified as folklore (this would include the potato cure), symptomatic relief that removes the warts but not the virus (including salicylic acid or duct

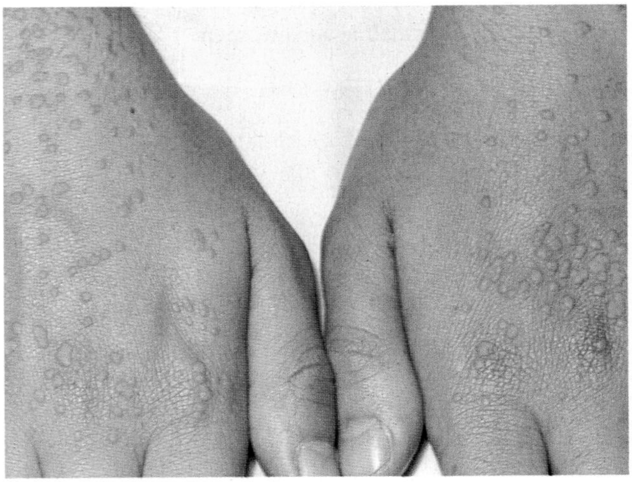

FIGURE 2.29 Flat warts

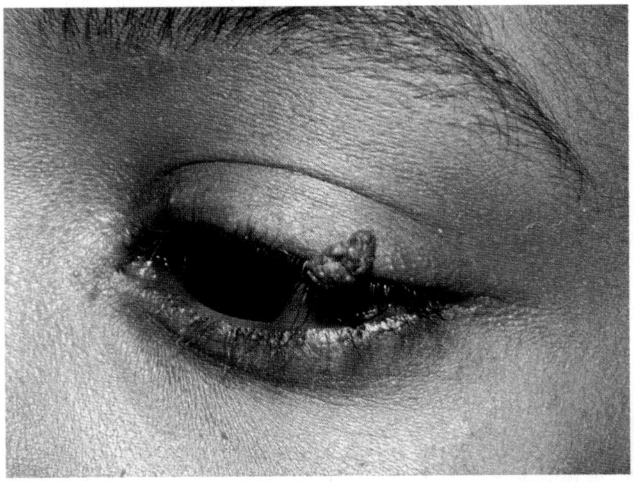

FIGURE 2.30 Filiform wart on an eyelid

tape application), destructive therapy (using lasers, surgery, or liquid nitrogen), virucidal therapy (using topical or oral antiviral medications), and drugs that interfere with cellular replication.

Medications

- Topical applications of salicylic acid or other irritants
- Antiviral medications (may be topical, injected or oral)
- Antimitotic therapy (drugs that inhibit cellular replication)

Massage Therapy Implications

RISKS	Warts locally contraindicate massage. A massage therapist is unlikely to pick up a new infection by gliding over them, but it is inappropriate to rub on or irritate these growths. Further, warts are often caught and torn around the edges, and if the skin is not intact, the client may be vulnerable to a secondary infection. Massage therapists who get warts on their hands, arms, or feet must be careful to keep these lesions covered if they contact the client during a massage.
BENEFITS	Massage probably has no direct impact on warts, but improved immune function in general may be a benefit for someone with a long-term viral infection.
OPTIONS	Warts are a local contraindication only, and only for specific, potentially irritating pressure. If the skin of the client and the therapist is intact, the affected area can be incorporated into the massage either directly or through a sheet.

Noncontagious Inflammatory Skin Disorders

Acne Rosacea

Definition: What Is It?

Acne rosacea is an idiopathic chronic skin condition. It affects the face, especially the middle third: the nose and cheeks. It can also affect the conjunctiva and the eyelids. It seldom develops elsewhere on the body.

Demographics

This condition is seen mostly in fair-skinned people between 30 and 60 years old. While women have rosacea about three times more often than do men, men tend to have more severe forms of the disease. It is estimated that about 16 million people in the United States have rosacea.

Etiology: What Happens?

The pathophysiology of acne rosacea is not well understood. It may be connected to a genetic predisposition: many patients appear to have superficial capillaries that dilate especially easily. Some researchers suggest that it may involve an overreaction to normally occurring skin bacteria, including those carried by common mites that colonize hair follicles (*Demodex folliculorum*).

Triggers for rosacea flares are fairly predictable. They include exposure to sunlight, wind, and cold temperatures; drinking hot liquids or alcohol; eating spicy food; perimenopause; the use of steroidal anti-inflammatories on the face; and emotional stress.

> **Papule:** A small, raised bump in the skin, similar to a pimple but without producing pus.

Types of Acne Rosacea

- ***Erythematotelangiectatic type rosacea***: This predominant sign of this type of rosacea is the presence of visible reddened capillary lines on the cheeks, nose, and forehead. Frequent flushing with a stinging sensation is a common symptom (Figure 2.31).
- ***Papularpustular rosacea***: This type of rosacea is marked by many small **papules** and pustules on the face. It is most common in middle-aged women.

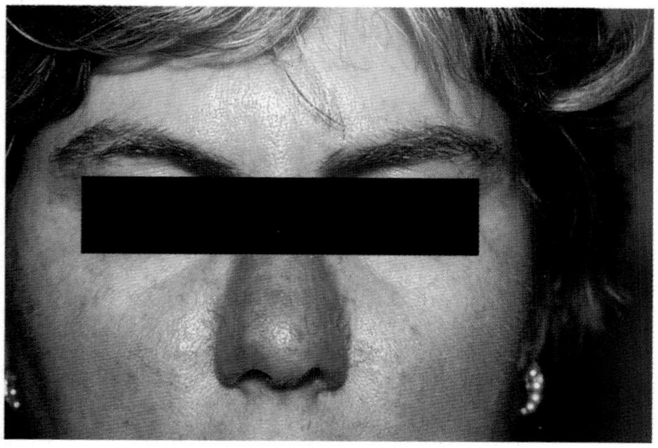

FIGURE 2.31 Mild acne rosacea, Erythematotelangiectatic type

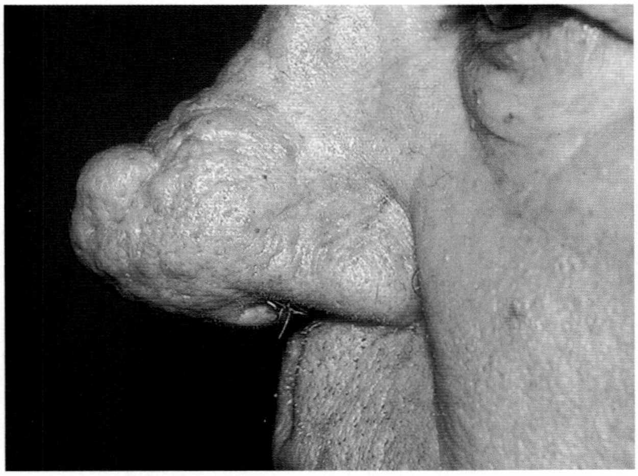

FIGURE 2.32 Severe rosacea: phymatous type

- ***Phymatous rosacea***: Rosacea that causes the nose to become distorted and bulbous fits into this category. It can also affect the chin, forehead, and ears (Figure 2.32). This version is more common in men than in women.
- ***Ocular rosacea***: Rosacea that affects the eye can cause painful, burning, and itching that affect the conjunctiva, tear ducts, and eyelids.

Signs and Symptoms

Acne rosacea occurs in flare and remission, on a spectrum from mild to severe symptoms. It is often but not always progressive without treatment. The subtypes of rosacea that have been identified by specialists who treat this condition are described under their individual headings.

An important issue for many people with acne rosacea is its consequences on self-esteem and public perception. Persons with this disorder may be sensitive to being judged by the appearance of their skin. Furthermore, a traditional but incorrect association between the bulbous nose seen with advanced acne rosacea and alcohol abuse can lead to social stigmas that are difficult to challenge.

Treatment

This is a condition that may not be curable, but it is usually controllable. Most people with rosacea must take extra care with soaps and lotions on their face, as they are hypersensitive to many products. In addition to identifying and avoiding triggers, patients may use topical or oral antibiotics. Photodynamic therapy (that combines specialized lights with medication), laser surgery, or dermabrasion may help the appearance of the skin and mask telangiectasias. Plastic surgery may be considered for a person with advanced **rhinophyma**.

Rhinophyma: A large, bulbous, and red nose often caused by rosacea.

NOTABLE CASES Comic W.C. Fields had rhinophyma, which unfairly contributed to his reputation as an alcoholic. Former President Bill Clinton has rosacea in a milder form.

Medications

- Oral antibiotics
- Topical antibiotics
- Topical antimite cream or gel

Massage Therapy Implications

RISKS	Acne rosacea may be exacerbated with stimulation of facial skin. Further, some clients may be sensitive to substances in the massage lubricant. It is important to consult with the client about his or her comfort in receiving massage to the face.
BENEFITS	Massage from a nonjudgmental therapist may provide welcome relief from the challenges to self-perception that many people with acne rosacea must deal with everyday.
OPTIONS	Consider inviting a client with acne rosacea to bring his or her own preferred moisturizer for the facial part of the massage session.

Acne Vulgaris

Definition: What Is It?

Acne is a condition in which a person develops many small, localized skin lesions. They usually appear on the face, neck, and upper back.

Demographics

Acne vulgaris, the most common skin disease in the United States, affects the vast majority of adolescents, although not everyone has it severely. About 40 to 50 million people in this country have had acne.

Etiology: What Happens?

Acne is a multifactorial condition. It has some factors in common with boils, but acne has a different etiology (see Compare & Contrast 2.2).

Several issues have been identified in the development of acne:

- Genetic predisposition
- Overactivity of sebaceous glands, plus the production of excess keratin that may contribute to blocking ducts
- Androgen production: this begins in puberty, and causes accelerated sebum production among other things

COMPARE & CONTRAST 2.2 Acne vs. Boils

Boils and acne have some characteristics in common: they are both bacterial infections that may begin at hair follicles. Indeed, if acne is unresponsive to usual treatment options, some dermatologists suggest testing for folliculitis: a rash of small boils. Here are some differentiating features:

CHARACTERISTICS	BOILS	ACNE
Appearance	One lesion at a time, or an interconnected group of pustules.	Spread over large areas (face, back, neck).
Virulence	Aggressive bacteria; attack healthy tissue.	Less aggressive bacteria; take advantage of hospitable growth medium.
Symptoms	Extremely painful.	Mildly painful.
Communicability	Can be communicable.	Communicable only with prolonged contact.
Special precautions for massage therapists	Local contraindication; may be systemic contraindication, if signs of general infection are present.	Local contraindication; no other precautions necessary.

- Colonization with *Propionibacterium acnes*, a bacterium that triggers inflammation
- Some environmental exposures, including hair products and some medications (especially steroids and other hormones, lithium, and some antiepileptic drugs)

In addition to these factors, hormonal shifts with the menstrual cycle or pregnancy can cause outbreaks, and anything that covers acne-prone skin (like headbands or shoulder pads) may make this condition worse.

Signs and Symptoms

The symptoms of acne are probably familiar to most people (Figure 2.33). It is most often found where sebaceous follicles are plentiful: on the face, upper chest, and back. It can be locally painful, but it is not usually associated with systemic infection. An exception to this rule is a rare form called acne fulminans: this condition involves fever, joint pain, and general illness.

Several types of acne lesions have been identified:

- *Pimples* are infections trapped below the surface of the skin; they are raised, red, painful bumps or papules. As they grow and accumulate purulent material (pus), they are called nodules.
- *Cysts* are infections trapped deep in the dermis. They can protrude into the subcutaneous layer, develop sinuses to drain to the surface of the skin, and cause permanent scarring. Cysts may or may not be inflamed (Figure 2.34).

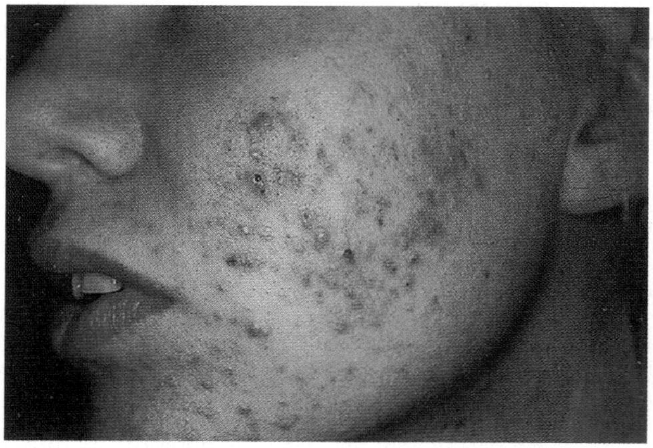

FIGURE 2.33 Acne vulgaris

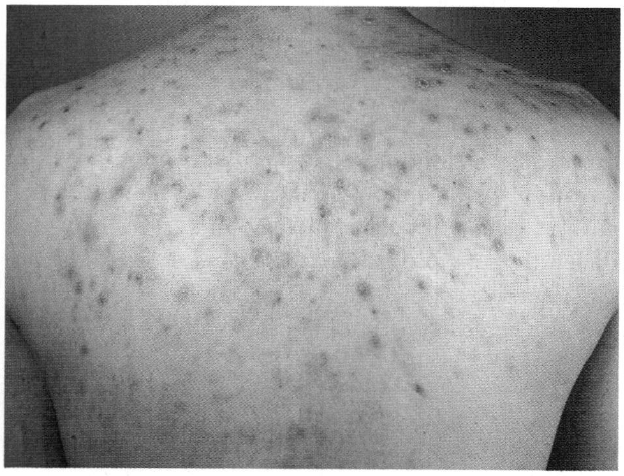

FIGURE 2.34 Cystic acne

- *Open comedones* are also called blackheads. **Comedones** are superficial, and the passage into the hair follicle is open to the air. This allows the trapped sebum to oxidize and turn dark. Blackheads are not, as popular belief would have it, trapped particles of dirt.
- *Closed comedones* are also called whiteheads or pustules. They are superficial infections that are covered with a thin layer of epithelium that traps the sebum and pus.

Treatment

It is important to point out that sebum serves a purpose: it keeps hair and hair shafts healthy, and it contributes to the acid mantle that discourages bacterial replication on the skin. If sebum is stripped away by harsh soaps or alcohol, the sebaceous glands work to replace it. Consequently, people who want to control their acne must find the fine line between keeping the skin healthily clean, but not completely stripped of its normal secretions.

The first treatment advice for people with acne is often the most difficult to follow: *don't touch the face*. Touching, scratching, and popping acne lesions does little except to spread the bacteria and create the possibility of permanent scarring.

Dietary interventions currently focus on links between a low glycemic index diet and improvement in acne symptoms (the reduction in insulin is linked to a reduction in androgenic hormones that stimulate sebum production), and a possible connection between increased acne symptoms and the use of hormone-supplemented milk products.

Washing the face twice daily with gentle soap and warm water is generally recommended before trying other interventions. Harsh soaps or scrubbing pads can make this condition much worse.

Medical interventions usually involve topical or oral antibiotics, often in combination with benzoyl peroxide, which appears to limit drug resistance in *P. acnes*. Low-dose contraceptives may reduce levels of sebum-stimulating hormones. More severe acne cases may be treated with a group of drugs called retinoids, which can be used topically or as an oral medication. They are associated with several potentially dangerous side effects, so their use is carefully controlled.

Nondrug treatments include manual extraction of comedones and chemical peels. Aesthetic options for acne-related scars are numerous. They include laser surgery, dermabrasion, and filling pockmarks with injected fat to smooth out their appearance.

Comedone: An acne lesion, a dilated hair follicle filled with bacteria and other material.

Medications

- Benzoyl peroxide alone or in combination with other medication
- Topical retinoids alone or in combination with other medication
- Oral antibiotics for moderate-to-severe acne
- Hormonal therapy and oral contraceptives if other interventions are not successful

Massage Therapy Implications

RISKS	Inflamed acne lesions locally contraindicate massage. Pimples are infections, and they are associated with a compromised shield: the skin is no longer intact, which means massage can make the infection worse. Further, lesions can be locally painful. And finally, the lubricant can block sebaceous glands, further aggravating an already irritable situation.
BENEFITS	Acne can have a devastating effect on self-perception. Massage from a nonjudgmental, welcoming therapist can be a wonderful experience for a person who lives with this disorder.
OPTIONS	If a client is concerned about massage lubricant, the best options are to use a water-based lotion instead of oil, or to recommend that the client shower with gentle soap as soon as possible after treatment. Do not attempt to remove excess lubricant with an alcohol-based application; this simply strips the skin of its natural protective sebum, and it is likely to work overtime to replace it.

Eczema, Dermatitis

Definition: What Are They?

Dermatitis is an umbrella term meaning skin inflammation, which is stunningly nonspecific. Many of the conditions in this chapter could be called dermatitis, although by convention the term is reserved for disorders that are not infectious. This section focuses on two issues: eczema and contact dermatitis, with some brief discussions of other types of skin inflammation (Figure 2.35).

Eczema is a condition connected to immune dysfunction and hypersensitivity reactions expressed in the skin. Contact dermatitis is a skin inflammation caused by an externally applied irritant or allergen. It is common to have aspects of both contact dermatitis and eczema simultaneously, especially on the hands of people who go through frequent cycles of wetting and drying the skin with exposure to chemicals and allergens.

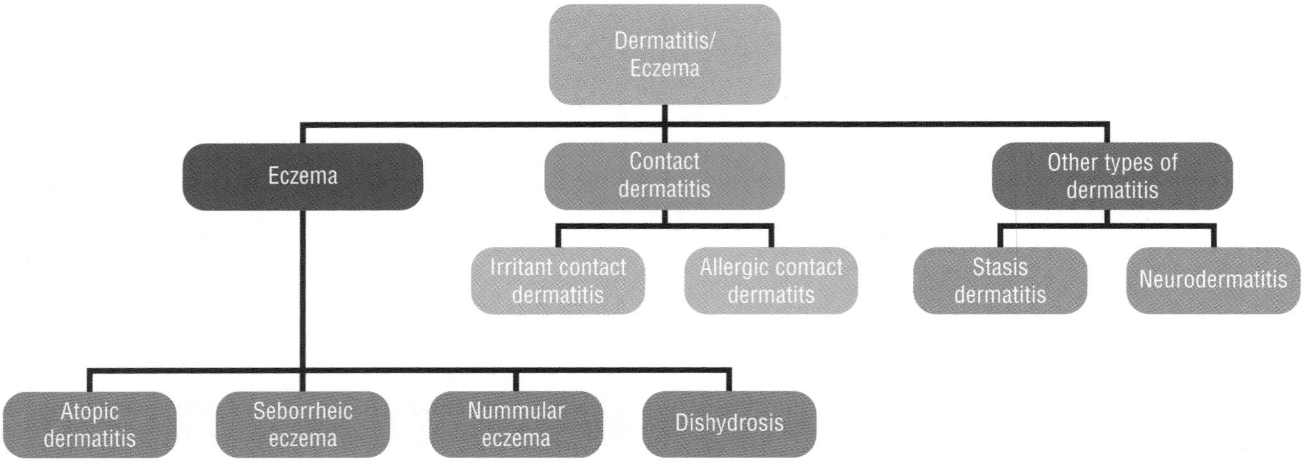

FIGURE 2.35 "Organizational chart" of dermatitis and eczema

Demographics

Atopic dermatitis, the most common version of eczema, is very common. It affects about 15% of children, but most grow out of it by puberty. It is estimated to affect about 18 million people in the United States.

Etiology: What Happens?

Many types of dermatitis are brought about by an overreaction in the immune system to some triggering substance. Hypersensitivity reactions are discussed in detail in the introduction to Chapter 6, but it is useful to look at an abbreviated version here.

The two types of hypersensitivity reactions that create skin symptoms are type I allergic reactions and type IV delayed reactions.

Eczema is a type I reaction. These are systemic immune system responses to nonthreatening stimuli. In this situation, mast cells release vasodilating chemicals, including histamine, and these create an inflammatory response. Eczema is frequently seen alongside or in the same family with allergic sinusitis (hay fever) and asthma. While many young children have signs of eczema, most grow out of it by puberty. For some people, however, this condition persists throughout adulthood.

Allergic contact dermatitis is a type IV delayed reaction, mediated by a several immune system agents. Poison oak, poison ivy, and local skin reactions to metals, soaps, dyes, and latex are examples of allergic contact dermatitis. With this type of reaction symptoms typically develop 12 to 48 hours after exposure.

Both contact dermatitis and eczema can begin a process by which a minor skin condition becomes a debilitating problem. When a person with dermatitis scratches the mildly itchy lesions, the lesions are stimulated and become much itchier. This leads to more scratching, more itchiness, and a vicious circle called the itch-scratch cycle.

People with dermatitis or eczema are particularly susceptible to secondary infection because their skin may be delicate and easy to invade. **Impetigo, herpes simplex, staphylococcal infections, fungal infections,** and **warts** are common complications of dermatitis and eczema.

Eczema

Factors in Eczema

Research into the causes of eczema is proceeding, but no single factor has been identified. In addition to a genetic predisposition, contributing factors include two main issues:

- *Fatty acid deficiency*: A deficiency in certain fatty acids compromises the lipid layer of the stratum corneum, leading to a high risk of damaged skin and immune dysregulation.
- *Excessive inflammatory responses*: Increased proinflammatory chemicals and allergy-related antibodies all contribute to inflammation with capillary dilation, redness, and itching.

Although it seems clear that eczema is connected to a genetically determined immune system dysfunction, flares can be triggered by local irritations such as rough textures, detergents, harsh chemicals, extreme temperatures, and excessive sweating.

Types of Eczema

- *Atopic dermatitis* is the most common variety of eczema, especially among children. It is usually itchy, red, flaky, and dry, occurring in the creases on the sides of the nose and other skin creases, such as knees, elbows, ankles, and hands (Figure 2.36). The skin may thicken and feel rough; this is called **lichenification**. On dark skin atopic dermatitis can take the form of flat papules (Figure 2.37).

> **Lichenification:** An area of thick and leathery skin *or* the process by which the epidermis becomes thick and leathery.

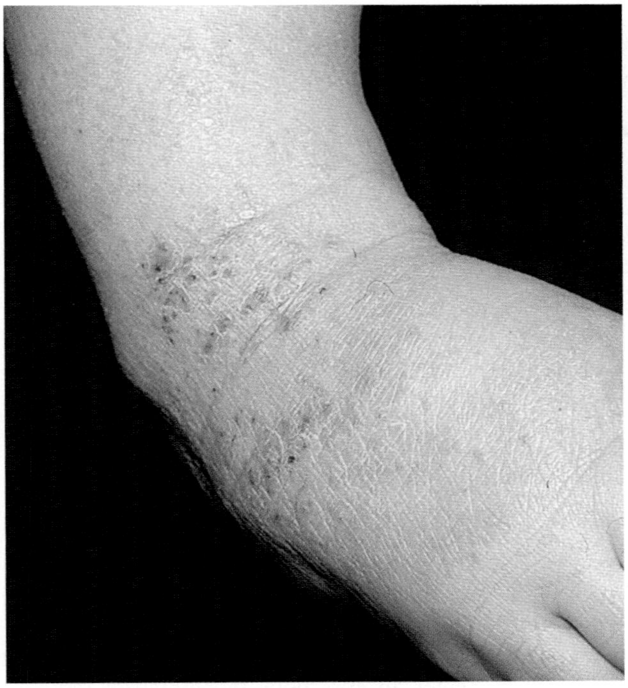

FIGURE 2.36 Atopic dermatitis on a person with light skin

People and families prone to atopic dermatitis are often also affected by allergic rhinitis (hay fever) and asthma.

- *Seborrheic eczema* in infants is called cradle cap. It produces yellowish, oily patches, usually in the skin folds around the nose or on the scalp, where it can cause extreme dandruff. Seborrheic eczema in adults is acutely itchy. Unlike other forms of eczema, this may involve cutaneous yeasts in the creation of the rash and other symptoms.
- *Dyshidrosis* produces blisters filled with fluid that appear mostly on hands and feet. It is sometimes described as looking like a combination of fungal infection and a contact allergy (Figure 2.38). It often occurs in response to hot weather or emotional stress. Because it involves weeping blisters, this form of eczema is a special caution for massage.

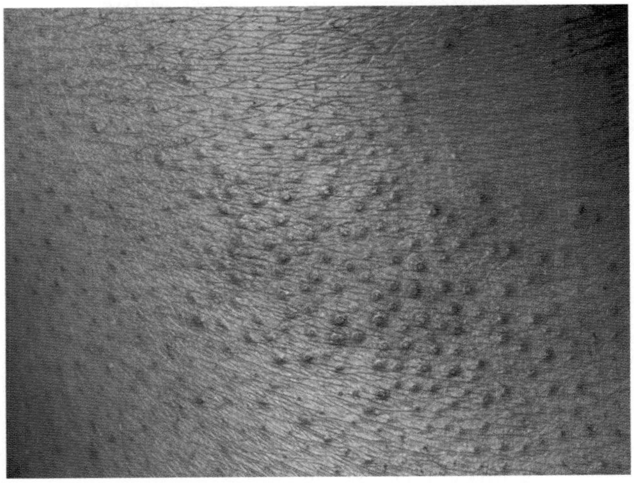

FIGURE 2.37 Atopic dermatitis on a person with dark skin

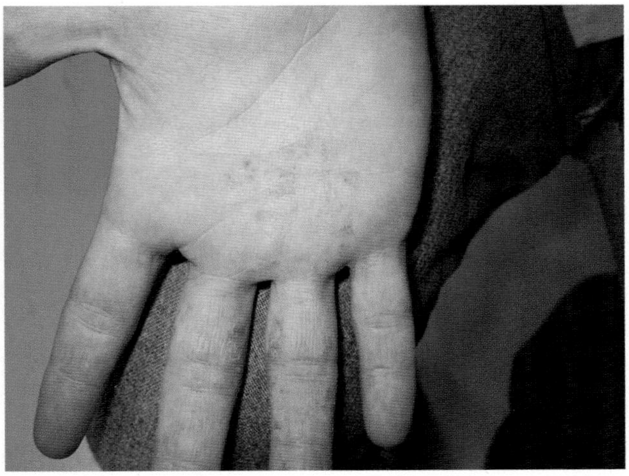

FIGURE 2.38 Dyshidrosis

- *Nummular eczema* appears in small circular lesions, often on the legs and buttocks (Figure 2.39). It can resemble ringworm, and it is often intensely itchy. Men have nummular eczema more often than women do, and it often accompanies some other form of eczema.

Signs and Symptoms of Eczema

Signs and symptoms of eczema vary according to what type is present, as described in the discussion of types of eczema. Most versions involve redness, itching, and the risk of secondary infection if the skin is damaged.

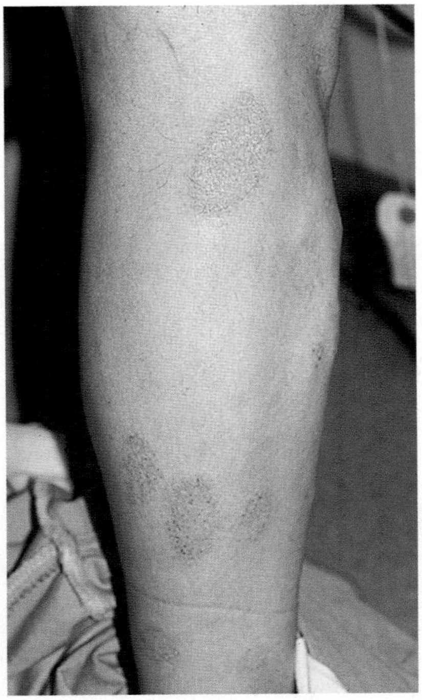

FIGURE 2.39 Nummular eczema: discrete circular lesions

Contact Dermatitis

Factors in Contact Dermatitis

Contact dermatitis can be a reaction to an allergen or a tissue irritant.

Types of Contact Dermatitis

- *Irritant contact dermatitis* is the result of using with some substance that would be irritating to anyone. Reliable triggers include prolonged working in water, exposure to harsh cleansers, solvents, and ongoing friction (Figure 2.40). All of these can damage even the healthiest skin, but cessation of the irritation relieves symptoms.
- *Allergic contact dermatitis* involves an immune response in the skin of the affected person; only people who are allergic have this reaction. Some common triggers include nickel (found in watchbands, snaps, the buttons on jeans, and earrings), preservatives used in lotions, the adhesive used in many medical bandages, some perfumes and dyes, latex, and urushiol: the allergenic substance in the sap of poison ivy (Figures 2.41 and 2.42). Allergic contact dermatitis tends to develop several hours after exposure to the trigger.

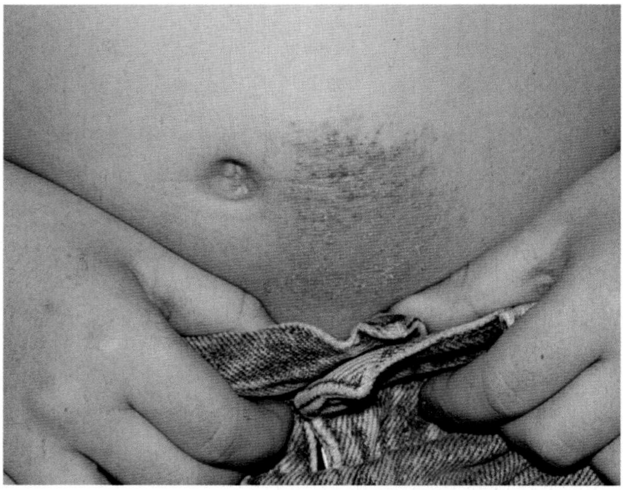

FIGURE 2.41 Allergic contact dermatitis: a nickel allergy

Signs and Symptoms of Contact Dermatitis

The symptoms of contact dermatitis vary according to the causative factors. Acute situations are typically locally red, swollen, and itchy or tender, showing exactly where the irritation took place. Long-lasting, low-grade reactions may not show signs of inflammation, although mild itchiness is common.

Other types of dermatitis show specific patterns but are not related to irritation or contact with allergenic substances.

Other Types of Dermatitis

- *Stasis dermatitis* usually appears on the lower legs in association with poor circulation, as seen with diabetes or heart failure. It is common in elders. Stasis dermatitis is red or purplish and may occur with small ulcers where the skin has been deprived of nutrition (Figure 2.43).
- *Neurodermatitis* involves a small injury, such as a mosquito bite, that creates an enormous inflammatory response and localized scaly patches of skin.

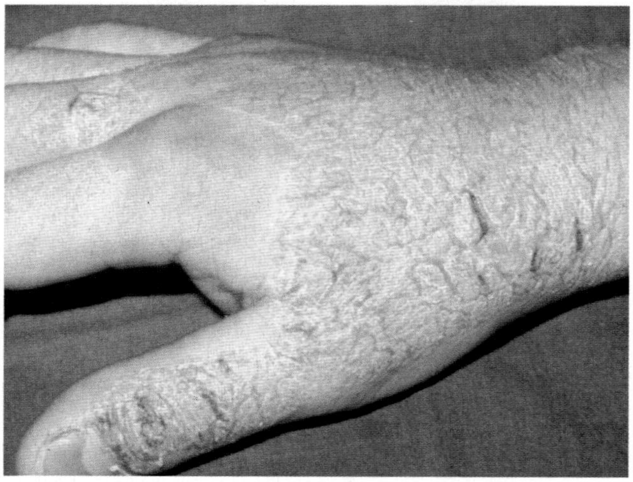

FIGURE 2.40 Irritant contact dermatitis with deep fissures

Complications of Eczema and Dermatitis

Any skin condition that results in cracked, bleeding or blistered skin carries a risk for secondary infection. Because eczema is frequently pruritic, and hands are seldom germ-free, *Staphylococcus* and *Streptococcus* infections are common. A condition called eczema herpeticum occurs when open lesions are infected with herpes simplex virus leading to a

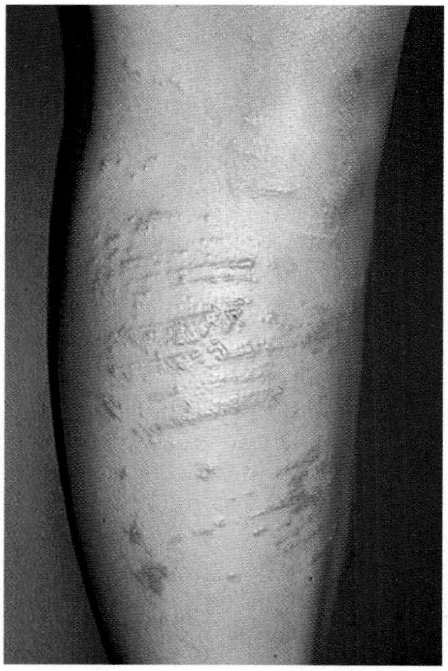

FIGURE 2.42 Allergic contact dermatitis: poison ivy

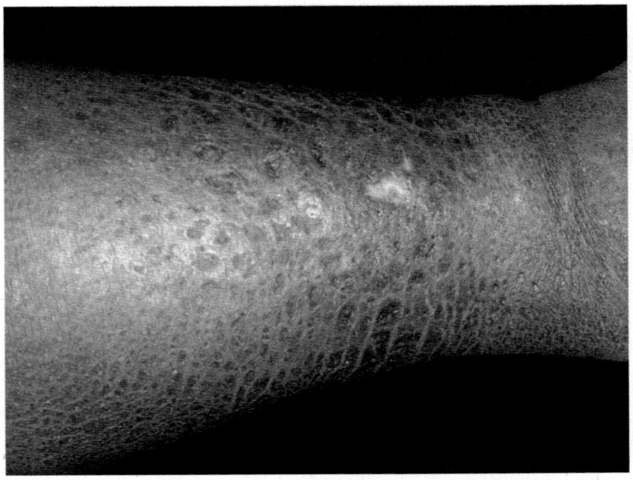

FIGURE 2.43 Stasis dermatitis with scaling and a clean ulceration

widespread and painful herpetic rash. Finally, repeated use of corticosteroid creams to control the rash and itching can lead to serious degeneration and atrophy of the skin. For more on skin, allergies, and stress, see Sidebar 2.2.

Treatment

Self-help measures for people with contact dermatitis and eczema begin with trying to identify their triggers, and then avoiding them carefully. Persons with eczema must also try to maintain adequate hydration of the skin, which means finding a moisturizer or emollient that doesn't contain any irritating substances, and applying it while the skin is still wet from bathing. Essential fatty acid supplements that help to strengthen the lipid layer in the skin may also be recommended. Acupuncture appears to decrease the symptoms of acute eczema, as well as decreasing the severity of subsequent flares.

Pharmaceutical management of dermatitis and eczema can vary from substances that suppress immune system activity to steroidal anti-inflammatories. Most of these interventions carry a risk of potentially serious side effects that require careful monitoring.

Medications

- Topical or oral steroidal anti-inflammatories
- Topical immunomodulators
- Topical or oral antihistamines
- Antibiotics for secondary infection, if necessary

Massage Therapy Implications

RISKS	Massage appears to temporarily boost local circulation. If an area is red, warm, and itchy, this could easily exacerbate symptoms of dermatitis or eczema. Further, people prone to these conditions may have an increased risk of having a hypersensitivity reaction to massage lubricants: this must be addressed before beginning a session. Finally, some of these conditions may involve blisters or scratching that damages the skin. These locally injuries contraindicate massage because of the risk of secondary infection.
BENEFITS	Clients with hypersensitive skin may find that careful massage with a hypoallergenic lubricant is soothing and deeply relaxing. As long as a therapist can find a way to work that does not increase itching or discomfort, the client can enjoy all the benefits that massage has to offer.
OPTIONS	Self-image can be a major factor for people who live with chronic skin conditions. Massage therapy can be a powerful positive experience, as long as the client is comfortable and safe. For areas that are compromised with scratching or scabbing, consider working gloved or through the sheet so that the "incorporating" aspects of a massage that can weave together a whole body experience are not lost.
RESEARCH	It is possible to theorize that massage may have an organizing influence on the immune system and strong stress-reducing properties that might help to manage these skin rashes, but the small amount of research that has so far been conducted on the effect of massage therapy for people with eczema has not shown significant positive results. Some research has found that massage has a potential adverse effect for people with these skin sensitivities, however, as some oils or oil additives may trigger a flare of dermatitis or eczema either in the client or in the therapist.[1–4] 1. Lakshmi C. Allergic contact dermatitis (type IV hypersensitivity) and type I hypersensitivity following aromatherapy with ayurvedic oils (dhanwantharam thailam, eladi coconut oil) presenting as generalized erythema and pruritus with flexural eczema. *Indianian Journal of Dermatology* 2014;59(3):283–286. http://www.e-ijd.org/article.asp?issn=0019-5154;year=2014;volume=59;issue=3;spage=283;epage=286;aulast=Lakshmi 2. Danby SG, AlEnezi T, Sultan A, et al. Effect of olive and sunflower seed oil on the adult skin barrier: implications for neonatal skin care. *Pediatric Dermatology* 2013;30(1):42–50. http://www.ncbi.nlm.nih.gov/pubmed/22995032 3. Larson D, Jacob SE. Tea tree oil. *Dermatitis* 2012;23(1):48–49. http://www.ncbi.nlm.nih.gov/pubmed/22653070 4. Adisen E, onder M. Allergic contact dermatitis from *laurus nobilis* oil induced by massage. *Contact Dermatitis* 2007;56(6):360–361. http://www.ncbi.nlm.nih.gov/pubmed/17577382

SIDEBAR 2.2 Stress, Allergies, and Cortisol

Stress can ripple through the body in a number of chemical ways. Massage therapists study some of these effects because they too have some influence over what chemicals are being released, and that influence should be informed and intentional.

For people who are prone to allergies, long-term stress creates some special problems. Cortisol is the hormone that is specifically related to long-term stress. When it is secreted over a long time, cortisol can damage the body by systemically weakening the connective tissues. But cortisol has one quality that makes it very, *very* useful: it is a powerful anti-inflammatory agent. When people undergo long-term stress, their cortisol supplies can be depleted. When cortisol is depleted, limited resources are available within the body to quell the inflammatory reaction. And for individuals subject to allergies, this means that they have a difficult time reducing the inflammation from immune system attacks against nonthreatening stimuli such as wheat, pollen, cat dander, and other irritants. If an immune reaction takes the form of a skin rash, it may be called dermatitis or eczema.

This is not to suggest that stress is the only cause of allergies or even the most important one; it's just to point out that long-term stress and cortisol depletion may make allergies worse.

Neoplastic Skin Disorders

Seborrheic Keratosis

Definition: What Is It?

SK is a benign skin growth in which epithelial cells proliferate in isolated areas.

Demographics

SK is the most common benign tumor seen in older adults. They are relatively rare in people younger than 40, but in some populations, they are found in 80% or more of older people. They are most common among fair-skinned people, but dark-skinned people may develop a similar benign lesion with an earlier onset called dermatosis papulosa nigra (Figure 2.44).

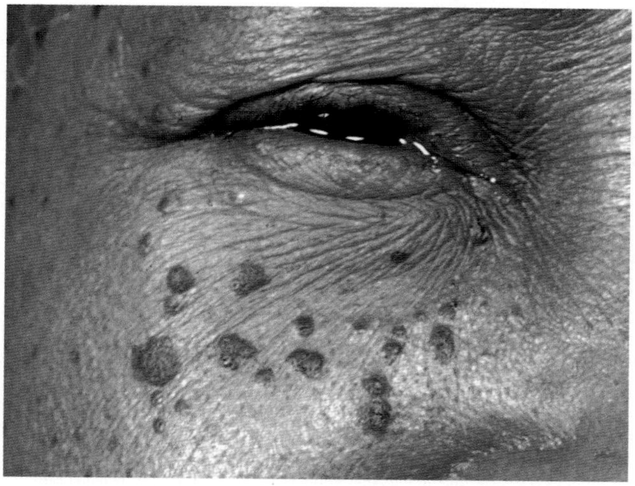

FIGURE 2.44 Individual lesions of dermatosis papulosa nigra may resemble typical seborrheic keratosis

Etiology: What Happens?

The etiology of SK is not well understood. Hyperproliferation of epithelial cells is evident, and a genetic predisposition seems clear, but other factors or triggers have not been identified. Lesions appear most frequently in people over 50 and in areas that have been exposed to sunlight: the chest, back, neck, face, and scalp. It is not seen on palms or soles. SK is not contagious.

SK is not skin cancer, but it can resemble actinic keratosis (a subtype of SCC) when lesions are relatively new, and malignant melanoma when lesions are advanced.

SK is usually considered a completely benign condition, but sometimes it has a dramatically rapid onset with multiple lesions. This phenomenon, called the Leser-Trélat sign, is associated with a risk of other diseases, especially cancer involving the gastrointestinal tract. The relationship between SK and internal cancers is unclear, however.

Signs and Symptoms

SK lesions typically appear singly or in groups as clearly edged soft light or dark brown spots on the trunk, face, or scalp. As they mature, they become thicker and often darker. Eventually, they develop a warty, "pasted on" appearance. They are sometimes described as looking like shiny spots of melted wax, or crusty barnacles adhered to the skin (Figure 2.45).

Complications

SK lesions can protrude from the skin and be caught on clothing. If they are irritated they can itch, bleed, and grow larger. Secondary bacterial infection at the injury is also a risk. It is possible for various types of skin cancer to begin within the borders of an SK lesion, and consequently escape early detection.

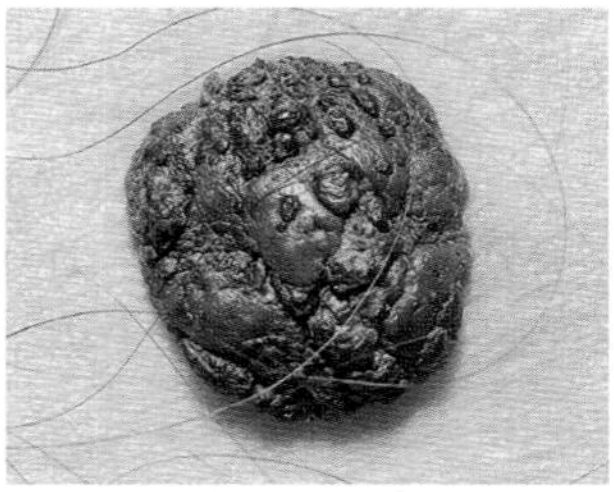

FIGURE 2.45 Seborrheic keratosis

Treatment

Most of the time SK isn't treated at all, because the lesions are completely benign and don't usually hurt. Some topical medications may reduce the thickness of the growths. When they are in a location to be irritated it may be worthwhile to remove the growths. This is usually accomplished with cryotherapy, but electrodissection and curettage may be suggested to cauterize and remove the growths surgically.

Medications

- Topical applications to reduce the thickness of SK lesions

Massage Therapy Implications

RISKS	Massage carries no risk for SK lesions, as long as they aren't irritated or bleeding. These can be considered local contraindications.
BENEFITS	Massage has no specific benefits for SK lesions; clients with this disorder can enjoy the same benefits from bodywork as does the rest of the population.

Skin Cancer

Definition: What Is It?

Cancer is the uncontrolled replication of cells. Usually, these cells accumulate into tumors that can invade and damage nearby tissues. Cells may also escape a primary tumor to travel elsewhere in the body and colonize a new area; this is metastasis.

Cells that are programed to replace themselves easily are particularly vulnerable to DNA damage that triggers uncontrolled and disorganized replication. Epithelial cells are highly labile; this explains why cancers of the skin, lungs, breast, prostate, and digestive tract (all epithelial tissues) are the most common cancer diagnoses.

Etiology: What Happens?

Skin cancer begins with a change in epithelial cell function. The trigger for this change is often attributed to a history of UV radiation (especially deep, blistering sunburns) or genetic predisposition, but exposure to other hazards has also been shown to increase the risk of various types of skin cancer. Arsenic, chronic skin inflammation and injury, and the use of immunosuppressant drugs are all associated with an increased risk for skin cancer.

Demographics

Skin cancer is by far the most commonly diagnosed form of cancer, accounting for about a million diagnoses each year; this is about one-half of all cancer diagnoses in the United States. People most at risk include those with a long history of sun exposure, those who are fair skinned, those with a personal or family history of skin cancer, and those who are immune suppressed.

Malignant melanoma is the least common and most dangerous form of skin cancer, and it is diagnosed in about 61,000 people each year in this country. Men slightly outnumber women. Each year close to 10,000 people in the United States die from melanoma.

Types of Skin Cancer

The major skin cancer types are usually divided into the three categories discussed here: BCC, SCC, and malignant melanoma. Another way to discuss them is in only two groups: nonmelanomas and melanoma. This is a useful delineation because it is easy to remember the key diagnostic features of each:

- The leading sign or symptom of nonmelanoma skin cancers is *a sore that doesn't heal, or that comes and goes in the same place.*
- The leading sign or symptom of melanoma is a mole that displays the *ABCDE* qualities described in the melanoma section.

Basal Cell Carcinoma

Definition: What Is It?

BCC is by far the most common type of skin cancer, accounting for about 80% of all skin cancer diagnoses. It is a slow-growing tumor of basal cells in the epidermis. It usually appears on the face or head. BCC only rarely metastasizes, but if a tumor is not treated it may invade and damage healthy tissues, including bones, blood vessels, and nerves.

Types of Basal Cell Carcinoma

- *Nodular BCC*: These lesions are sometimes called rodent ulcers. They have rounded pink pearly edges and a soft sunken middle (Figure 2.46). **Telangiectasias** may be visible. These lesions may itch and bleed easily, but they don't tend to be painful.

> **Telangiectasia:** Small dilated blood vessels, usually in the skin. "Spider veins."

2 Integumentary System Conditions

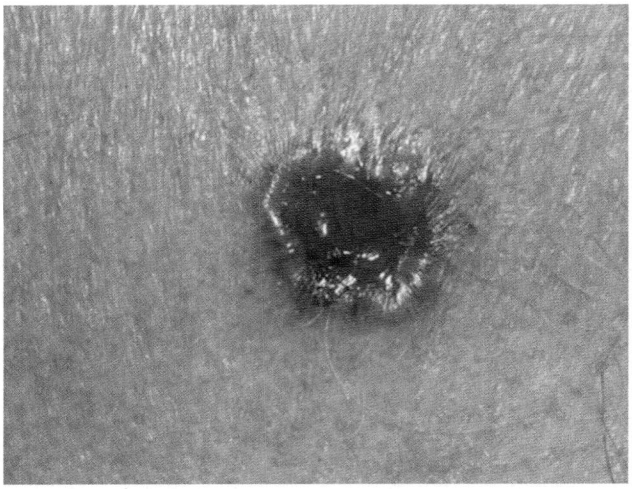

FIGURE 2.46 Nodular BCC: rodent ulcer

- *Pigmented BCC*: This form has darker lesions that may be flat and brown, bluish, or gray. It is easy to mistake it for malignant melanoma (Figure 2.47).
- *Superficial BCC*: This form resembles eczema or psoriasis, which means it could also be taken for AK: a type of SCC.
- *Micronodular BCC*: This type shows multiple well-defined white-yellow lesions.
- *Morpheaform BCC*: This is the most serious type. It tends to show only subtle scarlike lesions on the skin, while silently and aggressively invading deeper tissues (Figure 2.48).

Signs and Symptoms

BCC has several different presentations, but they have one common feature: the lesions don't heal, or they come and go in the same place. This is the cardinal sign of nonmelanoma skin cancer.

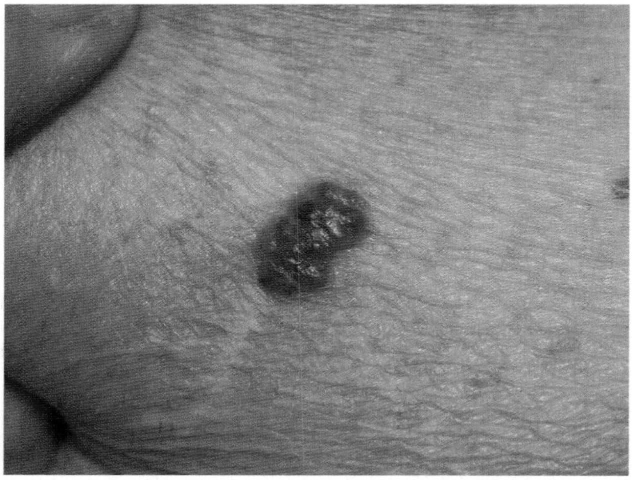

FIGURE 2.47 Pigmented BCC

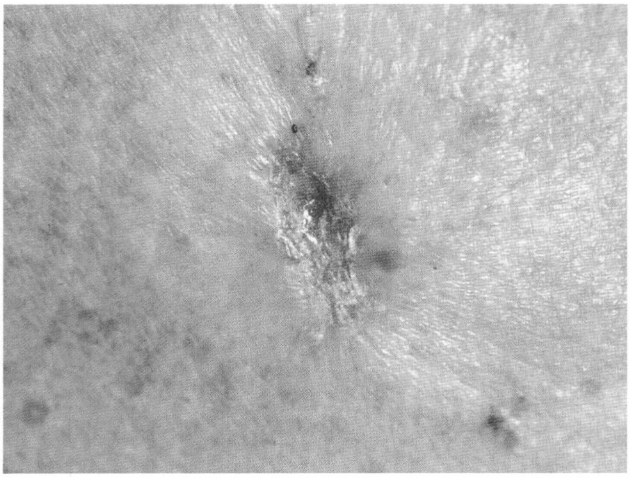

FIGURE 2.48 Morpheaform BCC: lesions may have a puckered appearance on the surface as they infiltrate deeper structures

Squamous Cell Carcinoma

Definition: What Is It?

SCC is a cancer of skin cells that arises in keratinocytes superficial to the basal layer. It often appears in areas exposed to sunlight, but unlike other skin cancers it also grows in the mouth, affecting the tongue, cheeks, and gums. SCC that grows on the penis or vaginal walls is associated with a history of genital warts.

Exposure to mid-range UV light is the main risk factor for SCC, but this condition can also develop in the presence of long-term skin injury or inflammation like decubitus ulcers, repeating boils, or draining sores.

It is rare but not impossible for SCC to metastasize to other places in the body. For this reason, lesions caught in early stages are typically removed as quickly as possible.

Types of Squamous Cell Carcinoma

- *Actinic keratosis (AK)*: Also called solar keratosis, this used to be discussed as a precancerous condition that may lead to SCC. However, the cellular changes seen with AK are identical to those seen with invasive SCC. Further, left long enough most AK lesions eventually develop aggressive characteristics, and they seldom spontaneously disappear. AK looks like brown or red scaly lesions in sun-exposed areas: forehead, ears, and hands (Figure 2.49).
- *Actinic cheilitis*: This is a form of AK that is found specifically on the lips (Figure 2.50).
- *Leukoplakia*: This form looks like gray and white patches on the tongue and inside the cheek that don't wipe or scrape off. It is most often associated with tobacco use. It isn't usually dangerous, but in rare cases can become malignant, especially when it appears next to raised, red patches.
- *Bowen disease*: Also called in situ SCC, Bowen disease is similar to AK except that the lesions tend to be larger and browner (Figure 2.51). A high frequency of HPV-16 infection within Bowen disease tumor cells suggests a link between this wart virus and skin cancer.

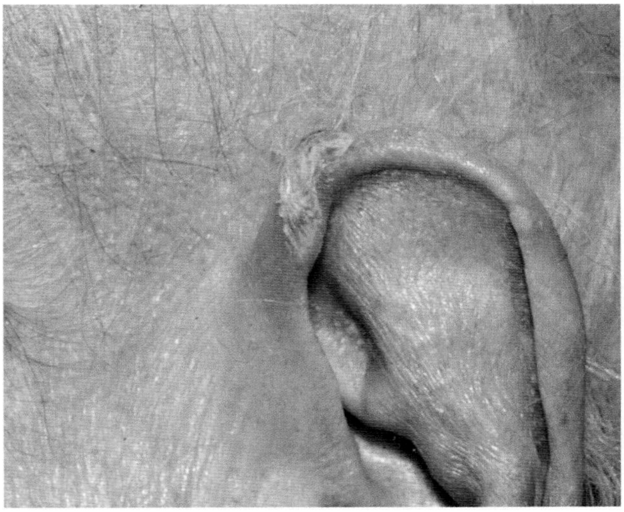

FIGURE 2.49 Actinic keratosis

Signs and Symptoms of Squamous Cell Carcinoma

SCC lesions often appear on preexisting injuries, inside the mouth, and in areas with a history of sun damage. They share the typical nonmelanoma skin cancer pattern; they appear as nonpainful sores that may itch or bleed, but they don't ever fully heal. SCC borders are often less distinct than those of BCC.

Melanoma

Definition: What Is It?

Melanocytes are the pigment cells deep in the epidermis that give skin its color. Melanin in skin cells offers some protection from UV radiation, but when melanocytes become overactive and replicate out of control, they can quickly become a life-threatening form of cancer.

Unlike other forms of skin cancer, melanoma metastasizes readily, often leading to tumors in the bones, liver, or central nervous system. It is the leading cause of death by skin cancer. Melanocytes are found in the eye, reproductive and digestive tracts, as well as the skin, so while it is rare, melanoma does have the potential to develop in these areas.

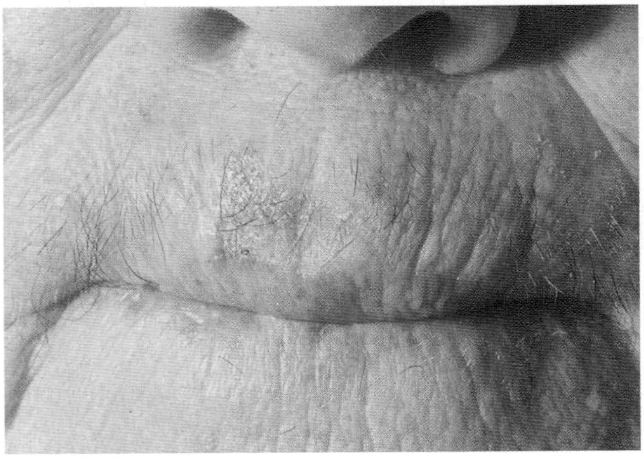

FIGURE 2.50 Actinic cheilitis

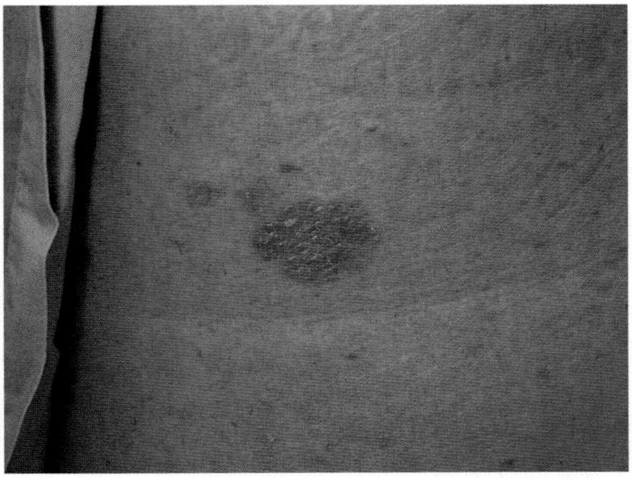

FIGURE 2.51 Bowen disease: back

Like other forms of cancer, melanoma has a good prognosis if it is found and treated early. An important part of the diagnosis is evaluating how deeply it has penetrated the layers of the skin. Lesions that are less than 0.7 mm deep typically have not yet spread, but lesions that have invaded 4 mm or more are often associated with distant metastasis.

Skin pigment variations take many forms. For a brief description of skin pigment issues that are not malignant melanoma, see Sidebar 2.3.

Types of Melanoma

- *Superficial spreading melanoma*: This is the most common variety. It spreads along the surface of the skin before invading deeper tissues. It may be multicolored and slightly elevated (Figure 2.52).
- *Lentigo melanoma*: This also begins as a superficial discoloration, usually in older people. Lesions are often deeply notched, which helps to distinguish them from simple round or oval "age spots" (Figure 2.53).
- *Acral lentiginous melanoma*: This type of skin cancer is as common in people of color as it is in Caucasians. It often begins under the nails or on the palms or soles (Figures 2.54 and 2.55).
- *Nodular melanoma*: This is the most aggressive type of skin cancer. It is significantly elevated from the skin, and it often penetrates deeper into the tissues than other types (Figure 2.56).
- *Uveal melanoma*: This is a rare subtype that affects the uveal tract, composed of the iris, ciliary body, and choroid of the eye. This is usually asymptomatic until it interferes with vision and is found by an optometrist or ophthalmologist.

Signs and Symptoms

Melanoma often starts from a preexisting mole that begins to change: it lightens, darkens, thickens, and may become

SIDEBAR 2.3 Skin Pigmentations

Age and the uneven distribution of melanin in the skin can give rise to several types of skin patches. Because massage therapists work so closely in this context, it is important to be familiar with the most common types of skin markings clients may have.

Moles
Moles, or nevi, are areas where melanocytes replicate without threatening to invade surrounding tissues. The melanocytes produce extra melanin, causing symmetrical brown, black, purple, blue, or reddish growths with well-defined borders.

Port-Wine Stains
Port-wine stains are a marking that affect blood vessels near the surface of the skin. They are often large, and are usually completely harmless, but may be treated to reduce their appearance.

Freckles
Freckles are simple concentrations of melanin in the skin. They can range from light tan to red, but are always darker than surrounding skin. They are small, but can blend together to form larger shapes. Freckles often darken in response to sun exposure, and fade when protected from UV radiation.

Lentigines
Lentigines (singular is lentigo) are similar to freckles, but they tend to appear on older people and they are much larger than freckles. They are sometimes called "liver spots," although they have nothing to do with liver function.

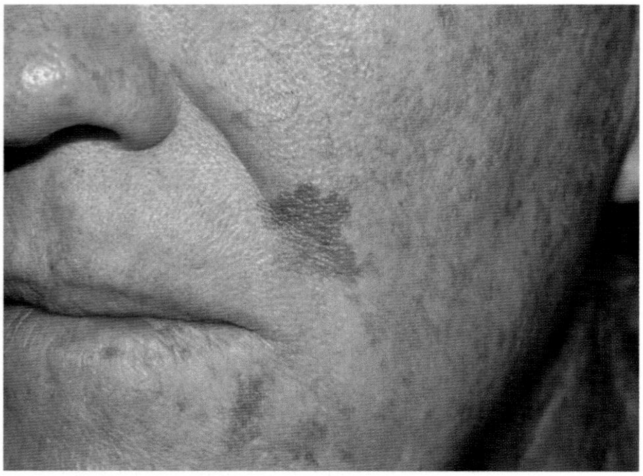

FIGURE 2.53 Lentigo melanoma: note notched border

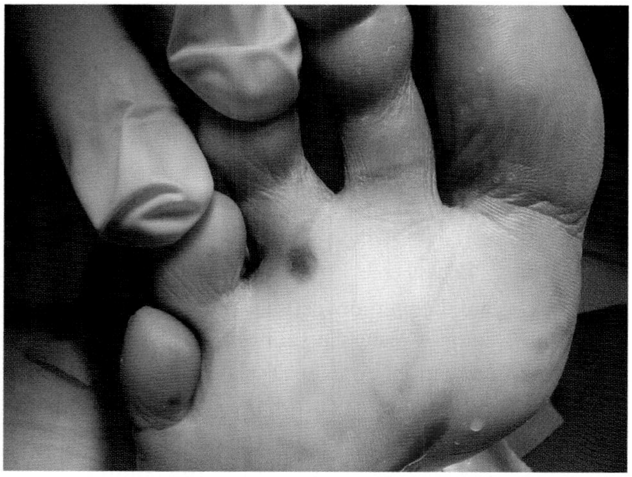

FIGURE 2.54 Acral lentiginous melanoma (small)

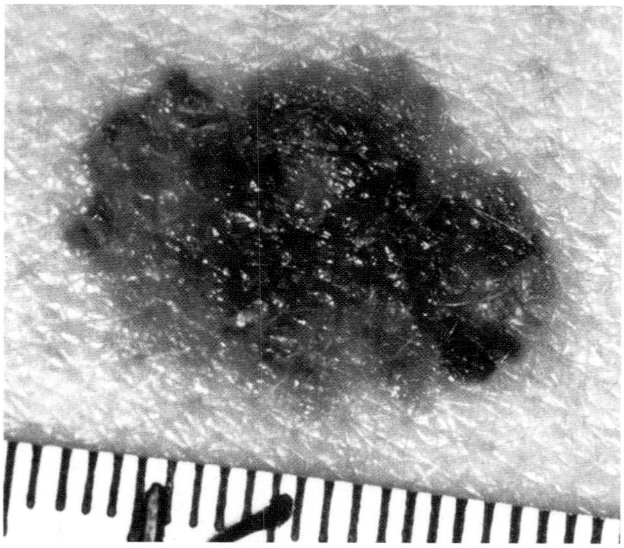

FIGURE 2.52 Superficial spreading melanoma

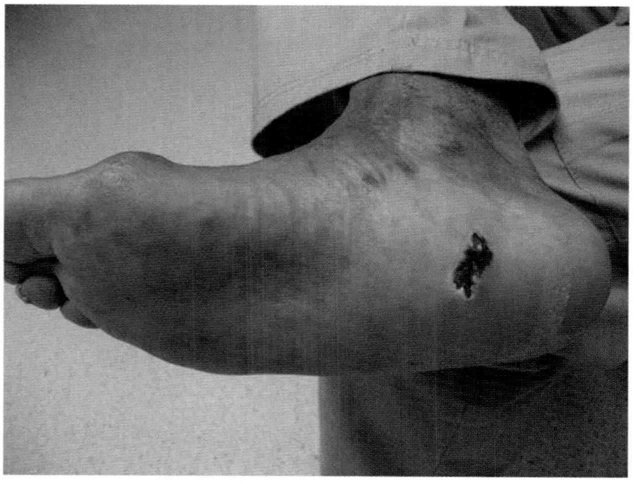

FIGURE 2.55 Acral lentiginous melanoma

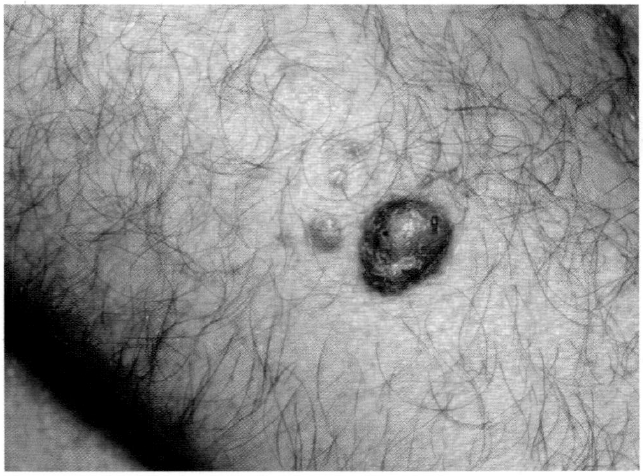

FIGURE 2.56 Nodular melanoma

elevated. It may itch or bleed around the edges. The color and texture may change. Many doctors rely on the "ugly duckling" principle: any mole that looks different from others should be examined.

Melanoma doesn't always start as a mole, however, nor does it always begin in places exposed to the sun.

Here is the traditional mnemonic to remember key features of melanoma (Figure 2.57):

- A = asymmetrical. Most benign moles are round or oval. Melanomas are irregular in shape.
- B = border. The borders of melanomas are often inconsistent; in some areas, they are clear, and in others on the same lesion they may be faded or hard to identify.
- C = color. Benign moles are black or brown or purple. Melanomas tend to be multicolored.
- D = diameter. Melanomas are typically larger than many moles. Any mole greater than 6 mm across should be examined by a dermatologist.
- E = elevated. The traditional usage refers to the fact that some melanomas, especially the nodular type, are elevated. Another way to use the E in this mnemonic is for "evolving," which refers to the fact that melanomas often change rapidly.

NOTABLE CASES Iconic reggae musician Bob Marley died of acral lentiginous melanoma at age 36. The cancer had metastasized to his lungs and brain. United States Senator John McCain is a melanoma survivor.

Treatment

Treatment for skin cancer depends on the type and stage at diagnosis (Sidebar 2.4).

Typically options are divided into cryotherapy, surgery, chemotherapy, photodynamic therapy, biological therapy, and radiation.

Medications

- Topical chemotherapy for shallow lesions
- Oral or injected chemotherapy for more invasive cancer
- Medication to cause cancer cells to become sensitive to specific light waves, followed by exposure to those lights
- Drugs that mimic cytokines to alter cell activity in and around tumors

Massage in the context of people living with and treating cancer has many benefits to offer; this is explored more thoroughly in Chapter 12.

Massage Therapy Implications

RISKS	The main risk for massage and clients with skin cancer is ignoring an important sign or symptom: a sore that doesn't heal, or a suspicious mole or other marking.
BENEFITS	Skin cancer is common, and, while not usually dangerous in the short run, it requires appropriate and timely care. Massage therapists are in a position to see possible lesions and bring them to their clients' attention. This must be done in a nondiagnostic and nonalarmist way, of course. Clients who have been fully treated for skin cancer can enjoy the same benefits from massage does as the rest of the population.
RESEARCH	Massage therapists are in a privileged position among healthcare providers, in that we have a chance to see skin that many other providers do not, and we frequently refer clients to primary care doctors when we see suspicious lesions. Research supports the need for massage therapists to be educated about skin cancer.[1,2] 1. Trotter SC, Louie-Gao Q, Hession MT, et al. Skin cancer education for massage therapists: a novel approach to the early detection of suspicious lesions. *Journal of Cancer Education* 2014;29(2):266–269. http://www.ncbi.nlm.nih.gov/pubmed/24407881 2. Campbell SM, Louie-Gao Q, Hession ML, et al. Skin cancer education among massage therapists: a survey at the 2010 meeting of the American Massage Therapy Association. *Journal of Cancer Education* 2013;28(1):158–164. http://www.ncbi.nlm.nih.gov/pubmed/22915212

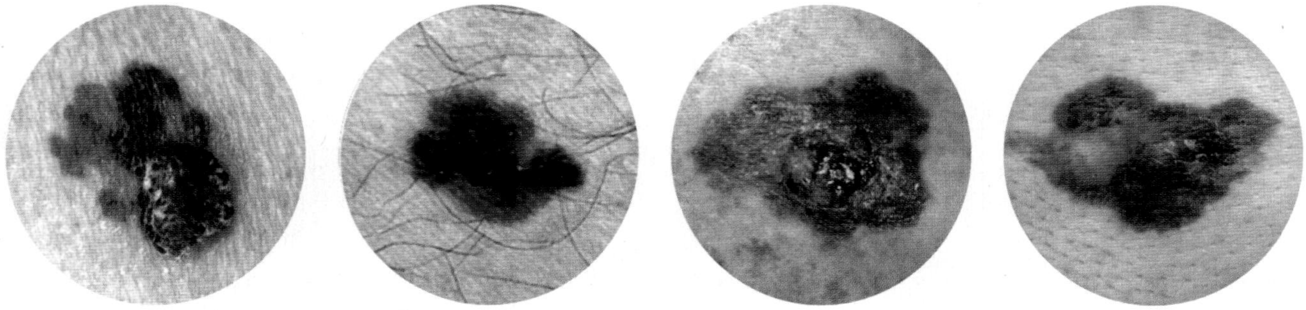

FIGURE 2.57 ABCDs of malignant melanoma

SIDEBAR 2.4 Melanoma Staging

Melanoma staging is a complicated process. It identifies how far the disease has progressed, which allows oncologists to choose treatment options that are most likely to be successful. Staging may be discussed as clinical or pathological:

- Clinical staging is based on a physical exam, imaging tests, and a biopsy of the lesion.
- Pathological staging is based on the biopsy of nearby lymph nodes or other organs.

Two other characteristics influence the seriousness of a melanoma diagnosis. One is the thickness of the tumor: anything less than 1/25th of an inch deep has an excellent prognosis. Another feature is the mitotic rate, that is, how many splitting cells are found within a sample of tissue.

The prognosis for melanoma is consistently worse when the lesion is ulcerated, so this feature is built into the staging protocol: "a" means without ulceration, and "b" means with ulceration.

TUMOR	DEFINITION
Tx	Can't be assessed
T0	No evidence of a primary tumor
Tis	In situ: epidermis only
T1a/b	Tumor is less than 1 mm deep
T2a/b	Tumor is 1.01–2 mm deep
T3a/b	Tumor is 2.01–4 mm deep
T4a/b	Tumor is more than 4 mm deep

N (node) clinical staging may be qualified by "a" or "b": "a" denotes that all growths are microscopic, while "b" denotes that growths are visible to the naked eye.

NODE	DEFINITION
Nx	Can't be assessed
N0	No spread to nodes
N1	Cancer cells are found in one node
N2	Two to three nodes are affected *OR* the tumor has enlarged with no spread to nodes
N3	Four or more nodes are affected, *OR* cells are found in groups of nodes, *OR* the tumor has spread and affected multiple nodes

M (metastasis) values determine whether cells have moved beyond the initial tumor.

METASTASIS	DEFINITION
Mx	Can't be assessed
M0	No distant metastasis
M1a	Distant metastases are found in skin and subdermis *OR* in distant lymph nodes
M1b	Distant metastases are found in lungs
M1c	Distant metastases are found in other organs

STAGE	DEFINITION	5-YEAR SURVIVAL RATE (%)
0	Tis, N0, M0	99
IA	T1a, N0, M0	97
IB	T1b or T2a, N0, M0	92
IIA	T2b or T2a, N0, M0	81
IIB	T3b or T4a, N0, M0	70
IIC	T4b, N0, N0	53
IIIA	T1a-4a, N1a, M0	78
IIIB	T1a/b-4a/b, N1a/b or N2a/b, N3, M0	59
IIIC	T any, N any, M0	40
IV	T any, N any, M1	15–20

It is important to remember that skin cancer is usually preventable. The single most important factor in reducing the risk of this disease is to be careful with sun exposure. The National Cancer Institute recommends the following steps:

- Stay out of direct sunlight between 10 A.M. and 4 P.M.
- Cover up with tightly woven clothing.
- Cover the ears and back of the neck.
- Use sunscreen with a minimum of SPF 15 that blocks both UVA and UVB radiation. Apply it 30 minutes before going outside, and reapply every 2 hours, and after swimming or perspiring.
- Use UV-absorbing sunglasses.
- Observe these precautions even on cloudy days, because UV radiation penetrates cloud cover. It can also reflect off of water, snow, ice, and pavement.

Skin Injuries

Burns

Definition: What Are They?

Many people think about burns in the context of touching a hot iron or brushing a hand across a broiler rack, but the world of burns goes far beyond household appliances. Burns are typically classified as thermal burns (this includes dry and wet heat), electrical burns, chemical burns, and radiation burns. Any one of these kills cells, essentially melting their proteins.

In addition to skin damage, burns may also injure other surfaces: the respiratory tract and digestive tract are both vulnerable to damage from overheated air, liquids, or corrosive chemicals. Burns to the face and neck are more serious than to other areas because the resulting inflammation can block breathing passages.

Demographics

An estimated 1.1 million people seek medical care for burns each year. Of those, 50,000 require hospitalization, and about 4,500 patients do not survive their initial injuries. An additional 10,000 people die each year from burn-related infections.

Etiology: What Happens?

The severity of burns is determined by how deep they go, how much surface area they cover, and what part of the body has been affected. Thermal burns occur at temperatures above 115°F (46°C); damage is determined by both temperature and the duration of contact. If a significant amount of skin function is lost, then its functions are compromised: the ability to regulate temperature, control fluid loss, provide a barrier against microbial invasion, and provide sensory information may all impaired. A burn that affects more than 15% of the skin's surface can put a person at risk for infection, shock, and circulatory collapse.

The severity of chemical burns is based on the pH of the substance, its concentration, duration of contact, and other factors. Because of the way these chemicals act on fat cells, acid burns tend not to penetrate deeply into the skin, but alkali burns, which can effectively melt through the protective fatty layer, can be much more serious.

Types of Burns

- *First-degree (superficial) burns*: These are a mild (but often quite painful) irritation of the superficial epidermis. They are red, but don't involve blisters. Nonblistering sunburns (Figure 2.58) are a common version of first-degree burns. They usually heal in 2 to 3 days, sometimes with flaking and peeling.

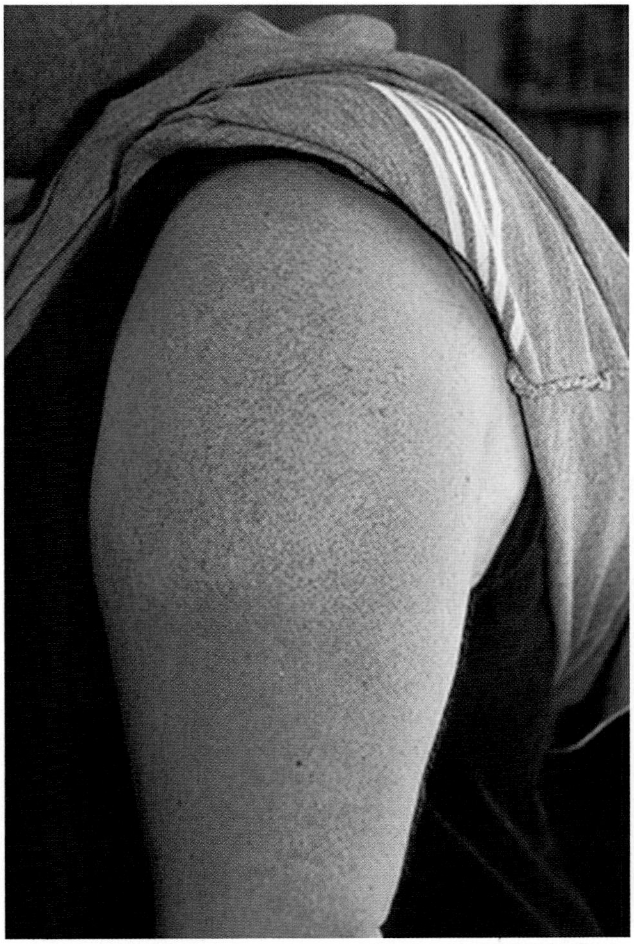

FIGURE 2.58 First-degree burn (sunburn) of an upper arm

- *Second-degree (partial thickness) burns*: These involve damage into deeper layers of the epidermis. They are red, with instantly appearing blisters. Second-degree burns often leave a permanent scar (Figure 2.59).
- *Third-degree (full thickness) burns*: These penetrate through the epidermis to the dermis or deeper. They destroy not only skin cells but glands, hair shafts, and nerve endings as well. They may present with white or black charred edges (Figure 2.60). If they penetrate into muscle tissue, proteins from the dead cells may accumulate to cause kidney damage. Third-degree burns tends to contract very extremely as they heal, which can cause disfiguring scars and limited mobility of the skin (Figure 2.61).

Signs and Symptoms

The symptoms of burn damage depend on what level of skin has been affected. Details on symptoms by degree of damage are listed with each description.

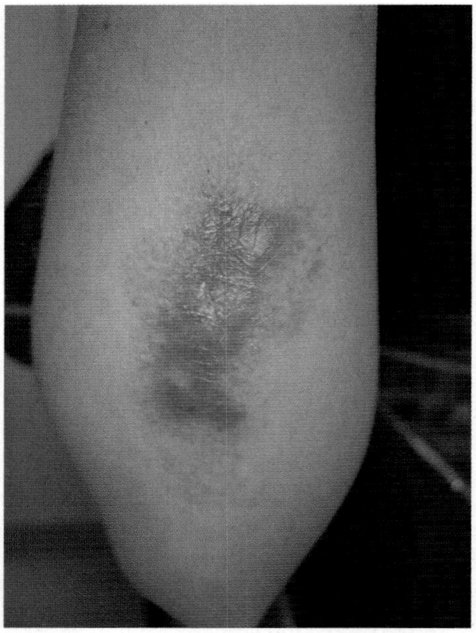

FIGURE 2.59 Second-degree burn: blistering and scarring

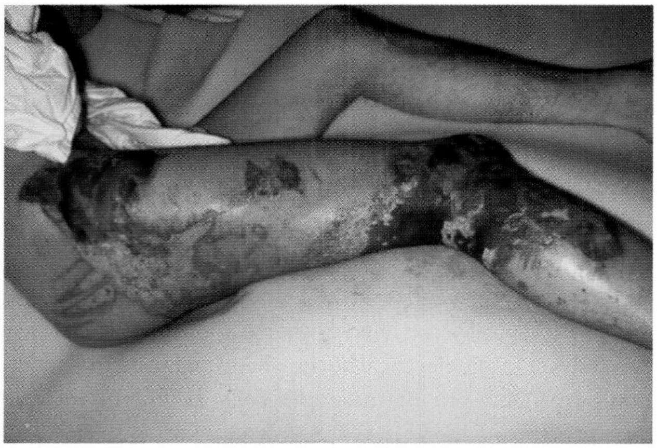

FIGURE 2.60 Third-degree full-thickness burn

Treatment

First- and second-degree burns are typically treated with soothing lotion. If blistering occurs, antibiotic cream may be recommended to prevent infection. Third-degree burns, however, must be treated with more care to minimize the accumulation of binding scar tissue. This often means wound cleansing and debridement (aggressive skin brushing to remove debris), as well as skin grafts and plastic surgery.

Medications

- Antibiotic cream, if necessary
- Analgesics for pain control

Massage Therapy Implications

RISKS	Most burns contraindicate massage when they are acute—not just for pain, but for infection risk. The only exception might be a very mild sunburn. A client with a history of severe burns might have impaired sensation in those areas; this requires extra care with massage to avoid overtreatment.
BENEFITS	A person who is recovering from third-degree burns may have to undergo painful treatments; relaxation massage can help to address the stress that accompanies that challenge. Some evidence also indicates that massage can improve itching, mood, range of motion, and the quality of scar tissue in burn survivors. Clients who have had burns with no long-term nerve damage can enjoy the same benefits from bodywork as does the rest of the population.
OPTIONS	Some researchers have developed specific massage protocols for skin rehabilitation. Bodywork practitioners interested in working with these populations can pursue this further at specialized burn treatment centers.
RESEARCH	Several studies on manual therapies for burns suggest that massage has significant benefits to offer this population. It has been seen to reduce itching and pain, and specific protocols for skin rehabilitation on mature scars was seen to reduce the thickness of the scarring while significantly improving elasticity and range of motion.[1–3] 1. Cho YS, Jeon JH, Hong A, et al. The effect of burn rehabilitation massage therapy on hypertrophic scar after burn: a randomized controlled trial. *Burns* 2014;40(8):1513–1520. http://www.ncbi.nlm.nih.gov/pubmed/24630820 2. Roh YS, Cho H, Oh JO, et al. Effects of skin rehabilitation massage therapy on pruritus, skin status, and depression in burn survivors. *Journal of Korean Academy of Nursing* 2007;37(2):221–226. http://kan.or.kr/kor/shop_sun/files/memoir_img/200702/221.pdf 3. Morien A, Garrison D, Smith NK. Range of motion improves after massage in children with burns: a pilot study. *Journal of Bodywork and Movement Therapies* 2008;12(1):67–71. http://www.ncbi.nlm.nih.gov/pubmed/19083657

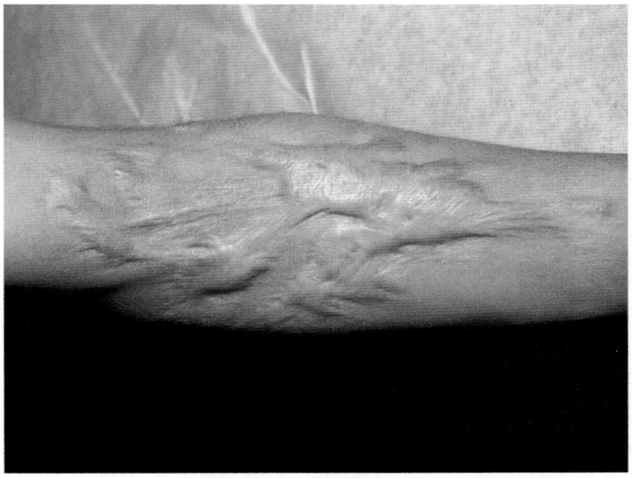

FIGURE 2.61 Hypertrophic burn scar with contractions

Decubitus Ulcers

Definition: What Are They?

Decubitus ulcers, also known as bedsores, pressure sores, and trophic ulcers, are problems massage therapists are most likely to see when working in a hospital, a nursing home, or some other setting with bedridden patients. They stem from inadequate blood flow to the skin that is compressed between bone and another surface (Figure 2.62).

Demographics

About 2.5 million people in the United States develop pressure sores each year. The highest risk groups include spinal cord injury patients, and those who are limited to wheelchair use or bedridden. They develop most readily in elders, but young people who are immobilized can also easily develop pressure sores.

Bedsores are one of the most expensive conditions to treat; it is estimated to cost about $70,000 to treat a single full-thickness pressure sore, and they cost the health care system up to $8 billion each year.

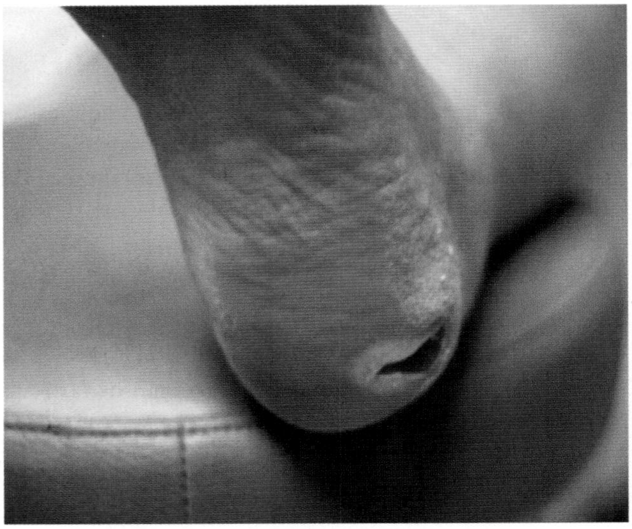

FIGURE 2.62 Stage III decubitus ulcer, heel

Etiology: What Happens?

All of the body's cells rely on unobstructed blood flow to deliver oxygen and nutrients, and to carry away wastes. If capillaries are compressed between two surfaces, it doesn't take long for cells to die. It's important to point out that the contacting surfaces don't have to be hard: pressure sores develop with contact to soft surfaces as well. Their damage can penetrate all the way down to the bone. Nearby bacteria may then take advantage of the situation and create a potentially life-threatening secondary infection. Finally, because bedsores involve long-term inflammation, they are also a significant risk factor for developing an aggressive form of SCC.

Pressure, friction, and shear are the external influences that set the stage for decubitus ulcers. Internal factors include impaired pain sensation, poor vasomotor responses in local capillaries, and extremely delicate skin. When these are present, the shearing and friction forces that occur with positional changes may actually increase the risk of pressure sores. This points out how important it is to prevent pressure sores before they happen.

The sacrum, ischial tuberosity, and elbows are the most common sites for decubitus ulcers, but they can develop virtually anywhere that tissue is compressed for more than 2 hours.

Signs and Symptoms

Stage I of pressure sores shows a marked change in skin temperature (it can become cooler or warmer than the surrounding area). Discoloration may appear to be red, purple, or bluish. Pain and itching may accompany these changes. It is difficult to estimate the amount of damage that has accrued at this point: often skin discoloration is the "tip of the iceberg," while extensive tissue loss has developed below.

> **NOTABLE CASES** "Superman" spinal cord injury patient Christopher Reeve died from complications related to pressure sores and subsequent infection.

In stage II, the wound can look like a full or ruptured blister. Part of the epidermis and dermis have been damaged.

In stage III, the wound is a deep open crater, often showing subcutaneous fat at its base.

Stage IV shows larger scale tissue loss, exposing muscles, bones, and tendons.

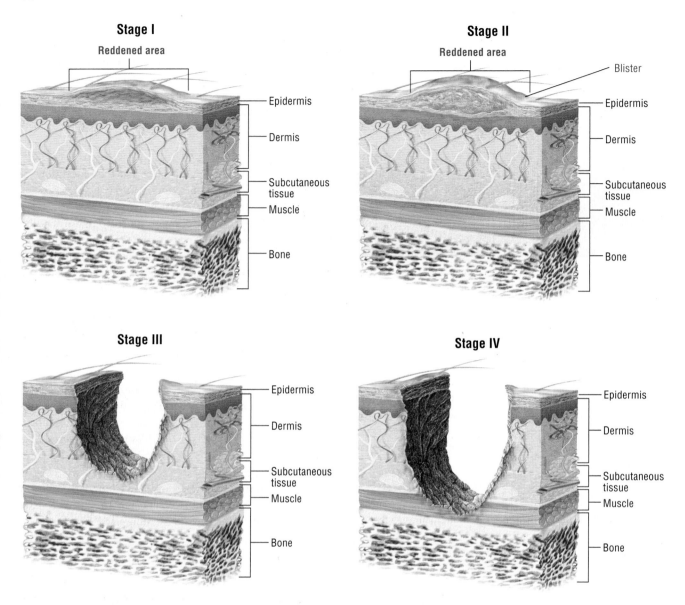

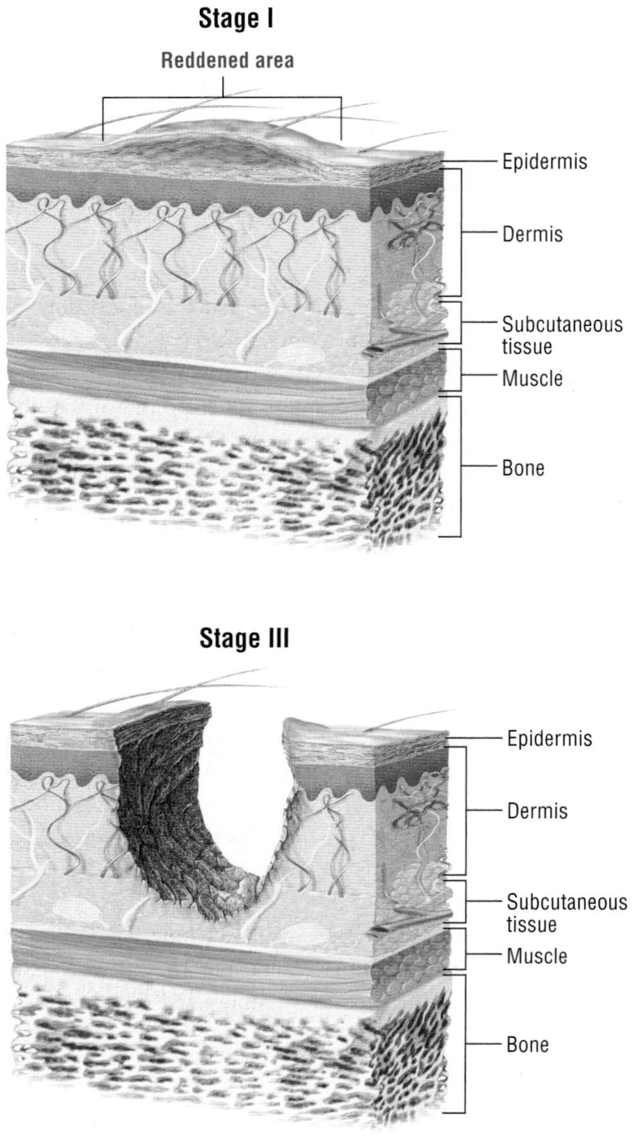

FIGURE 2.63 Stages of decubitus ulcer development

Ulcers differ from other types of sores because poor local circulation prevents a normal healing process. Eventually, ulcers can heal, but a permanent dip remains where the dead tissue never grows back (Figure 2.63).

Treatment

Bedsores are preventable through careful hygiene and frequent bed turning or other postural adjustments. Once they form, however, they are difficult and expensive to treat. Topical antibiotics and special dressings that promote tissue growth may be adequate for some; others may require extensive debridement and surgery to repair. Electrical stimulation may improve local blood flow. Whirlpool baths can support circulation and gentle removal of damaged tissue.

Medications

- Medicated dressings to promote cell growth
- Topical or systemic antibiotics for infection risk

Massage Therapy Implications

RISKS	The risk of infection is very high with decubitus ulcers, so any indication that an open ulcer has formed or is imminent at least locally contraindicates massage.
BENEFITS	Massage may help reduce the risk of pressure sores before they form, but only if the client has good sensation and the skin is resilient enough to accommodate the compression, friction, and shearing forces that even gentle massage may involve. Unfortunately, for many people vulnerable to bedsores, this is not the case.
RESEARCH	The research on massage for pressure sores is somewhat contradictory. Some caregivers promote massage as an early intervention because it appears to boost local circulation, but others cite the risks of massage because of pressure, shearing, and friction forces that may increase skin damage[1]. And some research suggests that massage makes little or no difference at all.[2] The general consensus appears to support gentle long strokes before the skin is compromised, and to avoid anything more intrusive, especially around bony prominences. 1. Duimel-Peeters IG, Halfens RJ, Berger MP, Snoeckx LH. The effects of massage as a method to prevent pressure ulcers. A review of the literature. *Ostomy Wound Management* 2005;51(4):70–80. http://www.o-wm.com/content/the-effects-massage-a-method-prevent-pressure-ulcers-a-review-literature?page=0,0 2. Duimel-Peeters IG, Rani JGH, Ambergen AW, et al. The effectiveness of massage with and without dimethyl sulfoxide in preventing pressure ulcers: a randomized, double-blind cross-over trial in patients prone to pressure ulcers. *International Journal of Nursing Studies* 2007;44(8):1285–1295. http://www.ncbi.nlm.nih.gov/pubmed/17553503

Scar Tissue

Definition: What Is It?

Scar tissue is the development of new cells and extracellular matrix where damage has occurred.

Scar tissue deposits are typically the outcome of trauma, burns, or surgery.

This discussion is limited to the regenerative capacities of the skin. For information on scar tissue associated with musculoskeletal injuries, see the section on **tendinopathies** in Chapter 3.

Etiology: What Happens?

The skin, made mostly of relatively delicate epithelial tissue, is our primary barrier against the outside world. Consequently, epidermal cells are genetically programed to heal fast. Imagine a minor scrape or abrasion: within seconds, clotting mechanisms allow a scab to begin to form. Under the new scab, basal cells detach from the basement membrane and migrate in a single-layered sheet across the wound. When they reach the other side and touch other epithelial cells, a process called contact inhibition makes them stop moving.

Back at the original site, stationary basal cells duplicate to build up the ranks of migrating cells. When the whole wound has been covered, the new sheet of basal cells begins dividing to form new strata. Finally, the superficial cells become keratinized, and the scab falls off. Then the wound is healed; the blood supply is protected from the outside world, and the wound is no longer vulnerable to infection. The whole process can take place within 24 hours to several days, depending on the size and location of the injury.

If the damage penetrates deeper than the dermis, or if the wound is complicated by any infectious risk, the healing process is more complicated. Fibroblasts migrate to the site, so beneath all that basal cell activity collagen and other extracellular matrices are deposited. Eventually, this delicate granulation tissue may become a dense accumulation of collagenous scar tissue.

For another look at this process, see the animation "Wound Healing" http://thePoint.lww.com/Werner6e. thePoint®

Types of Scar Tissue

- *Hypertrophic scars*: These are scars that overflow their boundaries but don't form permanently enlarged masses. They often appear a month or so after injury, and then stabilize or regress.
- *Keloid scars*: These are the result of overproduction of collagen, leading to a permanently raised mass of collagenous scar tissue. Keloids can be a complication of deep injury, piercing (see Figure 2.64), or surgery.
- *Contracture scars*: Occasionally, a skin injury can cover so much area that at the skin heals, it pulls together in a tight web of connective tissue that may limit the range of motion over joints. This is a potential complication of **burns** and some surgeries.

Signs and Symptoms

Scar tissue of superficial layers of the skin often leaves no mark after healing is complete. Common permanent scars like striae (stretch marks) and **acne** scars show where tissue damage that affects layers deeper than the

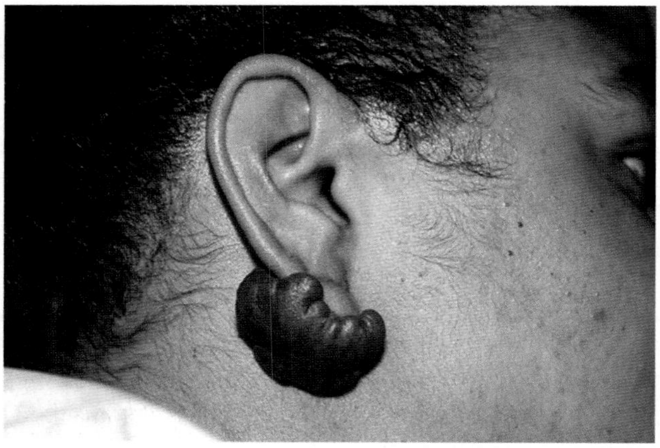

FIGURE 2.64 Keloid scar

epidermis has occurred. Deeper scars may be marked by discoloration, lack of pigmentation, and lack of hair follicles, sebaceous, and sweat glands. When the formation of scar tissue malfunctions, some other signs may be present.

Treatment

One of the challenges in scar tissue treatment is that no universally accepted rating scale for scar tissue exists, so it is difficult to demonstrate that an intervention is effective. Among the many characteristics that may be tracked with scar tissue treatment are pliability, firmness, color, vascularity, thickness, and elasticity.

People with obvious scars may treat them to reduce their appearance, but scars themselves can't be eradicated completely. Interventions include using collagen or fat injections to fill out dipped areas, dermabrasion, chemical peels, laser resurfacing, and small or larger skin grafts.

Hypertrophic and keloid scars are more challenging to treat because they often recur. Injections with cortisol to dissolve connective tissue, liquid nitrogen, pressure bandages, and other interventions may be applied.

Medications

- Injections of soft tissue fillers (collagen, fat cells, etc.)
- Application of tissue-engineered products for burns or ulcers
- Injections of cortisol to dissolve excessive collagen

Massage Therapy Implications

RISKS	Incompletely sealed wounds are obviously a local contraindication because of the risk for pain and infection. Very delicate scar tissue may also need to be treated carefully until it has become denser and stronger. Deep scarring may involve some loss of sensation; this requires some adjustments in bodywork.
BENEFITS	Fully formed scar tissue carries no risk for massage; clients can enjoy all the benefits of bodywork as does the rest of the population.
OPTIONS	Careful manipulation around the edges of new wounds and more aggressive manipulation of older scars may improve the elasticity and movability of tissue. Of course, all work must be conducted within client pain tolerance.
RESEARCH	The research on massage therapy for scars is not yet well developed, but massage shows some promise in certain situations. Some evidence suggests that massage improves several quality of life factors, including pain, anxiety, and muscle tension after surgery.[1] A systematic review of studies that look at the impact of massage for postsurgical scarring generally show stronger results than for those that look at massage for burns or other trauma.[2] Using massage to prevent or reverse keloid and hypertrophic scarring has not been shown to be significantly successful. 1. Wilk I, Kurpas D, Mroczek B, et al. Application of tensegrity massage to relive complications after mastectomy—case report. *Rehabilitation Nursing* 2014. http://www.ncbi.nlm.nih.gov/pubmed/24668661 2. Shin TM, Bordeaux JS. The role of massage in scar management: a literature review. *Dermatologic Surgery* 2012:38(3);414–423. http://www.ncbi.nlm.nih.gov/pubmed/22093081

Explore and Apply

LEVEL 1: Receive and Respond

1. Which is the list of animal parasites that live on their hosts?
   a. Scabies, fleas, chiggers
   b. Mites, ticks, mosquitoes
   c. Head lice, pubic lice, mites
   d. Crabs, scabies, mites

2. Which is the list of fungal infections of the skin?
   a. Ringworm, herpes, head lice
   b. Ringworm, athlete's foot, pubic lice
   c. Jock itch, athlete's foot, herpes
   d. Athlete's foot, jock itch, ringworm

3. What is the best description of herpes simplex?
   a. A very common viral infection of nerve endings in the skin
   b. A highly contagious bacterial infection of the face
   c. A mildly itchy fungal infection that appears at the lips
   d. A fairly painful lesion related to an animal parasite

4. Label the following conditions "staph" or "strep":
   a. MRSA
   b. Cellulitis
   c. St. Anthony's fire
   d. Pilonidal cyst
   e. Necrotizing fasciitis
   f. Sty

5. This condition involves a viral infection that causes hard, crusty growth on the skin. What is it?
   a. Wart
   b. Eczema
   c. Ringworm
   d. Boil

6. Which is a common contributing factor for acne rosacea?
   a. Fleas
   b. Mites
   c. Warts
   d. Fungi

7. A comedone is the principle lesion connected with which condition?
   a. Acne vulgaris
   b. Acne rosacea
   c. Dermatophytosis
   d. Tinea capitis

8. What is the most common form of eczema?
   a. Dyshidrosis
   b. Nummular eczema
   c. Atopic dermatitis
   d. Contact dermatitis

9. Seborrheic keratosis often looks like another skin condition. What is it?
   a. Malignant melanoma
   b. Actinic keratosis
   c. Verruca vulgaris
   d. Basal cell carcinoma

10. Which is the most commonly diagnosed skin cancer?
    a. Seborrheic keratosis
    b. Basal cell carcinoma
    c. Squamous cell carcinoma
    d. Malignant melanoma

11. Which is the most common cause of death by skin cancer?
    a. Seborrheic keratosis
    b. Basal cell carcinoma
    c. Squamous cell carcinoma
    d. Malignant melanoma

12. Which is the most accurate list of causes of burns?
    a. Radiation, electricity, corrosive chemicals
    b. Heat, friction, toxins
    c. Radiation, electricity, natural gas
    d. Heat, blisters, ice

13. Who is most likely to develop a decubitus ulcer?
    a. Someone who is obese and sedentary
    b. Someone who is underweight and sedentary
    c. Someone who is obese and active
    d. Someone who is underweight and active

14. How do keloid scars compare to hypertrophic scars?
    a. Keloids are larger and more permanent than hypertrophic scars
    b. Hypertrophic scars are larger and more permanent than keloids
    c. Keloids and hypertrophic scars are essentially the same thing
    d. Keloids form with surgery, while hypertrophic scars form with lacerations

Explore and Apply (continued)

LEVEL 2: Application of Concepts

1. A client has a large abrasion on her right knee that is crusted and dry. Does this situation contraindicate all massage? Why?

2. Your client has successfully treated his athlete's foot, and now he would like a massage. What is your best course of action?
   a. Conduct his foot massage wearing gloves or through the sheet to be extra sure about not contacting any residual pathogens
   b. Conduct his foot massage with no special precautions
   c. Conduct his foot massage after thoroughly inspecting his feet for signs of fungal infection
   d. Conduct his foot massage with antifungal essential oils in your lubricant

3. A client has an extremely dry and flaky eczema on her hands. Does this condition indicate or contraindicate massage? Why? What is an adaptation that could benefit this client?

4. A client reports that she has just had a basal cell carcinoma removed from her nose. She has a butterfly bandage over the wound. What is your best choice?
   a. Work normally but avoid any stretching or distortion of the unhealed skin
   b. Delay the session until you can confirm with her doctor that the tumor had not metastasized
   c. Suggest that she get a second opinion before undergoing chemotherapy
   d. Work normally but not within a 12-inch radius of the surgical site

5. Your 50-year-old client was involved in a kitchen fire when he was 7. His left shoulder is deeply invested with twisted, contracted scar tissue. What is a risk associated with working deeply in this area? How can you accommodate for that risk?

Note to educators: Due to space considerations, these review questions only address the most important material from Chapter 2. The Test Bank provides a much more comprehensive selection of questions, all of which are keyed to the relevant chapter objectives.

What Would *You* Do?

A Surprise

Your first-time, first-massage client is a 42-year-old woman who appears to be very nervous about her session. She reports having psoriasis on her intake form. When you fold back the sheet, you see that her back is covered with red and silver lesions, and in some places her skin is contracted and scarred, but no wounds are open or weeping. She has practically no skin on her back that has not been affected. You have never seen anything like this.

Knowing what you do about the risks and benefits of massage therapy in this situation, how will you proceed? Practice having this conversation with a partner, in the setting that has been described: the client is facedown on a massage table.

Where Can I Get More Information?

Let's say that you know you have been exposed to MRSA, but you have no current lesions. Is it safe for you to work with clients? List three resources where you can get current, accurate information on the communicability of MRSA.

Here are two good places to start:

- http://mrsa-research-center.bsd.uchicago.edu/timeline.html
- http://www.cdc.gov/mrsa/community/posters/index.html

Skin Cancer Concerns

- If a client has a skin lesion that makes you suspect some form of skin cancer, you have two important responsibilities:
  - To inform the client of your observation
  - To stay within your scope of practice for that conversation
- Work with a partner to role play being both a client and a therapist in this situation.
- Listen carefully for ways to misinterpret and overreact to what the therapist says.
- This situation will almost certainly come up in your practice. How will you respond?

An Ancient Scar

If a client had a major surgery several years ago, it is possible for residual scar tissue to alter his movement, balance, posture, or function. What might that look like? How might you make a treatment plan and track progress?

Explore and Apply (continued)

Suggested Activities

1. For each condition covered in your curriculum, write down the following on a card:
   - A brief definition
   - Most common cause or contributing factor(s)
   - Major signs and symptoms
   - Risks and benefits of massage therapy
     - Variables that contribute to risks and benefits
     - Appropriate adaptations

     Use these as flash cards as you study
2. For each condition covered in your curriculum, write one multiple-choice question. Share your questions with your classmates as you study together.
3. Quiz yourself using either the "labels off" feature in your enhanced e-book, or the labeling exercise on thePoint® for Figure 2.1. Identify the following structures: Dermis, Epidermis, Nerve endings, Subdermis, and Sweat gland
4. Use the student resources on thePoint® to find practice quiz questions and games.

3

Musculoskeletal System Conditions

CHAPTER 3 / Abbreviated Chapter Objectives

Having completed assignments and classroom time related to Chapter 3, the learner is expected to be able to…

- Identify definitions of the key terms in the introduction and those connected to the conditions covered in your curriculum.
- Describe the structure of long bones, with definitions of osteoblast, osteoclast, trabecular bone, and Wolff's law.
- Describe the structure of skeletal muscle, with the names of at least three connective tissue membranes found within them.
- Describe the purpose and location of articular cartilage.
- Name the cells that are found within fascial sheaths, and describe their functions.
- Provide the following information for each condition covered in your curriculum:
  - Identify the definition of the condition.
  - List the most common causes or contributing factors to the condition.
  - List major signs and symptoms of the condition.
  - Identify possible risks and benefits of massage therapy, with:
    - Variables that contribute to risks and benefits
    - Appropriate adaptations for massage therapy

For detailed chapter objectives for each condition in this chapter, consult the student resource page at http://thePoint.lww.com/Werner6e. thePoint®

Muscles, bones, joints, and fascia provide humans with shape, strength, and movement. They are composed almost entirely of the material that provides structure for working cells and permeates every part of the body: connective tissue. This chapter addresses disorders and injuries of these structures.

Injury to any of the connective tissue structures (except bone and sometimes cartilage) can be difficult for many medical professionals to identify. Soft tissues don't show well on x-rays, and while magnetic resonance imaging (MRI) can be useful, its ability to locate or identify injury is limited. Ultrasound technology to view structures in a conscious person is advancing, but this application is mostly limited to research settings. The upshot is that a thorough clinical examination still yields the most comprehensive information about injury to muscles, tendons, ligaments, and other connective tissues. Massage therapists, with their in-depth understanding of the musculoskeletal system, particularly with the formation of adhesions and scar tissue, are in a unique position to be able to help individuals with these types of injuries.

Bones

Bone Structure

The arrangement of living and nonliving material in bone is elegant and efficient. The collagen matrix on which solid bone is built is arranged as circles within circles. Calcium and phosphate deposits accumulate on this scaffolding in a similarly circular pattern, leaving holes for blood vessels. In addition, most long bones in the body grow in a slight spiral, much like evergreen tree trunks. The **diaphysis** of long bones is hollow, filled with red marrow in youth and yellow marrow in adulthood. All of these design features give bone remarkable properties: resilience and weight-bearing capacity alongside lightweight construction.

The commands to move rocklike calcium and phosphate salts around the collagen matrix are carried out by specialized cells. Osteoblasts, or "bone **b**uilders," help to lay new deposits, while osteo**cl**asts, or "bone **cl**earers," break them down. These cells are located in the **periosteum**, around the outside of the bone, the **endosteum**, which lines the central cavity, and in **trabecular** or spongy bone.

Osteoblasts and osteoclasts act according to hormonal command. Calcitonin from the thyroid lowers blood calcium by telling osteoblasts to pull calcium out of the blood and deposit it on bone tissue. Parathyroid hormone raises blood calcium by telling the osteoclasts to dismantle calcium deposits and put the valuable mineral back into the bloodstream. There, calcium is available to help with muscle contractions, nerve transmission, blood clotting, and maintenance of the appropriate pH balance in the blood and tissues. Consequently, the density of the bones depends partly on a person's physical activity, and also on whatever other chemical demands the body may make on its calcium banks. This is, in essence, Wolff's law: "Every change in the form and the function of a bone, or in its function alone, is followed by certain definite changes in its internal architecture and secondary alterations in its external conformation." In other words, bone is not inert; it is living tissue that remodels according to the stresses that are placed upon it.

Diaphysis: The shaft of a long bone.

Periosteum: The connective tissue membrane covering the outside surface of a bone.

Endosteum: The layer of cells lining the inner surface of bone in the central medullary cavity of long bones.

Trabecular bone: The less dense bone tissue generally found at the ends of long bones and in the interior of vertebrae. Also called spongy bone.

Myofiber: A muscle fiber.

Endomysium: The connective tissue membrane surrounding individual muscle fibers.

Fascicle: A band bundle of fibers. (Plural: fasciculi)

Perimysium: The connective tissue membrane surrounding a bundle of muscle fibers.

Epimysium: The connective tissue membrane surrounding a skeletal muscle.

Bone Function

The skeleton helps to define our shape, but it has many other functions as well. It provides a bony framework, protection for vulnerable organs, and points of leverage for efficient movement. Red and white blood cells are produced in the red marrow. Bones store calcium, phosphorus and other minerals for future use, including maintaining a narrow margin of tolerance for acid-base balance in the blood and other tissue fluids. Bones also secrete hormones that help to manage phosphate reabsorption in the kidneys, regulate blood sugar levels by boosting insulin-producing cells, and reduce fat deposition.

Muscles

Muscle Structure

Muscles are composed of specialized threadlike cells called **myofibers** that, with electrical and chemical stimulation, have the power to contract while bearing weight. Myofibers run the full length of the muscle, and each one is encased in a connective tissue envelope, the **endomysium**. Packets of wrapped myofibers are bound in another fascial envelope, creating bundles called **fascicles**. Fascicles are bound together by yet another membrane, the **perimysium** (Figure 3.1). Finally, some large muscle groups are further bound by an external connective tissue membrane (**epimysium**), which blends into

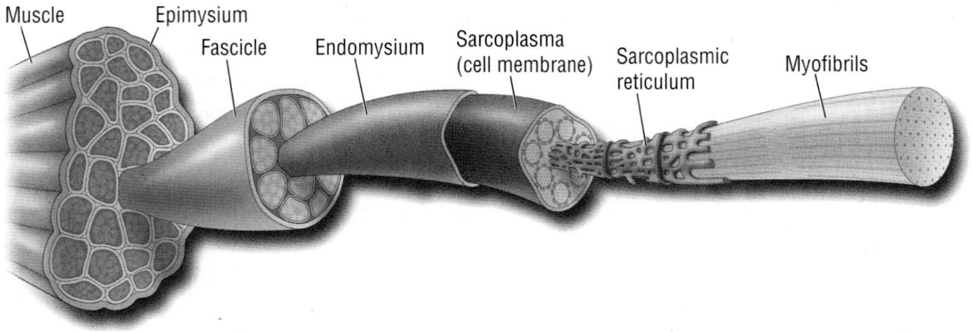

FIGURE 3.1 Muscles are composed of bundles within bundles, all enveloped by connective tissue membranes

the subcutaneous layer of the skin, the superficial fascia (which is—surprise!—another connective tissue membrane).

Muscle Function

Muscles work when a stimulus from a motor neuron crosses the synaptic cleft at the neuromuscular junction. This release of the neurotransmitter **acetylcholine** begins a sequence of events leading to the shortening of myofibers. Muscle contractions are typically classified as concentric (pulling the ends toward the center) or eccentric (preventing the uncontrolled lengthening of a muscle); or as isotonic (keeping the same tone or level of tension) or isometric (keeping the same length, while internal tone may change).

When muscles work, they consume fuel and produce both energy and wastes. What kinds of wastes are produced depends on how much work is done, how long it takes, and whether adequate oxygen is available during the process. Muscles that work with adequate supplies of oxygen burn very cleanly: the waste products of aerobic combustion are carbon dioxide and water. But when muscles work without adequate oxygen, a different chemical cascade occurs, which may produce irritants that can contribute to delayed-onset muscle soreness.

The role of lactic acid as an instigator in muscle soreness is no longer generally accepted, so the claim that massage reduces muscle soreness by removing lactic acid and other wastes from the tissues is probably inaccurate. Further, the question of massage and "toxin removal" is far from confirmed; to date, no research shows evidence of significant changes in the chemical makeup of urine following massage. While anecdotal and clinical evidence indicates that massage helps to improve recovery from muscle soreness and overuse, the mechanisms for how this might be accomplished have not been identified.

Acetylcholine: A common neurotransmitter that is necessary for the nervous system to stimulate muscle movement.

Chondroitin sulfate: An important component of cartilage, sometimes taken as a dietary supplement for joint health.

Joints

Joints are organized into three classes: synarthroses, amphiarthroses, and diarthroses. Of these classes of joints, the diarthrotic or synovial joints are by far the most vulnerable to injury. For this reason, it is worth a brief review of synovial joints in preparation for a discussion of what happens when they are injured.

Joint Structure

Synovial joints are constructed so that no rough surfaces ever touch, even in joints that bear an enormous amount of weight, like the knees and ankles (Figure 3.2). Articular cartilage, made of collagen fibers densely arranged around slippery **chondroitin sulfate** and water, caps the ends of bones where they meet. Maintaining the smoothness of that cartilage is crucial to maintaining the health of the joint. Each synovial joint is equipped with a synovial membrane, which produces synovial fluid, creating a generally slick, eggy environment; synovial means "with egg." As long as the membrane and cartilage stay

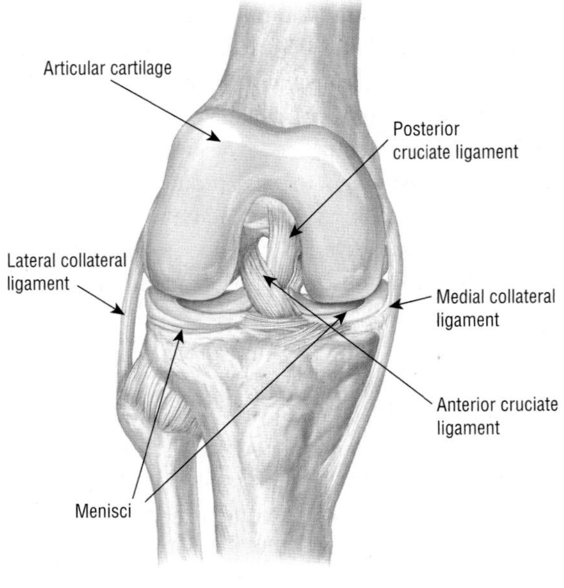

FIGURE 3.2 Synovial joint

moist and slick, the joint stays healthy. It takes only a very small amount of synovial fluid to lubricate the inside of a joint space.

Joint Function

Synovial joints help to produce movement between bones by providing the fulcrum that bones can use for leverage as the muscles pull on them in various directions.

Like most structures, joints are healthiest when they are used regularly. Healthy movement of the joint capsule stimulates the production of synovial fluid, which circulates through the joint space for the health of all joint components. Lack of movement results in a shortage of synovial fluid; too much movement can damage articular cartilage, or cause the bones to change shape in such a way that smooth surfaces are made rough, thus opening the door to irreversible arthritis. Other factors that can negatively impact joint health include trauma, dehydration, calcium metabolism, nutrition, and autoimmune disease.

Fascia

Until recently fascia was a profoundly understudied tissue. It was the material anatomists removed in order to see the "real" structures: muscles, tendons, ligaments or organs. It was considered simply to be packing material with little anatomical importance. But research into the function and form of fascia has revealed some surprising truths, and much of this information may impact our understanding of how movement and mechanical force is distributed through the body, and how pathologic changes in fascia may affect pain and mobility.

Fascial Structure

Layers of fascia have traditionally been assumed to be passive sheaths made of varying combinations of collagen, elastin, and other reticular fibers. Fascia is often discussed as being superficial or deep; dense or loose. The thickness, density, and elasticity of these layers are determined by the number and type of protein fibers that are present, and in what kind of liquid, gelid or solid matrix they are suspended. The living cells embedded in fascial sheaths were thought to only produce new protein fibers and matrix material. It turns out that some of those cells, called **myofibroblasts**, also have the capacity to slowly contract in the nature of smooth muscle cells. Mechanical force and some stress-related chemicals stimulate these contractions, leading to stiffness and rigidity in fascial sheaths. This appears to help distribute the force of muscle contraction across joints and planes to assist with movement, posture, and weight-bearing stress.

Another underappreciated aspect of fascia is its vast network of nerve supply. When neurons are irritated at the fascial level from compression, torsion, impingement, scar tissue, or other factors, it can lead to any number of complications with pain sensation. This pain sensation could be classified as a neurological problem, but fascial dysfunction may be at the root of it. Massage therapists are in a unique position to be able to unravel some of these factors for excellent client outcomes.

> **Myofibroblast:** An atypical type of fibroblast with some qualities of smooth muscle cells.
>
> **Proprioceptor:** A sensory neuron that conveys information about muscle tension and joint position.
>
> **Capsular ligament:** A ligamentous sac that surrounds the articular cavity of a freely moveable joint.
>
> **Bursae:** Fluid-filled sacs that reduce the friction where a muscle or tendon slides across bone. (Singular: bursa)

Fascial Function

The discovery of contractile cells within connective tissue sheaths changes our understanding of fascial function. Certainly fascia does the obvious job of separating layers of other tissues, providing lubricated gliding surfaces so that muscles can move easily, and acting as a protective covering to joints and organs. But in addition, it appears to play a role in maintaining long-term postural and movement patterns, especially in its largest structure, the lumbodorsal fascia.

Fascia's rich supply of sensory neurons includes the **proprioceptors** that help determine posture and resting tone. The feedback loops between fascial contraction and efficient skeletal muscular contraction are still being explored. As this new understanding of fascial function is explored, common conditions like **headaches**, low back pain, iliotibial band pain, or even **adhesive capsulitis** may be found to be at least partly related to fascial dysfunction.

For more of the author's insights into fascia, view the Ruth Werner video "Fascia" at http://thePoint.lww.com/Werner6e. thePoint®

Other Connective Tissues

Tendons connect muscle to bone, and they are an early line of defense when a joint undergoes traumatic stress. Ligaments are also frequently injured. The medial and lateral stabilizers outside the joint capsule and the internal stabilizers are generally damaged before the specialized **capsular ligament** that comprises the joint capsule itself. **Bursae** that cushion areas where two bones might otherwise knock heads or allow tendons to slide over sharp corners tend to become irritated with repetitive stress.

Connective Tissue Problems in General

Every part of the body is supported by connective tissue. It forms the fascial sheaths; it supports blood vessels and the tubes of the digestive tract. It is the framework on which bones grow. Connective tissue provides the scaffolding for the functioning cells of most organs. It gives strength and elasticity to most of the body's membranes. Indeed, connective tissue is such a large proportion of the human body that one way of evaluating a person's general health is by considering the strength, resiliency, and power of the connective tissues.

Our three-dimensional connective tissue web links every part of the body to every other part. It demonstrates that, contrary to traditional thinking, the body is not made of a series of interchangeable parts. When a car has a tire that keeps going flat, you replace the tire and the problem is solved. But when a person has an ankle that repeatedly sprains, or a back that is so fragile he can't pick up his child, or headaches that interfere with her day-to-day functioning, the answer isn't just in the ankle or the back or the neck. It's in the totality of how mental and emotional states ripple into physical experience. It's in how eating habits support or don't support growth and healing. It's in whether a person gets adequate amounts of high-quality sleep. Massage therapists who specialize in helping people with musculoskeletal problems must recognize all of these issues when clients have recurring, ongoing, or stubborn injuries that don't follow what might be considered a normal healing process.

The convenient feature in musculoskeletal problems, as far as massage therapists are concerned, is that most are not related to an infectious agent. A massage therapist can't catch or spread an epidemic of torn hamstrings or bunions. Nor do these injuries usually lead to permanent damage that massage can make worse: massage does not move bursitis throughout the body, for instance. But skillful, careful, knowledgeably applied massage administered in the appropriate stage of healing can help many musculoskeletal conditions to improve. Sometimes that improvement is just a temporary cessation of pain (which is a fine purpose in itself), but often this work can bring about the lasting changes that make structural massage an important factor in the healing process.

Musculoskeletal System Conditions

Muscle Disorders

- Muscular Dystrophy
  - Duchenne muscular dystrophy
  - Becker muscular dystrophy
  - Myotonic muscular dystrophy
  - Other forms of muscular dystrophy
    - Facioscapulohumeral; limb-girdle; Emery-Dreifuss; oculopharyngeal
- Spasms, cramps
- Strains

Bone Disorders

- Osteosarcoma
- Osgood-Schlatter disease
- Osteoporosis
- Postural deviations
  - Hyperkyphosis
    - Scheuermann disease
  - Hyperlordosis
  - Scoliosis/rotoscoliosis

Joint Disorders

- Adhesive capsulitis
- Baker cysts
- Gout
- Joint disruptions
  - Dislocations
  - Subluxations
  - Dysplasia
- Joint replacement surgery
- Lyme disease
- Osteoarthritis
- Patellofemoral pain syndrome
- Spondylolisthesis
  - Congenital spondylolisthesis
  - Isthmic spondylolisthesis
  - Degenerative spondylolisthesis
  - Traumatic spondylolisthesis
  - Pathologic spondylolisthesis
- Spondylosis
- Sprains
- Temporomandibular joint dysfunction

Fascial Disorders

- Compartment syndrome
  - Acute compartment syndrome
  - Chronic compartment syndrome
- Dupuytren contracture
  - Plantar fibromatosis
  - Peyronie disease
  - Garrod nodes
- Ganglion cysts
- Hammer toe
- Hernia
  - Direct inguinal hernia
  - Indirect inguinal hernia
  - Epigastric hernia
  - Paraumbilical hernia
  - Umbilical hernia
  - Incisional hernia
  - Hiatal hernia
- Morton neuroma
- Plantar fasciitis
- Pes planus, pes cavus

Neuromuscular Disorders

- Carpal tunnel syndrome
- Disc disease
  - Herniation
    - Bulge
    - Protrusion
    - Extrusion
    - Rupture
  - Degenerative disc disease
  - Internal disc disruption
  - Endplate junction failure
- Myofascial pain syndrome
- Thoracic outlet syndrome

Other Connective Tissue Disorders

- Bunions
- Bursitis
- Shin splints
  - Medial tibial stress syndrome
  - Periostitis
  - Stress fractures
- Tendinopathies
  - Tendinitis
  - Tendinosis
  - Tenosynovitis
    - Trigger finger
    - de Quervain tenosynovitis
- Whiplash

Muscle Disorders

Muscular Dystrophy

Definition: What Is It?

Muscular dystrophy (MD) is a group of several closely related neuromuscular diseases characterized by genetic anomalies that lead to the degeneration and wasting away of muscle tissue. It usually begins in skeletal muscles of the extremities, but ultimately it can affect the breathing muscles and the heart.

The two most common varieties of muscular dystrophy are X-linked inherited diseases. This means the affected gene is carried by the mother, but passed on only to her sons. Other types of muscular dystrophy are autosomal dominant or recessive; they may affect females as often as males (see Sidebar 3.1).

Demographics

MD occurs all over the world, affecting all races. Duchenne muscular dystrophy is the most common kind, and it affects 1 out of every 3,500 boys in the United States, and about a third of those are spontaneous genetic mutations; they appear in boys with no family history of this disease.

Becker MD occurs in 1 case out of every 30,000 births of boys. Other types of MD are much more rare than the Becker and Duchenne variants, and their distribution varies.

Etiology: What Happens?

Normal muscles convert fat or glycogen into fuel to do their work of pulling bony attachments together. They do this with the assistance of a protein called **dystrophin**, which is produced in muscle cells, just under the **sarcolemma**. Dystrophin also helps to maintain the health and stability of the sarcolemma. The most common versions of muscular dystrophy involve a genetic mutation that either prevents the production of dystrophin altogether or allows its production only at inadequate levels. Other forms of muscular dystrophy involve low production of other vital proteins.

In the absence of dystrophin the cell membrane degenerates, and muscle cells atrophy and die, to be replaced by fat and connective tissue. Antagonists to affected muscles have no resistance, and eventually their connective tissue shrinks, pulling bony attachments closer together in a permanent contracture.

Dystrophin: A protein found in skeletal muscle tissue; it is missing in people with some forms of muscular dystrophy.

Sarcolemma: The plasma membrane of a muscle fiber.

SIDEBAR 3.1 What's in Your Genes?

Genes are part of the building blocks of human cells. They are arranged along pairs of chromosomes, and each parent contributes one side of the pair. Some diseases are caused by anomalies in genetic structure. While these anomalies can be inherited from one or both parents, they can also occur with no family history as spontaneous mutations. Breakthroughs in the study of molecular genetics have revealed the specific anomalies responsible for various forms of muscular dystrophy, as well as other inherited disorders such as **sickle cell disease**, **Marfan syndrome**, **hemophilia**, and **osteogenesis imperfecta**.

Inherited diseases have three variations: they can be autosomal dominant, autosomal recessive, or X-linked disorders.

- **Autosomal dominant** inheritance means that one parent has a defective gene and the other does not. Each child has a 50% chance of inheriting the defective but dominant gene, which causes the disease. Males and females are at equal risk for autosomal dominant inheritance.
- **Autosomal recessive** inheritance means that each parent carries one defective gene, but it produces no symptoms. Each child has a 25% chance of inheriting both defective genes and developing the associated disease. Alternatively, each child has a 50% chance of inheriting only one gene and becoming a carrier for the next generation.
- **X-linked** inheritance means that a woman carries a defective gene on one X chromosome. Each of her sons has a 50% chance of inheriting the faulty gene from her. Each of her daughters has a 50% chance of carrying the faulty gene to her sons. It is rare for females to be severely affected by X-linked diseases. Women who carry these genetic defects are at increased risk for developing some but not all of the characteristics of the genetic disease. Men who have X-linked mutations may pass the genes onto their daughters, who may become carriers, but no sons are directly affected.

Muscular dystrophy may also affect the heart and breathing muscles, making patients vulnerable to cardiac and respiratory weakness.

Types of Muscular Dystrophy

- *Duchenne muscular dystrophy*: This X-linked genetic anomaly is the most common and most severe variety of the disease. Boys with this condition cannot produce any dystrophin at all.
- *Becker muscular dystrophy*: This is a less common and less severe form of MD that also affects only boys. In this version some dystrophin is produced, but not enough for normal function.

- *Myotonic muscular dystrophy*: This is the most common form of adult-onset muscular dystrophy, and it affects both men and women. Its primary symptom is **myotonia**: stiffness or spasm following muscular contraction. Myotonic MD appears in two slightly different forms, type 1 and type 2. It is a progressive disorder that affects many systems. It can cause cataracts, gastrointestinal dysfunction, and life-threatening heart problems, especially arrhythmia.
- *Other varieties of muscular dystrophy*:
  - Congenital muscular dystrophy includes several rare varieties that are diagnosed at birth or in early infancy.
  - Facioscapulohumeral dystrophy primarily affects the muscles of the face, shoulder, and upper arm.
  - Limb girdle dystrophy begins in the shoulders, upper arms, and pelvic area.
  - Emery-Dreifuss muscular dystrophy shows contractures of the Achilles tendon, elbow, and spine.
  - Oculopharyngeal muscular dystrophy affects the eyes and pharynx muscles first.

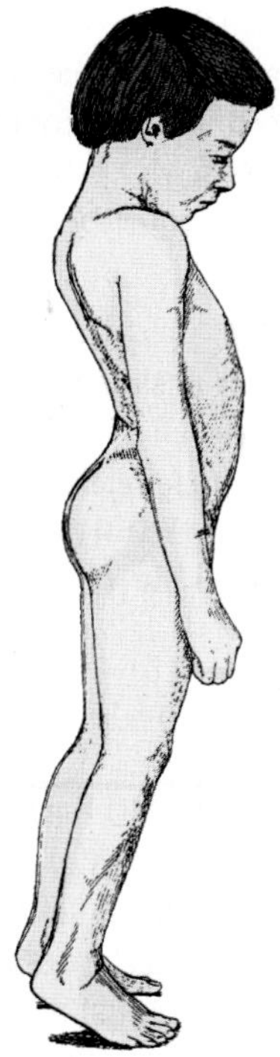

FIGURE 3.3 Characteristic posture of a child with Duchenne muscular dystrophy. Along with the typical toe gait, the child develops a lordotic posture as Duchenne dystrophy causes further deterioration.

Signs and Symptoms

Signs and symptoms of muscular dystrophy vary according to type, but the two most common varieties, Duchenne and Becker, are very similar in presentation: symptoms often begin during toddlerhood, when a little boy begins to have trouble walking or climbing stairs. He may complain of leg pain. He develops a waddling gait with an accentuated lumbar curve to compensate for the weakness in his legs. Eventually he may not put his whole foot down at all; instead, he walks on tiptoes (Figure 3.3). His calves may seem to become disproportionately large in a condition called pseudohypertrophy; in actuality the muscle mass is being replaced with fat and connective tissue.

MD can progress to affect the spine, joints, the heart, and the lungs. Many patients die at a young age of cardiac or respiratory failure.

Duchenne muscular dystrophy is usually diagnosed between 3 and 5 years of age, and an affected child will probably be in a wheelchair by his 12th birthday. Its progression is fairly dependable, and the best life expectancy is typically mid 20s.

Becker muscular dystrophy has a similar progression, but it is usually diagnosed later and has a less severe impact. The outlook may be a great deal brighter, depending on how much dystrophin individual patients may produce.

Muscular dystrophy is occasionally but not always accompanied by mental disability. Other conditions that accompany these diseases include contractures and severe **postural deviations** that develop as the skeletal muscles tighten and pull on the spine and rib cage. Severe scoliosis can in turn restrict lung capacity, which raises the risk for both cardiac impairment and respiratory infection.

Most MD patients experience pain as a consequence of immobility, **pressure sores**, and postural stress. This pain may be classified as neuropathic, but it can involve mechanical forces outside the central nervous system.

> **Myotonia:** Delayed relaxation of a muscle after a strong contraction.

Treatment

Because this is a genetic disorder, no treatment to reverse or cure muscular dystrophy exists. Some interventions work to prolong the use of muscles and limbs, including massage and physical therapy. Surgery is sometimes recommended to release tight tendons or to straighten a distorted spine. Gene therapies are in development, but nothing so far has improved the function or outlook for MD patients.

Outside of these interventions, a child with muscular dystrophy is supported to be as healthy, as comfortable, and as functional as possible. Exercise is recommended, as long as the patient isn't overstressed. Secondary infections are aggressively treated, and ventilation assistance is often used. Ultimately many patients need to learn to use leg braces, a standing walker, and finally a wheelchair.

Gene therapy for Duchenne and Becker MD may not be far off; human trials have already been conducted to examine the possibility of inserting a dystrophin-making gene into targeted muscle cells. Most MD patients are limited to traditional interventions at this point, however.

Medications

- Corticosteroids appear to slow progression of muscle loss in Duchenne MD
- Anticonvulsants or muscle relaxants for myotonic MD
- Nonsteroidal anti-inflammatory drugs (NSAIDs) for pain
- Tricyclic antidepressants for pain and depression

Massage Therapy Implications

RISKS	A person with MD may have general fragility, in the area of muscle contractures. Advanced cases of serious forms of MD may involve heart or respiratory weakness; any bodywork must allow for this fragility. Further, the drug regimen used may alter massage choices; steroids and muscle relaxants have specific cautions for bodywork.
BENEFITS	Massage and physical therapy may be recommended to preserve function, ease pain, and slow the process of contractures in muscles that are antagonistic to those weakened by the disease. Because sensation is intact with MD, massage is safe as long as systemic weaknesses are recognized and respected.
OPTIONS	Passive stretching to delay contractures and prolong muscle function is a key part of physical therapy for MD patients; this can be provided by a massage therapist as well.
RESEARCH	Caregivers of patients with MD are often willing users of complementary and integrative health care therapies, and massage for children with Becker and Duchenne MD is a common intervention.[1] Preventing or slowing the progression of fibrosis is considered a high priority, and massage is considered an option, along with yoga-like stretching, for this strategy.[2] 1. Zhu Y, Romitti PA, Conway KM, et al. Complementary and alternative medicine for Duchenne and Becker muscular dystrophies: characteristics of users and caregivers. *Pediatric Neurology* 2014;51(1):71–77. http://www.ncbi.nlm.nih.gov/pubmed/24785967 2. Klingler W, Jurkat-Rott K, Lehmann-Horn F, et al. The role of fibrosis in Duchenne muscular dystrophy. *Acta Myologica* 2012;31(3):184–195. http://www.ncbi.nlm.nih.gov/pubmed/23620650

Spasms, Cramps

Definition: What Is It?

A spasm or cramp is an involuntary contraction of a voluntary muscle. The difference between spasms and cramps is somewhat arbitrary; cramps are strong, painful, usually short-lived spasms. One could say that chronically tight, painful paraspinals are in spasm, while a gastrocnemius with a charley horse is a cramp. The severity of these episodes depends on how much of the muscle is involved. Spasms and cramps can be distinguished from muscle twitching or **fasciculations** by the scale of the tissues involved: twitching is typically a painless momentary contraction of a small number of superficial muscle fibers; spasms and cramps can be painful and involve whole muscles or muscle groups.

The terms "spasms" and "cramps" are sometimes used in reference to visceral muscle too (i.e., "spastic" constipation), but this discussion is restricted to the involuntary contraction of skeletal, or so-called voluntary muscle.

Etiology: What Happens?

It is not always clear why muscles contract involuntarily: this phenomenon is surprisingly understudied. Some of the most common situations are addressed here.

- *Nutrition*: Calcium, potassium, and magnesium deficiencies can make one prone to cramping, especially in the feet. Other important substances for efficient muscle contraction include water, glucose, and sodium. If any of these are in short supply, muscles can't work to their best potential.
- *Ischemia*: The **pain-spasm-ischemia cycle** presents one major theory behind involuntary muscle tightness. When a muscle, or part of a muscle, is suddenly or gradually deprived of oxygen, it can't function properly. Rather than becoming loose and weak, according to this theory, it becomes tighter and tighter (Figure 3.4). Often this is a gradual process, but sometimes it is a sudden and violent reaction to oxygen shortage. Long-term situations with tight postural muscles can become self-perpetuating in this way.
- *Exercise-associated muscle cramping*: Athletes often report problems with muscles cramping at or near the end of vigorous work. Dehydration, electrolyte imbalance, and hyperthermia may all be contributing factors, but a neurological component appears to be present as well. Whether messages are generated in the spine or in the muscles is a topic of debate. The target muscles usually cross two joints, and they cramp when they are contracted from a

Fasciculation: An involuntary twitching contraction of fasciculi.

Pain-spasm-ischemia cycle: A cycle traditionally thought to create trigger points: sensations of pain cause spasm, which limits blood flow, resulting in more pain, and so on.

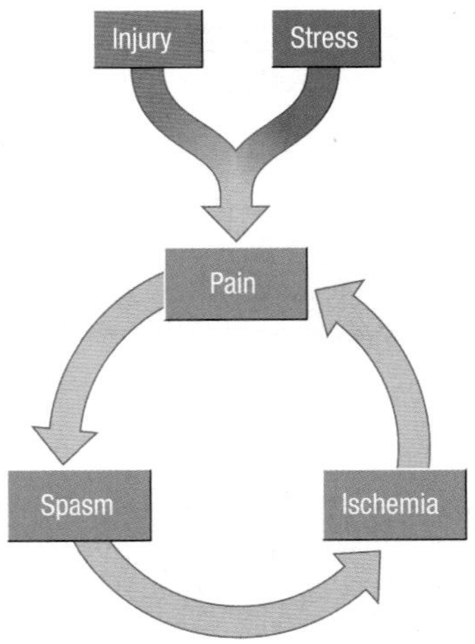

FIGURE 3.4 pain-spasm-ischemia cycle

shortened position. Being well warmed-up before exercising is often a good preventive strategy.

- *Splinting*: This is a reflexive reaction against injury. Consider an acute **whiplash**: the supraspinous and intertransverse ligaments have been severely wrenched, and the body senses a potentially dangerous instability in the cervical spine. The postural neck muscles contract in response; as far as they're concerned, they are keeping the head from falling off. This kind of spasm is an important protective mechanism, because it prevents movements that could cause further injury. The muscles create an effective splint, and the range of motion of affected joints is very limited.
- *Underlying conditions*: Other illnesses or conditions can contribute to muscle cramping and spasm, and some of these carry cautions for massage. Examples include **diabetes**, **anemia**, kidney disorders, **multiple sclerosis**, **peripheral neuropathy**, **dystonia**, or local nerve compression.
- *Medications*: Some medications have muscle cramps as a side effect. Diuretics like Lasix, several statins, some asthma treatments, and a few other more specialized drugs are associated with secondary cramping.

Treatment

Massage is a much-used strategy to manage long-term, low-grade muscle spasms. Muscle cramps and spasm may also be treated with heat or ice, or local applications of ointments that create hot and cold sensations to alter local blood flow. Ongoing mild but painful situations may be treated with analgesics, but muscle relaxants that affect the nervous system are usually reserved for very extreme situations.

Medications

- Analgesics for pain management
- Botulinum injections are sometimes prescribed for hypertonic muscles related to neurological problems
- Muscle relaxants for severe spasm, often in conjunction with trauma

Massage Therapy Implications

RISKS

Muscles that are chronically tight or cramping may not respond well to direct and aggressive bodywork delivered to the muscle bellies.

Underlying conditions or pathologies that contribute to involuntary contractions must be addressed if cramping is a frequent occurrence.

A client taking painkillers or muscle relaxants for muscle spasm will not be able to give accurate feedback to the massage therapist about pain or stretching limitations.

When muscles are splinting a new injury, it is important to respect this protective mechanism until the acute stage of injury has passed.

BENEFITS

Cramping muscles can respond well to bodywork that is not at the muscle belly, and muscles that have been in spasm or cramp may benefit from the circulatory turnover that massage can provide.

When a spasm that splints an injured area has outlived its usefulness, massage can help to reestablish efficient movement, but this is best done incrementally to avoid the risk of reinjury.

OPTIONS

Acute muscle cramps can often be relieved through stretching and massage to their attachment sites. After the cramp releases and pain is resolved, rigorous massage is safe and useful for local circulatory turnover.

RESEARCH

There is a surprising dearth of research on massage therapy in the context of common spasm and cramps. A small number of studies suggest massage for pain related to hypertonicity, and muscle spasms due to dystonia,[1–3] but as an intervention for exercise-related spasm, massage has not yet been scientifically demonstrated to be useful or not useful. It is an unexpected hole in the evidence base.

1. Halpin S. Case report: the effects of massage therapy on lumbar spondylolisthesis. *Journal of Bodywork and Movement Therapies* 2012;16(1):115–123. http://www.ncbi.nlm.nih.gov/pubmed/22196437
2. Albertin A, Kerppers II, Amorim CF, et al. The effect of manual therapy on masseter muscle pain and spasm. *Electromyography and Clinical Neurophysiology* 2010;50(2):107–112. http://www.ncbi.nlm.nih.gov/pubmed/20405786
3. Loyola DP, Camargos S, Maia D, et al. Sensory tricks in focal dystonia and hemifacial spasm. *European Journal of Neurology* 2013;20(4):704–707. http://www.ncbi.nlm.nih.gov/pubmed/23216586

Strains

Definition: What Are They?

Strains are injuries to muscle fibers involving the tearing of myofibers and production of scar tissue. They are sometimes difficult to distinguish from tendon injuries, which are discussed in the section on **tendinopathies** later in the chapter.

Etiology: What Happens?

Muscle strains and other soft tissue injuries may arise from specific trauma, but they often develop in the context of chronic, cumulative overuse patterns with no specific onset.

When a muscle is injured, myofibers are torn, the inflammatory process begins, and fibroblasts flood the area with collagen to knit the injury back together. The accumulation of scar tissue within contractile tissue is a normal process, but it has some potentially important implications:

- *Impaired* **contractility**: Scar tissue can impede the efficiency of uninjured muscle fibers. When the muscle cells try to contract, they bear the weight not only of their bony attachments, but also of the fibers that are disabled by the mass of collagen that binds them up. This increases the load on uninjured fibers, and raises the chance of repeated injury, more scar tissue, and further weakening of the muscle.
- *Adhesions*: Collagen that is manufactured around an injury isn't laid down in perfect alignment with the muscle fibers; instead it is deposited quickly but in haphazard form. Randomly arranged collagen fibers tend to bind up different layers of tissue that are designed to be separate. **Adhesions** can occur wherever layers of connective tissue come in contact with each other. They may occur within the muscle, as is frequently seen with the paraspinals, or between muscles, when muscle sheaths stick to other muscle sheaths. Hamstrings are a common place for this phenomenon. Wherever they occur, adhesions limit mobility and increase the chance of injury (Figure 3.5).

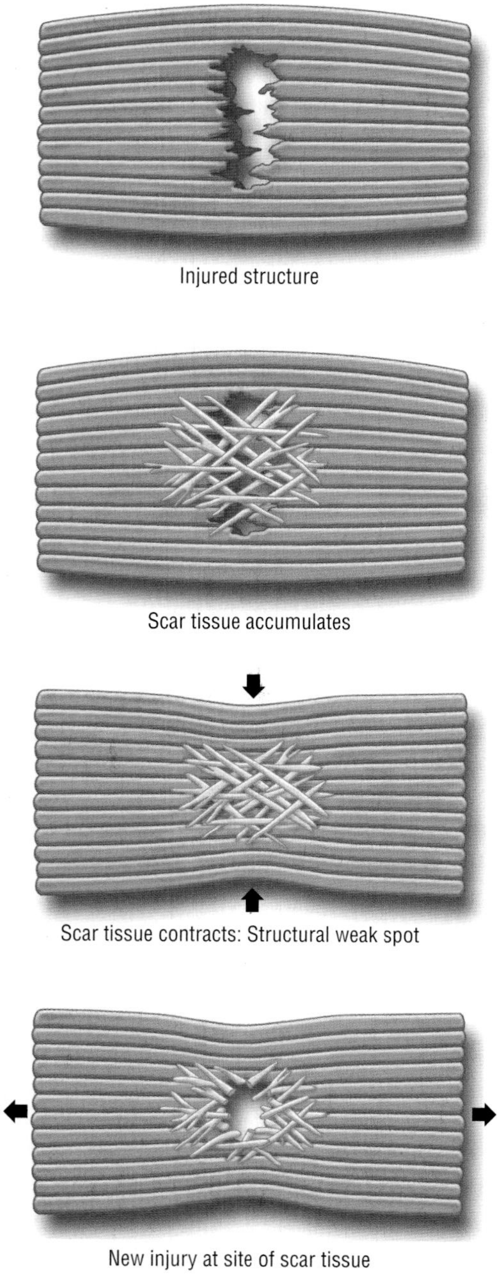

FIGURE 3.5 Strains and sprains: internal adhesions and the injury-reinjury cycle

Signs and Symptoms

Symptoms of muscle strain include mild or intense local pain, stiffness, and pain on resisted movement or passive stretching. Unless it is a very bad tear, no palpable heat or swelling is usually present.

Strains are graded by severity. First-degree strains are mildly painful but don't seriously impede function, while third-degree strains involve ruptured muscles and possibly the avulsion of bony attachments.

Contractility: The ability to contract.

Adhesion: An abnormal connection between one layer of tissue and another. Usually refers to the "gluing" of connective tissue layers.

Treatment

It is now generally recognized that early intervention in the healing process for injured muscles significantly improves the prognosis for full recovery. Although individual specialists approach musculoskeletal injuries with different tactics, several of their priorities are consistent:

- *Get an accurate diagnosis.* Evaluating muscular injuries requires a thorough patient history and a skilled clinical examination. Other diagnostic procedures (e.g., radiographs, bone scans, CT, MRI) may be recommended as well.
- *Control inflammation.* Inflammation is a valuable process, but it can outlive its usefulness and end up causing more

harm than good. Inflammation can often be controlled by RICE (rest, ice, compression, elevation), but some physicians now use the PRICES protocol, which adds protection and support to the list.

- *Rehabilitate damaged tissues.* This part of the treatment involves exercises that add incremental amounts of weight-bearing stress to the injured muscle to help the scar tissue realign with the original fibers and to gradually increase strength and fitness. This may be the most vulnerable time in the process, as athletes who are eager to resume training may try to go too fast and get injured again, and others may neglect the need to exercise and allow scar tissue to accumulate to inefficient levels.
- *Prevent further injury.* Most chronic muscle injuries are related to controllable factors that can be adjusted to help prevent future problems. These include dealing with muscle imbalances that make one area weaker while another may be tighter, improving technique in specific sports, making sure that equipment is appropriate and in good repair, adjusting training schedules so that changes are incorporated slowly, taping or bracing vulnerable areas, and being careful about good warm-up and cooldown procedures.

Medications

- NSAIDs for pain and inflammation

Massage Therapy Implications

RISKS	Vigorous, intrusive massage to a new or acute injury may exacerbate inflammation and tissue damage.
BENEFITS	Carefully performed massage at the appropriate stages of healing can be an important contributor to the recovery from a simple muscle strain, turning a potentially painful and long-lasting injury into a relatively trivial event with a successful outcome.
OPTIONS	In acute strains, lymphatic drainage or other work to limit edema is appropriate. Later, cross-fiber and linear friction along with passive stretching and carefully calibrated exercises can help the new scar tissue to align in the best possible formation for efficient contractions and range of motion.
RESEARCH	Best et al.[1] wondered if massage might speed healing by promoting angiogenesis in damaged muscle tissue, but the conclusions aren't yet clear. An animal model[2] suggests that massage following eccentric contractions has a positive effect on tissue repair, and a positive role for massage to influence inflammation in damaged tissue has been found by other researchers.[3,4]

1. Best TM, Gharaibeh B, Huard J. Stem cells, angiogenesis and muscle healing: a potential role in massage therapies? *British Journal of Sports Medicine* 2013;47(9):556–560. http://bjsm.bmj.com/content/early/2012/11/28/bjsports-2012-091685.short
2. Haas C, Butterfield TA, Zhao Y, et al. Dose-dependency of massage-like compressive loading on recovery of active muscle properties following eccentric exercise: rabbit study with clinical relevance. *British Journal of Sports Medicine* 2013;47(2):83–88. http://bjsm.bmj.com/content/47/2/83.short
3. Waters-Banker C, Dupont-Versteegden EE, Kitzman PH, et al. Investigating the mechanisms of massage efficacy: the role of mechanical immunomodulation. *Journal of Athletic Training* 2014;49(2):266–273. http://www.natajournals.org/doi/full/10.4085/1062-6050-49.2.25
4. Crane JD, Ogborn DI, Cupido C, et al. Massage therapy attenuates inflammatory signaling after exercise-induced muscle damage. *Science Translational Medicine* 2012;4(119):119ra113. http://www.ncbi.nlm.nih.gov/pubmed/22301554

Bone Disorders

Osteosarcoma

Definition: What Is It?

Osteosarcoma is a form of cancer that originates in bone tissue. It is most common in adolescents and young adults.

Demographics

Osteosarcoma is diagnosed about 400 times each year in this country. It is slightly more common in young men than young women, and the incidence is slightly higher among blacks than among whites.

Risk factors for osteosarcoma include exposure to radiation for other cancer treatment, genetic predisposition, and a period of rapid bone growth, as is seen in late adolescence.

Etiology: What Happens?

Cancer is the development of cells that replicate in a hyperactive and disorganized way. It most commonly affects cells that naturally grow fast, which is why epithelial cancers are more common than any other kind. Osteosarcoma is relatively rare because bone tends not to grow quickly—except in children

SIDEBAR 3.2 Staging Osteosarcoma

Until recently, osteosarcoma had no formal staging system, so treatment strategies were haphazard at best. Now a TNM system has been developed to track the progression of this disease, which allows doctors to design treatments to fit the stage of the disease.

Primary Tumor (T)

Tx	Cannot be assessed
T0	No evidence of a primary tumor
T1	Tumor <8 cm
T2	Tumor >8 cm
T3	Discontinuous tumors in the primary bone site

Regional Lymph Nodes (N)

Nx	Cannot be assessed
N0	No regional metastasis
N1	Regional metastasis

Distant Metastasis (M)

Mx	Cannot be assessed
M0	No distant metastasis
M1a	Lung only
M1b	Other distant sites

Histologic Grade (G)

Gx	Cannot be assessed
G1	Cells are well differentiated; low grade
G2	Moderately differentiated; low grade
G3	Poorly differentiated
G4	Undifferentiated

These delineations are translated into stages I to IV in this way:

STAGE	T	N	M	GRADE
IA	T1	N0	M0	Gx-G2
IB	T2	N0	M0	Gx-G2
	T3	N0	M0	G3
IIA	Any	N0	M0	G3-4
IIB	Any	N0	M0	G3-4
III	Any	N0	M0	G3
IV-A	Any	N0	M1a	Any
IV-B	Any	N1	Any	Any
IV-B	Any	Any	M1b	Any

and young adults: these are the people most vulnerable to this condition, especially during growth spurts.

It is important to delineate between osteosarcoma and metastatic carcinoma. Osteosarcoma begins in bone cells; metastatic carcinoma is the result of cancer that begins elsewhere (see Sidebar 3.2).

Osteosarcoma has some features in common with another bone cancer that usually affects young people: Ewing sarcoma. The main differences are in what part of the bones tends to be affected, and Ewing sarcoma doesn't always develop in bone tissue at all. Otherwise these two conditions are very similar and are treated in essentially the same way.

Osteosarcoma typically grows as one major tumor at a time, and it is most commonly found near the growth plates of the long bones: the femur, the proximal tibia, and the proximal humerus are the most common locations (Figure 3.6). Tumors can originate in either trabecular or **cortical bone** tissue. Left untreated, this cancer can destroy the bone and metastasize to other tissues: the lungs are the most frequent sites.

Cortical bone: The dense outer layer of bone. Also called compact bone.

Signs and Symptoms

Like many types of cancer, osteosarcoma tends to be silent until it is well established. The earliest symptoms include pain with activity, which progresses to pain at rest. Because this usually happens in an adolescent or young adult, it is easy to mistake these warning signs for growing pains or soft tissue injuries. A palpable mass eventually develops on the affected bone. The affected bone may **fracture**, and respiratory symptoms indicate metastasis to the lungs.

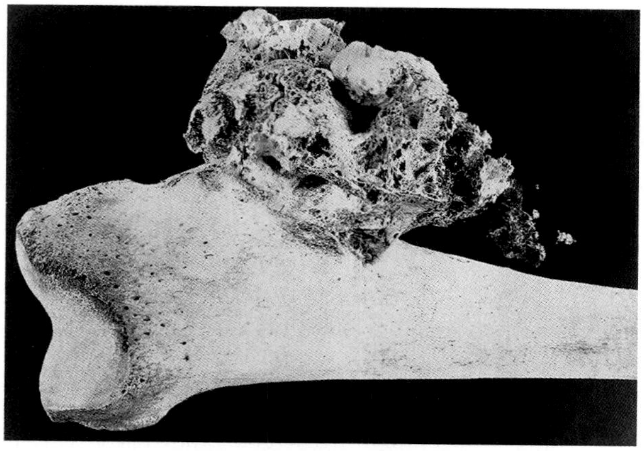

FIGURE 3.6 Osteosarcoma of the femur, from 5th Dynasty Egypt

Treatment

Osteosarcoma is typically treated with orthopedic surgery to biopsy the growth, to remove it with clean margins, and to support the remaining bone, sparing the limb if possible. Because the vast majority of osteosarcoma patients experience a relapse without further treatment, chemotherapy is a standard follow-up strategy.

Medications

- Chemotherapeutic drugs to minimize the risk of further cancer development
- Drugs to help manage the symptoms of chemotherapy

Massage Therapy Implications

RISKS	The symptoms of osteosarcoma can look like growing pains or simple soft tissue injury. This may lead patients to seek massage rather than medical treatment, which can delay an important diagnosis. Once the cancer has been identified, care must be taken around the damaged bone, because fractures are a possibility. And of course any massage or bodywork strategy must accommodate for the challenges of cancer treatment, which in this situation involves surgery and chemotherapy at least.
BENEFITS	Massage offers many benefits to cancer patients, including improving mood, lessening anxiety and depression, promoting good-quality sleep, and decreasing the negative side effects of cancer treatments. All this must be done in coordination with the rest of the health care team, of course. A client who has fully recovered from osteosarcoma can enjoy the same benefits of bodywork as does the rest of the population.
RESEARCH	One study[1] found that mice with induced osteosarcoma that were massaged directly on the tumor site twice a week had tumors that grew faster than did those in unmassaged mice with the same condition. This is good evidence for why massage therapists need to stay away from tumor sites and undiagnosed lesions of any kind. For patients who are going through cancer treatment, however, research suggests that carefully delivered massage therapy—away from the tumor site—has many benefits to offer. This is addressed in more detail in Chapter 12. 1. Wang JY, Wu PK, Chen PC, et al. Manipulation therapy prior to diagnosis induced primary osteosarcoma metastasis—from clinical to basic research. *PLoS One* 2014;9(5):e96571. http://www.ncbi.nlm.nih.gov/pmc/articles/PMC4013034/

Osgood-Schlatter Disease

Definition: What Is It?

Osgood-Schlatter disease (OSD) is irritation and inflammation at the site of the quadriceps attachment on the tibia. It can also be called tibial tuberosity **apophysitis**. It occurs when the quadriceps muscles are vigorously used in combination with rapid growth of the leg bones, typically during an adolescent growth spurt in athletic children.

Demographics

Adolescents are the prime demographic for OSD, especially those who engage in running and jumping sports. It affects as much as 21% of young athletes, as compared to less than 5% of nonathletic children. Boys with OSD outnumber girls by about 3 to 1. It usually affects girls between ages 8 and 12, and boys between 12 and 15.

Etiology: What Happens?

When children enter their teens, they begin a time of rapid bone growth, especially in their femurs and tibias: the bones that determine how tall they will be. The quadriceps group attaches at the tibial tuberosity, a bony landmark that doesn't fully calcify until late in adolescence. This structural weak spot is vulnerable to constant, repeated forceful contractions of the quadriceps that can lead to inflammation and injury.

With acute inflammation of the quadriceps attachment, the tendon can pull away from the bone, causing multiple tiny fractures and enlargement of the tibial tuberosity. In extreme cases, an avulsion can form: this is a separation of a part of the bone. It is common for OSD patients to develop a large, permanent bump at the tibial tuberosity; this is where the bone adapts to the constant pull of the quadriceps insertion. OSD is usually unilateral, but some athletes develop inflammation at both knees.

The severity of OSD varies greatly from one person to the next; one person may have to be careful warming up before playing soccer, while another athlete may have to quit the team altogether. It is generally a self-limiting condition, which means that when the connective tissue growth catches up with the bone growth, the pain and irritation subside even though a bone spur remains. Most cases subside when the tibia fully ossifies, late in adolescence.

Apophysitis: Inflammation of a bony process or outgrowth.

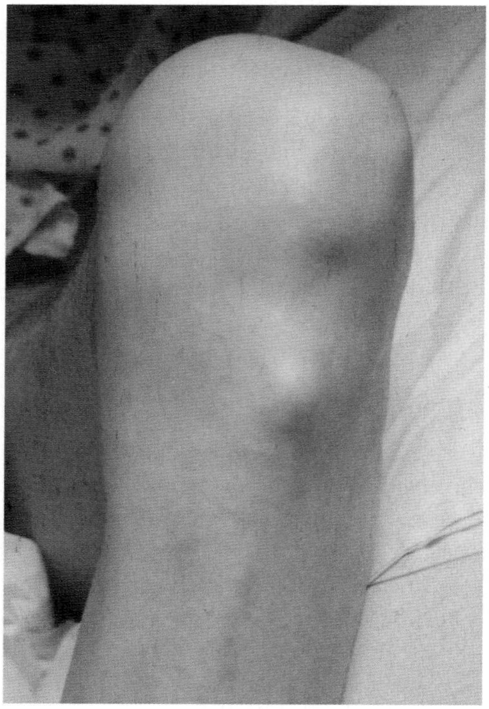

FIGURE 3.7 Osgood-Schlatter disease: a nontender enlargement of the tibial tuberosity

Signs and Symptoms

OSD is easy to identify because the people susceptible to it are such a well-defined group: athletic teens. In acute stages of OSD, the knee is hot, swollen, and painful just distal to the patella at the tibial tuberosity. Any activity that stresses or stretches the quadriceps aggravates symptoms.

When OSD is not acute, pain and inflammation are resolved, but the characteristic bump of the remodeled tibia may be permanent (Figure 3.7). A person who had OSD as a child may never be comfortable kneeling because of tibial distortion.

Treatment

Treatment for OSD focuses on reducing pain and limiting damage to the tibia. Mild cases can be managed by carefully warming up and stretching the quadriceps and hamstrings before exercise, and icing them afterward. Nonsteroidal anti-inflammatories may be suggested to help with pain and inflammation. A strap worn below the patella may ease pain during play, and kneepads can help if activities require kneeling.

Severe cases may require that the athlete suspend activity until the pain and inflammation have been gone for several weeks. In the meantime, the knee may be supported with a brace or cast. This period is followed by rehabilitative exercise to strengthen the muscles and reduce the chance of a recurrence when the athlete becomes active again.

In rare cases, the knee may need surgery to remove bits of the tibia that were pulled off and suspended in the tibial tendon.

Medications

- NSAIDs for pain and inflammation

Massage Therapy Implications

RISKS	Intrusive friction around the tibial tuberosity may exacerbate pain and inflammation during acute flares of OSD.
BENEFITS	Lymphatic work may help resolve acute inflammation. In nonflared cases, massage with careful stretching of the quadriceps may ease pain, improve flexibility, and reduce tension in the quadriceps. All of this may allow young athletes to safely return to play sooner than without treatment.
RESEARCH	No recent research supports massage therapy to manage or prevent OSD, but ice massage is mentioned in an older paper[1] as a strategy to manage pain. 1. Antich TJ, Brewster CE. Osgood-Schlatter disease: review of literature and physical therapy management. *Journal of Orthopaedic and Sports Physical Therapy* 1985;7(1):5–10. http://www.ncbi.nlm.nih.gov/pubmed/18802290

Osteoporosis

Definition: What Is It?

Osteoporosis literally means "porous bones." In this condition, calcium is pulled off the bones faster than it is replaced, leaving them thin, brittle, and prone to injury.

Demographics

Osteoporosis affects about 10 million Americans, but about 34 million others have a silent preosteoporotic condition called **osteopenia**. Women with osteoporosis outnumber men by about 4 to 1, for a variety of reasons. It

> **Osteopenia:** The condition of low bone density, but not low enough to be considered osteoporosis.

is more common among Whites and Asians than among other races. This condition is usually diagnosed in people over 60, but it is closely tied to events, habits, and activities of earlier years.

In the United States, about 1.5 million hip, spinal, and wrist fractures are identified as complications of osteoporosis each year.

Primary osteoporosis is almost exclusively seen in mature adults, unless a genetic condition or other problem interferes with bone density in childhood. Young people who fail to achieve good bone mass by early adulthood are very much at risk for problems with bone thinning later in life.

Etiology: What Happens?

Bones are composed of hard mineral deposits (mostly calcium phosphate) formed on an organized scaffold of collagen fibers. The volume of mineral deposits determines bone density. People normally accumulate most of their bone density by about age 20, but small gains are made until around age 30 to 35. After that point, either density is maintained at a stable level or withdrawals are made from this "calcium bank." The turnover of mineral deposits happens constantly, but this activity occurs in trabecular bone at a higher rate than in cortical bone. Osteoporosis develops when calcium is withdrawn from bone tissue faster than it is deposited.

Risk factors for osteoporosis are typically described as controllable or noncontrollable. Noncontrollable factors include gender (women are more at risk because of childbearing and breast-feeding, as well as having smaller bones to begin with), age, body size (smaller people are more at risk than are larger ones), ethnicity, and family history. Controllable factors include hormone levels, levels of calcium and vitamin D, medications, sedentary lifestyle, diet, and cigarette and alcohol use.

Osteoporosis can be the consequence of some other medical conditions, including **diabetes**, **anorexia** or **bulimia**, problems with absorption in the GI tract, and **hyper-** and **hypothyroidism**. **Rheumatoid arthritis** and **chronic obstructive pulmonary disease** can cause it. Dangerously weak bones are also a common and serious side effect of both radiation and the drugs used to treat many forms of **cancer**.

Logically, high calcium consumption should lead to high bone density, and high bone density should be linked to a low risk of osteoporosis and bone fractures. However, many factors beyond calcium influence bone health, including the accessibility of other vitamins and minerals, exercise habits, pH balance in the blood (especially as it is influenced by meat-based proteins), other diseases, medications, and even emotional state. The factors that help to determine a person's risk for osteoporosis boil down to variables in calcium absorption, calcium loss, and bone density maintenance.

- *Calcium absorption*: Calcium requires an acidic environment in the stomach to be absorbed into the bloodstream. If calcium enters the body in a form that impedes its contact with hydrochloric acid (for instance, in dairy products), the body has only limited access to this mineral. Similarly, if natural secretions of hydrochloric acid are reduced, as in older adults, it becomes harder to absorb whatever calcium is consumed.

  Some vitamins influence how the body uses calcium. Vitamin D controls absorption and retention of this important mineral. The body synthesizes vitamin D in response to direct sunlight (it takes about 15 minutes of exposure per day, depending on latitude), but vitamin D can also be easily supplemented. Vitamin K, found in many dark, leafy greens, also supports calcium absorption. Preformed vitamin A, however, can increase the risk of fractures if it is consumed in high quantities.
- *Calcium loss*: Calcium is constantly lost in sweat and urine. Some substances, specifically meat-based proteins, cause higher levels of calcium to be excreted in urine. So a person who takes in ample amounts of dietary calcium but who also eats a lot of meat tends to lose more calcium than does a vegetarian.

  The onset of **menopause** is another big factor in calcium loss. Low estrogen secretion causes osteoclasts to speed up, and osteoblasts to slow down. Ultimately women can lose 30% to 40% of their cortical bone and up to 50% of their trabecular bone density over a lifetime.

  Several other factors can lead to calcium loss. High caffeine consumption (more than three or four cups of coffee or servings of caffeinated soda per day) has been seen to have a negative impact. Other factors include medications (chemotherapeutic agents, corticosteroids, some diuretics, anticonvulsant drugs); **hyperthyroidism**; heavy alcohol use; smoking; inflammatory bowel disease (**Crohn disease, ulcerative colitis**); a history of **eating disorders**; and endocrine disorders, including **Cushing syndrome**, low testosterone, and low estrogen.
- *Bone density maintenance*: The shape and density of bones are determined by the activity of osteoclasts and osteoblasts. These cells work to remodel bones according to the commands of calcitonin, parathyroid hormone, estrogen, and progesterone. If hormones tell the osteoclasts to work faster than the osteoblasts, bone density declines. Osteoblasts and osteoclasts are most active in trabecular bone, which is found in epiphyses

of long bones and in vertebral bodies. The loss of key struts of calcium deposits in these areas can cause bones to collapse.

Bones are not the only part of the body that needs calcium. Calcium is consumed in nearly every chemical reaction that results in muscle contraction and nerve transmission, and it is essential to blood clotting. It also works as a buffer to help maintain the proper pH balance. The body has a strict prioritizing system for these important functions: chemical reactions that promote moment-to-moment survival are more important than maintaining the density of the vertebral bodies or femoral neck. Therefore, if calcium supplies are low, these bones lose some of their mineral structure.

NOTABLE CASES Many celebrities have shared their osteoporosis experiences with the public, including actress Sally Field and the late comedian Joan Rivers. Several influential men have had this condition as well, including Pope John Paul II, Winston Churchill, Clarence Darrow, and very possibly Benjamin Franklin.

When a person develops osteoporosis, it is usually because the balancing act between calcium absorption, calcium loss, and bone density maintenance is upset, and the calcium in the bones is pulled off faster than it is replaced. The bones, especially in the spine and femur, become progressively less dense, leaving the person vulnerable to the primary complications of this disease: spinal or hip **fractures** (Figures 3.8–3.10).

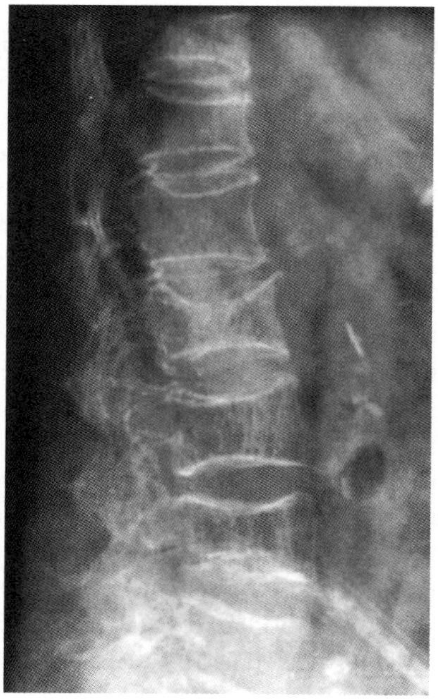

FIGURE 3.8 Demonstrable bone loss at vertebral bodies with osteoporosis

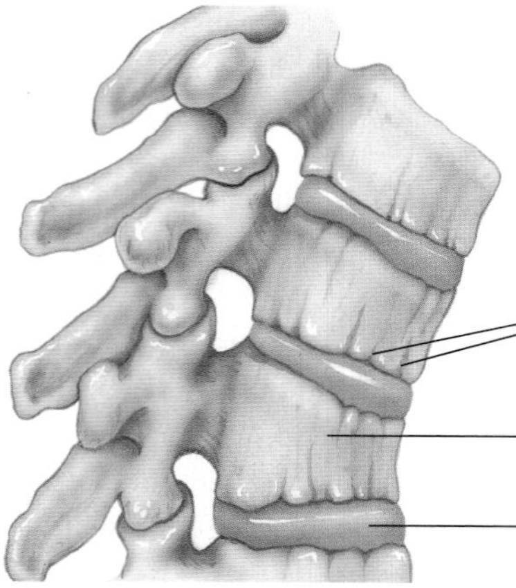

FIGURE 3.9 Vertebral bodies with compression fractures

Signs and Symptoms

Osteoporosis has no symptoms in its early stages. People who are at particularly high risk may undergo testing to try to identify it early, but it is often missed until complications, specifically fractures, develop.

Symptoms of osteoporosis center on pathologically weak bones. Thinned or collapsed vertebrae lead to a loss of height and the characteristic rounded "widow's hump" of **hyperkyphosis**. Chronic or acute back pain appears in this stage as the vertebrae continue to degenerate. Pain is worse with activity, and relieved by lying supine. Spasm of the paraspinal muscles is common, and patients may greatly limit their activity, even to becoming bedridden, to avoid exacerbating their discomfort.

Complications

People with osteoporosis are prone to fractures with little or no cause; these are called spontaneous or pathological fractures. Hips (usually the femoral neck rather than the ilium), vertebrae, and wrists are particularly vulnerable to breakage. Brittle ribs are often associated with osteoporosis due to corticosteroid use. And since in advanced age people are naturally low on both living **osteocytes** and growth hormone to support the healing process, it is difficult to recover from any injury of this severity. Most people who break a hip never return to prefracture levels of activity.

Treatment

Once osteoporosis has been recognized and rated for severity, a number of treatment options are available to keep it from getting worse. Pharmaceutical interventions include hormone replacement therapy to influence estrogen or

Osteocyte: A bone cell.

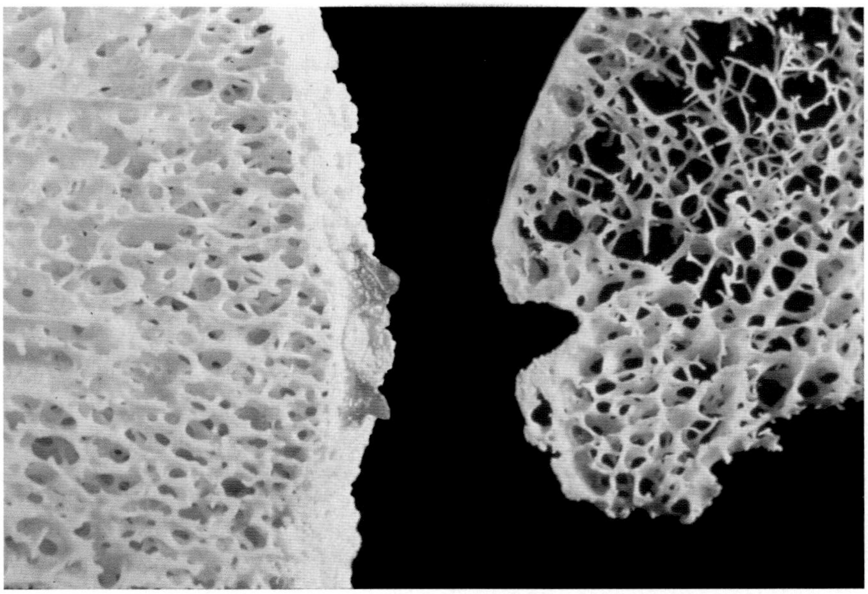

FIGURE 3.10 Loss of bone density in femoral head with osteoporosis

calcitonin, **bisphosphonates**, **SERMs** (selective estrogen receptor modules), and some others. None of these interventions is risk free, however, and osteoporosis patients must weigh risks and benefits of these medications carefully.

Exercise is almost always a part of the osteoporosis treatment strategy. Since bone remodels according to the stresses placed on it, weight-bearing stress ensures that maintaining healthy mass is a high priority. Diet also plays an important part in dealing with osteoporosis. Specific vitamins and other substances may improve calcium uptake, even for postmenopausal women, but that subject is outside the scope of this book.

Medications

- Vitamin and mineral supplements, including calcium, vitamin D, and others
- Hormone replacement therapy (including calcitonin) for slowed bone loss
- Selective estrogen receptor modules (SERMs) for slowed bone loss
- Bisphosphonates for slowed bone loss
- Parathyroid hormone analogues for accelerated bone growth
- **RANK ligand inhibitors** to interfere with osteoclast formation

Bisphosphonate: A class of drug used to restrict bone loss by reducing the number of bone-clearing cells.

SERMs: **S**elective **e**strogen **r**eceptor **m**odulators, a group of medications that reduce the risk of certain cancers as well as osteoporosis.

RANK ligand inhibitors: A class of drugs used to treat osteoporosis by interfering with bone resorption.

Prevention

It is possible to prevent osteoporosis, feasible to slow it down or halt it, and difficult to reverse it. The causes of this disease vary, but they center on one main theme: the time to build up calcium reserves is in youth and early adulthood. The skeleton grows in height until about age 20, but it continues to accumulate density until about age 30. After that point, it either stays stable or progressively demineralizes. Four main steps have been recommended to achieve and maintain optimal bone density and avoid osteoporosis:

- *Get dietary calcium from absorbable sources.* Dairy products are abundant and convenient, but not the most efficient source for all people. Other recommended calcium sources include beans and greens: legumes and most green leafy vegetables. (Spinach and chard, while rich in calcium and other nutrients, also have substances that limit calcium absorption.) Calcium supplements vary in absorbability; calcium carbonate, calcium phosphate, and calcium citrate are generally recognized to have good accessibility.
- *Exercise.* Weight-bearing stress makes it necessary for the body to maintain healthy bone density.
- *Get vitamin D.* The RDA for vitamin D is 200 units, or 5 μg/day. This can be ingested in supplement form or naturally synthesized by exposure to sunlight.
- *Avoid substances and behaviors that pull calcium off bones.* These include tobacco, excessive salt, animal-based proteins, and excessive caffeine and alcohol.

Massage Therapy Implications

RISKS	The primary risk for a person with osteoporosis who receives massage is that a fracture may occur because of undue pressure or problematic positioning on the table. It is important also to remember that elderly clients are unlikely to have only one pathology: this is a population that may have several problems in addition to osteoporosis that influence bodywork choices.
BENEFITS	Massage won't reverse osteoporosis, but it can be a powerful modality to help with pain and limited movement. Any work that respects a client's fragility while working for pain relief is welcome.
OPTIONS	Clients with osteoporosis may need imaginative bolstering to create a setting in which it is safe and comfortable to receive massage. Pillows, bolsters, rolled-up towels, or other tools may be needed to firmly "nest" them into the table for maximum comfort. In addition to extra bolstering, clients with osteoporosis may benefit from having extra help getting on and off the table.
RESEARCH	Guo et al.[1] report on a case in which an elderly man sustained a broken lumbar pedicle after receiving a back massage. This supports considering osteoporosis as a situation in which the risk of an adverse event is higher than with the general population. On the other hand, some evidence[2] indicates that even a single skilled massage may help elders with balance and postural stability, thus helping to prevent falls, which are a big risk for people with osteoporosis. 1. Guo Z, Chen W, Su Y, et al. Isolated unilateral vertebral pedicle fracture caused by a back massage in an elderly patient: a case report and literature review. *European Journal of Orthopaedic Surgery & Traumatology: Orthopedie Traumatologie* 2013;23(Suppl 2):S149–S153. http://www.ncbi.nlm.nih.gov/pubmed/23412164 2. Sefton JM, Yarar C, Berry JW. Six weeks of massage therapy produces changes in balance, neurological and cardiovascular measures in older persons. *International Journal of Therapeutic Massage and Bodywork* 2012;5(3):28–40. http://www.ncbi.nlm.nih.gov/pubmed/23087776

Postural Deviations

Definition: What Are They?

Although it is tempting to think about the spine like a ship's mast, a column, or a tent pole held erect by muscular tension, it is actually much stronger than any of those. The curves in the cervical, thoracic, and lumbar regions give the spine many times the resistance it would have if it were straight. Sometimes these natural curves are overdeveloped though, which reduces resiliency and strength rather than enhancing it. Hyperkyphosis (humpback), hyperlordosis (swayback), and scoliosis (S, C, or reverse-C curve) and rotoscoliosis (scoliosis with a twist) are the specific postural deviations addressed here (Figure 3.11).

Etiology: What Happens?

Postural deviations occur when the spine's normal curvature is overexaggerated or moves out of normal planes. Mild forms may not cause any visible signs or impairment in function, but more severe cases can interfere with pain-free posture, movement, and overall function.

The causes of most postural deviations are not fully understood, so the term **idiopathic** is often applied. As researchers continue to explore this problem, we may find that some situations are tied to several factors, including bone density, environmental exposures, genetic predisposition, and other postural compensations, especially at the cranium and sacrum.

> **Idiopathic:** Relating to a condition or disease of unknown cause.

Postural deviations may be discussed as functional or structural problems. In the early stages it may be that soft tissues pull the spine out of alignment: a functional problem. Functional deviations are often identified if observable curves disappear or are significantly reduced when the patient goes into trunk flexion or side flexion. The condition is most treatable at this point: muscles, tendons, and ligaments can be exercised, stretched, and manipulated into new holding and movement patterns.

Functional deviations can also be brought about by problems elsewhere in the body: unequal leg length, for instance, or a sacrum that isn't level. These are correctable, but if the soft tissues are left untreated and the bones are constantly pulled in one direction or another, they eventually change shape to adapt to those stressors. Vertebral bodies and discs adopt a wedge shape, and the facet joints may become distorted. At this point, the condition becomes a structural deviation, which is much harder to reverse. Some structural deviations are related to underlying conditions that affect the pattern of bone growth, so they are not preceded by a functional soft tissue problem.

Most cases of postural deviations are idiopathic, that is, of unknown origin. However, a small percentage of structural problems in the spine can be related to congenital or neuromuscular problems such as **cerebral palsy**, **polio**, **muscular dystrophy**, **osteogenesis imperfecta**, or **spina bifida**.

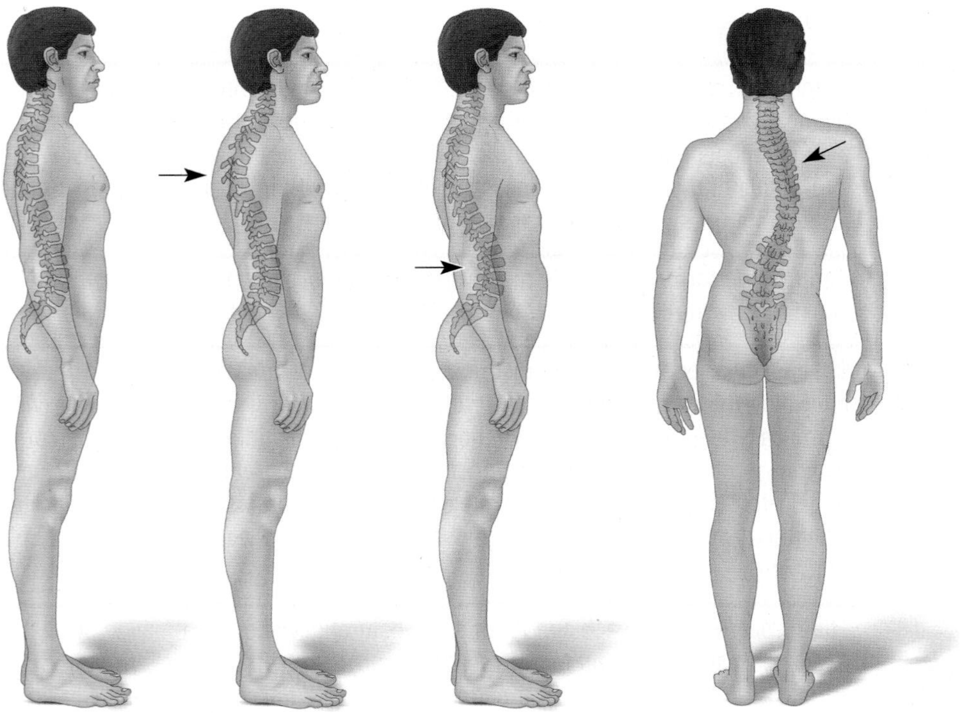

FIGURE 3.11 Postural deviations

Types of Postural Deviations

- **Hyperkyphosis**: Hyperkyphosis is an overdeveloped thoracic curve. In young people, it is very often a result of muscular imbalance. In older people, it may be due to muscular imbalance, but it can also be a complication of **osteoporosis** or **ankylosing spondylitis**. A kyphotic curve of 20 to 40 degrees is considered normal. Surgical intervention isn't usually suggested for anything under a 75-degree curvature.
    - **Scheuermann disease**: This is a type of hyperkyphosis that mostly affects young men. It involves uneven growth of the vertebrae and can create an extreme "hunchback" appearance. It is corrected with bracing, physical therapy, or surgery.
- **Hyperlordosis**: Hyperlordosis is an overdeveloped lumbar curve. The architecture and musculature of the low back makes it particularly vulnerable to this kind of imbalance. Hyperlordosis can often be much improved by exercise and physical therapy (including massage). Although not dangerous in itself, hyperlordosis can lead to serious low back pain.
- **Scoliosis, rotoscoliosis**: Scoliosis is a problem for approximately 1% to 2% of teenagers. It progresses in girls much more frequently than boys, and almost always involves a bend to the right. If it appears with a spinal rotation, the term rotoscoliosis is appropriate. This condition usually appears during the rapid-growth years of late childhood and early adolescence. Complications include nerve irritation as misshapen bones press on nerve roots, **spondylosis**, and serious heart and lung problems arising from a severely restricted rib cage.

Signs and Symptoms

Postural deviations range from being quite subtle to being painfully obvious. A visual examination can yield information about hyperkyphosis and hyperlordosis, and even mild scoliosis may be visible with a forward-bending test. Patients often report muscular tension and sometimes nerve impairment along with chronic ache and loss of range of motion. If the condition is very advanced, movement of the ribs may be impaired, leaving the patient vulnerable to cardiac and respiratory problems and lung infections.

NOTABLE CASES Actress Elizabeth Taylor had scoliosis that she credited with restricting her to a wheelchair. The recently exhumed skeleton of the "hunchback" King Richard III showed that he in fact had severe scoliosis in his thoracic vertebrae.

Treatment

Most postural deviations that are not related to underlying conditions are treated (if at all) with chiropractic or osteopathic manipulation, physical therapy, and exercise protocols. Bracing for external support may be recommended. When a deviation goes beyond a predetermined boundary, surgical intervention involving implants or bony fusions may be recommended. This is not always a permanent solution, however, many patients require follow-up procedures later in life.

Massage Therapy Implications

RISKS	Some postural deviations are the result of serious underlying conditions. These must be identified and accommodated as part of a massage therapy strategy. Of special note: hyperkyphosis may be related to osteoporosis and extremely brittle bones. Outside of these cautions, massage has few risks for a person with postural deviations that do not interfere with lung or cardiac function.
BENEFITS	Carefully performed massage that targets the complicated tangle of soft tissue stresses on the spine can be tremendously useful in addressing many postural deviations.
OPTIONS	The muscular component in most postural deviations presents a circular puzzle that must be explored by a massage therapist and client looking for long-term change. Addressing chronically lengthened as well as shortened muscles, adding hydrotherapy components, and being rigorous about tracking progress and adjusting strategies will help move toward the goal of pain-free posture and efficient movement. Many therapists and clients find the best results when bodywork is combined with movement training to learn new habits that preserve best function.
RESEARCH	The research on massage and functional postural deviations is small in scale but generally positive. Researchers find that massage therapy can help manage symptoms of muscle soreness and limited range of motion, and also with improved efficiency of breathing: an important function for lung health.[1,2] 1. Brooks WJ, Krupinski EA, Hawes MC. Reversal of childhood idiopathic scoliosis in an adult, without surgery: a case report and literature review. *Scoliosis* 2009;4:27. http://www.ncbi.nlm.nih.gov/pmc/articles/PMC2808297/ 2. LeBauer A, Brtalik R, Stowe K. The effect of myofascial release (MFR) on an adult with idiopathic scoliosis. *Journal of Bodywork and Movement Therapies* 2008;12(4):356–363.http://www.ncbi.nlm.nih.gov/pubmed/19083694

Joint Disorders

Adhesive Capsulitis

Definition: What Is It?

Adhesive capsulitis, or "frozen shoulder" is a poorly understood condition in which the connective tissues that surround the glenohumeral joint become first inflamed and then thickened and restrictive. This process typically takes several months to fully develop, then it is stable for several months, and then for most patients it eventually spontaneously resolves, and most or all of the lost range of motion is restored. For some, it leads to a lifetime of limited range of motion at the affected shoulder.

Demographics

Adhesive capsulitis is most common in people in their 50s and 60s. Women are slightly more likely to have it than are men. People with **diabetes, hyperthyroidism**, or pathologically high triglycerides appear to be most susceptible. It is also more common among people who have had recent shoulder injuries or chest or breast surgery, or who have been immobilized for other reasons. It is unusual for adhesive capsulitis to occur in both shoulders at one time, but many people who have in on one side may develop it on the other side later in life.

Etiology: What Happens?

The etiology of adhesive capsulitis is not at all clear. Some experts suggest that it always begins with an adhesion between the anterior aspect of the glenohumeral capsule to the head of the humerus; others propose that it begins in extracapsular tissues like local ligaments, the rotator cuff and biceps muscles, and the subacromial bursae; they suggest that the thickening that happens in the joint capsule is a secondary development.

Biopsies of the joint capsule of people with frozen shoulder show an anomaly in the quality of collagen fibers in the area, similar to that seen with **Dupuytren contracture**, although the prognosis for frozen shoulder is much better than that for other connective tissue contractures. The excessive pain signals that are recorded with this condition suggest some similarities to **complex regional pain syndrome (CRPS)**, a condition that involves a self-sustaining pain feedback loop between the central nervous system and peripheral tissues. Tissue changes seen with CRPS may be contributors to the damage seen with frozen shoulder joint capsules.

Signs and Symptoms

A typical presentation of adhesive capsulitis involves a person in her 50s or 60s who experiences pain in one shoulder, especially at night. Often, no precipitating event or factor is ever identified. The pain is severe and slowly progressive, and the shoulder gradually loses its range of motion: this is sometimes called the "freezing" phase. As the pain becomes constant regardless of activity, the shoulder becomes increasingly stiff. Over a period of several months, a person with adhesive capsulitis can lose up to 85% of normal joint mobility.

Eventually the progression stabilizes, and for several months the shoulder is extremely stiff, but no longer acutely painful. This is the "frozen" phase. Both active and passive motion is severely limited, especially in external rotation, abduction, and flexion.

Finally, for reasons that are still a mystery, the whole process reverses: pain is relieved, and full or nearly full range of motion is restored; this is the "thawing" phase. The whole cycle from beginning to end can take anywhere from 9 months to 3 years.

Treatment

Treatments for adhesive capsulitis are recommended depending on the stage of progression to manage pain and to restore mobility as much as possible. Many patients are unwilling to take the "wait and see" approach while their shoulder cycles through the stages. While some interventions may increase range of motion and decrease pain in the short term, no single treatment is consistently better in the long term than simply letting this condition run its course from "freezing" to "frozen" to "thawing."

Analgesics ranging from aspirin to narcotics may be recommended in the early stages, as this condition is extremely painful.

Injections of painkillers with corticosteroids are often used in the "freezing" or "frozen" stage, with and without physical therapy. If they are successfully administered, injections serve the double purpose of introducing anti-inflammatories into the affected area, and mechanically stretching and distending the joint capsule; sometimes this goal is accomplished with saline solution alone. If injections are unsatisfactory, some physicians recommend surgery to loosen the joint capsule. Other options include joint manipulation under anesthesia, or a nerve block to temporarily deaden the subscapular nerve.

Medications

- Analgesics, including NSAIDs and stronger drugs
- Corticosteroid injections to manage inflammation

Massage Therapy Implications

RISKS	Especially in the first "freezing" phase, adhesive capsulitis may be acutely painful and involve active inflammation. Direct and intense bodywork on and around the shoulder capsule at this time may only exacerbate symptoms. Furthermore, patients with adhesive capsulitis in its most painful presentation may be prescribed painkillers that mask important information. It is important that massage therapists don't overtreat this condition while symptoms are temporarily muffled.
BENEFITS	Manual therapies get generally good results with this condition, as long as care is taken not to exacerbate pain or inflammation. Physical therapy, exercise, and good self-care are often part of successful treatment plan as well. Muscles of the shoulder girdle are likely to be recruited to compensate for lost range of motion; massage therapists are in an excellent position to normalize muscle tone and posture as much as possible.
OPTIONS	Careful and specific work around the shoulder girdle with active participation from the client may be effective to help restore range of motion. It is important to work in a way that doesn't exacerbate inflammation, which may set the client back.
RESEARCH	A systematic review of manual therapies for shoulder problems[1] found that massage may be helpful for short-term relief. One study found that patients who received cross friction massage fared as well as or better than those receiving traditional physical therapy for their shoulders,[2] but another found the opposite, although it employed a different type of massage.[3] Most studies agree that frozen shoulder is a highly individualized situation that requires versatility and cooperation between specialists. 1. Ho CY, Sole G, Munn J. The effectiveness of manual therapy in the management of musculoskeletal disorders of the shoulder: a systematic review. *Manual Therapy* 2009;14(5):463–474. http://www.ncbi.nlm.nih.gov/pubmedhealth/PMH0028749/ 2. Guler-Uysal F, Kozanoglu E. Comparison of the early response to two methods of rehabilitation in adhesive capsulitis. *Swiss Medical Weekly* 2004;134(23–24):353–358. http://www.smw.ch/docs/pdf200x/2004/23/smw-10630.pdf 3. Jewell DV, Riddle DL, Thacker LR. Interventions associated with an increased or decreased likelihood of pain reduction and improved function in patients with adhesive capsulitis: a retrospective cohort study. *Physical Therapy* 2009;89(5):419–429. http://ptjournal.apta.org/content/89/5/419.long

Baker Cysts

Definition: What Are They?

Baker cysts are synovial cysts found in the popliteal fossa, usually on the medial side. They are also called popliteal cysts.

Demographics

These cysts are common in children, for whom the preferred treatment is to wait for them to resolve on their own. When they occur in adults, they usually accompany some other joint problem, and are typically seen in people over 40 years of age.

Etiology: What Happens?

Baker cysts form when the joint capsule or a bursa at the back of the knee develops a pouch at the posterior aspect. They usually protrude into a small gap between the medial head of the gastrocnemius and the tendon of the semimembranosus (Figure 3.12). Some experts theorize that Baker cysts are a protective mechanism to prevent too much fluid accumulation at the knee in the context of chronic inflammation. Many cysts have a one-way valve at the neck that directs the flow of excess fluid into the cavity and prevents it from returning to the joint capsule.

Baker cysts in adults are almost always connected to other joint problems: **osteoarthritis**, **rheumatoid arthritis**, **lupus**, **gout**, or knee injuries, including cruciate ligament tears or meniscus tears.

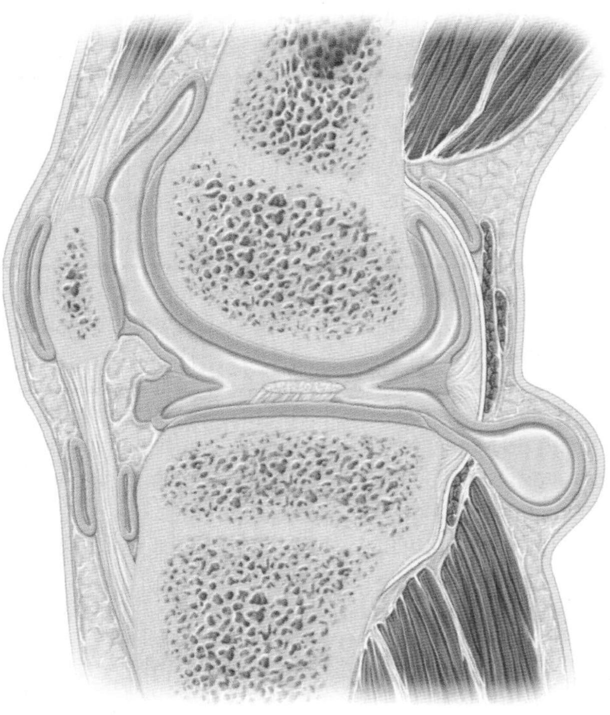

FIGURE 3.12 Baker cyst

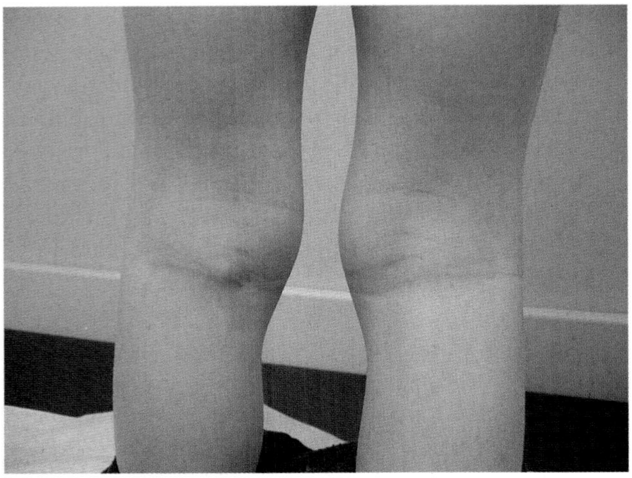

FIGURE 3.13 Baker cyst on left: a bulge on the medial aspect of the popliteal fossa

Baker cysts are not usually dangerous, but a cyst might become big enough impair blood flow through the lesser saphenous vein in the back of the leg. If that is the case, the patient is at risk for **thrombophlebitis** or **deep vein thrombosis** (DVT). Other complications include the risk of rupture (which creates symptoms that resemble DVT), bleeding into the joint, infection, or posterior **compartment syndrome** (blockage of fluid flow from the posterior compartment of the lower leg).

Signs and Symptoms

Baker cysts themselves are generally asymptomatic, but the affected knee may have pain from the underlying cause of inflammation. The cysts usually extend into the medial side of the popliteal fossa and may protrude down the leg, deep to the gastrocnemius. Patients with Baker cysts often report a feeling of tightness or fullness when the knee is in flexion, and mild pain on extension. Large cysts may create visually asymmetrical legs (see Figure 3.13).

Treatment

Most Baker cysts are first treated with ice and nonsteroidal anti-inflammatories in the hopes that they might resolve spontaneously. If this is unsuccessful, they may be aspirated, followed by cortisone shots to resolve joint inflammation. This is often an impermanent solution, however, as they easily recur until the underlying joint disruption has been resolved, often through surgery.

Medications

- NSAIDs for pain and inflammation control

Massage Therapy Implications

RISKS	Symptomatic Baker cysts present a local contraindication for massage, with the caution that if signs of thrombosis are present then medical intervention is called for.
BENEFITS	Massage elsewhere than the affected area is safe and appropriate. Clients who have successfully treated their Baker cyst can enjoy the same benefits from massage as the rest of the population.

Gout

Definition: What Is It?

Gout is a type of inflammatory arthritis that is relatively common in men between 40 and 50 years old and women who are postmenopausal. Its incidence appears to be increasing as baby boomers with long histories of problematic eating and drinking habits enter maturity. Gout is one of the oldest diseases in recorded medical history; treatment recommendations that are still in use date back to 580 A.D.

Demographics

About 6 million adults in the United States report having had gout at some point. Men between ages 40 and 50 are the most likely to develop this problem. Women can have gout, but it is rare before menopause.

Risk factors for gout include genetics, taking certain medications (especially diuretics, aspirin, and some Parkinson disease drugs), being overweight, and having a high consumption of alcohol and **purine**-rich foods. People with **psoriasis** or psoriatic arthritis appear to have a significantly higher chance of developing gout than does the rest of the population.

Etiology: What Happens?

Uric acid is a naturally occurring by-product of digestion. Foods and liquids that are high in a substance called purine are particularly potent sources of uric acid. Under normal circumstances, uric acid is extracted from the blood by the kidneys, and expelled through the urine. When this process is inefficient or overwhelmed, **hyperuricemia** develops: this is a predisposing factor for gout.

Hyperuricemia may develop for a couple of reasons. The kidneys may function normally, but if a person has high protein and alcohol intake, they can't keep up with demand. Alternatively, the uric acid load may be normal, but the kidneys are somehow impaired. This may be an inherited weakness, or related to other problems like **diabetes** or lead poisoning. And of course a person can have low-functioning kidneys and a high protein and alcohol intake: this is gout, waiting to happen.

The transition from hyperuricemia to an acute gouty attack is often precipitated by some specific event: binge eating or drinking (especially after fasting), surgery, sudden weight loss, or a systemic infection. When uric acid consolidates, it forms sharp, needlelike crystals that accumulate in and around the joint capsule, grinding on and irritating synovial membranes, bursae, tendons, and other tissues (Figure 3.14). The crystals attract neutrophils, and these white blood cells initiate an exaggerated inflammatory response. This can happen in a short period: typically a person goes to bed feeling fine, and wakes in the night with a foot that is red, throbbing, and painful; this is called **podagra** (Figure 3.15).

The joint between the first metatarsal and proximal phalanx of the great toe is the most frequent site for uric acid crystal accumulation. This is because of gravity, but it may also have to do with the lower temperature found in extremities that aids in the crystallization process.

NOTABLE CASES Gout has been known as the disease of kings, associated with rich diet and decadent living. This is witnessed by a list of some famous gout patients: Alexander the Great, Henry VIII of England, Charles V of Spain and his son Philip II, Dr. Samuel Johnson, Wolfgang von Goethe, and Benjamin Franklin.

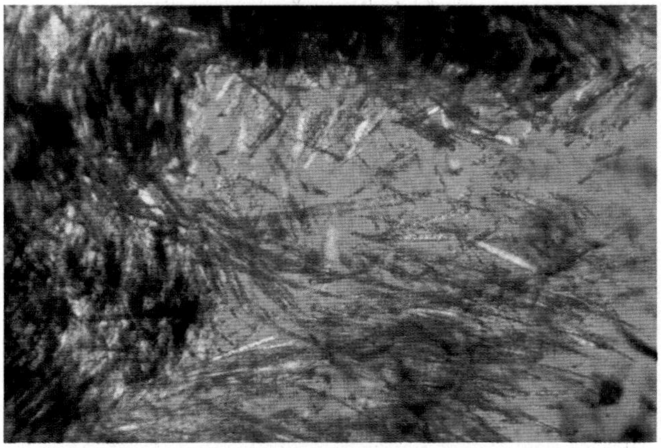

FIGURE 3.14 Gout crystals can erode joint capsules from the outside

Purine: A compound found in some foods, which can form uric acid. Meat, organs, and seafood are high in purine.

Hyperuricemia: An abnormally high concentration of uric acid in the blood.

Podagra: A painful condition of the foot (usually the great toe) caused by gout.

3 Musculoskeletal System Conditions

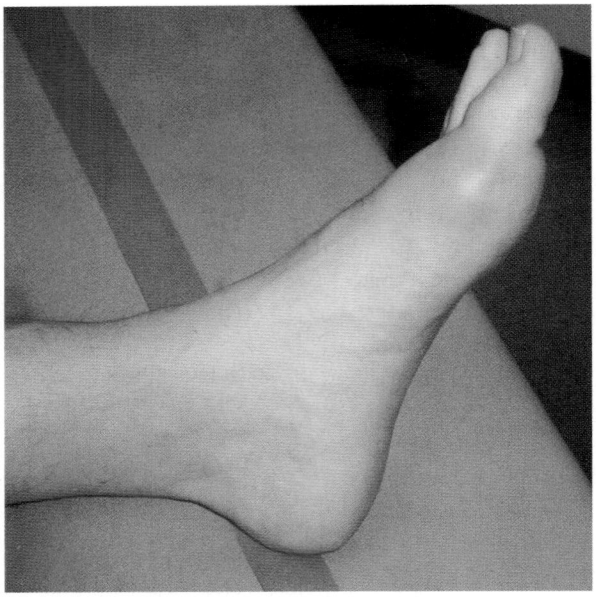

FIGURE 3.15 Gout: inflammation at the medial metatarsophalangeal joint (podagra)

In later stages of the disease, deposits of sodium urate called **tophi** may develop inside and around joints. These tophi erode the joint structures, leading to a complete loss of function. Tophi also grow along tendons, and in subcutaneous tissues on the ear, at the knees, and at the elbows (Figure 3.16).

Hyperuricemia is clearly connected to gout, but the cause and effect link is not always consistent. Many people have hyperuricemia without ever having gout. Conversely, some people with gout show normal or even below-normal levels of uric acid in the blood. Experts theorize that under normal circumstances the uric acid crystals are coated with serum proteins, and this quells any immune system response. When gout is triggered, the crystals are uncoated and can directly interact with local cells to stimulate pain and inflammation.

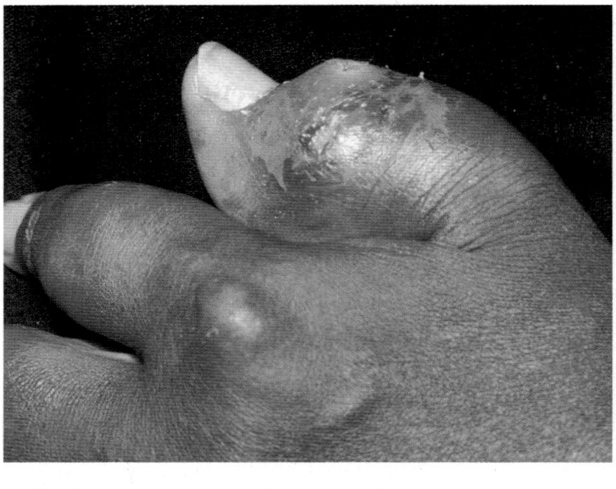

FIGURE 3.16 Gouty tophi and arthritis

Sometimes a person has just one attack of gout and then is never bothered by it again. If a second attack occurs, it usually comes several years later, and it may involve additional joints. The third attack happens after a shorter interval, and the fourth one, shorter still. Each event resolves itself in a few days or weeks. After 10 to 20 years, a patient may end up with almost constant acute attacks of this disease, but often by that time the associated complications are a much more important issue.

Signs and Symptoms

Acute gouty arthritis has some very predictable patterns. It has a sudden onset and almost always happens in the feet first, especially at the joints of the great toe. Cumulative damage creates a characteristic punched-out pattern of bony erosion. Gout may also appear elsewhere on the foot, or in other body areas.

An acute gouty joint shows all of the signs of extreme inflammation. The joint may swell so much that the skin is hot, red, dry, shiny, and exquisitely painful. This phase of inflammation is often accompanied by a moderate fever (up to 101°F, or 38.3°C) and chills.

Complications

While gout usually begins at a single joint, it doesn't usually stop there. Left untreated or incompletely treated, destructive uric acid deposits can accumulate at joints throughout the body, and eroded bones can fracture.

Further, gout indicates that kidneys are not functioning at adequate levels. Uric acid crystals may also cause **kidney stones**, which can contribute to **renal failure**. Impaired kidneys can't process fluid adequately. This stresses the rest of the circulatory system, causing **high blood pressure,** the end result of which can be **atherosclerosis** or **stroke**. All of these problems—hyperuricemia, kidney insufficiency, gout, high blood pressure, and cardiovascular disease—are closely related.

Treatment

It is important to get a reliable diagnosis to treat gout successfully. A similar condition called **pseudogout** has similar symptoms, but because it involves different chemical reactions, it requires different treatment options (see Compare & Contrast 3.1.)

A conventional medical approach to gout has three prongs: pain relief (with analgesics other than aspirin, which

Tophi: Deposits of uric acid and urates in tissue around joints and other areas. Often seen with gout. (Singular: tophus)

Pseudogout: A painful joint disease with symptoms similar to gout, but which does not involve uric acid.

COMPARE & CONTRAST 3.1 Gout vs. Pseudogout

Gout is a variety of arthritis brought about by the accumulation of uric acid (monosodium urate) crystals in and around joint capsules, especially in the feet. Calcium pyrophosphate dihydrate deposition, or pseudogout, has a very similar presentation, but since it doesn't involve uric acid or hyperuricemia, it requires a different treatment plan. Massage therapists are not required to be able to tell the difference between gout and pseudogout, but we can certainly counsel our clients to explore options if the treatment they receive doesn't seem to meet their needs.

CHARACTERISTICS	GOUT	CPDD (PSEUDOGOUT)
Prevalence	100:100,000	Unknown
Primary symptom	Exquisitely painful inflammation, usually around the great toe, instep or heel. May affect other joints as well.	Exquisitely painful inflammation, usually at the knee or wrist
Implications for massage	Most patients have hyperuricemia, a risk of kidney stones, or other urinary system challenges that may in turn impact the circulatory system.	CPDD is idiopathic, and may or may not be related to underlying problems. Clients must be screened for contributing factors, but none may be present.

inhibits uric acid excretion); anti-inflammatory drugs, and finally, drugs that modify metabolism and uric acid management to prevent future flares. Other preventive measures include increasing fluid intake (other than caffeine or alcohol, which act as diuretics), losing weight, and limiting purine-rich foods.

Medications

- NSAIDs, but not aspirin, for pain and inflammation
- Steroids (oral or injected) for inflammation
- Colchicine to treat or help prevent attacks
- Metabolic drugs (allopurinol, probenecid) to alter uric acid formation and excretion

Massage Therapy Implications

RISKS	Acutely inflamed gouty joints at least locally contraindicate massage. This situation often involves fever and general malaise, which contraindicates all but the gentlest bodywork systemically. Any joints that have had multiple gout attacks may be permanently distorted and vulnerable to irritation with pressure or movement: these are local cautions even when the acute stage has passed. Some massage therapists talk about "grinding out uric acid crystals" in the feet. For a person with a history of gout, work of this pressure and intent is not appropriate. A client who complains of pain and shows extreme inflammation around a joint should consult a doctor before applying ice: if it is gout, ice will promote the crystallization of uric acid, making the condition much worse.
BENEFITS	When gout is not acute and is successfully treated, patients can enjoy the same benefits from massage as do the rest of the population.

Joint Disruptions

Definition: What Are They?

Dislocations and associated joint disruptions describe situations where the articulating bones of a joint are not in correct relationship. In a full dislocation, the surfaces have no contact and the joint cannot be used. In a **subluxation**, the surfaces have partial contact; the joint may be functional but limited in range of motion. **Dysplasia** of a joint involves bony deformation that prevents a normal articulation. This happens most frequently at the hip.

Etiology: What Happens?

Synovial joints are composed of two or more bones with articulating cartilage, a synovial membrane, a ligamentous capsule, and varying types and amounts of supporting fascia, ligaments, tendons, and muscles. When the bones in a joint are not in their optimal relationship, joint function is impaired. This can happen because of specific trauma or because of a congenital problem with the shape of the bones, or it can be a slowly progressive chronic problem of instability without full dislocation.

Types of Dislocations and Joint Disruptions

- *Subluxation*: The bones are out of best alignment, but the joint capsule is intact. The joint is functional, but lacks a full range of motion. Joints that commonly subluxate include the intervertebral facet joints, the patellofemoral joint, and the radial head (this is sometimes called "nursemaid's elbow" from dangling a child by his or her forearm).
- *Dislocation*: The articulating bones are no longer touching; the shared surfaces have become disconnected, usually because of trauma. Dislocations are common for the shoulder, the fingers (especially the metacarpophalangeal joints), and the patella, although they can certainly occur elsewhere (Figures 3.17 and 3.18). A joint with a history of dislocation that is not surgically corrected is at increased risk for spontaneous dislocation in the future.
- *Dysplasia*: a congenital anomaly, dysplasia involves the formation of an abnormal acetabulum or femoral head. This can often be detected in early infancy, but if it causes no symptoms (usually this means it occurs bilaterally) it may require no treatment. Ultimately a person with hip dysplasia is has an increased risk for both subluxation and dislocation of the affected hip.

> **Subluxation:** An incomplete dislocation.
> **Dysplasia:** Abnormal tissue growth.

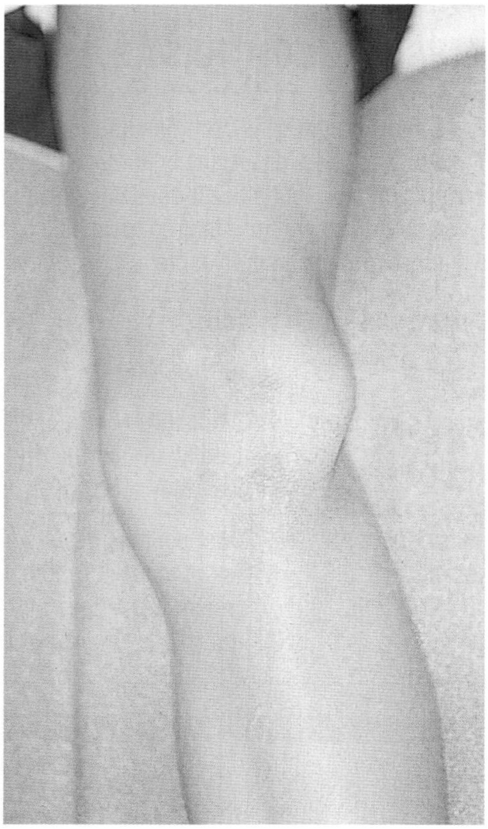

FIGURE 3.17 Dislocated patella

Signs and Symptoms

Joint disruptions can create various signs and symptoms, depending on the cause. Acute traumatic situations are obvious, with pain, swelling, and very often damage to other nearby tissues that may include bleeding, bone fractures, torn or irritated nerves, and damaged ligaments, muscles, and tendons.

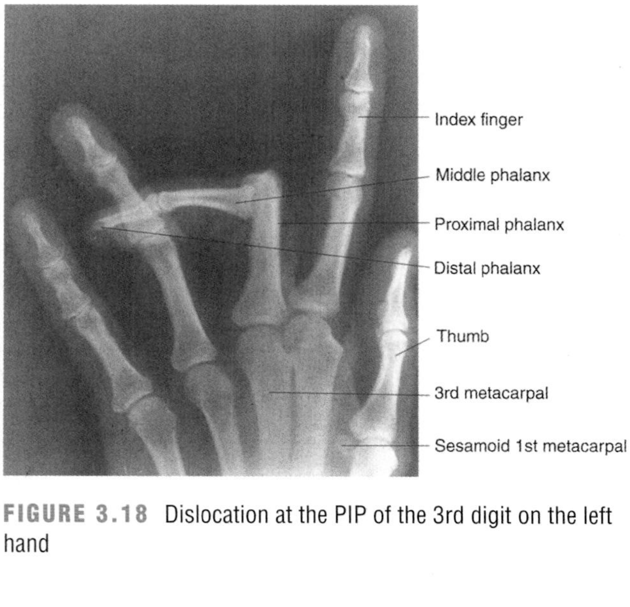

FIGURE 3.18 Dislocation at the PIP of the 3rd digit on the left hand

Subluxations can be related to trauma, but more often they involve low-level pain that is chronic and progressive. When they occur at the vertebrae, some experts suggest that they can put mechanical pressure on nerve roots, leading to referred pain and other symptoms in the extremities and viscera.

Hip dysplasia may be silent and undetected, or it may lead to uneven limb length and significant problems with walking in childhood.

Complications

A person with a history of dislocations may have permanently compromised ligaments, which can contribute to joint instability and an increased risk for both subluxation and **osteoarthritis**. In addition, the muscles that cross the affected joints may become hypertonic in an attempt to stabilize the nearby structures. This can lead to pain, trigger points, and limited range of motion.

Treatment

Treatment for joint disruptions depends on the cause. Traumatic situations that involve other tissue damage may call for surgery. Closed injuries and small-scale subluxations may be **reducible** through manipulation and traction of the affected joint. Chronic and congenital situations may be treated with splints, braces, physical therapy, and exercise to strengthen the muscles surrounding the compromised structures.

Medications

- NSAIDs to manage pain and inflammation for acute situations

Massage Therapy Implications

RISKS	Acute traumatic joint disruptions obviously contraindicate massage at least locally. For subacute or chronic problems, the practitioner must respect limitations in range of motion.
BENEFITS	Massage to the adjoining soft tissues around a weak or unstable joint may be helpful to manage pain, and to improve muscle and connective tissue function.
OPTIONS	Very specific protocols for work around the knee, hip, and shoulder may be applied specifically to these joints, with positioning adjustments to prevent spontaneous dislocations or subluxations. Additionally, any work that augments the goals of a physical therapy protocol may be helpful.

Joint Replacement Surgery

Definition: What Is It?

Joint replacement surgery, also called **arthroplasty**, is a procedure designed to repair articulating surfaces within a synovial joint. The goal is to restore pain-free (or pain-reduced) movement, although the range of motion at the joint may be permanently limited. Arthroplasty is not a condition in itself, but it is a common surgery; it carries some long-term consequences that may inform bodywork choices.

Demographics

About a million joint replacement surgeries are conducted in this country each year. Most of these procedures are for knees, hips, and shoulders. The distribution between men and women is about equal, and most arthroplasty patients are over 40 years old.

Etiology: What Happens?

The precipitating factor for most joint replacement surgeries is **osteoarthritis**, or "wear and tear" arthritis. **Rheumatoid arthritis**, **avascular necrosis**, or serious trauma (sometimes related to **osteoporosis**) may also contribute to reasons for an arthroplasty. In any case, this surgery is only conducted when all other options, including exercise, braces, anti-inflammatory medication, cortisone injections, and less invasive surgeries are no longer adequate interventions.

In a joint replacement surgery, the contacting bony surfaces are replaced by artificial components called **prostheses**. Historically, these have been made of various materials ranging from ceramic to titanium, but today they are most likely to include a highly polished ball made of cobalt chrome on one surface and a polyethylene cup or socket on the other. The average lifespan of a weight-bearing joint prosthesis is 10 to 15 years, at which time the components are likely to be worn down or loosened and in need of another replacement.

Several variables influence exactly how a joint replacement surgery is conducted. Older and less active patients may have their prostheses simply glued to their existing bone: this allows for a speedier recovery, but carries a risk of loosening and poor adherence between the bone and the implant. Younger or more active patients are better candidates for implants that have tiny pores where new bone tissue can

Reducible: Able to be reduced, or put back in proper position.

Arthroplasty: Joint replacement surgery.

Prostheses: Artificial body parts. (Singular: prosthesis)

grow to blend with the synthetic material. This means a longer recovery period, but the long-term strength of the joint tends to be much better.

The surgical approach through the soft tissues is another important variable in the prediction for how quickly or successfully a joint replacement surgery heals. Longitudinal approaches are less damaging to the muscles, but they may require a much longer incision than a lateral approach. The angle at which the socket is implanted and the size of the prosthesis are other important factors. Women obviously have differently sized and angled joints than those of men, but these differences have only recently been recognized by manufacturers of prostheses, which are now available in a range of sizes.

Types of Joint Replacements

- *Shoulders*: Arthroplasty of the glenohumeral joint is done when the joint is no longer competent: trauma, ongoing damage to the rotator cuff, or bone spurs have made the head of the humerus and the glenoid fossa incompatible in shape. Shoulder joint repairs can take two forms. The most common version replaces the ball of the humerus and the cup of the glenoid. Patients with advanced rotator cuff damage along with arthritis are candidates for a "reverse" shoulder replacement, in which a ball is attached to the scapula and the head of the humerus is replaced with a shallow cup, thus reversing the typical relationship between the bones.
- *Hips*: Hip joints are frequently replaced, either as a consequence of arthritis that wears away at this huge weight-bearing joint or as a result of femoral trauma. This situation, which combines femoral repair with joint resurfacing, is frequently associated with osteoporosis or other problems that make the femoral neck vulnerable to fracture (Figure 3.19).
- *Knees*: Knees are unique in that they combine a large range of motion with strict limitation in direction—that is, they flex and extend only (unless the knee is bent, in which position it can slightly rotate). Consequently, knees are vulnerable to shearing forces that can damage their stabilizing ligaments and put the internal cartilage at risk for permanent damage. Small repairs to the menisci can be made with arthroscopic surgery, but eventually the joint may be reduced to "bone on bone" contact. Knee joint replacements can sometimes involve resurfacing only one part of the joint, or they can involve replacing the ends of the tibia, femur, and the contacting surface of the patella (Figure 3.20). Cruciate ligaments may be replaced with polyethylene posts to help stabilize the new mechanism.
- *Other joints*: Arthroplasty can be conducted on ankles, various carpometacarpal and interphalangeal joints, the saddle joint of the thumb, and the temporomandibular joint.

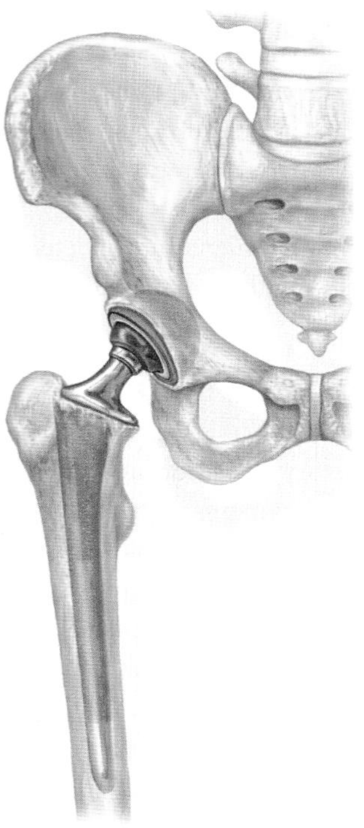

FIGURE 3.19 Joint replacement surgery: hip prosthesis

Signs and Symptoms

The symptoms that lead to a joint replacement are typically related to osteoarthritis or some other form of joint inflammation and damage. Most people report a deep ache that is made worse with movement, although it often progresses to the point of being painful all the time.

A person who has had arthroplastic surgery has a significant scar at the surgical site. The only other dependable sign is a loss of normal range of motion. People with

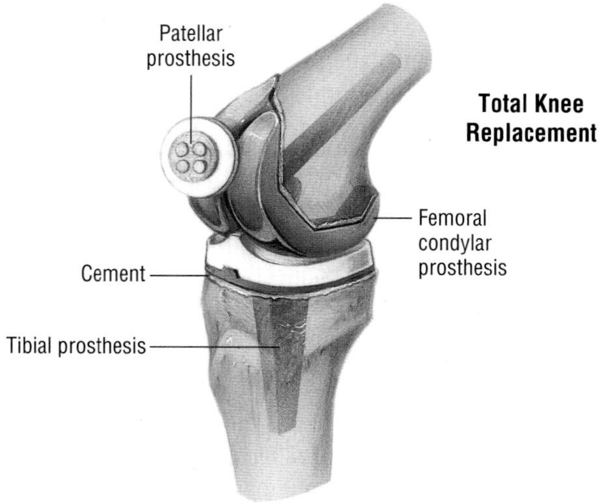

FIGURE 3.20 Knee prosthesis

reconstructed hips, knees, or shoulders are limited in the degree and direction of movement that is safe for their prostheses. Going beyond a safe range puts the implants at risk for loosening, which then requires surgical correction. And each successive surgery has a lower success rate and leads to a more limited range of motion.

Treatment

Joint replacement surgery is a major undertaking, involving general anesthesia, anywhere from 2 to 4 hours of surgery, and a 3- to 5-day hospital stay. Postsurgical treatment includes immediate mobilization (often starting on the same day as the surgery), pain medication, and because **DVT** is a common and dangerous complication, compression stockings and anticoagulant drugs. Knee surgery patients may also use a continuous passive motion machine that keeps the knee moving even when the patient is at rest. Physical therapy typically begins on the day after surgery, and may be recommended for several weeks following the procedure.

Complications

The possible complications that accompany any surgery are daunting. They include a reaction to anesthesia; arrhythmia; and the consequences of blood clots, including DVT, **pulmonary embolism**, and circulatory shock. Hospital-borne pathogens may lead to an infection in the joint, **urinary tract infection**, or **pneumonia**.

Complications related specifically to arthroplasty also include inadvertent fracture of the articulating bones, excessive scarring, and a loss of range of motion that is far beyond what was expected. Later complications can arise relating to a poorly seated prosthesis or failure to bond correctly with bone tissue.

Medications

- Analgesics for pain control
- Anticoagulants for blood clot limitation
- Antibiotics (if infection develops)

Massage Therapy Implications

RISKS

New joint replacements carry specific risks in relation to surgical complications. Older joint replacements must be carefully maneuvered to avoid stressing the joint and putting it at risk for loosening or failure. Always check with the client for limitations in range of motion.

BENEFITS

Evidence suggests that massage can improve the symptoms of some kinds of arthritis, which may delay the need for a joint replacement surgery: a definite benefit.

Massage can also reduce postsurgical pain and inflammation, and it can improve the quality of scar tissue for better mobility. For clients with older surgeries and no other complications, massage that respects their limited range of motion has the same benefits as it does for the rest of the population.

OPTIONS

It is important to determine why a client had a joint replacement surgery. Usually the reason is osteoarthritis, which means more than one joint may be affected. Look for postural compensation patterns that may cause pain and interfere with the most pain-free and efficient function possible.

RESEARCH

Massage therapy is frequently recommended following arthroplasty,[1] but there are no specific guidelines for how it is best applied in this context. Another study found that back massage helped with postoperative anxiety and pain management for arthroplasty patients, but it didn't look at massage for the joints themselves.[2] By contrast, Ebert et al.[3] found that manual lymphatic drainage at the knee, along with conventional physical therapy in the early postoperative period, led to improved knee flexion compared to conventional physical therapy alone for knee replacement patients.

1. Peter WF, Nelissen RG, Vlieland TP. Guideline recommendations for post-acute postoperative physiotherapy in total hip and knee arthroplasty: are they used in daily clinical practice? *Musculoskeletal Care* 2014;12(3):125–131. http://www.ncbi.nlm.nih.gov/pubmed/24497426
2. Buyukyilmaz F, Asti T. The effect of relaxation techniques and back massage on pain and anxiety in Turkish total hip or knee arthroplasty patients. *Pain Management Nursing* 2013;14(3):143–154. http://www.ncbi.nlm.nih.gov/pubmed/23972865
3. Ebert JR, Joss B, Jardine B, et al. Randomized trial investigating the efficacy of manual lymphatic drainage to improve early outcome after total knee arthroplasty. *Archives of Physical Medicine and Rehabilitation* 2013;94(11):2103–2111. http://www.ncbi.nlm.nih.gov/pubmed/23810354

Lyme Disease

Definition: What Is It?

Lyme disease is an infection with a spirochetal bacterium called *Borrelia burgdorferi*. This pathogen spreads through the bite of two species of ticks: deer ticks (*Ixodes scapularis*) and Western black-legged ticks (*Ixodes pacificus*). These ticks are very small, especially in the nymph stage, when they most frequently affect humans. This can make it difficult to find them on the skin. An unfed deer tick nymph is about as big as a sesame seed (Figure 3.21).

Demographics

Lyme disease has been reported in most states, but the highest concentrations are in the Northeast and Mid-Atlantic States, the upper Midwest, and Northern California. It is the most commonly reported vector-borne illness in the United States, with about 30,000 new cases reported each year, but the Centers for Disease Control considers the true infection rate to be much higher.

Persons most at risk for Lyme disease are those who work or play outside in grassy or wooded areas; the ticks don't thrive in sunny or arid environments.

Etiology: What Happens?

Deer ticks and Western black-legged ticks pick up the spiral bacterium *B. burgdorferi* from the blood of animal hosts, especially mice. If an infected tick subsequently bites a human, that bacterium may be transmitted to the human host. Immature nymphs and adults can both transmit the disease, but adults are easier to find and remove. Most human infections come from younger ticks.

It is the bacterial invasion, not the tick bite, that causes the damage seen with Lyme disease. The bacteria enter the bloodstream with the tick's saliva, and from there it can access joints and other tissues.

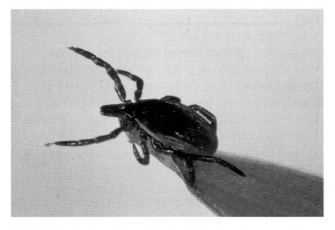

FIGURE 3.21 Deer tick on the tip of a blade of grass, waiting for a warm-blooded host to walk by

SIDEBAR 3.3 Other Tick-Borne Infections

Lyme disease is caused by tick-borne bacteria that infect joints and cause debilitating arthritis. Other tick-borne pathogens can cause serious infections as well. It is possible but rare to be coinfected with *Borrelia* and any of these:

- *Anaplasmosis* is an infection that can coexist with Lyme disease and is spread by the same ticks. It used to be considered a form of ehrlichiosis, but a different class of bacteria were found to be responsible for this condition. It causes fever, headache, chills, and muscle ache. It is sensitive to antibiotics.
- *Ehrlichiosis* is group of tick-borne bacterial infections usually spread by the lone star tick. Consequences of ehrlichiosis infection include low white blood cell and platelet counts. Symptoms can look like those of Lyme disease, with fever, headache, fatigue and muscle aches. This infection can be cleared with antibiotics, specifically doxycyclene.
- *Babesiosis* is caused by a parasite similar to the protozoan that causes malaria. Babesiosis can silent, or it can cause anemia and an enlarged spleen, as well as other serious problems, especially for immunosuppressed people. Babesiosis responds well to treatment.
- *Southern tick-associated rash illness (STARI)* is a condition endemic to southeast and south-central states. The pathogen that causes this illness has not been identified, but STARI appears to be treatable with antibiotics.
- *Rocky Mountain spotted fever (RMSF)* is an infection with the bacterium *Rickettsia rickettsii*, spread by hard ticks all over the United States. Early symptoms include fever, headache, muscle pain, and malaise, followed by a spotty rash (as opposed to a bull's-eye rash). Although RMSF is treatable with antibiotics, it is a potentially life-threatening infection that can affect blood and blood vessels all over the body, leading to serious long-term consequences.

Borrelia burgdorferi is a slow-growing bacterium. This creates several problems, including a delayed immune response and difficulties in getting accurate blood tests. So far three subspecies of the bacterium have been found, and up to 100 different strains of the infection are active in the United States. Further, *B. burgdorferi* is not the only tick-borne infection found in the United States; see Sidebar 3.3 for more on tick-borne infections.

Signs and Symptoms

Lyme disease moves in stages, with signs and symptoms particular to each.

- *Early localized disease*: This is the first stage of a Lyme disease infection. Ticks are slow feeders, so it may take several days for the bacteria to enter the body and some days after that for symptoms to appear. Early symptoms generally appear 7 to 30 days after an initial tick bite. A circular red "bull's-eye" rash called **erythema migrans** is hot and itchy, but not flaky or raised from the skin (Figure 3.22). This identifying feature of Lyme disease is found in fewer than 50% of all cases. Other signs include high fever, fatigue, night sweats, headache, stiff neck, and swollen lymph nodes. Without a telltale rash, these early symptoms may be mistaken for **flu**, **mononucleosis**, or **meningitis**.
- *Early disseminated disease*: This is the second stage, during which the infected person develops systemic symptoms of infection with *B. burgdorferi*. These include more bull's-eye rashes, cardiovascular symptoms (especially irregular heartbeat and dizziness), and neurological symptoms (chronic **headaches**, cranial nerve palsy that resembles **Bell palsy**, numbness, tingling, forgetfulness, and poor coordination), along with more general problems, including shooting pains and debilitating fatigue.
- *Late disease*: This is the final outcome of a Lyme disease infection. It is associated with extreme inflammation of one or more large joints. The knees are the most commonly affected area, but elbows and shoulders are often inflamed as well. Most patients don't have the infection in more than three joints at a time. The inflammation can be extreme enough to damage the joint permanently, especially if it is untreated.

NOTABLE CASES Authors Amy Tan (*Joy Luck Club*), Rebecca Wells (*Divine Secrets of the Ya-Ya Sisterhood*) and Alice Walker (*The Color Purple*) all have been affected by with Lyme disease.

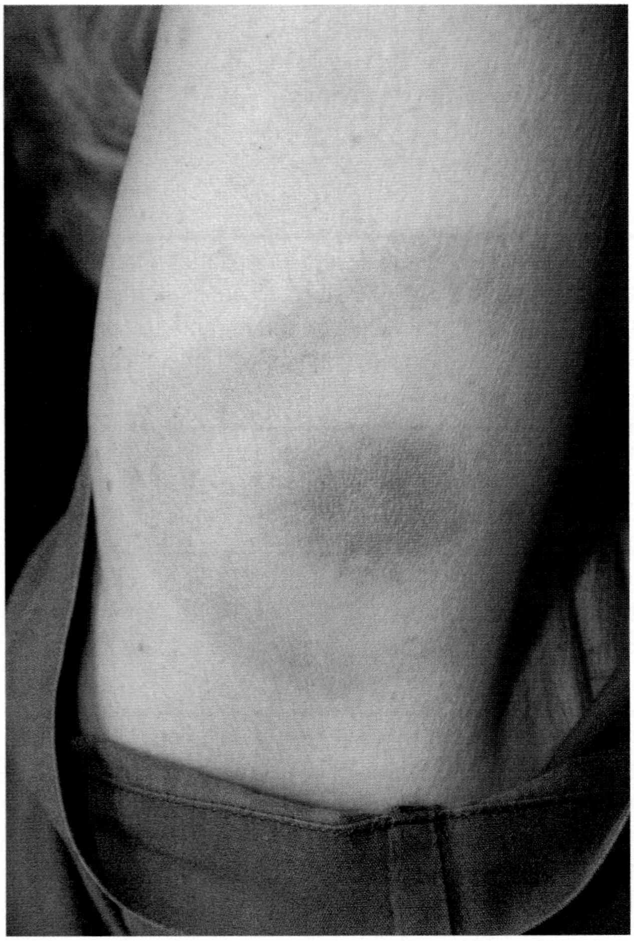

FIGURE 3.22 Bull's-eye rash: an indicator of Lyme disease

The tendency for Lyme disease to affect joints is what classifies it as an arthritic condition. In fact, the first cases of Lyme disease ever identified were among a group of children who were all initially misdiagnosed with juvenile **rheumatoid arthritis** (see Sidebar 3.4).

Most people with Lyme disease have symptoms for several weeks or months, and then they subside, but about 10% to 20% develop chronic muscle and joint pain that may persist for many months. This situation is now called **posttreatment Lyme disease syndrome (PTLDS)**. At one time, it was thought that these patients needed long-term antibiotic treatment, but research shows that this strategy is ineffective, as well as fraught with unnecessary complications. The current theory is that the *Borrelia* infection did some long-term tissue damage that could elicit some autoimmune responses; similar phenomena are seen with other pathogens: *Campylobacter* can lead to **Guillain-Barré syndrome**, and strep throat can cause **rheumatic heart disease**.

Treatment

Accurate diagnosis of Lyme disease is an ongoing challenge, as both false-positive and false-negative blood tests are common. Further, without the signature bull's-eye rash as an indicator, the signs of Lyme disease can resemble those of several

Erythema migrans: A "bull's-eye" rash, usually seen as an early symptom of Lyme disease.

Posttreatment Lyme disease syndrome: Chronic symptoms of pain and fatigue that may continue for months in some people after contracting Lyme disease.

SIDEBAR 3.4 History of Lyme Disease

Although Lyme disease was only definitively identified and named in 1982, it has probably been present for much longer.

In the early 20th century, doctors made note of target-shaped red rashes, which were named erythema migrans. People who developed these rashes seemed to have a high incidence of arthritis, but if they were treated with penicillin, their chances of developing arthritis were significantly lessened.

Then, in 1974, a group of children in Lyme, Connecticut, were diagnosed with juvenile rheumatoid arthritis. Parents were skeptical about such a high concentration of a disease that was not understood to be in any way communicable. This led to intensive research, during which a scientist named Burgdorfer isolated the spirochete now called *B. burgdorferi.* He found it in highest concentrations in the midgut of deer ticks. It lives here until ticks feed on a host, when it may exit the tick to invade new territory.

common chronic conditions. Doctors in endemic areas are encouraged to consider Lyme disease when investigating conditions like **fibromyalgia**, **chronic fatigue syndrome**, and **multiple chemical sensitivity syndrome**.

Borrelia burgdorferi is sensitive to antibiotics, so the outlook for someone who is accurately diagnosed with Lyme disease in the early stages is often hopeful. The type and duration of antibiotic treatment for Lyme disease is a topic of much debate, as some patients seem to require different treatment regimens than others.

The best protection against Lyme disease is protection from disease-bearing ticks. This means wearing long sleeves and long pants when working or playing in areas where tick infestation is high. Tucking pants into socks or boots may make it harder for ticks to gain access to skin. Wearing light-colored clothing is recommended, to make it easier to find and remove ticks. Using insect repellants can also reduce the risk of tick bites.

Examining the skin after being in a high-risk area is another important preventive measure. Ticks prefer to occupy warm, protected areas such as the groin, axilla, backs of knees, and insides of elbows. If a tick is found, it should be carefully removed with tweezers to keep the mouth parts intact, and then the person should report being bitten and take the tick to the doctor. If the tick is found and removed within 24 hours, the risk of infection is very low.

Medications

- Antibiotics for infection control

Massage Therapy Implications

RISKS	The arthritic phase of Lyme disease involves intermittently severe and painful inflammation of joints; this contraindicates massage, at least locally. Lyme disease can also affect the nervous and circulatory systems, and because treatment can take a long time to take effect, it is especially important for massage therapists to operate as part of a client's health care team.
BENEFITS	As long as sensation is present and inflammation is not acute, a person with Lyme disease may enjoy the relaxation, relief from anxiety, and general sense of well-being that massage can offer.
OPTIONS	Massage therapists who live and work in areas where Lyme disease is especially common should be aware of what deer ticks and Western black-legged ticks look like so that if they find these parasites during a session, they can counsel clients to receive appropriate medical care.
RESEARCH	One case study[1] looked at massage to manage symptoms of pain, fatigue, and poor concentration for a client with Lyme disease. Symptoms improved in periods when the client received massage, but when she stopped, the symptoms recurred. This is a strong finding, but with only one subject: more work must be done before it is possible to make definitive claims about massage therapy for people who have Lyme disease. 1. Thomason MJ, Moyer CA. Massage therapy for Lyme disease symptoms: a prospective case study. *International Journal of Therapeutic Massage and Bodywork* 2012;5(4):9–14. http://www.ncbi.nlm.nih.gov/pmc/articles/PMC3528190/

Osteoarthritis

Definition: What Is It?

Osteoarthritis (OA) is a condition in which synovial joints, especially weight-bearing joints, lose healthy cartilage. This condition is distinguished from other types of arthritis by being related to age and wear and tear, along with biomechanical factors and the consequences of inflammation. The etiology of osteoarthritis is restricted to synovial joints. Arthritis at the spine has some important differences, and is discussed in the section titled **spondylosis**.

Demographics

Osteoarthritis is the most common form of arthritis, affecting about 27 million people in the United States. It is diagnosed mainly by x-ray (radiograph), but these tests can show structural anomalies that don't necessarily cause symptoms. Radiographic criteria suggest that OA affects more than half of the population over 65 years old.

Etiology: What Happens?

Synovial joints, especially knees and hips, put up with tremendous weight-bearing stress and repetitive movements; their design is a marvel of efficiency and durability. But the environment inside a joint capsule is precarious; any long-lasting imbalance can have cumulative destructive impact. Once the process of arthritis has begun, it may be possible to stop it, but capacity for regeneration and repair inside a joint capsule is limited at best (Figure 3.23).

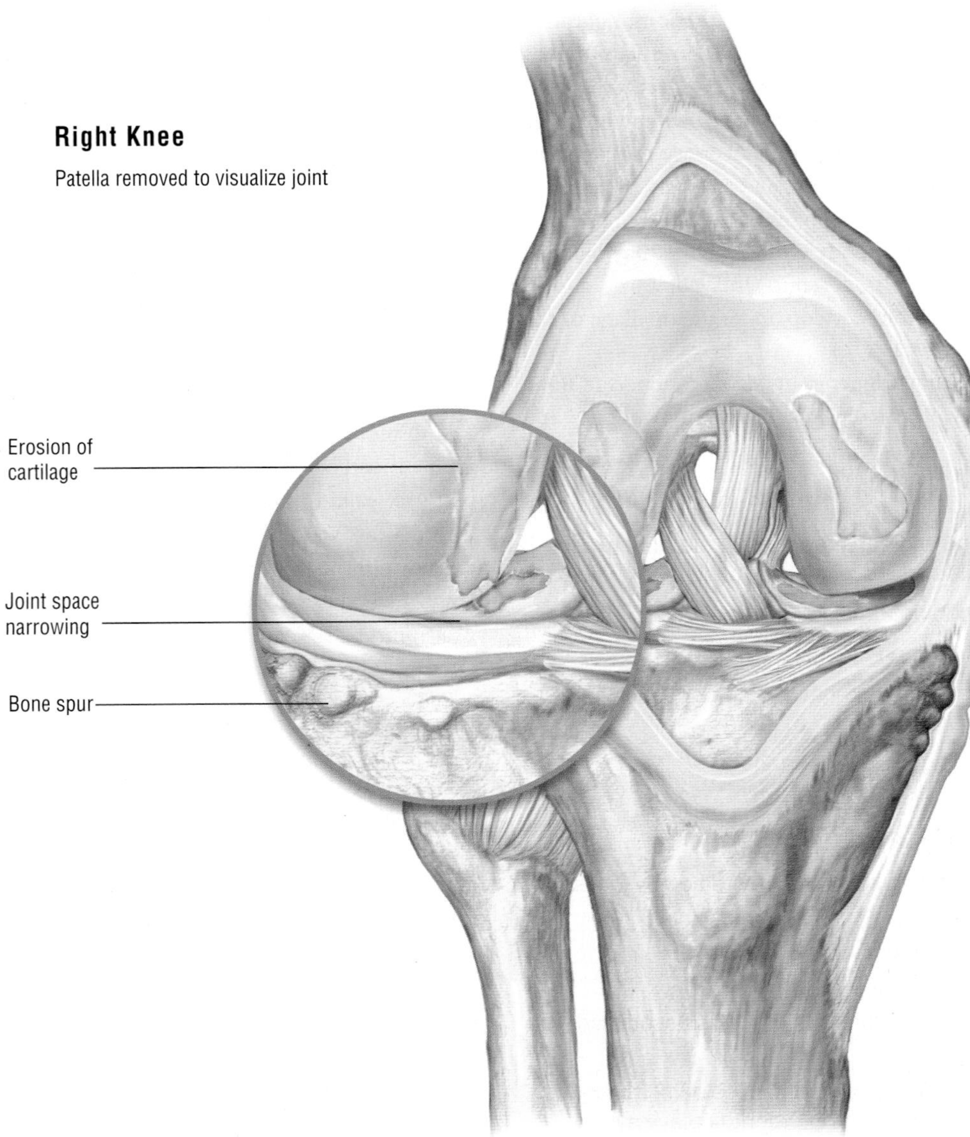

FIGURE 3.23 Osteoarthritis: progressive cartilage damage triggers bony adaptation

OA is understood to be a process of degeneration that begins with articular cartilage, but progresses to affect the **synovium** and the connecting bones. **Hyaline** or articular cartilage is constructed of a relatively small number of living **chondrocytes** that produce collagen (mostly type II fibers), along with **proteoglycans**: large negatively-charged molecules that attract water. The cells, protein fibers, and molecules of fluid are arranged in slightly different patterns, depending on whether they are superficial, intermediate, or attached directly to the **chondral** surface of the articulating bone. These varying zone densities give cartilage the ability to resist both shearing and compressive forces.

Chondrocytes remain active all through life, constantly replacing and rebuilding the cartilage surface, but they don't actively proliferate, and they don't migrate to damaged areas. Further, chondrocytes become less active with age. When chondrocytes make less fluid and collagen, the cartilage degenerates, and the whole structure of the joint degrades. The process is accelerated when local proinflammatory chemicals also inhibit normal chondrocyte activity. Local irritation can trigger the synovial lining to become inflamed and to produce yet more chemicals that damage the cartilage. Ultimately the breakdown, flaking, and cracking of cartilage stimulate osteocytes in the epiphyses of the affected bones to become more active: the condyle of the bone may become enlarged, **osteophytes** (bone spurs) may develop, and in some cases cystlike cavities develop under the cartilage of the affected bone (Figure 3.23).

Many changes may trigger joint degeneration. Age alone changes the quality of articular cartilage, making it drier and more prone to injury. Being overweight adds stress to knees and hips, and some evidence now points to a biochemical link between **adipocytes** and cartilage degeneration. If the ligaments that surround joints are chronically lax, the joint can become unstable, raising the risk of cartilage damage; this can be a long-term problem with joints that have been dislocated. A history of trauma or surgery (to remove pieces of the meniscus, for instance) is another predisposing factor. Repetitive pounding stress, such as running or jumping with inadequate support, can also open the door to problems. Hormonal imbalances and nutritional deficiencies, including dehydration, inadequate calcium metabolism, and foods that trigger inflammatory responses, may further compromise the health of joint structures.

Some features of osteoarthritis overlap with those of an etiologically different disease, **rheumatoid arthritis** (RA). The discussion of RA appears in Chapter 6, but a chart comparing the two conditions can be found in this chapter: see Compare & Contrast 3.2.

Synovium: The secreting membrane found between the joint capsule and the joint cavity of synovial joints.

Hyaline: Describing translucent articular cartilage.

Chondrocyte: A cartilage cell.

Proteoglycans: Large, negatively charged molecules that attract water.

Chondral: Having to do with cartilage.

Osteophyte: A bony outgrowth.

Adipocyte: A fat cell.

Crepitus: A crackling sound, often created by joints.

Heberden nodes: A bulging at the distal interphalangeal joints caused by arthritis.

Bouchard nodes: Enlargement of the proximal interphalangeal joints due to bone spurs associated with osteoarthritis.

Counterirritant: An agent that causes mild irritation or inflammation of the skin on order to relieve symptoms of inflammation in deeper tissues.

Signs and Symptoms

The symptoms of osteoarthritis are related to irritation of the joint structures. This condition is seldom hot, painful, or visibly swollen. More often, it lingers in a chronic stage in which the joints have ongoing deep pain and stiffness, especially when they are not warmed up, or when they have been overused. **Crepitus** is common for this population. Many osteoarthritis patients report that a change in weather triggers symptoms: this may be a reflection of ambient air pressure and its effect on joint capsules.

Osteoarthritis happens most often at weight-bearing joints. It can be crippling when it occurs at the hip or knee, because walking exacerbates the pain. Other common sites include the shoulders and knuckles. When osteoarthritis develops in the fingers, characteristic thickening of the phalangeal epiphyses is present. Bulges at the distal interphalangeal joints (DIPs) are called **Heberden nodes**. When they appear at the proximal interphalangeal joints (PIPs), they are called **Bouchard nodes** (Figure 3.24).

Treatment

The goals of treatment for osteoarthritis are to reduce pain and inflammation and to limit or reverse the damage to the joint structures. These are accomplished in a number of different ways, depending on how advanced the condition is.

NSAIDs may be recommended for pain control, but many patients find that the risk of negative side effects outweigh their benefits. Topical applications of **counterirritant** ointments can be helpful. Physical therapy and exercise address multiple goals by helping to maintain a healthy range of motion, increasing stamina, promoting weight loss, and improving the strength of muscles surrounding

COMPARE & CONTRAST 3.2 Osteoarthritis vs. Rheumatoid Arthritis

Of the 100 conditions that cause painful inflammation of joints, the two most common are osteoarthritis and rheumatoid arthritis. Osteoarthritis is a wear-and-tear disorder that could possibly be exacerbated by overenthusiastic bodywork but can't be spread through the body. Rheumatoid arthritis is an autoimmune disorder, and it can progress to affect additional joints.

The following is a brief list of the most common patterns seen with osteoarthritis compared with rheumatoid arthritis.

CHARACTERISTICS	OSTEOARTHRITIS	RHEUMATOID ARTHRITIS
Prevalence	Radiographs show bony deformation in 33%–90% of people over 65, although not all of them have symptoms.	Up to 1.5% of the population.
Demographics	Most common in people over 40. Men and women affected equally.	Women affected two to three times as often as men; men more likely to have systemic symptoms. May affect children.
Pain patterns	Spine, knees, hips most frequently affected. Distal finger joints, saddle joint (trapezium, first metacarpal) also at risk.	Proximal joints in hands and feet, ankles, wrists usually affected. Extreme distortion of joint capsules can cause joints to be visibly misshapen. Pain appears in flare and remission stages.
Other symptoms	None	In early stages and acute episodes, fever, malaise, lack of appetite, and muscle pain may be present.
Implications for massage	Can be useful to maintain range of motion and relieve pain in muscles that cross over affected joints, as long as inflammation is not acute.	Can be useful for joint function during remission.

affected joints. Nutritional supplements are sometimes recommended, including **glucosamine** and **chondroitin sulfate**. The research suggests that they are most effective for moderate to severe cases, and they do carry some risks of negative interactions with other substances, so they should be used with the advice of a primary care provider.

Glucosamine: A compound found in connective tissue, sometimes taken as a dietary supplement for joint health.

Chondroitin sulfate: An important component of cartilage, sometimes taken as a dietary supplement for joint health.

Viscosity: The degree to which a fluid resists flowing. Stickiness.

Lavage: The washing out of a hollow cavity.

Debridement: The removal of dead tissue and foreign matter from a wound.

Arthroscopic procedures include injections of corticosteroids to reduce inflammation (this can be done only a few times a year), injection of substances to improve joint fluid **viscosity**, aspiration of excess joint fluid, and joint **lavage** and **debridement** work to remove loose bits of cartilage (these are sometimes called "joint mice") and to smooth articulating surfaces.

Joint replacement surgery is addressed elsewhere in this chapter.

Medications

- Topical counterirritants and NSAIDs
- NSAIDs, including Cox-2 inhibitors, for pain control
- Tramadol, an analgesic, for pain control
- Injected steroidal anti-inflammatories

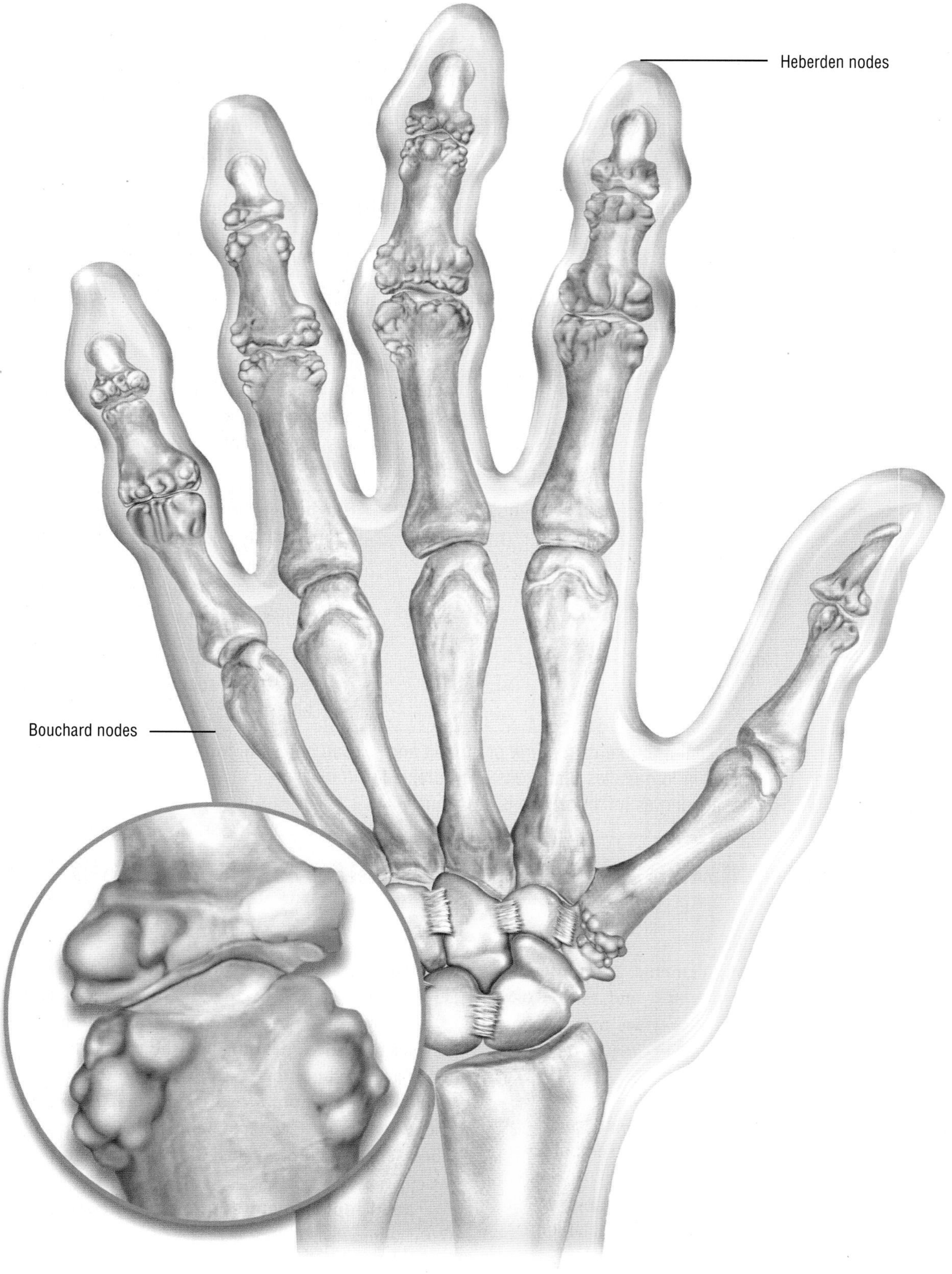

FIGURE 3.24 Osteoarthritis at the hand

Massage Therapy Implications

RISKS	Acute inflammation contraindicates massage that may exacerbate symptoms, but this is rare in osteoarthritis. As long as bodywork is well tolerated, it carries few risks for osteoarthritis patients.
BENEFITS	Carefully performed massage, including general work that does not specifically focus on affected joints, has been seen to reduce pain and stiffness and to improve function in osteoarthritis patients.
RESEARCH	Massage for osteoarthritis is well supported by research. Some findings[1] suggest that an overall relaxation massage provides effective pain relief, but other studies have looked at massage directly to the affected joints. One[2] examined self-massage of the knee as taught to residents of a senior home; another[3] compared traditional Thai massage with Swedish massage: both groups had improvement, but the changes were longer lasting in the Thai massage group.[3] The general consensus appears to be that massage therapy is a viable option for patients who want to manage their osteoarthritis symptoms. 1. Perlman AI, Sabina A, Williams AL, et al. Massage therapy for osteoarthritis of the knee: a randomized controlled trial. *Archives of Internal Medicine* 2006;166(22):2533–2538. http://archinte.jamanetwork.com/article.aspx?articleid=769544 2. Atkins DV, Eichler DA. The effects of self-massage on osteoarthritis of the knee: a randomized, controlled trial. *International Journal of Therapeutic Massage and Bodywork* 2013;6(1):4–14. http://www.ncbi.nlm.nih.gov/pmc/articles/PMC3577640/ 3. Peungsuwan P, Sermcheep P, Harnmontree P, et al. The effectiveness of Thai exercise with traditional massage on the pain, walking ability and QOL of older people with knee osteoarthritis: a randomized controlled trial in the community. *Journal of Physical Therapy Science* 2014;26(1):139–144. http://www.ncbi.nlm.nih.gov/pmc/articles/PMC3927027/

Patellofemoral Pain Syndrome

Definition: What Is It?

Patellofemoral pain syndrome (PFPS) is a group of conditions in which the patellar cartilage becomes irritated as it contacts the femoral cartilage. This situation can be a precursor of **osteoarthritis** at the knee.

PFPS is common, but its exact definition and etiology are not universally agreed upon. Most experts say that it is almost always associated with overloading or overuse of the patellofemoral joint, although it may also be precipitated by a specific injury or trauma.

Synonyms or subtypes of PFPS include **chondromalacia**, jumper's knee, moviegoer's knee, anterior knee pain syndrome, and overutilization syndrome.

Demographics

PFPS is extremely common; it is the most frequently documented knee injury in runners and other athletes. It is diagnosed among both adolescents and mature people.

> **Chondromalacia patellae:** A condition in which the cartilage behind the kneecap becomes irritated.
>
> **Chondroblast:** A cell that produces cartilage cells.

Etiology: What Happens?

When the knee is bent, whether or not it is bearing weight, the femur and the patella press together. The patella bone moves superiorly and inferiorly, but it can also move medially and laterally, and it can rotate or tip in any direction. Pressure must be evenly distributed across the back of the patella, or disruptions to the patellar cartilage can occur. Left unchecked, this can lead to damage at the femoral cartilage as well. This condition can be stopped or even reversed if it is caught early; **chondroblasts** in the hyaline cartilage can replace damaged tissue, especially in young people. But long-term irritation can ultimately lead to osteoarthritis at the knee, with damage to the cartilage on the patella, the femur, and the tibia.

Two main issues have been identified as contributors to PFPS: overuse or overloading, and poor alignment.

Overuse can be a result of percussive activities, especially with twisting and jumping. Overloading of the joint can occur even without repetitive percussive activity if the person is overweight, or if he or she has any anatomical anomalies that distribute pressure from the femur to the patella unequally.

Inefficient alignment at the knee can take many forms. Poor footwear or running on uneven surfaces can change how force moves up the leg into the knee. Flat feet, jammed arches, or problems in how the foot hits the ground can do the same thing. Unequal development of the medial and lateral quadriceps muscles is frequently identified as a factor;

PFPS almost always involves a lateral pull on the patella. Muscular imbalances between the quadriceps, hamstrings, and iliotibial band are also factors. An exaggerated **Q angle** is sometimes suggested in PFPS, but this has not been reliably demonstrated as a contributor.

Signs and Symptoms

Symptoms of PFPS include pain that is usually felt on the anterior aspect of the knee, stiffness after long immobility, difficulty walking down stairs, and a characteristic crackling, grinding noise on movement called crepitus.

One issue that makes this condition challenging is that it can be difficult to distinguish from—and frequently occurs concurrently with—another condition: patellar **tendinosis**. This is significant because while PFPS is not directly affected by massage, patellar tendinosis that is treated with skilled massage may respond well, with a virtually pain-free resolution. Consequently, it is important to have a very clear idea of what condition or conditions are present. One clue that is sometimes useful is that patellar tendinosis often hurts going up stairs (resisted extension of the leg) while PFPS may hurt more going down stairs (the weight of the femur pushing on the patella).

Treatment

The best treatment options for PFPS involve finding strategies to slow or stop the progression, while not becoming sedentary in the process. Running and jumping types of exercise may need to be replaced with swimming or cycling. Physical therapy often includes exercises to strengthen and balance tension in the muscles that cross the knee and that influence knee alignment. The quadriceps, hamstrings, tensor fasciae latae, and deep lateral rotators are often addressed in the challenge to improve alignment and stop the progression of damage that PFPS can cause.

Other interventions include ice, nonsteroidal anti-inflammatories for pain management, orthotics to improve alignment in the feet, and improved footwear. Some orthopedists recommend the use of a knee brace or sleeve to stabilize the patella, or special taping of the knee for the same purpose.

If noninvasive options aren't sufficient, surgery might be recommended. This may be in the form of **arthroscopy** to smooth out the articular cartilage, or a procedure called a "lateral release" that detaches a portion of the lateral stabilizing ligaments from the patella.

Medications

- NSAIDs for pain management

Massage Therapy Implications

RISKS	Massage carries no particular risk for a person with patellofemoral syndrome, but direct downward pressure on the patella may be irritating.
BENEFITS	Bodywork aimed specifically at the knee, but also systemically, can help to address the tension stiffness and chronic low-grade pain that many people with PFS experience.
OPTIONS	A good strategy might focus on equalizing tension on either side of the patella and retraining the knee extensors to track the patella appropriately over the joint.

Q angle: The angle formed by the line from the ASIS to the middle of the patella, and the line from the middle of the patella to the tibial tubercle.

Arthroscopy: A minimally invasive surgery in which the inside of a joint is examined using an arthroscope.

Intervertebral foramina: The openings between adjacent vertebrae. Through each intervertebral foramen passes a single spinal nerve.

Spondylolisthesis

Definition: What Is It?

Spondylolisthesis is a condition in which a structural problem in the lumbar spine allows one or more vertebral bodies to slip anteriorly (see Sidebar 3.5). This can involve tiny or large bone fractures, and put pressure on nerve roots at the **intervertebral foramina**, or on the spinal cord itself in the spinal canal.

Demographics

Different types of spondylolisthesis are associated with different ages. Congenital or isthmic cases may show up in adolescence or young adulthood during growth spurts combined with athletic pursuits. Athletes who lift heavy weights or who twist and hyperextend their spine: gymnasts, wrestlers, rowers, weight lifters, javelin throwers, pole-vaulters, and football players have a particularly high risk.

Degenerative spondylolisthesis is most likely to occur in adults over 40 years of age, and women outnumber men by about 5:1.

Etiology: What Happens?

The facet joints in healthy lumbar vertebrae occur on an essentially coronal plane. The superior facets of one lumbar vertebra contact the front sides of the inferior facets of its upstairs neighbor; this prevents the higher bone from sliding forward.

SIDEBAR 3.5 "Spondylo-" Tongue Twisters

The terminology used in the discussion of arthritis and **stenosis** in the spine can be puzzling. Here is a brief look at some of the most confusing terms:

- *Spondylosis.* A general term for any degenerative condition of the vertebrae. This comes from the Greek root *spondylo-*, for *vertebra.*
- *Spondylolysis.* A specific defect in vertebrae, usually in the lumbar spine, that impairs the weight-bearing capacity of the bone. The word roots are *spondylo-* and *lysis*, or *loosening.*
- *Spondylolisthesis.* An anterior displacement of the body of a lumbar vertebra onto its inferior vertebra or onto the sacrum. This is a combination of *spondylo-* and *olisthesis*, Greek for a *slipping and falling.*

All three of these conditions can contribute to stenosis, or a narrowing of the spinal canal that may involve nerve pressure.

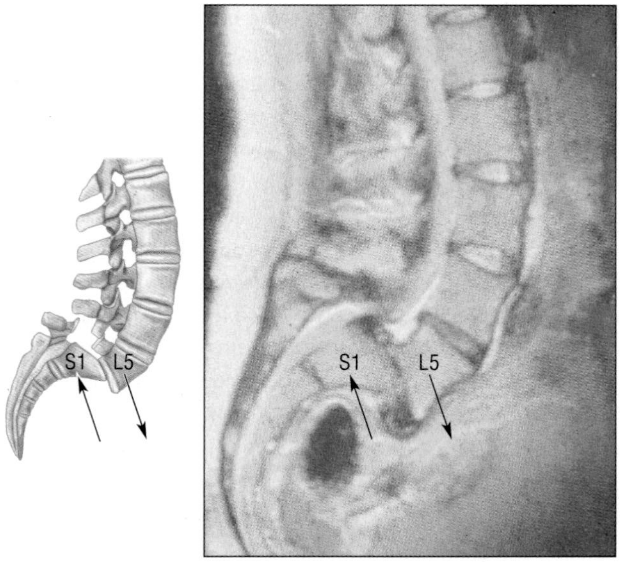

FIGURE 3.25 Spondylolisthesis

A structural weak spot in lumbar vertebrae can be found at the **pars interarticularis**, which forms the bridge between the lamina and the pedicle. Sometimes the pars is underdeveloped, and tiny microfractures allow for the anterior portion of the vertebra to shift forward. Alternatively, if the orientation of the facets is on a sagittal plane, or if the pars interarticularis has to accommodate for extreme shearing forces, the bone may fracture, allowing the vertebral body to slide forward (Figure 3.25).

Tiny microfractures of the pars interarticularis can have several outcomes. They can essentially heal with a false joint that allows permanent hypermobility; they can grow a bony bridge that lengthens the vertebral arch; or the fibrous bands that extend between the edges of the injury may never fully calcify.

Types of Spondylolisthesis

- *Congenital spondylolisthesis*: This occurs when a person is born with facets that are oriented on a sagittal rather than coronal plane in the lumbar vertebrae. This may never cause a problem, unless physical activity challenges the integrity of the facet joints.
- *Isthmic spondylolisthesis*: This involves a structural weakness at the pars interarticularis. While it may not create symptoms during childhood, adolescent growth spurts combined with athletic activities often create multiple microfractures of the bone, along with pain and loss of range of motion.
- *Degenerative spondylolisthesis*: This type is most common in mature adults. Unlike other forms, it may not involve any damage to the vertebral arch. Instead, it may begin with arthritis at the facet joints along with disc thinning that allows supporting ligaments to slacken and destabilize the lumbar joints. Then the joint capsule stretches as the bone is shifted forward.
- *Traumatic spondylolisthesis*: This is a rare situation where an accident or trauma damages the pars interarticularis.
- *Pathologic spondylolisthesis*: This occurs as a complication of some other event. It could involve tumors from metastatic cancer, an infection in the bone or joint capsule, or complications of a previous spinal surgery.

Stenosis: An abnormal narrowing of a tubular structure.

Pars interarticularis: The part of the vertebra between the superior and inferior articular process.

Signs and Symptoms

Anterior slippage of the lumbar vertebral body is usually described by degree of severity:

Signs and symptoms of spondylolisthesis generally correspond to the severity of the vertebral displacement. Grade

Grade 1	1%–25% slippage
Grade 2	26%–50% slippage
Grade 3	51%–75% slippage
Grade 4	76%–100% slippage
Grade 5	100% or more slippage

1 or 2 slippages are by far the most common, and they are associated with central low back pain, tight hamstrings, spasm of the lumbar paraspinal muscles, and in some cases pain that radiates into the buttock and thighs.

More severe cases may demonstrate a palpable shelf in the lumbar spine when the patient flexes the trunk. Nerve compression is more likely in this situation, which may result in pain, numbness, or weakness along the affected nerve pathways. Rarely, the damage to the spine may result in pressure directly on the spinal cord, which leads to an emergency situation called **cauda equina syndrome**. This can cause permanent loss of bladder and bowel control as well as other complications, so it is important to deal with this as quickly as possible.

One problem with degenerative spondylolisthesis is that it often has a slow onset, and it affects a population (people over 40 years of age) who may be at risk for other conditions that create a similar picture. The radiating pain and numbness that sometimes is seen with spondylolisthesis can easily be confused with symptoms of **peripheral artery disease** or **peripheral neuropathy**, and vice versa. These symptoms must be explored to be sure of their origin and the effectiveness of possible treatments.

> **Cauda equina syndrome:** A condition in which the inferior part of the spinal cord is damaged, resulting in loss of function.

Treatment

The majority of cases of spondylolisthesis cases can be treated with mild pain relievers, exercise to strengthen the abdominal muscles, and massage therapy to ease back pain and hamstring tightness. Back braces or corsets may be recommended for extra external support. Very severe cases involve a completely disrupted vertebral arch, and may indicate surgery for correction and stabilization.

Medications

- Nonsteroidal anti-inflammatory drugs for pain management

Massage Therapy Implications

RISKS

When a client's back is acutely painful, massage therapists must be careful not to exacerbate pain or inflammation. Any instability in the low back must be addressed with careful positioning. If symptoms include areas of numbness or reduced sensation, that needs to be pursued with a neurologist.

BENEFITS

The chronic low back pain, paraspinal spasm, and tightness in the psoas and hamstrings that many spondylolisthesis patients experience can all be addressed with massage. Bodywork won't correct structural problems with the vertebrae, but it can be an effective way to deal with the symptoms.

OPTIONS

Hyperextension of the back can be addressed by using bolsters under the abdomen and ankles when the client is prone, and under the knees when the client is supine.

RESEARCH

Not enough research has been done on nonoperative interventions for spondylolisthesis to identify a clear best choice,[1] but many specialists pursue conservative therapy first if possible. One case study points out the risk of pedicle fracture from massage,[2] while another found that massage therapy was effective for pain and hypertonicity for a client with isthmic spondylolisthesis.[3]

1. Garet M, Reiman MP, Mathers J, et al. Nonoperative treatment in lumbar spondylolysis and spondylolisthesis: a systematic review. *Sports Health* 2013;5(3):225–232. http://www.ncbi.nlm.nih.gov/pmc/articles/PMC3658408/
2. Guo Z, Chen W, Su Y, et al. Isolated unilateral vertebral pedicle fracture caused by a back massage in an elderly patient: a case report and literature review. *European Journal of Orthopaedic Surgery & Traumatology: Orthopedie Traumatologie* 2013;23 (Suppl 2):S149–S153. http://www.ncbi.nlm.nih.gov/pubmed/23412164
3. Halpin S. Case report: the effects of massage therapy on lumbar spondylolisthesis. *Journal of Bodywork and Movement Therapies* 2012;16(1):115–123. http://www.ncbi.nlm.nih.gov/pubmed/22196437

Spondylosis

Definition: What Is It?

Spondylosis is a form of degenerative arthritis, involving age-related changes of the vertebrae, discs, joints, and ligaments of the spine. It happens most frequently and most severely at the neck.

Demographics

Cervical spondylosis is very common in mature people; about 90% of men over 50 years of age and women over 60 years of age have some evidence of degeneration in the cervical spine, although many do not have symptoms.

Etiology: What Happens?

The section on **osteoarthritis** describes in some detail the changes that happen when damage occurs at synovial joints. Spondylosis has some features in common with osteoarthritis, but some important differences distinguish the two conditions.

The connections between the vertebral bodies and the intervertebral discs are not synovial joints, but they are vulnerable to some of the same problems that freely movable joints can develop. It can be a useful analogy to think of the vertebral bodies as articulating bones, the tough anulus fibrosus as a capsular ligament, and the softer gelatinous nucleus pulposus as the synovial fluid inside a joint. As the spine ages, especially if the connecting ligaments are lax or if the vertebrae are out of optimal alignment, shearing and compressive stresses can affect the joint. The disc thins, and bone spurs may develop around the vertebral body or on the facet joints (Figures 3.26 and 3.27).

Spinal osteophytes usually appear on the anterior or lateral aspects of the vertebral bodies but occasionally grow on the facets or in a place to put pressure on the nerve roots or spinal cord. Spondylosis causes back and neck pain only when the growths put mechanical pressure on nerve roots or the spinal cord, and this occurs only when the foramen is significantly less than its normal size.

In addition to excessive calcium deposits on vertebrae, advanced age may contribute to the ossification of the long vertical ligaments that stabilize the spine. The anterior longitudinal ligament runs on the anterior aspect of the vertebral bodies. **Diffuse idiopathic skeletal hyperostosis** is a common condition involving calcium deposits along this structure. This may be a major contributor to the gradual painless loss of range of motion that is frequently reported with spondylosis. The posterior longitudinal ligament runs along the posterior aspect of the vertebral bodies, on the anterior side of the spinal canal. Ossification may occur here as well; this carries a higher risk of spinal cord pressure. The **ligamentum flavum**, which runs on the posterior aspect of the spinal canal, often thickens and even buckles with age; this can contribute to stenosis that impinges the spinal cord. And finally, the blood supply to the CNS that is embedded in the dura mater is also vulnerable to the pressure exerted by this process (Figure 3.28).

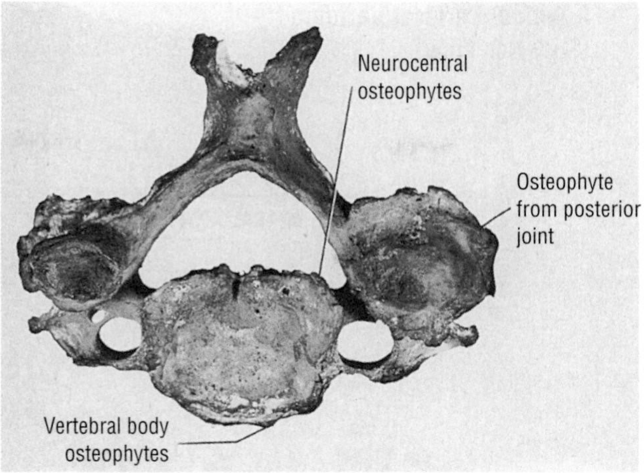

FIGURE 3.26 Osteophytic growths with spondylosis

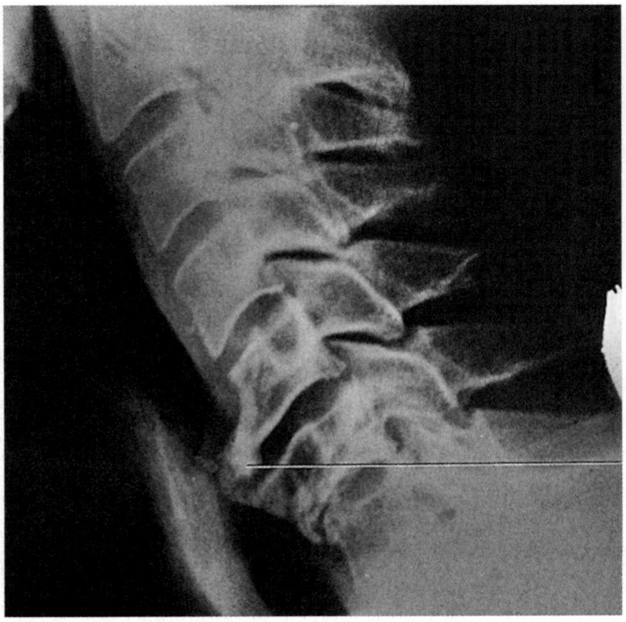

FIGURE 3.27 Fusion of vertebral bodies with spondylosis

Diffuse idiopathic skeletal hyperostosis: A bony hardening of ligaments that attach to the spine.

Ligamentum flavum: One of the ligaments of the spinal column that connect the laminae of adjacent vertebrae. (Plural: ligamenta flava)

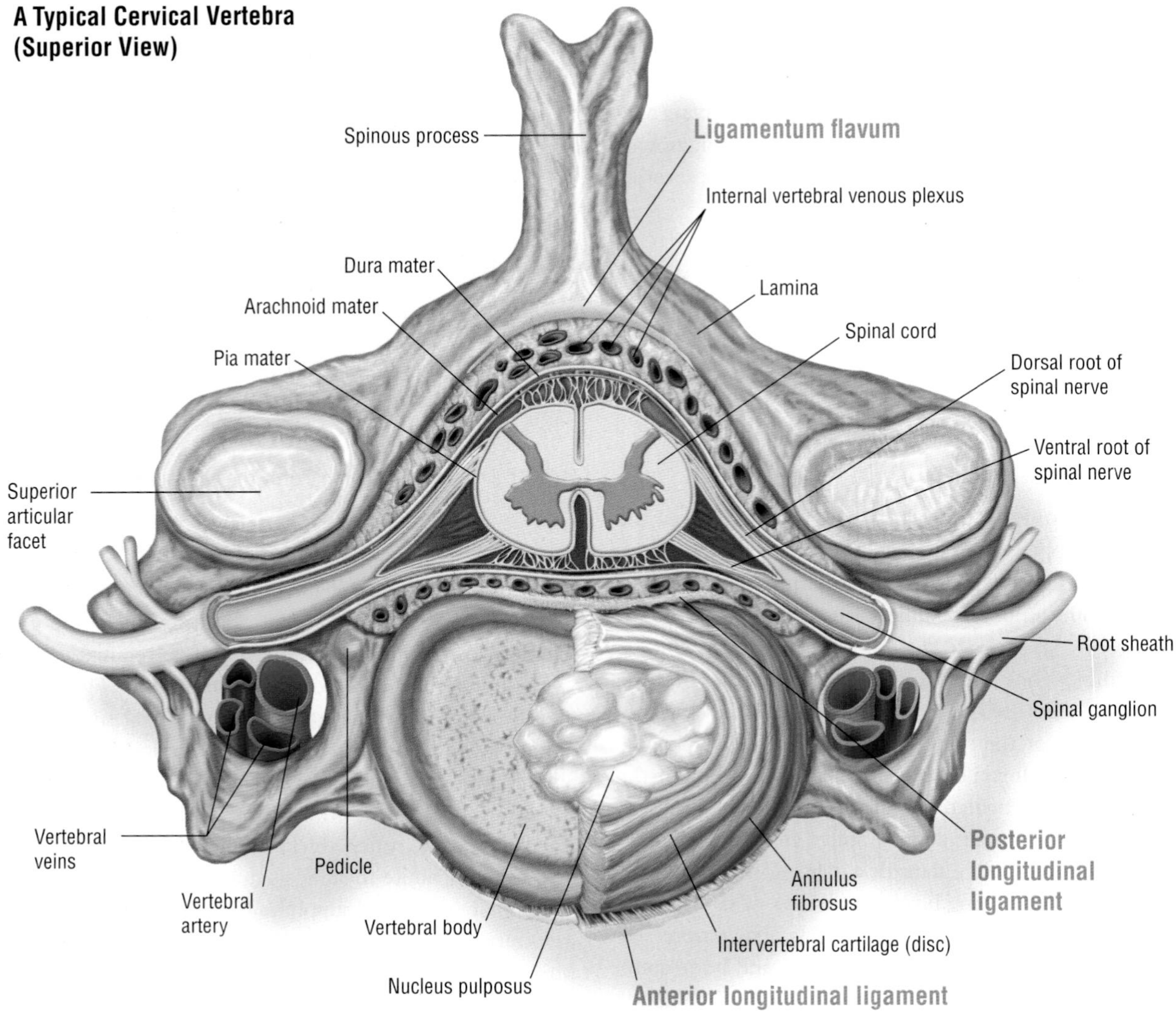

FIGURE 3.28 Thickening of the anterior longitudinal ligament; the posterior longitudinal ligament, and the ligamentum flavum can reduce spinal mobility and put pressure on the spinal cord

Signs and Symptoms

Spondylosis often has no painful symptoms whatever. If the bony changes do not press on nerve roots but grow somewhere that impedes movement, the main symptom is slow, painless, but irreversible stiffening of the spine.

When the osteophytes do press on nerve roots, the symptoms include shooting pain, tingling, pins and needles, numbness, and muscle weakness only in muscles supplied by the affected nerve. **Headaches** that begin at the back of the neck are frequent. If the pressure is on the spinal cord, myelopathy symptoms are bilateral and may include lost balance, trouble walking, and loss of bladder or bowel control.

One distinguishing feature of nerve pressure from osteophytes is that the pain is consistent; if the bone spurs are in a place to create pain when a person is in a certain position or posture, then that pain is predictable and tends to get worse over time instead of better.

Complications

Spondylosis is a slowly progressing condition that mostly affects middle-aged and elderly people. Usually it is not dangerous, but it can have some serious complications.

- *Spreading problems in the spine.* This is not a progressive disease that travels through the blood or lymph, but if two vertebrae become fused through bony remodeling, that puts much more stress on the joints above and below the fusion to provide mobility. Those joints can become unstable, develop arthritis, and undergo the same bony remodeling that created the first problem. Alternatively, the stress of hypermobility may cause disc problems. **Disc disease** can be both a predisposing factor and a complication of spondylosis.
- *Nerve pain.* This is the consequence of having osteophytes grow where they can put pressure on nerves as

they exit the spinal cord. The pain they cause is called radiculopathy, referring to the root (radix) of the affected spinal nerve.

- *Secondary spasm*. This accompanies nerve pain. Muscle spasm may be confined to the paraspinals, where it exacerbates the problem by compressing the affected joints, or it may follow the path of referred pain. Muscles may also work to protect the spine from movement that would otherwise be excruciatingly painful.
- *Blood vessel pressure*. Osteophytes in the neck sometimes press on the vertebral arteries as they go up the transverse foramina. If the head is turned or extended in a certain position, the patient may feel dizzy or have headaches or double vision from impaired blood flow into the head.
- *Myelopathy*. This is an extremely serious complication of spondylosis in the neck. Osteophytes may grow in a location to put pressure on the spinal cord itself, a condition called cervical spondylitic myelopathy. This is felt as progressive weakening down the body, potential loss of bladder and bowel control, and possible eventual paralysis.

Treatment

Treatment for spondylosis depends on which complications are present. Anti-inflammatories and pain control are the usual first recourse. Movement, bracing, and exercise can limit progression once the damage has begun. Massage therapy, acupuncture, and hydrotherapy are often recommended before more intrusive steps are tried.

If noninvasive measures are insufficient, local injections of steroids can provide temporary relief. A variety of surgeries can create more space for nerve roots or the spinal cord. These often involve spinal fusions, however, and they work best for younger patients who have not been having arthritic symptoms for a long time or in more than one joint.

Medications

- NSAIDs for pain control
- Narcotic or opioid drugs (Vicodin, Percocet) for pain control if NSAIDs are not sufficient
- Muscle relaxants for spasm
- Antiseizure drugs for paresthesia
- Injected steroidal anti-inflammatories

Radiculopathy: Any disorder of the spinal nerve roots.

Myelopathy: Disease or injury of the spinal cord.

Massage Therapy Implications

RISKS	The main risk for clients with spondylosis is that careless positioning may allow bone spurs to put pressure on nerves. Also, muscles that surround affected areas may be hypertonic for good reason: they could be protecting the spine from movement that may be painful.
BENEFITS	Massage can help reduce pain and stiffness, and improve the general quality of life for clients with spondylosis—as long as general cautions for frailty and positioning are observed.
RESEARCH	One systematic review supports massage therapy for neck pain in general, although spondylosis isn't necessarily the identified cause.[1] Sherman et al.[2] found a significant difference in the effectiveness of 60-minute massage sessions two or three times a week over the same frequency of 30-minute massage sessions to manage symptoms of chronic neck pain. 1. Cheng YH, Huang GC. Efficacy of massage therapy on pain and dysfunction in patients with neck pain: a systematic review and meta-analysis. *Evidence -Based Complementary and Alternative Medicine* 2014;2014:204360. http://www.ncbi.nlm.nih.gov/pmc/articles/PMC3950594/ 2. Sherman KJ, Cook AJ, Wellman RD, et al. Five-week outcomes from a dosing trial of therapeutic massage for chronic neck pain. *Annals of Family Medicine* 2014;12(2):112–120. http://www.annfammed.org/content/12/2/112.long

Sprains

Definition: What Are They?

Sprains are tears to ligaments, the fibrous connective tissue strapping tape that links bone to bone throughout the body.

Demographics

Sprains are extremely common in the United States; it is estimated that over 20,000 happen each day, just to ankles; this doesn't account for knee, elbow, wrist, and finger sprains.

Etiology: What Happens?

The traditional image of ligament tissue has been that it is composed mostly of linearly arranged collagen fibers, invested with a few fibroblasts, with the function of linking bone to bone. But ligaments are also highly invested with sensory neurons, many of which are proprioceptors that work with nearby muscles. This understanding has created new strategies in dealing with ligament injuries and the accompanying muscle adaptations that they inevitably involve.

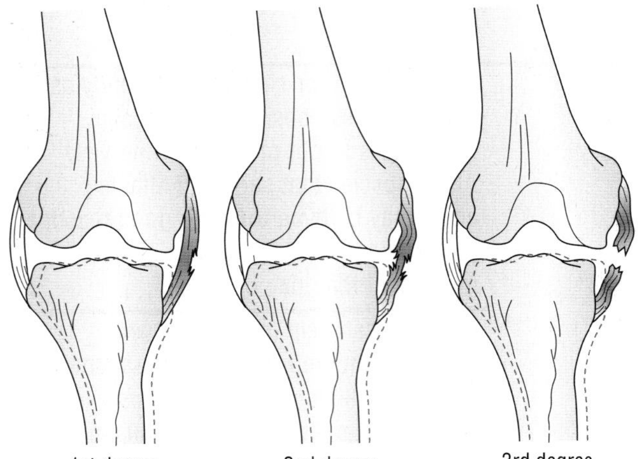

FIGURE 3.29 First-, second-, and third-degree sprains

Dense fibrous structures like ligaments are injured when some of their fibers are stretched or ripped. The severity of the injury depends on what percentage of the fibers is affected. First-degree injuries involve just a few fibers; second-degree injuries are much worse, and third-degree injuries are ruptures: the entire structure has been ripped through (Figure 3.29).

Injury to ligaments triggers an inflammatory response and the rapid production of new collagen fibers. These are laid down in a haphazard mass early in the healing process, similar to the process discussed in **muscle strains**. In the maturation phase, the perfect combination of movement, stretching, and weight-bearing stress helps to reorient the fibers in alignment with the uninjured structure. If this happens in the best possible way, the new scar tissue seamlessly blends with the uninjured portions of the ligament. But if a new injury is immobilized and kept from movement, the scar tissue may become dense and contracted, pulling on all the healthy fibers nearby and significantly hampering the weight-bearing capacity of the ligament. This situation can involve chronic, poor-quality scar tissue that slowly degrades the whole structure.

A few things distinguish sprains from strains and **tendinopathies,** which are discussed elsewhere.

- *Ligament structure*: The dense linear arrangement of collagen fibers in ligaments affords little stretch and almost no rebound. Further, the mechanics of ligament construction makes them vulnerable to injury under special circumstances: a sudden snap with no warming up or a prolonged but extreme stretch after activity can injure fibers. If a ligament becomes loose, it cannot stabilize the joint as well as it did before the injury. This ligament **laxity** contributes to chronic injury-reinjury situations and is a factor for the risk of **osteoarthritis**.

Laxity: Looseness.

- *Severity*: Sprains are more serious than strains and tendinosis. When a joint is injured, tendons and muscles are usually damaged before ligaments are.
- *Swelling*: With a few exceptions, acute sprains swell much more than do muscle strains or tendinosis; this is one way to differentiate between injuries. Ligaments are often contiguous with the joint capsules of the joints they stabilize, so an injury to them may signal the joint to swell too. Ligaments that are not attached to joint capsules swell much less than those that are.

Signs and Symptoms

Acute sprains show the usual signs of **inflammation**: pain, heat, redness, and swelling, along with loss of function because rapid swelling splints the unstable joint and makes it extremely painful to move. Inflamed ligaments are especially painful with passive stretches of the structure.

An acute sprain may mask the symptoms of a bone **fracture**, especially in the foot. This is important to clarify because the treatment and activity recommendations for sprains and for fractures are very different.

In the subacute stage signs of inflammation may still be present, but the joint begins to regain function. The physiological processes are no longer geared toward blood clotting and damage control; they have shifted toward clearing out debris and rebuilding torn fibers.

The amount of time that passes between acute and subacute stages varies with the severity of the injury, but 24 to 48 hours are typical. However, some injuries waver back and forth between acute and subacute, especially in response to overuse or intrusive massage.

Sprains can happen at almost any synovial joint, but the anterior talofibular ligament of the ankle is the most commonly sprained ligament in the body. Ligaments overlying the sacroiliac joint are also very commonly injured, as are various ligaments around the knees and fingers.

Treatment

At one time the recommendation for treating a sprain suggested soaking it in hot water and casting it to immobilize it during healing. Clearly, this was counterproductive: heat increases edema and the accumulation of scar tissue, while immobilization prevents the new fibers from aligning with the rest of the structure.

These days PRICE therapy (protection, rest, ice, compression, elevation) is considered the norm, with an emphasis on moving the joint within range of pain tolerance absolutely as soon as possible. The potential benefits are clear: ice keeps edema at bay, limiting further tissue damage from ischemia. Compression does the same. Elevation also encourages lymph flow out of an already congested area. Orthopedic specialists sometimes recommend modalities that may include ultrasound, exercise, and proprioceptive training to reduce the risk of a recurrence of injury.

The ideal amount of time to treat sprains with ice and rest after a sprain is debatable. The evidence suggests that the earlier a person uses the damaged joint without reinjuring it, the better. In the context of ankle sprains, adding balance training to the rehabilitation strategy is also important. Consequently some specialists recommend using the PRICE protocol for only a day or two, and then instituting the POLICE protocol: protection, optimal loading, ice, compression, and elevation.

Medications

- NSAIDs for pain and inflammation

Massage Therapy Implications

RISKS	Massage other than lymphatic work is not appropriate in the area of an acute sprain. Sprains that are not significantly better within a few days may be complicated by a bone fracture; this must be pursued with another medical professional.
BENEFITS	Massage can be extremely helpful for subacute or mature sprains. It can address poor-quality scar tissue and muscle holding around affected joints for improved local nutrition and efficiency of movement.
OPTIONS	Specific work on affected ligaments is appropriate in subacute or postacute situations: with-fiber and cross-fiber friction may be used, along with any variety of pin-and-stretch techniques that may work to improve mobility and work with proprioceptive affect on muscles.
RESEARCH	The use of massage therapy to treat the pain and swelling of ligament sprains has some documentation in the literature. A survey of 111 people with recent ankle sprains found that good recovery was associated with massage and proprioceptive training, as compared to those who received physiotherapy, weight training, and manipulative therapy.[1] Stecco et al.[2] found that focusing massage on the retinaculum of the ankle as well as the anteriofibular ligament led to improved outcomes in stability. 1. Guillodo Y, Le Goff A, Saraux A. Adherence and effectiveness of rehabilitation in acute ankle sprain. *Annals of Physical Rehabilitation Medicine* 2011;54(4):225–235. http://www.sciencedirect.com/science/article/pii/S1877065711000467 2. Stecco A, Stecco C, Macchi V, et al. RMI study and clinical correlations of ankle retinacula damage and outcomes of ankle sprain. *Surgical and Radiologic Anatomy* 2011;33(10):881–890. http://www.ncbi.nlm.nih.gov/pubmed/21305286

Prevention

Because a badly sprained ligament is easily reinjured, a lot of attention has been paid to preventing future trauma, especially at the ankle. Adding recovery components that address postural stability and proprioception appear to be an effective strategy to reduce the risk of future ankle sprains. Athletes are often counseled to treat new sprains as quickly as possible, and to wear low shoes with ankle braces to reduce the risk of injuries while playing.

Temporomandibular Joint Disorder

Definition: What Is It?

Temporomandibular joint disorder is an umbrella term that can refer to a multitude of common problems in and around the jaw. This collection of signs and symptoms is usually associated with malocclusion (a dysfunctional bite), **bruxism** (teeth grinding), and loose ligaments surrounding the jaw. These issues can lead to excessive movement between the temporal bone and mandible, damage to the internal cartilage, and possible dislocation of the joint. TMJ disorder is sometimes referred to as TMD: **t**emporo**m**andibular joint **d**isorder.

Demographics

TMJ disorders occur mostly in people between 30 and 50 years of age, and women diagnosed with this disorder outnumber men about 4:1. Some estimates suggest that about 10 million people in the United States have some kind of TMJ disorder.

Etiology: What Happens?

The TMJ is utterly unique. The left and right sides cannot move independently, but the joint still has a wide range of motion, allowing the mandible to move up, down, forward, back, and side to side. The jaw is unusually mobile, as the joint capsule stretches with the position of the mouth (Figure 3.30). A fibrocartilage disc cushions the temporal bone as it contacts the condyle of the mandible, but this disc is sometimes pulled awry or injured, which can lead to problems in the joint. *To explore the anatomy of the TMJ, watch the video "The Temporomandibular Joint" at* http://thePoint.lww.com/Werner6e. thePoint®

Furthermore, the muscles that work together to control jaw movement during chewing and speech are particularly prone to developing trigger points, which can refer pain into the jaw, into the face, over the head, and into the neck. Tension in the muscles of mastication (the masseter, the medial and lateral pterygoids, and the temporalis among others) can be both a symptom and trigger of TMJ disorders.

Bruxism: Habitual teeth grinding, especially while sleeping.

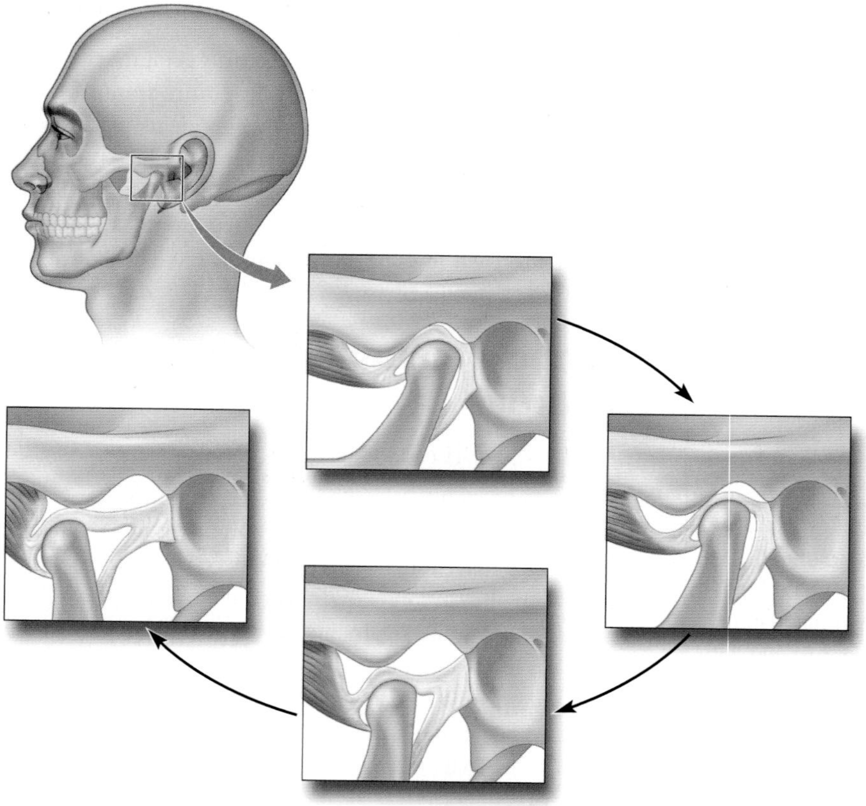

FIGURE 3.30 The TMJ allows great mobility as the jaw protracts

TMJ disorders are often categorized as three issues, but overlap can occur between these factors:

- ***Myofascial pain***: Trigger points in the jaw muscles can refer pain to the face, head and neck.
- *Internal derangement*: The cartilaginous disc or other structures may be abnormal or damaged.
- ***Osteoarthritis***: Progressive wear and tear at the jaw can lead to permanent remodeling of the joint (Figure 3.31).

TMJ problems are often circular—that is, the factors that cause TMJ disorders can also be the symptoms. In this way, tight muscles can lead to pain and tissue damage, which can lead to arthritis at the jaw, which reinforces muscle tightening. **Rheumatoid arthritis** occasionally occurs here, but osteoarthritis is a far more frequent contributor to TMJ problems. Other factors include misalignment of the bite and congenital malformations of the bones.

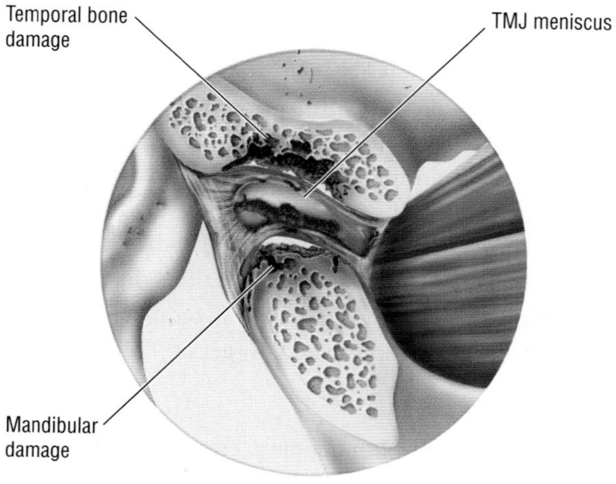

FIGURE 3.31 TMJ: joint damage

When the highly specialized joints at the jaw undergo chronic misalignment, trauma, or muscle tension, a person may find it difficult to open or close the mouth without pain. Chewing and swallowing become problematic, and pain in the jaw can reverberate systemically throughout the body.

Signs and Symptoms

The signs and symptoms of TMJ disorders include the following:

- *Jaw, neck, and shoulder pain*. This can be from deterioration of bony structures inside the capsule (arthritis), or it can be local and referred pain generated by tight, trigger point–laden muscles.
- *Limited range of motion*. Deformation or displacement of the cartilage inside the joint can make it difficult or impossible to open the mouth all the way or to move through a normal range of protraction, retraction, and side-to-side action.
- *Popping, clicking in the jaw*. This is usually attributed to having the disc or bone out of alignment, which interferes in jaw opening.
- *Locking of the joint*. Again, this is a result of having the fibrocartilage disc interfere with normal joint movement.

- *Bruxism*. Like many issues with this disorder, this symptom is also a possible cause of the problem. Chronically shortened jaw elevators contribute to clenching and grinding of teeth, especially during sleep, when the joint should be as relaxed as possible.
- *Ear pain*. Because of the location of the joint, pressure may be exerted directly on the eustachian tubes. Symptoms in this case include a feeling of stuffiness in the ears, and loss of hearing or tinnitus.
- *Headaches*. These can also be related to the pressure translated through the teeth to the cranium, to trigger points of muscles in spasm, and to cervical **subluxation**.
- *Chronic misalignment of cervical vertebrae*. This is probably a result of the muscular hypertonicity that is generated by this problem. As pain refers from the jaw to the neck and shoulders, the muscles there tighten up and pull asymmetrically on the neck bones. No matter how often the neck is adjusted or how brilliantly the neck muscles are massaged, this pain-spasm cycle is unlikely to resolve until the jaw situation is addressed.

Treatment

Several other injuries have similarities with TMJ disorder, and part of successful treatment is ruling these out. A short list includes Ernest syndrome (a **sprain** of a nearby ligament); **trigeminal neuralgia**, occipital neuralgia, and **osteomyelitis**, perhaps from an infected tooth.

Once a conclusive diagnosis is made, treatment options for TMJ disorders are typically divided into nonsurgical and surgical options. Nonsurgical options include applying heat or cold to painful areas, physical therapy, ultrasound and massage therapy for jaw muscles, anti-inflammatories, and local anesthetics. Special splints that reduce bone-to-bone pressure may be prescribed. **Proliferant** injections to tighten the ligaments that surround the jaw may also be effective. If these noninvasive techniques are successful, progression may be halted before permanent bony distortion or cartilage damage inside the joint occurs.

If these are not satisfactory, surgeries for TMJ disorders range from an outpatient procedure in which scar tissue and adhesions are cleared out or dissolved with injections into the joint, to arthroscopic surgery to manipulate the cartilage, to full prosthetic joint replacement.

Medications

- NSAIDs for pain and inflammation
- Steroidal anti-inflammatories, including injections into the joint
- Tricyclic antidepressants for pain and stress
- Muscle relaxants
- **Botulinum toxin** injections to temporarily paralyze jaw-clenching muscles (this has not been approved by the FDA, but some specialists use it)

Proliferant: A substance that stimulates the growth of tissues, in this case, connective tissue.

Botulinum toxin: A neurotoxic protein that interferes with acetylcholine activity to reduce muscle contraction.

Massage Therapy Implications

RISKS	Not all jaw pain is caused by TMJ disorder, and it is important to have an accurate diagnosis for the best outcome. Some of the disorders that mimic TMJ disorder contraindicate massage in certain circumstances.
BENEFITS	Massage can help reduce muscle tone, resolve trigger points, and improve client awareness of bruxism and other habits, all of which can improve the outlook for a person with TMJ disorder.
OPTIONS	Intraoral massage to the pterygoid muscles can be a successful part of TMJ disorder treatment, especially combined with specific work to address other jaw and neck muscles. This is not within scope in all massage therapy settings, however.
RESEARCH	A case report found that specifically targeted massage therapy had a positive impact on range of motion, muscle hypertonicity, pain, and stress in one TMJ disorder patient.[1] A study from Poland found that massage therapy for the myofascial pain component of TMJ disorders is effective, safe, and easy to apply in dental settings.[2] Another found that physiotherapy, including soft tissue massage, makes an effective partnership with dentistry in the treatment of TMJ disorders.[3] Researchers generally find that manual therapies are most effective for TMJ disorders if no damage to the disc or joint structures has yet accrued.

1. Pierson MJ. Changes in temporomandibular joint dysfunction symptoms following massage therapy: a case report. *International Journal of Therapeutic Massage and Bodywork* 2011;4(4):37–47. http://ijtmb.org/index.php/ijtmb/article/view/110/201
2. Miernik M, Wieckiewicz M, Paradowska A, et al. Massage therapy in myofascial TMD pain management. *Advances in Clinical and Experimental Medicine* 2012;21(5):681–685. http://www.advances.am.wroc.pl/pdf/2012/21/5/681.pdf
3. de Toledo EG, Jr., Silva DP, de Toledo JA, et al. The interrelationship between dentistry and physiotherapy in the treatment of temporomandibular disorders. *The Journal of Contemporary Dental Practice* 2012;13(5):579–583. http://www.ncbi.nlm.nih.gov/pubmed/23250156

Fascial Disorders

Compartment Syndrome

Definition: What Is It?

Compartment syndrome is a condition in which an injury or repetitive stress creates pressure inside a tight fascial compartment that can lead to the starvation and death of muscle and nerve cells. It usually happens in the lower leg, but it can develop elsewhere.

Demographics

The incidence of compartment syndrome is difficult to guess. Acute compartment syndrome is probably relatively rare, but it can occur as a complication of fractures (especially of the tibia) or crushing injury.

Etiology: What Happens?

Two forces operate to maintain fluid balance within tight fascial compartments, especially in the lower leg: **tissue pressure** (which is partly determined by the rate and volume of incoming fluid), and **perfusion pressure** (which describes the ratio of blood in the arteries compared to that in the veins within an enclosed space). When tissue pressure rises above perfusion pressure, then fluid enters the capsule, but the usual delivery system to move it out is compromised. The result is a vicious circle: fluid pours into the area, but cannot leave because exit routes are compressed; starving and damaged cells release proinflammatory chemicals that boost capillary permeability, and attract and retain yet more fluid (Figure 3.32). Eventually permanent damage may occur, including the death of muscle and nerve cells, muscle **contracture**, and rising levels of cellular debris in the bloodstream that could lead to **renal failure** and death.

Compartment syndrome can be acute or chronic.

- *Acute compartment syndrome*: this describes a sudden onset of massive swelling within an enclosed space. It is usually due to a crushing injury, a closed long bone contusion or **fracture**, or a penetrating injury that damages an artery (a gunshot or stab wound, for instance). Burns and venomous bites or stings can trigger this reaction, and it can also happen if arterial circulation is compressed and then suddenly restored: this is an occasional complication of surgery.
- *Chronic compartment syndrome*: this is a much less serious condition that is usually related to repetitive athletic activity. Also called exertional compartment syndrome, this describes a situation in which the increased circulation and normal muscle expansion that happens with exercise overwhelms the body's capacity to maintain proper fluid pressures within a fascial capsule. Chronic compartment syndrome may often be considered when an athlete complains of **shin splint** symptoms that are not resolved through other means.

Compartment syndrome usually affects one of the four fascial compartments of the lower leg, but it has been seen in other areas, including compartments of the foot, hand, forearm, buttocks, and abdomen. A special variant on the phenomenon of fluid-compressed nerves is seen in the lateral thigh with a condition called **meralgia paresthetica**: this version is usually related to weight gain, tight-fitting clothing, pregnancy, or seat belt injury.

> **Tissue pressure:** The pressure of interstitial tissue fluid in an enclosed space.
>
> **Perfusion pressure:** The gradient between arterial and venous pressure in a comparable location.
>
> **Contracture:** An abnormal contraction or shortening of a muscle. Can become permanent.
>
> **Meralgia paresthetica:** Paresthesia of the lateral thigh.
>
> **Tonometer:** An instrument for measuring pressure or tension.
>
> **Fasciotomy:** A surgical procedure to cut fascia in order to relieve internal pressure.

Signs and Symptoms

Acute compartment syndrome is usually related to some clear trauma, but in rare cases it can arise from intense exercise, or even from no discernable cause. It involves pain that is out of proportion to the extent of the injury; this is often described as "tight" or "burning" pain. Passive stretching of the tissues is especially painful. The area is hot and hard to the touch.

Chronic compartment syndrome is almost always a response to a repetitive athletic activity, and the symptoms may include pain, cramping, weakness, numbness, and changes in gait. Symptoms develop during exercise and subside when activity stops. However, many people report that this condition is progressive: it takes less and less exercise to elicit symptoms, and pain lingers for longer and longer afterward.

Treatment

Compartment syndrome of any kind is typically diagnosed with an instrument called a **tonometer**: this uses a needle to penetrate targeted muscles and measure internal pressure. In acute cases this is self-evident, but for chronic compartment syndrome, measures are taken at rest and immediately after exercise. If that pressure is reliably higher than 30 to 45 mm Hg, intervention is suggested, usually in the form of a **fasciotomy**: a surgical split of the affected fascial sheath to relieve internal pressure. Hyperbaric oxygen and drugs to support kidney health may also be recommended. Acute compartment syndrome is so extreme that if surgery is not performed within a few hours of the trauma, the patient may experience permanent loss of function, amputation, or potentially life-threatening kidney damage from debris released by dying muscle cells.

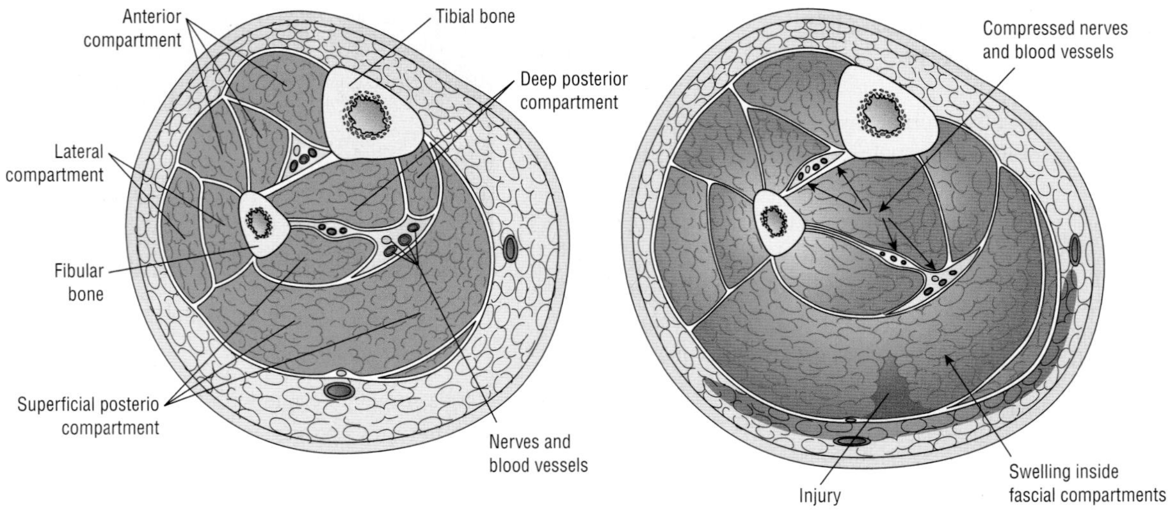

FIGURE 3.32 Swelling inside fascial compartments

A person with chronic compartment syndrome may also consider surgical release of the fascial sheath, but obviously this is not a medical emergency. Before reaching this point, patients are usually counseled to try orthotics or improving footwear, to stretch carefully, to warm up and cool down appropriately around exercise, to use massage therapy, which has been shown to delay the onset of symptoms but not to affect the pressure within internal compartments, and to add more variety to the exercise they do.

Medications

- For chronic compartment syndrome: anti-inflammatories to manage swelling and pain

Massage Therapy Implications

RISKS	Acute compartment syndrome is a medical emergency and must be treated quickly to avoid potentially life-threatening complications. Any clients presenting with these signs needs to be referred out immediately. Chronic compartment syndrome may respond well to massage when it is not active or irritated, but when the client is in pain, manipulating affected tissues with anything but the lightest touch is likely simply to interfere with the body's ability to compensate for increasing compartmental pressure.
BENEFITS	Chronic compartment syndrome in the lower leg may respond well to massage as a strategy to prevent or delay the onset of pain.
OPTIONS	In acute situations, it is important to secure medical care as soon as possible. Because the fascial compartments in the lower leg are so dense and inelastic, and because the normal range of motion at the tibiotalar joint prevents extensive stretching, massage with a "pin and pump" approach to the anterior and posterior lower leg muscles can be a powerful way to engage those muscles in preparation for activity, or as a postexercise protocol. If the leg is in a flared-up stage of chronic compartment syndrome, lymph drainage modalities may be useful to help move fluid appropriately through the area.
RESEARCH	Very little research about massage in the context of compartment syndrome has been conducted at this point. Bong et al.[1] found that massage therapy might help delay the onset of chronic exertional compartment syndrome symptoms, but not that it prevents it in people already affected. This confirmed findings of an earlier pilot study that found that massage and stretching increased the amount of work an athlete could do before having the onset of pain.[2] 1. Bong MR, Polatsch DB, Jazrawi LM, et al. Chronic exertional compartment syndrome: diagnosis and management. *Bulletin (Hospital for Joint Diseases (New York, N.Y.)* 2005;62(3–4):77–84. http://www.ncbi.nlm.nih.gov/pubmed/16022217 2. Blackman PG, Simmons LR, Crossley KM. Treatment of chronic exertional anterior compartment syndrome with massage: a pilot study. *Clinical Journal of Sport Medicine* 1998;8(1):14–17. http://www.ncbi.nlm.nih.gov/pubmed/9448951

3 Musculoskeletal System Conditions

Dupuytren Contracture

Definition: What Is It?

This condition, also called palmar fasciitis, is an idiopathic thickening and shrinking of the palmar fascia that limits the movement of the fingers. It is a type of **fibromatosis**: a benign soft tissue growth with a proliferation of fibroblasts and extracellular matrix. Usually the ring and little fingers are most severely affected, although the index and middle fingers may also be bent.

NOTABLE CASES Dupuytren contracture has affected several notable individuals, including US President Ronald Reagan, British Prime Minister Margaret Thatcher, playwright Samuel Beckett, and actors Bill Nighy and David McCallum.

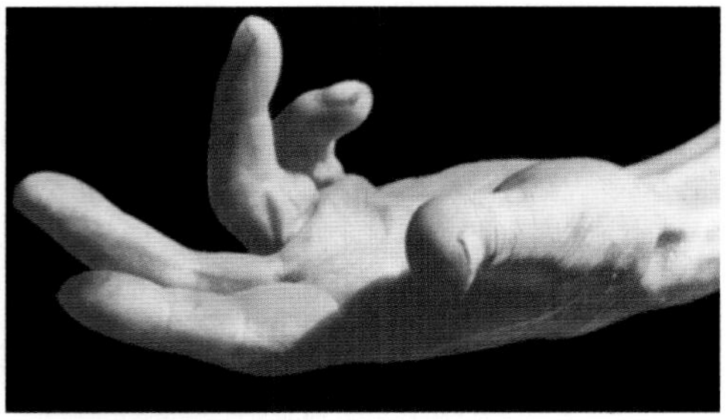

FIGURE 3.33 Dupuytren contracture

Demographics

Dupuytren contracture is most common among middle-aged white men of Northern European descent. Statistically it is seen most often along with physical labor that involves vibration, smoking, alcohol use, and type I and type II **diabetes**.

Etiology: What Happens?

It is unclear exactly what triggers the fascial changes seen with Dupuytren contracture, but it appears in three predictable stages. In the proliferative phase the myofibroblasts multiply, and a nodule develops, often at the base of the ring finger. This area often blanches when the affected finger is extended. During the **involutional** phase, a cord develops distally from the nodule toward the PIP joints. Symptoms may also develop in other fingers; the little finger is the second most common site. And in the residual phase, the cord tightens and the fingers bend into a permanent contracture.

Flexion of the fingers is normal for patients with Dupuytren contracture, but they cannot extend their fingers normally (Figure 3.33). When the extension is limited by 30 degrees or more, patients are considered to be candidates for corrective surgery. People with the most severe presentations are sometimes also susceptible other fibromatoses elsewhere in the body.

Fibromatosis: A condition in which connective tissue cells multiply into tumors called fibromas. Usually not cancerous.

Involutional: Describing something that is entangled or turned inward on itself.

Collagenase: A group of enzymes that help to dissolve collagen.

Needle aponeurotomy: A minimally invasive treatment for Dupuytren contracture, in which the offending band is weakened using microscopic punctures.

Types of Fibromatosis

- *Plantar fibromatosis* (Ledderhose disease): This is essentially the same as Dupuytren contracture, but it develops on the plantar aspect of the foot.
- *Peyronie disease*: This is a condition in which scar tissue develops under the skin of the shaft of the penis.
- *Garrod nodes* (knuckle pads): These are deposits of connective tissue at the interphalangeal joints of the hands. They are usually associated with a history of repetitive trauma related to sports or job-related activity.

Signs and Symptoms

The typical pattern of Dupuytren contracture is that a middle-aged man develops a mildly tender or painless bump just proximal to his ring finger on the palmar aspect of the hand. Over months or years, the nodule extends into a cord in his palm and out to the PIP joint. The little finger might develop a cord as well. The fingers are slowly drawn toward the palm, and they can't be straightened out. Dupuytren contracture is bilateral in almost half of cases, although one side is usually more extremely affected than is the other.

This condition may be mildly painful in early stages, but then often becomes painless. It is usually slowly progressive, although some people have a relatively fast onset. Some people have only the growth of tough, fibrous bumps on their hands, while others end up with severely bent, strangulated, unusable fingers. If the constriction to nerve and blood supply is very severe, the affected fingers may need to be amputated.

Treatment

If Dupuytren contracture is treated before too much atrophy occurs, corticosteroid injections can be effective to limit progression. Injections of **collagenase**, an enzyme that dissolves collagen, is another option, and release of the cord by way of tiny punctures (**needle aponeurotomy**) is a procedure with little risk of complications.

Surgical intervention is generally not recommended until fingers become bent and too stiff to move. At that point, the surgery involves making several zigzag cuts in the palm to release the fascia, followed by skin grafts, physical therapy, and massage to limit the growth of scar tissue. Even when surgery is successful, Dupuytren contracture recurs in about one-third of cases.

Medications

- Corticosteroid injection at the site of connective tissue overgrowth
- Enzyme injection at the site of connective tissue overgrowth

Massage Therapy Implications

RISKS	If nerves have been damaged, sensation could be impaired in the hand, and this requires special care. Steroid injections may alter the strength of the fascia, which may require adjustments in the intensity of treatment. Otherwise, massage within a client's pain tolerance has no specific contraindications for Dupuytren contracture.
BENEFITS	As long as sensation is intact, massage may be helpful in slowing the progression of Dupuytren contracture or in supporting the growth of healthy functional scar tissue after surgery.
RESEARCH	A case study using instrument-assisted cross-fiber friction massage and stretching reported good results with one client affected by Dupuytren contracture.[1] 1. Christie WS, Puhl AA, Lucaciu OC. Cross-frictional therapy and stretching for the treatment of palmar adhesions due to Dupuytren's contracture: a prospective case study. *Manual Therapy* 2012;17(5):479–482. http://www.ncbi.nlm.nih.gov/pubmed/22123331

Ganglion Cysts

Definition: What Are They?

Ganglion cysts are small connective tissue pouches filled with fluid that grow on joint capsules or tendinous sheaths. They usually appear on the wrist, the hand, or the top of the foot, but they have been found elsewhere as well.

Demographics

Ganglion cysts are found in women about three times more often than men. They are usually seen in children and young adults, with the exception of mucous cysts that often accompany **osteoarthritis** in older people.

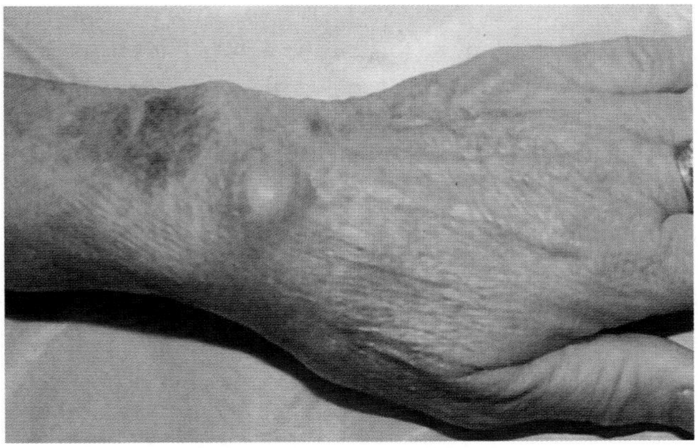

FIGURE 3.34 Ganglion cyst

Etiology: What Happens?

A ganglion cyst is essentially a connective tissue pouch filled with a viscous fluid. Cysts may have a single chamber, but many have multiple lobes that are connected by tiny channels. Some experts suggest that they are related to a long-term degeneration of fascia, leading to proliferation of collagen and other substances.

Ganglion cysts are not inherently dangerous, but they can grow in places that interfere with function. This can lead to pain and a loss of range of motion, among other problems. They usually grow on the wrist (Figure 3.34), hand, or foot, but have been found in many other locations.

One type of ganglion cyst is called a mucous cyst. This grows on the DIP, usually of older people with **osteoarthritis** at the same joints. Mucous cysts can damage the joint capsule or distort the growth of the fingernail (Figure 3.35).

Signs and Symptoms

Ganglion cysts may be too small to notice, or they may grow nearly to the size of a tennis ball, obstructing joint function and interfering with normal range of motion. They may have a gradual or sudden onset. Most ganglion cysts are not pain-

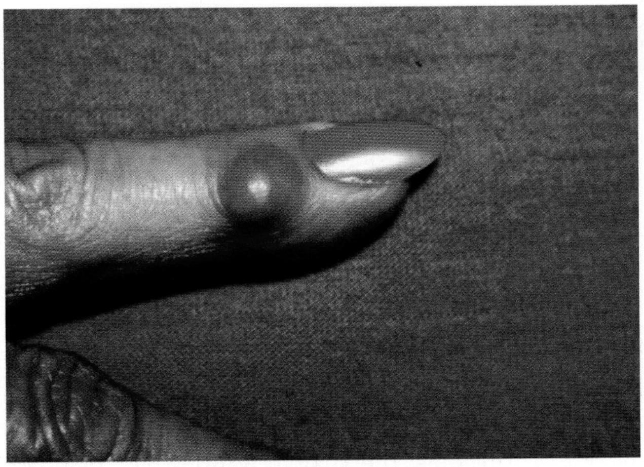

FIGURE 3.35 Mucous cysts grow near the DIP

ful, except when they grow in places where they can be easily irritated, such as on the fingers and around the wrists. This can put them in a state of chronic irritation, and it can be difficult for them to subside spontaneously.

Treatment

Generally the treatment for ganglion cysts is to leave them alone: they often resolve without interference. They may be aspirated to relieve internal pressure, but they often grow back. The traditional home remedy for ganglion cysts used to be to smash them with a Bible. Patients are not advised to use this option, however, as smashing a ganglion cyst with a book or any other heavy object can obviously cause a lot of other soft tissue damage.

Cysts may be excised through open surgery or arthroscopy if they are big enough to be a significant problem. If they grow back, they are usually not as large as the original cyst.

Massage Therapy Implications

RISKS	While massage is unlikely to rupture a cyst, deep specific work in the area may be irritating. Of course, undiagnosed bumps need to be evaluated by a primary provider.
BENEFITS	Bodywork is not likely to improve a client's ganglion cyst, but massage elsewhere is safe and appropriate: these clients can enjoy the same benefits from massage as does the rest of the population.

Hammer Toe

Definition: What Is It?

Hammer toe is a foot deformity that affects the lateral toes. The second toe is most commonly affected, especially when this digit is longer than the great toe. In this situation, the muscles and tendons that cross the foot joints become permanently shortened, and their fascial wrappings shrink to fit. The result is hyperextension at the metacarpophalangeal joint and distal interphalangeal joint, and flexion at the PIP (Figure 3.36).

Closely related deformities include claw toe (with flexion at both interphalangeal joints), mallet toe (with flexion only at the DIP), and curly toe (with flexion at all interphalangeal joints).

Etiology: What Happens?

Hammer toe and other toe problems are multifactoral conditions. They are seen most often in people with second toes that are longer than the great toe, and they occur frequently along with **bunions** and **pes cavus**. The main contributing factor is usually footwear that causes the second toe to curl over, but other issues include the use of high heels that force pressure onto the long second toe, trauma, underlying disease (**diabetes**, **rheumatoid arthritis**, and **osteoarthritis** are sometimes seen with hammer toe), and a genetic predisposition for this condition to develop, as seen with **Charcot-Marie Tooth syndrome**.

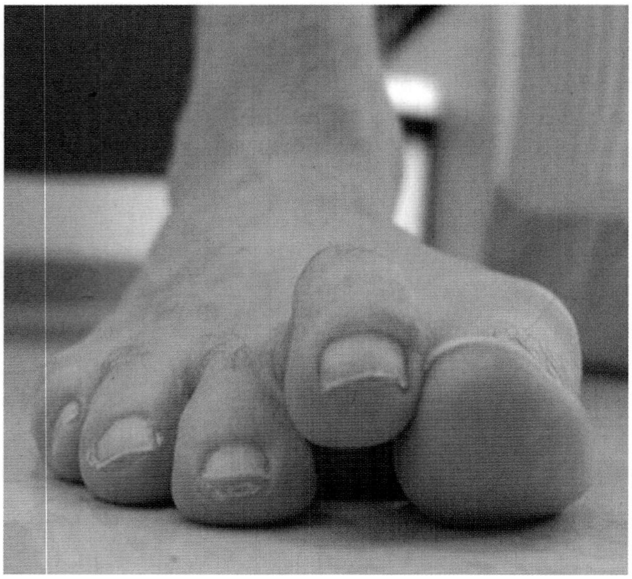

FIGURE 3.36 Hammer toe

Hammer toe is a progressive condition. It generally starts with an involuntary contracture as the normal balance between toe flexors and extensors is lost, but the tissues are soft and malleable. It gradually becomes rigid as the connective tissues thicken and shrink around the contracted muscles.

Signs and Symptoms

The primary signs of hammer toe and other toe problems include a visible deformity, involuntary contraction of the foot muscles, and pain where the toe is irritated by friction. This often results in corns or callus on the dorsal aspect of the toe joints, where they rub against shoes. Left untreated, this can lead to open sores and the risk of infection.

Hammer toe in its early stages can be flexible, but it becomes progressively more rigid over time.

Treatment

Changing footwear, using pads to treat corns and callus, orthotics, and using tape or splints to straighten toes are the first recommendations for a person with hammer toe. Some specialists may suggest steroid injections for inflammation and to address connective tissue thickness. If these are insufficient, surgery may be recommended. Surgeries vary according to whether the tissues are soft or rigid, but most involve opening and correcting the involved joints. If a bunion is present, this can be corrected at the same time.

Medications

- Nonsteroidal anti-inflammatory drugs to manage pain and inflammation
- Corticosteroid injection

Massage Therapy Implications

RISKS	If a client's foot is hot and inflamed, this is obviously a local caution for any but the lightest touch. Otherwise as long as sensation is intact and work is not painful, hammer toe has no specific contraindications for massage.
BENEFITS	If a client's hammer toe is rigid, massage may have little immediate or local impact. However, if this situation is still passively malleable, massage may work along with taping, splints, or other devices and stretching to help restore balance between the musculotendinous forces in the foot.
OPTIONS	A client with hammer toe in any form is likely to compensate for a loss of foot strength in both posture and gait. Massage can be used to address these issues to reduce pain and improve efficiency of movement.

Hernia

Definition: What Is It?

Hernia means "hole." A variety of hernias can occur in the body: muscles may herniate through fascial walls; vertebral discs may herniate; the brain may even herniate through the cranium. This discussion focuses on abdominal hernias: holes or weak spots in the abdominal wall or diaphragm, through which contents may protrude or become trapped.

Demographics

Hernias are common: about 5 million are diagnosed each year in this country, and about 1 million surgeries are conducted to correct them. Inguinal hernias account for about 77% of hernia surgeries.

Men have abdominal hernias much more frequently than do women; about 25% of men and 2% of women will develop an inguinal hernia in their lifetimes.

Etiology: What Happens?

Abdominal hernias can be classified as fascial disorders because they involve weakness in the connective tissue layers that normally form strong containers. When the fascia is challenged through mechanical forces or congenital flaws, a hole forms and the abdominal contents—usually fat or loops of small intestine encased within a peritoneal sac—can be forced through.

Many hernias are **reducible**, which means that the contents can be put back where they belong without surgery. But they may progressively get worse, bulging more often, while a bigger hole develops. Therefore, once a hernia has been identified, surgery to tighten up or close the hole is recommended sooner rather than later. Where a hernia develops and what it feels like depend mainly on gender and what forces push the abdominal contents against their walls. A hernia that cannot be reduced is said to be **incarcerated**, and the entrapped structures are at high risk for strangulation and infection.

Men are more prone to inguinal hernias than are women, because women's inguinal canals are not as large as men's. Further, the broad ligament that supports the uterus provides some extra protection against the mechanical forces that cause inguinal hernias.

Reducible: Able to be reduced, or put back in proper position.

Incarcerated: Describing a hernia that is entrapped to the degree that it cannot be repaired without surgery.

Linea alba: A fibrous band that runs down the center of the abdomen. The name literally means "white line."

Umbilicus: The navel.

Types of Hernia

- *Direct inguinal hernia*: This is a hole in the abdominal wall at the inguinal ring: the top of the inguinal canal. A sudden change in internal abdominal pressure, like coughing, sneezing, or heavy lifting (especially with simultaneous twisting) may force a section of small intestine to protrude into this structural weak spot (Figure 3.37).
- *Indirect inguinal hernia*: In this situation, structures protrude into the inguinal canal and, in men, down into the scrotum. This is usually present at birth.
- *Epigastric hernia*: This is a bulge superior to the umbilicus. The **linea alba** splits, and a portion of the omentum pushes through. The symptoms, besides a visible lump above the navel, may include a feeling of tenderness or heaviness in the area but seldom extreme pain. This hernia happens with women and men, but it is more common in men.
- *Paraumbilical hernia*: This is another split of the linea alba, this time right at the navel. It is sometimes a complication of childbirth. This type of hernia is almost exclusive to women.
- *Umbilical hernia*: This occurs at the **umbilicus**, and it is a common condition in newborn babies. It usually closes without intervention by age 2. In adults, umbilical hernias may occur with obesity or ascites, or as a result of multiple pregnancies.

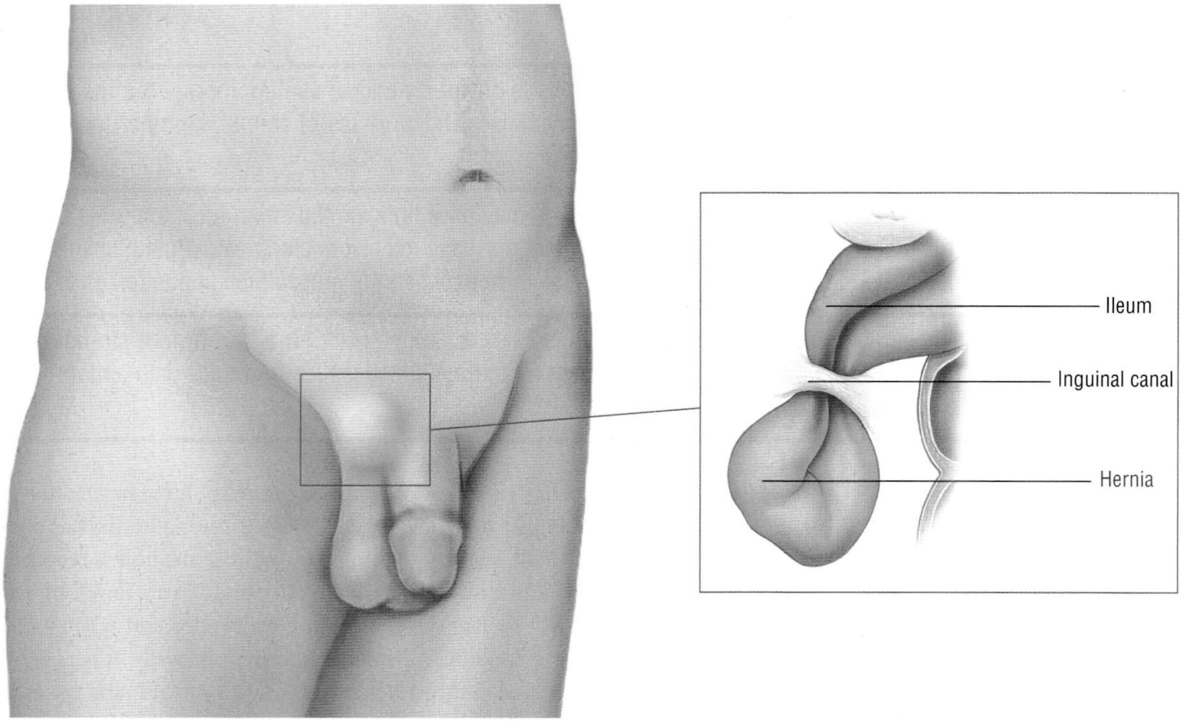

FIGURE 3.37 Inguinal hernia

- *Incisional hernia*: This is a surgical complication in which scar tissue at an incision site breaks down, and the tissues underneath bulge into the weak area.
- *Hiatal hernia*: This is an enlargement of the diaphragmatic **hiatus**: the opening in the dome of the diaphragm where the esophagus and other structures pass from the thorax to the abdomen. When this opening is enlarged, the stomach can protrude up into the thoracic cavity (Figure 3.38). Hiatal hernias are often a contributor to **gastroesophageal reflux disorder** (GERD). It is usually related to the depletion of elastin fibers in the local connective tissue structures.

  Hiatal hernias may be classified as types I to IV. Type I is most common, and involves a gastroesophageal junction that can slide above the diaphragm. A type II hernia has a junction that stays in the correct position, but the fundus of the stomach protrudes into a widened opening at the diaphragmatic hiatus. Type III is a combination of I and II; and a type IV hiatal hernia can involve tissues other than the stomach (i.e., the small or large intestine) protruding through the hiatus.
- *Other hernias*: These are rare. Femoral hernias involve a bulge inferior to the inguinal ligament into the femoral canal. Obturator hernia is a bulge of pelvic contents into the obturator foramen. Spigelian hernia is a bulge at the lateral aspect of the rectus abdominis.

Hiatus: A natural opening.

Signs and Symptoms

Signs and symptoms of hernias depend on the location and size of the bulge. Sharp or mild pain, a feeling of fullness, and a palpable bulge are common indicators. Hiatal hernias are recognized by the signs of GERD, along with shortness of breath as the stomach protrudes between the lungs.

The seriousness of a hernia is determined by how big it is. Paradoxically, the bigger the hernia, the safer it is, at least for the short term. Small holes can be more dangerous because structures can become trapped and strangulated. Signs of this complication range from discomfort and vomiting to an area becoming red, enlarged, and excruciatingly painful.

Treatment

Surgery is frequently recommended even for mild hernias because they tend to get worse as time goes on, and a small repair is less risky than a large one. The standard surgical technique entails inserting a small piece of mesh at the site of the tear. This helps to distribute the force of abdominal pressure more evenly than do stitches or staples alone, reducing the risk of a recurrence. This procedure can be conducted as open or laparoscopic surgery.

A variety of surgeries to repair hiatal hernias have been developed.

If a person doesn't need immediate surgery, a special corset or truss may be recommended to prevent sudden changes in abdominal pressure, but trusses are considered only temporary measures, not a solution to the problem.

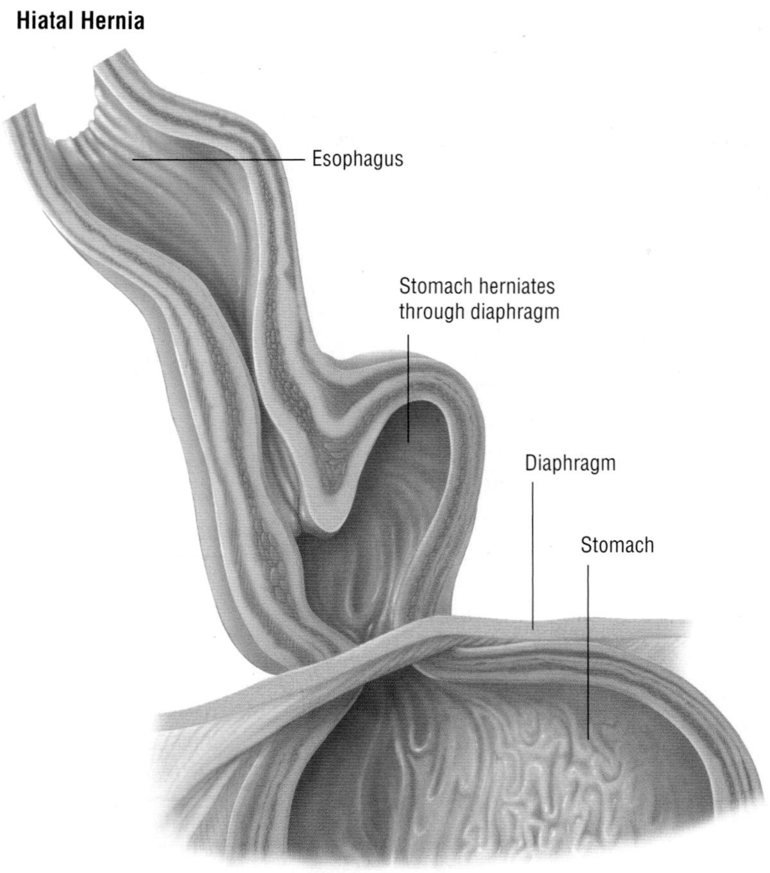

FIGURE 3.38 Hiatal hernia: the stomach protrudes through the diaphragm

Medications

- Antibiotics if strangulation of internal structures occurs
- Medications to manage acid reflux for hiatal hernias

Massage Therapy Implications

RISKS	Untreated hernias are local contraindications for specific massage, because the fascial wall is already compromised: any extra pressure or stretching would not be helpful.
BENEFITS	Gentle massage around the edges of new postoperative scars, and directly applied to older scars, may be helpful in scar tissue organization. Clients who have successfully treated a hernia in the past can enjoy all the benefits of bodywork as does the rest of the population.

Morton Neuroma

Definition: What Is It?

Morton neuroma is a situation in which the connective tissue sheath that encases the common digital nerves of the toes becomes thickened. The term "neuroma" is a misnomer; this is not a nerve tumor. Instead, it is perineurial fibrosis: a pathologic condition of the **perineurium**.

Demographics

The incidence of Morton neuroma isn't tracked, but it is generally regarded as a common condition. Women are diagnosed with Morton neuroma about five times more frequently than are men.

Etiology: What Happens?

The bones in the long part of the foot are the metatarsals, numbered 1 to 5 from medial to lateral. Their distal heads form the "ball" of the foot.

The common digital nerves supply sensation and motor control for the distal foot. Their branches converge between the superior aspects of the metatarsal heads. At this location, they can be squeezed from all sides when pressure is translated across the bottom of the foot and toward the toes, as during the "toe-off" phase of walking.

Perineurium: Connective tissue wrapping around bundles of nerve fibers.

3 Musculoskeletal System Conditions

Several issues can contribute to nerve irritation in the ball of the foot. The nerve is embedded in thick fascia, the perineurium, all the way down the leg. If that fascia is tight and restrictive, it inhibits the ability of the nerve to function well, and increases the risk of entrapment or stretching of the nerve. Additionally, muscle tightness in the hamstrings or plantarflexors can pull on or compress the medial and lateral plantar nerves that eventually become the common digital nerves. People who spend a lot of their day in heels put pressure at the metatarsal heads, just where the nerves are compressed under the intermetatarsal ligaments.

The net result is that the fascial sheath around the irritated nerves becomes fibrotic, which only puts more pressure exactly where it is already a problem. Any other foot problem that alters the gait or puts extra weight on the ball of the foot can contribute to the pattern. **Plantar fasciitis**, **bunions**, **hammer toe**, **pes planus**, and **pes cavus** are frequent contributors to Morton neuroma.

Signs and Symptoms

The irritation that occurs with Morton neuroma creates a characteristic electrical shooting pain that travels distally from the ball of the foot to the toes, usually between the third and fourth metatarsals (Figure 3.39). This happens mainly with walking or other weight bearing, rather than at rest.

Treatment

If Morton neuroma is identified early, it can be treated with a change in footwear, orthotics, and pads for the metatarsal heads. Careful stretching and massage therapy may also be a part of this strategy.

More invasive options include steroid injections to reduce the bulk of the fibroma, or injections to kill the sensory neurons if the pain is intractable. Surgery may be conducted to remove the connective tissue mass, but the risk of complications is fairly high.

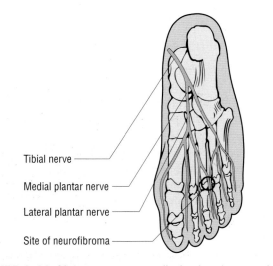

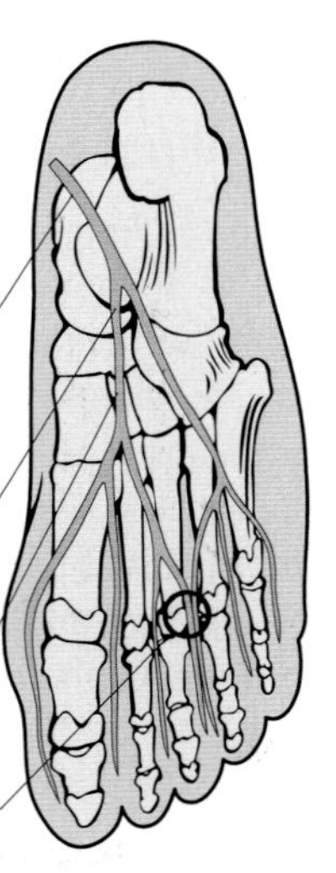

FIGURE 3.39 Morton neuroma usually develops between the 3rd and 4th metatarsals

Massage Therapy Implications

RISKS	Squeezing the metatarsal heads may elicit symptoms. Avoid this maneuver, and most other types of massage are safe and appropriate for clients with Morton neuroma.
BENEFITS	Massage therapy appears to offer some benefits to clients with Morton neuroma, as is evidenced by the natural response to rub our tender feet when we are in pain. As long as symptoms are not exacerbated, most types of massage are safe, and some could be helpful in reducing the irritation both at the compression site in the foot and along the length of the sciatic nerve where the affected branches begin.
OPTIONS	Work directly on the foot to create space between the affected metatarsals is helpful as long as symptoms are not made worse. This can be coupled with massage and stretching to the whole posterior aspect of the leg, where the source of the common digital nerves can be freed from fascial restrictions.
RESEARCH	One case report found that a client with Morton neuroma had less pain and more ability to exercise with massage.[1] This is worthwhile in itself, but it is especially so because this client had not had success with other noninvasive therapies and was contemplating surgery. 1. Davis F. Therapeutic massage provides pain relief to a client with Morton's neuroma: a case report. *International Journal of Therapeutic Massage and Bodywork* 2012;5(2):12–19. http://www.ncbi.nlm.nih.gov/pmc/articles/PMC3390214/

Plantar Fasciitis

Definition: What Is It?

Plantar fasciitis (PF) is a common condition involving pain at the plantar fascia, which stretches from the calcaneus to the proximal phalanges on the plantar surface of the foot. While the suffix "-itis" implies that this is an inflammatory condition, PF is related to the degeneration of collagen more than to chronic inflammation. Consequently it is more accurately termed "fasciosis," but this terminology is not yet commonly used.

Demographics

PF is the most common cause of heel pain. It is diagnosed in about a million adults every year, in both sedentary and athletic people. It is associated with foot pronation, excessive running, and prolonged standing. Women are diagnosed about twice as often as are men.

Etiology: What Happens?

The plantar fascia is a tough band of connective tissue that supports the medial longitudinal arch of the foot. It is thickest in the middle of the band and thinner on the medial and lateral aspects. It is vulnerable to damage through anatomic and repetitive biomechanical forces.

Plantar fasciitis often occurs in conjunction with the growth of bone spurs on the calcaneus. While these spurs were once assumed to be the source of heel pain, that assumption is no longer taken for granted.

Excessive running, especially in worn-down shoes, is a contributor to PF. Being overweight can predispose some people to plantar fasciitis, as can sudden changes in activity levels. Unequal leg length, flat or pronated feet, and jammed arches are associated with this problem. Very tight calf muscles are also contributing factors, especially for runners. And plantar fasciitis may occur as a secondary complication to an underlying disorder such as **gout**, **rheumatoid arthritis**, or **diabetes**. It is frequently bilateral.

When the plantar fascia is overused or stressed, its fibers tend to fray or become disorganized (Figure 3.40). The quality of the tissue degrades, fibroblasts become large, and they produce excessive, disorganized collagen. Function of the plantar fascia as an effective spring and shock absorber is gradually lost. Imaging studies show that the disorganized fascia is thicker than healthy structures, but plantar fasciitis is not an inflammatory condition. Rather, it is the result of degeneration of the collagen matrix of the plantar aponeurosis. The absence of acute inflammation has some implications for determining the best treatment options, so it is an important point to consider.

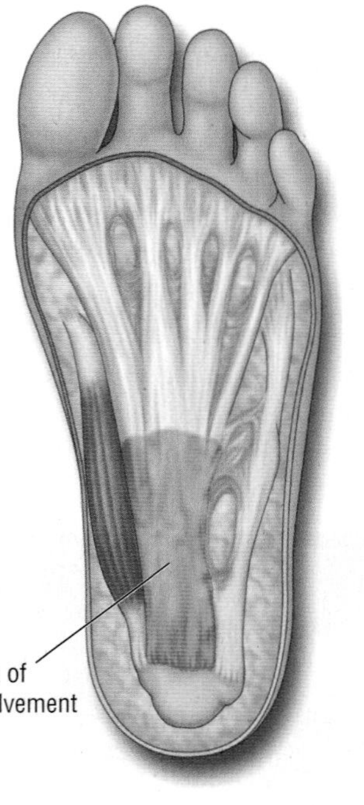

FIGURE 3.40 Plantar fasciitis

Signs and Symptoms

Plantar fasciitis follows a distinctive pattern that makes it easy to identify: it is acutely painful for the first few steps after a period of immobility. Then the pain subsides or disappears altogether, but becomes a problem again with prolonged standing, walking, or running. A sharp bruised feeling either just anterior to the calcaneus on the plantar surface or deep in the arch of the foot often marks this disorder.

Treatment

The most important thing to do for PF is to manage the tensions that cause the plantar fascia to be irritated after periods of immobility, especially first thing in the morning. Warming and massaging the foot and lower leg before getting out of bed can make the tissue more flexible. Orthotics or heel cups can keep the foot from going into deep dorsiflexion. Some experts suggest that heel cups in particular are better targeted at heel fat pad degeneration rather than PF. Another device that many patients find helpful is a night splint that holds the foot in a slightly dorsiflexed position. This allows the plantar fascia fibers to heal in a way that won't be stressed and irritated so easily.

Ice, stretching, and deep massage to the calf muscles and at the site of the irritation are frequently prescribed as a first strategy for plantar fasciitis. Corticosteroid injections are sometimes given if other interventions are unsuccessful, but steroids damage the fat pads on the heels and may weaken the collagen fibers and increase the risk of plantar fascia rupture, so they are used only sparingly. Proliferant or Botox injections may be employed, and **extracorporeal shockwave lithotripsy** is used with some success for plantar fasciitis, and may also be directed at some of the calf muscles that are involved. As a final option, surgery may be performed to divide sections of the plantar fascia.

No single treatment is universally effective; each patient must experiment with the treatments that meet his or her own needs. Most people eventually find relief, but it may take 6 to 18 months before all symptoms are resolved.

Medications

- NSAIDs for pain management
- Cortisone injection for anti-inflammatory and collagen-dissolving effect

Extracorporeal shockwave lithotripsy: A treatment for kidney stones and gallbladder stones using focused ultrasound energy.

Massage Therapy Implications

RISKS	If a client has used cortisone injections to treat his or her PF, massage at the site should be avoided until the tissues have stabilized. Acute inflammation (which is rare) should be locally avoided in order to not exacerbate symptoms. Otherwise, massage for PF is safe and appropriate.
BENEFITS	Massage is often suggested both to decrease tension in nearby muscles and to have an organizing influence on collagen fibers within the plantar fascia itself.
OPTIONS	A bodywork focus not only on the affected foot but also on the deep calf muscles that control foot alignment is often recommended.
RESEARCH	While massage therapy is often mentioned as a treatment option in studies on PF[1,2] no studies have undertaken looking at massage as a stand-alone treatment option for this condition. 1. Goff JD, Crawford R. Diagnosis and treatment of plantar fasciitis. *American Family Physician* 2011;84(6): 676–682. http://www.aafp.org/afp/2011/0915/p676.html 2. Schwartz EN, Su J. Plantar fasciitis: a concise review. *The Permanente Journal* 2014;18(1):e105–e107. http://www.ncbi.nlm.nih.gov/pmc/articles/PMC3951039/

Pes Planus, Pes Cavus

Definition: What Are They?

Pes planus ("flat feet") is the technical term for feet that lack the medial arch between the calcaneus and the great toe, the lateral arch between the calcaneus and the little toe, and the transverse arch that stretches across the ball of the foot. Another name for this condition is adult-acquired flatfoot deformity.

Pes cavus ("caved feet") is the term for feet with jammed arches, or a hyperaccentuated arch that does not flatten out with each step, but instead stays high and immobile.

Etiology: What Happens?

The feet are architecturally complex. Each one has 26 bones, 33 joints, and more than 100 muscles, tendons, and ligaments to mediate our relation to gravity when we stand. Imbalance at the forefoot, midfoot, or hindfoot can lead to problems in how weight is distributed over the whole surface and how the stress of weight bearing is translated to the rest of the body.

Tarsal coalition: An abnormal fusion of two or more tarsal bones; usually involves the calcaneus and talus or navicular.

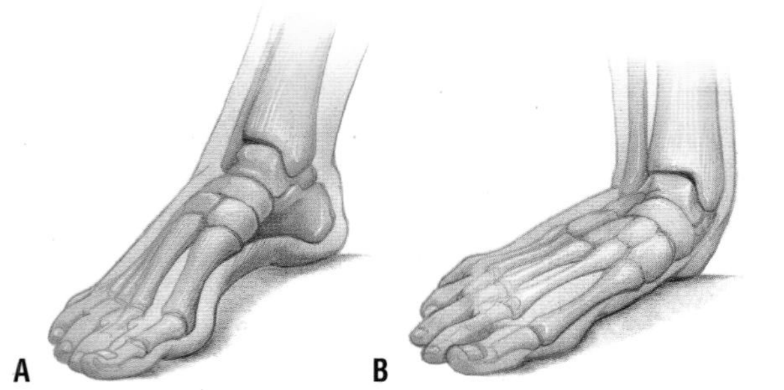

FIGURE 3.41 **A:** Pes cavus. **B:** Pes planus

Pes planus and pes cavus may develop for several reasons. A congenital problem in the shape of the foot bones or the strength of the foot ligaments is one cause. Foot trauma and malunion fractures of the calcaneus or talus may alter the shape of the foot. Problems may also arise from the ongoing battle between the deep flexors and everters, combined with poorly functioning ligaments and footwear that offers little or no support.

Whatever the source of distortion, if the foot bones lack spring and mobility, shock absorption is lost (Figure 3.41). Each time the foot hits the ground, thousands of pounds of downward pressure that should be softly distributed through the tarsal bones reverberates through the rest of the skeleton. In this way, flat feet or jammed arches can lead to **arthritis** in the feet, **plantar fasciitis**, **neuromas**, and then knee problems, hip problems, back pain, even **headaches** and **TMJ disorders**. Furthermore, foot problems can be especially dangerous for people with poor peripheral circulation, because chronic friction and irritation at isolated spots can lead to sores on the feet.

Pes Planus

Pes planus in particular has been studied in relation to an imbalance between the active and passive arch stabilizers, with a particular focus on weakness at the tibialis posterior tendon. This leads to hypertonicity and imbalanced pulling, especially at the peroneus muscles on the lateral aspect of the foot. A failure of ligaments that support the arches of the feet contributes to symptoms. Ultimately, while the medial arch is flattened, the foot veers laterally, putting excessive pull on the medial deltoid ligament (Figure 3.42).

Pes planus in young children is not pathologic; it is normal that the arch-supporting structures tighten later in life. But when children have flat feet and foot pain, it may be due to an abnormal fusion of foot bones called **tarsal coalition**.

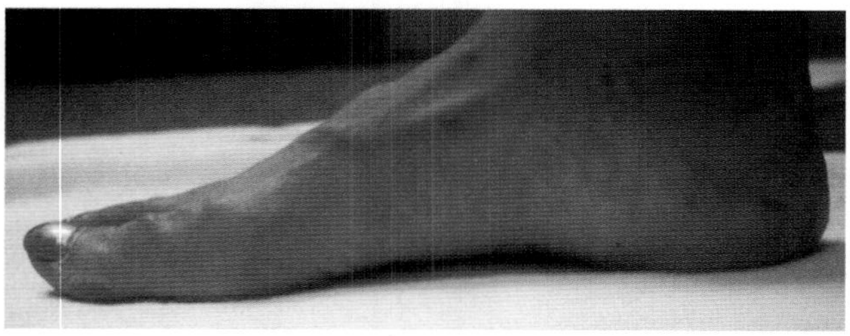

FIGURE 3.42 Pes planus: flatfoot

Pes Cavus

Pes cavus, when it is serious enough to interfere with function, is often examined as a complication of an underlying or preexisting disorder. Malunion **fractures** and **compartment syndrome** are often considered. Neuromuscular disorders, such as **Charcot-Marie-Tooth syndrome**, **muscular dystrophy**, **polio**, or **cerebral palsy**, may contribute to jammed arches. It can be a postsurgical condition following a correction for clubfoot.

When pes cavus has a sudden onset and is bilateral (i.e., not related to a specific trauma), it is likely to have a neurological cause. It could be related to a tumor or other problem in the central nervous system, leading to spasticity in lower leg muscles.

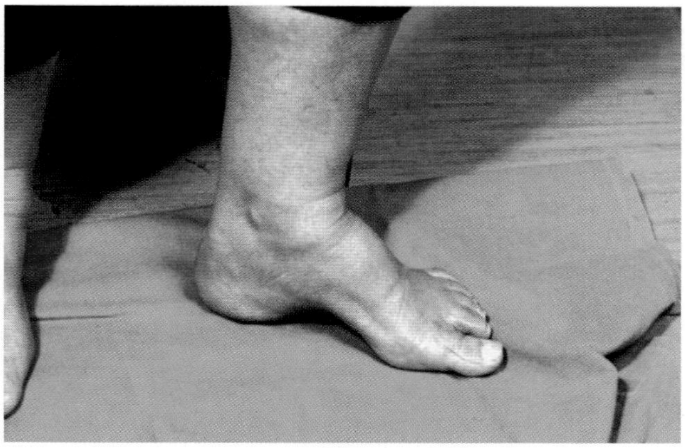

FIGURE 3.43 Pes cavus: rigidly arched foot

Signs and Symptoms

Pes planus signs may be subtle until complications develop. Pain, a visible lack of an arch while standing, and a laterally deviated heel are typical indicators. Pes cavus tends to be more severe and dramatic, especially when it is related to an underlying neuromuscular condition. Along with a rigid arch, patients experience lateral foot pain, extensive callus, and ankle instability (Figure 3.43).

Treatment

A person who is aware that the alignment of his or her feet is a problem may be recommended to switch to highly supportive shoes. Physical therapy to rebalance the peroneus longus and tibialis posterior muscles may be suggested. Orthotics or braces to improve foot alignment can help with pain and dysfunction. Rarely, surgery may be performed to repair injured tendons that can contribute to flat feet, to reshape foot bones, or to fuse foot joints for reduced pain and improved stability.

When pes cavus is related to an underlying condition and function could be restored by surgically releasing tight tissues, this may be considered a viable choice.

Massage Therapy Implications

RISKS	Pes cavus is often connected to an underlying disorder that may require modifications in bodywork. Outside of this caution, massage has little risk for a person with flat feet or jammed arches.
BENEFITS	Deep specific massage to the feet and muscles of the lower legs may improve the local environment to the extent that secondary symptoms are decreased and function improves.

Neuromuscular Disorders

Carpal Tunnel Syndrome

Definition: What Is It?

Carpal tunnel syndrome (CTS) is a set of signs and symptoms brought about by entrapment of the median nerve between the carpal bones of the wrist and the transverse carpal ligament that holds down the flexor tendons (Figure 3.44). The median nerve supplies sensation to the thumb, forefinger, middle finger, and half of the ring finger (Figure 3.45). If it is caught, pinched, or squeezed in any way, it creates symptoms in the part of the hand the nerve supplies. *To explore the anatomy involved, view the video "Median and Ulnar Nerves in the Forearm and Hand," at* http://thePoint.lww.com/Werner6e. thePoint®

Demographics

CTS is the most common peripheral nerve compression syndrome. It is an occupational hazard for massage practitioners and anyone else who performs repetitive movements for several hours every day, including people who work with keyboards, string musicians, bakers, assembly line workers, and checkout clerks. Women with CTS outnumber men; this may be because their carpal tunnels are smaller to begin with, so less irritation may lead to symptoms.

Etiology: What Happens?

The source of the pain associated with CTS is debatable. While some experts claim that pressure directly on the nerve causes pain, others suggest that pressure impedes blood flow to the nerve, and that is the source of the problem.

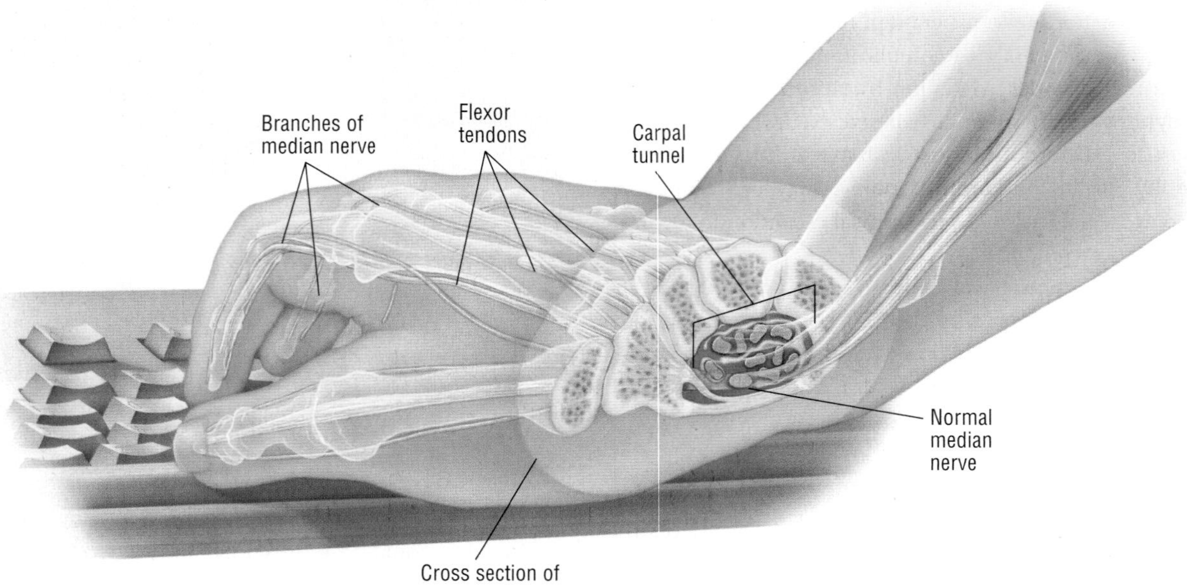

FIGURE 3.44 Carpal tunnel syndrome: median nerve compression can be exacerbated by extension at the wrist and repetitive motion

Whether the damage is to the nerve itself or to its blood supply, irritation within the carpal tunnel may arise from several sources. To develop a treatment strategy (and to assess the appropriateness of massage), the aggravating factors must be determined. These factors include edema, subluxation of a carpal bone, or what is probably the most common situation: fibrotic buildup of connective tissues in the wrist due to repetitive use.

What makes CTS especially challenging to identify and treat, however, is that many things can mimic or contribute to nerve pain in the hand, and these must also be addressed for successful outcomes. The possibilities include but are not limited to the following:

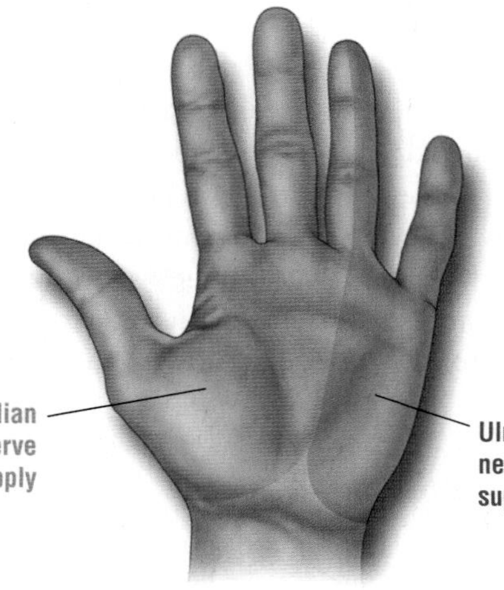

FIGURE 3.45 Nerve supply to the hand

- *Neck injury*. **Herniated discs** and irritated neck ligaments refer pain distally. The worse the irritation, the further the pain refers.
- *General nerve impairment*. When a nerve is irritated, the flow of nutrients and wastes can be impaired along its entire length. This puts it at risk for irritation at multiple sites in addition to the wrist, all of which must be addressed for successful treatment. Cervical disruption, disc pressure, **thoracic outlet syndrome**, or entrapment or elongation elsewhere in the arm can all irritate the median nerve, which can then also become compressed at the carpal tunnel. This is sometimes referred to as **double crush**, or **multiple crush syndrome**.
- *Other wrist injuries*. These can include **osteoarthritis**, **rheumatoid arthritis**, **tendinosis**, and sprains, all of which can cause pain in the wrist and hand and none of which will be affected by any of the standard treatments for CTS.

CTS can also be a symptom or consequence of several other systemic diseases. **Diabetes**, **hypothyroidism**, lymphedema associated with cancer staging, **acromegaly**, **rheumatoid arthritis**, and **gout** can all involve pressure at the carpal tunnel.

Double crush syndrome: Irritation of peripheral nerves at multiple sites, leading to confusing signs and symptoms. Also called "multiple crush syndrome."

Multiple crush syndrome: Irritation of peripheral nerves at multiple sites, leading to confusing signs and symptoms. Also called "double crush syndrome"

Signs and Symptoms

Depending on the source and severity of the problem, CTS can manifest as tingling; pins and needles; burning, shooting pains; intermittent numbness; and weakness as innervation to the hand muscles is interrupted. The thenar pad may flatten out as the thumb muscles atrophy. It is often worse at night, when people may sleep on their arm, or turn their wrist into awkward positions. It can be painful enough to wake someone out of a deep sleep.

Commonly used tests for CTS include the **Phalen test** and **Tinel sign**. These are simple to do, and yield some information about pressure at the wrist; they do not reveal anything about nerve compression happening elsewhere, however.

To explore this further, you can view the following videos: "Tinel's Sign for Median Nerve Pathology" and "Phalen's (Wrist Flexion) Test," both available at http://thePoint.lww.com/Werner6e. thePoint®

If pressure is taken off the nerve promptly, CTS symptoms may completely disappear: this is a best-case scenario. But the other end of the spectrum is permanent damage to the median nerve, resulting in loss of muscle function and sensation in the hand.

Treatment

Treatment for CTS often begins with a wrist splint. The goal is to keep the carpal tunnel in a neutral position (in which it is as spacious as possible) and to require less work from the supportive tissues. Anti-inflammatories may be recommended or prescribed. Corticosteroid injections into the wrist may also be recommended to reduce inflammation and dissolve excess connective tissue. Exercises to stretch and mobilize tight wrist tendons may be recommended. Acupuncture, chiropractic, low-level laser treatments, and yoga may be suggested as other noninvasive strategies to deal with CTS symptoms.

If no other interventions are successful, CTS treatment culminates with surgery. The transverse carpal ligament is split, and some of the accumulated connective tissue is scraped away. This may be done as an open or endoscopic procedure. Surgery isn't entirely successful, however, if other sites of nerve irritation aren't addressed.

Medications

- NSAIDs for pain and inflammation
- Injected steroids for connective tissue dissolution and anti-inflammatory action
- Injected lidocaine for pain relief

Phalen test: A common test for carpal tunnel syndrome in which the wrists are held in flexion for 60 seconds or longer.

Tinel sign: A test used to detect an irritated nerve (such as in carpal tunnel syndrome) by tapping directly over the nerve.

Massage Therapy Implications

RISKS	Any work that creates CTS symptoms should be modified immediately. Otherwise, CTS is only a local caution that may be appropriate for careful work that doesn't cause pain.
BENEFITS	Massage that doesn't exacerbate symptoms has been shown to contribute to improvement in strength, function, and symptoms for CTS patients.
OPTIONS	Specific work within pain tolerance on the hand, wrist, forearm, and shoulder of a person with CTS may have some success at decompressing the median nerve.
RESEARCH	The evidence in favor of massage therapy as an effective, low-risk, noninvasive strategy for CTS is fairly consistent. Elliot and Burkett[1] found that massage coupled with trigger point therapy helped to reduce symptoms and improve function. Madenci et al.[2] developed a self-massage protocol for use with nighttime splinting that compared favorably to the use of a hand splint alone in a group of 80 patients. Moraska et al.[3] compared general full-body massage to specifically targeted massage to the wrist, arm, and shoulder of CTS patients; while both groups reported an improvement in subjective measures, only the targeted massage group showed an improvement in grip strength.

1. Elliott R, Burkett B. Massage therapy as an effective treatment for carpal tunnel syndrome. *Journal of Bodywork and Movement Therapies* 2013;17(3):332–338. http://www.ncbi.nlm.nih.gov/pubmed/23768278
2. Madenci E, Altindag O, Koca I, et al. Reliability and efficacy of the new massage technique on the treatment in the patients with carpal tunnel syndrome. *Rheumatology International* 2012;32(10):3171–3179. http://www.ncbi.nlm.nih.gov/pmc/articles/PMC3456919/
3. Moraska A, Chandler C, Edmiston-Schaetzel A, et al. Comparison of a targeted and general massage protocol on strength, function, and symptoms associated with carpal tunnel syndrome: a randomized pilot study. *Journal of Alternative and Complementary Medicine* 2008;14(3):259–267. http://www.ncbi.nlm.nih.gov/pubmed/18370581

Disc Disease

Definition: What Is It?

Disc disease is an umbrella term referring to a collection of problems in which the nucleus pulposus and/or the anulus fibrosus of an intervertebral disc extends beyond its normal borders. Pain is present if the disc presses on the spinal cord or spinal nerve roots. If the bulge or crack doesn't happen to interfere with nerve tissue, no symptoms may be present at all.

Another term for the general label of disc disease that is finding usage among specialists is "intervertebral disc degeneration," or IDD. This term is often used alongside a closely related problem, intervertebral disc displacement. In this section we will use the more familiar term "herniated disc" for that delineation.

Demographics

It is estimated that up to 80% of the population will experience low back pain at some point, and disc disease is a common contributor. Not surprisingly, lumbar disc degeneration is most common among overweight and obese adults over 40 years of age. Factors in disc injury include overuse patterns, but studies of disc disease in twins reveal that genetics may play an even bigger role in how well the disc structures maintain their internal integrity.

Etiology: What Happens?

A typical intervertebral disc is a complex package. It has an outer wrapping of very tough, hard material called the anulus fibrosus. This wraps around a soft, gelatinous center called the nucleus pulposus. Ideally, the nucleus should be roughly spherical, with the harder annulus layers forming a firm surface around the ball. Cartilage endplates attach the disc to the adjoining vertebral bodies. This combination of textures gives the disc the ability to resist both compressive and shearing forces (Figure 3.46). *To explore the anatomy of the spinal column, view the video "Ligaments of the Vertebral Column, Intervertebral Disks" at* http://thePoint.lww.com/Werner6e. thePoint®

The anulus fibrosus is an arrangement of concentric circles of collagen fibers. These fibers are arranged so that when they are pulled, as in the posterior part of the disc during flexion of the spine, they become stiffer. On the other hand, the closer the vertebrae are, the looser and weaker the annulus is—this is what happens on the anterior side of the spine during flexion. This pattern has important implications for the nucleus pulposus, which relies on a tight, solid exterior wall for support.

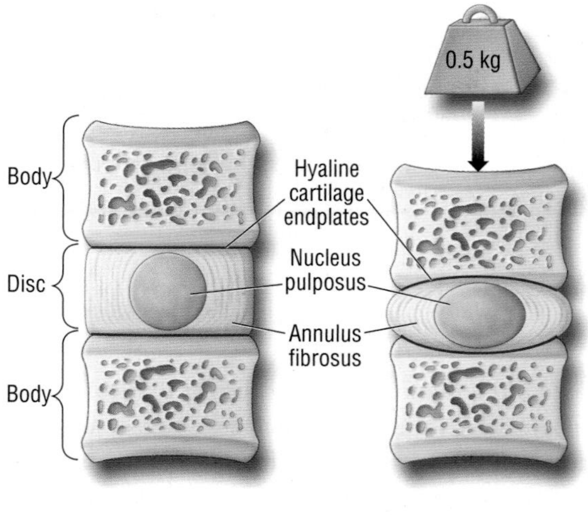

FIGURE 3.46 Intervertebral discs increase the weight-bearing capacity of the spine

The nucleus pulposus often becomes thinner and dryer with age. This means the annulus must bear more weight and absorb more shock and shearing. Consequently, as we age, the annulus has an increased risk for developing cracks or fissures. The cartilage endplates may ossify as the connecting vertebrae respond; osteophytes frequently develop on the lip of the vertebral bodies or around the facet joints. In this way, disc disease is closely aligned to **spondylosis**.

Causes of disc injury may vary according to the general resiliency and age of the connective tissues of the person involved. For some people, it takes a major trauma such as a car accident or a bad fall to damage a disc. But some people with weak, loose intervertebral ligaments have a risk of disc damage from ordinary everyday activity. The classic scenario for this kind of disc damage is an incident that involves simultaneous lifting and twisting:

- A person bends over to pick up something heavy: a big basket of laundry, for instance. Trunk flexion flattens the anterior portion of the nucleus and opens up a posterior space, while stretching the posterior fibers of the annulus, making them taut and strong.
- The person jerks into an erect posture, possibly twisting at the same time, while carrying a heavy load. Suddenly coming into extension, especially while carrying something heavy, quickly redistributes the nucleus and shoots it into that posterior space with great force. The posterior annulus fibers are now at their weakest, most lax position.
- The nucleus presses against the weakest part of the posterior annulus, and breaks through, putting pressure on nerve roots. Or the force of the motion, combined with the brittleness of the annulus, causes the annulus to crack and put pressure on nerve tissue.
- The injury triggers an inflammatory response that can be a major contributor to the nerve pain that accompanies these injuries.

The kind of lifting-and-twisting injury described here usually affects the discs below L4 and L5. Cervical disc lesions can occur with sports injuries, **whiplash**, and similar trauma, usually at the disc below C5 or C6. Thoracic injuries are possible but rarer, since the ribs make the thoracic spine much more stable than its cervical and lumbar counterparts.

Discs that cause pain usually bulge posterolaterally, because that is the path of least resistance in the tight space they inhabit, but they can also go to the left or the right side (Figures 3.47 and 3.48).

Most injured discs are temporarily painful but don't lead to permanent or serious problems. The most serious complication of a disc injury is the threat of pressure exerted directly posteriorly. In the neck, this means the spinal cord is

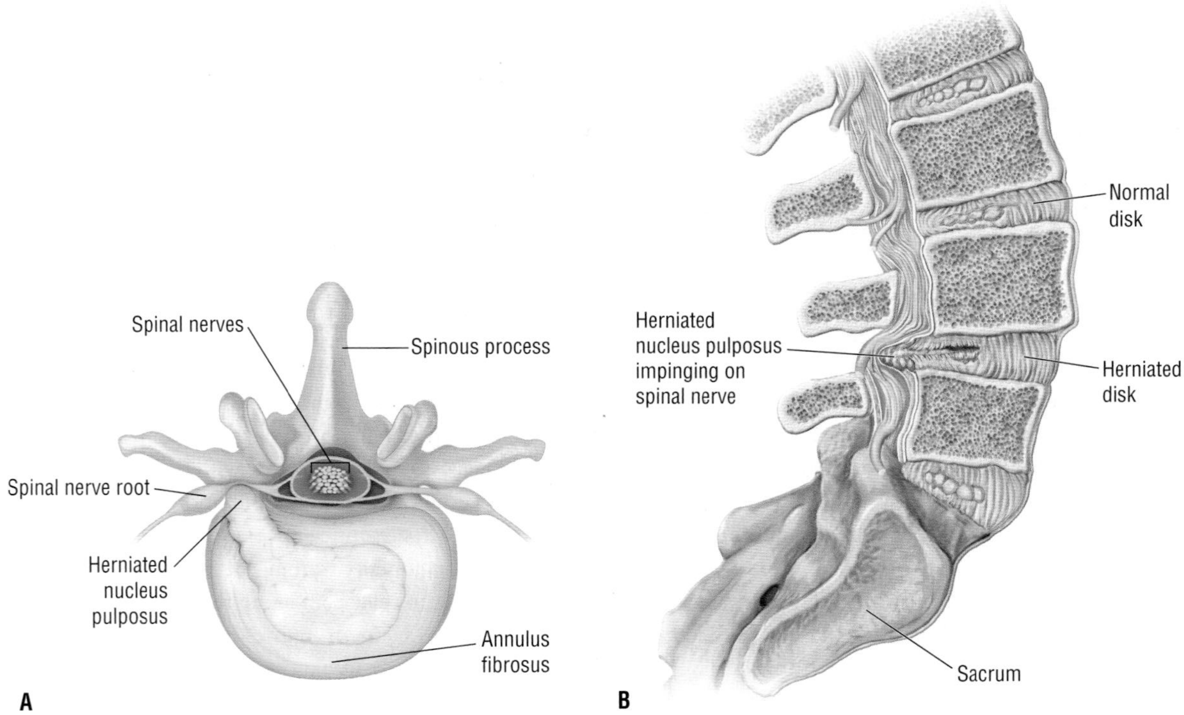

FIGURE 3.47 Herniated disc

compressed; in the lumbar spine it is called **cauda equina syndrome** because the disc material presses on the extensions of spinal nerves between T1 and S5 called the cauda equina. Direct spinal cord compression leads to some specific signs, including hyperactive reflexes; bilateral pain, **paresthesia**, or numbness in a "saddle" distribution; and the loss of bladder or bowel control. Any of these problems can become permanent, or paralysis can develop, if pressure is not resolved quickly.

Types of Disc Problems

It is useful to be able to recognize the terminology for disc problems that may turn up in a diagnosis. Disc problems are generally discussed as three major issues: herniated discs with several subtypes, degenerative disc disease, and internal disc disruption. A fourth possibility, endplate junction failure, has recently been added to this list.

- *Herniated disc*: The nucleus pulposus extends beyond the margin of the vertebral body. These injuries are most common in young adults. The nucleus may be damaged in these ways:

> **Cauda equina syndrome:** A condition in which the inferior part of the spinal cord is damaged, resulting in loss of function.
>
> **Paresthesia:** An abnormal sensation, such as burning, prickling, tickling, or tingling.

- *Bulge*. The entire disc protrudes symmetrically beyond the normal boundaries of the vertebral body.
- *Protrusion*. The nucleus pulposus extends out of the annulus at a specific location. If it protrudes posterolaterally (the most common version), it may press on

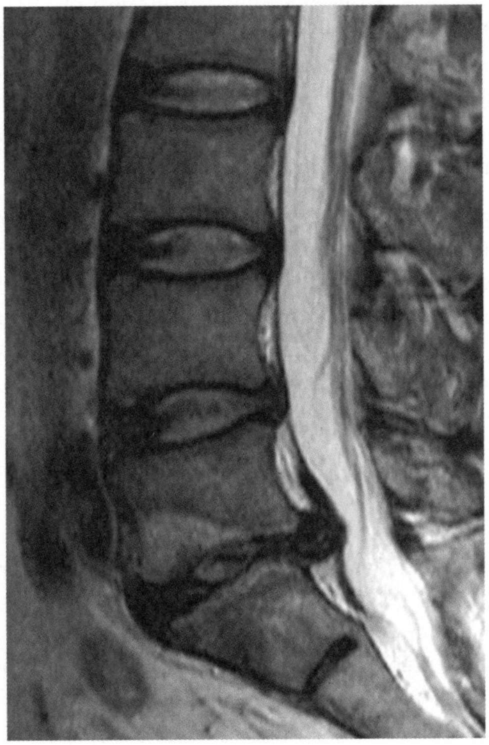

FIGURE 3.48 Herniated disc at L5-S1

nerve roots. If it protrudes straight back, it may press on the spinal cord or cauda equina.
  - *Extrusion*. A small piece of the nucleus protrudes, with a narrow connection back to the body of the nucleus. In some cases, the protrusion can separate from the nucleus altogether; this is called a sequestration.
  - *Rupture*. The nucleus pulposus has burst and leaked its entire contents into the surrounding area.
- *Degenerative disc disease*: This refers to small, cumulative tears of the annulus, along with decreased disc height and dehydration of the nucleus. Eventually the annulus may press against a nerve root or the spinal cord. Alternatively, the disc can degenerate and shrink in place without symptoms, but the adjoining vertebrae may fuse together.
- *Internal disc disruption*: This condition is often related to trauma in addition to degenerative disc disease. In this case, the nucleus protrudes through the annulus but stays within the boundaries of the whole disc.
- *Endplate junction failure*: Careful study of the images of many disc disease surgical patients has led to the identification of another feature present in many cases: failure of the connection between the cartilage endplate and the adjoining vertebral body. Avulsions of the cartilage or bone fragments were found in many of the images. This discovery changes the point of focus for orthopedists and surgeons for helping patients with this condition.

Signs and Symptoms

It is important to point out that disc degeneration can occur without major symptoms. When symptoms do occur, they usually arise from pressure on nerve tissue or from an extreme inflammatory response that occurs when the nucleus pulposus leaks. Nerve pressure can come and go as the patient's position and alignment shift, and so once the initial inflammation subsides, pain may be intermittent.

- *Local and radicular pain*: pain that radiates along the dermatome of the affected nerve root. Pain is often described as shooting, burning, or electrical. When pain originates from a lumbar disc injury, it may cause pain through the buttock and down the back of the leg: this is often called **sciatica**, although other professionals use that term to mean irritation of the sciatic nerve elsewhere than at the spinal roots.

Sciatica: Irritation of the sciatic nerve. Often causes pain that radiates down the leg through the buttox.

Papain: An enzyme derived from papayas that is used to dissolve connective tissue. Also used as a meat tenderizer.

Discectomy: The surgical removal of some or all of a vertebral disc.

- *Specific muscle weakness*: weakness or even atrophy in the muscles that are affected by irritated nerves. (This is different from general muscle weakness that can arise from overall deconditioning.)
- *Paresthesia*: "pin and needles" in the affected dermatome.
- *Reduced sensation*: (This can also be a sign of ligament damage instead of or in addition to disc damage.)
- *Numbness*: Total numbness is one distinguishing factor between disc problems and ligament injuries.

Treatment

The most successful treatment outcomes for disc injuries depend on an accurate diagnosis. Red flags that must be ruled out include the possibility of cancer, infection, spinal **fracture** and, in the cervical spine, problems with the structure or function of the vertebral artery. One situation that mimics a disc problem but is actually much less serious is a ligament **sprain**: irritated spinal ligaments running between spinous or transverse processes can refer pain along the same dermatomes as the nearby discs. Ligament injuries do not cause total numbness or specific muscle weakness, however, and they respond well to specific types of massage. Another factor in this equation is the presence of stenosis due to spondylosis, and bone spurs that may exert pressure on the spinal cord or nerve roots.

It is difficult to determine if any given treatment option is better than allowing time to do its work; this often results in relief of symptoms without long-term problems.

The main goal of disc disease treatment is to create a situation where pressure on nerve roots is relieved. Chiropractors and osteopaths work to correct bony alignment and to create a maximum of space for the nucleus to retreat back to its normal boundaries. Medical doctors recommend short-term bed rest or traction, followed by movement within tolerance, for the same reason. Physical therapy and education on correct posture and body mechanics are often recommended to people recovering from disc problems.

If noninvasive strategies are insufficient, a variety of other options exist. Injections of cortisone to deinflame the area are sometimes used. Injected **papain** (derived from papaya enzymes) may be used to dissolve some of the disc material. Surgery to remove the disc (**discectomy**), with or without spinal fusion of the connecting vertebrae, is also possible, but most research suggests that this should be used only in cases that don't respond to less invasive strategies.

Medications

- NSAIDs for pain and inflammation control
- Short-term narcotic analgesics if necessary
- Antiseizure drugs or tricyclic antidepressants for nerve pain
- Steroidal anti-inflammatories, including injected cortisone, for inflammation control
- Injected papain to help dissolve displaced proteins
- Injected lidocaine to myofascial trigger points causing pain around injured discs
- Muscle relaxants

Massage Therapy Implications

RISKS	Disc problems can be complex and difficult to pin down; these are situations where massage therapists can benefit most by working as part of a health care team. Acute inflammation and muscle splinting to guard an unstable area call for bodywork that respects these processes rather than interfering with them.
BENEFITS	Massage therapy for low back pain in general is often successful for symptom management. Bodywork with the intent to create space for a disc to retreat and to reduce muscle spasm and inflammation (after the acute stage has passed) may be especially useful for clients with disc problems.
OPTIONS	People with disc problems may have difficulties with any position that puts their back into hyperextension. Bolsters or body cushions may be needed to avoid aggravating symptoms.
RESEARCH	Small-scale studies and case reports support the use of massage therapy for back and neck pain in general, and some studies have targeted postsurgical degenerative disc disease clients[1] and clients hoping to avoid surgery.[2] A larger-scale review[3] didn't find enough evidence to endorse massage therapy for disc problems, but that doesn't mean it is ineffective; it means that not enough research has been done to come to a conclusion about this question. 1. Keller G. The effects of massage therapy after decompression and fusion surgery of the lumbar spine: a case study. *International Journal of Therapeutic Massage and Bodywork* 2012;5(4):3–8. http://www.ncbi.nlm.nih.gov/pubmed/23429839 2. Avery RM. Massage therapy for cervical degenerative disc disease: alleviating a pain in the neck? *International Journal of Therapeutic Massage and Bodywork* 2012;5(3):41–46. http://ijtmb.org/index.php/ijtmb/article/view/146/232 3. Jordan J, Konstantinou K, O'Dowd J. Herniated lumbar disc. *Clinical Evidence (Online)* 2011;2011. http://www.ncbi.nlm.nih.gov/pmc/articles/PMC3275148/

Myofascial Pain Syndrome

Definition: What Is It?

Myofascial pain syndrome (MPS) is a condition that is identified when a person develops many trigger points: pain-generating spots in muscles that are palpable as knots or taut bands.

Demographics

The incidence of myofascial pain syndrome is unknown, but it is reported equally among men and women. It is estimated that over 14% of the United States population has chronic musculoskeletal pain in which MPS may be a factor. Even in asymptomatic people, latent trigger points are found 25% to 54% of the time.

Sedentary people appear to develop active trigger points more often than do physically active people.

Etiology: What Happens?

Myofascial trigger points probably develop as a multifactorial process. Traditionally it was thought that they began as microscopic injuries to individual muscle fiber, and these fibers descend into a pain-spasm-ischemia cycle. This may be the situation with some trigger points, but many trigger points are more closely related to problems with the synapse between the motor neuron and the motor endplate of the myofiber: this makes myofascial pain syndrome (MPS) primarily a neuromuscular condition.

The main issue in a trigger point is a sustained, involuntary contraction of an isolated group of **sarcomeres** (the overlapping units of myofibrils that create the striations seen in skeletal muscle cells). If this occurs close to the neuromuscular junction, it is called a central trigger point. Contractions that develop close to the tenoperiosteal junction may also involve folded and dehydrated collagen fibers; these are called attachment trigger points.

When a microscopic contraction of the sarcomeres pulls on the rest of the myofiber, it creates a taut band. This gives rise to two simultaneous problems: an increased need for fuel, and a decreased supply of blood due to local ischemia. This situation is sometimes called an **ATP energy crisis** (Figure 3.49). Chemicals that increase sensitivity and pain are released, including prostaglandins, bradykinin, serotonin, substance P, and others: this helps to generate and reinforce pain sensation. In response to pain, more of the muscle attempts to tighten, causing more secretion of acetylcholine (ACh). Poor local circulation limits the availability of ACh-neutralizing enzymes, it keeps irritating chemicals present, and it inhibits the movement of calcium back into channels in the cell membrane.

Sarcomere: The contracting part of a myofibril.

ATP energy crisis: The cycle of involuntary muscle cell contraction that leads to an increased need for fuel and a decreased supply of blood.

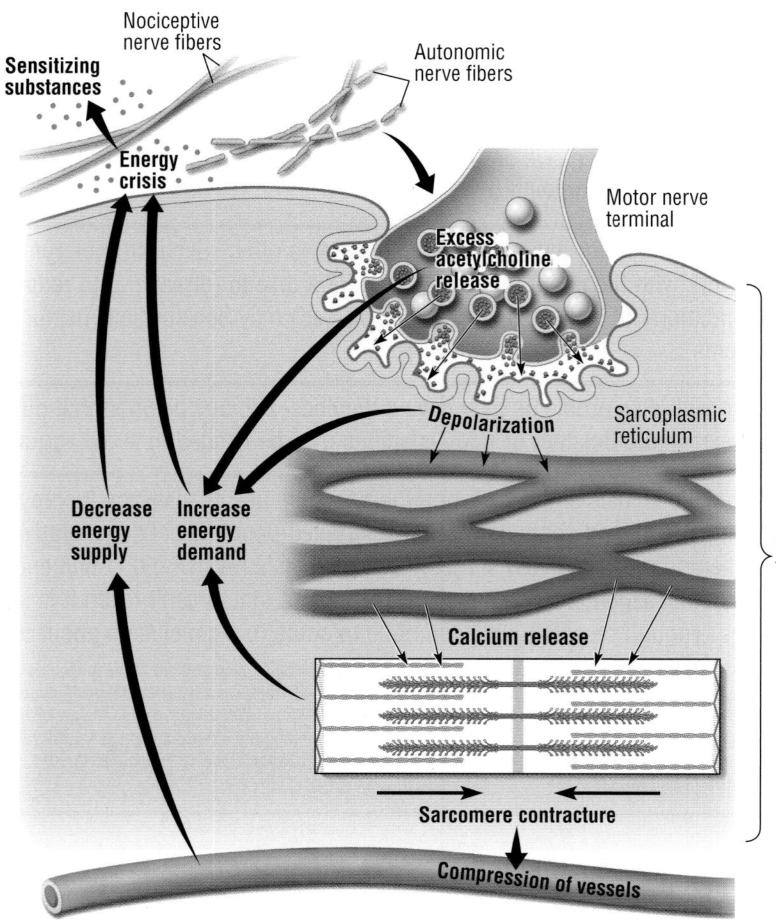

FIGURE 3.49 ATP energy crisis

The consequence: a tiny, involuntary, but prolonged and painful contraction of one part of a muscle cell.

Prolonged exposure to pain-causing chemicals takes a toll on local sensory neurons. Some research suggests that the neurons become locally demyelinated, which may contribute to the unique referred pain pattern seen with trigger points (Figure 3.50). Further, the sensory neurons in the spinal cord that receive signals from the neurons in the peripheral system can become sensitized, that is, excessively reactive to pain inputs from trigger points.

Trigger points that are not frequently irritated may become latent: they are not painful, and they do not refer pain, but they are functionally tight. Latent trigger points are associated with restricted range of motion and muscle weakness. Further, very little stimulus can turn a latent trigger point into an active one, which is locally and distantly painful even when the muscle is at rest.

Satellite points are trigger points that form as secondary issue to primary trigger points. They may develop in areas where referred pain is perceived, in areas where muscle fibers are overloaded because of compensation patterns to protect a primary trigger point, in the antagonists to muscles with active trigger points, or in muscles that are referred pain areas for the heart or other organs.

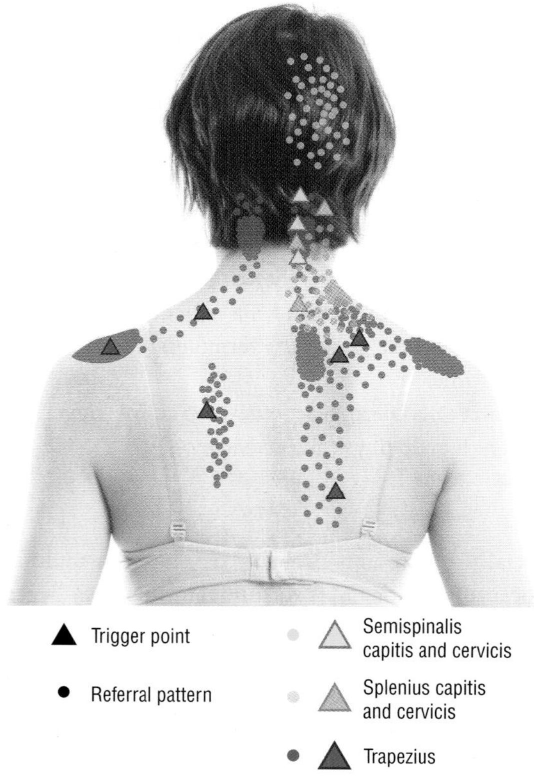

FIGURE 3.50 Referred pain from trigger points

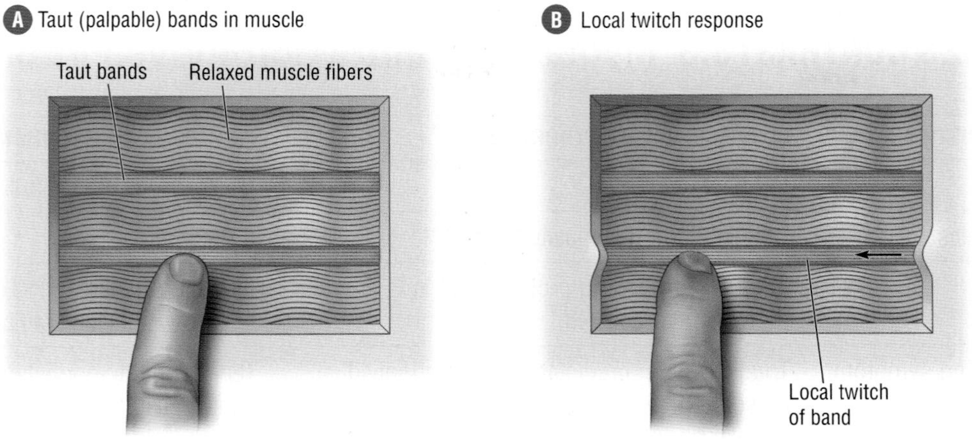

FIGURE 3.51 **A:** Taut bands are easily palpable. **B:** Local twitch response creates a visible contraction.

Signs and Symptoms

Trigger points have some qualities that make them unique among muscle disorders.

- *Taut bands or nodules*. Trigger points can be palpated in muscle tissue as taut, hypertonic bands of fibers within a mass of muscle that is less tight (Figure 3.51) or as small nodules that dissipate under static or pulsing manual pressure. A muscle flicker, or twitch response, is often seen when a trigger point is palpated.
- *Predictable trigger point map*. Each skeletal muscle in the body has an area or group of areas where trigger points are most likely to form. These areas have been extensively mapped. Interestingly, over 70% of mapped trigger points correspond to acupuncture points used to treat pain.
- *Referred pain pattern*. Active trigger points are always locally painful under digital pressure, but they often refer pain to other areas in the body as well. Their referred pain patterns are consistent from person to person.
- *Regional pain*. MPS is seldom a whole-body dysfunction. More often, trigger points flare up in specific regions, often around the neck and shoulders. Jaw muscles are notorious for developing trigger points, which refer pain all over the face and head. This variety of MPS is often discussed in the context of **temporomandibular joint disorders**.

Other symptoms of MPS are less predictable than is trigger point development. **Sleep disorders** occur occasionally but not consistently. **Depression** and **anxiety** are also possible, especially when a person has little success in getting an accurate diagnosis and effective treatment. These make MPS resemble another chronic pain syndrome, **fibromyalgia**. It is important to distinguish between the two conditions, however, because while tender points (fibromyalgia) and trigger points (MPS) can occur in the same areas, their treatment protocols—especially for bodywork—are different (see Compare & Contrast 3.3).

> **Vapocoolant spray:** A topical anesthetic aerosol spray.

Treatment

The top priority for MPS treatment is to eradicate both active and latent trigger points. This is accomplished in a number of ways, including the use of **vapocoolant spray**, local injections of anesthetics, dry needling, and acupuncture. Injections of botulinum toxin have been explored to block ACh release at the neuromuscular junction. All of these approaches work to interrupt the pain-spasm cycle or the ATP energy crisis, allowing the tight fibers to relax while the muscle is stretched.

Manual therapies in several forms have been seen to have success in the resolution of trigger points. Prolonged ischemic pressure has been the traditional strategy, but approaches to trigger points typically find that pulsing pressure that follows the taut band of the muscle may also be effective, while being somewhat less painful.

For another look at trigger point massage, see the video Abdominal Trigger Points available at http://thePoint.lww.com/Werner6e. thePoint®

Because MPS often develops out of chronic overuse or poor ergonomics, the patient's movement and work habits are often examined and adjusted so that perpetuating factors may be eliminated.

Medications

- NSAIDs for pain management
- Tricyclic antidepressants for pain management
- Injected anesthetics or Botox
- Muscle relaxants
- Transdermal lidocaine patches

3 Musculoskeletal System Conditions

COMPARE & CONTRAST 3.3 Myofascial Pain Syndrome vs. Fibromyalgia

CHARACTERISTICS	MYOFASCIAL PAIN SYNDROME	FIBROMYALGIA SYNDROME
Prevalence	Unknown.	Up to 3% of U.S. population.
Demographics	Women and men equally affected.	85% women.
Prognosis	Can be a short-term problem that is permanently resolved.	Lifelong problem; can be managed, but may never be eradicated.
Distinguishing symptom	Trigger points: predictable spots in individual muscles, areas of hypertonicity. May be nodular or appear as a taut band that generates a twitch response. Manual pressure on active trigger point elicits pain locally, and also in predictable patterns of referral.	Tender points: predictable areas; light pressure yields intense, diffuse pain. Tender points are often hypotonic, and are not always in muscle tissue.
Implications for massage	Responds well to massage; rhythmic pressure can interrupt pain-spasm cycle to eradicate trigger points.	Massage can help, but manual pressure exacerbates tender points.

Massage Therapy Implications

RISKS	A person with many active trigger points not only experiences chronic pain, but may be easy to overtreat because of an abundance of pain-sensitizing chemicals in the tissues. Massage can help to resolve trigger points, but it must also address the residual "cleanup" that must follow.
BENEFITS	Careful massage can be effective to resolve MPS, by addressing the pain-spasm cycle and the ATP energy crisis that occurs where trigger points develop. Various subspecialties of bodywork have been developed to address these issues, and evidence shows both efficacy and safety for their application.
RESEARCH	Many experts accept that massage is effective, but it hasn't been tested rigorously, except in the context of how trigger points contribute to other problems. Several trials suggest that addressing trigger points with massage therapy in the process of treating something else (CTS, headaches, etc.) can be more effective than is treating those conditions without addressing the trigger points.[1–3] 1. Bodes-Pardo G, Pecos-Martin D, Gallego-Izquierdo T, et al. Manual treatment for cervicogenic headache and active trigger point in the sternocleidomastoid muscle: a pilot randomized clinical trial. *Journal of Manipulative and Physiological Therapeutics* 2013;36(7):403–411. http://www.ncbi.nlm.nih.gov/pubmed/2384520 2. Elliott R, Burkett B. Massage therapy as an effective treatment for carpal tunnel syndrome. *Journal of Bodywork and Movement Therapies* 2013;17(3):332–338. http://www.ncbi.nlm.nih.gov/pubmed/23768278 3. Moraska A, Chandler C. Changes in clinical parameters in patients with tension-type headache following massage therapy: a pilot study. *Journal of Manual & Manipulative Therapy* 2008;16(2):106–112. http://www.ncbi.nlm.nih.gov/pmc/articles/PMC2565109/

Thoracic Outlet Syndrome

Definition: What Is It?

Thoracic outlet syndrome (TOS) is a neurovascular entrapment. The nerves of the brachial plexus or the blood vessels running to or from the arm (or some combination thereof) are impinged or impaired at one or more of three places: between the anterior and medial scalenes, between the clavicle and the first rib, or under the coracoid process (Figure 3.52).

Demographics

People who habitually carry heavy loads, who do a lot of repetitive movements with their arms and shoulders, and who spend a lot of time with their arms in the air (electricians,

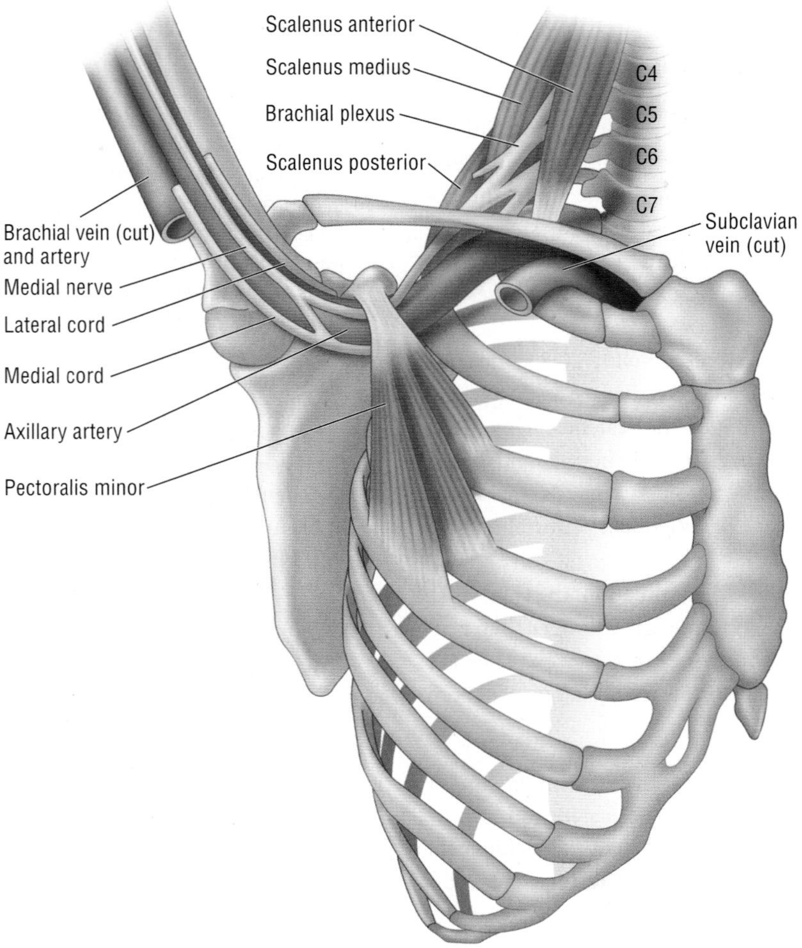

FIGURE 3.52 Thoracic outlet syndrome

plumbers, painters, and so on) are more at risk for thoracic outlet syndrome than is the general population. Women have this more often than men, perhaps because their passageways are smaller and it is easier for structures to be impinged or irritated.

Etiology: What Happens?

The brachial plexus, the network of nerves that supplies the arm with sensation and motor control, consists of spinal nerves C5 to T1. These nerves travel from intervertebral foramina through the anterior and medial scalenes, between the clavicle and the first rib, under the pectoralis minor, and around the humerus. If some part of the plexus is somehow compressed along the way, symptoms develop along the distance of that nerve. The nerve roots C8 and T1, both of which contribute to the ulnar and median nerves, are most at risk for compression with TOS. *To explore the anatomy involved in TOS, view the video Nerves of the Shoulder Region: The Brachial Plexus, available at* http://thePoint.lww.com/Werner6e. thePoint®

Pinched nerves are only one aspect of TOS. This is a neurovascular entrapment, and the vessels at risk are the subclavian vein and the axillary artery, which is a distal portion of the subclavian artery. These vessels can be mechanically obstructed when muscles in small spaces get too tight.

TOS is discussed in many ways in medical literature. It is labeled as neurogenic TOS if it involves only nerve compression. This the most common form of TOS, accounting for 85% to 90% of all cases. It is called vascular TOS if it involves only blood vessels; this condition may be further classified as venous or arterial TOS. Often it is called disputed TOS, because while the patient may have severe symptoms, the exact point of nerve or vascular impression may not be identified. And the term neurovascular TOS suggests that all structures might be involved; this is usually due to a specific trauma.

TOS can be caused by anything that impinges brachial plexus nerves or blood vessels, anywhere from the anterior neck to the anterior chest. Although postural habits and bony growth patterns can make a person susceptible to TOS, it often seems to be precipitated by a specific traumatic event: a hyperextension injury, or a repetitive stress situation similar to the factors seen with **carpal tunnel syndrome**.

The most common contributing factors to TOS include the following:

- *Muscle imbalance*. The anterior and medial scalenes and the pectoralis minor are the muscles most immediately involved with TOS. These tight muscles tend to become shrunken and fibrotic, while their antagonists (rhomboids, trapezius, neck extensors) become stretched out and weak. This leads to a characteristic stooped or caved-in posture that significantly raises the risk of TOS.
- *Connective tissue bands*. Many people with TOS symptoms are found to have excessive connective tissue accumulation around the attachments of the scalenes. This material can put mechanical pressure on nerves and blood vessels. Whether the connective tissue bands are a congenital problem or a result of long-term postural habit is debatable.
- *Cervical ribs*. In about 1% of the population, the transverse processes of the cervical vertebrae grow longer than normal, extending into the soft tissues of the neck. They are usually unilateral, and C7 is the vertebra that grows them most frequently.

Although TOS is diagnosed only when the impingement occurs at the scalenes, at the **costoclavicular space**, or under the coracoid, other factors can contribute to identical symptoms. To treat this condition successfully, it is important to find out exactly where that interference is happening. Some possibilities include misalignment at the cervical vertebrae; **spondylosis**; rib misalignment; injuries to the wrist, elbow, or shoulder (including CTS); or nerve entrapment in the arm that causes the whole nerve to become inflamed. In rare cases, serious nonorthopedic conditions can create symptoms that look like TOC. Lung tumors in the apex of the lung, **aneurysm**, **thrombus**, or nerve damage from surgery can all lead to the collapse of the shoulder girdle and pressure on delicate structures.

Signs and Symptoms

Symptoms of TOS include all signs of nerve irritation: shooting pains, numbness and similar sensations, weakness, tingling, and pins and needles (see Sidebar 3.6). Spinal nerves C8 and T1 are affected most often; these contribute to the ulnar nerve. Vascular symptoms include a feeling of fullness when blood return from a vein is blocked, or cold and weakness when blood flow to the axillary artery is impaired. In rare cases, a throbbing lump above the clavicle may be palpated. A difference in color or temperature of the affected arm may also be noticeable. Neurologic and vascular symptoms tend to be worst at night, when the patient lifts the affected arm over the head, or when the person is tired from other activities. Exposure to cold temperatures tends to make symptoms worse for most people with TOS.

> **Costoclavicular space:** The space between the clavicle and the first rib.

SIDEBAR 3.6 TOS Tests

Several tests for TOS have been developed that are available for massage therapists to use, although a client with positive tests must still be diagnosed by a primary care provider.

One of the most dependable tests for TOS is the **EAST** (elevated arm stress test). The patient is seated, and the arms are abducted to 90 degrees. The elbows are flexed, and the hands point toward the ceiling. He or she opens and closes fists for 3 minutes. Most people with TOS are unable to complete this task before their symptoms interfere.

In the **Wright test**, the arm is moved up and back as the pulse is felt. If this exacerbates symptoms or reduces the strength of the pulse of the affected side, impingement to the axillary artery and lower brachial plexus nerves is suspected.

For **Adson test**, the head is extended and rotated toward the affected side. The client takes a deep breath, and the radial pulse on the affected side diminishes or even completely disappears.

TOS that is due to muscle atrophy may show best when a client lies on his or her affected side and the pulse is diminished by axillary artery compression.

Treatment

TOS is typically treated conservatively. Analgesics, gentle physical therapy, and stretching are the first lines of strategy. If these don't work, surgery to correct a bony anomaly or to remove connective tissue bands may be suggested. If the obstruction is found to interfere with blood flow, treatment may be more aggressive to avoid the risk of **embolism**.

Medications

- NSAIDs for pain
- Opioids if NSAIDs are not sufficient
- Muscle relaxants for spasms
- Antiseizure drugs (including gabapentin or clonazepam) for intractable nerve pain
- Antidepressants for nerve pain
- Anticoagulants with vascular compression to reduce the risk of thromboembolism

Massage Therapy Implications

RISKS	Some forms of TOS are related to anatomical anomalies, and massage will not resolve this situation. Careful positioning and sensitive work are important to avoid exacerbating impingement of delicate nerves or blood vessels. Therapists must be aware of what drugs the client may be using to make appropriate adjustments.
BENEFITS	Massage along with postural and movement education can drastically improve TOS for a person with symptoms due to muscular imbalances. Even in cases where the impingement is not muscular, massage may be able to lessen fascial restrictions and lift the pressure from inflamed nerves in the arms, leading to improved function.
OPTIONS	Focus on the shoulder girdle, the scalenes, and the postural muscles of the neck is key to unlocking the postural pattern that contributes to this condition.
RESEARCH	Massage for TOS has only been studied in individuals so far. A case study[1] suggests that massage may reduce weakness and pain in the setting of neurogenic TOS. Another case report found excellent results that lasted over a year without additional treatments for one patient.[2] 1. Streit RS. NTOS symptoms and mobility: a case study on neurogenic thoracic outlet syndrome involving massage therapy. *Journal of Bodywork and Movement Therapies* 2014;18(1):42–48.http://www.ncbi.nlm.nih.gov/pubmed/24411148 2. Wakefield M. Case report: The effects of massage therapy on a woman with thoracic outlet syndrome. *International Journal of Therapeutic Massage and Bodywork* 2014;7(4):7–14. http://www.ncbi.nlm.nih.gov/pmc/articles/PMC4240700/

Other Connective Tissue Disorders

Bunions

Definition: What Are They?

Bunions are also known as hallux valgus, which means "laterally deviated big toe." The first phalanx of the great toe is distorted toward the lateral aspect of the foot. The joint capsule stretches, a bursa grows at the irritated site, and callus grows over the protrusion. A smaller version of the same problem sometimes appears at the base of the little toe; this is called "tailor's bunion" or "bunionette."

Demographics

Women have bunions about 10 times more often than do men. High-heeled, narrow-toed shoes are factors, but a genetic weakness in the toe joints may predispose some people to bunions regardless of footwear. Bunions appear to run in families, and they are more common in adults who wore shoes that were too small during their childhood.

Etiology: What Happens?

Several factors can contribute to the misalignment between the first metatarsal and the proximal phalanx of the great toe. Feet with **pes cavus** or **pes planus** can force pressure onto the targeted spot. Muscle imbalances within the foot and the lower leg can influence how force is distributed through the joint. Further, the shape of the head of the first metatarsal determines the stability of the metatarsophalangeal joint: the rounder the head, the less stable the joint and the more prone it is to valgus stress.

Any of these issues, in combination with footwear that squeezes the toes or forces weight onto the medial aspect of the foot (i.e., high-heeled, narrow-toed shoes or cowboy boots), can open the door to the painful distortion that bunions involve.

Pressure at the metacarpophalangeal joint can cause erosion and irritation, but the acute pain of bunions is also often related to local friction **bursitis**. Ultimately, if this misaligned weight-bearing joint is not corrected or supported in a way that limits erosion of the joint structures, the bunion patient can also develop bone spurs and **arthritis**, which can make it prohibitively painful to walk.

Signs and Symptoms

Bunions look like a large lump on the medial side of the metatarsophalangeal joint of the great toe. If the bunion is not irritated, a simple protrusion, often covered with a thick layer of callus, is obvious (Figure 3.53). If the bursa is inflamed, the area is red, hot, and extremely painful (Figure 3.54).

Treatment

The highest priority in treating a bunion is to remove whatever irritants contribute to the problem. This may mean switching footgear or even cutting holes in shoes to make room for

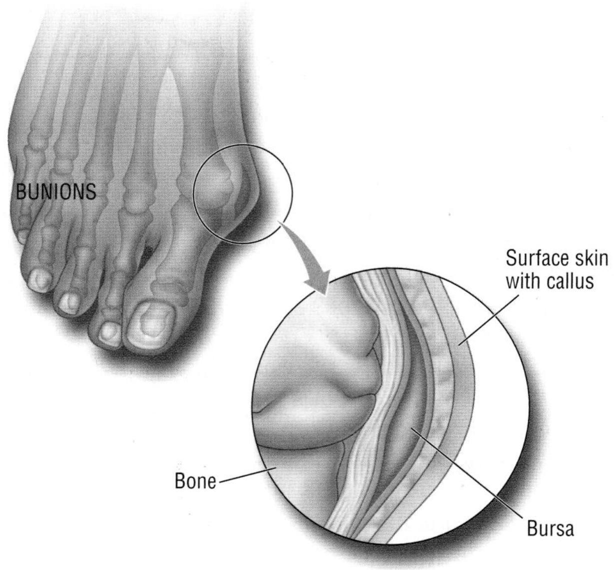

FIGURE 3.53 Bunion with friction bursitis

the protrusion. Other noninvasive strategies include massage and exercise: range-of-motion stretches, gentle traction, and friction around (not on) the affected area are recommended to limit pain and slow progression, but these interventions do not necessarily realign the toe.

Elevating the heel to an appropriate height can relieve some pain, and a corticosteroid injection can reduce inflammation. But if damage has developed inside the joint and if the bunion is painful enough to limit the patient's activity, surgery may be recommended. A variety of surgeries have been developed to remove the bunion, reshape the foot bones, or fuse the joint. The need for surgery is determined by the angles of distortion in the foot bones and the expectations of the patient.

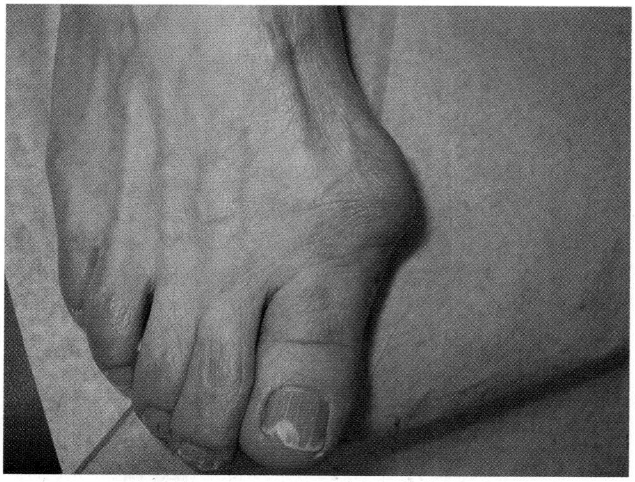

FIGURE 3.54 An inflamed, painful bunion

Medications

- NSAIDs for pain and inflammation management
- Injected cortisol for inflammation

Massage Therapy Implications

RISKS	Acutely inflamed bunions locally contraindicate deep, specific massage, which may exacerbate swelling and pain.
BENEFITS	Massage won't reverse a bunion, but it can certainly improve the quality of life for a person with this painful condition.
OPTIONS	Focus on intrinsic foot muscles and other postural and gait compensation patterns that arise when walking is painful may improve efficiency of movement and reduce overall pain.

Bursitis

Definition: What Is It?

Bursae are small closed sacs made of connective tissue. They are lined with synovial membrane and filled with synovial fluid. Bursitis is inflammation of the bursae. When these fluid-filled sacs are irritated, internal cells proliferate and generate excess fluid, which causes pain and limits mobility.

The human body has about 160 bursae, but new ones can be generated in areas that need protection. Most bursae are very small, but the ones that protect the knee, shoulder, and hip can be quite large.

Bursitis comes in all shapes and forms, some of which have descriptive names, like *housemaid's knee* and *student's elbow*, which occurs on the point of the olecranon. *Weaver's bottom* is bursitis on the ischial tuberosity. Bursitis at the greater trochanter is a common variety, as is bursitis at the insertion of the iliopsoas on the lesser trochanter and at the calcaneus. Subacromial bursitis (Figure 3.55) is probably the most common presentation.

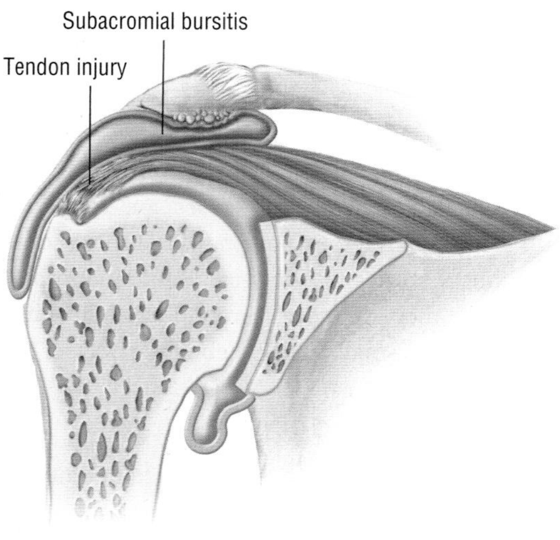

FIGURE 3.55 Subacromial bursitis

Demographics

Bursitis is most common among physically active people. Some locations of bursitis are more common in certain populations; for instance, knee bursitis may be more common in people whose occupations involve carrying heavy loads and kneeling.

Etiology: What Happens?

Imagine stretching a rubber band over the sharp edge of a table. Now imagine moving it back and forth for several minutes. In a short time, the rubber band frays and then breaks. But if you put a tiny water balloon between the rubber band and the edge of the table, the rubber band has freedom to move without the friction from the table: the water balloon protects it from damage. Bursae are the water balloons; they serve to ease the movement of tendons (rubber bands) over bony angles (table edge) (see Figure 3.56). Bursae also cushion the bones where they would otherwise collide. Bursae pad people's sharpest corners: they are on elbows, knees, heels, and ischial tuberosities, and between layers of fascia. Some bursae are present at birth, but others grow in response to wear and tear.

Repetitive stress is the most common bursitis trigger. Ongoing irritation leads to changes in the synovial lining: the walls of the bursa thicken, and the inflammatory process stimulates a massive production of fluid. Nearby muscles contract to splint the perceived injury, limiting the range of motion of the affected joint. Sometimes the muscles may aggravate and prolong an episode of bursitis by compressing the joint and the bursa at the same time. In the long run, structural changes to the walls of the bursa may become permanent: the bursal lining, which should be synovial membrane, can be replaced by tough fibrous tissue. The fluid inside can also change, to become thick and protein rich.

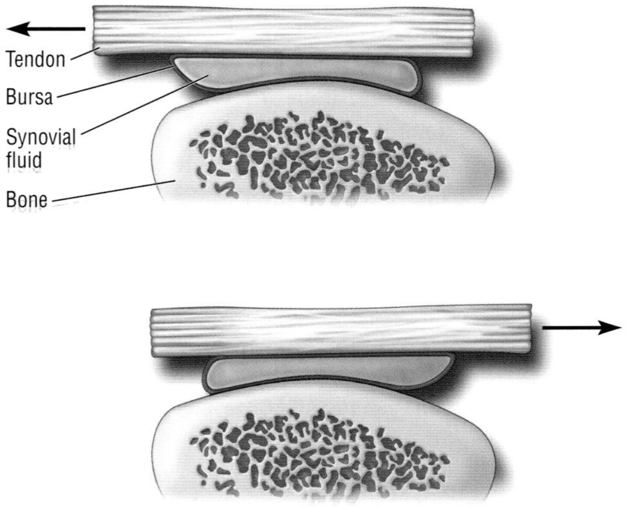

FIGURE 3.56 Bursae allow tendons to move freely over bony prominences

Bursitis often occurs in concert with other inflammatory conditions. It tends to accompany general area inflammation, so if a person has a **tendon injury**, bursitis is often present as well. It also attends **gout, rheumatoid arthritis,** and **tuberculosis**.

The most common sites of bursitis are at the subacromial bursae, several of the 11 bursae around the knees, at the greater trochanter, and at the ischial tuberosities. Bursae can also be inflamed through a local infection, usually with *Staphylococcus aureus*. This happens most often with superficial bursae, especially at the elbow and the knee; this is called septic bursitis.

Signs and Symptoms

The symptoms of bursitis include pain on passive and active movement, along with extremely limited range of motion because of muscular splinting. Superficial bursitis or septic bursitis may also show palpable heat and swelling.

Treatment

Left untreated, most cases of bursitis resolve by themselves. However, once bursitis has occurred, it is likely to happen again.

Treatment strategies for bursitis include rest, oral anti-inflammatories, hot or cold packs, aspiration of excess fluid, and corticosteroid injections. Surgery may be considered if other options fail.

Medications

- NSAIDs for pain and inflammation management
- Injected cortisone for inflammation
- Antibiotics for septic bursitis

Massage Therapy Implications

RISKS	Acute bursitis can be exacerbated if deep specific massage is applied to the irritated area. Any infection must be resolved before bodywork is applied as well.
BENEFITS	Massage that respects the limitations of acute inflammation is safe for clients with bursitis. Clients who have a history of bursitis can enjoy the same benefits of bodywork as does the rest of the population.
OPTIONS	Careful work to muscles that cross the affected joint may help to restore a normal range of motion, decompress the area, and reduce some of the bursal irritation.

Shin Splints

Definition: What Are They?

Shin splints is a term that refers to a variety of lower leg problems. Medial tibial stress syndrome is the injury most commonly associated with shin splints, but closely related problems include periostitis and stress fractures. Chronic or acute **compartment syndrome** can be related injuries, but they are discussed elsewhere in this chapter.

Demographics

People who are physically very active are more prone to shin splints than are others. Military personnel, runners, gymnasts, and dancers are frequently affected.

Etiology: What Happens?

Several features make the lower leg susceptible to certain injuries. One of them is the fact that the lower leg muscles have long attachments. Their endomysial sheaths blend directly into the deep **crural fascia**, and the periosteum and **interosseous membrane** of the tibia and fibula. This means any irritation of these muscles and fascia easily translates into irritation of the attaching periosteum and other nearby structures (Figure 3.57).

Another key to lower leg function is the shock-absorbing capacity of the feet. Feet are designed to spread out and rebound with each step. If the foot has inadequate shock absorption—because of flat feet or jammed arches (**pes planus** or **pes cavus**, respectively), worn-out shoes, hard surfaces, or any combination thereof—the tibia and the muscles in the lower leg, especially the soleus, tibialis anterior, and tibialis posterior, absorb a disproportionate amount of the shock. They are not designed for this job, and ongoing stress may cause the periosteum to become irritated, the bone to crack, and the muscles to fray and become inflamed.

Shin splints often develop when a training routine is suddenly changed, or in relation to worn-out footwear, or running consistently on hard surfaces. Running all uphill or all downhill can also be triggers.

Types of Shin Splints

- *Medial tibial stress syndrome*: This may be the most common presentation of shin splints. It involves muscular injury on the medial side of the tibia, specifically to the soleus and tibialis anterior. It is typically painful at the distal third segment of the medial tibia.
- *Tibialis anterior, tibialis posterior injury*: The pain associated with these injuries often runs most of the length of the tibia on the lateral side (for tibialis anterior) or deep in the back of the calf (for tibialis posterior).
- *Periostitis*: This inflammation of the periosteum may develop with damage to the soleus, anterior tibialis, or posterior tibialis muscles. That seamless connection of membranes begins to rip apart, and the fibers of the muscles pull away from the bone.
- *Stress fractures*: These hairline **fractures** of the tibia can be extremely painful, and they don't heal unless activity is suspended. They are frequently the result of "running through the pain." Stress fractures of the tibia often don't show up well on radiographs: they are best diagnosed by bone scan, which looks for areas of increased circulatory activity.

Crural fascia: The deep fascia (connective tissue) of the leg.

Interosseous membrane: A thin membrane of connective tissue extending from one bone to another. The interosseous membrane of the leg is also called the middle tibiofibular ligament.

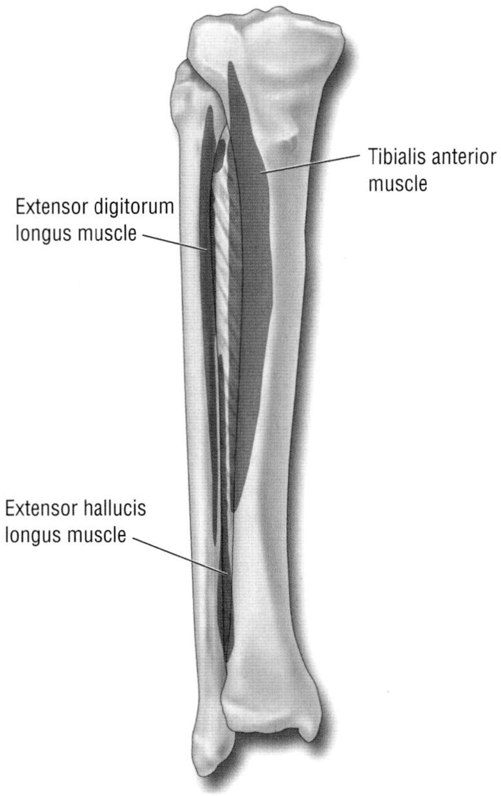

FIGURE 3.57 Shin splints: anterior leg muscles blend into the tibial periosteum

Signs and Symptoms

Pain from shin splints can be mild or severe, and the location varies according to which of the structures has been damaged. It gets worse with whatever actions the affected muscles do: dorsiflexion, inversion, or **plantar flexion**. Simple muscle injuries are rarely visibly or palpably inflamed, but palpation of the shin muscles is painful. If the anterior lower leg is red, hot, and puffy, compartment syndrome may be present.

Treatment

The typical approach to mild shin splints is to reduce activity and to alternate applications of heat and cold to the affected area. Changing footwear and analyzing inefficient movement or training patterns are helpful. Patients may be counseled to replace their normal activity with nonpercussive exercise while their legs recover. If pain is intense or long-lasting, further evaluation for stress fractures or compartment syndrome may be necessary.

Medications

- NSAIDs for pain and inflammation control

Massage Therapy Implications

RISKS	Any palpably hot or inflamed situation in the lower leg musculature requires medical attention before massage is appropriate. If a case of shin splints seems particularly long-lasting, evaluation for a stress fracture is important: a massage therapist may be in a position to give good advice in this situation.
BENEFITS	Mild muscle injury or periosteum irritation can respond well to massage, which may allow the client to return to pain-free activity sooner than otherwise.
OPTIONS	Pin-and-stretch techniques that focus on the accessible shin muscles can target structures that are otherwise difficult to stretch and mobilize.
RESEARCH	A systematic review of physical therapy interventions for MTSS found that ice massage can be helpful along with several other options, but it didn't stand out as being more effective than any other intervention.[1] 1. Winters M, Eskes M, Weir A, et al. Treatment of medial tibial stress syndrome: a systematic review. *Sports Medicine* 2013;43(12):1315–1333. http://www.ncbi.nlm.nih.gov/pubmed/23979968

Tendinopathies

Definition: What Are They?

Tendinopathy is an umbrella term that covers injury and damage to tendons and tenosynovial sheaths. These conditions can include acute tears and ruptures, but are most often related to chronic degeneration due to injury, repetitive use, age, nutrition, and other factors.

> **Tenocyte:** A tendon cell.
>
> **Type I collagen:** The most common form of collagen in the body, found in places including tendons, skin, artery walls, and scar tissue.
>
> **Ground substance:** The gel-like substance that surrounds connective tissue cells.

Demographics

Tendinopathies can happen to anyone, active or sedentary. They appear to occur most often in active people who are mature; the aging process makes tendons less elastic and more prone to injury.

People who live with **rheumatoid arthritis**, **lupus**, or **chronic renal failure** develop tendinopathies more readily than does the general population. People who have taken quinolone-type antibiotics are also at increased risk; these drugs may interfere with **tenocyte** activity. And people who have used oral or injected steroids are more likely to develop tendon problems than are those who have not.

Etiology: What Happens?

When tendons are injured, a number of changes in the tissue occur. Acute injuries prompt the secretion of proinflammatory chemicals, leading to edema and pain; the correct term in this situation is tendinitis. But most tendinopathies do not involve acute inflammation. Rather, they are conditions in which the collagen degenerates faster than it can be replaced, and the tendon loses its weight-bearing capacity. This situation is more correctly termed tendinosis: pathologic condition of the tendon.

Tendons are made mostly of **type I collagen** fibers suspended in liquid **ground substance**. A small number of elastin fibers are woven into the structure to lend some limited stretch and rebound, but the bulk of the tissues are dense, linearly arranged collagen fibers. Healthy tendons look hard, shiny, and white. By contrast, tendons with chronic degeneration look dull, gray or brown, and soft or shaggy (Figure 3.58).

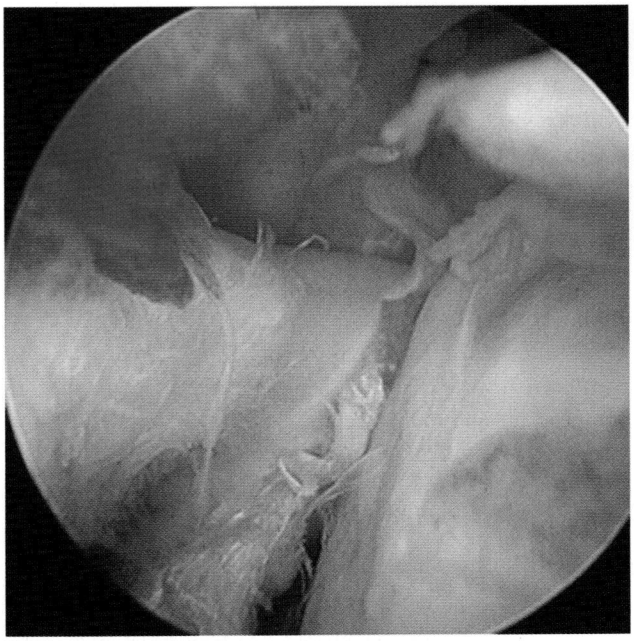

FIGURE 3.58 Arthroscopy of tendinopathy at the long head of the biceps: note the frayed, disorganized appearance of the structure

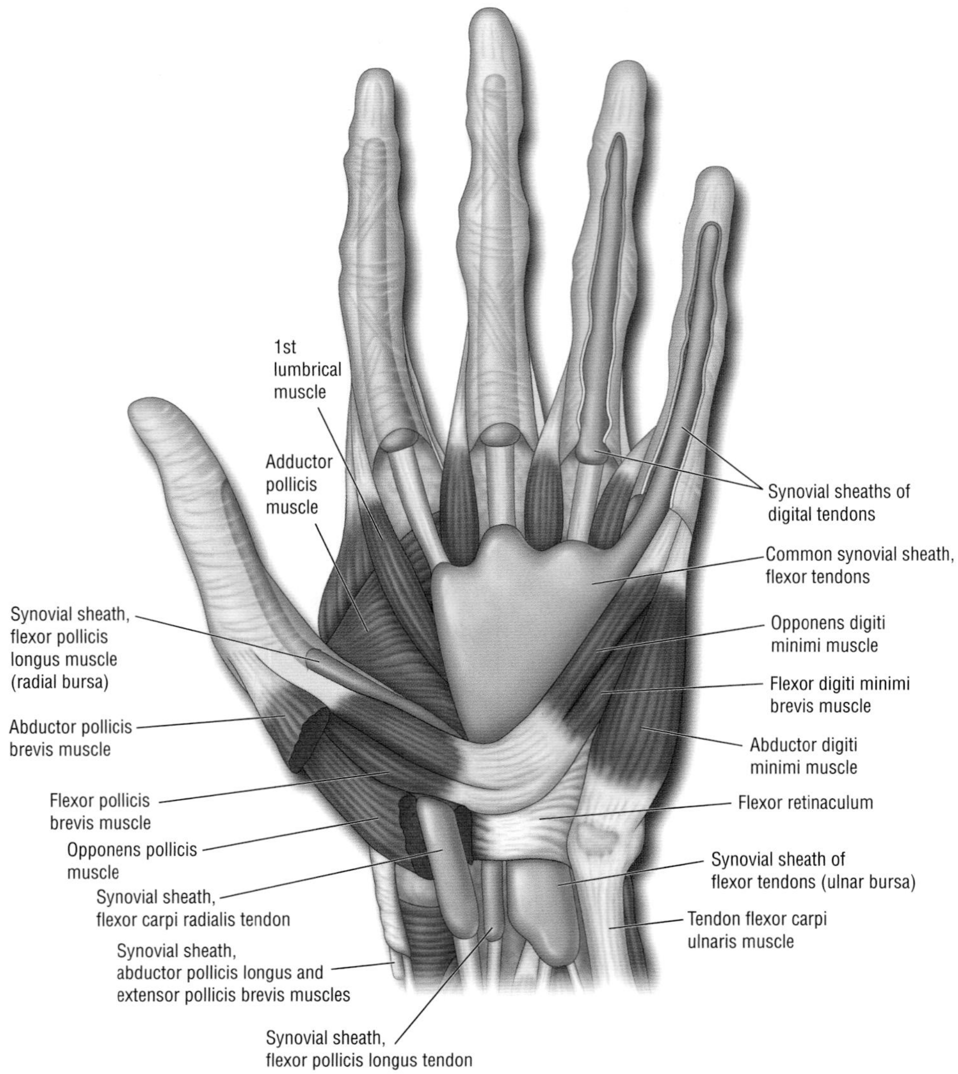

FIGURE 3.59 Tenosynovitis: synovial sheaths should allow tendons to slide easily over each other

The causes for the chronic degenerative processes of tendinosis can be discussed as a combination of intrinsic and extrinsic factors. Intrinsic factors include direct or shearing forces transferred through the tendon, overuse without recovery time, poor flexibility, underlying disease, or a history of corticosteroid injection. Extrinsic factors can include training errors of athletes, problems with equipment, or a fall or blow that damages the tendon from the outside.

Tendinopathies occur most often at the rotator cuff and biceps tendons, at the medial and lateral epicondyles of the humerus, around the patella, at the distal attachment of the iliotibial band, and at the Achilles tendon.

Types of Tendinopathies

- *Tendinitis*: This is a new injury that leads to the classic signs of inflammation: pain, heat, redness, and swelling.
- *Tendinosis*: In this condition of long-term degeneration, microscopy shows more liquid ground substance in than in a healthy tendon, and the collagen fibers are disrupted and discontinuous. Fibroblasts are active, and new blood vessels are present. The new tissue is composed mainly of **type III collagen** fibers, which are thinner and weaker than are the normal type I fibers of healthy tendons.
- *Tenosynovitis*: In this condition, irritation develops where tendons slide through their synovial sheaths. It happens most often at the wrist and flexor aspect of the fingers and is often characterized by gritty crepitus during movement (Figure 3.59).
  - *"Trigger finger"*: This describes tenosynovitis at any of the fingers other than the thumb. It usually happens in

Type III collagen: A form of collagen that is thinner and weaker than Type I.

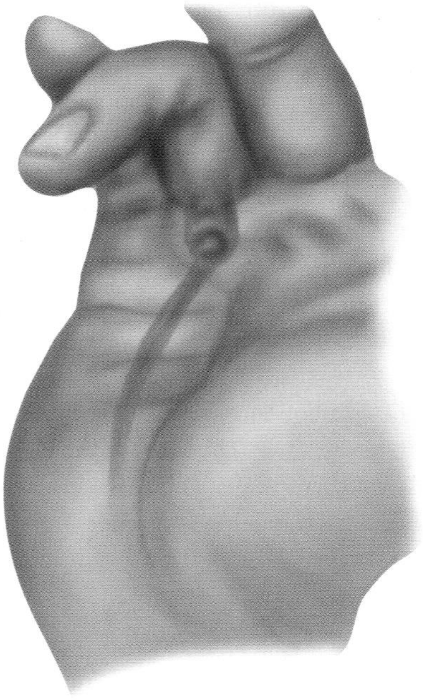

FIGURE 3.60 Trigger finger: a type of tenosynovitis

the dominant hand. The ring, middle, and little fingers are affected most often. The finger can become stuck in flexion or extension, depending on where the tendon gets caught in the sheath (Figure 3.60).

- *de Quervain tenosynovitis*: This is tenosynovitis specifically of the abductor and extensor pollicis tendons. It is often acutely inflamed, and may be related to a systemic bacterial infection.

Signs and Symptoms

The symptoms of tendinopathies are very similar to those of **muscle strains**, though they may be more intense. The acute stage may show heat and swelling, depending on which tendons are affected. Most tendon swelling is not visible or palpable with a few exceptions: the Achilles tendon and the posterior tibialis tendon at the medial ankle may swell significantly with injury. In all stages of tendinosis, stiffness and pain are present, especially with resistive movements and in stretching.

Tenosynovitis has an added feature of resistance and crepitus as the affected tendon moves through its sheath.

Treatment

The quality of the healing of a damaged tendon or sheath depends largely on what happens with the production of new collagen fibers. Because inflammation turns out not to be a significant issue in most long-lasting tendon injuries, the use of anti-inflammatories and steroid injections is no longer standard.

A combination of rest, ice, stretching, and carefully gauged exercise turns out to be an effective treatment option for many of these injuries. Ultrasound or extracorporeal shock wave therapy also get good results, especially in combination with exercise. Eccentric contractions appear to be particularly useful to rebuild a damaged tendon. Some orthopedists recommend that patients wear a splint or brace to help bear some of the force of a damaged tendon, especially with de Quervain tenosynovitis.

Medications

- NSAIDs for pain (but usually not for anti-inflammatory action)
- Steroid injections (this is now controversial, but they may be appropriate in some circumstances)

Massage Therapy Implications

RISKS	Acute injuries locally contraindicate deep massage until the inflammation has begun to resolve, but lymphatic work during this phase may be helpful.
BENEFITS	Various types of massage can contribute to the healing process for chronically irritated tendons. Whether that comes about because of impact on circulation, the mechanical impact of movement and stretching, or neurological soothing isn't clear, however.
OPTIONS	With-fiber friction and cross-fiber friction may help promote the production of good-quality scar tissue, but the most important part of the healing process for these injuries may be getting the right amount of the right kind of weight-bearing stress.
RESEARCH	Research about the role of massage, particularly various types of specific friction, is fairly robust in the context of tendinopathies.[1–3] Most studies and reviews conclude that massage therapy is an appropriate conservative intervention for several tendinoses in several locations, and that conservative interventions should be pursued before surgery is considered. 1. Cook JL, Khan KM. What is the most appropriate treatment for patellar tendinopathy? *British Journal of Sports Medicine* 2001;35(5):291–294. http://www.ncbi.nlm.nih.gov/pmc/articles/PMC1724394/ 2. Wilson JJ, Best TM. Common overuse tendon problems: a review and recommendations for treatment. *American Family Physician* 2005;72(5):811–818. http://www.aafp.org/afp/2005/0901/p811.html 3. Joseph MF, Taft K, Moskwa M, et al. Deep friction massage to treat tendinopathy: a systematic review of a classic treatment in the face of a new paradigm of understanding. *Journal of Sport Rehabilitation* 2012;21(4):343–353. http://www.ncbi.nlm.nih.gov/pubmed/22234925

3 Musculoskeletal System Conditions

Whiplash

Definition: What Is It?

Whiplash, or CAD (cervical acceleration-deceleration) is a broad term used to refer to a mixture of injuries, including **sprains**, **strains**, and **joint disruptions**. Bone **fractures**, **herniated discs**, nerve damage, and **traumatic brain injuries** are commonly seen along with these soft tissue injuries and so are often addressed simultaneously. Whiplash injuries are usually, but not always, associated with motor vehicle accidents (MVAs) in which the head whips backward and then forward in rapid succession (Figure 3.61).

Demographics

More than a million whiplash injuries due to MVAs happen each year in this country, and it is estimated that about 15.5 million people have whiplash-related injuries.

Etiology: What Happens?

The nature of damage incurred by whiplash accidents depends on many variables. In MVAs, some of the most important factors are the direction of impact, the speed with which the vehicles were moving, the relative weight of the vehicles involved, whether the individual was wearing a seat belt, the position of the individual's head, and whether the person was aware of the impending impact and had time to brace. Analysis of rear-impact accidents shows that as the momentum of the car seat forces the thorax forward, the head initially stays in the same place, which means it functionally goes into extension. About 100 milliseconds later, the head is propelled into flexion. The momentum of this movement is magnified by the leverage of the neck.

While MVAs account for the majority of diagnosed whiplash cases, it is important to remember that other injuries can create the same scenario. Sports injuries and falls can involve a similar process, especially when a collision affects the neck and head.

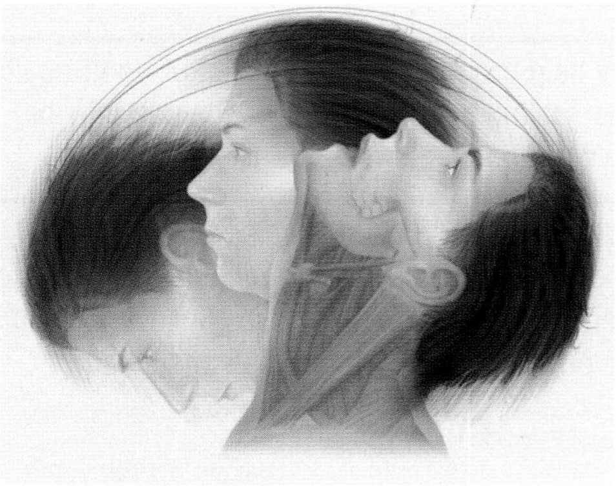

FIGURE 3.61 Cervical acceleration and deceleration: whiplash

Accidents of this nature put the cervical muscles (especially the sternocleidomastoid, scalenes, and splenius cervicis) at risk for strains. Supraspinous and intertransverse spinal ligaments are frequently sprained. The anterior and posterior longitudinal ligaments may also be traumatized. Other damage may affect the capsules of the facet joints; the esophagus and larynx; intervertebral discs; vertebrae, which may subluxate or fracture; the temporomandibular joint; spinal nerve roots; the spinal cord, which may be compressed or stretched; and the brain, which is vulnerable to concussion.

Long-term consequences of whiplash can range from being minor to devastating. The force of the trauma does not always correlate to symptoms, and the multifactorial nature of the injuries can be difficult to untangle. Long-lasting neck pain with central sensitization is not an unusual outcome for whiplash patients.

Signs and Symptoms

A lot of crossover exists between whiplash-related injuries and subsequent complications; both are discussed here. Basic signs and symptoms include head and neck pain, which may radiate into the trunk or arms; loss of range of motion; and paresthesia. One of the curious aspects of whiplash is that it is common for symptoms to be delayed for days, weeks, and occasionally months before coming to full intensity. This phenomenon is not well understood.

- *Ligament sprains*: The supraspinous and intertransverse ligaments are at risk for injury in a whiplash type of accident. These ligaments can refer pain up over the head, into the chest, and down the arms: this can be difficult to distinguish from nerve pain. Ligament sprains often take a long time to heal, and they tend to accumulate excessive scar tissue.
- *Damaged facet joint capsules*: Joint capsules are often irritated in CAD events and they, like spinous ligaments, can refer pain to the head. Furthermore, these joint capsules are richly equipped with nociceptors that may intensify pain messages sent to the spinal cord. They also have proprioceptors that can send confusing messages to the brain, leading to dizziness or disorientation.
- *Subluxated cervical vertebrae*: Vertebrae may be displaced to the front, back, or side or rotated one way or another. In some very extreme cases, fractures may occur. Left untreated or incompletely treated, misaligned vertebrae with lax ligaments and lack of structural support may develop **spondylosis**.
- ***Damaged discs***: This is not inevitable, but it may happen that the force of trauma causes the anulus fibrosus of the discs to crack, allowing the nucleus pulposus to bulge or herniate.
- ***Spasm***: When a neck injury is acute, the paraspinals and other neck muscles go into spasm to splint the stretched

CASE HISTORY 3.1 Whiplash

A massage therapist met with a first-time client approximately 1 year after the client was in a car accident. The client was still in considerable pain. He was diagnosed with whiplash and was seeking massage under prescription from his doctor.

The therapist worked slowly and carefully, and was encouraged by the client to go deeper into his neck muscles, all the way down to the transverse processes of the neck vertebrae. He felt better after the massage; his muscles were looser, and he had an improved range of motion.

Several hours later, the client sneezed. The force of the motion wrenched his neck and reinjured the tissues so that he was in greater pain and more spasm and had much less range of motion than he had before his massage. He returned for another session, but it was ineffective at reducing his pain and dysfunction. He never sought massage again.

What is the moral here? It is utterly unclear whether the first massage put the client at risk for reinjuring himself just by sneezing. The therapist followed all the rules of good sense, worked with a doctor's recommendation, and let the client guide her into how much pressure felt comfortable. Yet it is necessary to entertain the possibility that the massage somehow did put the client at risk, even though the therapist was well informed and made what seemed to be the right decisions. No two people go through the same kind of healing process, and no two people respond to massage the same way. Massage therapists must weigh the benefits and risks of their work on a case-by-case basis. It is impossible to rely only on books and rules to make decisions about whether to give massage.

neck ligaments. But this reaction has a tendency to outlive its usefulness. Spasm of neck muscles significantly limits range of motion (Case History 3.1).

- *Trigger points*: Traumatized muscles often develop trigger points: local tight areas that refer pain, often into the head, causing chronic headaches. This is one form of **myofascial pain syndrome**.
- *Neurological symptoms*: These can include dizziness, blurred vision, abnormal smell or taste, tinnitus (ringing in the ears), or loss of hearing. These signs indicate cranial trauma: the brain has been bruised and may have some internal bleeding. This is usually the result of a specific blow, but concussion and postconcussion syndrome can also happen without direct impact.
- ***TMJ disorders***: Direct impact of the jaw can damage the temporomandibular joint, but it is possible that the joint can be traumatized simply through the rapid acceleration and deceleration that accompany whiplash injuries. This is sometimes called "jawlash."
- ***Headaches***: These arise for a variety of reasons, including but not limited to referred pain and trigger points from spasms in the neck, sprained ligaments that refer pain up over the head, irritated facet joint capsules, cranial bones that may be out of alignment, stress and its autonomic action on blood flow, muscle tightness in the neck and head, TMJ problems, and concussion.

Treatment

Neck collars are used for acute whiplash patients to take the stress off their wrenched ligaments and to try to reduce muscle spasm. But the sooner the injured structures are put back to use, the less scar tissue is likely to accumulate. Therefore, collars are strictly for short-term use, as this kind of immobilization has been seen to create more long-term problems than benefits.

Other treatment recommendations for whiplash patients include heat, ice, electrical stimulation, massage therapy, traction, and stretching and strengthening programs.

Medical intervention typically focuses on pain relievers, anti-inflammatories, and muscle relaxants. These substances can change the quality of the tissues and sensory responses, so massage therapists should be aware when clients use them.

Medications

- NSAIDs for inflammation and pain control
- Narcotic analgesics for pain control
- Tricyclic antidepressants for sleep aid, pain control, and sedation
- Muscle relaxants for pain and spasm
- Injected steroids for inflammation
- Injected analgesics for pain
- Injected botox into cervical trigger points for pain
- Oral steroids for inflammation

Massage Therapy Implications

RISKS	The risk of exacerbating inflammation or inappropriately disrupting damaged tissues with vigorous massage during the acute phase of whiplash is important to respect. Further, because damage can affect the vertebrae, central nervous system, and structures in the anterior neck, it is important for a client with a recent neck trauma to be fully evaluated by a primary care provider before using bodywork as a treatment strategy.
BENEFITS	In the subacute and postacute phases of whiplash recovery, massage can be an excellent strategy to deal with pain, proprioception, muscle tone, movement patterns, and dysfunctional scar tissue. Massage in combination with bony manipulation can be an especially powerful combination.
RESEARCH	One observational study[1] of over 1,000 whiplash patients found that the unifying features were damage at the muscular attachments (especially the trapezius—including its attachments to the scapula), and reduced ROM at the neck. The researchers suggest that rehabilitation for these patients focused specifically on these features. Another study[2] found that anxiety and depression were predictors of pain relief and function for whiplash patients. Because massage therapy has demonstrated value in range of motion improvement, pain management, and mood disorders, it is a logical component of a whiplash management strategy. 1. Bismil Q, Bismil M. Myofascial-entheseal dysfunction in chronic whiplash injury: an observational study. *JRSM Short Reports* 2012;3(8):57. http://www.ncbi.nlm.nih.gov/pmc/articles/PMC3434435/ 2. Angst F, Gantenbein AR, Lehmann S, et al. Multidimensional associative factors for improvement in pain, function, and working capacity after rehabilitation of whiplash associated disorder: a prognostic, prospective outcome study. *BMC Musculoskeletal Disorders* 2014;15(130). http://www.medscape.com/viewarticle/825023

Explore and Apply

LEVEL 1: Receive and Respond

1. What is the best description of muscular dystrophy?
   a. A genetic disorder that leads to the wasting of muscle tissue
   b. A chronic pain syndrome characterized by trigger points
   c. Involuntary contraction of voluntary muscle cells
   d. Idiopathic thickening and shrinking of fascial sheets

2. What kind of muscle spasm serves an important function in healing?
   a. Splinting
   b. Ischemic
   c. Spastic
   d. Nutritional

3. In which situation is massage therapy likely to have the best results?
   a. Strain
   b. Subluxation
   c. Rupture
   d. Dislocation

4. What is the most reliable sign of early-stage osteosarcoma?
   a. Pain with activity, and at rest
   b. Nothing: this condition is silent in the early stage
   c. Trouble breathing as tumors invade the lungs
   d. A palpable mass on the primary affected bone, and others nearby

5. What is the best description for Osgood-Schlatter disease?
   a. A genetic disorder involving the degeneration of muscle tissue
   b. A synonym for patellofemoral pain syndrome
   c. Inflammation at the tibial tuberosity
   d. A subtype of osteosarcoma

6. What is a synonym for hyperlordosis?
   a. Widow's hump
   b. Swayback
   c. Bamboo spine
   d. Brittle bone disease

7. What is a synonym for adhesive capsulitis?
   a. Jumper's knee
   b. Student's elbow
   c. Frozen shoulder
   d. Lockjaw

8. What serious condition can a Baker cyst mimic?
   a. Cellulitis
   b. ACL tear
   c. MRSA infection
   d. Deep vein thrombosis

9. Your client has excruciating pain at the base of the great toe. The skin is red, shiny, hot, and throbbing. What condition is probably present?
   a. Bunion
   b. Gout
   c. Hammer toe
   d. Morton neuroma

10. Which is the best description of osteoarthritis?
    a. A type of joint inflammation related to the accumulation of sharp crystals around synovial joints
    b. A type of joint inflammation related to autoimmune dysfunction
    c. A type of joint inflammation that is limited specifically to synovial joints
    d. A type of joint inflammation that can spread through the bloodstream to other joints

11. Which is the best description of patellofemoral pain syndrome?
    a. Chronic degeneration of the tissues that connects the quadriceps to the tibial tuberosity
    b. Wearing down of the cartilage on the posterior aspect of the patella
    c. Neuromuscular disorder involving trigger points in the quadriceps expansion
    d. A pouch develops at the posterior aspect of the popliteal fossa

12. This condition may involve bone fractures, pressure on nerve roots, and instability in the low back. What is it?
    a. Spondylosis
    b. Spondylolisthesis
    c. Spondylitis
    d. Spondylolysis

13. What is a common feature of spondylosis that distinguishes it from other types of arthritis?
    a. Bone spurs that can impinge on spinal nerve roots
    b. An inflamed capsular ligament at risk for rupture
    c. A close association with rheumatoid arthritis
    d. Absence of damage to the articular cartilage

14. What are common symptoms of temporomandibular joint disorder?
  a. Swollen tongue, inflamed lymph nodes, lockjaw
  b. Headaches, shooting pain down the arm, limited range of motion
  c. Locking of the joint, hypotonicity of the jaw muscles, weakness
  d. Bruxism, popping, ear pain

15. What is the best description of compartment syndrome?
  a. Pressure inside a tight fascial compartment can lead to tissue damage
  b. Constant percussive stress causes the periosteum to pull away from the tibia
  c. The tibialis posterior develops tears at the musculotendinous junction
  d. Byproducts of dying muscle accumulate in the kidneys and lead to renal failure

16. Match the following terms to their primary symptoms:

a. Ganglion cyst	___shooting pain between the all third and fourth toes
b. Dupuytren contracture	___a painless bump, often on the hand or the foot
c. Morton neuroma	___the medial fingers curl into permanent flexion
d. Plantar fasciitis	___contracture of toe muscles leading to permanent deformity
e. Hammer toe	___pain on the bottom of the foot, just distal to the calcaneus

17. What does "herniated" mean?
  a. Strangulated small intestine
  b. Enlarged diaphragmatic hiatus
  c. Broken
  d. Pushed through a hole or weak spot

18. Your client has electrical pain and weakness in the hand, especially at the thumb and lateral three fingers. What condition is probably present?
  a. Thoracic outlet syndrome
  b. Carpal tunnel syndrome
  c. Myofascial pain syndrome
  d. Compartment syndrome

19. Which muscles tend to be shortened in the context of thoracic outlet syndrome?
  a. Trapezius, rhomboids, splenius cervicis
  b. Pectoralis major, latissimus dorsi, biceps
  c. Pectoralis minor, scalenes, serratus anterior
  d. Sternocleidomastoid, scalenes, external intercostals

20. Your client has excruciating pain at the base of the great toe. The skin is thick and callused, and a large bump protrudes medially. What condition is probably present?
  a. Bunion
  b. Gout
  c. Hammer toe
  d. Morton neuroma

21. Which condition has subtypes called "student's elbow," "housemaid's knee," and "tailor's bottom"?
  a. Bunions
  b. Bursitis
  c. Baker cyst
  d. Bone spurs

22. What condition is associated with the accumulation of trigger points?
  a. Fibromyalgia syndrome
  b. Thoracic outlet syndrome
  c. Myofascial pain syndrome
  d. Compartment syndrome

Explore and Apply (continued)

LEVEL 2: Application of Concepts

1. Osteoporosis is more likely to affect trabecular bone than cortical bone. Explain why that increases the risk for bone fractures.

2. Your 54-year-old client has severe Schuermann disease, with back pain and limited lung capacity. What are reasonable expectations for how massage might help?
   a. He may experience temporary pain relief but no permanent changes
   b. He may experience a reversal of his kyphosis and improved lung capacity
   c. He may experience compression fractures of his vertebrae with any touch
   d. He may experience exacerbation of his pain and muscle spasm due to neurologic insufficiency

3. Your 16-year-old, backpack-carrying client has hyperkyphosis with pain between her scapulae. Describe the benefits massage can offer her, and outline a treatment plan for your first session together.

4. At the finish line of a marathon in hot, humid weather, your client limps to your table and complains of cramps. What is your best course of action?
   a. Ice the affected calf while heating the unaffected calf
   b. Stretch the affected calf and work on the muscular attachments
   c. Recommend a hot bath followed by ice packs
   d. Refer to the medical tent

5. Your 75-year-old physically active client had a successful hip replacement last year. What is the most important accommodation to make for him?
   a. Don't use lubricant near his scar
   b. Don't expect a normal range of motion at his hip
   c. Don't leave him alone to get on the table
   d. Don't overdo the massage because he is probably taking painkillers

6. Your client has a subluxated vertebra that he traces to a recent car wreck. What does this mean?
   a. You need to call an ambulance immediately
   b. He needs permission from a doctor to work safely
   c. He has an abnormally wide range of motion
   d. He probably has some pain and loss of range of motion

7. Your client has been diagnosed with Lyme disease. What extra hygienic measures do you need to take to prevent contracting this infection?
   a. None; Lyme disease is not contagious from human to human so normal hygienic measures are adequate
   b. Observe standard plus universal precautions against this blood-borne infection
   c. Isolate her linens to be either washed with bleach or discarded
   d. Wear gloves to protect yourself from potential contamination

8. Your client has a 3-week-old ankle sprain. It is still painful, but not palpably hot or swollen. Is he a good candidate for massage?
   a. Yes, he can receive massage, but not on the ankle until the pain is resolved
   b. No, he cannot receive massage until all risk of deep vein thrombosis has passed
   c. Yes, he can receive massage within pain tolerance on the sore ankle
   d. No, he cannot receive massage without a doctor's note

9. Briefly explain how pes planus can lead to headaches.

10. Your client has been diagnosed with degenerative disc disease at the L4–L5 disc. What accommodations is he likely to need?
    a. Extra bolsters to be sure he doesn't hyperextend his low back
    b. Extra bolsters to be sure he doesn't flex his neck
    c. A table-warmer so he doesn't get chilled
    d. A step-stool to make getting on and off the table easier

11. Your client reports that she has just started a new training program, and it yesterday she ran 2 miles, almost all of it uphill. Today she has bilateral pain at the anterior and lateral aspects of her lower legs. What condition is probably present?
    a. Shin splints
    b. Compartment syndrome
    c. Stress fractures
    d. Interosseous ligament sprain

Explore and Apply (continued)

12. Your client was in a motor vehicle accident 2 days ago, and has been diagnosed with whiplash. Name three possible associated injuries that must be ruled out before it is safe to proceed with massage.

Note to educators: Due to space considerations, these review questions only skim over the most important material from Chapter 3. The Test Bank provides a much more comprehensive selection of questions, all of which are keyed to the relevant chapter objectives.

What Would *You* Do?

Consider each of the four types of muscle contractions. Name some examples of how you do concentric, eccentric, isometric, and isotonic contractions every day. Then make a list of activities in which those contractions could lead to muscle injury.

Massage for Unstable Joints?

No published research has yet documented any effect of massage for people with joint instability at the spine, shoulder, sacroiliac joints, or elsewhere. If you were to create a research project on this topic, how would you study it?

Write a proposal identifying the problems with joint instability, your target population of subjects, the intervention you would recommend, what your control group would receive, and how you would measure and document results to see if massage is effective.

Your client has a tick

Your client has just returned from vacation in an area where deer ticks are common. As you work on her legs, you notice a speck at the back of her knee. Closer inspection reveals that it is a tick.

Work with a partner to role-play this scenario, taking turns being the therapist and the client. Feel free to use Internet resources to help you through this, including these:

- http://www.cdc.gov/lyme/stats/maps/map2012.html
- http://www.cdc.gov/ticks/removing_a_tick.html.

Under what circumstances would you be willing to remove a tick?

What are the realistic worst-case scenarios that you can imagine in this situation?

Suggested Activities

1. For each condition covered in your curriculum, write down the following on a card:
   - A brief definition
   - Most common cause or contributing factor(s)
   - Major signs and symptoms
   - Risks and benefits of massage therapy
     - Variables that contribute to risks and benefits
     - Appropriate adaptations

   Use these as flash cards as you study
2. For each condition covered in your curriculum, write one multiple-choice question. Share your questions with your classmates as you study together.
3. Quiz yourself using either the "labels off" feature in your enhanced e-book, or the labeling exercise on thePoint® for Figures 3.1 and 3.2. For Figure 3.1, be sure you can label each of the following: Epimysium, Fascicle, Endomysium, Sarcoplasmic reticulum, and Myofibrils. For Figure 3.2, be sure you can label each of the following: Synovial membrane, Articular cartilage, Collateral ligament, and Internal ligaments.

4

Nervous System Conditions

CHAPTER 4 / Abbreviated Chapter Objectives

Having completed assignments and classroom time related to Chapter 4, the learner is expected to be able to…

- Identify definitions of the key terms in the introduction and those connected to the conditions covered in your curriculum.
- Name the purpose of myelin and neurilemma.
- Identify the most widely accepted definition of pain.
- Describe why it is important for massage therapists to be familiar with concepts about chronic pain.
- List three major cautions about working with clients who have nervous system problems.
- Provide the following information for each condition covered in your curriculum:
  - Identify the definition of the condition.
  - List the most common causes or contributing factors to the condition.
  - List major signs and symptoms of the condition.
  - Identify possible risks and benefits of massage therapy, with:
    - Variables that contribute to risks and benefits
    - Appropriate adaptations for massage therapy

For detailed chapter objectives for each condition in this chapter, consult the student resources page at http://thePoint.lww.com/Werner6e. thePoint®

By the time most massage therapists finish their core education, they probably know more about the nervous system than they ever suspected existed, and they may still feel like rank amateurs on the subject. That feeling is common to most people who study this topic: it is a complex system about which we are still learning, so detailed information changes often. Fortunately, only a passing familiarity with the structure and function of this system is needed to make educated decisions about massage and many nervous system disorders.

Many of the conditions considered here affect the peripheral nerves rather than the central nervous system (CNS), so this introductory discussion focuses mainly on the structure and function of the parts of the nervous system massage therapists can reach—which, not coincidentally, are also the parts of the system that are most vulnerable to injury.

Nervous System Function and Structure

Nerves are bundles of individual neurons: fibrous cells capable of transmitting electrical impulses from one place to another. At their most basic level, the function of neurons is to transmit information from the body to the brain (sensation) and responses from the brain to the body (motor control). Interconnecting neurons in the brain also provide the potential for consciousness, learning, creativity, memory, and other fascinating abilities, but they are beyond the scope of this book.

Peripheral nerves are composed of bundles of long filaments (neurons) that run from the spinal cord to the area in the body for which they supply sensation or motor control. Each neuron is a single living cell. Neurons in the CNS may be tiny, but the neurons that signal when we stub our toe run from the toe up the leg, through the buttock, into the spine, and up to the spinal cord, which terminates around T_{12} to L_1. Each of these cells is several feet long.

Neurons have three functional parts: the **dendrite** (which picks up signals), the cell body with a nucleus, and the **axons** (fibers that carry signals). Sensory neurons have exceptionally long fibers that begin with treelike dendrites located in the skin or other tissues. Dendrites are sensitive to stimuli, and they initiate an electrochemical signal. Long axons carry signals from the peripheral dendrites toward the cell body in the dorsal root ganglia, and short axons leave the cell body to carry that impulse into the spinal cord. By contrast, motor neurons have dendrites and cell bodies inside the spinal cord and very long axons to carry messages out to their terminating sites in the muscles and glands.

Neurons connect via **synapses**, where axons and dendrites meet. Motor and sensory neurons sometimes use combinations of central, or association, neurons to pass messages. When a stimulus enters the spinal cord via a sensory neuron, the message can cross the synapse to multiple neurons simultaneously. Some carry the message up to the brain to be consciously processed, but other neurons immediately exit the spinal cord to appropriate muscles, so we have an even faster response to the stimulus. This stimulus/response loop is called a **reflex arc** (Figure 4.1).

Most axons in the peripheral and central nervous systems have a waxy insulating coating called **myelin**. This layer of material speeds conduction along the fiber and also prevents the electrical impulses from jumping from one fiber to another. In the peripheral nervous system, neurons have another protective feature in **neurilemma**, an outside layer of myelin that can help to regenerate damaged tissue. Each neuron has a connective tissue covering (endoneuron). Finally, layers of connective tissue wrap bundles of neurons together in a structure called the epineuron (Figure 4.2).

It is a convenient analogy to think about nerves as bundles of electrical wires. The similarities are obvious: here are thousands of filaments carrying electrical impulses, each one wrapped by an insulating layer of myelin, and they are bundled together in fascial packages. The analogy stops, however, when one considers the effect of external pressure on nerve fiber transmission. Nerves function with a combination of electrical and fluid flow; this flow may be severely limited by external pressure. Squeeze an electrical cord, and it still works. But when a femoral nerve is compressed by a psoas in spasm, or the brachial **plexus** nerves are stretched in the tangled maze of scalenes and pectoralis minor muscles, signals may be blocked or interrupted.

General Neurological Problems

Most of the nervous system disorders that massage can mechanically affect involve some kind of pinching or distortion of peripheral nerves as they wend their way from the spinal cord to their destination in the body. Some of these conditions (**carpal tunnel syndrome, thoracic outlet syndrome**) are discussed in the neuromuscular section of

Dendrite: The process of a nerve cell that carries impulses toward the cell body.

Axon: The long process of a nerve cell that conducts impulses away from the cell body.

Synapse: The junction between two nerve cells.

Reflex arc: A neural pathway for an action reflex, which bypasses the brain.

Myelin: The insulating cover surrounding the axons of nerve cells.

Neurilemma: The outermost sheath surrounding nerve cells.

Plexus: A network of interwoven nerves; can also refer to blood vessels or lymphatic vessels. Plural is plexi.

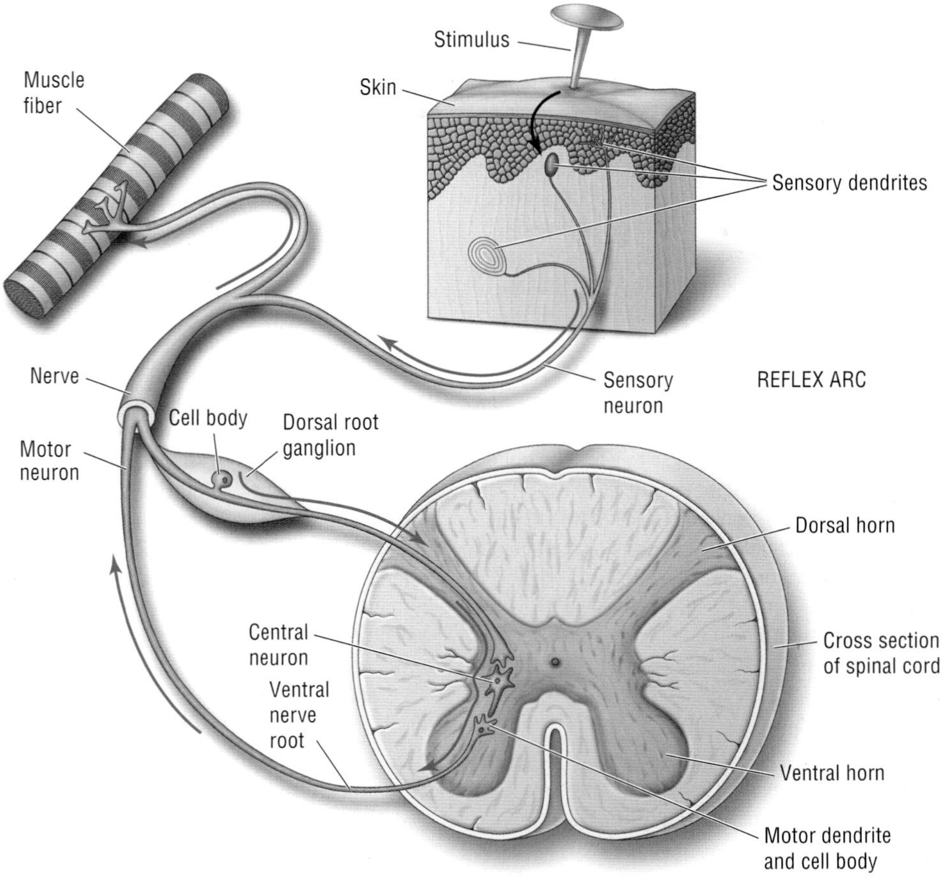

FIGURE 4.1 The reflex arc: connecting sensation to motor response at the spinal cord level

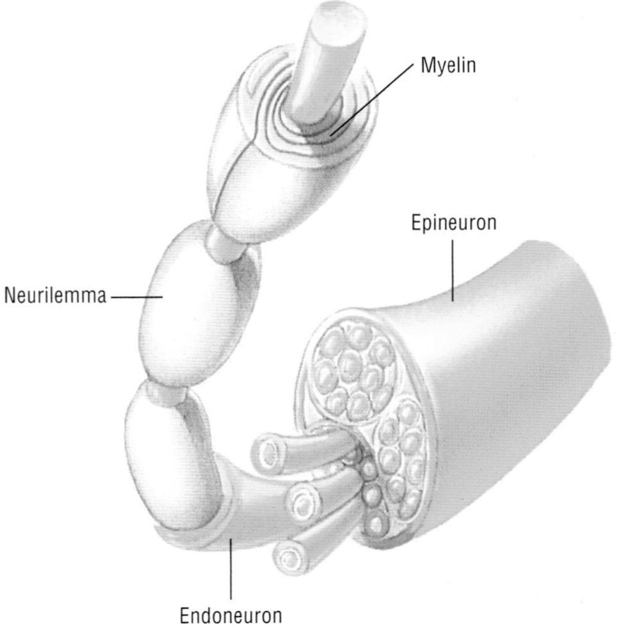

FIGURE 4.2 Nerve coverings: myelin, neurilemma, endoneuron, epineuron

Chapter 3. Peripheral nerve damage often has a good prognosis because of the regenerative properties provided by the neurilemma.

Other neurological problems involve the CNS, which has more limited ability to regenerate and which massage obviously cannot directly access. But even when the spinal cord has been injured, overlapping patterns of innervation created by the plexi often allow at least partial motor and sensory function of what would otherwise be a totally useless limb. This remarkable advantage shows the benefits of the complicated interweaving patterns of spinal nerves that supply the extremities. The best plan, when faced with a client who has sustained CNS damage, is to address the symptoms of these disorders as within our skill sets, looking for sensation where it is present, and to create as hospitable an internal environment as possible.

Various kinds of CNS damage often lead to the progressive loss of motor function. This has traditionally been viewed as an inevitable consequence of CNS injury, but it turns out not always to be accurate. In many cases, the loss of motor function may be an issue of peripheral proprioceptive adaptation more than true nerve loss. In other words, a **stroke** or **traumatic brain injury** (TBI) survivor may lose some strength in an arm or a leg, and the compensatory

SIDEBAR 4.1 The Stress Response System

The stress response system is the link between the CNS and the endocrine system that allows humans to respond to both short-term and long-term stressors. It is controlled by the **HPA axis**, the communication loop between the hypothalamus, the pituitary gland, and the adrenal glands. A healthy stress response system allows immediate reactions that are appropriately gauged to the circumstances: big reactions to big threats, small reactions to small threats. And when the stress response system works well, the chemical changes it brings about are transitory and quickly neutralized once the threat has passed.

Some people have a stress response system that doesn't work well. The chemical messages issued first from the hypothalamus, then by the pituitary gland, are slow to leave the brain and reach the adrenals. This takes longer to have an effect on the body, decreasing the ability to respond quickly to threat. But the stress reaction, once it takes hold, is tenacious, and aftereffects linger much longer than for someone who has a healthy stress response system. Furthermore, people who have a sluggish stress response system also tend to have more stress responses with less threatening stimuli. This is a person who fumes in a long checkout line, who frets in heavy traffic, and who blows up when the kids leave their bikes in the driveway. This is someone who may have a sluggish but overactive stress response, and this person has a high propensity to develop several diseases, including **depression** and **anxiety disorders**.

What determines the health of the stress response system? Studies with animals reveal one reliable predictor for a sluggish stress response: lack of tactile stimulation, or touch. Understimulated animals have consistently slower, longer-lasting, and more frequent stress responses than do animals that were regularly petted and fondled. Consider what this means for the average undertouched person in our society: low-functioning but long-lasting stress reactions that occur with unnecessary and unhealthy frequency.

A solid body of evidence supports the use of massage for several psychiatric conditions, including depression and some types of anxiety. The mechanism for how massage helps in these situations isn't yet clear, but it seems possible that welcomed, educated touch can be an important link between physical experience and psychiatric health.

movement patterns allow for further degeneration of affected muscle fibers. Massage, stretching, and careful exercise may help make it possible to interrupt and even reverse this type of progressive loss. Further, the phenomenon of **neuroplasticity**, the ability for CNS structures to change and adapt, is being employed in new and imaginative ways in the treatment of CNS injuries.

Organic and mechanical problems with the central and peripheral nervous systems are one class of neurological problem massage therapists encounter. Psychiatric disorders, which can also be classified as neurological problems, are another matter altogether. Many people have a bewildering array of mental or psychological qualities that set them apart from what is labeled "normal." Some of these people seek massage as a way to deal with some of the difficulties that their conditions create. This is often a good impulse; touch is an integral part of physical and psychological health. Research on massage and mood disorders shows a strong and reliable positive effect. Indeed, it could be said that touch is an important link between physical and psychological health (Sidebar 4.1). Further, the stress response systems don't always work perfectly. This leaves us vulnerable to a host of conditions that are linked to living in chronic stress (Sidebar 4.2)

HPA axis: The hypothalamic-pituitary-adrenal axis, consisting of the complex interactions between these three glands.

Neuroplasticity: The ability of the central nervous system to change functionally and structurally as a result of injury or damage.

The *Diagnostic and Statistical Manual of Mental Disorders* (DSM) is the reference that doctors around the world use to study and treat psychiatric patients. It has recently been updated as DSM-V. This project has reorganized the way some of the psychiatric conditions are classified and discussed. So that users of MTGP 6e are up to date with the health care profession, we have reorganized relevant sections of the nervous system chapter to be in alignment with the DSM-V.

Chronic Pain and Massage Therapy

Pain, according to the International Association for the Study of Pain, is *"an unpleasant sensory and emotional experience associated with actual or potential tissue damage, or described in terms of such damage.*[1]*"*

It is usually a useful signal, letting us know that we are at risk of or actually undergoing tissue damage, so we'd better stop doing whatever it is that is causing that signal. But sometimes pain signals can be dysfunctional. Our brain can make mistakes about the location of the initiating stimulus, or the signals themselves can become distorted. One of the complications of conditions that involve long-term pain is that the complex connections from sensors in the body to sensors in the spinal cord and brain can change: they can become hypersensitive to smaller signals, and our innate ability to fil-

[1]https://www.iasp-pain.org/Education/Content.aspx?ItemNumber=1698

SIDEBAR 4.2 "Stress": The Predisease

The term "stress" originally entered the language as a way to describe an architectural principle: stress on roof beams must be equally distributed, for instance, or the building will collapse. Now, of course, "stress" is commonly used to describe a long-term sense of physical, mental, or emotional strain arising from demanding circumstances.

It is important to point out that stress in and of itself is not a bad thing. Humans have mechanisms that help us to cope with a sense of imminent or far-off danger, and we also have mechanisms to help us recover from that sense of threat. Some people seem to do this very well, and the stress of everyday life does not inevitably lead to negative outcomes for them.

Stress becomes a health problem when our physical and mental and emotional reactions develop dysfunctional patterns—often they perpetuate the sense of near or distant threat. Lying in bed with insomnia, and being worried because you're not sleeping is a good example of this. Locked in this vicious circle, the hormones we secrete, the sleep we lose, the food we don't digest well, the resistance we add to our circulatory systems, and the bad habits we indulge in for temporary relief can have a cumulative negative effect on health. In this way, unmanaged or poorly managed stress can be called a predisease state.

It is not a stretch to see how this takes a toll on health. From suppressed immunity that makes us more susceptible to **colds** and **flu**, to a change in neuroendocrine function that opens the door to depression, stress can make us weak and vulnerable. Other common stress-related conditions include **peptic ulcers**, **hypertension**, **heart attack**, **stroke**, **irritable bowel syndrome**, **fibromyalgia**, **dysmenorrhea**, **headache**, and many others. Further, anyone diagnosed with a chronic non–stress-related disease is vulnerable to the added burden that the stress of living in that circumstance adds. Thus the disease itself may take a backseat to the depression, anxiety, or other complications that stress carries.

Every year, more than 30 million people pay for a professional massage in this country. The ones who say they're doing it purely for pampering are in a distinct minority. The vast majority of massage therapy users (typically 80% to 90%) report that the reason they see a massage therapist is to help them manage a disease or condition, *or to help them reduce stress.*

Human experience supports the use of educated, experienced touch as a way to manage stress. The research supports it too: studies find with some consistency that massage therapy is a safe, cost-effective, and efficacious way to reduce the perception of stress related to work, related to other health concerns, in postsurgery recovery, and for caregivers, children, elders, and others. This doesn't suggest that massage therapy has the power to undo the results of long-term stress, but it does support the use of this intervention for people who are looking for a noninvasive, nonpharmaceutical option to include in their stress management strategies.

ter out or modulate pain signals can become impaired. In this way, many kinds of stimuli can cause the perception of pain, and the perception of pain is more extreme and long lasting. This altered processing is sometimes referred to as **central sensitization**. Conditions as diverse as **complex regional pain syndrome**, **postherpetic neuralgia**, and **fibromyalgia syndrome** may all involve central sensitization.

Chronic pain and central sensitization are important topics for massage therapists and other health care providers. They present one of the most expensive, risk-laden, challenging situations for our health care system. The research on massage therapy for people who live with chronic pain is in its infancy, but it is promising. As we learn more about this condition and the factors that contribute to it, we may also learn how massage may effectively interrupt or reverse some of those factors.

Central sensitization: A change in the central nervous system in response to repeated incidences of pain, leading the person to feel more pain in response to the same stimulus, or even to feel pain in response to a stimulus that would not normally be considered painful.

Major Cautions for Massage Therapists

In the context of nervous system problems and massage, a few cautions emerge as common themes:

- *Numbness.* When a client can't feel part of his or her body, it is inappropriate to try to change the quality of those tissues. It is appropriate to include the numb area as a part of the incorporating aspect of massage, but extra care must be taken not to damage tissues where the client has no sensation.
- *Verbal communication.* Some types of nervous system problems make it difficult or impossible for clients to communicate verbally. While massage can still be safe and supportive, it is especially important for therapists to be sensitive to nonverbal cues about comfort and pain from these clients.
- *Medications.* Clients who take medication to help manage their mood or other mental states may find that massage is especially helpful—so much so that they want to change or stop taking their medication altogether. While this sounds like wonderful progress, it must only be done with the guidance of the prescribing physician.

Nervous System Conditions

Chronic Degenerative Disorders

- Alzheimer disease
- Amyotrophic lateral sclerosis
  - Sporadic ALS
  - Familial ALS
  - Mariana Islands–type ALS
- Huntington disease
- Peripheral neuropathy

Movement Disorders

- Dystonia
  - Focal dystonia
    - Cervical dystonia
    - Vocal dysphonia
    - Oromandibular dystonia
    - Blepharospasm
  - Multifocal dystonia
  - Segmental dystonia
    - Meige syndrome
    - Upper limb dystonia
    - Lower limb dystonia
  - Hemidystonia
  - Generalized dystonia
    - Paroxysmal dystonia
    - Torsion dystonia
    - Tardive dystonia
  - Parkinson disease
  - Tremor
    - Essential tremor
    - Secondary tremor

Infectious Disorders

- Encephalitis
- Herpes zoster
  - Chickenpox
  - Shingles
  - Herpes zoster ophthalmicus
  - Postherpetic neuralgia
  - Ramsay Hunt syndrome
  - Sine herpete
- Meningitis
  - Bacterial meningitis
  - Viral meningitis
- Polio, postpolio syndrome

Psychiatric Disorders

- Addiction
  - Alcoholism
- Anxiety disorders
  - General anxiety disorder
  - Panic disorder
  - Agoraphobia
  - Phobias
    - Social phobia
    - Specific phobias
  - Separation anxiety
- Attention deficit hyperactivity disorder
- Autism spectrum disorder
  - Autistic disorder
  - Asperger syndrome
  - Pervasive development disorder, not otherwise specified
- Bipolar disorder
  - Bipolar disorder type I
  - Bipolar disorder type II
  - Cyclothymia
  - Mixed bipolar disorder
  - Rapid-cycling bipolar disorder
- Depression
  - Major depressive disorder
  - Persistent depressive disorder
  - Psychotic depression
  - Seasonal affective disorder
  - Premenstrual dysphoric disorder
  - Postpartum depression
- Eating disorders
  - Anorexia
  - Bulimia
  - Binge-eating disorder
- Obsessive-compulsive and related disorders
  - Obsessive-compulsive disorder
  - Body dysmorphic disorder
  - Excoriation disorder
  - Trichotillomania
  - Hoarding disorder
- Trauma- and stressor-related disorders
  - Posttraumatic stress disorder
    - Dissociative PTSD
  - Acute traumatic stress disorder
  - Adjustment disorder
  - Reactive attachment disorder

Nervous System Injuries

- Bell palsy
- Complex regional pain syndrome
- Spinal cord injury
- Stroke
  - Ischemic stroke
    - Stenosis
    - Transient ischemic attack
    - Cryptogenic
  - Hemorrhagic stroke
- Traumatic brain injury
- Trigeminal neuralgia

Nervous system birth defects

- Spina bifida
  - SB occulta
  - SB meningocele
  - SB myelomeningocele
- Cerebral palsy
  - Spastic CP
  - Athetoid CP
  - Ataxic CP
  - Dystonic CP
  - Mixed CP

Other Nervous System Conditions

- Fibromyalgia
- Headaches
  - Tension type
  - Migraine
  - Cluster
  - Rebound
- Ménière disease
- Seizure disorders
  - Epilepsy
- Sleep disorders
  - Insomnia
  - Obstructive sleep apnea
  - Central sleep apnea
  - Restless leg syndrome
  - Narcolepsy
  - Circadian rhythm disruption
- Vestibular balance disorders
  - Benign paroxysmal positional vertigo
  - Labyrinthitis
  - Acute vestibular neuronitis
  - Perilymph fistula

Chronic Degenerative Disorders

Alzheimer Disease

Definition: What Is It?

Alzheimer disease (AD) is a progressive degenerative disorder of the brain causing memory loss, personality changes, and eventually death.

Demographics

Alzheimer disease affects more than 5 million Americans and causes about 500,000 deaths each year; those numbers are expected to triple by 2050. AD costs the country about $214 billion a year in direct and indirect medical expenses.

The incidence of most cases of AD is strongly tied to age: 10% of people over 65 have it, and about 50% of those over 85 have been diagnosed. It affects many more women than men, but that may be as much tied to life expectancy as to a gender-based predisposition. Another way in which AD disproportionately affects women is that most of the caregivers that provide the 17.7 billion hours of unpaid round-the-clock care for Alzheimer patients each year are women. A version of this condition can affect younger people: about 200,000 of the 5 million AD patients in the United States are under age 65.

Etiology: What Happens?

AD is named for a German doctor, Alois Alzheimer, who first documented the typical lesions in the brain seen with this disorder in 1906. He performed an autopsy on a female patient who died in a mental institution in her mid-50s, and he noticed two specific changes in her brain tissue: plaques and tangles. These observations are now the primary postmortem diagnostic features of this disease.

- *Plaques.* Sticky deposits of a naturally occurring cellular protein called **beta amyloid** have been noted on neural cells of people with AD. Beta amyloid is produced by many cells in the body, and it occurs in various lengths and qualities, depending on where it is found. In the brain, it seems to be particularly sticky. When it accumulates in sufficient amounts, the deposits stimulate an inflammatory response in the brain that kills off not only the cells affected by the plaques, but also the nearby unaffected cells. Plaques are found in the hippocampus and throughout the cerebral cortex of AD patients.
- *Neurofibrillary tangles.* Another Alzheimer-related protein is called **tau**. This substance helps to physically support long fibers in the CNS so they can connect at synapses. When tau proteins in AD patients degenerate, the long fibers collapse and become twisted and snarled together: **neurofibrillary tangles**. Eventually, the cells, which are no longer capable of transmitting messages to each other, shrink and die. The brain of a person with AD shows predictable patterns of atrophy, with deeper **sulci** (Figure 4.3), a smaller hippocampus, and larger ventricles than the brains of people without AD.

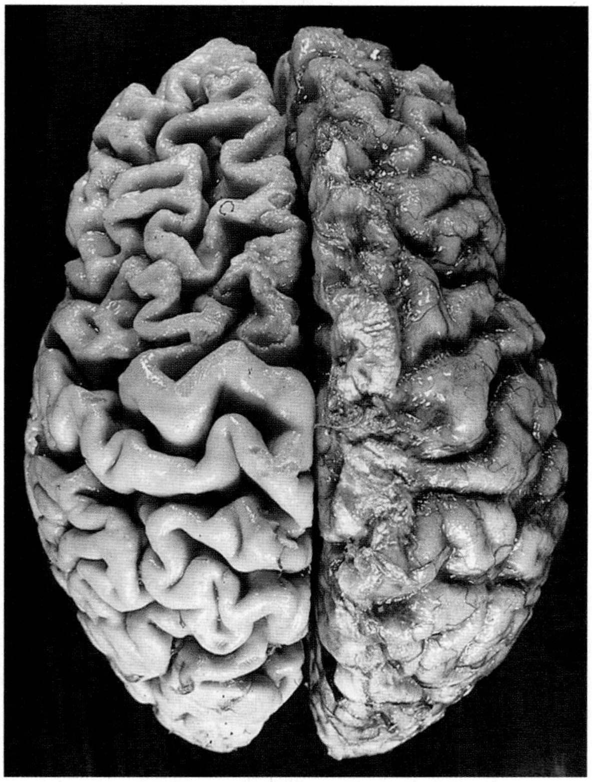

FIGURE 4.3 Visible atrophy associated with Alzheimer disease

The presence of beta amyloid plaques and tau-related tangles means that fewer brain cells function at normal levels. With the loss of neural tissue, levels of many

Beta amyloid: A type of protein associated with formation of plaque in the brain.

Tau: A protein that helps to maintain the structure of the cytoskeleton. Found in the plaques of people with Alzheimer disease.

Neurofibrillary tangles: Intraneural accumulations of filaments with twisted, contorted patterns. Associated with Alzheimer disease.

Sulci: The grooves or furrows on the surface of the brain. (Singular: sulcus)

neurotransmitters in the brains of AD patients become pathologically low. This makes it difficult for the functioning nerve cells that remain to communicate with each other. Further, the **hippocampus** (the part of the brain that processes and stores new information and knowledge) also shrinks and loses function. Consequently, the AD patient loses access to memories and loses the ability to process new information.

Plaques and tangles were the first features associated with Alzheimer disease. Other contributing factors include genetics, chronic inflammation, a history of head injury, exposure to environmental toxins, high cholesterol levels, low estrogen levels (in women), the presence of cardiovascular disease and diabetes, and many other variables. These discoveries reveal many new possibilities for treatment and prevention of this disease.

While the exact causes of Alzheimer disease remain a mystery, it seems clear that some choices influence the chance of developing this disease. Regular physical activity, a healthy diet, frequent interactions with others, and a habit of lifelong learning are factors that appear to lessen the risk of developing this disease.

SIDEBAR 4.3 What Is Dementia?

Dementia is not a freestanding disease; it is an umbrella term describing cognitive degeneration that mostly affects older adults. It is not a synonym for Alzheimer disease, but it is one of the symptoms.

Dementia, or "neurocognitive disorder" (NCD), as it is now labeled in the DSM-V, can also occur with several other neurodegenerative diseases, including **Parkinson disease**, **Lewy body disease**, **Creutzfeldt-Jakob disease**, vascular dementia, and others.

NCD is expensive; it costs in the neighborhood of $230 billion each year to care for the people diagnosed with some form of this condition, and the incidence is expected to rise significantly in the next decades.

Recognizing NCD early is an important clinical factor, because its course may be influenced by medication and early intervention. Diagnosing it in early stages has historically been challenging, however. The DSM-V has now published a full set of criteria that evaluate various cognitive domains (i.e., learning and memory, word finding and fluency, and executive function), along with looking at the patient's ability to engage in simple and complex activities of daily living. Ruling out other possible causes of cognitive loss is also important; cognitive impairment can be a result of other treatable diseases or B_{12} deficiency.

Signs and Symptoms

The degeneration associated with AD can occur across a wide spectrum over many years, and it can be difficult to delineate between the mild loss of memory that occurs for many aging people and the early signs of AD-related dementia (see Sidebar 4.3). Key changes include loss of recent memory, including conversations and misplacing possessions; poor judgment in decision making; disorientation and loss of spatial and temporal awareness; increasing difficulty in word finding in both written language and spoken language; and difficulty in performing complex and simple tasks like dressing and cooking. As the disease progresses, more functions are lost, including the ability to walk, communicate, or do any self-care. Ultimately, a person in late-stage Alzheimer disease becomes vulnerable to infection like **pneumonia** or to progressive organ failure.

Hippocampus: A structure in the brain located within the temporal lobe. Part of the limbic system and involved in the consolidation of information from short- to long-term memory.

Lewy body disease: A multisystem disease involving abnormal proteins in the brain that contribute to dementia and Parkinson disease symptoms.

Creutzfeldt-Jakob disease: A degenerative and fatal neurological disease caused by prions. Commonly known as mad cow disease.

In addition, Alzheimer disease can affect parts of the brain that influence personality and behavior. The consequences can include depression, anxiety, paranoia, aggressiveness, emotional lability, and loss of inhibitions.

Treatment

Because Alzheimer disease is a complex condition that is not fully understood, no single treatment can address all the symptoms, and no intervention either prevents or reverses this disease. Treatment strategies focus on slowing the process and dealing with the other conditions that frequently occur alongside, especially depression and anxiety.

Medications

- Cholinesterase inhibitors for memory improvement
- Antidepressants
- Antianxiety medication
- Nonsteroidal anti-inflammatory drugs (NSAIDs) (excluding aspirin and acetaminophen) to limit inflammatory responses to plaques

Massage Therapy Implications

RISKS	Clients with Alzheimer disease may have a collection of other long-term diseases that require adaptations in bodywork: it is important to be fully informed about a client's health profile. Further, AD patients may be not able to communicate verbally, and they may become disoriented and confused. For this reason, it is especially important for a massage therapist working in this setting to be sensitive to nonverbal signals about their client's sense of safety and well-being.
BENEFITS	Although bodywork doesn't slow or reverse Alzheimer disease, it may improve the quality of life for patients, in that they become less disruptive, show a better sense of orientation, and have more positive interactions in nursing home settings.
RESEARCH	Massage therapy is one intervention among many that experts recommend for Alzheimer disease[1]; it has been seen to help with orientation, restlessness, and combativeness.[2] While not specifically targeted to Alzheimer disease patients, Harris and Richards[3] found that slow-stroke back and hand massage was extremely relaxing and well received among older patients.

1. Behrman S, Chouliaras L, Ebmeier KP. Considering the senses in the diagnosis and management of dementia. *Maturitas* 2014;77(4): 305–310. http://www.ncbi.nlm.nih.gov/pubmed/24495787
2. Rowe M, Alfred D. The effectiveness of slow-stroke massage in diffusing agitated behaviors in individuals with Alzheimer's disease. *Journal of Gerontological Nursing* 1999;25(6):22–34. http://www.ncbi.nlm.nih.gov/pubmed/10603811
3. Harris M, Richards KC. The physiological and psychological effects of slow-stroke back massage and hand massage on relaxation in older people. *Journal of Clinical Nursing* 2010;19(7–8):917–926. http://www.ncbi.nlm.nih.gov/pubmed/20492036

Amyotrophic Lateral Sclerosis

Definition: What Is It?

Also known as Lou Gehrig disease in the United States and motor neurone disease in Great Britain, amyotrophic lateral sclerosis (ALS) is a progressive and fatal condition that destroys motor neurons in the central and peripheral nervous systems, leading to the atrophy of voluntary muscles. The cells most at risk are the large motor neurons in the lateral aspects of the spinal cord. These are replaced by fibrous **astrocytes**, which make the spinal cord hard and scarlike. "Amyotrophic" refers to muscle atrophy, "lateral" refers to the parts of the spinal cord that are affected, and "sclerosis" refers to the hardening of the spinal cord tissue.

Demographics

ALS is diagnosed in about 5,600 people each year in this country, and between 20,000 and 30,000 people live with this condition. Its incidence is higher among the Chamorro population of Guam and the Marianas Islands and in some isolated areas in Japan. It is more common in men than women, although that ratio isn't completely unbalanced; it is about 1.5:1. After age 50, the incidence in men and women is about the same.

Astrocytes: Star-shaped glial cells in the central nervous system.

Microglia: Glial cells that act as on-site macrophages in the central nervous system.

Motor unit: A motor neuron and the skeletal muscle fibers it innervates.

Etiology: What Happens?

The cause or causes of ALS are unknown. When the disease develops, motor neurons in the central and peripheral nervous system die. Nearby **microglia**, which would normally be protective, change their qualities to contribute to the degeneration of motor neurons. Inflammation develops throughout the spinal cord and brain. Many ALS patients also have damage in the parts of the frontal lobe that are involved in the planning and execution of movement. This may also lead to some cognitive changes, which can contribute to some of the emotional aspects of this disease. All of these discoveries have led to the conclusion that ALS is not a disease of motor neurons alone, but a combination of multicellular and multisystemic influences.

Surviving neurons in the peripheral system grow new axon branches to supply deprived muscle fibers, which increases the size of each **motor unit**. When those neurons ultimately fail, progressive and irreversible atrophy of voluntary muscle occurs (Figure 4.4). About one-third of the motor

NOTABLE CASES First baseman "Iron Horse" Lou Gehrig was diagnosed with ALS after he began dropping catches and tripping over his own feet. In his 1939 farewell speech, he famously declared, "Today I consider myself the luckiest man on the face of the earth." He died 2 years later.

Physicist and author of *A Brief History of Time* Stephen Hawking (and subject of the film *The Theory of Everything*) is one of the longest-lived and most famous ALS patients. He has had this condition for many years and has built a rich career while being paralyzed with this disease.

The massage therapy community lost a great friend and resource when Nina McIntosh, author of *The Educated Heart*, died of ALS in 2010. She is greatly missed. This section is for you, Nina.

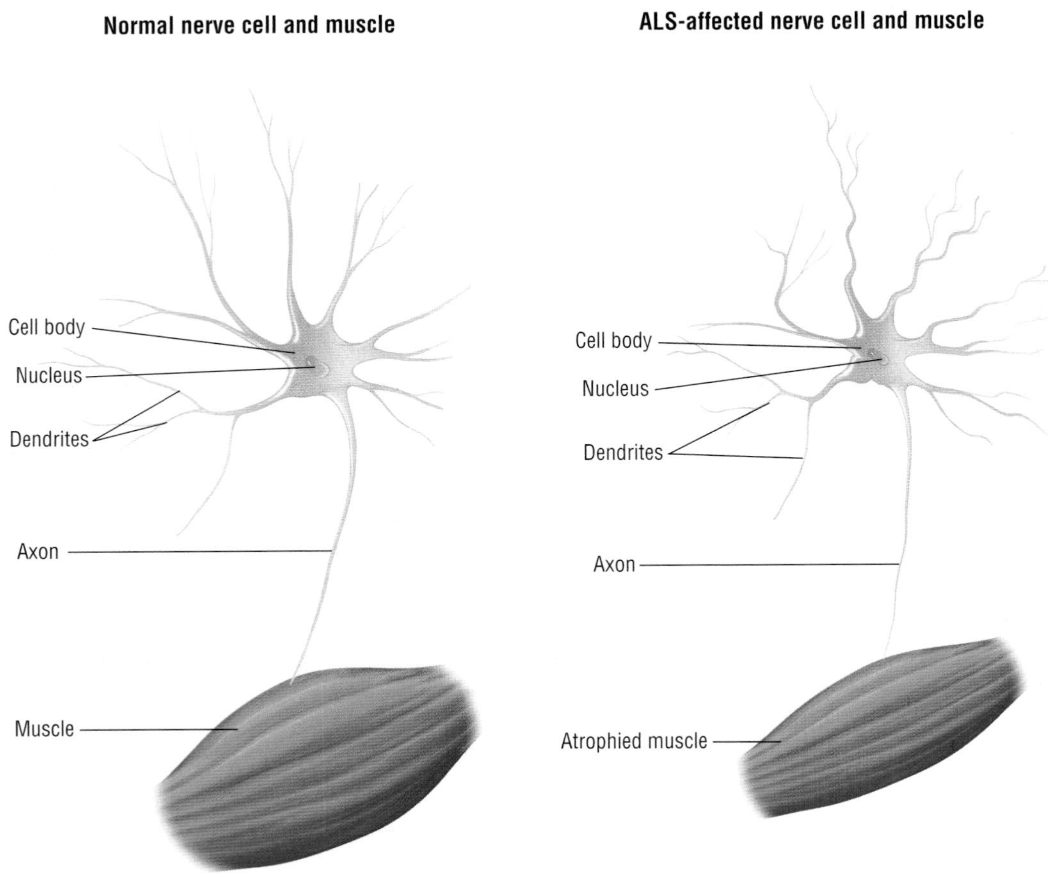

FIGURE 4.4 ALS: Nerve damage leads to muscle atrophy

neurons that supply a muscle must be destroyed before atrophy becomes noticeable.

Several possible contributing factors for ALS have been identified, including genetic predisposition, oxidative injury, mitochondrial dysfunction, premature cell death, glial cell pathology, and the presence of too much glutamate. Glutamate is a neurotransmitter that, for reasons that are not clear, is not neutralized or reabsorbed by presynaptic neurons, and it eventually damages and even kills the motor neuron it is meant to stimulate, in a situation called glutamate **excitotoxicity**.

Types of Amyotrophic Lateral Sclerosis

- *Sporadic ALS*: This is the most common type, accounting for 90% to 95% of all cases in the United States.
- *Familial ALS*: This form shows a genetic link for ALS. It accounts for about 5% to 15% of all cases in the United States and is characterized by an earlier onset than the sporadic variety of ALS.
- *Mariana Islands–type ALS*: This is endemic to a specific population in the Western Pacific Islands, especially Guam. It may be related to food sources that are limited to that region.

> **Excitotoxicity:** A pathologic state in which nerve cells are damaged by excessive exposure to excitatory neurotransmitters.
>
> **Upper motor neurons:** Motor neurons that originate in the brain and carry signals to lower motor neurons.
>
> **Lower motor neurons:** Motor neurons that link upper motor neurons and skeletal muscles.
>
> **Bulbar:** Bulb shaped.

Signs and Symptoms

Symptoms of ALS are sometimes classified by whether the disease affects spinal nerves or cranial nerves and whether the symptoms demonstrate damage to **upper motor neurons** or **lower motor neurons**.

About 75% of ALS cases are diagnosed as the spinal variation, with early symptoms in the arms or legs. Difficulty with fine motor skills in the hands (writing, buttoning a shirt) may be the first sign of a problem. When early symptoms occur in the legs, frequent tripping or stumbling may be the first indication of the disease. Both sides may be affected, but one side is typically worse than the other. Fatigue, cramping, stiffness, and weakness move proximally up the limb and eventually affect the voluntary trunk muscles that control breathing.

About 25% of ALS cases first present as difficulties with speech, swallowing, or motor control of the tongue. This is the **bulbar** form, and it is often more serious, with a faster progression, than the spinal form of the disease. Bulbar ALS is also associated with extreme and rapid mood swings, or "emotional incontinence."

Upper motor neuron problems manifest as progressive **spasticity**, exaggerated reflexes (including the gag reflex), and a positive **Babinski sign**. Lower motor neurons are involved when weakness, atrophy, muscle cramps, and **fasciculations** (uncontrolled twitching) are present. Both upper and lower motor neurons are damaged in ALS.

The nerve damage seen with this disease affects motor neurons only; sensory neurons are left intact. This can be a painful process, however, with wracking muscle spasms, constipation, and the gradual collapse of the body as gravity puts demand on muscles that have no power to respond.

Treatment

Drug treatment for ALS is designed to deal with general fatigue, muscle spasms, and secondary infections. In addition, some drugs can limit the amount of glutamate in the CNS, so motor nerves function for a longer period. Interventions that limit saliva production (low-dose radiation or botulinum toxin injections to the salivary glands) can help with swallowing problems and lower the risk of aspiration-related **pneumonia**. These are not a cure for ALS, but they may significantly prolong the lives of people affected by this disease.

Nonpharmacological treatment for ALS includes moderate exercise along with physical and occupational therapy to maintain muscle strength for as long as possible. Heat and whirlpools are used to control muscle spasms, and speech therapy helps with difficulties in swallowing and speech. Assistive devices such as leg braces, arm braces, wheelchairs, voice aids, and computers can improve a patient's ability to function. A healthy diet is critical for as long as patients can eat easily. In advanced cases, swallowing may be so difficult that the insertion of a stomach tube (gastrostomy) may be recommended. Breathing support can help with both lung function and fatigue. Psychological therapy for ALS patients and their families to deal with anxiety and depression is an important part of the treatment plan.

Treatment options for ALS can delay the inevitable, but once diagnosed, this disease, which has no known cure, usually results in death within 2 to 10 years. Most ALS patients die of pneumonia or **cachexia**. Some ALS patients, however, have survived for decades, and it is unclear how (Case History 4.1).

Spasticity: A state of increased muscle tone with exaggerated muscle tendon reflexes.

Babinski sign: An abnormal reflexive extension of the great toe, indicating an injury to the central nervous system.

Fasciculations: Involuntary twitching of fasciculi.

Cachexia: Dramatic weight loss and muscle atrophy seen in people with chronic, often terminal diseases.

Medications

- Riluzole to reduce neuron damage due to glutamate excitotoxicity
- Muscle relaxants for spasm and spasticity
- Antidepressants for depression
- Anxiolytics for anxiety
- Dextromethorphan and quinidine to ameliorate involuntary emotional responses seen with bulbar-type ALS

Massage Therapy Implications

RISKS	Many ALS patients struggle with painful cramping, and any massage must be designed to minimize that symptom. Advanced patients become very frail and vulnerable to secondary infection, so bodywork must be careful about those risks.
BENEFITS	ALS is treated with heat, exercise, and physical therapy. Any bodywork that fits within these parameters is also appropriate, especially when delivered as part of a coordinated health care strategy. Massage has been used with some success to help with the pain of muscle spasms and the stress of living with a fatal disease.
OPTIONS	ALS patients can find special value in massage that focuses on pain and strong breathing.
RESEARCH	The use of Complementary and Integrative Health (ICIH) therapies, including massage therapy, is popular among some ALS patients to help manage some of the symptoms of the disease, along with side effects of some of the medications.[1,2] Some studies suggest the usefulness of massage therapy in the context of constipation[3,4] and massage therapy for spasticity,[5] although these have looked at other CNS dysfunctions rather than ALS specifically.

1. Pan W, Chen X, Bao J, et al. The use of integrative therapies in patients with amyotrophic lateral sclerosis in Shanghai, China. *Evidence-Based Complementary and Alternative Medicine* 2013;2013:613596. http://www.ncbi.nlm.nih.gov/pmc/articles/PMC3865630/
2. Blatzheim K. Interdisciplinary palliative care, including massage, in treatment of amyotrophic lateral sclerosis. *Journal of Bodywork and Movement Therapies* 2009;13(4):328–335. http://www.ncbi.nlm.nih.gov/pubmed/19761955
3. Coggrave M, Norton C, Cody JD. Management of faecal incontinence and constipation in adults with central neurological diseases. *Cochrane Database of Systematic Reviews* 2014;(1):CD002115. http://www.ncbi.nlm.nih.gov/pubmed/24420006
4. McClurg D, Lowe-Strong A. Does abdominal massage relieve constipation? *Nursing Times* 2011;107(12):20–22. http://www.ncbi.nlm.nih.gov/pubmed/21520798
5. Negahban H, Rezaie S, Goharpey S. Massage therapy and exercise therapy in patients with multiple sclerosis: a randomized controlled pilot study. *Clinical Rehabilitation* 2013;27(12):1126–1136. http://www.ncbi.nlm.nih.gov/pubmed/23828184

CASE HISTORY 4.1 Amyotrophic Lateral Sclerosis

Six months after he married the love of his life and built her a home, Eric was diagnosed with ALS. Rather than succumb to sadness, the couple decided to go to Paris for a vacation and try to conceive a child. Nine months later, a baby girl joined the household.

For the past 2 years, I have treated Eric for 90 minutes in his home every week. Before he lost control of his facial muscles, I could understand his slurred speech; he sounded like a poststroke patient or a fellow hammered with too many whiskeys. Now, all he can do is grunt and point, so he communicates with the aid of a small computer keyboard through which a stilted robotic male voice "speaks" as he types. He can no longer walk, and he moves about his huge home with a fancy battery-operated wheelchair.

In these 2 years, he has changed from being a hearty, muscular chiseled strong man to a man who leans on one entire side of my body as he takes slow, uneven steps from his wheelchair to the massage table.

Eric says that without the weekly massage sessions, his medication level would be much higher, he would have more muscular spasms, and the pain in his shoulder would be unbearable.

Approaching a body with ALS is more than a little tricky. Spasms occur without warning; the beginning of slow, even, medium-pressure effleurage while applying lotion to a lower extremity can result in a board-hard leg that extends as if levitating off the table of its own accord. All I can do is place my hand on the leg and slowly coax it back down to the table. Arms that used to open wide to hug those around him would contract against his body were it not for the slow, sometimes painful range-of-motion exercises we perform on all arm joints each week. Every bit of therapy takes twice as long as working on a "normal" body: if he's not stretched, he contracts; if I go too fast, he spasms; communication is cumbersome; and causing pain, though unintended, is always a possibility.

The end of life for an ALS patient is often related to diaphragm function. It can slow down to the point that the decreased lung capacity invites pneumonia, which is the ultimate threat to any sedentary human. For this reason, aggressive (though careful) resisted breathing exercises are part of every session. This means I have to get up on the table and place my hands just at his tenth rib, trying not to dislodge his feeding tube or the dressing around his diaphragmatic monitor. Then, I encourage him to push against me with his breath while I'm wobbling all over and trying hard not to fall off the table. This brings on a lot of laughter—therapeutic in itself for someone with limited lung capacity. I hover above him while he laughs and tries to take a deep breath. I watch as he deems himself victorious if he can take at least one deep inhale and exhale; it's enough to bring a strong woman to tears. The victory is minuscule to most of us, but this effort could help extend his life.

Presently, there is no cure for this frustrating and frightening disease. But massage therapy can make a profound difference in the patient's pain and in the progression of muscular contractions. Every case is different, but the intelligent and dedicated therapist can adapt her skills to these very special patients and help make the damnable progression of ALS more tolerable as it is accompanied by loving touch.

—Charlotte Versagi

To view a portion of the diagnostic process of a person who may have ALS, see the video "Amyotrophic Lateral Sclerosis at" http://thePoint.lww.com/Werner6e. thePoint®

Huntington Disease

Definition: What Is It?

Huntington disease (HD) is a progressive degenerative disease of the CNS that is ultimately terminal. It is brought about by an autosomal dominant genetic mutation. This means that only one gene must be present for the disease to manifest; it can be passed to children by both mothers and fathers; and every child of a parent with the HD gene has a 50% chance of having the gene and therefore developing the disease.

Demographics

Statistics vary but most suggest that in the United States, HD has been diagnosed in 15,000 to 30,000 Americans, and 150,000 to 250,000 people may carry the HD gene. Most people experience the onset of symptoms between age 35 and 44, but it can affect much younger and much older people. It appears equally in men and women, although men are more likely to have a quickly progressive version of this disease. HD is seen in every country.

Etiology: What Happens?

Symptoms of what was probably HD have been in the medical record since the Middle Ages, but it wasn't until 1872 that a British doctor named George Huntington put together a comprehensive list of signs and symptoms of this genetic disorder. Since then, it has been known as dancing mania, hereditary chorea, Huntington chorea, and finally HD.

This disorder is the result of a genetic mutation that alters the behavior of neurons in the **basal ganglia** and the cerebral cortex, leading to cell death and irreversible and progressive loss of brain function. Intensive research has revealed that the mutation occurs when a gene has an abnormal number of repeating base pairs in a section of the DNA molecule. HD symptoms are most likely to develop when the repeating "stutter" of abnormal base pairs is over 40. The more repeating pairs that are present, the earlier symptoms tend to develop. Each successive generation of HD patients shows an increasing number of repeating pairs, especially among males: children who inherit the HD gene from their father are likely to develop symptoms earlier than do those who inherit the gene from their mother.

It is unclear exactly how these mutated genes lead to HD symptoms. Theories include the secretion of an abnormal protein that damages neurons, mitochondrial dysfunction, the presence of oxygen free radicals, and a disruption in how the brain accumulates cholesterol. Understanding the process will create better treatment options in the future, but regardless of the mechanism, predictable patterns of neuron damage are demonstrable. Degeneration of neurons stimulates **astrocytes** to multiply, which can further interfere with neuron function. Damage appears to concentrate in certain areas of the basal ganglia that have to do with organizing motor control. Sections of the frontal lobes and cerebral cortex are also vulnerable to damage, and many HD patients have abnormally large ventricles: the hollow areas inside the brain where cerebrospinal fluid circulates. When key neurons in the brain die, they not only lose their own function, but the neurotransmitters they would have secreted are also in short supply, which affects normal nearby neurons; this imbalance may account for some HD symptoms.

Ultimately, every person who carries the HD gene will develop the disease, and the disease is progressive, degenerative, and terminal, usually from **pneumonia**, complications of an injury, or suicide. New tests that identify the HD gene early are available, but they don't predict the time of onset or life expectancy. Children of a parent with HD are now faced with the difficult decision of finding out whether they are positive for the gene and whether to risk passing that gene along to their own children.

Most people with HD have a life span of 10 to 20 years after symptoms first develop.

> **NOTABLE CASES** Iconic American activist and folk singer Woody Guthrie ("This Land is Your Land," "This Train is Bound for Glory") may be the most familiar face of HD. For many years, it was assumed that Guthrie was an alcoholic or schizophrenic; he was not appropriately diagnosed until 1954, and he died in 1967—a month before his son Arlo released his own signature album, "Alice's Restaurant."

> **Basal ganglia:** Large masses of gray matter at the base of the cerebral hemispheres.
>
> **Astrocytes:** Star-shaped glial cells in the central nervous system.

Signs and Symptoms

A person's age at the onset of HD symptoms has been recorded as young as 3 years old and as old as 80, but most patients report the beginning of symptoms between ages 35 and 50. Typically, the younger a person is when symptoms develop, the more rapid the progression of the disease is likely to be.

Early signs and symptoms vary widely from one patient to another, but all of them can be categorized into three main types: changes in motor function, changes in emotional stability, and changes in cognition.

- **Motor function**: Some HD patients begin their symptoms with mild clumsiness and occasional loss of balance. Twitching, tics, and **dystonia** may start at the extremities and face, but may progress to involve the whole body. "Chorea" (from the Greek root word for dance, as in choreography) refers to the involuntary writhing, twisting movements of the face, trunk, and arms many HD patients experience.

When HD occurs in children, they may experience muscular rigidity, slow movement, tremors, and **seizures**.

Advanced HD patients have extreme balance and coordination problems, and the risk of falls can be extremely threatening. Loss of facial coordination can make swallowing and speaking prohibitively difficult.

- **Emotional stability**: Personality changes are sometimes the first sign of HD onset. These can include rapid and very extreme mood swings, irritability, apathy, hostility, and extreme depression.

  Depression is a common complication of HD, as it is of many progressive and terminal diseases. Unfortunately, depression and suicidal ideation is a common side effect of some HD medications, making this aspect of the disease particularly difficult to manage.
- **Cognition**: Most HD patients experience significant cognitive decline as their disease progresses. Unlike the dementia seen with **Alzheimer disease**, HD dementia is centered on attention, learning, judgment, and decision making rather than on language and memory loss.

Treatment

As a genetic mutation, HD is not treatable at this time. Drug therapies are aimed at controlling the worst symptoms and complications. Outside of drugs, HD is treated with psychiatric counseling, speech therapy, occupational therapy, and physical therapy designed to preserve maximum motor functioning for as long as possible.

Genetic counseling is available both for children of HD-positive parents and for HD patients who are considering being a parent themselves.

HD is a potential future target for stem cell therapy to help replace the damaged tissue in the brain. The research on this prospect is revealing a lot of information about stem cell function in the brain, but it is still a long way from human trials.

Medications

- Tetrabenazine to treat chorea symptoms; it raises the risk of depression, however, which is already a risk for HD patients
- Antipsychotic medications for delusion and psychosis
- Tranquilizers for anxiety and paranoia
- Antidepressants

Massage Therapy Implications

RISKS	A client with HD may experience any combination of motor problems, emotional volatility, and cognitive decline. If that person becomes disoriented and confused during a session, massage may feel unwelcomed at best and actively threatening at worst: this situation obviously contraindicates any bodywork that the client does not desire. Clients in an advanced state may be physically frail and vulnerable to infection; any bodywork must be gauged to their ability to adapt to the internal changes that massage brings about.
BENEFITS	Because HD affects motor control and may lead to a high risk of falls and other injuries, many patients are counseled to exercise and stay physically fit for as long as possible. Massage may be a helpful part of this strategy. Also, any symptoms that are aggravated by stress may be at least mitigated by massage, as long as it is welcomed. Finally, depression is a predictable complication of this disorder, and massage therapy has a strong evidence base for being effective for this condition. Massage therapy obviously won't address the HD itself, but it may serve to improve the quality of life for the person who lives with this condition.
OPTIONS	HD can involve involuntary muscle contractions, including twitching, tics, and jerking. Depending on how any individual receives the stimulus of massage, it may be safer and more comfortable to work with a massage chair than on a table. This situation requires flexibility and imagination to keep the client safe and comfortable.

Peripheral Neuropathy

Definition: What Is It?

Peripheral neuropathy (PN) is usually not a disease in itself, but a symptom or a complication of other underlying conditions. In this situation, peripheral nerves, either singly or in groups, are damaged through lack of circulation, chemical imbalance, trauma, or other factors.

Etiology: What Happens?

PN can affect one nerve at a time (**mononeuropathy**) or multiple nerves (**polyneuropathy**). It is typically classified by whether it affects sensation, voluntary muscle control, or autonomic function.

PN is occasionally related to a genetic anomaly, but it is usually a consequence of some other injury, infection, or systemic disease; this is called acquired PN. Some common causes of acquired PN include the following:

- *Injury*. **Carpal tunnel syndrome**, **thoracic outlet syndrome**, **Bell palsy**, **disc disease**, and **trigeminal neuralgia** are all examples of PN related to acute or chronic injury.
- *Infection*. **Herpes simplex**, **herpes zoster** (shingles), **HIV/AIDS**, **Lyme disease**, **hepatitis**, **syphilis**, and Hansen disease (leprosy) can all cause damage and irritation to peripheral nerves. The PN seen with HIV/AIDS can be from the virus itself, the drugs that treat the infection, or both. Each version tends to affect different sets of nerve fibers.
- *Systemic disease*. **Diabetes** (type 1 or type 2), **renal failure**, vitamin B_{12} deficiency, cancer, and other tumors can all contribute to nerve damage, as can some autoimmune diseases, including **lupus**, **Sjögren syndrome**, **sarcoidosis**, and **Guillain-Barré syndrome**. The sequelae for how PN develops from these diseases are still being explored. The better the process is understood, the more effectively this complication can be avoided or treated.
- *Toxic exposure*. Chronic alcoholism; sniffing glue; some medications, including chemotherapy; and exposure to heavy metals (especially lead and mercury), solvents, and other environmental contaminants can damage peripheral nerves. PN affects up to half of all heavy alcohol users, partly because of the effect alcohol has on nerve tissue and partly because severe long-term alcoholism often goes hand-in-hand with various nutritional deficiencies.

> **Mononeuropathy:** A disorder of a single nerve.
>
> **Polyneuropathy:** A condition affecting multiple peripheral nerves.
>
> **Capsaicin:** The compound that gives hot peppers their hotness. Also used topically in diluted form for pain relief.
>
> **TENS unit:** A transcutaneous electrical nerve stimulation device, used to control pain.

Signs and Symptoms

Most cases of PN begin subtly and slowly, and symptoms depend on what combinations of sensory, motor, and autonomic nerves are damaged. Injury to sensory neurons produces burning pain or tingling in the hands and feet, which gradually spreads proximally into the limbs and finally the trunk. Extreme sensitivity to touch (hyperalgesia or allodynia) can follow, but this may eventually be replaced by reduced sensation (people feel like they are always wearing socks or gloves, even when they're not), or numbness. Numbness is problematic because if a person who can't feel something—a toe, for instance—he or she can't tell if it's been injured or infected. Secondary infections and ulcers are common complications of numbness with any disease.

Damage to motor nerves can lead to twitching, cramps, and eventually to atrophy of the affected muscles.

Damage to autonomic nerves is often the most serious; this can interfere with digestion, maintaining heart and respiratory rates, sweating, blood pressure, and control of the bladder or bowel.

Treatment

Treatment for PN depends entirely on the underlying pathology that is causing the nerve damage: controlling the primary disease can help to control associated nerve pain. Topical ointments with lidocaine or **capsaicin** sometimes offer some relief. Other therapies include **TENS units**, biofeedback, acupuncture, relaxation techniques, and massage to improve circulation in the affected extremities.

The good news is that if PN is interrupted before damage affects the neuronal cell bodies, the peripheral nerves may be able to heal and regenerate.

Medications

- Analgesics for pain control
- Anti-inflammatories, especially for autoimmune disease
- Immunoglobulins to suppress immune system response
- Antiseizure drugs
- Tricyclic antidepressants

Massage Therapy Implications

RISKS	Undiagnosed pain, tingling, or numbness needs to be evaluated by a primary care provider before massage can be known to be safe. Numbness and reduced sensation can interfere with a client's ability to know when pressure is sufficient. Other clients with PN may experience that any touch is irritating, so massage may have to be adjusted or even delayed until the contributing factors to PN have been addressed.
BENEFITS	Massage, through soothing touch, relief of general stress, or improvements in local circulation, may improve the quality of life for a person with PN, but this can only be determined on a case-by-case basis.
RESEARCH	The benefits of massage therapy for carpal tunnel syndrome and thoracic outlet syndrome are discussed in Chapter 3; other nerve compression situations are described in this chapter. Chemotherapy-induced PN is a particularly serious form of this condition, as it can interfere with the ability of a person with cancer to tolerate treatment. Massage in this context has been found to be profoundly helpful.[1] 1. Cunningham JE, Kelechi T, Sterba K, et al. Case report of a patient with chemotherapy-induced peripheral neuropathy treated with manual therapy (massage). *Supportive Care in Cancer* 2011;19(9):1473–1476. http://www.ncbi.nlm.nih.gov/pubmed/21766161

Dystonia

Definition: What Is It?

Dystonia is a common condition that involves repetitive, involuntary, sometimes sustained contractions of skeletal muscles. Symptoms often reach a peak and then stabilize or subside in intensity, but they may recur. Dystonia can develop without an identifiable cause, as a result of a genetic anomaly, or as a secondary symptom of an underlying disorder or drug reaction.

NOTABLE CASES National Public Radio talk show host Diane Rehm is affected by vocal dysphonia, a form of dystonia. Other influential people who have had dystonia include late actress Katharine Hepburn, Supreme Court Justice Sandra Day O'Connor, the late Senator Robert Byrd, and Founding Father Samuel Adams.

Demographics

Dystonia is found among all ages and races, but women are affected more often than men.

Dopamine: A neurotransmitter in the basal ganglia,associated with attention and pleasure.

GABA: A neurotransmitter in the central nervous system.

Serotonin: A chemical found in many tissues, functioning as a neurotransmitter in the brain and a vasoconstrictor, stimulator of smooth muscle contractions, and gastric secretion inhibitor in other parts of the body.

Acetylcholine: Cholinergic neurotransmitter that conveys motor commands from the central nervous system to the muscles.

Etiology: What Happens?

Like other movement disorders, dystonia appears to be linked to problems with the basal ganglia. In many cases, it appears to involve an inability to process certain neurotransmitters, including **dopamine**, **GABA**, **serotonin**, and **acetylcholine**. The result is prolonged bursts of electrical activity in the affected muscles. This distinguishes it from other movement disorders such as **Parkinson disease** or **tremor**, which result in rhythmic, oscillating shaking on one plane of movement.

Causes of dystonia vary. Genetic predisposition, underlying neurological disorders, and reactions to medications are the most frequent triggers. Symptoms of dystonia can be seen as part of other neurological diseases like **cerebral palsy** and **Huntington disease**, but these situations have a different etiology.

Dystonia can be classified by age of onset (childhood, adolescent, or adult) or by cause (primary, secondary, or dystonia-plus syndromes). Most often, however, dystonia is described by what part or how much of the body is affected.

Types of Dystonia

- *Focal dystonia*: These conditions affect specific muscles or muscle groups.
  - *Cervical dystonia*: This is the most common form of dystonia. Also called spasmodic torticollis, it involves unilateral involuntary contractions of neck rotators, usually the sternocleidomastoid. For other types of torticollis, see Sidebar 4.4. To see the videos "Cervical Dystonia 1" and "Cervical Dystonia 2," showing a patient with cervical dystonia before and after treatment, visit http://thePoint.lww.com/Werner6e. thePoint®
  - *Vocal dysphonia*: This affects the vocal cords, leading to difficulty with speech and a shaky, hoarse, or whispery

SIDEBAR 4.4 Other Types of Torticollis

Spasmodic torticollis is classified as a type of dystonia, a movement disorder that starts in the CNS. Other forms of torticollis are related to musculoskeletal problems, which of course have very different implications for massage.

- *Congenital torticollis.* A genetic anomaly results in the development of only one sternocleidomastoid muscle. Because so many other muscles can rotate and flex the head, this problem may be dealt with through physical therapy.
- *Infant torticollis.* In the late stages of pregnancy, the fetus may lie with the head twisted to one side. This can create a shortened or weakened sternocleidomastoid and cranial bone distortion. This condition is usually successfully treated with exercise and a special helmet designed to reshape the cranial bones.
- *Wryneck.* This is a simple stiff neck, often caused by irritation of the intertransverse ligament at C7. A cervical misalignment may also create the problem, which will not be relieved until both the muscles and the bony alignment have been addressed. Trigger points and spasm in the splenius cervicis are another possible cause. Short-lived cases of wryneck may be brought about by sleeping in a bad position or some other event or trauma that might cause irritation in the neck muscles.

Torticollis can, on rare occasions, be the earliest presenting sign of a more serious condition. In some documented cases, it was the first symptom of bone cancer in the spine (the tumor may affect the motor and/or sensory neurons), bone infection, and even a bad infection of the adenoids.

quality to the voice. It is sometimes called laryngeal dystonia.

- *Oromandibular dystonia*: This affects the face and lower jaw muscles. It can lead to problems with eating and swallowing.
- *Blepharospasm*: This leads to repetitive, forceful blinking and squinting of the eyes. It can be severe enough to cause functional blindness, even though the eyes themselves are not affected (Figure 4.5).
- *Multifocal dystonia*: This affects disconnected parts of the body: the left leg and the face, for instance.

- *Segmental dystonia*: This is seen in contiguous areas of the body, like the neck and shoulder (Figure 4.6).
  - *Meige syndrome*: This is a combination of blepharospasm and oromandibular dystonia.
  - *Upper limb dystonia*: The most common example of this is writer's cramp: a condition in which the dominant hand and arm develops painful cramps during writing, but not necessarily other activities. Similar problems are seen with musicians and other hand-intensive professionals; it has been documented in 55 professions.
  - *Lower limb dystonia*: This is a rare disorder, mostly seen in children.
- *Hemidystonia*: This affects the left or right side of the body. It is an occasional repercussion of **stroke**.
- *Generalized dystonia*: This is the most severe form of this disorder. It usually starts in the leg and progresses to affect the whole body.

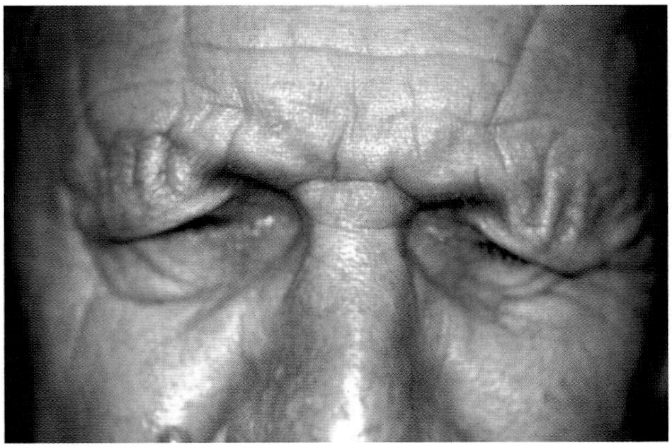

FIGURE 4.5 Blepharospasm, a type of focal dystonia

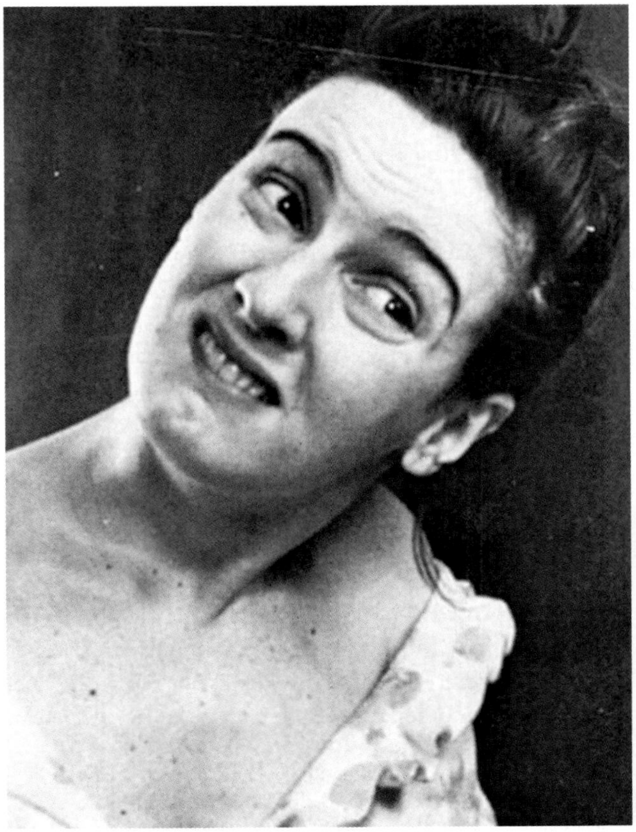

FIGURE 4.6 Spasmodic torticollis with some dystonia of facial muscles: a form of segmental dystonia

- *Paroxysmal dystonia*: In this version, symptoms can affect multiple parts of the body. An episode can resemble a grand mal seizure, but the patient never loses consciousness. Attacks can last several minutes or hours.
- *Torsion dystonia*: This can affect the trunk and limbs with twisting, writhing spasms.
- *Tardive dystonia*: This generalized dystonia is a complication of long-term use of antipsychotic drugs. Not all psychosis patients develop it, and it can be reversed if the drug use stops in time, but in some cases, it becomes permanent.

Signs and Symptoms

Signs and symptoms of dystonia are related to what type is present and at what age symptoms began.

People who develop this disorder in childhood tend to have it in more severe forms than do those who develop dystonia in maturity.

The primary symptom is involuntary contraction of an area. Contractions may be quick or sustained, and they often involve multiplane movement and twisting. Episodes tend to be exacerbated by stress or fatigue. Contractions are often related to specific tasks and disappear when other tasks that use the same muscles are substituted: walking backward instead of forward, for instance. Many dystonia patients develop a habit of repeatedly touching the affected area, which serves to reduce local contractions. This pattern is called **geste antagoniste**.

Dystonic contractions may not be painful, but they can lead to painful consequences. **Headaches** can result from spasmodic torticollis or facial contractions. Muscle irritation and **arthritis** may develop in areas where contractions are continually sustained. Eventually, the muscle fibers may shrink and the connective tissue sheaths around them thicken into a permanent contracture. Another complication is the functional blindness that occurs when blepharospasm interferes with normal eyelid contractions.

Treatment

Treatment options for dystonia work to modulate motor function in the affected muscles. Physical therapy and gentle stretching are often recommended. Oral or injected medications can affect neurotransmitter secretion or uptake. Injections of botulinum toxin can block the acetylcholine receptors in the affected muscles. A device can be implanted in the brain to help regulate motor function (deep brain stimulation). If no other interventions are satisfactory, surgery can disrupt portions of the basal ganglia or interrupt nerve transmission to the muscle or in the spinal cord.

> **Geste antagoniste:** The habit of touching an area of the body to relieve symptoms of dystonia.

Medications

- Levodopa (synthetic dopamine) to test for and treat one subtype of dystonia
- Benzodiazepines to limit messages to motor neurons
- Baclofen to reduce spasticity and spasm
- Anticholinergic medications to block acetylcholine activity
- Injected botulinum toxin to locally affect acetylcholine uptake

Massage Therapy Implications

RISKS

Some of the treatment interventions for dystonia may impact choices for massage. When a client uses a drug that makes muscles less responsive, the therapist must accommodate by limiting the intensity of the pressure or the extent of any passive stretching that is part of the session.

BENEFITS

Dystonia is exacerbated by fatigue and stress, so patients may seek massage as a coping mechanism.

RESEARCH

One study found that self-massage for hemifacial spasm was an effective intervention to reduce the severity of muscle spasms.[1] Another study looking at careful, 1-finger massage for infants with muscular torticollis was effective enough to predict a shorter treatment and recovery time compared to the infants who did not receive massage.[2]

1. Loyola DP, Camargos S, Maia D, Cardoso F. Sensory tricks in focal dystonia and hemifacial spasm. *European Journal of Neurology* 2013;20(4):704–707. http://www.ncbi.nlm.nih.gov/pubmed/23216586
2. Kang Y, Lu S, Li J, et al. Primary massage using one-finger twining manipulation for treatment of infantile muscular torticollis. *Journal of Alternative and Complementary Medicine* 2011;17(3):231–237. http://www.ncbi.nlm.nih.gov/pubmed/21381962

Parkinson Disease

Definition: What Is It?

Parkinson disease (PD), first discussed by the British physician James Parkinson in 1817 as the "shaking palsy," is a movement disorder involving the progressive degeneration of nerve tissue and a reduction in neurotransmitter production in the CNS.

Demographics

PD is one of the most common neurologic diseases. It affects about 1.5 million people in the United States, which is about 1% of all people older than age 60. It is diagnosed about 500,000 times each year. Men with PD outnumber women by about 3 to 2.

Etiology: What Happens?

The basal ganglia are small pockets of gray matter deep in the brain that work with several other structures to provide learned reflexes, motor control, and coordination: smooth movement that is balanced between prime movers and their antagonists.

Healthy basal ganglia cells are supplied with a vital neurotransmitter, **dopamine**, by cells in a nearby structure, the **substantia nigra** (aka "black stuff"). In PD, the substantia nigra cells die off, depriving the basal ganglia cells of dopamine. Without dopamine, the basal ganglia cells cannot do their job, so coordination and controlled movement degenerates. Further, the presence of Lewy bodies in the basal ganglia cells and other areas is now considered an important contributor: these protein deposits are not cleared appropriately, and they can trigger premature apoptosis. Experts believe that Lewy bodies begin to accumulate long before PD becomes symptomatic.

It is not clear how or why PD begins in most cases. Environmental agents may be found to be one cause; risk factors for PD include exposure to many pesticides, herbicides, fertilizers, and other industrial chemicals. Mitochondrial dysfunction is a factor for some individuals, along with a loss in protection from free radicals in the brain. In some families, a genetic connection is clear, and specific sites of genetic abnormality have been located. In these cases, the age of onset is usually younger than the typical 60 years or more.

The net result of impairment of basal ganglia function is an inability to balance out nerve impulses to muscular prime movers and antagonists for given tasks. Sixty to 80% of substantia nigra cells are lost before symptoms develop, but then, movement is ultimately suppressed and muscles, especially flexors, progressively tighten.

> **Dopamine:** A neurotransmitter in the basal ganglia, associated with attention and pleasure.
>
> **Substantia nigra:** A large mass in the brainstem, composed of pigmented cells. Synthesizes dopamine.

Signs and Symptoms

Symptoms of PD can be divided into primary and secondary problems. Primary symptoms arise from the disease itself, while secondary symptoms are results of primary symptoms. The three most clearly indicative symptoms of PD are rigidity, bradykinesia, and resting tremor.

Primary Symptoms

- *Resting tremor.* This phenomenon is present in most PD patients and is often one of the first noticeable symptoms. A rhythmic shaking or pill-rolling action of the hand is often seen. Tremor may also affect the foot, head, and neck. This tremor is most noticeable when the patient is at rest, but not sleeping. It often disappears entirely when the patient is engaged in some other activity. This distinguishes it from essential **tremor**, which is discussed elsewhere.
- *Bradykinesia.* This is difficulty in initiating or sustaining movement. It can take a long time to begin a voluntary movement of the arm or leg; movement may be halting and interrupted midstream. PD patients with bradykinesia sometimes report feeling rooted to the floor when they can visualize moving a leg, but it doesn't happen without sustained effort.
- *Rigidity.* Because of changes in motor function, flexor muscles become chronically tight. This can give rise to a characteristically stooped posture, as the trunk flexors contract more strongly than the paraspinals. This is particularly obvious when PD accompanies osteoporosis, as it often does in elderly patients. Rigidity also makes it difficult to bend or straighten arms and legs and can cause a particular masklike appearance as the facial muscles lose flexibility and ease of movement (Figure 4.7). Rigidity also accounts for a reduced rate of blinking, increased drooling, and difficulty with eating, swallowing, and digestion: painful constipation is a frequent result.
- *Nonspecific achiness, weakness, and fatigue.* PD has a slow onset and is most common in elderly people, so these early symptoms are often missed.
- *Poor postural reflexes.* Disruption in the activity of basal ganglia cells results in uncoordinated movement and poor balance. PD patients are particularly susceptible to falling.

> **NOTABLE CASES** Perhaps the most recognized spokesperson for PD at present is actor Michael J. Fox who was diagnosed at age 41 with this disease. Other well-known PD patients include "The Man in Black" Johnny Cash, heavyweight boxing champion Mohammed Ali (who has pugilistic parkinsonism), and Pope John Paul II.

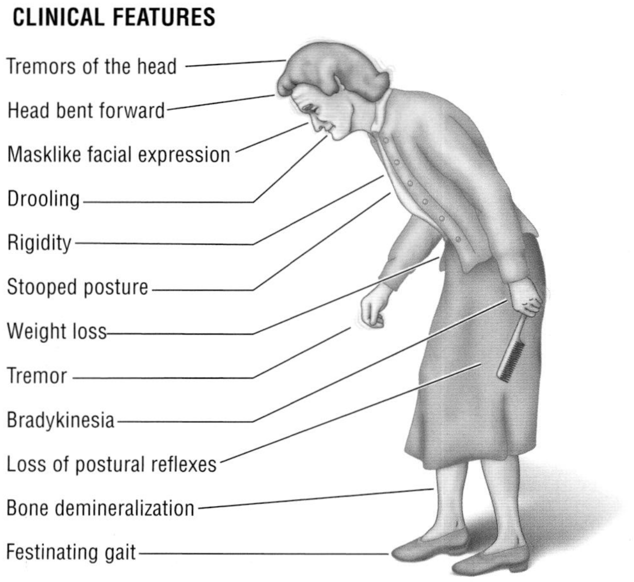

FIGURE 4.7 Clinical features of Parkinson disease

Secondary Symptoms

- *Shuffling gait.* Difficulty in bending arms and legs makes walking a special challenge. Often, the ability to swing the arm is noticeably diminished on one side. The patient takes small steps and may then have to stumble forward to avoid falling. This is called a **festinating gait**.
- *Changes in speech and eating.* PD causes progressive rigidity of the muscles in the larynx that control vocalization. The speech gradually becomes monotone and expressionless. Muscular changes in the mouth and throat also create problems with swallowing and drooling, particularly while lying down.
- *Changes in handwriting.* The loss of coordination in fine motor muscles changes the ability of a PD patient to write by hand. **Micrographia**, or progressively shrinking, cramped handwriting, is one of the later symptoms of this disease.
- *Sleep disorders.* PD patients are subject to a variety of **sleep disorders**, from a complete reversal of normal sleeping schedules, to extra-active REM sleep, to chronic sleeplessness.
- *Depression.* The progressive nature of PD makes anxiety and **depression** a very predictable part of the disease process. Depression can also be related to insomnia, or it can be a side effect of medication. Sometimes, the symptoms of depression can outweigh the symptoms of the disease, and treatment for depression can lessen PD symptoms as well.
- *Mental degeneration.* Advanced PD patients may have memory loss and deterioration of cognition, but these can also be side effects of PD drugs.

> **Festinating gait:** The small, shuffling steps characteristic of Parkinson disease.
>
> **Micrographia:** Handwriting that grows progressively more cramped.
>
> **Levodopa:** The biologically active form of dopa; a precursor of dopamine.
>
> **Carbidopa:** A drug used to treat symptoms of Parkinson disease.

Parkinson-like symptoms can arise with other conditions that have very different etiologies. The term parkinsonism refers to this presentation. Some of these cases can be traced to specific issues, including certain drugs, repeated head trauma (pugilistic parkinsonism affects boxers, for instance), and neurovascular disease.

Treatment

Pharmacologic treatment for PD patients is a complicated subject. Doctors must balance the benefits of early intervention to slow the progression of this disease with the many unacceptable side effects that accompany long-term drug use. Choosing which drugs to prescribe, in which sequence, and in which combinations is an ongoing challenge.

Because PD is related to a lack of dopamine in the basal ganglia, the most common strategy is to supplement a synthetic form of this neurotransmitter. **Levodopa** (L-dopa) can cross the blood-brain barrier, especially with a companion drug called **carbidopa**, but it tends to have a lot of negative side effects, and many patients develop resistance, so it is a temporary solution.

Other drug therapies include substances that slow the metabolism of dopamine so that whatever is available stays for a longer time and medications that stimulate dopamine receptors in the basal ganglia so that uptake of the neurotransmitter happens more easily. Anticholinergic agents work to limit muscle contraction. None of these is a permanent solution however, and all of them carry risks of serious side effects. Doctors working with PD patients must monitor their medications carefully and make frequent adjustments.

Physical, speech, and occupational therapies are often employed to maintain the health and general functioning levels of PD patients for as long as possible. Psychotherapy and support groups are recommended to cope with the effects of depression.

Some PD patients find that deep brain stimulation (an electrode activates the thalamus by way of a magnet implanted under the skin) can help to control tremors. Other neurosurgery options have worked to modulate motor dysfunction at other locations in the brain. These interventions are typically employed only when other options have failed.

Medications

- Levodopa and carbidopa to cross the blood-brain barrier and supplement dopamine to the brain
- Catechol-O-methyltransferase inhibitors (COMT inhibitors) to prolong the effects of levodopa and carbidopa therapy
- Monoamine oxidase B inhibitors to protect damaged neurons, act as antioxidants
- Anticholinergics to block acetylcholine and manage muscle rigidity

Massage Therapy Implications

RISKS

Many PD patients have difficulty getting on or off a table and may need assistance to do so. Because this is usually a disease of the elderly, other disorders may be present along with PD; these must also be addressed for the safety of massage.

BENEFITS

Massage can help with many aspect of PD, including sleep quality, muscle rigidity, anxiety, and depression. Because it is an option with little risk of negative side effects, massage is one of the most frequently used complementary therapies by PD patients.

OPTIONS

Some massage therapists report that they see the best benefits for their clients with PD when massage sessions are short but frequent, as opposed to longer and less frequent.

RESEARCH

Chronic and painful constipation is one aspect of PD that is often underaddressed. Research supports careful abdominal massage for older adults with central neurological disorders to treat this symptom.[1] A case series[2] examined traditional Japanese massage for PD patients and found improvements in gait, range of motion, and subjective scores for quality of life. Svircev et al.[3] found that neuromuscular therapy could be helpful for some symptoms, especially tremor. One relatively early study[4] looked at Trager therapy (a technique involving loose and gentle shaking of joints) to address PD-related rigidity; they found that the approach had some potential to be developed into a protocol specifically designed for PD patients.

1. Coggrave M, Norton C, Cody JD. Management of faecal incontinence and constipation in adults with central neurological diseases. *Cochrane Database of Systematic Reviews* 2014;(1):CD002115. http://www.ncbi.nlm.nih.gov/pubmed/24420006
2. Donoyama N, Ohkoshi N. Effects of traditional Japanese massage therapy on various symptoms in patients with Parkinson's disease: a case-series study. *Journal of Alternative and Complementary Medicine* 2012;18(3):294–299. http://www.ncbi.nlm.nih.gov/pubmed/22385078
3. Svircev A, Craig LH, Juncos JL. A pilot study examining the effects of neuromuscular therapy on patients with Parkinson's disease. *Journal of the American Osteopathic Association* 2005;105(1):26. http://www.jaoa.osteopathic.org/content/105/1/26.1.long
4. Duval C, Lafontaine D, Hebert J, et al. The effect of Trager therapy on the level of evoked stretch responses in patients with Parkinson's disease and rigidity. *Journal of Manipulative and Physiological Therapeutics* 2002;25(7):455–464. http://www.ncbi.nlm.nih.gov/pubmed/12214187

Tremor

Definition: What Is It?

The term tremor refers to involuntary oscillating movements on a fixed plane. This can be a freestanding disorder, or a symptom of a number of different types of CNS problems. The key characteristics of tremor disorders are that the movements are rhythmic back-and-forth movements of antagonistic muscle groups and the movement occurs in a single plane: this distinguishes tremor from **dystonia**, which may involve involuntary movement in multiple planes. Tremors vary by velocity, amplitude, and body parts involved.

Demographics

Up to 10 million people in the United States have essential tremor, although it is frequently initially misdiagnosed as **Parkinson disease**, a much more complicated condition that requires very different treatment.

Essential tremor is most often diagnosed among older people, but it has been seen to affect people of all ages, including infants. Up to 50% of all cases show a familial link, indicating a possible genetic component.

Etiology: What Happens?

Tremors can occur in a variety of ways. Most situations appear to be related to dysfunction in the links between the brainstem, the cerebellum, and the thalamus, although these are not always fully understood.

Tremors affect the hands, face, and head more often than other areas. They are sometimes classified by whether they are physiologic or pathologic. Physiologic tremors are exacerbated by stress, fear, or underlying problems like alcohol withdrawal, hypoglycemia, hyperthyroidism, or drug reactions. Pathologic tremors are either idiopathic or caused by some other condition.

Types of Pathologic Tremor

- *Essential tremor*: This is an idiopathic chronic tremor that is not secondary to any other pathology. This condition is slowly progressive and potentially debilitating. It typically involves low-amplitude tremor with high frequency, mostly during action rather than rest. Onset can occur as early as adolescence, but essential tremor most often shows up at about 45 years of age. It can be an inherited disorder.

- *Secondary tremor*: This is a situation where tremor develops as a part of some other CNS disorder. **Parkinson disease, multiple system atrophy, dystonia**, and **Huntington disease** all list tremor among their symptoms.

Signs and Symptoms

Tremors, whether they are pathologic or physiologic, generally show symptoms in three patterns. These are described as resting tremor, action tremor, or psychogenic tremor.

- *Resting tremor*: Oscillations occur when the person is at rest, but not during sleep.
- *Action tremor*: This has three subtypes.
  - *Postural tremor*: Oscillations occur when the patient attempts to hold a limb against gravity, that is, holding an arm out in front of him.
  - *Isometric tremor*: Shaking occurs with isometric contractions, that is, squeezing the examiner's fingers.
  - *Intention tremor*: This is worst when the patient attempts to use the hands for fine or complex tasks.
- *Psychogenic tremor*: This is present in everyone, but is usually so subtle it is unnoticeable. When it becomes pronounced, it is often stress related and disappears when the person is distracted.

Treatment

Several medications, including moderate alcohol consumption, can help control tremor symptoms. Surgical interventions may be used if the tremor is debilitating and unresponsive to medication; these include implanting a deep brain stimulation device or creating interruptions at the thalamus or **globus pallidus**.

Medication

- Beta-blockers appear to inhibit receptors in muscle spindles
- Tranquilizers, including benzodiazepines or phenobarbitals to inhibit muscle function
- Antiseizure medications
- Botulinum toxin (specifically for muscles of the face or head)
- Controlled doses of alcohol

Massage Therapy Implications

RISKS	Tremor can occur as part of serious underlying disorders. These must be identified before massage can safely proceed. Some clients may find that the physical challenges of getting on or off a massage table or chair may make them feel unstable. In these situations, it is important to be in attendance during transition times.
BENEFITS	A client with essential tremor that is exacerbated by stress may find that his or her symptoms are lessened with massage.

See the video "Intention Tremor" available at http://thePoint.lww.com/Werner6e. thePoint®

Infectious Disorders

Encephalitis

Definition: What Is It?

Encephalitis is an infection of the brain, usually caused by any of a variety of viruses. It frequently occurs along with inflammation of the spinal cord (myelitis) and/or inflammation of the meninges (**meningitis**). While some strains of infection-causing pathogens used to be found only in certain geographical areas, the ease of worldwide travel has made the phenomenon of **endemic** infections less limiting than they used to be (Sidebar 4.5).

> **Endemic:** Present in a given community or people.
>
> **Globus pallidus:** The inner and lighter gray portion of the lentiform nucleus in the brain. Literally "pale globe."
>
> **Parenchyma:** The functional tissue of an organ.
>
> **Arbovirus:** A virus transmitted by arthropods, such as mosquitoes, ticks, and midges.

Demographics

The Centers for Disease Control and Prevention suggest that encephalitis is diagnosed about 20,000 times each year in the United States, although most cases are mild.

Etiology: What Happens?

Most cases of encephalitis are viral. Viral infections can be primary (a direct attack on the nervous system) or secondary (a complication of viral infection elsewhere in the body).

Encephalitis infections affect the **parenchyma** of the brain and sometimes the meninges and spinal cord. Inflammation is an inevitable result. Infections are often mild and do not always lead to long-lasting damage, but occasionally, and especially if the patient is very young or very old, encephalitis infections cause permanent neurological damage, cognitive changes, **stroke**, **seizures**, paralysis, or even death.

Herpes simplex is the most common pathogen that causes encephalitis in the United States: it is responsible for about 10% of all cases. Other common infections involve **herpes zoster** virus, **influenza** viruses, and a variety of **arboviruses**: vector-borne pathogens that are spread via the bites of animals, usually insects. West Nile virus is an example of a type of encephalitis that

SIDEBAR 4.5 West Nile Encephalitis: Watching a Virus Take Hold

In August 1999, six residents of Queens, New York, checked into local hospitals with high fever in combination with debilitating headaches. Five of them also developed alarming neurological symptoms: weakness, paralysis, and even coma.

Initial tests suggested an outbreak of Saint Louis encephalitis, a mosquito-borne viral infection. But patients showed a different pattern from that usually seen with St. Louis encephalitis; several of them were much sicker than medical professionals expected to see. Within days, several more people in the area were reporting similar symptoms.

At the same time, a few miles away from the epicenter, birds in the Bronx Zoo were dying at a startling rate. Crows all over the city were dying, too. Horses in nearby suburbs were falling to a mysterious brain fever.

It took some time, but epidemiologists finally put the phenomena together and realized that the viruses attacking humans were the same as those attacking the birds and horses. It was firmly established that the infectious agent was one never before seen in the United States: West Nile encephalitis virus was being transmitted from horses and birds to humans by common mosquitoes.

By the time the first frost killed the mosquito population, 56 confirmed cases were identified among humans, with 7 deaths. The people who died of encephalitis were all over 68 years of age.

It has never been firmly established exactly how the West Nile virus got to New York. One of the patients had been to Africa the previous June and might have been infected then, or it is possible that one of the birds in the Bronx Zoo carried the virus into the United States. Aggressive mosquito abatement programs limited the spread of the disease for that season, but studies of both mosquitoes and birds indicate that the virus has now expanded over much of the continent.

The virus continues to be watched closely, but mortality rates are now generally low. This suggests that most people now have been exposed and developed resistance to the virus. It is still important to be vigilant about this infection, which can be life threatening, but the initially aggressive phase appears to be over.

rapidly moved across the continent. Now, **dengue fever**, another arbovirus that is diagnosed up in a 100 million cases each year worldwide, may be making an appearance here as well. These are still relatively rare, however; arboviruses account for fewer than 3,000 infections each year in this country. **Enteroviruses** are introduced through fecal-oral contamination and move from the digestive tract to the CNS: **hepatitis** and **polio** are examples.

It is possible for other pathogens like fungi or bacteria to cause encephalitis, but this is rare in this country.

Dengue fever: A disease transmitted by mosquitoes that is characterized by fever, aches, and a measles-like rash.

Enterovirus: A group of viruses that attack the intestines.

Signs and Symptoms

Symptoms of encephalitis can range from so mild they are never identified to extremely severe. How the disease presents depends on the pathogen and the age and general health of the patient. Infants, the elderly, and immune-suppressed people are most vulnerable to the very extreme forms of the disease, while others only rarely have any lasting damage from the inflammation.

The mild end of the symptomatic scale includes a sudden onset of fever with headaches, drowsiness, irritability, and disordered thought processes. In severe cases, brain inflammation causes drowsiness that can progress to stupor and then coma. The patient may also have double vision, confused sensation, impaired speech or hearing, convulsions, and partial or full paralysis. Changes in personality, intellect, and memory may develop, depending on which parts of the brain are inflamed and subsequently damaged.

Treatment

Viral encephalitis is treated with antiviral medications, along with steroids to limit inflammation, sedatives to moderate convulsions, and "supportive therapy," which is to say, rest, good nutrition, and adequate hydration. Speedy treatment is critical to avoid the risk of permanent brain damage or death.

Medications

- NSAIDs, especially acetaminophen, for fever and headache relief (mild cases only and no aspirin for infants)
- Antiviral medication to interrupt viral replication
- Anti-inflammatories, including steroids, to limit inflammation in the CNS
- Antiseizure drugs
- Sedatives

Massage Therapy Implications

RISKS	A client with an acute infection of any kind needs to reschedule a massage appointment, but if along with fever he or she has headache, confusion, and changes in speech, sensation, or motor control, it is important to seek immediate medical attention.
BENEFITS	A client who has fully recovered from an encephalitis infection can enjoy the same benefits from massage as the rest of the population. If permanent damage occurs, accommodations can be made accordingly.

Herpes Zoster

Definition: What Is It?

Herpes zoster is an infection of the nervous system caused by the varicella zoster virus (VZV). In this case, the virus targets the dendrites at the receiving ends of sensory neurons, which leads to painful, fluid-filled blisters on the nerve endings of a specific dermatome.

Chickenpox is usually the first interaction people have with VZV, but subsequent outbreaks are called shingles. This comes from the Latin *cingulum*, which means girdle or belt. This describes the typical distribution of blisters around the chest or abdomen along a dermatomal line.

Demographics

In the United States, about 95% of adults carry VZV colonies and so are vulnerable to a reactivated bout of shingles. Those who are vaccinated against chickenpox are also susceptible to a later outbreak of shingles, but the rate is much lower than among the population exposed to wild VZV.

About 4% of adults experience shingles at some point, but that number is much higher among people with suppressed immunity for any reason, especially among cancer patients, people who use steroidal anti-inflammatories, who are HIV positive, and organ transplant recipients. Shingles is diagnosed about a million times each year.

Most people have shingles only once, but immune-suppressed people may have multiple outbreaks.

Etiology: What Happens?

VZV is a virus in the herpes family that attacks sensory nerve cell endings, leading to painful, itchy blisters on the skin. Most people's first exposure to this pathogen is through a childhood bout of chickenpox. Like other herpes viruses, VZV is never fully expelled from the body. Instead, it goes dormant, in this case in the dorsal root ganglia (the meeting point for all the sensory neurons in each dermatome) or the **geniculate ganglion** of the trigeminal nerve. Later in life, when circulating antibodies are low, the virus may reactivate, this time as shingles.

VZV is initially spread through mucous secretions. Triggers for later reactivations can be difficult to pin down. Contributing factors include stress, age, and impaired immunity because of other diseases. Shingles is notorious for accompanying HIV, Hodgkin lymphoma, advanced tuberculosis, pneumonia, chemotherapy, or having had an initial infection before 18 months of age. Shingles occasionally occurs after severe trauma or as a drug reaction.

Although the fluid in zoster blisters carries live virus, among adults, it isn't particularly contagious because most people are exposed to chickenpox in childhood and have immune system protection. This does not hold true, however, for a person who comes in contact with shingles while his or her immune system is suppressed or who has never been exposed to the virus in the first place. In this case, an adult may get either shingles or chickenpox, but shingles is probably more likely.

> **Geniculate ganglion:** A cluster of sensory fibers of the facial nerve, running through the facial canal.

Types of Herpes Zoster

- *Chickenpox*: This is the first infection with VZV that most people experience, although with the development of a vaccine for this condition, this is becoming rarer (Sidebar 4.6). Chickenpox involves itchy blisters on a red base, but unlike shingles, they are spread all over the body.
- *Shingles*: This is a resurgence of VZV, usually later in life. It involves the outbreak of painful blisters along the dermatome that is colonized by virus from an earlier infection (Figure 4.8).
- *Herpes zoster ophthalmicus*: This occurs when the site of reactivation is the trigeminal nerve. This can involve conjunctivitis, corneal ulcers, and inflammation of other eye structures, leading to temporary or permanent vision loss (Figure 4.9).
- *Postherpetic neuralgia*: In this situation, the pain generated by the viral infection outlives the blisters by a minimum of 3 months and may persist for years. The risk for developing postherpetic neuralgia (PHN) rises significantly with age: 60% of 60-year-old patients with shingles develop PHN, while 75% of 70-year-old patients

SIDEBAR 4.6 Vaccines for Chickenpox and Shingles

A chickenpox vaccine for young children was licensed in the United States in 1995. Many schools now require that children entering kindergarten be vaccinated against this infection. While this protects children from an uncomfortable time (and a small but significant risk of dangerous complications), perhaps, the greater incentive is for their parents, who would otherwise have to miss a week of work to stay home with a sick child.

But two unexpected consequences came out of this vaccination campaign. One is that the chickenpox vaccine wears off within several years, leaving vaccinated children vulnerable to breakout infections with the virus, although these tend to be less severe than typical infections. Another consequence is that adults now seldom spend time with children who have chickenpox. Without this additional exposure, the incidence of shingles among older adults has gone up.

This has led to the development of an adult booster vaccine for varicella zoster that can prevent the outbreak of shingles and its painful complication, PHN.

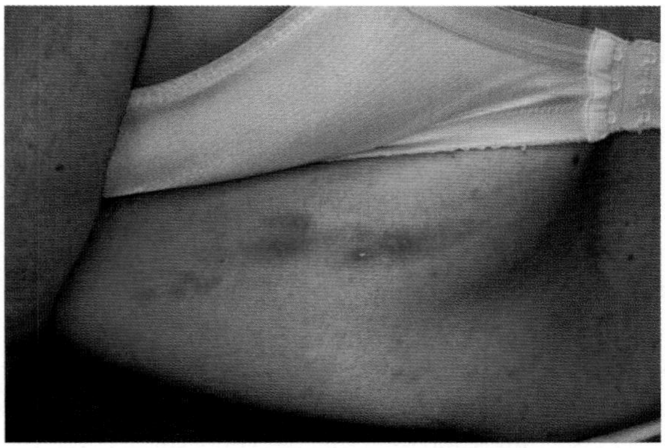

FIGURE 4.8 Shingles: blisters on a red base along a dermatomal line

have this complication, which is believed to be a **central sensitization** phenomenon.

- *Zoster sine herpete*: Occasionally, a person can have a reactivation of VZV with all the pain sensation, but with no visible lesions. This condition is called zoster sine herpete ("sine" means "without," so this means "zoster without herpes lesions"). It can be easily misdiagnosed as a herniated disc, a heart attack, or multiple other painful but invisible conditions.
- *Ramsay Hunt syndrome*: When the site of a herpes zoster infection involves facial and auditory nerves, hearing loss, and temporary or permanent facial paralysis resembling Bell palsy can occur.

Signs and Symptoms

Pain and itching are the primary symptoms of a zoster infection. In chickenpox, an outbreak can take several days to resolve, but in shingles, pain is present for 1 to 3 days before the blisters break out and for the 2 to 3 weeks in which blisters develop, erupt, and scab over. Pain often persists even after the lesions have healed and the skin is intact again.

Chickenpox blisters can be all over the skin, and some people report blisters inside the mouth and down the digestive tract as well. Shingles blisters may grow along the entire dermatome of the host dorsal root ganglion, but more often, they appear along an isolated stretch, with disconnected patches of painful blisters. It is nearly always a unilateral attack. Sensory nerves that supply the trunk and legs are the most frequently affected, although the trigeminal nerve may also be attacked.

Treatment

Herpes zoster infections are treated mainly palliatively. Cool baths and soothing lotion are recommended for chickenpox.

> **Central sensitization:** A change in the central nervous system in response to repeated incidences of pain, leading the person to feel more pain in response to the same stimulus, or even to feel pain in response to a stimulus that would not normally be considered painful.

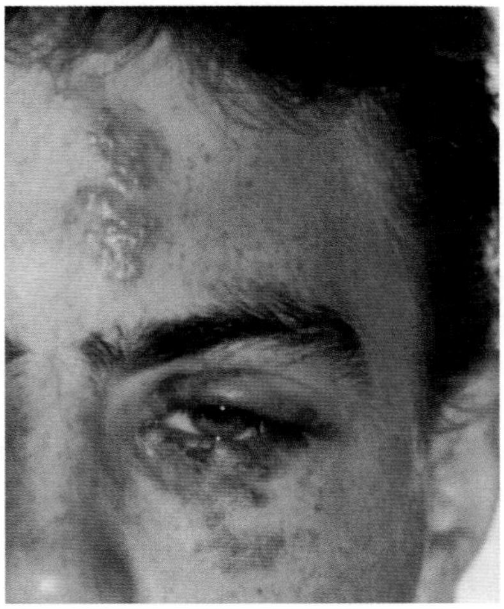

FIGURE 4.9 Herpes zoster ophthalmicus: note the dermatomal distribution of the blisters

More aggressive painkillers may be required for shingles and PHN.

Medications

- NSAIDs for pain and inflammation (no aspirin for children)
- Steroidal anti-inflammatories for inflammation
- Antiviral medications to shorten the outbreak
- For PHN:
  - Opioid analgesics
  - Tricyclic antidepressants
  - Antiseizure medication
  - Topical lidocaine or capsaicin patches

Massage Therapy Implications

RISKS	A client with an active case of chickenpox or shingles is unlikely to seek massage, simply because touch is uncomfortable. Cautions for this condition center around both the client's pain and the risk of spreading infection, although most people have been exposed to VZV by adulthood so that risk is relatively low. Clients with PHN may want to avoid touch, but that is unpredictable; others may find careful touch to be soothing.
BENEFITS	Any client who has fully recovered from shingles or chickenpox can enjoy the same benefits from massage as the rest of the population. Clients with PHN may seek the soothing qualities that massage can offer.

To see a patient in recovery from this condition, view the video "Herpes Zoster" available at http://thePoint.com/Werner6e. thePoint®

Meningitis

Definition: What Is It?

Meningitis is inflammation of the meninges that surround the brain and spinal cord. The pia mater and arachnoid are the layers most often affected; collectively these are called the **leptomeninges**. Meningitis is distinguished from **encephalitis** or spinal cord infection (myelitis) by the lack of involvement of nerve tissue; the infection is limited to the connective tissue membranes. When multiple structures are infected, the term meningoencephalitis or meningomyelitis might be applied.

Demographics

Most meningitis infections are found within three groups: children under 5 years old; young adults living in dormitories, barracks, or other close quarters; and elderly people. It is most threatening for the very young and very old.

Viral meningitis is reported about 10,000 times each year, but an unknown number of cases are never documented. Most cases of viral meningitis are reported in infants.

Bacterial meningitis is rarer, but potentially much more serious. Roughly 4,100 cases are recorded each year, with about 500 deaths.

Etiology: What Happens?

Meningitis is usually caused by bacterial or viral infection. Fungi and amoebae can also cause it, but this is relatively rare in the United States. It is important to find the causative factor because the severity and treatment options vary according to the pathogen.

When a pathogen enters the CNS, it causes a number of changes that can be very dangerous. Infection in the cerebrospinal fluid increases the permeability of the blood-brain barrier. This in turn leads to cerebral edema and invites an influx of waste products that would otherwise be filtered out. Intracranial pressure can damage cranial nerves. CN VIII is especially at risk, and damage here can lead to permanent hearing loss or deafness. Obstructive **hydrocephalus**, which limits the normal circulation of cerebrospinal fluid within the brain and spinal cord, can also occur, and inflammation of internal blood vessels can lead to blood clots and ischemic damage to brain cells: a type of **stroke**. Left unchecked, the body's autoregulating centers are damaged, and the person may die of diffuse brain injury.

The pathogens that cause meningitis can infect other tissues as well. Most people with pneumococcal infections of the CNS concurrently have **pneumonia**, for instance. And bacterial infections of the blood can lead to the distinctive reddish-purple rash associated with meningitis, along with a risk of blood clotting in capillaries, which opens the door to gangrene in the extremities.

Bacterial meningitis can be contagious. Its mode of transmission is much like the common cold: an infected person sneezes or coughs and then touches some surface, such as a doorknob or light switch. An uninfected person touches the surface and then touches his or her eye or mouth. Meningitis brought about by the intestinal **enterovirus** family can also be spread by oral-fecal contact, which is an issue when it occurs in young children or in day care settings.

Some parts of the world are subject to epidemics of meningitis. The "meningeal belt" of sub-Saharan Africa has seasonal outbreaks of a severe bacterial version of this disease.

CNS infections can also be complications of various kinds of trauma. Open skull fractures, neurosurgeries, and cerebrospinal shunts can introduce contaminants to this environment.

> **Leptomeninges:** The inner two meninges, the pia mater and arachnoid layers.
>
> **Hydrocephalus:** A condition marked by the excessive accumulation of cerebrospinal fluid.
>
> **Enterovirus:** A group of viruses that attack the intestines.

Types of Meningitis

- *Bacterial meningitis*: This infection is usually due to an invasion of *Streptococcus pneumoniae* (also called pneumococcus) or *Neisseria meningitides* (also called meningococcus). Other agents include **tuberculosis** and **staphylococcus** bacteria.

  Bacterial meningitis tends to be more severe than the viral infection, and the risk of long-term CNS damage, specifically hearing loss or loss of mental function, is much higher. It does respond to antibiotics if the correct ones are administered early in the disease process. Meningeal infection with drug-resistant forms of bacteria has presented a new treatment challenge recently.
- *Viral meningitis*: The viruses that can cause meningitis are many and varied, including coxsackievirus, a number of enteroviruses (usually associated with intestinal infections), **herpes simplex**, **herpes zoster**, **HIV**, and others. Viral meningitis tends to be less severe than bacterial meningitis and seldom causes permanent damage. When the patient is a very young child however, complications can include **seizure disorders**, hydrocephalus, hearing loss, weakness, paralysis, learning disabilities, blindness, behavioral disorders, and speech delay.

Signs and Symptoms

The symptoms of an acute meningitis infection include a rapid onset of high fever and chills, a deep red or purple rash, extreme headache, irritability, aversion to bright light, and a stiff, rigid neck—this is because any stretch or pull of the meninges is acutely painful. Confusion, drowsiness, slurred speech, nausea, delirium, and convulsions may accompany severe infections.

Incubation between exposure to a disease-causing organism and the development of symptoms can be anywhere from several hours for bacterial infections to 3 weeks for viral ones. Symptoms typically peak and then taper off over a period of 2 to 3 weeks.

Treatment

The most common forms of bacterial meningitis can be prevented with the *Haemophilus influenzae* type B (HiB) vaccine. Vaccines for viral types can be obtained, but are recommended only for people traveling to areas where the infections are endemic.

Once an infection has developed, if the pathogen is identified as a bacterium, large doses of antibiotics are administered immediately to forestall the possibility of CNS damage. Steroids may also be prescribed to limit inflammation in the brain. Viral meningitis is generally treated with supportive therapy consisting of rest, fluids, and good nutrition while the patient's immune system fights back.

Medications

- Oral and/or intravenous antibiotics for bacterial infection
- Antiviral medication for viral infection
- Steroidal anti-inflammatories for inflammation control
- Antiseizure medications if necessary

Massage Therapy Implications

RISKS	Meningitis is inflammatory, potentially communicable, and has the possibility of creating very severe damage. One of the leading signs is a stiff neck. It contraindicates massage while it is acute.
BENEFITS	Clients who have fully recovered from meningitis can enjoy the same benefits from bodywork as the rest of the population.

Polio, Postpolio Syndrome

Definition: What Are They?

Poliomyelitis, or infantile paralysis, as it used to be known, is a viral infection. The poliovirus targets intestinal mucosa first and motor nerve cells in the anterior horn of the spinal cord later. Polio has become a rare disease, especially in developed countries (see Sidebar 4.7), but many survivors of childhood infections are still alive.

SIDEBAR 4.7 Polio: It's Almost Extinct

In 1988, the Global Poliomyelitis Eradication Initiative combined efforts by the World Health Organization (WHO), UNICEF, Rotary International, and the Centers for Disease Control and Prevention in the largest public health effort for the eradication of a disease. As a result of this initiative, the last new case of wild poliovirus in the Western Hemisphere was diagnosed in Peru in August 1991. The Western Pacific Region was certified polio-free in October 2000. The last reported case in Europe was in 1998.

At this time, Afghanistan, Nigeria, and Pakistan are the only countries where wild virus causes new infections, and the total number of cases reported to the WHO in 2013 was 406—down from 350,000 in 1988. Countries with little or no incidence of polio infection are still vulnerable to invasion with the virus, especially those along borders with countries where the virus is still active. Therefore, it is recommended that even "safe" countries maintain their vaccination schedules until the globe is free of the poliovirus.

Postpolio syndrome (PPS) is a progressive muscular weakness that develops 10 to 40 years after an initial infection with the poliovirus.

Demographics

About 1.6 million people in the United States have PPS. Women have it more often than men. Most patients are identified at 30 to 35 years after their initial infection.

Etiology: What Happens?

Wild poliovirus occurs in three subtypes. It can be spread through airborne droplets, but the most efficient mechanism is oral-fecal contamination. It usually enters the body through the mouth in contaminated water and sets up an infection in the intestine. New virus is concentrated and released in fecal matter, possibly to contaminate water elsewhere.

For over 99% of people exposed to the poliovirus, nothing else happens. But in a small portion of people, the virus travels through the bloodstream into the spinal cord, where it targets and destroys motor nerve cells in the anterior horn. This impedes motor signals leaving the spinal cord, which in turn leads to rapid deterioration and atrophy of muscles and motor paralysis (Figure 4.10).

The paralysis caused by polio is motor only; sensation is still present. And because the motor nerves overlap muscle groups in the extremities, some muscle fibers still function, even though many motor neurons may have been damaged.

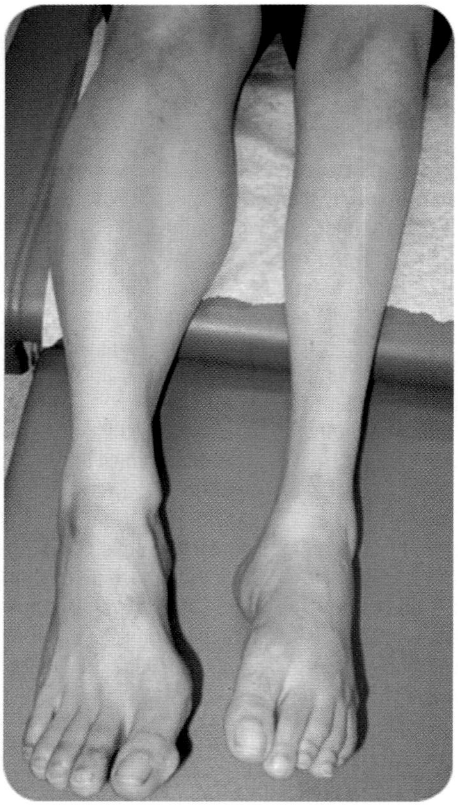

FIGURE 4.10 Polio: motor paralysis and muscle wasting

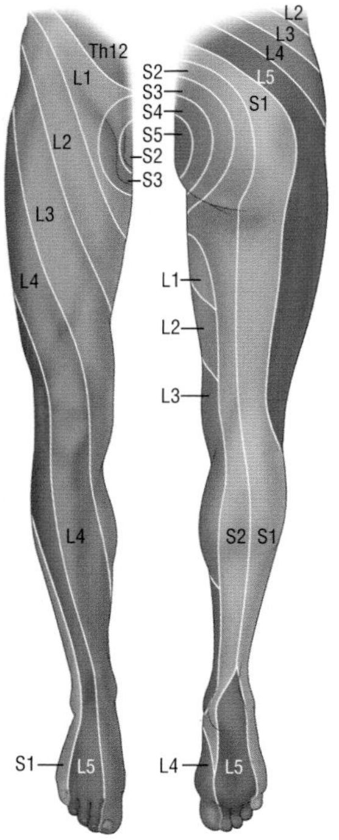

FIGURE 4.11 Dermatome patterns in the leg muscles allow multiple nerves to supply muscle groups; if one nerve root is damaged, the muscle group is still usable

For example, consider the dermatomes for the quadriceps. Even if all of the impulses to the motor neurons in L_2 have been eliminated, L_3 supplies other motor neurons to the same muscle group (Figure 4.11). Furthermore, nerve cells that survive the initial attack can grow new terminal axons to enervate muscle cells that were otherwise cut off. This increases the size of each motor unit and puts excessive demand on the cell body of the enlarged motor neuron to supply the long fiber with nutrition. Eventually, these motor neurons wear out and die, leading to muscle weakness and possible atrophy: this is PPS.

NOTABLE CASES The list of well-known people who have had polio is long and diverse. It includes musicians Joni Mitchell and Neil Young; actors Donald Sutherland, Alan Alda, and Mia Farrow; science fiction novelist Arthur C. Clarke; professional golfer Jack Nicklaus; artist Frida Kahlo; and President Franklin Delano Roosevelt.

Some specialists now suggest that PPS could also be related to a reactivation of a persistent latent poliovirus, or some other enterovirus that attacks the weakened motor neurons. This theory is connected to the finding of pro-inflammatory indicators in tissue biopsies of PPS patients.

Polio is rarely seen now because two inexpensive, stable, easy-to-administer vaccines have enabled eradication efforts in most countries. It is important to note, however, that the Sabin vaccine, which is given orally, introduces weakened viruses into the digestive system, where they stimulate the production of polio antibodies. The virus is concentrated in the feces, and people who handle the diapers of recently vaccinated infants need to be aware of this. Immune-suppressed people should avoid contact with infants who are undergoing this treatment.

Signs and Symptoms

A new infection of polio is unlikely to occur in this country, but PPS is common among childhood polio survivors. This is marked by a sudden and sometimes extreme onset of fatigue, pain, and weakness. Spinal changes, including the onset of **spondylosis** and **postural deviations**, are common. Many patients report a decreased tolerance for cold. Breathing difficulties, sleep disturbances, and trouble swallowing may also develop. These symptoms usually begin 10 to 40 years after the original infection. They tend to run in cycles in which function is progressively lost, followed by periods of stability, and then more loss of function.

Treatment

Moist heat applications, physical therapy, and massage have been used to treat polio survivors once the initial infection has subsided. Together, hydrotherapy and massage can help to keep functioning muscle fibers healthy and well nourished.

PPS is treated by reducing muscular and neurological stress: adjusted walking braces or crutches, changing activity levels, and exercise programs that encourage the use of muscles not supplied by the damaged nerves are often suggested. People with PPS need to avoid excessive use of affected muscles, since exercise to these compromised tissues can cause permanent damage to the working fibers.

Massage Therapy Implications

RISKS	Because polio is a motor paralysis with full sensation, the only caution for massage is that it should not take place during acute infection, and this is unlikely to happen if the therapist practices in a developed country.
BENEFITS	PPS indicates massage that may help improve the efficiency of weakened muscles, improve sleep, reduce fatigue, and add to the quality of life for these patients.
RESEARCH	A survey of PPS patients about their quality of life found that many of them use acupuncture and massage to help manage the symptoms of their condition.[1] 1. Atwal A, Spiliotopoulou G, Coleman C, et al. Polio survivors' perceptions of the meaning of quality of life and strategies used to promote participation in everyday activities. *Health Expectations* 2014. http://www.ncbi.nlm.nih.gov/pubmed/24438097

Psychiatric Disorders

Addiction

Definition: What Is It?

Addiction is a complex topic. While definitions of chemical use, abuse, and dependency are relatively clear, the whole issue is clouded by the legal status of the substance in question. For instance, a person may become addicted to caffeine or to crack, but caffeine is not generally considered an addiction problem, while crack certainly is. Alcoholism is a form of addiction that, because of its prevalence in the culture and the profound effects it has on virtually every system of the body, is discussed as a specific subset in this section.

One way to discuss addiction is as an arc of three patterns: use, abuse, and dependency.

- *Use*: If a person ingests a substance specifically to change mood or physical experience, it is substance use.
- *Abuse*: Abuse is the use of a substance in a way that is potentially harmful to the user or to other people. It is further identified when substance use leads to impairment or distress, and when within a 12-month period at least one of the following facts is true: the user finds that he or she cannot fulfill obligations to work, family, or school; recurrent use puts the user in dangerous situations; the user has legal problems in relation to substance use; or the user has social or interpersonal problems in relation to substance use. Abuse is also identified when prescribed drugs are used by someone else or out of the context for which they were intended.
- *Dependency*: The line between use, abuse, and addiction is sometimes blurry, and it is not always connected to length of time or amount of substance ingested. Dependency occurs when three or more of the following are true: the user develops increasing tolerance for the substance; the user has withdrawal symptoms when access to the substance is interrupted; increasing amounts of the substance are used; the user cannot voluntarily limit use; the user devotes significant time to using or recovering from use; the user replaces other activities with substance use; or the user continues to abuse the substance even when fully aware of the dangers involved.

The phenomenon of being addicted to something is not limited to the ingestion of substances. Gambling can be an addiction, as can shopping, or having sex, or using the Internet. These behaviors can be pathologic, but they aren't discussed in this section, which is specifically focused on the introduction of substances to the body.

Demographics

It is difficult to gather statistics on addiction and drug abuse, especially since much of it happens in privacy. It is estimated that 5% to 17% of the US population has a substance abuse problem of some type. Some illicit drug use appears to have gone down in recent years, but it has been replaced with prescription drug abuse: use of prescribed drugs nonmedically. Most of this happens in the home or between friends, so it is under the radar of legal or health care observation.

Alcohol abuse is a leading cause of illness and death in the United States. It is estimated that excessive drinking contributes up to 10% of all adult premature deaths: about

SIDEBAR 4.8 Drinking Definitions

Alcohol consumption is often measured by the number of drinks a person has, but the most reliable information also stipulates the type of alcohol. Equivalencies of beer to wine to liquor are shown in Figure 4.12.

"Moderate drinking" means no more than 4 drinks per day or 14 per week for men. It means no more than 3 drinks per day and 7 drinks per week for women. This is due to a number of factors, including that women usually weigh less than men and that women's blood alcohol rises faster than men's.

"Binge drinking" means drinking enough over a course of 2 hours that the blood alcohol concentration is over 0.08 g/dL. For women, this is about four drinks. For men, this is about five drinks.

No specific research has been conducted to identify "safe" drinking limits for a person who wants to receive massage, but many therapists report that clients who arrive intoxicated for a session often feel nauseated or even vomit during a massage: a good reason to delay an appointment.

88,000 deaths, taking an average of 30 years off of a normal life span. For specific information on what constitutes "a drink," see Sidebar 4.8.

Etiology: What Happens?

The process of developing dependency on a particular substance depends on the chemical makeup of that product and the susceptibility of the user. Some drugs work in the CNS by slowing the rate at which neurotransmitters are reabsorbed at key synapses. This can lead to an increase in the numbers of neurotransmitter receptors, which is then perceived as an increased need for the drug. This is the process seen with nicotine exposure, and it is why cigarette smoking is one of the most difficult addictions to overcome. Other disruptions in neural pathways and neurotransmitter relationships have been noted as well, and brain studies have revealed that some people are genetically predisposed for addiction, even without a history of exposure. Some of these people appear to have a fault in their brains' "reward pathway." Normally, the brain would put out signals of satiation when some specific need or drive is satisfied, but this population lacks that process, so they keep trying to achieve the sense of "enough."

12 fl oz of regular beer
8–9 fl oz of malt liquor
5 fl oz of table wine
1.5 fl oz of 80-proof liquor

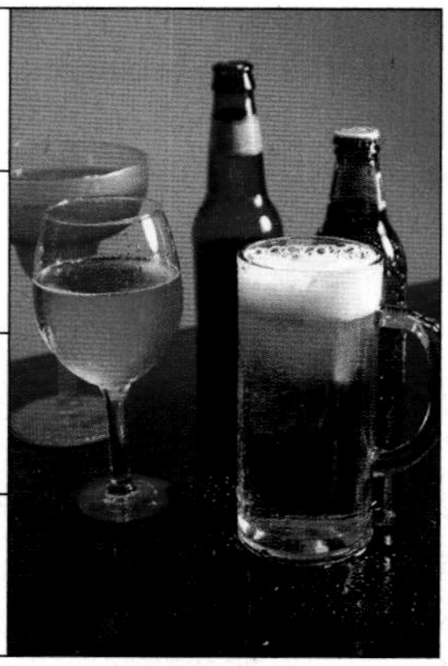

FIGURE 4.12 Equivalencies of different alcoholic drinks (Photo credit: CDC/Debora Cartagena)

Alcohol and sedatives such as tranquilizers and barbiturates work by depressing CNS arousal. While alcohol is technically a depressant, the loss of inhibitions felt by the drinker can give the impression that it is a stimulant. Some people have a genetic susceptibility to alcohol addiction, but many alcoholics develop the disease over many months or years of repeated use that finally and permanently changes the chemistry in the brain.

Once a person becomes dependent on a substance, two things happen: it takes more and more to achieve the desired affects, and to stop using the substance can create physical responses that are daunting to contemplate. Addiction is defined in two categories: psychological and physical. Psychological addiction is dependency on the pleasurable or satisfying sensations that some substance provides—in other words, the addict loves the feeling the drug gives. Physical addiction is a dependency arising from the need to avoid withdrawal symptoms, which can include general physical pain, hallucinations, nausea, vomiting, seizures, and, in extreme cases, death.

In addition to the psychological and physical aspects of addiction, this condition occurs in two distinct phases: active and recovering. Active addiction describes a person in the throes of his or her dependency, with all the associated symptoms and risks. Recovering addicts are still and always will be at risk for relapse, but their general state is likely to be more functional and healthy. Special challenges arise for the treatment of pain in recovering addicts: if their pain isn't satisfactorily managed, they may relapse into illicit drug use. But if their pain is aggressively managed, they have to start their rehabilitation process all over again once the injury is resolved.

Risk Factors

Several risk factors contribute to a person's susceptibility to addiction.

- *Genetic predisposition.* The rate of drug abuse and alcoholism is demonstrably greater in the families of other addicts than in the general population. This is partly an environmental and availability issue, but studies have shown that even children who are not raised with their chemically dependent parents have a higher than average incidence of addiction.

- *Other mental illness*. Depression and/or anxiety disorders increase the risk of a person becoming a substance abuser, as he or she may attempt to self-medicate to cope with problems.
- *Environmental factors*. These include availability of the substance in question, peer pressure, low self-esteem, a history of physical or sexual abuse, being a child in the household of a substance abuser, and other stressors that may make drug use look like an attractive choice.
- *Type of drug being used*. Some drugs are simply more addictive than others, but many drugs can cause dependency if they are used consistently enough.
- *Age*. The younger a person is at the beginning of use of an addictive substance, the more likely he or she is to develop a long-term dependency on it.
- *Medical reasons*. A patient's need for medication sometimes outlives the problem that required the initial prescription. Addictions to painkillers and sleeping pills are examples of this phenomenon.

Complications

Drug addiction

Complications of drug addiction can range from inconvenience to paranoid delusions to coma or even death. Some of the worst effects of drug use are not limited to the users, however. People close to substance abusers are also at risk. Drug-related violent crime, car accidents, industrial accidents, impaired judgment leading to the spread of **sexually transmitted infections**, and high rates of domestic violence and child abuse are other complications of chemical dependency that affect many people beyond the user.

Alcoholism

The complications of alcoholism can be progressive and insidious, and its use affects virtually every system of the body.

- *The digestive system*: Alcohol irritates the stomach lining, and high levels of consumption are responsible for a specific type of **gastritis**. It is also very rapidly absorbed through the gastric mucosa into the portal system. The portal vein dumps the alcohol directly into the liver, where it enters the rest of the bloodstream. The effects of alcohol are felt until the liver has finished neutralizing it.

  People who have preexisting gastrointestinal problems are especially vulnerable to the worst effects of alcohol. It is implicated in the development of cancer in the upper gastrointestinal tract, especially in the esophagus, pharynx, larynx, and mouth. Alcoholism can cause **ulcers**, internal hemorrhaging, **pancreatitis**, and **cirrhosis**.
- *The cardiovascular system*: Alcohol use decreases the force of cardiac contractions and can lead to irregular heartbeat, or arrhythmia. Alcohol is also toxic to myocardial tissue and can lead to alcoholic **cardiomyopathy**. Alcohol tends to **agglutinate** red blood cells, making them stick together. This leads to the possibility of **thrombi**, not only in the brain but also in the coronary arteries. Alcohol use can also have the opposite effect: liver damage can lead to reduced clotting factors and poor vitamin K synthesis, which may result in uncontrollable bleeding.

  By contrast, for some people, moderate alcohol consumption may help prevent cardiovascular disease by increasing high-density lipoprotein levels (the "good" cholesterol) in the blood.
- *The nervous system*: Memory loss frequently occurs for biochemical reasons as well as from agglutinated red blood cells blocking cerebral capillaries, causing brain cells to starve to death. Even some social drinkers sustain measurable brain damage from repeated agglutination. In the short term, alcohol slows reflexes, slurs speech, impairs judgment, and compromises motor control. In the long term, the same effects can happen on a permanent basis, often

NOTABLE CASES The list of famous people who have battled addiction is too long to explore. Rather than lingering on the many creative souls lost to the complications of alcoholism and drug abuse, in this context, it is more fitting to wonder what works of art we might have enjoyed if their lives had not been shortened by this disease.

Gastritis: Inflammation of the stomach.

Cardiomyopathy: Disease of the myocardium.

Agglutinate: To stick together, as when red blood cells form clumps.

due to a thiamine deficiency. This is also known as **Wernicke-Korsakoff syndrome**. In advanced stages of cirrhosis, the blood accumulates levels of metabolic wastes that can cause brain damage.

- *The immune system*: Prolonged alcohol use severely impedes resistance, especially to respiratory infections. People who are alcoholics are especially vulnerable to **pneumonia**.
- *The reproductive system*: Alcoholism can cause reduced sex drive, erectile dysfunction, menstrual irregularities, and infertility. Babies of alcoholic women are susceptible to **fetal alcohol syndrome**, the most common type of environmentally caused developmental disorder in the United States.
- *Alcoholic families*: Children raised in homes with one or more alcoholic adults have an increased risk of becoming substance abusers themselves. Their chances of developing **depression**, **general anxiety disorder**, and **phobias** are higher than in the general population. Further, their health costs are higher than those of other children, and many children in foster care settings are from alcoholic homes.
- *Other complications*: Alcohol is frequently a factor in traffic injuries, drownings, falls, **burns**, and shootings.

Signs and Symptoms

Symptoms of chemical dependency vary according to the substance, but main features are consistent:

- The person feels a persistent craving for the substance.
- The person goes to great lengths, including actions that could be illegal, to ensure that the substance is always available.
- The person cannot voluntarily control the use of the substance.
- The person develops an increasing tolerance to the effects of the substance and so must consume more to achieve the same results; the substance is necessary for the person to feel "normal."
- The person puts himself or herself and others at risk for harm while under the influence.
- Cessation of use creates unpleasant, alarming, and even physically dangerous withdrawal symptoms.

In addition to these signs, an addict or alcoholic may devote a significant amount of time to using and then recovering from substance use. He or she may neglect responsibilities to family, job, friends, and other relationships while distracted by substance use. And finally, the addict often denies that substance use seriously impedes or endangers his or her life: "I'm not dead yet, so obviously, I'm okay."

Treatment

The first and most important step in treating any kind of addiction is for the addict to accept that a problem exists. Once a person has reached that point, many treatment programs have good success rates, although the recurrence rate is high until a person reaches about 5 years of sobriety. Treatment goals for addiction are threefold: abstinence, rehabilitation, and prevention of relapses.

Most programs begin with detoxification, during which, the drugs are expelled from the body. This may be ameliorated with sedatives, tranquilizers, or less potent versions of the drug in question until all chemical remnants have been processed out of the body. The time this takes varies according to the substance in question.

Detoxification is followed by rehabilitation, during which the patient is taught about the effects of chemical use and trained in avoidance behaviors to provide some tools to handle the temptation to fall back into old habits.

Aftercare has been shown to be the most important part of treatment for chemical dependency. This sets up the patient with a support system that will carry him or her throughout a lifetime choice of abstinence.

Some medications can help to suppress the craving for alcohol or can cause violent physical illness when alcohol is consumed, but this doesn't eradicate the effects of alcohol. The potential for relapse into substance abuse lasts indefinitely, so this is a condition that is treated most successfully with long-term coping skills rather than short-term patches.

Medications

- Benzodiazepines in low doses to mitigate the stress of withdrawal symptoms
- Neurotransmitter receptor blockers to lessen the "reward" response in the brain and reduce craving for alcohol or narcotics
- Disulfiram to create negative physical responses (nausea, vomiting, headache) to alcohol use

Wernicke-Korsakoff syndrome: A combination of conditions related to prolonged alcohol abuse and thiamine deficiency, including tremor, psychosis, confusion, memory loss, and delirium tremens.

Fetal alcohol syndrome: A pattern of health problems that arises in children of mothers who consume excessive amounts of alcohol during pregnancy.

Massage Therapy Implications

RISKS	A client with a history of drug or alcohol abuse is at higher-than-average risk for secondary health problems, including liver damage, bacterial infections, HIV/AIDS, hepatitis, and heart problems. All of these require adjustments in bodywork choices if they impact a client's general health and resilience.
BENEFITS	Some rehabilitation facilities employ massage therapists to help ameliorate withdrawal symptoms, speed detoxification, and reduce the need for tranquilizers and other drugs. Clients who are in long-term recovery and good health can enjoy the same benefits from bodywork as the rest of the population.
OPTIONS	Current alcohol or other drug use at the time of an appointment contraindicates massage, mainly because of the risk of overwhelming the system leading to nausea and vomiting. This guideline can be a judgment call, based on the level of intoxication (one glass of wine is different from a fifth of vodka), the setting of the massage session, the behavior of the client, and the boundaries set by the therapist.
RESEARCH	Massage therapy has been used as an alternative or in addition to tranquilizers to soften the process of withdrawal and detoxification for various types of substance abuse. One study found that compared with rest, a seated massage was connected to more positive withdrawal symptom scores for an alcohol rehabilitation program.[1] Another found that massage was an effective way to manage withdrawal-related anxiety for people transitioning off of psychoactive drugs, including alcohol, cocaine, and opiates.[2] An emphasis at the National Institutes of Health on finding ways to manage pain without the risk of addictive drugs may lead to increasing interest in massage therapy for this population. 1. Reader M, Young R, Connor JP. Massage therapy improves the management of alcohol withdrawal syndrome. *Journal of Alternative and Complementary Medicine* 2005;11(2):311–313. http://www.ncbi.nlm.nih.gov/pubmed/15865498 2. Black S, Jacques K, Webber A, et al. Chair massage for treating anxiety in patients withdrawing from psychoactive drugs. *Journal of Alternative and Complementary Medicine* 2010;16(9):979–987. http://www.ncbi.nlm.nih.gov/pubmed/20799900

Anxiety Disorders

Definition: What Are They?

Anxiety disorders are a collection of distinct psychiatric disorders that have to do with irrational fears. These conditions often overlap, so a person can meet the diagnostic criteria for multiple conditions. Anxiety disorders range in severity from mild to completely debilitating.

Demographics

Various types of anxiety disorders affect up to 40 million Americans, although only a minority of those affected receive treatment.

Etiology: What Happens?

"Am I safe?" At this moment, every person who is alive and awake is asking this question at some level of consciousness. The answer for people with anxiety disorders is *"Probably not."* This interpretation of environmental signals is reflected in emotional and physical experiences that can be completely debilitating. Contributing factors include genetic vulnerability, a history of traumatic events, and situations or circumstances that trigger a stress response that is out of proportion to the actual threat.

To aid in the investigation of these conditions, careful distinctions have been drawn between the terms arousal, fear, and anxiety. *Arousal* is preparation for the possibility of a stressful event. It is directly linked to a perceived trigger or stressor (the deer that might dart across the darkened highway; the tsunami warnings on TV). *Fear* occurs when the possibility of a stressful event is confirmed. The deer has jumped front of you; the waves are rising quickly—evacuate now. *Anxiety*, by contrast, is a state of prolonged heightened arousal or fear, but with no discernible immediate or significant threat: no deer, no tsunami, but all the physical and emotional reactions that accompany the feeling of impending disaster.

Anxiety disorders take a huge toll on a person's ability to complete school or hold a job. Consequently, a disproportionately high percentage of people with anxiety disorders never earn a high school diploma and are in the lowest end of socioeconomic ranking. Furthermore, complications of anxiety disorders include an increased risk for **addiction**, **sleep disorders**, **eating disorders**, cardiovascular disease, and **depression** (with an increased danger for suicidal thoughts or behaviors).

Studies of people who live with anxiety disorders reveal some predictable neurotransmitter disruptions. The neurotransmitters most commonly involved are serotonin, dopamine, norepinephrine, and GABA. In addition, the sympathetic nervous system, with all its influence on the action of the organs, is engaged in anxiety disorder reactions to triggers.

It is important to point out that some medication use and overuse, including some herbal remedies, can mimic anxiety disorders and lead to a misdiagnosis. It is important to rule out this possibility before proceeding on to other treatment options.

Types of Anxiety Disorders

- *General anxiety disorder (GAD)*: GAD consists of chronic, exaggerated, consuming worry and the constant anticipation of disaster. It does not cause the person to avoid stressful situations, but he or she lives in a constant state of anxiety that makes it difficult to accomplish many tasks. It appears earlier and develops more slowly than other anxiety disorders.

  GAD is diagnosed when at least three of the following symptoms persist for 6 months or longer: restlessness or a feeling of being on edge, easy fatigability, poor concentration, irritability, muscle tension, and sleeping problems.
- *Panic attack, panic disorder*: Panic disorder is characterized by the sudden onset (often with no identifiable trigger) of very extreme sympathetic symptoms: a pounding heart, chest pain, sweatiness, dizziness, faintness, and alternating flushing and chilling. Hyperventilation causes numbness and tingling in the lips and extremities. A feeling of being smothered, of impending doom, and the nearness of death usually lasts for about 10 minutes but may persist for many hours. This describes a panic attack.

  A person can have a single panic attack without having panic disorder. But when episodes repeat, especially if they are associated with a certain place or situation, panic disorder is diagnosed.

  Panic disorder is one of the most successfully treated of all anxiety disorders, but treatment is most successful if it is initiated before the onset of agoraphobia.
- *Agoraphobia*: About one-third of panic disorder patients develop agoraphobia: a situation where people avoid any situations that they feel might trigger a panic attack. Agoraphobia is sometimes defined as a fear of open spaces, but in the context of panic disorder, it really means fear of anywhere that a panic attack might occur. Gradually, a person's perceived safety zone shrinks to the point where he or she becomes reluctant to leave the immediate environment
- *Phobias, Social and Specific*
  - *Social phobia*. Also called social anxiety disorder, social phobia is characterized by intense, irrational fears of being judged negatively by others or of being publicly embarrassed. Social phobia is sometimes described as simple shyness that has been over medicalized, but this condition can be debilitating. Physical symptoms include blushing, sweating, trembling, and nausea, but many social phobia patients display no outward signs of their disorder. While many people feel shy or nervous among strangers, patients with social phobia are significantly distressed and even disabled by their fear, which can interfere with work, school, or relationships.

    Social phobia is the most common anxiety disorder, and it has a relatively early age of onset: about half of all people with this condition develop symptoms by age 11, and 80% develop symptoms by age 20. Women are affected more often than men.
  - *Specific phobias*. A phobia is an intense, irrational fear of something that poses little or no real danger. Some common phobias include fear of animals (including larger animals such as dogs, cats, or birds, but also insects and spiders); closed-in places (claustrophobia), heights (acrophobia), flying, elevators, and blood. Untreated phobias can severely restrict a person's ability to hold a certain kind of job, to live in a certain kind of building, or to perform mundane tasks, such as grocery shopping. Persons with this disorder often respond better to controlled desensitization and relaxation techniques than they do to medication.
- *Separation anxiety*: This condition is usually associated with young children, but it is increasingly diagnosed among adults. It is often missed because it occurs with other anxiety disorders or depression, but it can be debilitating. Standard therapy for other anxiety disorders that does not address separation anxiety for these patients may not be as successful. Adults who develop this condition did not necessarily have it as young children.

NOTABLE CASES Many historical figures left records of their struggles with anxiety disorders, although they were never officially diagnosed. Abraham Lincoln, Sir Isaac Newton, Emily Dickenson, and John Steinbeck may be among the most influential figures to show signs of problems ranging from social phobia to GAD to disabling agoraphobia.

Signs and Symptoms

Signs and symptoms of anxiety disorders vary according to type. While they usually involve irrational fears and inappropriate sympathetic nervous system responses, they present differently by variety and patient. Brief descriptions of their signs and symptoms are included in the descriptions.

Treatment

Most anxiety disorders are treated with a combination of medication and psychotherapy. Some varieties respond better to psychotherapy and the development of coping skills alone, while others also require chemical intervention to reestablish neurotransmitter balance in the CNS. Most patients with anxiety disorders can find some combination of therapies that successfully treat their problem—if they seek treatment. Sadly, many patients are inadequately treated, or never seek treatment at all.

Psychotherapeutic techniques used for anxiety disorders vary from controlled exposure to frightening stimuli for people with specific phobias to various forms of behavioral-cognitive therapies to help patients learn ways to address and often overcome the irrational fears that limit their lives.

Other interventions have been shown to improve the quality of life for anxiety disorder patients, including relaxation techniques, meditation, yoga, acupuncture, and massage.

Medications to treat anxiety disorders fall in three classes: antidepressants, antianxiety drugs, and beta-blockers.

Medications

- Benzodiazepines for sedative effect (these carry a high risk for dependence)
- Buspirone for sedative effect
- Antidepressants, including selective serotonin reuptake inhibitors (SSRIs), tricyclics, and MAO inhibitors
- Beta-blockers to control symptoms of panic disorder

Massage Therapy Implications

RISKS	Some anxiety disorder patients have a history of physical or sexual abuse; this can create problematic reactions to touch. It is vital that these clients feel safe and in control of a massage environment.
BENEFITS	Massage has been documented to help clients with anxiety disorder feel calmer and more able to cope with the everyday stresses that life offers, as long as the client feels safe and in control.
OPTIONS	It is vital to be flexible to meet the needs of clients with anxiety disorders. Adjustments like working through clothing, with another person in the room, or with the office door open may help them to feel safer. It is also important to remember that progress is not a smooth curve, and clients' needs may fluctuate from one session to the next.
RESEARCH	From simple facial massage[1] to an extensive randomized controlled trial for massage therapy in the context of GAD,[2] to massage administered soon after cardiac surgery,[3] massage therapy as an intervention for anxiety has been well examined. Most studies find that massage therapy is helpful in this situation, although how it compares to controls varies from study to study. But as a low-risk intervention for a complicated and potentially debilitating condition that often accompanies other difficult situations, it shows a great deal of promise. 1. Hatayama T, Kitamura S, Tamura C, et al. The facial massage reduced anxiety and negative mood status, and increased sympathetic nervous activity. *Biomedical Research* 2008;29(6):317–320. https://www.jstage.jst.go.jp/article/biomedres/29/6/29_6_317/_pdf 2. Sherman KJ, Ludman EJ, Cook AJ, et al. Effectiveness of therapeutic massage for generalized anxiety disorder: a randomized controlled trial. *Depression and Anxiety* 2010;27(5):441–450. http://www.ncbi.nlm.nih.gov/pmc/articles/PMC2922919/ 3. Cutshall SM, Wentworth LJ, Engen D, et al. Effect of massage therapy on pain, anxiety, and tension in cardiac surgical patients: a pilot study. *Complementary Therapies in Clinical Practice* 2010;16(2):92–95. http://www.ncbi.nlm.nih.gov/pubmed/20347840

Attention Deficit Hyperactivity Disorder

Definition: What Is It?

Attention deficit hyperactivity disorder (ADHD) is a neurodevelopmental disorder resulting in difficulties with attention, movement, and impulse control. It has been recognized in children since the early 1900s, but was not discussed in medical literature as an issue for adults until 1976, and adult ADHD was not acknowledged in the Diagnostic Statistical Manual of Mental Disorders until 1987.

An argument can be made that the ADHD label is a misnomer. In this condition, a person pays attention to matters that are peripheral to a central task and may not be able to filter what is important from what is trivial in any moment. This is not attention deficit; rather, it is too much attention to too many things.

Demographics

A reliable estimate suggests that some 5% to 8% of children in this country meet the diagnostic criteria for ADHD, and about one-half of the people diagnosed in childhood will have symptoms that persist into adulthood. It is diagnosed much more often in boys than in girls, but the real distribution may be more equal because girls tend to present with symptoms that are more acceptable in classroom settings.

Etiology: What Happens?

ADHD is a neurochemically mediated disorder. It has been traced to problems with dopamine production, transportation, and reabsorption and with noradrenaline disruption in the frontal cortex, basal ganglia, and cerebellum: areas in the brain that have to do with decision making and movement.

While the causes of ADHD are still unclear, some contributing factors have been identified. Genetic predisposition is certainly an issue; many ADHD patients have a first-degree relative with the same disorder. Altered brain function is observable, as motor control and planning centers in the brain are affected by disturbed chemical levels. Maternal behaviors (smoking and alcohol consumption) and exposure to toxins (lead, **dioxins**, and **PCBs**) have been seen to increase the risk of ADHD in children. Some experts also suggest that this condition may arise as an adaptive measure to early childhood stress responses, which cause the brain to be overstimulated by epinephrine and norepinephrine and other excitatory neurotransmitters.

Dioxin: A toxic, carcinogenic compound that is the byproduct of some herbicides.

PCBs: Polychlorinated biphenyls, chemicals that were banned in the United States when their harmful impact on human health and the environment was discovered.

Signs and Symptoms

Three specific patterns of behavior indicate ADHD: inattentiveness, hyperactivity, and impulsivity. A person with ADHD may be primarily inattentive, or primarily impulsive and hyperactive, or have a combination of these features, but behaviors are consistent in multiple settings, for instance, at school or work, at home, and in social situations.

Signs of inattention include becoming easily distracted by irrelevant sights and sounds, failing to pay attention to details and making careless mistakes, having difficulty with following instructions carefully and completely, and losing or forgetting things such as toys, pencils, books, and tools needed for a task.

Some signs of hyperactivity and impulsivity include feeling restless, fidgeting with hands or feet, or squirming; running, climbing, or leaving a seat when sitting or quiet behavior is expected; blurting out answers before hearing the whole question; and having difficulty waiting for others to complete a task.

Adults with this disorder often manage to develop coping skills for many of their childhood symptoms, but they may have long-term problems with concentration and prioritizing actions so that relationships and occupational tasks are affected.

NOTABLE CASES Olympic swimming champion Michael Phelps was diagnosed with ADHD at age 8 and was able to turn his "hyperfocus" to a gold medal-winning goal. It is not surprising that people with ADHD are known as class clowns; other celebrities diagnosed with this condition include actors Jim Carrey and Will Smith.

Treatment

Diagnosis and treatment of ADHD in children and adults is complicated by the fact that several disorders commonly occur along with it, including **sleep disorders**, oppositional defiant disorder, **depression**, and **anxiety disorders**.

At this moment, the most common treatment for ADHD is psychostimulants, usually from classes of drugs called methylphenidates or dextroamphetamines. These drugs work by stimulating areas in the brain where activity is diminished. Another option is a norepinephrine reuptake inhibitor; this is not a stimulant; instead, it works to keep norepinephrine available in some synapses for a longer period.

Research suggests that ADHD responds best to medication, but that when medication is coupled with family counseling or parental training, the average required dosage is smaller than for children who are treated with medication alone. In adults, an expanded version of counseling called metacognitive therapy has been found to be effective.

Side effects of ADHD medications are a concern, especially if the patient is a young child. They can include appetite suppression, increased blood pressure and heart rate, sleep problems, and sometimes the development of facial or vocal tics. These signs indicate that a medication is poorly tolerated or the dosage needs to be adjusted. Some ADHD medications cannot be combined with some asthma medications.

Other approaches for ADHD include the use of nutritional supplements and adjusting the diet to avoid sugar, caffeine, and other stimulants.

Untreated or undertreated ADHD carries the risk of several serious consequences. Children with this disorder have difficulty with self-esteem, maintaining relationships, and performing well with schoolwork or other jobs. Later in life, untreated or unsuccessfully treated ADHD patients have a higher-than-average rate of automobile accidents and an elevated risk of developing **substance abuse** or other addictive behaviors (i.e., gambling, shopping, engaging in sexual encounters) in attempts to self-medicate to manage their disease.

Medications

- Psychostimulants
  - Methylphenidate
  - Dextroamphetamine
- Norepinephrine reuptake inhibitors
- Antidepressants

Massage Therapy Implications

RISKS	Massage holds no risks for children or adults with ADHD, except that some people are uncomfortable trying to be still for as long as a typical massage may take.
BENEFITS	Bodywork has been seen to improve anger control, sleep quality, classroom behavior, mood, and interpersonal relationships in people diagnosed with ADHD.
OPTIONS	While some clients with ADHD love the stimulation of a rigorous, fast-paced sports massage type of bodywork, others prefer the chance to achieve the stillness found with subtler techniques.
RESEARCH	A number of studies have looked at massage therapy for ADHD patients, most with positive results. A study of German children[1] found that massage along with other active therapies was only slightly less effective than medication, and it was extremely well regarded by the parents. This reinforced the findings from a 2003 Canadian study[2] that reported better focus at school, less disturbed sleep, and better anger control than before the intervention, which was 6 weeks of massage therapy.

1. Hamre HJ, Witt CM, Kienle GS, et al. Anthroposophic therapy for attention deficit hyperactivity: a two-year prospective study in outpatients. *International Journal of General Medicine* 2010:3239–3253. http://www.ncbi.nlm.nih.gov/pubmed/20830200
2. Maddigan B, Hodgson P, Heath S, et al. The effects of massage therapy & exercise therapy on children/adolescents with attention deficit hyperactivity disorder. *Canadian Child and Adolescent Psychiatry Review* 2003;12(2):40–43. http://www.ncbi.nlm.nih.gov/pmc/articles/PMC2538473/

Autism Spectrum Disorder

Definition: What Is It?

Autism spectrum disorder (ASD) is a complex developmental disorder characterized by problems with interpersonal interaction, communication, and learning. ASD patients often have difficulty connecting emotionally with other people, including parents and family members; communication difficulties; restricted interests; specific and predictable movement patterns; and sensory problems. Signs of ASD turn up in early childhood. It is usually diagnosable by age 3, although many children with ASD aren't identified until they start kindergarten.

Demographics

The numbers of people diagnosed on the autism spectrum have been climbing for several years. It is unclear however whether this represents a true increase in the incidence of the disorder, or improved screening and diagnostic protocols, or overdiagnosis of nonpathologic but sometimes inconvenient behavior in children. Estimates of the prevalence of ASD in the United States suggest that it affects 1 out of every 88 children and that some 400,000 individuals in this country are on the spectrum. It appears to affect boys more than girls, although the exact ratios in diagnosed populations vary from region to region.

Etiology: What Happens?

The difference in CNS function between people with ASD and people without it is the subject of intense study. Abnormalities are present within various neural systems linking the brainstem, limbic system, basal ganglia, cerebellum, corpus callosum, and cerebral cortex of people with ASD, but no predictable pattern is present for all patients.

The most easily distinguishable factor behind some cases of ASD is a genetic anomaly. **Fragile X syndrome** is a condition in which a pinch appears in the X chromosome; this is the most common form of inherited mental disability, and it affects many ASD patients. **Tuberous sclerosis**, another genetic anomaly, involves the growth of benign tumors in the CNS and other vital organs. Children with tuberous sclerosis have a higher chance of also being on the autism spectrum. Siblings of children with ASD have a much greater chance of being on the spectrum than the general public (and the chance for identical twins is much higher still). This clearly points to a genetic factor, although the specific mutations are not always identifiable.

> **Fragile X syndrome:** A condition in which a pinch appears in the X chromosome, leading to mental disability.
>
> **Tuberous sclerosis:** A rare genetic disease that causes nonmalignant tumors to grow in the brain and other vital organs.
>
> **Savant:** A condition in which a person with developmental disorders shows one or more areas of unusually strong ability or skill.

Types of Autism Spectrum Disorders

Until recently, these subtypes were addressed as separate, freestanding disorders, which led to inconsistent diagnoses and treatment plans. These are now all considered part of one condition: ASD. Understanding autism spectrum in this way allows clinicians to recognize that an individual's symptoms can be mild in one area, but more extreme in others. Although the disorder is now seen as one issue, labels can help give a snapshot of symptom severity.

- *Autistic disorder*: This may also be called "severe autism" to distinguish it from the milder form. It is characterized by the three basic traits associated with ASD: impairment in communication skills; poor social interactions; and restricted, repetitive patterns of movement.
- *Asperger syndrome*: This is ASD at the milder end of the spectrum, involving difficulties with socializing, but language skills and mental development are often normal or above normal. Some people classify Asperger syndrome as an entity distinct from mild autism, but not all experts agree on this. Many people with Asperger syndrome develop a consuming interest in some subject that completely engages them.
- *Pervasive developmental disorder, not otherwise specified*: This is a condition in which a child exhibits several ASD signs, but in an unusual or unique pattern.

Signs and Symptoms

Signs and symptoms of ASD vary according to what type is present. Three major issues are present for most types: deficits in verbal and nonverbal communication, problems with social interaction, and repetitive behaviors or movements. These occur in varying combinations and severity for each person. In addition, many ASD patients show unusual reactions to some sensory stimuli: they often seem to be impervious to cold or pain, while some sounds and textures, even soft ones, appear to be unbearable.

ASD frequently occurs with other conditions. About 25% of ASD patients also have **seizures**, and most have some level of cognitive disability. By contrast, of ASD patients with an IQ of 35 or above, many show signs of **savant** characteristics, that is, extremely highly developed skills with some narrow set of interests, such as numbers, music, reading, or other talents.

Early indicators of ASD include some movement anomalies during infancy; a lack of babbling, pointing, or smiling at 12 months; no word use at 16 months; no word linkage at 24 months; no response to the child's name; and observable regression in language and social skills. Other signs include little or no eye contact, limited imaginative play with toys, obsessive lining up of objects, extreme attachment to one object, and the appearance of a hearing deficiency. Many children show restricted, repetitive behaviors, such as hand wringing, rocking, or other movements, especially when they are tense or upset.

NOTABLE CASES Perhaps, the most notable spokesperson for ASD is Temple Grandin, a writer and animal behavior consultant who invented a "hug machine" to help calm hypersensitive people. You can find a TED talk with Ms. Grandin at http://www.ted.com/talks

Treatment

ASD is treated according to type and the individual characteristics of the child. Experts agree that children on the spectrum do best in highly structured, specialized settings that reinforce positive behaviors and work to reduce negative ones.

Applied behavioral analysis is an intensive one-on-one intervention that occurs for many hours every week. Children who undergo this kind of therapy, especially in early years (preschool is preferable), often have significant improvement in function. Sensory integration therapy uses touch, pressure, vibration, massage, and lots of play equipment to help patients better organize their sense of touch.

Many ASD patients also have symptoms of other disorders, especially **attention deficit hyperactivity disorder**, **obsessive-compulsive disorder**, and **depression**. Treating these can improve the possibility that other ASD interventions are successful.

Some parents find that dietary adjustments help their children. Avoiding gluten and casein (a protein found in dairy products) reduces symptoms for some, but not all, ASD patients. Supplementing vitamin B6 with magnesium has similar results: some people benefit, and others have no response.

In addition to these interventions, medication may be prescribed to help manage seizures, anxiety, and depression, but no medication addresses the issue of autism itself.

Medications

- Antipsychotics to manage anger, irritation, or aggressive or self-destructive behaviors
- Antidepressants, especially SSRIs for depression and anxiety
- Psychostimulants for ADHD symptoms
- Antiseizure drugs for seizures

Massage Therapy Implications

RISKS	The most important caution for working with clients who have ASD is that the sensation of touch is not always welcome. Therapists may have to be patient and imaginative to create an environment where the best outcomes can occur.
BENEFITS	If the ASD patient is comfortable receiving touch, massage can have a profound impact on a person's ability to connect with the world in a positive way.
OPTIONS	A person on the spectrum, child or adult, can enjoy many benefits of massage as long as he or she can feel in control of the choice to receive touch or not. It may take patience and imagination to entice a person on the spectrum onto the table, but once there, they often enjoy the experience of firm, predictable contact.
RESEARCH	A surprising amount of research documents benefits of massage therapy for people on the autism spectrum. It has been seen to help with disrupted sleep,[1] and a qigong massage protocol may help with tactile disturbances so that parents and children can more meaningfully connect.[2] A systematic review[3] found several studies with positive outcomes, but a strong bias toward a successful intervention brings their accuracy into question. Like many conditions, this calls for more high-quality research.

1. McLay LL, France K. Empirical research evaluating non-traditional approaches to managing sleep problems in children with autism. *Developmental Neurorehabilitation* 2014. http://www.ncbi.nlm.nih.gov/pubmed/24724691
2. Silva L, Schalock M. Treatment of tactile impairment in young children with autism: results with qigong massage. *International Journal of Therapeutic Massage and Bodywork* 2013;6(4):12–20. http://www.ncbi.nlm.nih.gov/pmc/articles/PMC3838308/
3. Lee MS, Kim JI, Ernst E. Massage therapy for children with autism spectrum disorders: a systematic review. *Journal of Clinical Psychiatry* 2011;72(3):406–411. http://www.ncbi.nlm.nih.gov/pubmed/21208598

Bipolar Disorder

Definition: What Is It?

Bipolar disorder has also been called manic depression. It is marked by mood swings on a continuum from major depression to mania (Sidebar 4.9).

Demographics

Bipolar disorder affects about 2.6% of the US adult population: about 2.3 million people. Of those, 83% have a severe form of this condition. Bipolar disorder can be diagnosed at almost any age, but it usually appears between late adolescence and early adulthood.

Men and women are affected by bipolar disorder about equally, but this condition is often misdiagnosed in its early manifestations. Consequently, women are far more likely to be originally diagnosed with **major depressive disorder** (also called unipolar depression), while men are most likely to be initially diagnosed with schizophrenia.

Etiology: What Happens?

The development of bipolar disorder is not well understood. It runs in families, so a genetic component is probably at least one factor among many in this disorder. Differences in brain development that occur during adolescence may trigger some symptoms; this could explain why this condition is often identified in the teenage years.

People with bipolar disorder also show some differences in myelination in various brain regions. These differences resemble some findings with schizophrenia, suggesting that these two conditions may be closely related. Some of this damage occurs in centers for regulating emotion. It is hypothesized that mood-stabilizing drugs and antidepressants work by stimulating cellular function and resilience in these areas.

SIDEBAR 4.9 Arc of Mood States

Depression is sometimes discussed in the context of a continuum of moods. Bipolar disorder in particular refers to swings from one place on the scale to another, and the extremity of mood determines the subtype of bipolar disorder that is diagnosed.

The descriptors for moods along this continuum are these:

- Severe depression (as seen with **major depressive disorder**)
- Moderate depression
- Mild low mood (as seen with **persistent depressive disorder**)
- Balanced mood (no pathology is present)
- Hypomania
- Severe mania (as seen with the most extreme version of bipolar disorder)

Types of Bipolar Disorder

- *Bipolar type I*: This is the most common form of bipolar disorder. It is diagnosed when a person experiences a manic episode that lasts at least a week and a depressive episode that lasts at least 2 weeks. Hospitalization and impaired social function are common. Psychotic delusions and hallucinations can occur in both the manic and depressive phases.
- *Bipolar type II*: This is a milder form, with mood swings between the narrower extremes of mild depression and hypomania. It does not involve psychosis or social and occupational impairment.
- *Cyclothymia*: This describes type II mood swings that last for 2 years or more.
- *Mixed bipolar disorder*: This extremely disruptive disorder involves some manic and depressive symptoms occurring either simultaneously or in rapid succession.
- *Rapid-cycling bipolar disorder*: This very severe form shows four or more cycles in a year. It has a younger onset than other forms of bipolar disorder.

Signs and Symptoms

The manic phase of bipolar disorder is marked by heightened energy, elation, irritability, racing thoughts, increased sex drive, decreased inhibitions, and unrealistic or grandiose ideas that lead to decisions made on poor judgment. Someone in a manic state might undertake a huge new project, spontaneously quit a job, buy a car, or make some other major life change without realizing the long-term implications—which will linger after the manic phase subsides.

The depressive phase has all the depth and severity of major depressive disorder, which is discussed elsewhere.

NOTABLE CASES Artist Vincent Van Gogh probably lived with bipolar disease, as well as gonorrhea, absinthe addiction, and possible poisoning from the paints he was using. In one manic period of 2 months, he produced 90 spectacular paintings, none of which found a buyer in his lifetime. He died at age 37 of a self-inflicted gunshot wound.

Treatment

One of the reasons bipolar disorder has been separated from other depressive disorders is that it responds best to a different line of treatment. Further, bipolar disorder presents some challenges to manage because it almost always requires a complicated mix of medications to address manic, depressive, and possible psychotic symptoms. Even when a successful combination is found, some of these drugs have unpleasant side effects and bad interactions with other commonly used medications like hormone supplements and birth control pills.

Rather than addressing the uptake of serotonin or dopamine, bipolar disorder treatment works to out mood swings with mood-stabilizing medications built on a mineral called lithium. These drugs can tamp down manic symptoms, but they may not address depression. Lithium and its analogues can be helpful, but these medications are also potentially toxic, so it is important that they be prescribed and used with great care.

Antidepressants are also used for patients with bipolar disorder, but they can precipitate a manic episode if they are used alone. Consequently, they are usually prescribed along with antipsychotic or mood-stabilizing drugs.

Medications

- Mood stabilizers (lithium and lithium analogues)
- Antidepressants
- Anticonvulsants (to manage manic symptoms)
- Antipsychotics (for hallucinations or delusions)

Massage Therapy Implications

RISKS	The risks of working with a client who has bipolar disorder center on two issues: side effects of medications and the client-therapist relationship. If the client is able to exercise and engage in normal activities of daily living, massage is probably not too taxing physically. On the other hand, if the client feels lethargic and irritable, it may not be appropriate to challenge him or her with a rigorous massage. The client-therapist relationship, with all appropriate boundaries, is especially important in working with any client who lives with psychiatric challenges. Clients can invest too much authority in their massage therapists, which can lead to many problems. Practitioners must be especially careful to be as sure as possible that their communications are clear and trustworthy.
BENEFITS	Bipolar disorder patients are counseled to maintain good social connections and to get good quality sleep; massage therapy may help with both of those goals.

Depression

Definition: What Is It?

Depression is a group of disorders that involve negative changes in emotional state. One of the best descriptions of this disease is "a genetic-neurochemical disorder requiring a strong environmental trigger whose characteristic manifestation is an inability to appreciate sunsets."[2]

[2]Sapolsky R. Why Zebras don't get ulcers. 3rd ed. © 2004, Holt Paperbacks, p. 272.

In other words, depression is a CNS disorder involving a genetic predisposition, chemical changes, and a significant triggering event that results in a person losing the ability to enjoy life. Depression is more than a temporary spell of the blues; it can be a long-lasting, self-propagating, and ultimately debilitating—even life-threatening—disease.

Demographics

About 20% of all American women and some 12% of American men will experience a depressive episode at some point. This prevalence is about the same in other developed countries. Depression rates are highest among people between 25 and 45 years old, but this condition has been observed in young children and elders as well. The older the individual is at onset, the harder depression seems to be to treat, and the longer each episode appears to last.

Etiology: What Happens?

The pathophysiology of depression is not well understood. Several distinctive features have been noted in the brain and endocrine system of depressive individuals, but whether these features cause the problem or are caused by the problem is still a mystery. The most significant and consistent distinguishing features of depression is a neurotransmitter imbalance, especially with serotonin, norepinephrine, and dopamine: these may be in short supply, or receptor sites for them may not function well. Either way, the drugs most often prescribed for depression work to increase the accessibility of these important chemicals.

The hypothalamus-pituitary-adrenal (HPA) axis is another factor in depression and chemical imbalances. The HPA axis describes the tight connection between the CNS and the endocrine system: the pituitary gland, under the control of the hypothalamus, controls the adrenal glands by way of corticotrophin-releasing hormone (Figure 4.13). Depressive people tend to secrete excessive amounts of corticotrophin-releasing hormone, meaning that they create stress responses to minimal stimuli, and those responses tend to have a longer-lasting effect on the body.

Many factors contribute to depressive episodes. Some of them are controllable, but many are not. Whether or not someone develops depression depends on personal chemistry, genetics, emotional and environmental triggers, and unique personality qualities and problem-solving tendencies. Other psychiatric conditions commonly overlap with depression, especially **posttraumatic stress disorder** and **obsessive-compulsive disorder**. In addition, chronic illness increases the risk for this disorder. This is easy to understand, as chronic pain, or the prospect of sliding into inevitable disability naturally deprives a person of a sense of hopefulness or investment in life. Often, the symptoms of depression outweigh the symptoms of the chronic illness: if

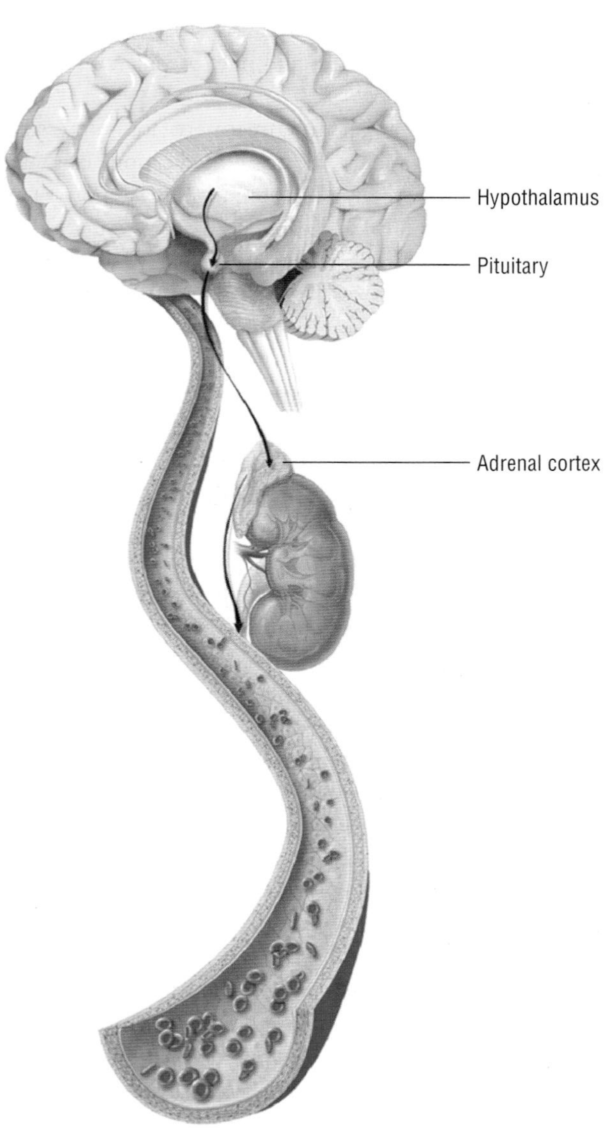

FIGURE 4.13 HPA axis: the link between the hypothalamus, the pituitary gland, and the adrenal cortex regulates circulating stress hormones in the bloodstream

the depression can be resolved, coping skills for the illness may also improve.

Several other problems can contribute to depression, but these are often much more easily controlled than the ones so far discussed. **Hypothyroidism**, smoking, alcohol, drug use, or side effects of medication can all create depressive symptoms. Also, certain nutritional deficiencies, notably vitamin B_{12} and folate, can contribute to depressive symptoms.

Complications

The most obvious and serious complication of depression is suicide. About 30,000 people successfully commit suicide each year in the United States, and up to 200,000 suicide attempts are recorded. It is estimated that half of those attempts are related to depressive episodes. Although men have depression about half as often as women, they are four times more likely to successfully commit suicide.

In addition to suicide risk, a history of depression is now found to be a risk factor for several other conditions, including **addiction**. Notably, **stroke**, **heart attack**, and other forms of cardiovascular disease show a link with depression. Further, the severity of the preexisting depression can be a predictor for how well a person recovers from a stroke or heart attack. Although the cause-and-effect relationships between depression and cardiovascular disease have not been fully identified, an obvious connection can be made between depression and the physical manifestations of long-term stress.

Finally, depression frequently accompanies other long-term diseases. The symptoms of depression can make the consequences of other conditions worse (e.g., pain sensation is amplified, sleep is disrupted), and people who are depressed are not likely to take good care of themselves by eating well, taking medication according to prescription, and staying in contact with supportive friends and loved ones.

NOTABLE CASES *Sophie's Choice* author William Styron was a depression patient whose eloquence is haunting. This comes from his memoir, *Darkness Visible*: "Mysteriously and in ways that are totally remote from normal experience, the gray drizzle of horror induced by depression takes on the quality of physical pain ... it is entirely natural that the victim begins to think ceaselessly of oblivion." He did eventually recover to become a vocal advocate for mental health issues. He died of pneumonia at age 81 in 2006.

Types of Depression

Experts recognize several etiologically distinct types of depression. This is a short list.

- *Major depressive disorder*: This is classic debilitating clinical depression. It is recognized when very severe symptoms persist for periods longer than 2 weeks. Left untreated, episodes of major depression may last anywhere from 6 to 18 months and on average recur anywhere from four to six times over a lifetime. Each successive episode can be triggered by a less important event: in other words, the person becomes increasingly vulnerable. Ultimately, someone who doesn't seek treatment for a major depressive disorder can expect to spend many years feeling hopeless, helpless, and worthless.
- *Persistent depressive disorder*: This is a depressed mood that lasts for at least 2 years. It can be less severe than major depressive disorder, but many people experience fluctuations of severity within this long-term problem. This condition is sometimes called dysthymia.
- *Psychotic depression*: This is major depressive disorder with **psychosis**: that is, hallucinations (a distortion of

Psychosis: A mental and behavioral disorder affecting a person's ability to recognize reality.

perception with a powerful sense of reality) and/or delusions (beliefs that are not changed by reason or contradictory evidence).

- *Seasonal affective disorder*: This is depression related to the absence of sunlight. Its incidence goes up according to distance from the equator. It is thought to be related to low levels of melatonin, a neurotransmitter stimulated by exposure to sunlight. In the Northern Hemisphere, it is most prevalent during December, January, and February.
- *Premenstrual dysphoric disorder*: This form of **premenstrual syndrome** involves very severe PMS symptoms along with monthly depressive cycles.
- *Postpartum depression*: This is the depression that affects new mothers, usually developing within the first few months after giving birth. It is related to several factors, including vast hormonal shifts, a sense of inadequate social support, and biologic vulnerability: women with a history of other types of depression, especially bipolar disorder, are at increased risk. A woman with postpartum depression has all of the symptoms of major depression, along with the deep-rooted fear of having harm come to or of actually doing harm to her baby. A different condition, called postpartum psychosis, involves hallucinations or delusions that may put the mother or her children in danger.

Signs and Symptoms

The signs and symptoms of depression depend partly on what type is present. The two leading symptoms include a persistent sad or empty feeling and experiencing less enjoyment from usual activities and hobbies. Other common symptoms include a deep sense of guilt or disappointment with oneself, a feeling of hopelessness—that things will never get better—irritability, and a change in sleeping habits: the person either sleeps very little or sleeps much more than usual.

Additional signs and symptoms can include a decreasing ability to concentrate, weight changes (the person either eats much more than usual or loses all interest in food), a loss of energy, a feeling of helplessness, persistent physical pain that is unresponsive to treatment (especially headaches, backache, and digestive discomfort), and suicidal thoughts, plans, or attempts. A person is typically diagnosed with depression when five or more of these symptoms are present for in a new pattern for a minimum of 2 weeks.

Treatment

Most types of depression are treatable, although finding the right combination of therapies can be time-consuming, frustrating, and expensive. Several different classes of antidepressant medications have been developed, each with advantages and disadvantages, and new medications are in development all the time.

The success of a person's treatment for depression depends largely on patience, as many medications can take several weeks to achieve their full potential. It is important to try to treat depression fully, because when people find relief but have lingering symptoms, they are at high risk for recurrent episodes.

Medications used for major depressive disorder usually fall into one of four categories: **SSRIs** (including Prozac and Zoloft), **SNRIs** (including Effexor and Cymbalta), **MAOIs** (including Nardil), and **tricyclic antidepressants** (including Elavil). All of these classes of medication aim to make neurotransmitters more easily accessible in the mood-determining areas of the brain.

Antidepressants work by making targeted neurotransmitters more available in brain synapses, often by inhibiting the reuptake of those chemicals. They are effective for most people, but they have two major disadvantages: they take several weeks to establish any noticeable mood changes, and they tend to produce unpleasant side effects during that initial adjustment period. Side effects usually include dry mouth, dizziness, constipation, skin rashes, sleepiness or sleeplessness, sexual dysfunction, and restlessness. These symptoms generally subside within 4 to 6 weeks, which is about when the benefits of the medication begin to be felt.

Psychologists and psychiatrists may also employ various types of talk therapy to help patients improve coping skills and reduce both the effects and the recurrence of depressive episodes. Some evidence suggests that talk therapy along with medication leads to more successful outcomes. Three major approaches have been found to be most useful, depending on the personality and needs of the affected individual. **Cognitive-behavioral therapy** focuses on the patient's skills at managing life and making beneficial

SSRI: Selective serotonin reuptake inhibitors, a type of drug used to relieve depression.

SNRI: Serotonin and norepinephrine reuptake inhibitors, a type of drug used to relieve depression.

MAOIs: Monoamine oxidase inhibitors, group of chemicals used in the treatment of depression.

Tricyclic antidepressants: An early class of antidepressant that works to alter neurotransmitter reuptake; these have more side effects than more recent options.

Cognitive-behavioral therapy: A technique in psychotherapy whereby negative patterns of thought are challenged in order to alter them.

choices. **Interpersonal therapy** focuses on how relationships color a person's life for better or worse. And **psychodynamic therapy** looks at how unresolved inner conflicts can affect the way a person makes choices and lives with those choices.

Other therapies for depression include:

- *Light therapy*. Persons living with seasonal affective disorder may not need medication or talk therapy; they need sunlight. Exposure to broad-spectrum lights can help to reduce symptoms.
- *Electroconvulsive therapy*. Some major depressive disorder patients don't respond to medication, and they are at high risk for suicide. Electroconvulsive, or shock, therapy may be the best choice for these patients. It is not entirely clear why it works, but it can be a highly effective intervention for people who don't get relief from other options.
- *St. John's wort*. This herbal extract has received a lot of attention as a mood enhancer without the side effects that other antidepressants carry. While some studies indicate that it can be effective for mild depression, it has been shown to be ineffective as a treatment for major depressive disorder. St. John's wort has some risks; if a person takes medication to control HIV or any cytotoxic drugs (to reduce the risk of organ rejection, for instance), St. John's wort has been seen to make these medications less effective.
- *Others*. A number of other interventions for depression continue to be explored, including SAM-e (S-adenosylmethionine), omega-3 fish oil, 5-hydroxytryptophan (a supplement that provides the building blocks for serotonin), and others.

Transcranial magnetic stimulation is sometimes suggested for treatment-resistant depression, as is **vagus nerve stimulation**.

Acupuncture, massage, and exercise have also been seen to be helpful to manage depression symptoms.

> **Interpersonal therapy:** A type of psychotherapy focused on interpersonal relationships and skills.
>
> **Psychodynamic therapy:** A form of psychotherapy that focuses on how unresolved inner conflicts affect one's decision making.
>
> **Transcranial magnetic stimulation:** A treatment using magnetic fields to stimulate nerves in the brain in order to relieve depression
>
> **Vagus nerve stimulation:** A treatment for depression that does not respond to other interventions. Also used for control of epileptic seizures.

Medications

- Antidepressants, including SSRIs, SNRIs, TCAs, and MAOIs
    - Note: MAOIs carry a high risk of dangerous interactions with other drugs, but new application strategies minimize that danger.
- Antianxiety medication if needed for postpartum depression and others

Massage Therapy Implications

RISKS No specific physical risks exist for a person with depression who wants to receive massage. It is important to bear in mind however that massage may be so well received that the client may want to reduce or completely abandon his or her medications. It is vital that this not happen without the oversight of the prescribing physician.

BENEFITS Although the mechanisms for how it works are not understood, massage has a powerful positive influence on mood, anxiety, and the perceived ability to deal with the stressors of daily life. Depression of any kind indicates massage.

RESEARCH Massage has been shown to have a positive effect on depression both as a freestanding condition[1] and in the context of many other conditions, including fibromyalgia,[2] cancer,[3] perimenopause,[4] recent surgery,[5] and chronic pain.[6]

1. Hou WH, Chiang PT, Hsu TY, et al. Treatment effects of massage therapy in depressed people: a meta-analysis. *Journal of Clinical Psychiatry* 2010;71(7):894–901. http://www.ncbi.nlm.nih.gov/pubmed/20361919
2. Li YH, Wang FY, Feng CQ, et al. Massage therapy for fibromyalgia: a systematic review and meta-analysis of randomized controlled trials. *PLoS One* 2014;9(2):e89304. http://www.ncbi.nlm.nih.gov/pmc/articles/PMC3930706/
3. Falkensteiner M, Mantovan F, Muller I, et al. The use of massage therapy for reducing pain, anxiety, and depression in oncological palliative care patients: a narrative review of the literature. *ISRN Nursing* 2011;2011:929868. http://www.ncbi.nlm.nih.gov/pmc/articles/PMC3168862/
4. Oliveira DS, Hachul H, Goto V, et al. Effect of therapeutic massage on insomnia and climacteric symptoms in postmenopausal women. *Climacteric* 2012;15(1):21–29. http://www.ncbi.nlm.nih.gov/pubmed/22017318
5. Babaee S, Shafiei Z, Sadeghi MM, et al. Effectiveness of massage therapy on the mood of patients after open-heart surgery. *Iranian Journal of Nursing and Midwifery Research* 2012;17(2 suppl 1):S120–S124. http://www.ncbi.nlm.nih.gov/pmc/articles/PMC3696961/
6. Munk N, Kruger T, Zanjani F. Massage therapy usage and reported health in older adults experiencing persistent pain. *Journal of Alternative and Complementary Medicine* 2011;17(7):609–616. http://www.ncbi.nlm.nih.gov/pubmed/21668368

Eating Disorders

Definition: What Are They?

Eating disorders are a variety of unhealthy eating habits that become difficult or even impossible to reverse. Eating disorders often arise in response to emotional or physical stressors. They may begin as a short-term coping mechanism, but they can become a serious long-term impairment to health. The disorders discussed here include anorexia, bulimia, and binge-eating disorder.

Demographics

Most anorexia and bulimia patients are young women, although men can deal with these as well. Demographics on binge-eating disorder are difficult to gather, but given the fact that about two-thirds of the adults in the United States are overweight, and 60 million adults are classified as obese (with a body mass index of 30 or above), it is reasonable to suggest that many people in this country have a dysfunctional relationship with food.

Etiology: What Happens?

The personality profiles of anorexia and bulimia patients point toward adolescents and young adults with high expectations of themselves. They are often eager-to-please overachievers who do well in school and may be involved in athletics that emphasize thinness or strength-to-weight ratios: dancing or gymnastics among girls, for instance, and wrestling for young men.

Anorexia and bulimia tend to center on control among a population that often feels powerless: adolescent girls in a culture that bombards them with impossible standards to live up to. A young woman may not be able to control how people treat her, but she can at least control what goes into her mouth. For many, that feels like a major victory, at least in the short run.

NOTABLE CASES Many public figures have battled eating disorders, some of them unsuccessfully. Princess Diana of Wales struggled with bulimia related to the stress of her public position. Singer Karen Carpenter died of complications due to anorexia at age 32. Supermodels Isabella Caro and Ana Carolina Reston both lost their battles with anorexia. Olympic hopeful gymnast Christy Henrich died of multiple organ failure related to anorexia at age 22, opening the way for many gymnasts to share their struggles with anorexia and bulimia.

In addition, some neurotransmitter levels appear to be different among eating disorder patients compared to the general population. Whether this is a cause or a result of anorexia and bulimia is debatable, but it does open the door to some treatment options.

When a person begins to pathologically limit her diet in order to stay thin, ultimately it doesn't matter whether it's because of a neurotransmitter imbalance or because she's desperate to get on the gymnastics team or to feel her hipbones sticking out. Her choices eventually change the way her body functions. If this persists for long enough, she may reach the point at which it's impossible for her digestive system to work properly: she can lose the ability to break down nutrients, absorb nutrition, or to eliminate waste. Anorexia and bulimia can be terminal illnesses.

The phenomenon of binge eating can also be linked to a sense of a lack of control, but has a number of other physical and psychological factors, many of which are not well understood. It has significance for massage therapists for several reasons, but touch and protection are perhaps the most immediately pertinent.

The experience of welcomed touch is a basic human need, and its presence or absence has an impact on overall health. In this culture, nonsexual touch between adults is almost exclusively limited to greeting and leave-taking, sports and violence, and personal care, that is, health care or aesthetician services. Consequently, if a person doesn't get touch on the outside, she can at least get touch on the inside: the sensation of eating past the point of satiation can be perceived as an internal "hug." Eating for comfort can become a vicious circle, as our culture places a high premium on physical attractiveness (i.e., being slender), which means that overweight people may have a harder time making and keeping supportive touch-rich relationships. This can drive them to the short-term comfort measure of overeating more frequently. Massage therapists are in a position to provide nurturing, restorative, educated, and nonjudgmental touch to a population of people who may have little or no other access to this important sensory nourishment.

Weight gain creates a physical barrier between a person and the world. This protective device may be a person's conscious or subconscious attempt to create distance between herself and experiences she wants to avoid. It is common to see overeating and weight gain, for instance, in people who are subject to physical, verbal, or sexual abuse. Survivors may use overeating as a strategy to discourage their abusers. Many survivors of touch abuse are binge eaters. Many survivors of abuse also eventually explore massage as a way to experience touch that is positive and nurturing. Massage therapists who work with this population must be aware of how closely these clients' emotional state may be reflected in their physical state.

The complications associated with eating disorders can be divided into mental/emotional issues and physical issues. Many eating disorder patients struggle with **depression**, irritability, **sleep disorders**, **anxiety disorders**, and **obsessive-compulsive disorder**.

Physical complications can include a slow heart rate (**bradycardia**), low blood pressure, and arrhythmia.

Bradycardia: Slow heart rate.

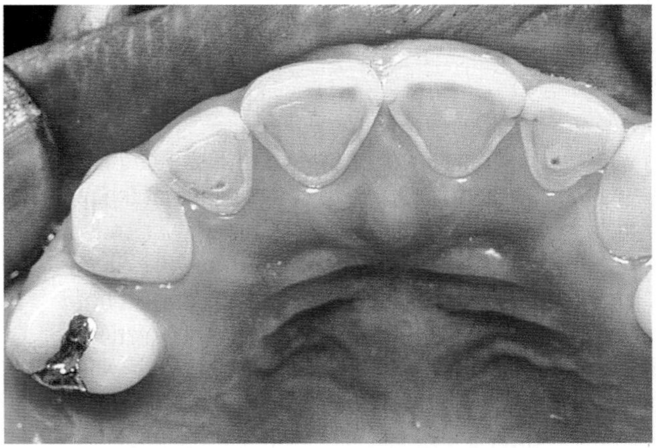

FIGURE 4.14 Erosion caused by chronic vomiting in bulimia

Changes in hormone secretion with **amenorrhea** can cause early-onset menopause, with osteopenia or even **osteoporosis**—exactly at a time when young adults should be adding to their total bone mass instead of losing it. This happens often enough in young women athletes that the symptomatic pattern of disordered eating with low energy plus menstrual dysfunction and low bone density has a name: **female athlete triad**.

Other physical complications involve the overuse of laxatives, which can cause colon dysfunction. Self-induced vomiting can lead to tooth damage (Figure 4.14), esophageal erosion and scarring, and dangerously imbalanced electrolytes. Eventually, a person who regularly induces vomiting may find it difficult to keep food down, even if she wants to.

Binge eaters are at risk for cardiovascular disease, **osteoarthritis**, **type 2 diabetes**, gallbladder disease, and other physical problems associated with being overweight if their eating habits are never modified. However, these patients do not accrue the same life-threatening chemical imbalances that anorexic or bulimic patients do. If eating behaviors are changed, binge eaters may sustain few if any long-term problems.

This is a short list of well-recognized eating disorders, but many other dysfunctional eating patterns exist. One is a special risk for health care providers, called orthorexia (see Sidebar 4.10).

SIDEBAR 4.10 Eating Too Healthy? Or Too Healthy to Eat?

Some people invest a lot of time and energy in planning and executing healthy eating patterns, and they are happy and strong. Some people invest so much time and energy in this pursuit that they end up risking their own well-being. Their interest becomes a preoccupation, and finally an obsession. The net result is a condition that is now being called orthorexia nervosa.

Orthorexia is not recognized as an official label in DSM-5, but many clinicians are documenting this behavioral pattern, which has several features in common with **obsessive-compulsive disorder**. Interestingly, many people in health care, including medical students and nutritionists, appear to be especially prone to developing these habits. Many massage therapists might fit this description as well.

Investing in healthy eating is not pathological, but the consequences of orthorexia include very stringent dietary restrictions and intense anxiety, guilt, and shame—even self-loathing—when those standards are not upheld. This is the aspect of the condition that interferes with the quality of life, and it is important to address it.

Types of Eating Disorders

- *Anorexia nervosa*: This is a situation in which a person drastically limits his or her caloric intake. It is essentially self-starvation. It may be restrictive, in which a person simply doesn't take in enough calories to sustain her, or purge type, in which calorie intake may be adequate for sustenance, but it is negated by compensatory activities, including vomiting; use of laxatives, diuretics, and/or enemas; and excessive exercise (Case History 4.2).
- *Bulimia nervosa*: Bulimia translates literally to "ox hunger." This is a disorder in which a person may appear to eat normally in public, but then in private binges on "forbidden" or self-indulgent foods. This behavior then leads to compensatory activity including self-induced vomiting, laxative use, or excessive exercise. Many patients fluctuate between anorexic and bulimic behaviors.
- *Binge-eating disorder*: This describes a situation where a person engages in overeating that is accompanied by a distressing sense of loss of control. This may be mitigated by follow-up dieting and exercise, but often, it is not—or unsuccessful attempts to diet bring on more bingeing episodes.

Amenorrhea: Absence of menses.

Female athlete triad: The combination of disordered eating, amenorrhea, and osteopenia or osteoporosis that is sometimes seen with women athletes and is predictive of later serious health problems.

Signs and Symptoms

Signs and symptoms of eating disorders obviously depend on which type is present. Diagnostic criteria for anorexia include intense fear of gaining weight, distorted self-perception

CASE HISTORY 4.2 Eating Disorders

I think my eating problems began when I was around 12 years old. I was an only child and a gymnast, working hard in my program. All my coaches wanted muscle, muscle, muscle—no flab. At that time I got in the mindset that the more I worked out, the more muscle I'd have, so I started skipping meals to have more body-building time. Having muscles and doing my routines perfectly were the only things on my mind.

I went on a pretty much just rice diet. Rice doesn't have any fat but lots of carbs to burn for energy. I'd have a bowl of rice and some water, which would make me feel really full. I think because of that my stomach shrank; just eating regular foods became really hard. Since I was always by myself, my parents didn't realize my problem. I always wore baggy clothes because I was constantly cold, and if I wore something tighter, my mother would say I looked fat; but in truth I was barely 5 feet tall and about 70 or 75 pounds.

JESSICA, AGE 19:
"Food was the one thing I thought I could control completely."

When I was 15 my grandfather, who had been the center of my life, died. I went into a deep depression. I had already lost gymnastics because of an injury. So I'd just go to school, go home, go to sleep, get up for a little bit to eat, and go back to sleep to do it all over again. When I slept, I had terrible dreams, and I heard voices when I was awake. I started to lose a lot of hair and have irregular menstrual cycles.

At this time and up until I turned 18, I felt like my parents controlled everything: what I wore, who I spent time with, where I was, every minute of the day. Food was one thing I thought I could control completely. Sometimes, I'd get up in the middle of the night and eat and eat like I was about to die. I would feel awful later, but I would never make myself throw up. I saw a movie on bulimia once and saw how much damage it caused, so instead I would not eat for a day or two after I binged. I still do that sometimes, but not as severely as I used to.

Now I'm in massage school. I eat about two and a half meals a day. I was kind of surprised that getting massage was so easy for me. I did have some fears about lying supine on the table, but I'm over it. I have chronic back pain, and I enjoy deep massage.

I know I was lucky. I was able to control my eating before it got so bad that I needed to be admitted to the hospital. My whole sense of who I am and what makes me feel good is different now. I still really like getting compliments. If I hear "You look great" or "That shirt looks good on you," then I feel like I can eat a chicken sandwich or a bowl of ice cream without feeling guilty later. But for the most part, for stuff like the grades I get in school or what courses I take, no one decides what I need now. I am my own person, and I am in control of my life once again. It feels really good.

(Figure 4.15), and a loss of the menstrual cycle. Advanced anorexics, in addition to being extraordinarily thin, sometimes develop lanugo: fine, downy hair usually seen only in early infancy. This grows all over the body, possibly as an effort to compensate for the absence of any insulating fat in the superficial fascia.

Bulimia patients experience recurrent episodes of binge eating coupled with damaging compensatory behaviors that include self-induced vomiting, laxative use, and excessive exercise.

Binge-eating disorder is characterized by bouts of uncontrollable, rapid eating that occur at least once a week for 3 months or more. These episodes are marked by the sense of a lack powerlessness and significant distress. It is important to distinguish between habitual overeating and binge-eating disorder; binge eating is much more severe and is connected to serious psychological problems.

Treatment

Treatment for eating disorders is most successful when the emphasis is less on gaining or losing weight than on resolving the issues that lead to the behaviors. While it is important to stabilize weight and support patients with healthy eating habits, these interventions are generally unsuccessful until the patient's psychological and emotional issues have been addressed. If a patient has progressed to the point where he or she is at risk for very serious complications or death, then treatment may begin in a hospital setting.

Research revealing neurotransmitter imbalances in the brain of many eating disorder patients has opened the door to medications that may help. Medication with individual or group psychotherapy support often leads to successful outcomes for all types of eating disorders.

Medications

- Antidepressants, especially SSRIs
- Mood stabilizers, including antiseizure drugs

Massage Therapy Implications

RISKS Anorexia and bulimia can lead to changes in body function that affects the gastrointestinal tract, the cardiovascular system, and bone density. A frail client requires accommodation for bodywork to respect these challenges.

The main risk for overweight clients is the sense of being judged when they receive massage. It is imperative to create physical and emotional environment where people of all body shapes are welcomed with unconditional positive regard.

BENEFITS Clients who struggle with eating disorders tend to have a distorted and strongly negative perception of their physical being. Massage can be a powerful way to experience their bodies as safe, strong, and healthy.

RESEARCH Because eating disorders often appear with anxiety disorders and obsessive-compulsive disorder, it is reasonable to suggest that the success that massage therapy has in those contexts may cross over. One exception to that generalization is the struggle many people in this population have with body image and self-worth. Studies comparing acupressure with acupuncture[1,2] found that the key factor in treatment was the value of the therapeutic relationship: the level of trust between the practitioner and the patient.

1. Fogarty S, Smith CA, Touyz S, et al. Patients with anorexia nervosa receiving acupuncture or acupressure; their view of the therapeutic encounter. *Complementary Therapies in Medicine* 2013;21(6):675–681. http://www.ncbi.nlm.nih.gov/pubmed/24280477
2. Smith C, Fogarty S, Touyz S, et al. Acupuncture and acupressure and massage health outcomes for patients with anorexia nervosa: findings from a pilot randomized controlled trial and patient interviews. *Journal of Alternative and Complementary Medicine* 2014;20(2):103–112. http://www.ncbi.nlm.nih.gov/pubmed/24102480

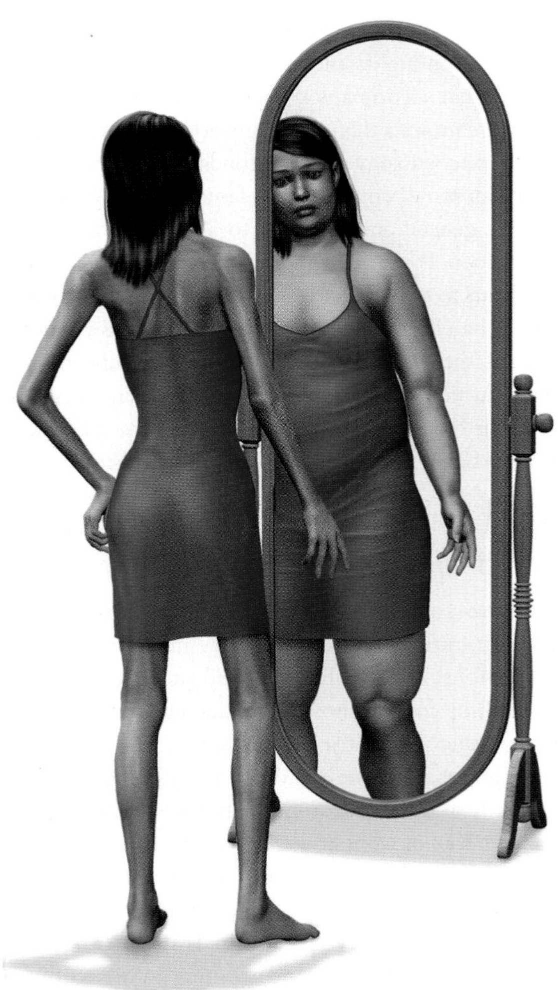

FIGURE 4.15 Anorexia: distorted body image

Obsessive-Compulsive and Related Disorders

Definition: What Are They?

Obsessive-compulsive and related disorders are a group of conditions that used to be classified as anxiety disorders, but have been designated as unique because of their predictable pattern of obsessive preoccupations and repetitive behaviors.

Demographics

These disorders affect about 2.2 million American adults. They are usually diagnosed in late adolescence or early adulthood. Men and women are affected about equally.

Etiology: What Happens?

Obsessive-compulsive and related disorders used to be considered types of anxiety disorders, but the latest edition of DSM-5 has separated them into their own section, because they have some features that other anxiety disorders do not share, and treatment strategies are different. The focus on unwelcomed thoughts and repetitive, sometimes destructive behaviors that accompany those obsessions, respond best to different treatments than other anxiety disorders.

The exact etiology of these conditions may vary. It seems clear that for some people, a strong family tendency exists, which suggests a genetic predisposition to a fundamental change in brain function. For others, a specific event like an illness or surgery appears to be a trigger that sets off a whole new behavioral pattern. The effectiveness of serotonin reuptake inhibitors for patients of these disorders points to some dysfunction in serotonin production or uptake. New imaging techniques can identify areas of the brain that are unusually active in people with these disorders, and these areas normalize with successful treatment.

Types of Obsessive-Compulsive and Related Disorders

- *Obsessive-compulsive disorder (OCD)*: OCD is a combination of intrusive, uncontrollable, unwelcome thoughts (obsessions) and highly developed rituals designed to try to quell or control those thoughts (compulsions). Unlike many other psychiatric disorders, OCD can come and go throughout a lifetime and is not always progressive.

  Some of the most common obsessions of OCD patients include fear of contamination by dirt, germs, or sexual activity; fear of violence or catastrophic accidents; fear of committing violent or sexual acts; and fears surrounding disorder or asymmetry. The rituals used to battle these fears include repeated hand washing (often to the point of damaging the skin); refusing to touch other people or contaminated surfaces; repeatedly checking locks, stoves, irons, or other appliances; counting telephone poles; carefully and symmetrically arranging clothes, food, or other items; and persistently repeating words, phrases, or prayers. While many people occasionally engage in some of these behaviors, OCD patients often devote hours every day to the rituals that are designed to keep them safe.
- *Body dysmorphic disorder*: This is a condition in which a person experiences extreme anxiety and unhappiness because of a real or imagined physical flaw. This goes beyond common insecurity to become a pathologic disorder that interferes with the ability to function in society. It has been seen to lead to excoriation disorder and hair pulling, as well as **depression**.
- *Excoriation disorder*: Also called skin-picking disorder, this behavior involves picking at the skin, often on or around the face, to the point of self-injury, which may lead to more picking. A diagnosis requires that attempts to stop the behavior have been unsuccessful and that it leads to impairment in social and occupational functioning. Infection and permanent scars are frequent complications of this self-perpetuating disorder.
- *Trichotillomania*: This is hair-pulling disorder, closely related to excoriation disorder. Patients pull their hair as a stress management mechanism: they feel anxious; they pluck at their hair; they feel better—until they feel anxious again. Head hair, eyebrows, eyelashes, beard hair, and body hair are all possible targeted areas. Occasionally, this complicates to hair eating, which can lead to serious intestinal problems.
- *Hoarding disorder*: This is a situation in which a person becomes reluctant to part with possessions, regardless of any inherent or objective lack of value. It reaches the point of pathology when it causes significant distress to patients or their partners, interferes with normal daily activities, and creates physical dangers of clutter, fire hazard, or poor hygiene.

Signs and Symptoms

The signs and symptoms of OCD and related disorders are discussed under their individual descriptions.

Treatment

OCD and related disorders are typically treated with a combination of psychotherapy and medication. A branch of therapy called "exposure and response prevention" is especially designed to address the behaviors seen with OCD-type disorders.

Medications

- Antidepressants, especially SSRIs
- Antianxiety medication

Massage Therapy Implications

RISKS	If the disorder in question is triggered by body image or by fears about hygiene, the massage therapist is in a position to inadvertently say or do something that may not be well received by the client. Extra care and compassion in all communications with this population is essential.
BENEFITS	As with most psychiatric disorders, welcomed massage therapy may help to instill a stronger sense of self-efficacy and ability to cope with everyday challenges for clients with OCD and related disorders.
OPTIONS	Flexibility and versatility are valuable qualities to help clients who struggle with these disorders, who may have different needs from one appointment to the next.
RESEARCH	Studies specifically about massage therapy and OCD are few, but because these disorders often overlap with other anxiety disorders, it is useful to point out that massage therapy is well accepted as a strategy to promote good self-care and relief from stress.

Trauma- and Stressor-Related Disorders

Definition: What Are They?

This is a collection of conditions that used to be considered subtypes of anxiety disorders. Because they have some different and very specific diagnostic criteria, they are now described as their own set of disorders in the Diagnostic and Statistical Manual of Mental Health Disorders (DSM-5).

Some advocates for military personnel suggest that posttraumatic stress disorder (PTSD) should be called posttraumatic stress injury, in an attempt to lessen the stigma attached to "disorders."

Demographics

Trauma- and stress-related disorders can happen at any age. Special diagnostic criteria have been developed to recognize these conditions in children, among whom prevalence is almost 4% of all boys and 6% of all girls. Approximately 30% of men and women who spend time in a war zone develop PTSD. Women appear to be more susceptible to PTSD than men are.

Etiology: What Happens?

When a person goes through a life-threatening ordeal, specific changes in brain function may occur. Exposure to traumatic stimuli leads to activation of the **amygdala**, hypothalamus, and several other structures, leading to sympathetic responses with accompanying changes in hormone secretions. Then, for various reasons, these reactions recur and persist. Normal factors that would inhibit the sympathetic response don't appear to function well in people with trauma- and stress-related disorders.

Other factors that influence whether an ordeal leads to a long-term change in function include the nature of the event (how close it was, how long it lasted, how severe it was); characteristics of the individual (whether he or she had a history of similar experiences, other psychiatric conditions, and gender); and what happens in the posttrauma time period (whether support is available, and how severe early symptoms are).

Types of Trauma- and Stressor-Related Disorders

- *Posttraumatic stress disorder (PTSD)*: This is a disorder experienced by a person who was exposed to death, actual or threatened injury, or violence, either as a participant or as an in-person witness. It may also affect close relatives or friends of the person in the trauma. Professionals who are repeatedly exposed to the effects of violence, like first responders or caregivers to the victims of child abuse, may also be vulnerable to PTSD.
  - *Dissociative PTSD*: This subtype of PTSD describes a person who feels detached from his mind or body, or as though the world is unreal and distorted. Scientists believe that this **disassociation** may be modulated by inhibition of **limbic system** activity. This distinction may allow for more effective treatment options.
- *Acute traumatic stress disorder*: This has the hallmarks of all stressor-related disorders, but symptoms develop more quickly after an ordeal than they do with PTSD.
- *Adjustment disorder*: This reaction to a traumatic or nontraumatic stressor can be acute (symptoms persist for less than 6 months) or chronic (symptoms are present for more than 6 months) after the termination of the stressor. It has the typical signs of stressor-related conditions and may be a precursor to PTSD.
- *Reactive attachment disorder*: This is a childhood stressor-related disorder that leads to a person being pathologically withdrawn and inhibited: a pattern that lasts through adulthood. Patients have reduced responses to their environment, and they tend to neglect themselves and their responsibilities.

Amygdala: One of two groups of nuclei in the brain (one in each hemisphere) involved in the processing of emotional memories.

Dissociation: Psychological detachment from one's surroundings.

Limbic system: A group of brain structures that exert major influence on the endocrine and autonomic nervous systems.

Signs and Symptoms

PTSD, which is the centerpiece for this group of conditions, usually shows symptoms within 3 months of the traumatic event, but for some patients, the onset of symptoms may be delayed for much longer. The symptoms for these conditions are classified as belonging to four specific groups: reexperiencing, avoidance, negative cognitions and moods, and arousal.

Reexperiencing-based symptoms include persistent, spontaneous, and upsetting memories and severe, violent nightmares.

Avoidance-based symptoms include behaviors to avoid possible triggers, including trauma-related thoughts and feelings and trauma-related objects, people, or activities.

Negative beliefs and moods encompass the tendency to self-blame for the ordeal, or to not trust the environment to be safe; feeling alienated and disconnected from other people; and an inability to experience positive emotions.

Arousal-based symptoms include hypervigilance, sleep disruption, aggressive or destructive behavior, and an exaggerated startle response.

Treatment

Treatment for this set of disorders usually involves some combination of group, individual, and family therapy along with medication, but treatment can have a better chance of success if the timing and focus is appropriately targeted. PTSD and associated disorders frequently occur with other psychiatric problems, including **addiction** and **depression**, so these must also be addressed.

Another nonpharmacologic intervention that is effective with this population is eye movement desensitization and reprocessing, which combines psychotherapy and eye movements to influence the way the brain processes information.

Medications

- Antidepressants
- Beta-blockers
- Sleep aids to decrease nightmares and sleep disturbance

Massage Therapy Implications

RISKS	The primary risk for a client with one of these disorders is having something in the massage session trigger a flashback or other kinds of reaction. If the therapist can control for this and be present and appropriate with a client in the event of a dissociative episode, a person with PTSD should be able to enjoy the experience of receiving massage.
BENEFITS	Massage has been demonstrated to be helpful for people with PTSD and related disorders as a way to feel connected to themselves and to others. The act of trusting another person to have one's best interests at heart is a commitment of great courage.
RESEARCH	Collinge et al.[1] created a program teaching veterans and their partners how to do massage to promote their reintegration and ability to connect with each other with good success. Massage therapy has also been recommended in the treatment of refugees and survivors of torture, if the recipients are comfortable with being touched.[2] 1. Collinge W, Kahn J, Soltysik R. Promoting reintegration of National Guard veterans and their partners using a self-directed program of integrative therapies: a pilot study. *Military Medicine* 2012;177(12):1477–1485. http://www.ncbi.nlm.nih.gov/pmc/articles/PMC3645256/ 2. Longacre M, Silver-Highfield E, Lama P, et al. Complementary and alternative medicine in the treatment of refugees and survivors of torture: a review and proposal for action. *Torture* 2012;22(1):38–57. http://www.irct.org/Files/Filer/TortureJournal/22_1_2012/Complementary-alternative-1-2012.pdf

Nervous System Injuries

Bell Palsy

Definition: What Is It?

Bell palsy is the result of damage to or impairment of CN VII, the facial nerve. This nerve is composed almost entirely of motor neurons and is responsible for providing facial expression, blinking the eyes, and providing some taste sensation (Figure 4.16). It travels a complicated route from its origins in the brain to the face and exits the cranium through a small foramen just behind the earlobe. Bell palsy is usually a temporary condition.

Demographics

Bell palsy is fairly common. It is most often seen among people who are pregnant, those with **diabetes**, those who are immune-compromised, and those who had recently dealt with a **cold** or the **flu**. It is diagnosed about 40,000 times each year in this country.

Etiology: What Happens?

Bell palsy is a type of peripheral neuritis, that is, inflammation of a peripheral nerve. The facial nerve (CN VII) begins in the brain and passes through several narrow spaces before emerging to supply the tongue with some taste sensation and the muscles of the face with motor control. When the nerve is inflamed in a tight passageway, it sustains damage that affects both sensory and motor functions.

Several possible factors may contribute to Bell palsy, but most cases are linked to the **herpes simplex** virus. This pathogen, which lies dormant in the nervous system, stimulates the production of antibodies when it reactivates. This elicits an inflammatory response against the facial nerve. Other causative agents for Bell palsy can include **Lyme disease**, Epstein-Barr virus, and cytomegalovirus.

Bell palsy can range from mild to severe. A mild case may cause damage only to the myelin sheath, but a more serious episode can damage the facial nerve fibers. Since CN VII provides motor control for muscles of facial expression and the platysma, damage results in weakness or total paralysis of the face on the affected side. Fortunately, the facial nerve has the potential to regenerate, so the prognosis for Bell palsy is generally very good: about 85% of people who have it regain full or nearly full function within a few months.

One serious complication of Bell palsy can develop if the lubrication and cleaning of the eyeball provided by blinking is impaired. Another rarer complication occurs when the facial nerve forges some new and inappropriate connections as it heals. The result may be unpredictable muscle activity in

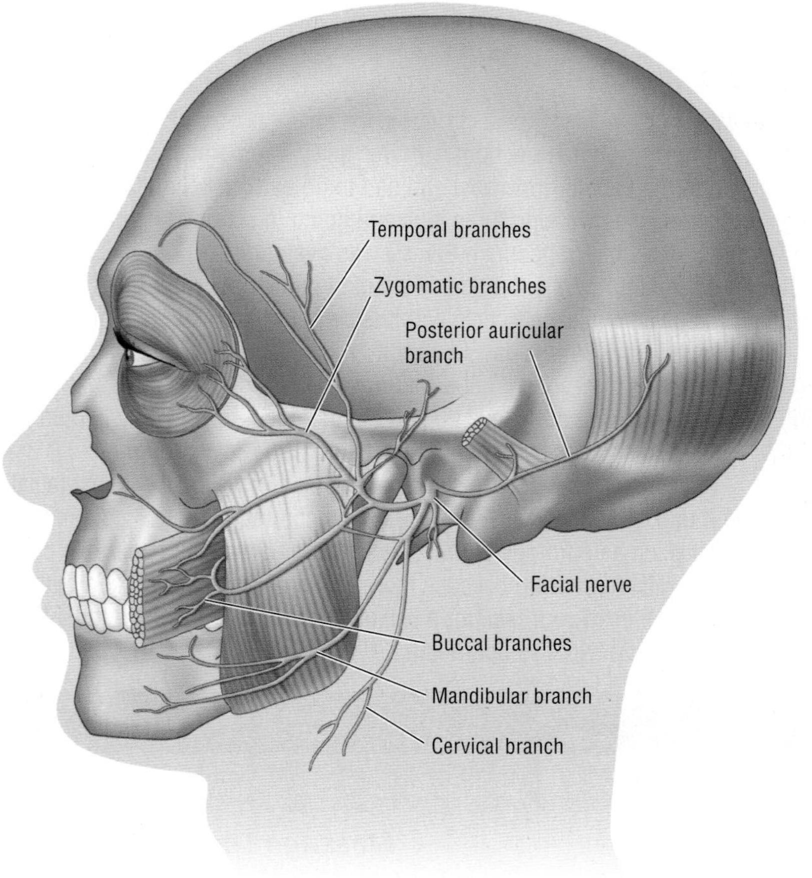

FIGURE 4.16 The facial nerve provides most of the motor function to facial muscles

the face (**synkinesis**), or secretion of excessive tears during salivation.

Signs and Symptoms

Symptoms of Bell palsy are brought about by loss of nerve supply to the muscles on one side of the face. Classic signs include a sudden onset (often overnight) of flaccid paralysis of the muscles of the upper and lower face (Figure 4.17). It is difficult to eat, drink, and close the eye of the affected side. Production of saliva may be increased or decreased, and taste may be distorted. Sometimes, the ear on the affected side becomes hypersensitive, because a muscle connected to the eardrum (the **stapedius**) is paralyzed; this is called **hyperacusis**. The affected side may have pain, but it is more likely to be in the form of headaches or an ache behind the ear than electrical nerve pain. This is motor, not sensory, paralysis (except for some taste buds that may be affected), so sensation throughout the face stays intact.

Synkinesis: An involuntary movement that follows a voluntary one.

Stapedius: A muscle in the ear that stabilizes the stapes bone. The smallest skeletal muscle.

Hyperacusis: Abnormally acute hearing due to irritability of sensory nerves.

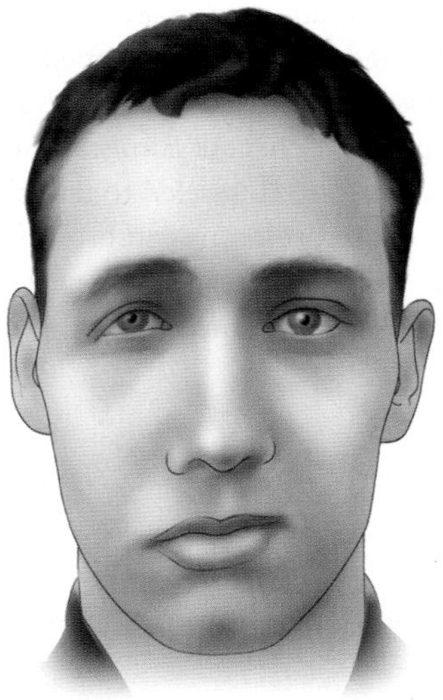

FIGURE 4.17 Bell palsy: flaccid paralysis on one side of the face

CASE HISTORY 4.3

JIM S: "No dimple for a year!"

When I think about what may have precipitated my bout with Bell palsy, I remember one of the most stressful years of my life. I had recently moved to the Pacific Northwest and had to go back to school to receive Washington State licensure as a massage practitioner. I was working three jobs and going to school. I had also spent some days plunging into the cold water of a tributary of the Breitenbush River. I was overcooked!

When the paralysis started, I thought it was a temporary effect of some bodywork I had received. I was told to take Advil and ice my neck. I was given massage to help with the pain. But nobody recognized the seriousness of the symptoms. Within a day, I had full-on Bell palsy complete with hyperacusis (abnormal acuteness of hearing), full facial muscle paralysis, an eyelid that would not blink (with the inherent rolling of the eye up and out of danger when the lid would normally blink), and a distorted soapy beer taste on the affected side of my tongue.

Because I neglected to see a neurologist for over a week, my facial nerve degenerated, and it took almost a year for nearly full function to resume. I couldn't use my dimple for a year! I'm adamant about people seeing a neurologist immediately these days when I hear of a case of Bell palsy.

The whole experience was generally frustrating because there's a lot of poor information out there, but it was a great emotional process; when you've used your face for a calling card all your life and suddenly it's not available to you anymore, you have to really deal with what's underneath.

Treatment

Treatment for Bell palsy depends on the causative agent, which means it is important to have an accurate diagnosis. Facial paralysis can also be related to **multiple sclerosis**, **Guillain-Barré syndrome**, **sarcoidosis**, or tumors on or around CN VII or CN VIII. Ramsay-Hunt syndrome is a complication of **herpes zoster** (shingles) that can affect the facial nerve, but it tends to be much more painful and longer-lasting than Bell palsy.

Bell palsy treatment is usually conservative because most cases are self-limiting, that is, they resolve without interference. Steroids and antiviral medications are the typical prescription, but research suggests that steroids are helpful but no particular benefit comes from using antiviral medications. Patients are counseled to tape the affected eye closed at night and to use drops and protect it from drying and dust during the day. Massage is often recommended to stretch and mobilize facial muscles until the nerve repairs itself (Case History 4.3).

Medications

- Steroidal anti-inflammatories to manage nerve inflammation
- Acyclovir or other antiviral medications to shorten the duration of attack
- NSAIDs for pain relief

Massage Therapy Implications

RISKS	If the underlying cause of facial paralysis doesn't contraindicate massage, then massage has no specific risks for Bell palsy.
BENEFITS	Massage keeps the facial muscles elastic and the local circulation strong. This sets the stage for a more complete recovery when nerve supply is eventually restored.
RESEARCH	Many professionals recommend massage therapy as part of treatment for Bell palsy.[1,2] The general consensus is that while no rigorous research has been done on massage therapy in this context, it appears to be helpful in some cases, and to not be harmful: this is an important finding. 1. Shafshak TS. The treatment of facial palsy from the point of view of physical and rehabilitation medicine. *Europa Medicophysica* 2006;42(1):41–47. http://www.ncbi.nlm.nih.gov/pubmed/16565685 2. Teixeira LJ, Valbuza JS, Prado GF. Physical therapy for Bell's palsy (idiopathic facial paralysis). *Cochrane Database of Systematic Reviews* 2011;(12):CD006283. http://www.ncbi.nlm.nih.gov/pubmed/22161401

To view a person with this condition, see the video "Bell Palsy," available at http://thePoint.lww.com/Werner6e. thePoint®

Complex Regional Pain Syndrome

Definition: What Is It?

Complex regional pain syndrome (CRPS) is a collection of signs and symptoms including long-lasting pain and changes to the skin, muscles, joints, nerves, and blood vessels of the affected areas. CRPS 1 is the most current label for what used to be called reflex sympathetic dystrophy syndrome (RSDS); this is abnormal pain and other signs related to soft tissue or other injuries, usually to a distal portion of the arm or leg. CRPS 2 (formerly known as causalgia) is pain related to a nerve injury that again outlives a normal process and often exceeds the boundaries of the affected nerve (Sidebar 4.11). CRPS is a progressive disorder that is potentially debilitating.

Demographics

Because it is frequently misdiagnosed, it is difficult to estimate how many people in the United States have CRPS. Experts suggest that 1% to 2% of people with fractures and 2% to 5% of people with peripheral nerve injury may develop this chronic pain syndrome. It appears to be much more common in women than in men.

Etiology: What Happens?

When a person receives a stimulus, a sensory neuron carries that information to the spinal cord. That efferent neuron has a synapse with ascending sensory neurons that carry the stimulus to the brain where it is interpreted, but it also communicates with motor neurons right in the spinal cord to elicit a faster response: this is the reflex arc in a nutshell.

If the stimulus is something soothing and welcomed (a smooth, confident effleurage stroke, for instance), the result is a relaxation response in the tissues. But if the stimulus is threatening or painful, the brain-mediated response is a sympathetic reaction, with associated changes in blood flow.

In CRPS, an initial trauma (often to a hand or foot, but anywhere on the body can be affected) begins a pain sensation that is mediated by the sympathetic nervous system. This disorder is often associated with high-velocity trauma like bullet or shrapnel wounds, but it has also been seen with minor strains and sprains, as a postsurgical complication, with fractures, at injection sites, following strokes, as a consequence of disc disease, and sometimes with no identified causative trauma at all.

Regardless of the trigger, pain creates a sympathetic response, which reinforces pain sensation: a **positive feedback loop** with an exaggerated inflammatory response. In addition, pain sensors in the affected area and in their connections in the spinal cord become increasingly sensitive. In other words, the pain becomes a self-fulfilling prophecy: a person hurts, which causes stress and which makes the pain worse, and the healing processes that should interrupt this sequence are unable to overcome the power of the vicious circle.

Eventually, the physiologic changes that occur when a specific part of the body is stuck in a sympathetic loop cause their own damage, which may eventually be irreversible: circulation affects the skin, the bones become thin, and joints may fuse.

Part of this chronic pain scenario involves structural changes to the sensory neurons in the extremity and in the spinal cord. As they develop new connections, they become more sensitized to pain. This can increase the perception of the sensory field: it feels like a larger and larger area of the body is affected, and this leads to more sympathetic responses. This maladaptation of the CNS means that the pain cycle seen with CRPS has the potential to spread proximally on the affected limb, to the contralateral limb, and elsewhere.

> **Positive feedback loop:** A process in which a response intensifies the stimulus causing it.
> **Hyperalgesia:** Extreme sensitivity to painful stimuli.

SIDEBAR 4.11 Pain by Any Other Name...

In October 1864, a group of doctors compared their observations of Civil War soldiers recovering from gunshot wounds. Their comments were remarkably astute, and they provide a vivid picture of the experience of the condition eventually termed causalgia, from the Greek *kausis* (burning) and *algia* (pain).

"In our early experience of nerve wounds, we met with a small number of men who were suffering from a pain that they described as 'burning' or as 'mustard red-hot' or as 'red-hot file rasping the skin' . . . . Its intensity varies from the most trivial burning to a state of torture, which can hardly be credited, but which reacts on the whole economy, until the general health is seriously affected . . . ."[3]

Over the years, this condition, now called CRPS, has been known by many names. Sympathetic maintained pain syndrome is another term, along with shoulder-hand syndrome and Sudeck atrophy. Causalgia itself is now considered to refer to pain related to any peripheral nerve injury (CRPS 2), while RSDS refers to pain that begins in the extremities (CRPS 1).

American RSDHope, (c) 2014. URL: http://www.rsdhope.org/crps-or-rsds.html.

Signs and Symptoms

Signs and symptoms of CRPS vary widely, but three major issues are usually present: one is burning pain around the site of initial injury. Another is autonomic dysfunction that shows as changes in skin temperature and texture, edema, hair and nail growth, and changes in local blood supply that can lead to bone density loss. Third is motor dysfunction that begins as weakness and spasms in local muscles along with joint stiffness but may progress to contracture and atrophy of muscle, bone, and joint structures. In any case, **hyperalgesia** (excessive pain sensation) and **allodynia** (pain reaction to any sensory signal) are dependable symptoms.

CRPS has been discussed as three loosely defined stages. Not all experts agree on the sequence of progression, as this disorder is experienced differently by every person who has it, but these constructs can provide a useful organizing principle to understand the process of the problem.

- *Stage I*: These signs and symptoms are prevalent during the first 1 to 3 months of pain. They include severe burning pain at the site of the injury; muscle spasm; reduced range of motion, excessive hair and nail growth if the injury is on a hand or foot; and shiny, hot, red, sweaty skin (Figure 4.18). Stage I is sometimes called the acute stage.
- *Stage II*: This is characterized by changes in the growth pattern of the affected tissues. The swelling spreads proximally from the initial site, the hair stops growing, and the nails become brittle and easily cracked. Skin that was red in stage I takes on a bluish cast in stage II. In this intensely painful stage, the muscles begin to atrophy from underuse, and the nearby joints may thicken and become stiffer. Stage II usually lasts 3 to 6 months. It is also called the dystrophic stage.
- *Stage III*: At this point, irreversible changes to the affected structures have occurred. The bones are thin and brittle, the joints are immobile, and the muscles tighten into permanent contracture. The condition may spread proximally up the limb, to the contralateral limb, or anywhere else in the body, including internal organs. At this point, the pain sensation is a self-sustaining phenomenon and not responsive to most treatments. This is known as the atrophic stage.

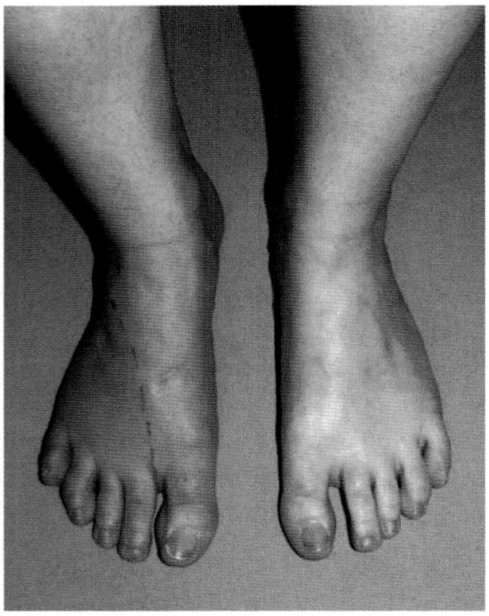

FIGURE 4.18 Acute CRPS type I after foot surgery: *dotted line* on foot shows the border of allodynia; hyperalgesia was present to midtibia. The patient went into remission with pharmacological treatment and physical therapy.

Treatment

Treatment for CRPS is a challenging process. Evidence suggests that the best outcomes occur when treatment is instituted early, but it can be difficult to distinguish this condition in early stages. Physical and occupational therapy are recommended to preserve function and prevent or delay atrophy of the affected areas, and massage therapy is sometimes suggested in this context as well. This can be problematic for many people who are in significant pain that is exacerbated by movement or exercise. Other noninvasive therapies include recreational therapy, hydrotherapy (within tolerance), biofeedback training, topical analgesics, and **TENS units** to block some pain perception.

> **Allodynia:** A condition in which a normally painless stimulus causes pain.
>
> **TENS unit:** A transcutaneous electrical nerve stimulation device, used to control pain.
>
> **Intrathecal:** An injection directly into the central nervous system.
>
> **Sympathectomy:** The surgical removal of a section of sympathetic nerve or one or more of the sympathetic ganglia.

Psychotherapeutic intervention is useful, as the pain and disability involved with this condition can lead to extreme forms of depression, anxiety, and sleep disorders, and these complications can make CRPS symptoms worse.

Chemical nerve blocks are often used to block nerve transmission at the sympathetic ganglia near the spinal cord and other locations. These are often useful, but they are temporary and cannot be used indefinitely. Implanted devices to "crowd out" pain sensation may also be used with varying levels of success.

Intrathecal pumps that deliver painkilling medications directly into the spinal cord allow patients to manage their own pain. These bypass the blood-brain barrier to allow the same results with smaller doses of drugs.

Some patients undergo a full **sympathectomy**, that is, their sympathetic motor neurons are surgically severed. While it has been effective for some, others find that this extreme intervention is also temporary and has many serious possible complications.

Pharmacologic approaches to CRPS run the gamut from NSAIDs to antidepressants to muscle relaxants. Because this is such a painful condition, doctors and their patients tend to be willing to try many options, although many of these are strictly experimental at this point.

Medications

- NSAIDs for early-stage CRPS to control pain and inflammation
- Oral analgesics, including opioids, narcotics, and ketamine for pain control; although these drugs carry many risks and potential side effects, they can be useful for CRPS
- Antidepressants, especially tricyclics, for pain relief and improved sleep
- Antiseizure drugs for pain control

Massage Therapy Implications

RISKS	CRPS locally contraindicates most massage because touch is so painful. It is important to know what treatment options clients with CRPS use, because some medications or medical devices may require adaptation with bodywork.
BENEFITS	If massage can be offered in a way that doesn't exacerbate symptoms, it could be a wonderful addition to the quality of life of someone who lives with this extremely challenging condition—even for short-term benefit.
RESEARCH	Little research has been done on massage therapy for CRPS patients, but one case study using manual lymphatic drainage got good results.[1] An earlier study of lymphatic massage found improvement in pain and edema compared to a control group, but the benefits did not last through the follow-up period.[2] Some doctors recommend self-massage to keep sensation healthy, especially in the early stage of CRPS.[3]

1. Safaz I, Tok F, Taskaynatan MA, et al. Manual lymphatic drainage in management of edema in a case with CRPS: why the(y) wait? *Rheumatology International* 2011;31(3):387–390. http://www.ncbi.nlm.nih.gov/pubmed/19823831
2. Duman I, Ozdemir A, Tan AK, et al. The efficacy of manual lymphatic drainage therapy in the management of limb edema secondary to reflex sympathetic dystrophy. *Rheumatology International* 2009;29(7):759–763. http://www.ncbi.nlm.nih.gov/pubmed/19030864
3. Lee J, Nandi P. Early aggressive treatment improves prognosis in complex regional pain syndrome. *Practitioner* 2011;255(1736):23–26, 23. http://www.ncbi.nlm.nih.gov/pubmed/21370711

Spinal Cord Injury

Definition: What Is It?

The definition of spinal cord injury (SCI) is self-evident: this is damage to nerve tissue in the spinal canal. How that damage is reflected in the body depends on where and how much of the tissue has been affected.

Traumatic SCI falls into one of five categories:

- *Concussion*: Tissue is jarred and irritated, but not structurally damaged.
- *Contusion*: Bleeding in the cord damages nerve tissue.
- *Compression*: A disc, bone spur, or tumor puts mechanical pressure on the cord.
- *Laceration*: The cord is partially cut, as with a gunshot wound.
- *Transection*: The cord is severed completely.

Transections are rare, and their mortality rate is high. Most people with SCI have a partial injury.

An injury that affects nerve supply to the lower abdomen and legs but leaves the supply to the chest and arms intact is called **paraplegia**. An injury that affects the body from the neck down is called **tetraplegia** or **quadriplegia**. For more terminology in the context of CNS injuries, see Sidebar 4.12.

Demographics

An estimated 12,000 new spinal cord injuries happen each year. About 275,000 people in the United States live with this condition, and males outnumber females by about 4:1.

The main cause of SCIs in this country is motor vehicle accidents (37%). This is followed by falls (29%), which cause the majority of injuries among people over 65. Acts of violence (14%) and sporting accidents (9%) are the other major causes. About 11% of injuries occur without a recorded cause. Alcohol plays a role in about 25% of all spinal cord injuries.

Etiology: What Happens?

A primary injury to the spinal cord is usually a crushing blow (Figure 4.19), but a penetrating injury like a gunshot injury or knife wound can do equal or worse damage.

A newly injured spinal cord goes through an initial period called **spinal cord shock**. During this time, the cord swells, and many body functions are severely impaired: blood pressure is dangerously low, the heart beats slowly, peripheral blood vessels dilate, and the patient is susceptible to hypothermia. In this acute phase of injury, the affected muscles may be hypotonic. Then, when the inflammatory process begins to subside, the muscles supplied by damaged axons begin to tighten, and their reflexes become hyperreactive. Spasticity along with **autonomic dysreflexia** is a hallmark of SCI. If muscles stay flaccid and reflexes are dull or nonexistent, the damage is probably to the nerve roots or peripheral nerves, rather than to the spinal cord itself. Depending on the nature of the accident, it is perfectly possible to sustain injury to both the spinal cord and the nerve roots, especially in the

Paraplegia: Paralysis of both lower extremities and (usually) the lower trunk.

Tetraplegia: Quadriplegia.

Quadriplegia: Paralysis of all four limbs. Called tetraplegia in Europe.

Spinal cord shock: The period immediately following a spinal cord injury, characterized by swelling of the spinal cord and impairment of various bodily functions.

Autonomic dysreflexia: A condition in which an ordinary stimulus results in an uncontrollable sympathetic reaction. Caused by a spinal cord injury above T6.

SIDEBAR 4.12 Nerve Damage Terminology

Nerve damage can manifest in several ways. Familiarity with some of the vocabulary of nervous system damage can make it much easier to "talk shop" with clients and doctors dealing with these problems.

- *Paresthesia* is any abnormal sensation, particularly the tingling, burning, and prickling feelings associated with pins-and-needles sensation.
- *Hyperkinesia* is excessive muscular activity.
- *Hypokinesia* is diminished or slowed movement.
- *Hypertonia* is a general term for extreme tension, or tone, in the muscles.
- *Hypotonia* is an abnormally low level of muscle tone, as seen with flaccid paralysis.
- *Spasticity* is a situation in which the stretch reflex is overactive. The flexors want to flex, but the extensors don't want to give up. Finally, the extensors are stretched too far, and they release altogether. This phenomenon is called the clasp-knife effect.
- *Paralysis* is loss of any function controlled by the nervous system. The word comes from the Greek for loosening.
- *Paresis* is partial or incomplete paralysis.
- *Flaccid paralysis* is typically a sign of lower motor neuron, that is, peripheral, damage. Flaccid paralysis occurs with muscles in a state of hypotonicity.
- *Spastic paralysis* is the result of brain or upper motor neuron damage. It combines aspects of hypertonia, hypokinesia, and dysreflexia. It is never resolved, which distinguishes it from simple spasm. These are types of spastic paralysis:
  - *Hemiplegia* means the left or right side (or hemisphere) of the body is affected. This is the variation that most often accompanies stroke.
  - *Paraplegia* means the bottom half of the body or some part of it has been affected. These patients still have at least partial use of their arms and hands.
  - *Diplegia* is symmetrical paralysis of upper or lower extremities resulting from injuries to the cerebrum.
  - *Tetraplegia*, or *quadriplegia*, means that the body has been affected from the neck down. Tetraplegics can eat, breathe, talk, and move their head because these functions are controlled by the cranial nerves, which are usually protected from injury.

cauda equina. You can see this area in the Acland video "Spinal Cord From Behind Nerve Roots" online at http://thePoint.lww.com/Werner6e). thePoint®

A person's ultimate level of function after sustaining an SCI is related to how much tissue damage accrues. A significant portion of the damage to delicate CNS tissue is incurred not by the trauma, but by posttraumatic reactions that damage tissue adjacent to the injury site. This understanding opens the possibility for treatments that provide a much-improved prognosis for SCI survivors.

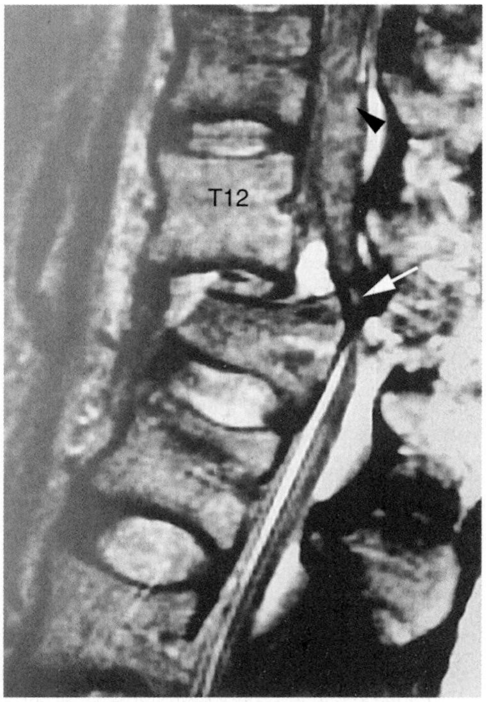

FIGURE 4.19 Spinal cord injury due to crushing blow

Some of the most serious posttraumatic reactions include these:

- Excessive bleeding in and around the spinal cord; this can also contribute to circulatory shock, dangerously low blood pressure, and slowed heart rate.
- Free radical activity that destroys cell membranes.
- The secretion of excessive glutamate, leading to excitotoxicity and myelin damage.
- Immune system activity with inflammatory cytokines that contribute to cell damage and the accumulation of scar tissue in the spinal cord.
- Accelerated apoptosis, or cell death. This process seems to affect the **oligodendrocytes** in particular: these are glial cells that form myelin in the CNS. When they degenerate, CNS cells are stripped of the covering that would otherwise speed transmission and provide electrical insulation from other fibers.
- Scarring: astrocytes attempt to wall off the injured area, but this prevents injured axons from reconnecting with the rest of the system.

Cauda equina: Bundle of spinal nerve roots at the base of the spinal column. Literally "horse tail."

Oligodendrocytes: A type of glial cells found in the central nervous system.

Complications

Spinal cord injuries can lead to many serious long-term complications. An SCI patient must invest a lot of time and energy in working to prevent, manage, or recover from these secondary problems:

- *Respiratory infection*. When the chest can't fully expand and contract and the cough reflex is limited (as is often seen with injuries higher than T_{12}), it is difficult to expel pathogens from the body. **Pneumonia** is almost inevitable.
- ***Deep vein thrombosis, pulmonary embolism***. The formation of blood clots in the venous system is a high risk for new SCI patients, and the risk decreases only slightly with the passage of time.
- ***Urinary tract infection***. SCI patients who must use a catheter to urinate are at high risk for contamination and infection of the urinary tract. Left untended, the risk of these infections invading the kidneys is significant.
- ***Decubitus ulcers***. Also known as bedsores or pressure sores, these can arise anywhere circulation is limited by mechanical compression of the skin. Because these wounds don't heal quickly or easily, they are highly susceptible to infection, which can easily complicate to **septicemia**.
- *Heterotopic ossification*. This is the formation of calcium deposits in soft tissues. It typically occurs around the hips or knees, where it can be acutely painful. It can be corrected only with surgery.
- *Autonomic dysreflexia*. Damage to the spinal cord above T_6 raises the risk of developing autonomic dysreflexia, in which a minor stimulus (e.g., a full bladder or bowel, a ridge of cloth caught under the skin, menstrual cramps) creates an uncontrollable sympathetic reaction. It causes a pounding headache, increased heart rate, flushing, sweating, and other symptoms, including dangerously high blood pressure. Autonomic dysreflexia can be a medical emergency.
- *Cardiovascular disease*. Suddenly changing from an active life to confinement in a wheelchair means a significant reduction in physical activity for most SCI patients. The risk of developing **hypertension, atherosclerosis**, and other cardiovascular problems is high for this sedentary population.
- *Numbness*. Most SCI patients have some numbness or reduction in sensation, depending on which part of the spinal cord has been damaged. The absence of pain is dangerous, because it allows damage to occur without warning. Small cuts or abrasions can become infected, and an SCI patient may never know.
- *Pain*. Many SCI patients have various kinds of pain along with numbness and lack of sensation. Some chronic pain is generated in the nerve tissue, but refers to the damaged limbs. Nerve root pressure may refer pain along the associated dermatome. Pain may be generated by the development of calcium deposits. Also, pain may be related to musculoskeletal injury, as a person must learn to use the arms and shoulders in new ways to propel the wheelchair and get into and out of it.
- *Spasticity, contractures*. As the muscles supplied by damaged motor axons begin to tighten, an SCI patient progressively loses range of motion. Chronically tight muscle fibers eventually atrophy, to be replaced by thick, tough layers of connective tissue; this is called a contracture. If any sensory or motor function is left in the limb, temporary episodes of spasticity may also be a problem. These may be caused by any kind of stimulus; the reflexes of active muscle fibers in SCI patients are very extreme and sensitive.

> **Septicemia:** Systemic disease caused by the spread of microorganisms and their toxins in the circulating blood.

> **NOTABLE CASES** When "Superman" Christopher Reeve fell off his horse in 1995, the world of SCI treatment and prognosis radically changed. Having such a high-profile and charismatic advocate brought attention, funding, and research to this field. Mr. Reeve died in 2004 from cardiac arrest, a sequence of septicemia from an infected decubitus ulcer.
>
> Mark Beck, the author of *Theory and Practice of Therapeutic Massage*—one of the first contemporary textbooks for the massage therapy profession—had a catastrophic skiing accident at age 42: "I caught a tip, flew down the hill and landed on my head." He shattered the lamina of C_6 and it dislocated anteriorly over C_7, crushing the spinal cord. Over 20 years later, he is thriving as a quadriplegic, still writing, teaching, and deeply involved in the industry. He credits regular bodywork with range-of-motion exercises, skin brushing, lymphatic work below the injury level, and clinical massage where sensation is present for his longevity.

Signs and Symptoms

The motor and sensory impairment caused by SCI is determined by what parts of the cord are damaged and at what levels. The higher the damage, the more of the body is affected. Injuries to the anterior cord affect motor function, while damage to the posterior aspect affects the senses of touch, proprioception, and vibration. Damage to the lateral parts of the cord interrupts sensations of pain and temperature. Most SCIs involve damage to multiple areas.

Treatment

If something presses directly on the spinal cord or cauda equina, emergency surgery to remove it is indicated. The other very important early intervention with these traumas is to limit secondary reactions that may damage uninjured tissue, so powerful anti-inflammatories and other medications are usually administered as quickly as possible.

Some later treatments for SCI include procedures to implant electrodes that can help with movement or transplantation of tendons for improved strength. Another line of treatment focuses on spinal reflexes for walking and other movements. Even when the patient needs extensive help, going through the motions on a treadmill or stationary bike improves motor function, exercises functioning muscles, and benefits the cardiovascular system. Furthermore, these interventions appear to improve reflexes in general, which leads to an overall better prognosis.

SCI survivors must learn new skills to live as fully as possible. Physical and occupational therapists specialize in helping these patients gain the skills they need to function; mental/emotional therapists are also essential, especially for those who are adapting to their paralysis as a new way of life.

Medications

- For recent spinal cord injuries:
  - Steroidal anti-inflammatories
  - Anticoagulants (usually heparin) to control blood clot risk
- For long-term SCI patients:
  - Anticoagulants (usually heparin) to control blood clot risk
  - Fast-acting antihypertensives for autonomic dysreflexia
  - Antibiotics for respiratory and urinary tract infections
  - Muscle relaxants for spasm and spasticity
  - Botulinum toxin injections for spasm and spasticity
  - NSAIDs for pain
  - Opioids for pain
  - Antiseizure drugs for pain
  - Antidepressants, if necessary

Massage Therapy Implications

RISKS	Massage carries many potential risks for SCI patients, including numbness that interferes with accurate feedback and a host of possibly life-threatening complications. Still, as long as these are addressed, massage can be safely administered in this context.
BENEFITS	It is hard to overstate the benefit of non–task-related touch for a person who lives with a medically complicated condition. Massage may help maintain function for SCI patients, but it is also a powerful positive physical experience for people who live with a great challenge. Some research suggests that SCI patients use massage more than any other alternative health care modality and report that it is consistently helpful for dealing with pain.
OPTIONS	In addition to working for pain relief, focus on proprioceptors and muscle tone may forestall muscle tightness due to habit rather than to CNS damage; this may allow a SCI patient to maintain a level dexterity and postural strength that would not otherwise be achievable.
RESEARCH	A feasibility study with nurses giving broad compression massage to SCI patients found that massage was safe and well tolerated[1]; this opens the door to future research in efficacy. Physiotherapy and massage were found to be among the most effective strategies to manage chronic pain for SCI patients,[2] and Cardenas and Felix[3] report that massage therapy, acupuncture, and meditation are just as successful as several medications for treating pain after SCI. A case report[4] found substantial changes in gait, spasticity, and range of motion when massage therapy was added to a client's care. Healthy bowel function after SCI is considered to be a high priority, and several studies support manual or mechanical abdominal massage to achieve this goal.[5–7]

1. Chase T, Jha A, Brooks CA, et al. A pilot feasibility study of massage to reduce pain in people with spinal cord injury during acute rehabilitation. *Spinal Cord* 2013;51(11):847–851. http://www.ncbi.nlm.nih.gov/pmc/articles/PMC3815956/
2. Heutink M, Post MW, Wollaars MM, et al. Chronic spinal cord injury pain: pharmacological and non-pharmacological treatments and treatment effectiveness. *Disability and Rehabilitation* 2011;33(5):433–440. http://www.ncbi.nlm.nih.gov/pubmed/20695788
3. Cardenas DD, Felix ER. Pain after spinal cord injury: a review of classification, treatment approaches, and treatment assessment. *PM & R* 2009;1(12):1077–1090. http://www.ncbi.nlm.nih.gov/pubmed/19797006
4. Manella C, Backus D. Gait characteristics, range of motion, and spasticity changes in response to massage in a person with incomplete spinal cord injury: case report. *International Journal of Therapeutic Massage and Bodywork* 2011;4(1):28–39. http://www.ijtmb.org/index.php/ijtmb/article/view/108/157
5. Janssen TW, Prakken ES, Hendriks JM, et al. Electromechanical abdominal massage and colonic function in individuals with a spinal cord injury and chronic bowel problems. *Spinal Cord* 2014;52(9):693–696. http://www.ncbi.nlm.nih.gov/pubmed/24937700
6. Coggrave M, Norton C, Cody JD. Management of faecal incontinence and constipation in adults with central neurological diseases. *Cochrane Database of Systematic Reviews* 2014;(1):CD002115. http://www.ncbi.nlm.nih.gov/pubmed/24420006
7. Coggrave M, Norton C. Management of faecal incontinence and constipation in adults with central neurological diseases. *Cochrane Database of Systematic Reviews* 2013;(12):CD002115. http://www.ncbi.nlm.nih.gov/pubmed/24347087

SIDEBAR 4.13 Depression →Stroke →Depression . . .

The relation between stroke and depression is fascinating and complicated. It is well established that depression is an independent risk factor for stroke, but the mechanism is not well understood. One theory suggests that a low serotonin level changes the function of platelets and increases inflammation. This is also an issue for heart attack and atherosclerosis. Interestingly, while cognitive-behavioral therapy is effective to relieve the symptoms of depression, it does not reduce the risk of other vascular problems—but antidepressants that improve the uptake of serotonin have been seen to reduce the risk of future vascular problems, especially heart attack.

Massage therapists should be interested in this phenomenon, since one of the most consistently measured effects of massage is an increase in the secretion of serotonin. Wouldn't it be interesting if massage and bodywork had an influence on the risk of depression-related stroke?

Many stroke survivors develop depression after their incident; this is called poststroke depression. This number is not separated from the people who had depression before their stroke, however. Depression tends to make all stroke treatments less effective and significantly affects the prognosis for recovery.

Stroke

Definition: What Is It?

Stroke, also called brain attack or cerebrovascular accident (CVA), is damage to brain cells due to oxygen deprivation brought about by **thrombosis** (a clot forms onsite), **embolism** (a clot travels from elsewhere), or hemorrhage (internal bleeding). It is the single most common type of CNS disorder.

Demographics

Stroke is the fourth leading cause of death in the United States. It is the leading cause of adult disability. Men have more strokes than do women, but women are more likely to have an incident at an older age and consequently to die from stroke.

About 795,000 people have a stroke each year in this country. Of them, 610,000 will have their first attack, while 185,000 will have a repeat stroke. About 160,000 Americans die of stroke each year. About 5 million stroke survivors are alive in this country today.

Worldwide, it is estimated that 15 million people have a stroke each year. Of these, 5 million die and 5 million are disabled.

Etiology: What Happens?

Oxygen deprivation in the cranium kills brain cells, leading to dysfunction in the rest of the body. The oxygen shortage can come about either because of a blockage, which is a form of ischemic stroke, or because of bleeding, in which case it is a hemorrhagic stroke. *You can see the animation "Stroke" at* http://thePoint.lww.com/Werner6e. thePoint®

The amount of damage a stroke causes is determined primarily by the location and number of neurons that are damaged by oxygen deprivation, along with secondary responses. Inflammatory reactions, free radical activity, and other factors can cause tissue damage that far exceeds the oxygen deprivation brought about by the stroke itself. The injured area around the site of the stroke is called the **ischemic penumbra**. Interrupting the cascade of secondary responses with appropriate treatment can limit the extent of this area and improve the overall prognosis.

Motor damage from strokes can result in partial or full paralysis of one side of the body; this is called **hemiparesis** for weakness or **hemiplegia** for complete loss of function. The side of the body is opposite to the side of the brain affected by the stroke. **Aphasia** (loss of language), **dysarthria** (slurred speech), memory loss, and mild or severe personality changes may also occur. Sensory damage may result in permanent numbness and/or vision loss. **Depression** is another complication that is frequently seen after stroke; this condition has a complex intersection with stroke that is discussed in Sidebar 4.13.

Risk Factors

Although a person can have a genetic predisposition toward a CVA, many of the factors that contribute to stroke are well within the reach of personal control. When a person has any single risk factor for stroke, that risk is considerably amplified by adding another factor: for instance, hypertension with cigarette smoking is a much higher risk profile than either of the two issues separately.

Risk Factors That Can Be Controlled

- *High blood pressure.* Untreated **hypertension** is the biggest single contributing factor to the risk of stroke.
- *Smoking.* Nicotine constricts blood vessels and raises blood pressure.

Ischemic penumbra: The area surrounding an ischemic stroke.

Hemiparesis: Muscle weakness of one side of the body.

Hemiplegia: Paralysis of one side of the body.

Aphasia: A loss of language and communication skills due to brain damage.

Dysarthria: Difficulty articulating words.

- ***Atherosclerosis,*** *high cholesterol*. These conditions also contribute to high blood pressure and raise the risk of emboli.
- *C-reactive protein*. This substance is present with long-term low-grade inflammation. A high C-reactive protein level is a dependable predictor for both ischemic stroke and atherosclerosis.
- *Atrial fibrillation*. Left untreated, this condition can help to form the emboli responsible for some ischemic embolic strokes.
- *High alcohol consumption*. This is generally considered to be more than two drinks per day, or an episode of binge drinking.
- *Drug use*. Cocaine and methamphetamines have been seen to increase stroke risk.
- *Obesity and sedentary lifestyle*.
- ***Diabetes***. Untreated, this condition can contribute to high blood pressure and atherosclerosis. Poorly treated diabetes triples the risk of stroke.
- *High-estrogen birth control pills*. These pose a risk especially when used by a person who smokes.
- *Hormone replacement therapy*. Some women who supplement estrogen and progesterone as a way to manage symptoms of menopause have a significantly increased risk of stroke.
- *Depression*. Depression has been seen to be a predictive factor for stroke: one-third of stroke patients are diagnosed for depression before their CVA.
- *Overall stress*.
- ***Sickle cell disease***.
- ***Obstructive sleep apnea***.

Risk Factors That Cannot Be Controlled

- *Age*. Three-quarters of stroke patients are over 65 years of age. The risk of stroke doubles each decade after 55.
- *Gender*. About 25% more men than women have strokes, but strokes kill more women than men.
- ***Migraines***. For reasons that are not yet clear, people who have migraines—especially migraines with auras—have a twofold risk of subclinical brain infarction (transient ischemic attacks [TIAs] with small areas of damage), as compared to the general population.
- *Race*. African Americans have a higher incidence of hypertension than do Whites. They are about twice as likely to have a stroke as whites, and they are almost twice as likely to die of it.
- *Family history*. Having a family history of stroke and cardiovascular disease can be a predisposing factor. Structurally weak blood vessels can be an inherited problem.
- *Previous stroke*. Having one stroke usually predisposes a person to having another. Predisposition is not predestination, however; by taking control over whatever factors are within reach, a person can take big steps toward reducing the chances that he or she will have another stroke.

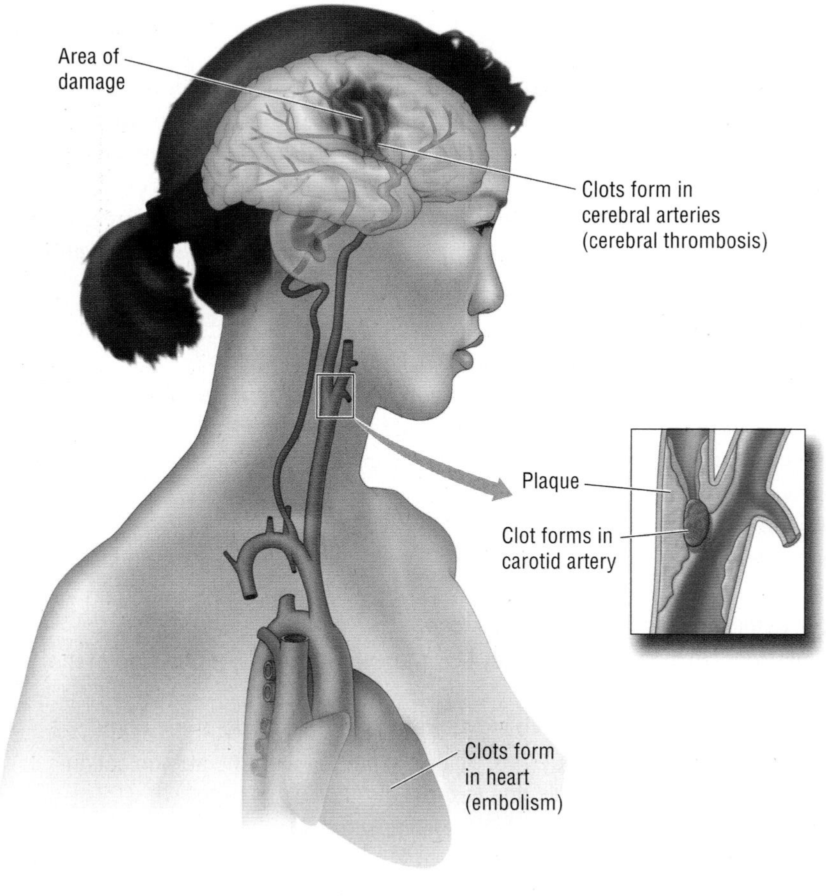

FIGURE 4.20 Ischemic stroke can originate on-site in the brain, in the carotid artery, or in the heart

Types of Stroke

- *Ischemic stroke*: These are the most common version of CVA. The ischemia can be caused by cerebral thrombosis (a blood clot or blockage forms inside a vessel in the brain) or embolism (a clot forms somewhere else and travels to the brain to create a blockage) (Figure 4.20). Thrombotic strokes are further classified by whether they are large vessel thrombi or small vessel disease with tiny areas of damage called **lacunar infarctions**.

  Emboli that cause strokes may originate in the carotid artery (Sidebar 4.14) or in the chambers of the heart, especially if valves are damaged or the heartbeat is unsteady so blood can pool and thicken. (See Animation at http://thePoint.lww.com/Werner6e. thePoint®)
  - *Stenosis*: This describes a narrowing of a brain artery with the same process that is seen in **atherosclerosis**. If the artery is completely occluded, brain damage will occur.
  - *Transient ischemic attack (TIA)*: Also called a "ministroke," this occurs when the blockage is due to a small clot that melts within a few hours. Damage may be mild, but cumulative: a person may have many TIAs, and they can serve as a warning signal for the risk of a more serious event: a full stroke or heart attack. Someone who has had many TIAs may also appear to have dementia (Figure 4.21).
  - *Cryptogenic stroke*: This is a CVA with no known cause. It may be connected to a **patent foramen ovale**. This is especially likely when a stroke occurs in a person younger than 55 years of age.
- *Hemorrhagic stroke*: These account for about 20% of all strokes. They can involve bleeding deep inside the brain (intracerebral hemorrhage) or on the surface of the brain (subarachnoid hemorrhage) (Figure 4.22). These strokes are often associated with **aneurysms**, which may be a result of genetic anomaly, chronic **hypertension**, bleeding disorders, head trauma, or a malformation of blood vessels called **arteriovenous malformation**.

  An overview of these strokes is found in Figure 4.23.

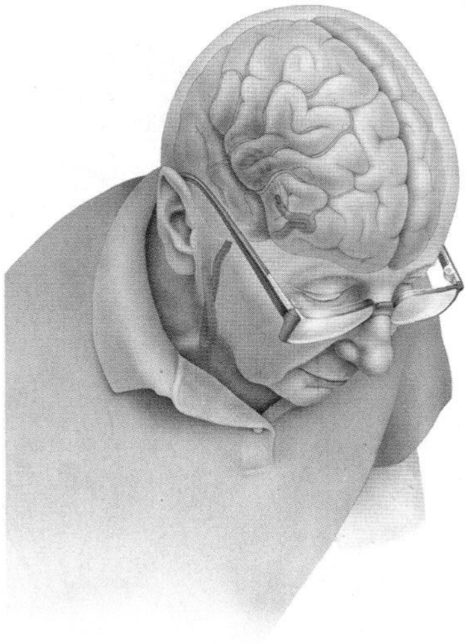

FIGURE 4.21 TIA: a tiny clot is trapped but quickly dissolves

SIDEBAR 4.14 Carotid Artery Disease: Nowhere to Go but Up

The discussion of **atherosclerosis** points out that because of chronically high blood pressure, both the aorta and coronary arteries are particularly prone to the development of atherosclerotic plaque. The carotid arteries, which emerge from the aortic arch, are similarly vulnerable. Although they are farther from the heart, blood pressure in the arteries that supply the head is ordinarily high to ensure adequate blood flow to the brain. This puts the carotid arteries at risk for the same endothelial damage and plaque development seen with the aorta and the coronary arteries; this is called carotid artery disease.

The problem with carotid artery disease is that if any fragment of plaque or blood clot should break free, it has only one direction to go: straight up into the brain. When this happens in very tiny increments, it is called transient ischemic attack, or TIA. But the presence of carotid artery disease significantly raises the risk of a major stroke—so much so that identifying this disorder often leads to aggressive treatment, in the shape of carotid **endarterectomy**.

Massage therapists working with clients who know they have carotid artery disease must stay away from the neck, especially the anterior triangle, which is bordered by the sternocleidomastoid muscle, as it runs superficially over the carotid arteries.

Signs and Symptoms

It is important to be able to recognize the signs of stroke; the sooner treatment is administered, the less damage will occur. The signs of someone having a stroke are these:

- Sudden onset of unilateral weakness, numbness, or paralysis on the face, arm, leg, or any combination of the three
- Suddenly blurred or decreased vision in one or both eyes; asymmetrical dilation of pupils
- Difficulty in speaking or understanding simple sentences; confusion
- Sudden onset of dizziness, clumsiness, and vertigo
- Sudden extreme headache
- Possible loss of consciousness

Lacunar infarction: Tiny areas of damage caused by stroke occurring in a small vessel.

Patent foramen ovale: A condition in which the valve in the atrial septum of the heart does not fully close after birth.

Endarterectomy: Removal of diseased layers of an artery.

Arteriovenous malformation: An abnormal connection between veins and arteries, usually found in the cranium.

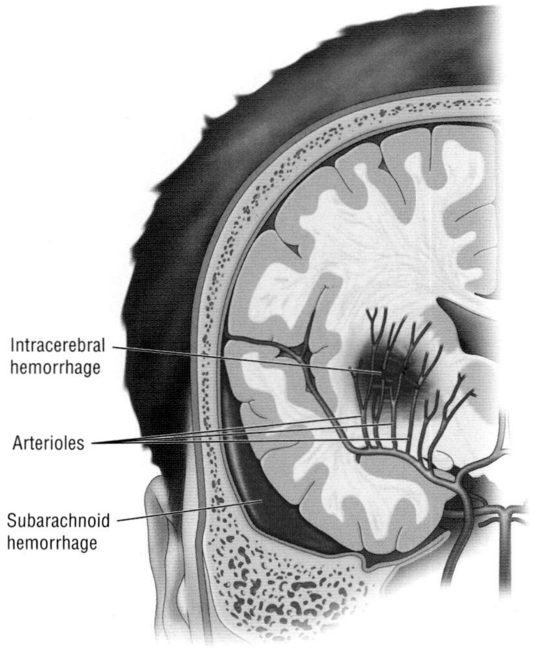

FIGURE 4.22 Hemorrhagic strokes can occur within the brain (intracerebral hemorrhage) or on the surface (subarachnoid hemorrhage)

SIDEBAR 4.15 Neuroplasticity

Neuroplasticity refers to the potential for neurons to grow and adapt. Contrary to traditional belief, it has been found that nerve cells in the CNS have the capacity to change under the right circumstances, even after catastrophic injury. This can happen in several ways: they may sprout new axon terminals to establish new synapses, redundant nerve pathways may be recruited postinjury, or latent nerve pathways may become newly viable.

One of the most exciting aspects of this discovery is that some brain chemicals appear to promote neuroplasticity. Introduced at the key moments in CNS injury, they may significantly improve the prognosis for a stroke, TBI, or SCI patient. Using neuroprotective drugs in the context of CNS injury is a new field that is still undergoing testing, but it may become the industry standard.

Another way to remember this is the mnemonic FAST: **Face** (Does one side of the face droop when the person tries to smile?); **Arms** (When you ask the person to raise both arms, is one much weaker?); **Speech** (Can the person repeat a simple phrase clearly, or is speech slurred?); **Time** (If any of these are positive, it's time to call emergency services).

Treatment

Treatment for stroke is typically broken into three categories: prevention, acute care, and postacute or long-term care.

Prevention includes identifying people at high risk for stroke and encouraging preventive measures. This may include exercise and diet changes, antiplatelet or anticoagulant drugs, or surgery on the carotid artery. Intracranial aneurysms may also be surgically corrected or reinforced before they rupture.

The treatment of choice for acute ischemic stroke is thrombolytic medication to melt existing clots, but this must be administered within the first few hours of onset to be effective.

If the CVA was from a hemorrhage on the other hand, thrombolysis could be dangerous or even deadly. Hemorrhagic strokes are treated by working to relieve pressure in the brain as quickly as possible.

Once it is clear how much function was lost during a stroke, postacute care begins. The patient must relearn how to do basic tasks, including walking, speaking, eating, and self-care. At one time, the main focus with physical and occupational therapy was to teach the patient how to do self-care with the unaffected side of the body, but a growing understanding of

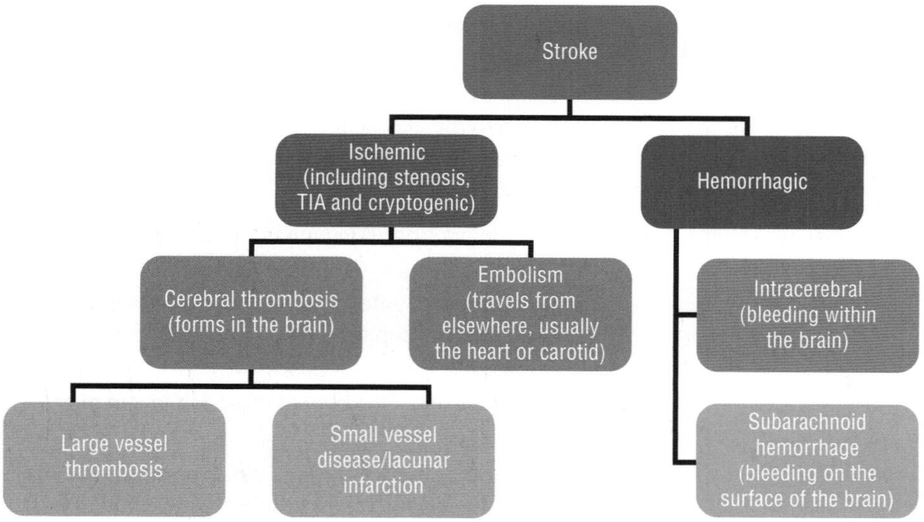

FIGURE 4.23 Types of strokes

neuroplasticity (see Sidebar 4.15) has led to rehabilitation programs that focus on strengthening the function of the weakened side of the body, with much better results.

Medications

- Thrombolytics for ischemic stroke to dissolve blood clots
- Anticoagulants and antiplatelet drugs for ischemic stroke to limit the formation of new clots
- Insulin for blood glucose management (high blood glucose is associated with poor outcome for stroke patients)
- Antihypertensive medications to control blood pressure

Massage Therapy Implications

RISKS	The main risks for stroke patients who want to receive massage concern the possibility of other cardiovascular compromise and the threat of another CVA. If these concerns are addressed, careful massage can be helpful and appropriate. The drugs these patients take and the complications to which they are vulnerable also require adaptation for bodywork.
BENEFITS	Much of the lost function for stroke patients is related to changes that happen outside the CNS: consistent tightness and lack of use allow any functioning muscle fibers finally to degenerate. Massage and other therapies that challenge this process through gentle stretching, exercises, and building awareness may help to minimize unnecessary loss of function, along with pain and other lingering challenges.
RESEARCH	Massage therapy and other CIH therapies are willingly used by many stroke patients.[1] A cohort study using Thai massage with other CIH interventions[2] found that activities of daily living, mood, pain, and sleep patterns were all substantially improved, but because they didn't use a control group, it isn't possible to compare this to conventional treatment. 1. Pandian JD, Toor G, Arora R, et al. Complementary and alternative medicine treatments among stroke patients in India. *Topics in Stroke Rehabilitation* 2012;19(5):384–394. http://www.ncbi.nlm.nih.gov/pubmed/22982825 2. Sibbritt D, van der Riet P, Dedkhard S, et al. Rehabilitation of stroke patients using traditional Thai massage, herbal treatments and physical therapies. *Zhong Xi Yi Jie He Xue Bao* 2012;10(7):743–750. http://www.jcimjournal.com/articles/publishArticles/pdf/jcim20120704.pdf

For the author's perspective on massage therapy, proprioceptors, and CNS injury recovery, see the video "Proprioception" at http://thePoint.lww.com/Werner6e. thePoint®

Traumatic Brain Injury

Definition: What Is It?

TBI is an insult to the brain, not brought about by congenital or degenerative conditions, that leads to altered states of consciousness, cognitive impairment, and disruption of physical, emotional, and behavioral function.

Demographics

TBI is the leading cause of death and disability for people between the ages of 1 and 44 in the United States. They are identified about 1.4 million times and cause 52,000 deaths in this country each year. About 2% of the population, over 5 million people, live with long-term disabilities related to TBI today.

Within the United States, motor vehicle accidents, falls, and assaults are leading causes of TBI. For soldiers in war zones, exposure to blasts is the leading cause. Some veterans' advocates estimate that 10% to 20% of Iraq veterans (up to 300,000 returning service members) have had at least one TBI.

Etiology: What Happens?

When brain tissue is injured, it goes through the same inflammatory process as every other part of the body. The problem is that the brain is enclosed in a rigid casing, so any swelling of blood vessels, glial cells, or neurons, threatens damage to working tissue. When pressure inside the cranium rises, normal nutrient supply through the blood flow and cerebrospinal fluid movement are impaired. This leads to even more edema, in a positive feedback loop that can lead to permanent damage.

Several classifications for head injuries have been created to try to organize the vast number of ways the brain can be injured. Head injuries are sometimes distinguished as primary or secondary issues. Primary injuries are related to the mechanical force that causes damage. Secondary injuries are the consequences or complications of primary injuries.

Primary injuries include these:

- *Skull fracture* occurs when the bones around the skull are broken, usually by a direct blow. Surprisingly, the prognosis for an open head injury is often better than for a closed head injury, because the risk of damage from intracranial pressure is less.

Thrombolytic: Related to the therapeutic dissolving of blood clots.

Neuroplasticity: The ability of the central nervous system to change functionally and structurally as a result of injury or damage.

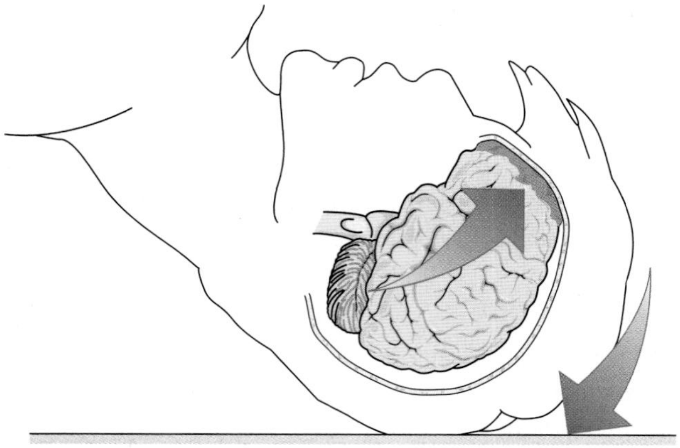

FIGURE 4.24 Concussion: a blow to the head makes the brain hit against the opposite side

- *Penetrating injury* is usually due to a gunshot wound, but may also be from a knife or other objects. Penetrating injuries are the leading cause of death among TBI patients.
- *Concussion* is any temporary loss of brain function. Concussion is the most common type of TBI. It often involves a blow followed by temporary damage at the opposite side of the brain (Figure 4.24). When it occurs in an athlete, it is essential that the tissues heal completely before the athlete returns to play. If he or she has another head injury too soon, **postconcussion syndrome** can develop: a much more serious condition than a simple concussion.

NOTABLE CASES Professional American football players are, not surprisingly, particularly prone to TBI and postconcussion syndrome, sometimes building to a condition called chronic traumatic encephalopathy (CTE): brain damage due to multiple injuries that causes dementia, mood swings, and other severe symptoms. CTE is difficult to diagnose in a living person, but it was identified posthumously in many professional football players who committed suicide, including Junior Seau, Ray Easterling, Dave Duerson, Andre Waters, and Terry Long.

Postconcussion syndrome: A condition in which concussion symptoms last for weeks or months after the concussion itself.

Contusion: A bruise.

Coup-contrecoup: A brain injury that occurs both directly beneath the impact and also on the opposite side of the head.

Diffuse axonal injury: Injury to white matter in the central nervous system, often associated with a persistent vegetative state.

- ***Contusion*** is bruising inside the cranium. When a contusion happens at the point of impact and also where the brain hits the opposite wall, it is a **coup-contrecoup** injury.
- ***Diffuse axonal injury*** is internal tearing or shearing of nerve tissue throughout the brain. It is often related to acceleration/deceleration accidents, as seen with **whiplash** or shaken baby syndrome.

Secondary injuries include these:

- *Anoxic brain injury* is complete lack of oxygen in the brain. It can be brought about by airway obstruction or sudden apnea.
- *Hypoxic brain injury* is an inadequate supply of oxygen, often associated with ischemic stroke, edema, or toxic exposure, especially carbon monoxide poisoning.
- *Hemorrhage* is bleeding inside the brain, often associated with ruptured **aneurysms**.
- *Hematoma* is development of a large amount of coagulated blood, pressing outside or within the brain.
- *Intracranial pressure* is a secondary inflammatory response that can follow any or all of the causes of TBI. The swelling of brain tissue and action of free radicals against healthy tissue may ultimately be responsible for more damage than the original source of the trauma.

Preventive measures to guard against the risk of TBI are self-evident but worth repeating. Most TBIs happen as a transport injury, that is, in an event involving cars, motorcycles, bicycles, scooters, skates, or skateboards. Driving only while alert and sober, using a seat belt, and wearing a helmet can reduce the risk and severity of these accidents. Other preventive measures include making sure the home is safe for young children and elderly people to reduce the risk of falls, and ensuring the appropriate storage of firearms.

Signs and Symptoms

Signs and symptoms of a TBI vary according to what areas of the brain are affected and how severe the injury is. Trauma to the frontal lobes is most common and may result in language and motor dysfunction; trauma to structures close to the brainstem is more likely to lead to massive loss of autonomic function.

Symptoms of an acute TBI include leakage of cerebrospinal fluid from the ears or nose; dilated or asymmetrical pupils; visual disturbances; dizziness and confusion; apnea or slowed breathing; nausea and vomiting; slow pulse and low blood pressure; loss of bowel and bladder control; and possible seizures, paralysis, numbness, lethargy, or loss of consciousness. In infants, chronic crying, lethargy, or unusual sleep patterns are cause for concern. Symptoms may occur immediately or grow in severity over a course of days or even weeks.

Long-term consequences of TBI are sometimes referred to as postconcussion syndrome. They include mild to severe cognitive dysfunction, especially with memory and learning skills. Movement disorders may range from hypertonicity to spasticity. Seizures are a frequent complication. Permanent changes in behavioral and emotional function are also common; many TBI survivors are emotionally volatile and may develop new patterns of aggressiveness and hostility.

One outcome of long-term, repeated head injury is a condition called **chronic traumatic encephalopathy**: permanent brain damage with dementia, personality changes, and other symptoms. Severe cases of TBI (usually ones that affect the brainstem) may lead to stupor, coma, **locked-in syndrome**, **persistent vegetative state**, or brain death.

Treatment

TBI is treated with surgery to remove pressure on the brain if necessary, followed by intensive physical, recreational, occupational, and speech therapy to preserve or recover function. The prognosis with children is generally best, since their brains seem to be most capable of establishing new pathways to relearn skills. Nonetheless, our understanding of neuroplasticity grows daily and continues to brighten the outlook even for mature TBI survivors.

Medications

- Antiseizure medication
- Antidepressants
- Antipsychotic medications
- NSAIDs to manage pain
- Muscle relaxants for spasm and spasticity
- Cholinesterase inhibitors for memory improvement

Massage Therapy Implications

RISKS	TBI is a complicated, serious problem, and a massage therapist working with a client who has this condition is best doing so as part of an integrated health care team. If a client has numbness or is noncommunicative, massage or other stroking techniques may be performed to help preserve the health of the tissues and prevent some complications, but this must be performed with caution, since the client cannot give feedback.
BENEFITS	If sensation is present and the client is able to communicate clearly about comfort, massage can be an important part of a rehabilitation strategy to maintain healthy muscles and connective tissues.
OPTIONS	As with other CNS injuries, massage or bodywork that focuses on proprioception and muscle tone may be especially helpful to maintain strength and flexibility in affected areas.
RESEARCH	People with TBI frequently seek care from multiple providers, including massage therapists[1]: a good reason to build relationships with integrative providers. The Defense and Veterans Brain Injury Center includes massage therapy in its studies of rehabilitation techniques for returning soldiers.[2] 1. Hartvigsen J, Boyle E, Cassidy JD, et al. Mild traumatic brain injury after motor vehicle collisions: what are the symptoms and who treats them? A population-based 1-year inception cohort study. *Archives of Physical Medicine and Rehabilitation* 2014;95 (3 Suppl):S286–S294. http://www.ncbi.nlm.nih.gov/pubmed/24581914 2. Hoffman SW, Shesko K, Harrison CR. Enhanced neurorehabilitation techniques in the DVBIC Assisted Living Pilot Project. *NeuroRehabilitation* 2010;26(3):257–269. http://www.ncbi.nlm.nih.gov/pubmed/20448315

Trigeminal Neuralgia

Definition: What Is It?

Trigeminal neuralgia (TN) is neuro-algia ("nerve pain") along one or more of the three branches of cranial nerve V, the trigeminal nerve (Figure 4.25). It is also called tic douloureux, which is French for painful spasm or "unhappy twitch."

Demographics

TN is diagnosed roughly 4,000 times each year and affects about 15,000 people in the United States. This condition is usually seen in people over 50 years old. In younger adults, it may be linked to **multiple sclerosis**. It is more common in women than in men, by about 2:1.

Etiology: What Happens?

TN is usually classified as primary or secondary. In either case, the trigeminal nerve is irritated, and the result is brief,

> **Chronic traumatic encephalopathy:** A degenerative condition of the brain resulting from multiple head injuries.
>
> **Locked-in syndrome:** A condition in which the body and most of the face are paralyzed, but consciousness remains.
>
> **Persistent vegetative state:** A state characterized by normal levels of arousal (including sleep-wake cycles), but complete lack of awareness.

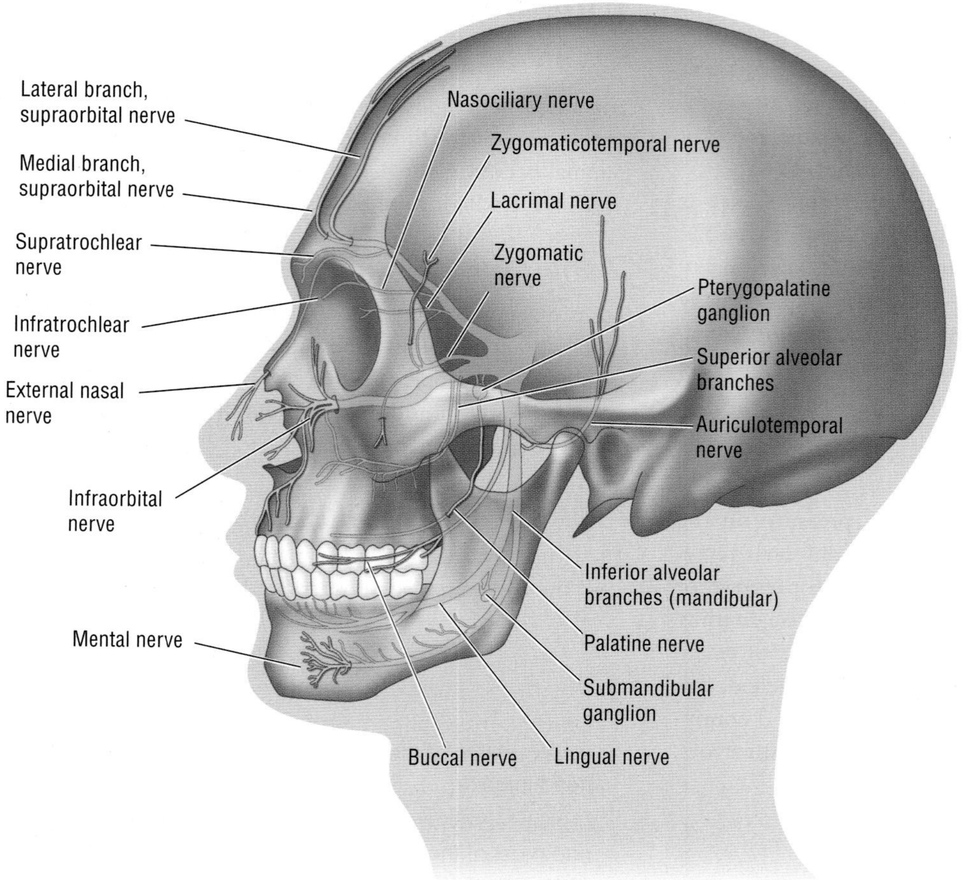

FIGURE 4.25 Trigeminal nerve: main sensory supply for the face

repeating episodes of sharp, electrical, burning, or stabbing pain on one side of the face.

The most typical presentation of primary TN happens when a blood vessel wraps around or irritates the trigeminal nerve where it emerges from the **pons** at the base of the brain. This vessel may wear away the myelin covering on some of the fibers, which allows the nerve to misfire. Autopsies of people with TN are not always consistent about this, however, and many people have this structural anomaly with no painful symptoms. Ultimately, the source of the pain may be a combination of factors.

Secondary TN is due to some other problem that leads to irritation of the trigeminal nerve, which could include accidents and injuries, tumors, bone spurs, recent infection, complications of sinus or dental surgery, or multiple sclerosis.

Signs and Symptoms

Some people call the pain of TN among the worst in the world. It's often described as a sharp, electrical, stabbing, or burning sensation. These episodes may last for 10 seconds to 2 minutes, or several jabs may occur in rapid succession. A muscle tic or grimace goes along with the nerve pain.

In the most common form of TN, sometimes called TN1, episodes take the form of sharp blasts of pain on one side of the face in response to some mild trigger. A rarer version, called TN2, involves a constant ache or burning sensation that may be interrupted by bolts of electrical stabbing or burning pain.

Episodes of trigeminal nerve pain can be triggered by speaking, chewing, swallowing, sitting in a draft, a light touch to the wrong spot, and sometimes by no stimulus at all. Episodes may happen several times a day for days, weeks, or months and then suddenly disappear—only to begin again months or years later. In some cases, it is progressive: attacks become both more frequent and more severe. TN can be a debilitating lifelong condition if it is not treated.

TN is not painful during sleep, nor does it cause numbness, muscle weakness, or hearing loss. It is usually unilateral, and the right side is affected about five times more often than the left. All of these factors help to differentiate TN from other conditions that might cause similar symptoms, including **migraine** or **cluster headaches**, Ramsay-Hunt syndrome, **stroke**, or other cranial nerve problems (Sidebar 4.16).

Pons: A part of the brainstem, located between the medulla oblongata and the thalamus.

SIDEBAR 4.16 Other Cranial Nerve Disorders

Any damage or irritation to a cranial nerve may lead to symptoms in the face. TN and **Bell palsy** are two of the most common disorders that may cause facial symptoms. But a few other cranial nerve disorders can create confusion, so they are listed here:

- *Postherpetic neuralgia* is a complication of **herpes zoster**. It may occur wherever the shingles blisters appeared but can outlast the visible lesions by several weeks or months. When the herpes infection affects the optic nerve, PHN can create extremely painful facial symptoms.
- *Glossopharyngeal neuralgia* is etiologically identical to vascular compression on the trigeminal nerve, but this condition affects CN IX, which supplies sensation to the back of the throat.
- *Atypical face pain* is a condition similar to TN and in some cases may be a predecessor to it. It is characterized by pain that is less severe than TN, but it tends to involve continuous rather than intermittent pain. The pain may go up over the back of the head and into the scalp, and it may involve the occipital as well as the trigeminal nerve.
- *Hemifacial spasm* creates a painless tic that is related to blood vessel compression of the facial nerve rather than the trigeminal nerve.

Treatment

A conventional medical approach to TN starts with medication, but typical analgesics are ineffective. Antiseizure drugs that inhibit nerve conduction are often successful in the short run, but many patients don't tolerate them well, or they experience "breakthrough pain" that requires a change in dosage or a combination of drugs. Muscle relaxants and tricyclic antidepressants may also be prescribed.

Several other interventions have been developed to treat TN. These usually involve the controlled destruction of part of the nerve with lasers, radiation, a heated probe, or injected chemicals. These options often provide some relief, with the understanding that the patient may have permanent numbness and some facial muscle weakness as a result. Microvascular surgery to relieve pressure on the trigeminal nerve is the most invasive procedure. It entails unwrapping the strangulating blood vessel from around the trigeminal nerve. This process leaves sensation intact and has the longest-lasting success, but it carries more risks of complication than other approaches.

Medications

- Antiseizure medications for pain control (TN1)
- Muscle relaxants
- Tricyclic antidepressants for pain control (TN2)
- Botulinum toxin injections to reduce trigeminal nerve activity

Massage Therapy Implications

RISKS	TN contraindicates any bodywork that might elicit symptoms, which means that touching the face or head is probably off-limits unless the client can guide the therapist into work that is soothing instead of irritating. Further, the pressure of a face cradle may trigger symptoms, so prone work may not be possible.
BENEFITS	A person with TN often has musculoskeletal consequences that can be successfully addressed by massage. Tension in the neck and shoulders is predictable, as people chronically guard against the possibility of an episode.

Nervous System Birth Defects

Spina Bifida

Definition: What Is It?

Spina bifida (literally, "cleft spine") is a **neural tube** defect in which the vertebral arch fails to close completely over the spinal cord. Sometimes, this defect is so subtle it is found only through incidental radiography or MRI, but in other cases, it can be so severe that the spinal canal is open and the baby may not survive the birth.

> **Neural tube:** An embryonic structure from which the brain and spinal cord eventually develop.

Demographics

In the United States, the incidence of spina bifida is estimated at about 166,000 people. Rates have been going down with improved access to prenatal health care. Genetic predisposition and maternal **diabetes** and exposures to heat or toxins are contributors, but the greatest risk factor for spina bifida is folic acid deficiency.

SIDEBAR 4.17 Other Neural Tube Defects

The neural tube is composed of fetal cells that fold in on themselves during the earliest days of development. Under normal circumstances, the tube is complete and closed by day 28, when the fetus is about the size of a grain of rice.

Sometimes those cells, which are the starting material of the vertebrae, skull, spinal cord, spinal nerves, and brain, deform. SBO, meningocele, and myelomeningocele describe problems with the spinal cord, but the brain can also be affected. Some neural tube defects that can occur apart from or along with spina bifida include the following:

- *Encephalocele.* In this condition, the bones of the skull don't develop properly. A cyst protrudes from the head, containing cerebrospinal fluid and possibly brain tissue as well.
- *Anencephaly.* In this condition, the brain forms incompletely or doesn't form at all. These babies tend to be stillborn or die soon after birth.
- *Arnold-Chiari malformation.* This is a rare disorder except in the presence of myelomeningocele, with which it is relatively common. In this situation, the brainstem and some of the cerebellum protrude into the spinal canal in the neck. This leads to hydrocephalus, difficulties with swallowing and breathing, and impaired coordination of the arms.

Etiology: What Happens?

Several types of neural tube defects may occur between day 14 and day 28 after conception (Sidebar 4.17). At this time, the woman may not know she is pregnant, and the fetus is about the size of a grain of rice, but the cells that eventually differentiate into connective, muscle, and epithelial tissue at various levels of the spinal cord are in place. If something interrupts their development, spina bifida may occur.

Spina bifida is a complex disorder with several possible complications. **Meningitis** is a threat if the CNS is exposed. **Hydrocephalus** affects about 85% of children with spina bifida diagnosed at birth. The insertion of a shunt that drains cerebrospinal fluid down the neck and into the abdominal cavity prevents hydrocephalus from damaging the brain. Hydrocephalus is sometimes related to **Chiari II formation**: a defect in which the brain protrudes into the spinal canal, blocking off the flow of cerebrospinal fluid. While most children with spina bifida have normal intelligence, some have mild to severe learning disabilities that may make it difficult to function in a mainstream classroom. Many spina bifida patients develop a very severe latex hypersensitivity, possibly as a result of having multiple intrusive surgeries and other medical procedures. This allergy may create a dangerous anaphylactic reaction later in life.

Hydrocephalus: A condition marked by the excessive accumulation of cerebrospinal fluid.

Chiari II formation: A malformation of the brain in which part of the brain protrudes through the foramen magnum.

Tethered cord: A group of malformations that all involve the restriction of the movement of the spinal cord within the spinal canal.

Spina bifida patients who are born with obvious cysts experience lower limb paralysis and sensory loss: the higher the cyst, the more function is lost. Other common complications include **tethered cord**, **decubitus ulcers**, bowel and bladder problems with a high risk of **urinary tract infection** and **renal failure**, obesity, and muscle imbalances that can lead to severe **scoliosis**.

Types of Spina Bifida

- *Spina bifida occulta (SBO).* In this situation, the vertebral arch, usually in a lumbar vertebra, does not completely fuse, but no signs or symptoms are obvious. A person with SBO may never be aware of the condition unless a low back radiograph is taken for another reason. Some people with SBO have a small dimple, birthmark, or tuft of hair on the spine at the location of the abnormality, but they have no dysfunction because of it. While SBO is usually inconsequential, it can be serious. Two or more vertebrae may be affected, and the person may develop a tethered spinal cord. This can manifest as problems in the feet (especially pes cavus) and problems with bladder and bowel control. These often arise during puberty, when the child goes through a growth spurt that stretches the spinal cord.
- *Spina bifida meningocele.* This is the rarest type of cystic spina bifida. Only the dura mater and arachnoid layers of the meninges press through at the site of the vertebral cleft, forming a cyst that is visible at birth. It is easily reparable with surgery and generally has few or no long-term consequences for the baby.
- *Spina bifida myelomeningocele.* This is the most common and most severe version of cystic spina bifida, accounting for about 94% of diagnosed cases. In this case, the spinal cord or extensions of the cauda equina protrude along with the meninges through several incompletely formed vertebral arches. Occasionally, the skin doesn't cover the protrusion, raising a serious risk of CNS infection if no immediate intervention takes place.

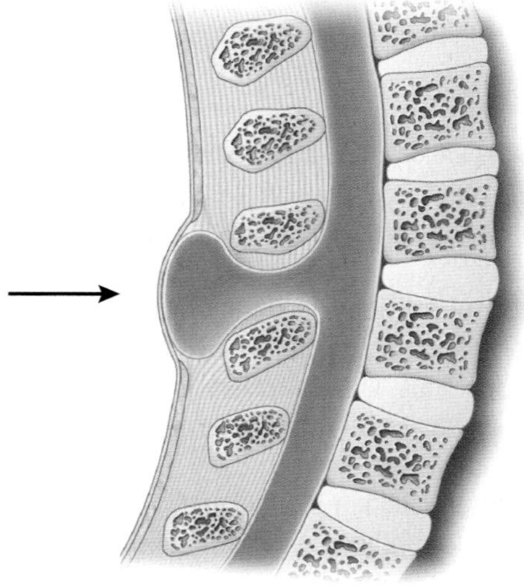

FIGURE 4.26 Spina bifida occulta. The vertebral arch is incompletely fused; no external sac is present.

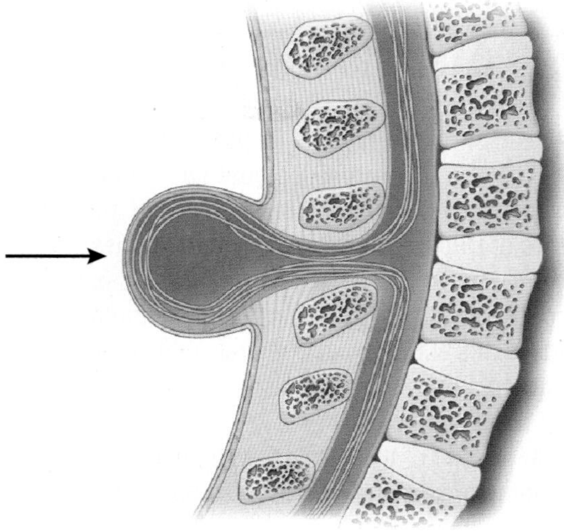

FIGURE 4.28 Spina bifida myelomeningocele. An external sac contains the meninges and cerebrospinal fluid, peripheral nerves, and spinal cord tissue.

Signs and Symptoms

SBO is not obvious at birth, although it sometimes causes a birthmark, patch of hair, or a dimple at the site of the abnormality. Cystic spina bifida is obvious, because a sac containing meninges and/or spinal cord material protrudes on the back of the newborn infant. It usually occurs in the lumbar spine, and the sac is often red and raw looking (Figures 4.26–4.28).

The severity of cystic spina bifida is determined by the location and size of the cyst: nerve function below the cyst is severely impaired or absent. Most cases present in the thoracic or lumbar spine (Case History 4.4).

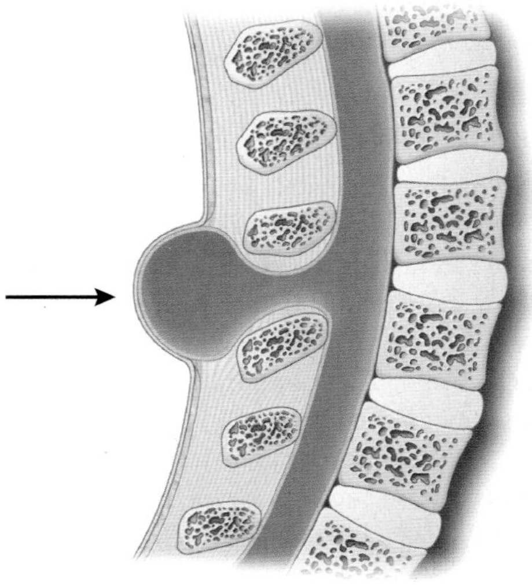

FIGURE 4.27 Spina bifida meningocele. An external sac contains the meninges and cerebrospinal fluid.

Treatment

A baby born with cystic spina bifida needs surgery to reduce the cyst and preserve as much spinal cord function as possible. Many surgeries are even conducted in utero at 26 weeks, well before the baby is born: this is associated with improved outcomes, but also with higher risks. Afterward, even tiny babies are supported with rigorous physical therapy and exercises to maintain function in the leg muscles as much as possible. As children mature and their functional level becomes clear, they may be taught to use crutches, braces, wheelchairs, or other equipment as necessary.

NOTABLE CASES Musician Hank Williams Sr. had SBO, which probably contributed to a lifelong struggle with back pain leading to alcohol and drug abuse problems. World-renowned athlete and motivational speaker Jean Driscoll is a spina bifida patient and wheelchair rider who has won eight championships in the Women's Wheelchair division of the Boston Marathon.

Many spina bifida patients undergo multiple surgeries, not only to reduce the protruding cyst but also to correct a tethered cord, to deal with the complications of hydrocephalus, and to address complications brought about by severe scoliosis

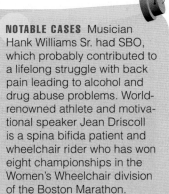

CASE HISTORY 4.4 Spina Bifida

With an effortless motion, he pulled himself onto the table. He grasped his lifeless legs and twisted his whole body until he was lying prone. To gaze on his body was to grasp two opposing realities at once. His legs, clad in a loose-fitting pair of sweatpants, were shriveled and limp. Even his hips and buttocks were hollowed out and gaunt after years of frustrated growth and nearly useless service to the greater whole.

Yet, beginning with his lower back and especially with the lower border of his rib cage, a transformation of epic proportions occurred. The sides of his torso tapered out dramatically to accommodate his thickly muscled back. Indeed, his entire upper body resembled that of a professional bodybuilder. Thus, while the lower half of his body revealed a life of disease, death, and despair, his upper body reflected a life filled with drive, determination, ambition, and hope.

At the end of the session, when my client had gotten off my table, dressed, and left the building, I reflected on the meaning of wholeness. It dawned on me that wholeness is not a disease-free condition, at least in this life, in this reality.

Instead, wholeness is a realized and used connection between the human will and a greater purpose, a greater goal. This athlete thrives because his sights are set on goals that diminish the significance of his lower body and magnify the significance of his upper body, including and especially his mind. Similarly, I thrive when my sights are set on goals that are adorned in truth and immersed in love—on my best days and even on my worst days.

—Jan Fields, observations on the 2002 Paralympic Games

Medications

- Anticholinergic drugs to help with bladder function
- Alpha adrenergic drugs to help with bladder function
- Tricyclic antidepressants

Massage Therapy Implications

RISKS	The risks related to massage for people with spina bifida revolve around paralysis, numbness, and complications like decubitus ulcers or scoliosis.
BENEFITS	As long as risks are addressed, massage can be helpful and supportive for spina bifida patients.
RESEARCH	Parents of children with spina bifida, like those of children with other chronic conditions, often seek out CIH therapies to complement conventional medical approaches. Massage therapy is dependably a popular choice.[1] 1. Samdup DZ, Smith II RG, Song S. The use of complementary and alternative medicine in children with chronic medical conditions. *American Journal of Physical Medicine and Rehabilitation* 2006;85(10):842–846. http://www.ncbi.nlm.nih.gov/pubmed/16998432

Cerebral Palsy

Definition: What Is It?

Cerebral palsy (CP) is a collective term for many possible injuries to the brain during gestational development, birth, and early infancy. Several types of CP have been identified, each involving damage to different parts of the brain at different moments in development.

Demographics

In spite of improved prenatal care, the incidence of CP in the United States has remained unchanged for several decades and in some areas has even gone up. This may be related to the fact that more premature babies are surviving than ever before, and they are especially vulnerable to these problems. Other high-risk populations are hard to identify, but statistics are highest among children of mothers who smoke, who live in poverty, who don't receive prenatal care, and who have previously had preterm babies.

About 764,000 children and adults in the United States have cerebral palsy.

Etiology: What Happens?

CP is the result of brain damage, usually to motor areas of the brain, specifically the basal ganglia and the cerebrum.

Intracranial hemorrhage, damage to the white matter around the ventricles, and toxicity due to extreme infantile **jaundice** are leading factors in CP. Causes of CP can fall into three groups, according to when they occur.

- *Prenatal causes*. Many cases of CP can be traced to maternal illness during pregnancy. Contributing factors include infection with rubella or toxoplasmosis, **hyperthyroidism**, **diabetes**, **Rh sensitization**, toxic exposure, or abdominal trauma. Pregnancy-induced hypertension and infection of the placental membrane can also increase the risk of CP. Other prenatal causes involve random mutations of genes that affect brain growth.
- *Birth trauma*. CP can result if the child undergoes **anoxia** or **asphyxia** during birth. Respiratory distress and head trauma (often from a difficult presentation or the use of forceps in delivery) may also increase the risk of brain damage.
- *Acquired CP*. This is CP that develops in early infancy. Causes include very extreme jaundice that can lead to brain damage and deafness, head trauma (often from car accidents or child abuse), infection with **meningitis** or **encephalitis**, brain hemorrhages, or neoplasms in the brain that may lead to brain damage.

Regardless of the cause of the brain damage, a child with CP has some impairment of function. The problem may be subtle, or it may be completely debilitating both physically and mentally, or somewhere in between: it all depends on what part and how much of the brain has been affected.

Complications of CP include several other serious challenges. Seizures, hearing loss, and **strabismus** are common. Digestive difficulties, including **gastroesophageal reflux disease**, poor gastrointestinal **motility**, and urinary incontinence, are common, as are low bone density and heart disease. CP is also associated with excessive drooling and a high risk of dental cavities.

Rh sensitization: A complication that occurs when a person with Rh-negative blood becomes pregnant with an Rh-positive child for the second time, in which the mother's antibodies attack the fetus' red blood cells.

Anoxia: The absence of oxygen.

Asphyxia: Impaired or absent exchange of carbon dioxide and oxygen in the respiratory system. Suffocation.

Strabismus: A lack of parallel alignment of the eyes.

Motility: The ability to move.

Clasp-knife effect: An abnormal reflex in which passive flexion of a joint is resisted at first, but gives way suddenly with continued pressure.

Although it doesn't always involve cognitive problems, about two-thirds of all CP patients have some level of mental disability, and fully mentally able patients may have challenges in communicating clearly. Many CP patients have **seizure disorders**, which can require very powerful medication to control.

The muscles of CP patients can become so chronically tight that they are replaced with tight, restrictive contractures. Contractures can pull on the skeleton so constantly and so powerfully that the patient is at risk for developing **osteoarthritis**, hip **dislocation**, or extreme **scoliosis** that can make it painful to sit or stand and difficult to breathe. Finally, although the damage in the CNS is stable, adults with CP find that their strength, stamina, and general resilience all decrease with age, so that every kind of activity becomes progressively more difficult to do.

Perhaps the most pervasive and least studied complication of CP is the pain that these children and adults must deal with on a daily basis. The disorder itself can be painful as it twists the body into stressful postures and positions, but the treatments, from frequent surgeries, to aggressive rehabilitation exercises, can also be severely painful.

NOTABLE CASES Irish author, painter, and poet Christy Brown had cerebral palsy. He was the subject of the award-winning film *My Left Foot*, which chronicled his life from infancy, when it was assumed he was hopelessly disabled, through the discovery that he could write and draw with his toes, to his recognition as a leading artist in his country.

While CP is discussed as the types described below, it may also be classified by what part of the body is affected. These terms are consistent with those used for other CNS disorders: hemiplegic CP means the left or right side is affected, diplegic CP means either the arms or the legs are affected, and quadriplegic CP means all the extremities are affected to some extent.

Types of Cerebral Palsy

- *Spastic CP*. This is the most common form of the condition, accounting for 60% to 75% of all cases. In some areas, muscle tone is so high that the tight muscle's antagonists have completely let go. This is called the **clasp-knife effect**.
- *Athetoid CP*. This involves very weak muscles and frequent involuntary writhing movements of the extremities, face, and mouth.
- *Ataxic CP*. This is a rare variety of the disorder, involving chronic shaking, intention tremors, and very poor balance.
- *Dystonic CP*. This involves slow, involuntary twisting movements of the trunk and extremities.
- *Mixed CP*. This is a combination of the forms, and it affects many CP patients.

Signs and Symptoms

Signs and symptoms of CP vary according to the location and extent of brain injury. They typically develop between age 6 months and early toddlerhood. Some of the most common features of CP include hypotonicity, hypertonicity, problems with walking, poor coordination and voluntary muscle control, unusually weak muscles, random movements, and early hearing and/or vision problems.

Adults with CP tend to age faster than others; it takes much more energy and effort to move for someone with CP than for someone without. Simple activities are more draining, and adult patients tend to be prone to fatigue, exhaustion, and overuse syndromes.

Treatment

The CNS damage that occurs with CP is incurable and irreversible. CP is therefore managed, rather than treated, by providing skills and equipment to live as fully and functionally as possible. For some CP patients, this means braces, crutches, or orthotics; for others, it means intensive occupational, physical, and speech therapy for many years. Computers have become an important tool for many patients with CP; these appliances can improve communication and open many new opportunities for this population.

Speech therapy helps with communication and safe swallowing. Intensive physical and occupational therapy, often combined with massage, is used to maintain and improve muscle function and elasticity.

Medication for CP is prescribed to help manage seizures and to reduce muscle spasm. Botox injections can limit excessive salivation and involuntary muscle contractions for several months at a time. Some surgical interventions have been developed to correct hip dislocations, to lengthen contracted muscles, to realign vertebrae that have become distorted by scoliosis, to sever some motor neurons to the legs, and to alter nerve pathways in the brain to reduce the severity of tremors.

Most CP treatments focus on children, but an increasing percentage of CP patients (now 65% to 90%) live well into adulthood, and their treatment needs are different. This is a new population of patients who have special needs related to premature aging. These concerns have mostly not yet been successfully addressed with medication or surgical protocols.

Medications

- Oral or injected muscle relaxants for spasticity
- Injected botulinum toxin to reduce spasticity
- Injected antispasmodic medication to reduce spasticity
- Antiseizure medications for seizures and chronic pain
- Bisphosphonates for improved bone density

Massage Therapy Implications

RISKS

Some people with CP may not be able to verbally communicate easily; massage therapists must be sensitive to nonverbal signals from these clients. In addition, any numbness contraindicates intrusive massage that may overchallenge the tissues, and care must be taken not to trigger seizures, if that is part of a client's symptomatic profile. Finally, the combination of medications used by a client may require massage therapy adaptations.

BENEFITS

Massage can be a wonderful addition to the health care strategy of a person with CP: it can be used to help with pain and stress, muscular efficiency, digestive function, and muscle tension. These are all problems that affect both children and adults with CP.

OPTIONS

Bodywork that focuses on muscle tone and proprioception can be especially useful for clients with CNS problems.

RESEARCH

Parents of children with CP often look for massage therapy as part of a strategy to maximize function and minimize pain.[1] Children who receive massage generally enjoy it, finding it helpful with relaxation, mobility, pain, and bowel regularity.[2] One study[3] found that pain-free, slow, cross-fiber strumming of the calves of children with diplegia led to substantial changes in the muscles, although those changes were different from one subject to another.

1. Glew GM, Fan MY, Hagland S, et al. Survey of the use of massage for children with cerebral palsy. *International Journal of Therapeutic Massage and Bodywork* 2010;3(4):10–15. http://www.ncbi.nlm.nih.gov/pmc/articles/PMC3088521/
2. Powell L, Cheshire A, Swaby L. Children's experiences of their participation in a training and support programme involving massage. *Complementary Therapies in Clinical Practice* 2010;16(1):47–51. http://www.ncbi.nlm.nih.gov/pubmed/20129410
3. Macgregor R, Campbell R, Gladden MH, et al. Effects of massage on the mechanical behaviour of muscles in adolescents with spastic diplegia: a pilot study. *Developmental Medicine and Child Neurology* 2007;49(3):187–191. http://www.ncbi.nlm.nih.gov/pubmed/17355474

Other Nervous System Conditions

Fibromyalgia

Definition: What Is It?

Fibromyalgia syndrome (FMS) describes a multifactoral condition involving problems with neurotransmitter and hormone imbalances, sleep disorders, and ultimately chronic pain in muscles, tendons, ligaments, and other soft tissues. FMS is frequently seen with **chronic fatigue syndrome**, **irritable bowel syndrome**, **migraine headaches**, **temporomandibular joint disorders**, and several other chronic conditions.

Demographics

It is estimated that according to diagnostic criteria, the prevalence of fibromyalgia in the United States is about 6.4%, encompassing roughly 7.7% of women and 4.9% of men. It is the second most commonly seen disorder among rheumatologists (osteoarthritis is first).

This condition can affect anyone, but its prevalence increases with age, peaking for among women between 60 and 70 years old.

Etiology: What Happens?

Fibromyalgia is a relatively common disorder, but it is not well understood. While the etiology of this condition is not clear, several issues are consistent among people who meet the diagnostic criteria for this disorder:

- *HPA axis dysregulation*. The HPA axis is one line of connection between the autonomic nervous system and the endocrine system. Its dysregulation appears to be a factor for many fibromyalgia patients. This means they tend to secrete more stress-related hormones for longer periods of time than other people. HPA axis dysregulation is also a factor in several other disorders, including depression and chronic fatigue syndrome—both of which are often seen in people with FMS.
- *Sleep disorder*. Most people with FMS seldom or never enter the deepest level of sleep, stage IV. It is in this stage that adults secrete growth hormone, which stimulates the production of new cells and extracellular matrix for healing and recovery. People with FMS have reliably lower-than-normal levels of human growth hormone.
- *Central sensitization*. Fibromyalgia pain is perceived in muscles and soft tissues, but it is not generated there. The pain signals are generated, often spontaneously, by malfunctioning pain receptors. Signals travel to neurons in the spinal cord, and their receptors grow extra dendrites to become increasingly sensitive to pain, which appears to amplify the sensation. These processes are supported by changes in neurotransmitter activity and balance.
- *Neurotransmitter imbalances*. The cerebrospinal fluid of many FMS patients has unusually high levels of two neurotransmitters: substance P and nerve growth factor. These substances are believed to stimulate nerve activity, cause vasodilation, and increase pain sensation. At the same time, FMS patients tend to have low levels of important inhibitory neurotransmitters, specifically norepinephrine and serotonin.
- *Tender points*. Many fibromyalgia patients eventually develop tender points that are distributed all over the body, but they are most numerous around the neck, shoulders, and low back (Figure 4.29). Tender points themselves are not well understood. Histological studies of affected tissue have yielded little useful information about how these areas develop. Tender points are unique indicators of fibromyalgia, but not all patients experience them as a leading symptom.

While FMS is not a life-threatening disease, it certainly threatens quality of life. The pain it causes is "invisible": it doesn't show on imaging tests, in blood analysis, or by visible signs. Doctors, employers, and even friends and family may easily dismiss a person with this syndrome as a faker or malingerer. By the time a patient has reached a definitive diagnosis, her experience with the medical community has often been frustrating and overwhelmingly negative. It is not surprising, then, that **anxiety** and **depression** are common complications of FMS.

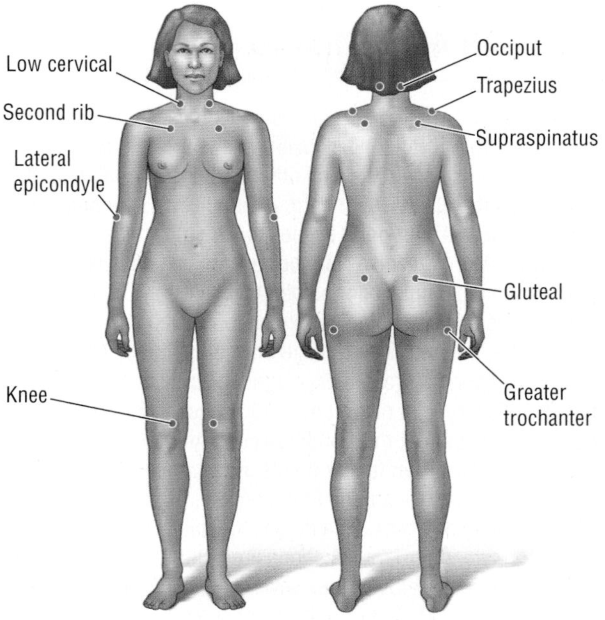

FIGURE 4.29 Tender point map: one feature of fibromyalgia

Signs and Symptoms

The signs and symptoms of FMS vary widely from one person to the next. Some of the most common indicators include the following:

- Stiffness after rest.
- Poor stamina.
- Fatigue.
- Memory problems and poor concentration; this is sometimes called "fibro fog."
- Widespread pain in shifting locations that is extremely difficult to pin down. The intensity of the pain can be inconsistent, and it can range from a deep ache to burning and tingling.
- Tender points. Nine predictable pairs of these are distributed among all quadrants of the body. Tender points are painful, and that pain may appear to be diffused around the area, but they do not refer pain to distant sites.
- Sensitivity amplification and low pain tolerance. All kinds of sensation become more intense and likely to cause pain. This includes light, sound, and smells but is true especially of cold, texture, and pressure.

Treatment

Treatment for FMS begins with a good diagnosis, which is a challenge (see Sidebar 4.18). This condition is typically diagnosed by ruling out other diseases with similar signs and symptoms, including **Lyme disease**, **multiple sclerosis**, **rheumatoid arthritis**, **lupus**, **hypothyroidism**, **candidiasis**, and several others. Several of these diagnostic differentials are also made by ruling out similar-looking conditions, and it is quite possible for a person to have more than one of these conditions at a time. Further, a long history of confusion between FMS tender points and **myofascial pain syndrome** (MPS) trigger points continues to cloud the issue. A side-by-side comparison of FMS and MPS is provided in the table in Compare & Contrast 4.1.

For most people, FMS is a lifelong condition, all though it often goes through phases of remission and relapse. Treatment focuses on finding ways to manage the disorder so that the patient may lead as normal a life as possible and so that the patient feels empowered to take control of his or her health rather than relying on other people. This includes patient education, lifestyle choices that include careful exercise, good diet and good quality sleep, and, for many, cognitive-behavioral therapy.

Drug therapies for FMS include mild antidepressants to reduce levels of depression, to manage pain, and to improve the quality of sleep. Painkilling drugs are generally avoided, because they interfere with sleep and can be habit forming. A line of antiseizure drugs has been successful with pain management without some of the side effects that these medications may involve.

Medications

- Analgesics, including NSAIDs (have varying effectiveness)
- Antidepressants to aid with sleep, pain, and mood
- Antiseizure drugs to help with pain
- Antiparkinsonian drugs

For more on the author's point of view about fibromyalgia syndrome, see the video at http://thePoint.lww.com/Werner6e. thePoint®

SIDEBAR 4.18 Diagnosing Fibromyalgia Syndrome

The history of FMS identification and diagnosis is long and confusing. This condition has been called myositis, fibromyositis, myofibrositis, and several other names. It wasn't until the mid-1980s that tissue biopsies revealed that no inflammation was present in tender point tissue, so the suffix "-itis" was a misnomer. More recently, histological studies of fascial wrappings around painful tender points do show signs of inflammation, so this understanding continues to evolve.

In 1990, the American College of Rheumatology (ACR) determined some fibromyalgia diagnostic criteria, including the identification of a minimum of 11 active tender points. As our understanding of this condition continued to progress, it has become clear that tender points are a common, but not universal, experience among FMS patients. Consequently, the ACR updated its fibromyalgia diagnostic guidelines in 2010, relying on two important questionnaires: the Widespread Pain Index (WPI) and the Symptom Severity Scale (SS). Because many specialists still refer to the 1990 criteria, both are provided here.

1990 Criteria:
- The patient reports chronic pain for a minimum of 3 months.
- The patient shows at least 11 of 18 mapped tender points to be active (i.e., significant diffuse pain with digital pressure of about 4 kg must be elicited).
- The active tender points are widely distributed, with some from each quadrant of the body.
- The patient reports persistent fatigue.
- The patient reports nonrefreshing sleep and awakens with morning stiffness.

2010 Criteria:
- WPI score of 7 or higher and SS score of 5 or higher
  - OR
- WPI of 3 to 6, SS of 9 or more, *and* pain pattern that persists for 3 months or more
  - AND
- Other possible sources of pain have been ruled out.

COMPARE & CONTRAST 4.1 Fibromyalgia versus Myofascial Pain Syndrome

Fibromyalgia and MPS are frequently confused. Because they call for quite different treatment options, it is important to be able to recognize both their similarities and their unique qualities.

CHARACTERISTICS	FIBROMYALGIA SYNDROME	MYOFASCIAL PAIN SYNDROME
Prevalence	Up to 3% of the US population	Unknown
Demographics	85%–90% of all diagnoses are in women.	Women and men are equally affected
Prognosis	Lifelong problem; can be managed	Can be a short-term problem that is permanently solved
Primary symptoms	Tender points: predictable areas; light touch elicits intense, diffuse pain at the site	Trigger points: predictable areas in muscles; may be nodular or appear as a taut band that generates a twitch response with pressure. Manual pressure elicits pain locally and at distant areas
Implications for massage	Careful massage can help, but patients are often hypersensitive and easy to overtreat.	Responds well to massage: rhythmic pressure and release can interrupt dysfunctional signals at trigger point sites

Massage Therapy Implications

RISKS	People with fibromyalgia live with chronic, invisible, widespread, and unpredictable pain. It is important that their pain not be exacerbated by massage that is insensitive or too aggressive.
BENEFITS	Massage has much to offer to fibromyalgia patients in terms of pain relief, sleep quality, improved mood, and reduced anxiety. Massage as part of an emphasis on good self-care is frequently part of a successful treatment strategy.
OPTIONS	Research suggests that while many kinds of massage improve fibromyalgia symptoms, lighter and gentler work is more effective than deeper, more intrusive types of bodywork, especially for clients new to massage.
RESEARCH	Some excellent research has been conducted to investigate the usefulness of massage therapy for FMS, using techniques including myofascial release, Swedish massage, shiatsu, vibration massage, and others. Castro-Sanchez et al.[1] looked at several variables and found that myofascial release was useful for pain, anxiety, and quality of life, and its impact on sleep lasted for several months. A systematic review[2] found modest support for massage in the context of FMS. This researcher also concluded that the best results were achieved when massage was painless and delivered 1 to 2 times per week. Kalichman's paper was supported by a 2014 systematic review[3] that concluded that when massage therapy was delivered for a minimum of 5 weeks, it shows beneficial effects on pain, anxiety, and depression.

1. Castro-Sanchez AM, Mataran-Penarrocha GA, Granero-Molina J, et al. Benefits of massage-myofascial release therapy on pain, anxiety, quality of sleep, depression, and quality of life in patients with fibromyalgia. *Evidence-Based Complementary and Alternative Medicine* 2011;2011:561753. http://www.ninds.nih.gov/disorders/spina_bifida/detail_spina_bifida.htm
2. Kalichman L. Massage therapy for fibromyalgia symptoms. *Rheumatology International* 2010;30(9):1151–1157. http://www.ncbi.nlm.nih.gov/pubmedhealth/PMH0029074/
3. Li YH, Wang FY, Feng CQ, et al. Massage therapy for fibromyalgia: a systematic review and meta-analysis of randomized controlled trials. *PLoS One* 2014;9(2):e89304. http://www.ncbi.nlm.nih.gov/pmc/articles/PMC3930706/

Headaches

Definition: What Are They?

Headaches are one of the most common physical problems in the range of human experience. Although they can be symptoms of other problems, most headaches are self-contained, temporary issues.

Many experts discuss headaches as primary or secondary issues. Primary headaches are unrelated to underlying pathology, while secondary headaches are symptoms of other problems, some of which may be serious.

The topic of headaches is enormous and could be an entire text in itself. What follows is a very brief overview of the most important concepts.

Demographics

About 90% of all people will have a headache at some point, and most of them will be tension-type headaches.

In this country, about 30 million people have at least 1 migraine each year; it is seen in 18% of all females and 6% of males. Migraines are most common in children and young adults; many people find that they subside by middle age, except for women in perimenopause.

Cluster headaches are rare, affecting less than 1% of the population. Men are much more at risk than women; about 80% of those diagnosed with cluster headaches are men.

Etiology: What Happens?

Headaches have been organized into dozens of subtypes of primary and secondary phenomena. Among primary headaches, some unifying features that are frequently observed include hypersensitivity among specific nerve pathways, irritability of the trigeminal nerve, and dilation of cranial blood vessels with subsequent edema, which also causes pain. A phenomenon called **cortical spreading depression** may be enlisted in this process: it is a wave of increased brain activity that usually begins in the occipital lobes and spreads anteriorly. Some research suggests that some headache patients don't go through the internal chemical reactions that would normally inhibit pain signals in the brain. The most important distinctions between types of headaches, therefore, may simply be the triggers and the presence or absence of a throbbing sensation.

> **Cortical spreading depression:** A wave of increased brain activity that usually begins in the occipital lobes and spreads anteriorly.

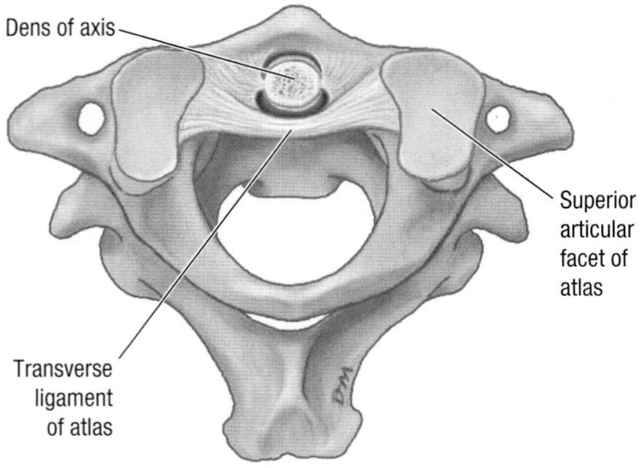

FIGURE 4.30 The cranium is balanced on the surface area of the superior articular facets of the atlas

Types of Primary Headaches

The International Headache Society (IHS) has created a comprehensive classification system for every type of headache on record. In it, they separate primary from secondary headaches, and within the primary headaches, they list tension-type, migraine, cluster headaches, and headache attributed to head and/or neck trauma. Several subtypes are listed under each heading, but an abbreviated description of the IHS classification system is this:

- *Tension-type headaches*: The average head weighs about 10 to 11 pounds, and the area of bone-to-bone contact between the occipital condyles and the facets of C_1 is about the same as two pairs of fingertips touching (Figure 4.30). The whole mechanism is kept in balance by tension exerted by muscles and ligaments around the neck and head. The muscles primarily responsible for the stability of the cranium are easily influenced by hypertonicity and postural problems, and they can entrap the occipital nerve (Figure 4.31). It

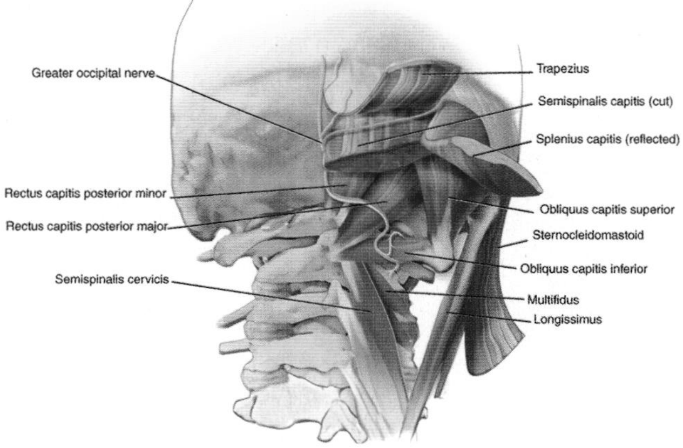

FIGURE 4.31 Imbalance in the muscles that help to stabilize the cranium, along with occipital nerve entrapment, can contribute to tension-type headaches

is not surprising, then, that when this delicate balance is a little off, the resulting pain reverberates throughout the whole structure.

Similarly, when postural or movement patterns elsewhere in the body exert force on the spine, the end result can be tension at the occipital connection. In this way, a foot that strikes the ground too hard on the lateral side may pull on the knee, which may then demand compensation in the hip. The sacrum moves to adjust to the tip in the os coxae. This creates a slight twist in the lumbar vertebrae, which reverberates all the way up the spine to the head. The result: headaches because the feet are not in alignment or shoes are worn down.

Tension-type headache triggers can include soft tissue injury, muscle tightness and trigger points, temporomandibular joint disorders, subluxation or misalignment of cervical vertebrae, eyestrain, poor ergonomics, and ongoing mental or emotional stress that exacerbates inefficient postural and movement patterns.

Tension-type headaches can be frequent or infrequent and episodic or chronic. They are often bilateral or nonfocused in area. Many patients describe a tight band around the head or a deep, dull ache rather than a precise focal point for pain.

- *Migraine headaches*: The word migraine originated from the Greek "hemikrania" to describe pain in one-half of the head. Migraine headaches, like tension-type headaches, involve hyperexcitability within pain-sensitive nerves of the cranium. When these nerves are irritated, a complex cascade of reactions occurs that lead to vasoconstriction followed by vasodilation. Common triggers include hormonal shifts with pregnancy or menstruation; food sensitivities, especially to red wine, aged cheese, and chocolate; excessive exercise; too much or too little sleep; and stress.

  Many subtypes of migraine have been identified, but the two most common are called migraine with aura (which accounts for about 20% of all diagnoses) and migraines without aura, which is much more common. Migraine with aura may involve blurred vision, the perception of flashing and jagged lights or auras, and auditory hallucinations.

  Migraines can occur in children, in whom they may not be immediately identifiable because the symptoms can be unpredictable. Symptoms of juvenile migraine range infantile colic, to feeling faint, to torticollis, to vomiting.

  Most adult migraine patients experience throbbing pain on one side of the head, which may cause the ipsilateral eye and nostril to water. Hypersensitivity to light and noise, along with nausea, and vomiting are common in this scenario. Some patients have tingling or other sensation changes in their extremities. Migraine pain can persist for several hours to several days.

  Migraines can have several important complications. They can become chronic, ongoing problems with long-term changes leading to central sensitization; they can trigger seizures (this is sometimes called migralepsy), and it is important to point out that people who have migraine with aura, especially women under 45, have an increased risk for stroke.
- *Cluster headaches*: These are a fairly rare, not well-understood variety of headache. Like migraines, they involve unilateral pain that can cause the eye and nostril of the affected side to water. They may also cause facial swelling and unilateral sweating. Each headache lasts a few moments to several hours, and in an episode, a person may have one to four headaches every day for 4 to 8 weeks. They may occur seasonally, once or twice in a year, or just once in a lifetime. Cluster headaches affect men much more often than women. They usually occur at night, with pain severe enough to wake a person out of a sound sleep. Unlike migraines, which tend to make patients want to rest in a dark quiet room, cluster headaches tend to cause restlessness; stillness seems to exacerbate the pain.
- *Rebound headaches*: The IHS classifies rebound or medicine-overuse headaches under the "headache due to neck or head trauma" section, because they are common in people who have preexisting tension-type headaches. They are related to increasing tolerance for headache medication, which means more painkiller is needed to achieve the same level of relief. Rebound headaches can be present on waking in the morning, and they can include nausea, anxiety, restlessness, and irritability. The only way to eradicate them is to stop taking headache medication altogether, which can be a daunting prospect.

Types of Secondary Headaches

Secondary headaches are symptoms of underlying pathologies that can range from a mild fever with cold or flu to a stroke, brain injury, or tumor. Symptoms indicate a serious underlying condition when headaches are severe and repeating and have a sudden onset ("thunderclap headache"), when they appear in a new pattern after age 50, or when they have a gradual onset but no remission. This is true particularly if the headache is accompanied by slurred speech, numbness anywhere in the body, and difficulties with motor control: any of these signs indicate a medical emergency. The first things to investigate in cases like this are **encephalitis**, **meningitis**, **stroke**, tumor, or **aneurysm**.

Signs and Symptoms

The signs and symptoms of headaches are self-evident, but they may have specific characteristics in terms of location, triggers, duration, severity, and frequency, as discussed above.

Treatment

Occasional headaches respond well to rest and NSAIDs, but if they are a recurring problem, then avoiding or managing headache triggers is the most proactive and least invasive solution. People who have recurrent headaches of any type are often encouraged to keep a headache journal to try to pin down specific triggers.

Medication for headaches falls into two categories: prophylactic treatment, which works to prevent the headache from beginning, and abortive treatment, which works to end the headache once it has begun.

Prophylactic Medications

- NSAIDs
- Beta-blockers and calcium channel blockers
- Antidepressants, including tricyclics and SSRIs
- Serotonin (5 HT1) agonists (triptans)
- Antiseizure medications
- Injections of botulinum toxin

Abortive Medications

- Serotonin (5 HT1) agonists (triptans)
- Ergot alkaloids
- Analgesics
- NSAIDs
- Antiemetics to manage nausea

Massage Therapy Implications

RISKS	Any headache that is accompanied by fever, confusion, numbness, or other CNS signs contraindicates massage and may be a medical emergency. Many migraine or cluster headache patients don't seek massage until after the pain has subsided, because the experience just doesn't seem appealing.
BENEFITS	Tension-type headaches indicate massage, which can help to address the musculoskeletal and stress-related holding patterns that contribute to inefficient movement and pain.
OPTIONS	It is important to be cognizant of all the factors that can contribute to headaches, including distortions that may occur far away from the head. Massage therapists are in a better position than many care providers to untangle the clues that can lead to long-term improvement.
RESEARCH	A study comparing traditional Thai massage to sham ultrasound for TTH and migraine patients found that both groups had improvement, but the massaged subjects had much more improvement in their pressure pain threshold.[1] Cervicogenic headache is a subtype of headache involving restricted ROM; researchers found that soft tissue massage to the upper cervical muscles led to improved range of motion that persisted after the sessions had completed.[2] Another study of cervicogenic headache compared massage therapy to spinal manipulation. Both groups had improvement for intensity, duration, and frequency of headaches, but the manipulation group had better responses for every score except the functional Neck Disability Index, in which the massage therapy subjects fared better.[3] Massage therapy appears to be useful for migraines, when subjects are able to receive it: a study found that cervical and upper thoracic massage plus spinal manipulation reduced migraine pain intensity by almost 69%.[4] Moraska and Chandler[5] determined that massage therapy was helpful in lowering various stress and anxiety scores for subjects with chronic headaches; this is helpful to know for people in chronic pain in general. 1. Chatchawan U, Eungpinichpong W, Sooktho S, et al. Effects of Thai traditional massage on pressure pain threshold and headache intensity in patients with chronic tension-type and migraine headaches. *Journal of Alternative and Complementary Medicine* 2014;20(6):486–492. http://www.ncbi.nlm.nih.gov/pubmed/24738648 2. Hopper D, Bajaj Y, Kei Choi C, et al. A pilot study to investigate the short-term effects of specific soft tissue massage on upper cervical movement impairment in patients with cervicogenic headache. *Journal of Manual and Manipulative Therapy* 2013;21(1):18–23. http://www.ncbi.nlm.nih.gov/pmc/articles/PMC3578191/ 3. Youssef EF, Shanb AS. Mobilization versus massage therapy in the treatment of cervicogenic headache: a clinical study. *Journal of Back and Musculoskeletal Rehabilitation* 2013;26(1):17–24. http://www.ncbi.nlm.nih.gov/pubmed/23411644 4. Noudeh YJ, Vatankhah N, Baradaran HR. Reduction of current migraine headache pain following neck massage and spinal manipulation. *International Journal of Therapeutic Massage and Bodywork* 2012;5(1):5–13. http://www.ncbi.nlm.nih.gov/pmc/articles/PMC3312646/ 5. Moraska A, Chandler C. Changes in psychological parameters in patients with tension-type headache following massage therapy: a pilot study. *Journal of Manual and Manipulative Therapy* 2009;17(2):86–94. http://www.ncbi.nlm.nih.gov/pmc/articles/PMC2700492/

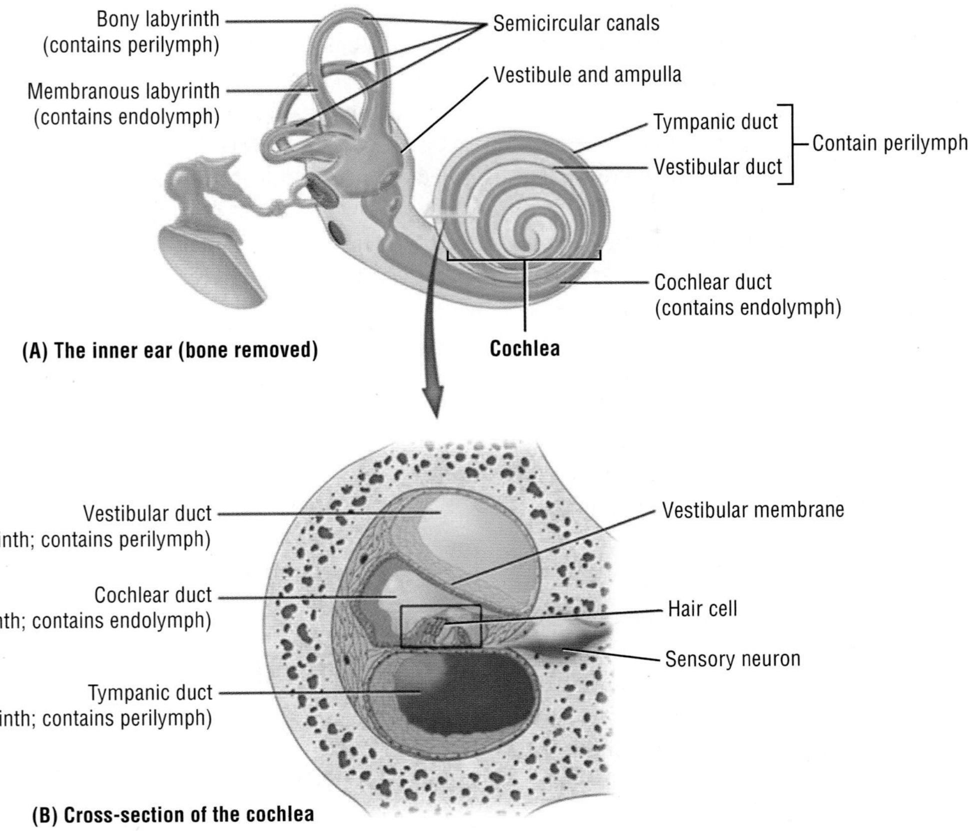

FIGURE 4.32 **A:** Inner ear: *yellow area* is the bony labyrinth, containing perilymph; *green area* is the membranous labyrinth, containing endolymph. It is important that these do not mix. **B:** Inside the cochlea, the hair cells are suspended in endolymph.

Ménière Disease

Definition: What Is It?

Ménière disease is a group of signs and symptoms that center on inner ear dysfunction, leading to **vertigo**, **tinnitus**, and hearing loss. It was first described and documented by French physician Prosper Ménière in 1861.

Demographics

This is a surprisingly common condition; about 615,000 people in the United States have it, and an additional 45,500 are diagnosed each year. Most new diagnoses are in people between 40 and 60 years old.

Etiology: What Happens?

The inner ear is composed of several structures that conduct sound and provide a sense of position in relation to gravity. The **bony labyrinth** forms the semicircular ducts leading to the **ampulla**, the **vestibule**, and the snail-shaped **cochlea**. The bony labyrinth is filled with a sodium-rich fluid called **perilymph**. Inside the bony labyrinth, the **membranous labyrinth** floats in the perilymph. The membranous labyrinth is filled with a potassium-rich fluid called **endolymph** (Figure 4.32). Together, the endolymph and perilymph, separated by the membranous labyrinth, help to conduct sound vibrations.

Nerve endings from the vestibulocochlear nerve begin in the ampulla, an enlarged space where the semicircular canals converge. These nerve projections, call hair cells, are suspended in endolymph and move like seaweed in water whenever the head changes position. Signals from the

Vertigo: A sensation of being spun around.
Tinnitus: Ringing in the ears.
Bony labyrinth: The rigid outer wall of the inner ear.
Ampulla: The dilated end of a duct
Vestibule: The central part of the bony labyrinth of the ear.
Cochlea: The coiled part of the inner ear where sound is converted into nerve impulses.
Perilymph: The fluid surrounding the membranous labyrinth of the ear.
Membranous labyrinth: An organ of the ear lying within the bony labyrinth. Filled with endolymph.
Endolymph: The fluid filling the membranous labyrinth of the ear.

vestibulocochlear nerve coordinate with the eyes and proprioceptors throughout the body to help orient us in space.

The exact causes or sequence of events that lead to Ménière disease are not well understood. Most specialists agree that it has to do with the accumulation of excess endolymph inside the membranous labyrinth. This is called **idiopathic endolymphatic hydrops**. Possible factors include allergic reactions, head trauma, genetic predisposition, autoimmune activity, or viral infection. Swelling causes the membranous labyrinth to rupture, which allows the endolymph and perilymph to mix. This abnormal mixture of fluids causes the nerve endings of the vestibulocochlear nerve to misfire, sending incorrect messages about our position in space: this leads to sudden and severe vertigo. In addition, the distension of the membranous labyrinth can cause changes to hearing; this may account for loss of hearing and tinnitus.

Signs and Symptoms

Ménière disease has four classic symptoms, all of which appear intermittently and in any combination. It usually affects only one ear, but it can progress to affect the other ear as well. Onset of an episode is typically fast and unpredictable, and any given attack can last 20 minutes to 24 hours. Many patients find that their symptoms fluctuate in frequency, duration, and severity.

- *Hearing loss*. Hearing loss typically involves low-frequency sound. It is worst during flares, but eventually becomes permanent.
- *Tinnitus*. Patients often describe noise like a million crickets or like the whine of a jet engine. It can feel loud enough to interfere with the ability to sleep or concentrate.
- *Aural fullness*. A feeling of fullness or pressure in the middle ear (similar to the sense of descent in an airplane) may come and go.
- *Rotational vertigo*. This may be the most disabling symptom of Ménière disease: the person perceives that the world is spinning, or the floor is sloping. **Nystagmus** (an abnormal rhythmic oscillation of the eyes) is observed as well. Nausea and vomiting are common results. This can last for several minutes or hours and is aggravated by any movement of the head.

Treatment

Because Ménière disease is an idiopathic condition, treatment options focus on symptomatic control. Some patients are able to identify triggers that increase their risk of having an episode. Many people are counseled to avoid foods and habits that raise blood pressure and increase fluid retention. A low-salt diet, avoiding monosodium glutamate, limiting caffeine and alcohol, and quitting smoking are usually recommended as early interventions. Medications to manage vertigo and nausea may be prescribed.

If diet and medications are unsuccessful, some patients explore more intrusive options to interfere with the sensation of vertigo. This can be accomplished by essentially disabling the vestibulocochlear nerve and relying on the unaffected side to compensate for the lost function. This is an option only when Ménière disease has not progressed to affect the contralateral side.

Idiopathic endolymphatic hydrops: The accumulation of excess endolymph inside the membranous labyrinth.

Nystagmus: Abnormal involuntary eye movements.

Medications

- Antiemetics for nausea control
- Steroidal anti-inflammatories
- Diuretics
- Antihistamines
- Anticholinergics to suppress nerve activity
- Benzodiazepines for vertigo and nausea

Massage Therapy Implications

RISKS	Massage has no specific risks for clients with Ménière disease, as long as they are comfortable getting on and off a table, and lying down. Clients may appreciate a massage chair instead of a table. Any bodywork that exacerbates symptoms must be avoided, of course.
BENEFITS	Ménière disease is an extremely stressful condition, with sudden, unpredictable episodes of debilitating vertigo, and other symptoms that radically interfere with quality of life. While massage therapy is unlikely to improve Ménière disease, it may address some of the anxiety of a person who lives with it, as long as he or she is comfortable receiving bodywork.

Seizure Disorders

Definition: What Are They?

A seizure disorder is any kind of problem that causes seizures. Epilepsy is a subtype of seizure disorders. Epilepsy is one of the oldest conditions recorded in medical history. It was first described about 2,000 years BCE, but it was not studied as a specific problem other than "demonic possession" until the mid-19th century.

Demographics

Many people have seizures, but not all of them have epilepsy.

It is estimated that 2.3 million adults and 447,000 children in the United States have epilepsy. About 150,000 new diagnoses are made each year.

Etiology: What Happens?

When interconnecting neurons in the brain are stimulated in a certain way, a tremendous burst of excess electricity may stimulate the neighboring neurons. The reaction is repeated, and soon millions of neurons in the brain are giving off electrical discharge. This is the CNS "lightning storm" of a seizure, and it affects the rest of the body in a number of ways.

Seizure triggers vary from person to person. They can include sudden changes in light levels; flashing, flickering, or strobe lights, or the effect created by a ceiling fan or the sun shining through moving leaves; watching television or playing video games; certain sounds; or even particular notes of music. Anxiety, sleep deprivation, hormonal changes, and fever can also lead to seizures.

Whatever the trigger, the result is uncoordinated neuronal activity that allows electrical signals to become increasingly extreme, sometimes to the point of collapse and loss of consciousness. Some seizures are linked to underactive inhibitory neurotransmitters, overactive excitatory neurotransmitters, or both. The permeability of nerve cell membranes may also be a factor, as this has influence on the speed and strength of electrical signals.

In some cases, the cause of seizures can be definitively linked to a mechanical or chemical problem in the brain. Birth trauma, **traumatic brain injury**, **stroke**, and brain tumors can all cause repeating seizures, as can exposure to some toxins (lead, carbon monoxide, and others), and extreme hypotension or hemorrhage. **Alzheimer disease** is a leading cause of seizures among the elderly.

Other conditions can cause nonepileptic seizures that don't involve the same "lightning storm" of activity in the brain. These situations can include extreme hypotension or hemorrhage, hypoglycemia, drug and anesthetic reactions, and some other medical emergencies.

Febrile seizures are a common childhood event that can be triggered by fever related to an upper respiratory infection, ear infections, and other mild problems. Most of these events are uncomplicated. A child with a more serious infection can also have more serious seizures, and these children may have a substantially increased risk for epilepsy.

A person with a history of simple febrile seizures has a slightly higher chance of developing epilepsy than the rest of the population.

Febrile seizure: Seizures brought on by sudden increase in body temperature. Most common in infants and young children.

Types of Seizure Disorders

- *Epilepsy*: This is identified as a diagnosis when a person has two or more nonfebrile seizures, at least 24 hours apart. Seizures can take several forms.

Signs and Symptoms

Seizures take very different forms in each person they affect. More than 30 classes of seizures have been identified, according to the parts of the brain they affect. Generalized seizures affect the whole brain, while partial seizures involve abnormal activity in isolated areas. The most common types of seizures are described here.

Partial seizures These seizures involve abnormal activity only in isolated areas. The motor cortex and the temporal lobes are the sites most often affected. Partial seizures can sometimes spread throughout the brain to become generalized. Partial seizures come in two subtypes:

NOTABLE CASES Russian novelist Fyodor Dostoyevsky had epilepsy and used his experience in the development of various characters. Actor Danny Glover, musician Neil Young, and track and field athlete Florence Griffith Joyner were all diagnosed with epilepsy. "Flo-Jo" died in 1998 when she asphyxiated during a tonic-clonic seizure in her sleep.

- *Simple partial seizures*. In this type of seizure, the patient doesn't lose consciousness. He or she may become weak or numb, may smell or taste things that aren't present, and may have some changes in vision or temporary vertigo along with some muscular tics or twitching.
- *Complex partial seizures*. This type of seizure is specifically associated with temporal lobe dysfunction. The patient may exhibit repetitive behaviors such as pacing in a circle, rocking, or smacking the lips. He or she may laugh uncontrollably or experience fear. Visual and olfactory hallucinations are other symptoms of complex partial seizures.

Generalized seizures. These seizures involve electrical signals that occur all over the brain. They may be very subtle or dramatic. These are the major types:

- *Absence seizures*: These involve very short episodes of loss of consciousness. The patient may simply "check out" for 5 to 10 seconds and have no memory of the lapse.
- *Clonic seizures*: These consist of jerking movements with or without loss of consciousness in both upper and lower extremities.
- *Tonic seizures*: These show a sudden onset of tight muscles leading to flexion of the head, trunk, and extremities for several seconds.

- *Tonic-clonic seizures*: These are what have traditionally been called grand mal seizures. They involve uncontrolled movement of the face, arms, and legs followed by loss of consciousness, loss of bladder control, and loss of all muscle tone. Events may last for 5 to 20 minutes, and the patient is usually tired and disoriented after an episode.
- *Myoclonic seizures*: These involve bilateral muscular jerking, which may be very pronounced or almost unnoticeable. They are usually seen among very young patients.
- *Atonic seizures*: These involve a brief but complete loss in muscle tone, leading to falls and a risk of injury.
- *Status epilepticus*: These are a life-threatening variation of tonic-clonic seizures; they last for a long period and can put such a strain on the body that they can cause brain damage or death. Status epilepticus, or static seizures, are a medical emergency.

Treatment

Seizures are treated with antiseizure medication, which acts to make neurons in the brain harder to stimulate. It can be difficult to find the right dosage of these powerful medications, and while most patients can find a strategy that works for them, some patients don't tolerate them well. It is important to try to treat and prevent seizures, because they can cumulatively change cardiovascular autonomic reflexes: in other words, it can become progressively more difficult for a person with seizures to maintain appropriate heart rate and blood pressure. Failure to treat this successfully may lead to a complication called SUDEP: sudden unexplained death in epilepsy.

Some epilepsy patients find that their seizures are less frequent and less extreme when they follow a strict high-fat, low-fiber **ketogenic** diet.

Surgical intervention for seizure disorders is reserved for when an isolated and expendable mass (i.e., a tumor or clump of scar tissue) can be determined to be the cause of the seizures. Some patients with tonic-clonic seizures can control them when their corpus callosum is severed.

One device that is successful for some patients for whom medications don't work is a vagus nerve stimulator. This mechanism is implanted in the vagus nerves in the neck and sends pulses of electrical stimulation to the vagus nerve. It is believed that stimulating the vagus nerve in this way helps to activate some of the inhibitory neurotransmitters that seizure disorder patients lack.

Medications

- Antiseizure drugs
- Barbiturates and tranquilizers

Ketogenic: Giving rise to ketones in the metabolism.

Massage Therapy Implications

RISKS	It is inappropriate to try to massage someone who is in the midst of a seizure of any kind, and it is important to try to minimize the chances of triggering a seizure for clients who know they are vulnerable. This may mean adjusting lighting, turning off a ceiling fan, or being careful what kinds of scents or music are present in the treatment room. It is wise to discuss ahead of time how a client with seizure disorders would like an episode to be managed. Antiseizure medication may make a client feel fatigued or dizzy; massage must accommodate for that, with extra time to recover, or stimulating strokes to finish, or both.
BENEFITS	While massage is unlikely to change the course or prognosis for a client with a seizure disorder, bodywork can certainly add to his or her quality of life. Someone recovering from a tonic-clonic seizure is likely to be sore and may have soft tissue injuries that massage can help to address.
OPTIONS	Antiseizure medication may make a client feel fatigued or dizzy; massage must accommodate for that, with extra time to recover, or stimulating strokes to finish, or both.
RESEARCH	Not much evidence has been accrued about massage therapy for seizures, but one study looked at 77 participants who were not candidates for surgery and who were not responsive to antiepileptic drugs. One group continued with their drugs (treatment as usual), and the other got their drugs and reflexology treatments to the hands and feet. In the massaged group, median baseline seizure frequency decreased from 9.5 to 2. There was a decrease in the medicated group, but it was a fraction of what was seen with the massaged group.[1] 1. Dalal K, Devarajan E, Pandey RM, et al. Role of reflexology and antiepileptic drugs in managing intractable epilepsy—a randomized controlled trial. *Forschende Komplementarmedizin (2006)* 2013;20(2):104–111. http://www.ncbi.nlm.nih.gov/pubmed/23636029

Sleep Disorders

Definition: What Are They?

Sleep disorders are any disorders that interfere with the ability to fall asleep, to stay asleep, or to wake up feeling refreshed. More than 70 sleep disorders have been defined, and DSM-5 has recently reclassified several to reflect how often sleep disorders are stand-alone problems that need to be addressed specifically rather than as an add-on to other problem.

This discussion covers the disorders that massage therapists are most likely to see: insomnia, types of sleep apnea, circadian rhythm disruption, restless leg syndrome, and narcolepsy.

Demographics

About 30% of the population complains about inadequate or nonrestorative sleep, and about 10% have symptoms of daytime limitations because of it. Sleep disorders become more severe with age, especially when overlapping health concerns interrupt normal sleep patterns.

Etiology: What Happens?

The need for sleep is determined partly by the accumulation of metabolic byproducts in the blood and by the hormone **melatonin**, a secretion of the pineal gland, deep within the brain. Melatonin contributes to a feeling of drowsiness. A standard rotation of wakefulness and sleepiness usually runs on a 24- to 25-hour cycle called the **circadian rhythm**. Most healthy adults sleep about 8 to 8.5 hours per night, if not interrupted by an alarm clock or other disruption.

Chronic sleep deprivation can lead to a multitude of short-term and long-term problems, including higher pain sensitivity, slowed reflexes, lower cognitive skills, poor immune system efficiency, **fibromyalgia syndrome**, **depression**, hallucinations, and psychosis. Poor sleep is now linked to weight gain, high blood sugar, and an elevated risk of developing heart disease and type 2 **diabetes**. Sleep apnea is associated with an increased risk for **stroke**. Drowsy driving now rivals drunk driving for causes of motor vehicle accidents. In addition, fatigue and sleep deprivation contribute dangerously to on-the-job injuries that affect not only the sleep-deprived person but many others as well.

Melatonin: A hormone secreted by the pineal gland that is associated with cycles of sleeping and waking.
Hypnic myoclonia: A muscular jerk experienced at the onset of sleep that may replicate the feeling of falling.
Parasomnia: Disruption of the sleep cycle.
Dyssomnia: A category including sleep disorders that involve difficulty falling asleep or remaining asleep.

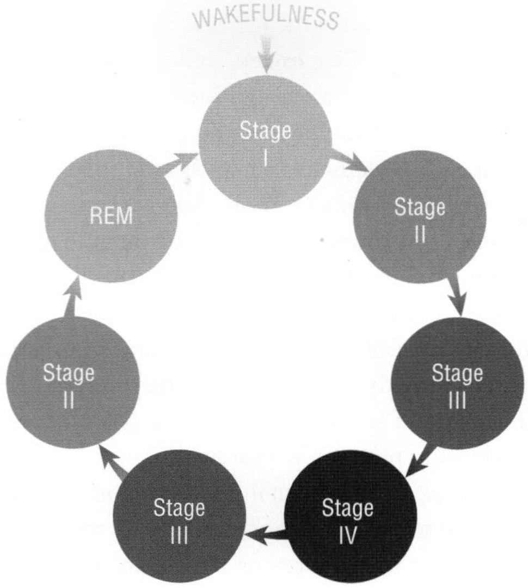

FIGURE 4.33 Sleep cycle

Stages of Sleep

Sleep occurs in five distinct phases or stages:

- *Stage I*. In this light sleep, a person is easily wakened. Eye movement is slow. A phenomenon called **hypnic myoclonia** sometimes occurs in this stage.
- *Stage II*. The eyes stop moving. Brain waves slow down but still show occasional bursts of activity called sleep spindles.
- *Stage III*. Brain waves are much slower. A deep-sleep pattern called delta waves is intermixed with slightly faster brain waves during this stage.
- *Stage IV*. Only delta waves are emitted from the brain. The body secretes growth hormone that enables new growth for children and adolescents and repair and regeneration for adults during this stage.
- *REM sleep*. In REM (rapid eye movement), sleep breathing is rapid, shallow, and irregular. Eyes move quickly, but muscular activity in the limbs is usually absent. Heart rate and blood pressure approach waking levels. REM sleep is the stage in which dreams occur.

During normal sleep, a person cycles through each of the five stages and back again (Figure 4.33). It takes about 90 to 100 minutes to complete a sleep cycle, although the amount of time spent in each stage varies according to the time of night. Overall, a healthy, organized sleep session allows an adult to spend 20% to 25% of his time in REM sleep, 50% of his time in stage II, and 30% of his time in the other stages.

Types of Sleep Disorders

Sleep disorders are loosely classified as **parasomnias** and **dyssomnias**. Parasomnias include night terrors, sleep talking, and sleepwalking; they won't be discussed here. The most common dyssomnias among adults are the following:

- *Insomnia*: Literally, this means lack of sleep. Insomnia can involve difficulty falling asleep, difficulty staying asleep, or difficulty sleeping long enough for the body to get the rest it needs. Insomnia can be transient, in which case it occurs for less than 4 weeks at a time, or chronic, in which a person can't sleep most nights for more than a month at a time.

  Transient insomnia is usually attributable to habits or environmental issues that are controllable. Caffeine taken too close to bedtime, alcohol, and some medications, including diet pills, antihistamines, and antidepressants, can interfere with sleep or reduce the time spent in REM stage. Cigarette smoking can cause a person to wake up too early from nicotine withdrawal.

  Unhelpful environmental conditions include having a room that is too cold, too hot, too loud, or too light; having a bed partner who snores or moves around a lot in the night; exercising too late in the day; or not exercising at all.

  Emotional stress is of course another major contributor to sleep loss. Ironically, the longer a person lies in bed feeling the need to sleep, the less likely he or she is to drop off: the stress of be impatient for sleep ensures that it doesn't come.

  Chronic insomnia is usually examined as a sign of a medical or psychological problem. **Hyperthyroidism**, fibromyalgia, depression, **kidney failure**, heart problems, and **chronic fatigue syndrome** are all possible factors when a person doesn't sleep well or long enough.
- *Sleep apneas*:
  - *Obstructive sleep apnea or hypopnea* is a mechanical problem in which the air passage collapses when muscles relax, so that oxygen cannot enter during inhalation (Figure 4.34). When oxygen levels fall sufficiently, muscles tighten slightly, and air reenters the passageway with a loud snort or gasp. Repeated episodes may occur dozens or even hundreds of time each night. People with obstructive sleep apnea tend to have excessive daytime sleepiness and morning headache from oxygen deprivation.
  - *Central sleep apnea* is a neurologic problem involving decreased respiratory drive. A rise in carbon dioxide in the blood is the signal to waken and breathe again. In some extreme cases, central sleep apnea has caused brain damage or even death from respiratory arrest during sleep. This condition is often linked to heart disease.
- *Circadian rhythm sleep-wake disorders*: The circadian rhythm is the normal cycle of drowsiness and wakefulness that all humans experience. Most people run through this cycle every 24 to 25 hours. They feel drowsy as the sun goes down and wider awake as it rises. When people are forced to be physically or mentally active in a different cycle, their circadian rhythms are disrupted and the quality of their sleep, as well as the quality of their waking hours, is compromised.

  Circadian rhythm disruption can occur in response to variable shift work, losing a night's sleep, or changing time zones through travel. Short-term difficulties associated with this problem are excessive sleepiness along with the degenerating reflexes and mental functioning that accompany exhaustion. Longer-term problems can include depression and other physical and psychological disorders brought about by sleep deprivation.
- *Restless leg syndrome* often runs in families, and it can also be associated with several other conditions, including **pregnancy**, **diabetes**, **anemia**, **fibromyalgia**, and **ADHD**. It involves a constant crawling, prickling, and tingling sensation in the extremities, especially the legs, that is relieved only by rubbing and movement. It is closely related to another disorder called **periodic limb movement disorder**. Although restless leg syndrome is present at all times, its symptoms are most pronounced when a person lies still in an effort to sleep. It is relieved by movement, massaging the affected areas, or warm baths. Symptoms tend to subside in the morning.
- *Narcolepsy*: This chronic neurological dysfunction gets its name from the Greek *narco* for stupor and *lepsis* for seizure. It involves unpredictable "sleep attacks" at inappropriate times, often in response to intense emotional reactions such as laughing or anger.

  One identified contributor to narcolepsy is a deficiency of **hypocretin**: a neurotransmitter that promotes

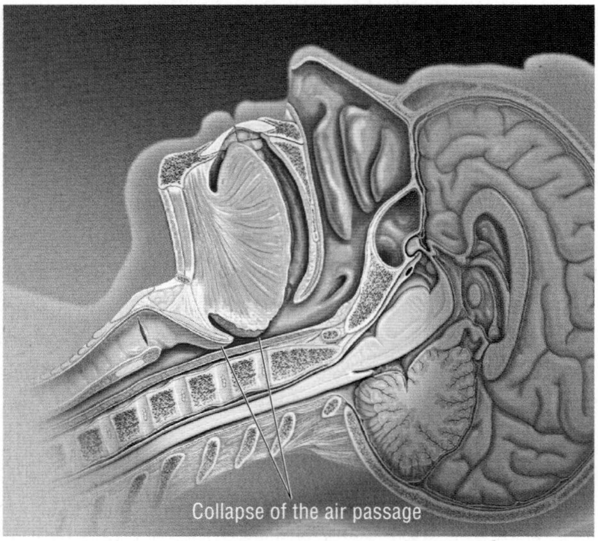

FIGURE 4.34 Obstructive sleep apnea: notice where the air passages collapse

Circadian rhythm disruption: A disruption of the biological 24 hour cycles that occur within the body.

Periodic limb movement disorder: A disorder characterized by problematic episodes of limb movements during sleep.

Hypocretin: A neurotransmitter produced by the hypothalamus that regulates wakefulness and appetite. Also called orexin.

wakefulness. Some patients have fewer hypocretin-producing cells, and this may lead to "sleep attacks." This can occur as a genetic problem, or autoimmune dysfunction.

Narcolepsy has three basic symptoms, which can appear in any combination for a positive diagnosis. **Cataplexy** refers to a sudden loss of muscle tone, even during waking hours. These events can last anywhere from several seconds to 30 minutes. Sleep paralysis is a phenomenon in which a person temporarily cannot speak or move while dozing. **Hypnagogic hallucinations** occur while drifting off to sleep. Narcolepsy patients don't sleep any more than others, but they often have poor nighttime sleep, which adds to a general problem with drowsiness during the day.

Signs and Symptoms

The primary sign of a sleep disorder is excessive daytime sleepiness. Chronic sleep deprivation can also cause irritability, decreased ability to focus or concentrate, mood changes, and poor short-term memory. Other symptoms are associated with specific disorders, as described above.

Treatment

Cases of transient insomnia are treated with lifestyle changes that better support healthy sleep, including changes in diet and exercise habits, quitting smoking, adjusting temperature or sound levels in the bedroom, or other simple interventions.

The active ingredient in many over-the-counter sleep aids is usually an antihistamine, which has a diminishing effect over time. Prescription sleep aids can be helpful for short periods, but several of them are habit forming, so short-term use to reestablish a healthy sleep cycle is the preferred strategy.

Sleep apnea can be treated in a variety of ways. A mask to provide oxygen or continuous positive airway pressure (CPAP) may be used, or surgery to keep airways open may be conducted. Apnea patients should not sleep on their back, and if they are overweight, they should work to lose weight and reduce their risk of apnea complications. It is especially important that sleep apnea patients not drink alcohol or use sleep aids at night; these substances may interfere with their already challenged breathing mechanisms.

Restless leg syndrome is believed to be associated with dopamine deficiencies in certain brain areas. It is managed with dopamine agents, tranquilizers, and, for very extreme cases, opioids and anticonvulsants. Less severe cases of restless leg syndrome can be managed with mild exercise, warm baths, and massage.

Narcolepsy is treatable with some medications and increasing exercise, which has been seen to reduce the number of sleep attacks.

Cataplexy: A transient attack of extreme generalized muscular weakness, often precipitated by an emotional reaction or surprise.

Hypnagogic hallucinations: Vivid hallucinations that occur while transitioning from wakefulness to sleep or vice versa.

Polysomnography: Continuous monitoring of physiological functioning during sleep.

Medications

- Over-the-counter sleep aids
- Benzodiazepines
- Nonbenzodiazepines
- Antianxiety medications
- Antidepressants
- Barbiturates (rarely)
- Parkinson drugs for restless leg syndrome
- Stimulants and depressants for narcolepsy

Massage Therapy Implications

RISKS	Massage has no particular risk for clients with sleep disorders.
BENEFITS	Massage has been shown to assist people who are anxious or in pain to get to sleep and to increase the amount of time spent in deep sleep. In addition, a massage therapist may be able to identify the risk of obstructive sleep apnea through the characteristic lack of breath followed by a gasping snore pattern in dozing clients.
RESEARCH	Massage has been well demonstrated to help with sleep in the context of many underlying conditions like cancer, chronic pain, and fibromyalgia. A pilot study with postmenopausal women complaining specifically of insomnia found that those who got massage fell asleep faster and they reported feeling better on awakening. **Polysomnography** also showed that they spent more time in stages 3 and 4.[2] This is consistent with findings on massage therapy for sleep quality in other settings as well. A case report on a person with narcolepsy used several self-measuring devices for quality of sleep and found that massage made a very substantial difference for this client, who received one 45-minute session once a week.[2] 1. Oliveira D, Hachul H, Tufik S, et al. Effect of massage in postmenopausal women with insomnia: a pilot study. *Clinics (Sao Paulo)* 2011;66(2):343–346. http://www.ncbi.nlm.nih.gov/pmc/articles/PMC3059875/ 2. Hill R, Baskwill A. Positive effects of massage therapy on a patient with narcolepsy. *International Journal of Therapeutic Massage and Bodywork* 2013;6(2):24–28. http://ijtmb.org/index.php/ijtmb/article/view/205/256

Vestibular Balance Disorders

Definition: What Are They?

Vestibular balance disorders (VBDs) are a group of conditions that can cause the vestibular branch of cranial nerve VIII to dysfunction, leading to debilitating vertigo that may last anywhere from a few seconds to many hours.

Demographics

The prevalence of balance disorders in the general population isn't known, but it is estimated that 12.5 million Americans over 65 live with balance problems that limit their activity. This is especially significant, given that about one quarter of all seniors will have a fall at some point, and the risk of injury or accidental death from balance-related falls is high.

Etiology: What Happens?

The vestibulocochlear nerve (CN VIII) begins in the inner ear in two segments, each of which takes sensation to the brain for interpretation. The cochlear branch begins in the cochlea, where sound vibrations are transmitted: it is solely dedicated to hearing. The vestibular branch relays information about balance and orientation. It begins in the vestibule, an area of the inner ear where the semicircular canals converge. Vestibular nerve endings are like tiny hairs suspended in masses of jelly called **cupulae**, and they sway like seaweed whenever the head moves or tilts in any direction (Figure 4.35). This information, when correlated with sensation from the eyes and general proprioceptors all over the body, provides our sense of position in relation to gravity and the horizon.

Changes in the vestibule or other problems with the vestibular branch of CN VIII can lead to vertigo: a sensation of uncontrollable spinning. These changes can be related to fluid pressure as seen with **Ménière disease**, which is discussed elsewhere, or to inflammation, injury, calcium deposits that fall out of place, or other factors.

Less common causes of VBDs focus on the CNS. These include **stroke**, **tumors**, **multiple sclerosis**, **aneurysm**, or **migraine headaches**. **Allergies** that block the eustachian tubes can interfere with fluid in the inner ear. Drugs, including alcohol, barbiturates, antihypertensives, diuretics, and cocaine, can also cause vertigo.

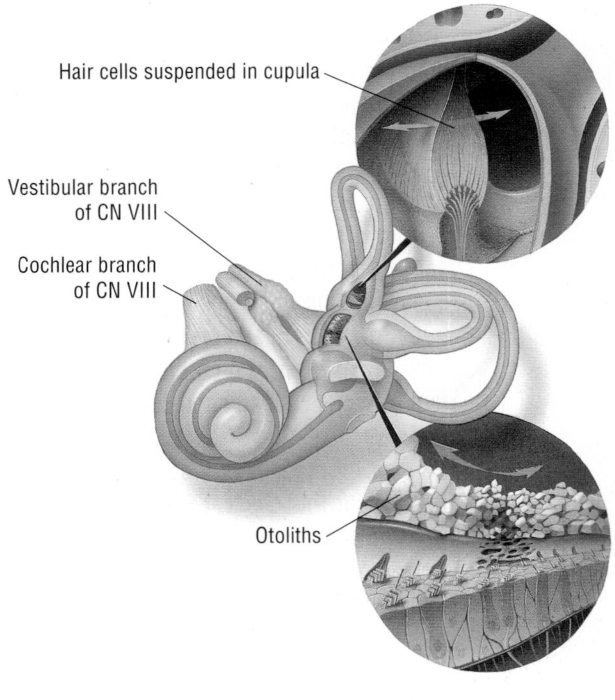

FIGURE 4.35 Hair cells and otoliths in the inner ear

Types of Vestibular Balance Disorders

- *Benign paroxysmal positional vertigo* (BPPV): In this common condition, small grains of calcium called **otoliths** that are normally located on the cupulae are displaced into the semicircular canals. This causes a sudden onset of extreme vertigo that may last a few seconds to a few minutes. Special maneuvers of the head allow the otoliths to move back into the vestibule. *To see a patient with BPPV receiving one of these maneuvers from a doctor, view the video "Vestibular Balance," available at* http://thePoint.lww.com/Werner6e. thePoint®
- *Labyrinthitis*: This is inflammation within the bony or membranous labyrinth. It is usually related to a self-limiting viral infection, sometimes with **herpes zoster**. This condition typically lasts a few days or weeks and then gradually subsides.
- *Acute vestibular neuronitis*: This is inflammation of the vestibular portion of CN VIII. If the cochlear branch is affected, hearing loss may develop along with vertigo. This can be a complication of a viral or bacterial infection or of autoimmune activity.
- *Perilymph fistula*: Blows to the head, violent sneezing, or whiplash-type accidents can cause inner ear fluid to leak into the middle ear in a condition called perilymph fistula. This can also occur while scuba diving, when it is a part of **barotrauma**.

Cupula: The gelatinous mass inside the ampulla that senses spatial orientation. (Plural: cupulae)

Otolith: A tiny ear stone of hardened material found in the vestibule of the inner ear.

Barotrauma: An injury to the inner ear resulting from rapid changes in pressure. Most often seen in scuba divers.

Signs and Symptoms

VBDs cause vertigo (a sensation of spinning), dizziness (a sensation of disequilibrium), light-headedness (a sensation of floating or faintness), blurred vision, and sometimes nausea and gastrointestinal upset. Nystagmus (abnormal rhythmic oscillations of the eyes) is predictable as well. Changes to blood pressure and heart rate sometimes occur.

Treatment

Treatment for VBDs depends on what the contributing factors are determined to be. BPPV is treated with appropriate head maneuvers; medication is usually not necessary. Labyrinthitis and acute vestibular neuronitis are treated with drugs to control nausea and vomiting and **vestibular rehabilitation** exercises to help the CNS adapt to changes in sensation. These exercises have been found to be extremely helpful in managing vertigo and have the added benefit of giving elders more confidence to avoid falls. Other forms of vertigo are treated according to underlying causes.

> **Vestibular rehabilitation:** A program of exercises designed to improve balance and decrease dizziness.

Medications

- Benzodiazepines to suppress vertigo symptoms
- Antiemetics to manage nausea
- Antivirals for viral infection
- Antibiotics for bacterial infection
- Steroidal anti-inflammatories for autoimmune dysfunction

Massage Therapy Implications

RISKS	The biggest threat for a person with VBD who wants to get a massage is getting on and off the table and rolling over. Any of these postural changes may trigger an attack, so the client and therapist must work together to strategize how to minimize this risk.
BENEFITS	People who live in fear of "dizzy spells" may develop postural habits that are inefficient and that cause pain. Massage, as long as it doesn't threaten to cause an episode of vertigo, may help with some of these compensatory patterns.
OPTIONS	Trigger points in neck muscles have been seen to create symptoms of vertigo and dizziness; this is treatable with focused massage.

Explore and Apply

LEVEL 1: Receive and Respond

1. Match the terms to their best description.

a. Central sensitization	__Interwoven network of peripheral nerve fibers
b. Neuroplasticity	__Nervous system becomes especially receptive to pain signals
c. HPA axis	__Neuroendocrine aspect of stress response system
d. Plexi	__Nervous system structures grow and adapt according to environmental influences.

2. The primary symptom of this condition is memory loss.
   a. Amyotrophic lateral sclerosis
   b. Alzheimer disease
   c. Ataxia
   d. Adjustment disorder

3. Match the condition to the best description.

a. Huntington disease	__Involuntary contractions of an area of the body
b. Tremor	__Symptom of other conditions with hyperalgesia and allodynia
c. Peripheral neuropathy	__Rhythmic oscillations of a body part on a fixed plane
d. Dystonia	__Twitching, tics, writhing of face and trunk

4. Which is a symptom indicative specifically of meningitis?
   a. Headache and irritability
   b. Fever and body ache
   c. Itchy, painful blisters that appear in a stripe
   d. Stiff neck and red rash

5. Psychological addiction means that…
   a. The person likes how the substance makes him or her feel
   b. The substance makes the person feel sad
   c. The substance makes the person feel manic
   d. The person hates how the substance makes him or her feel

6. Physical addiction means that…
   a. The person uses to avoid feeling sad
   b. The person uses to feel good
   c. The person uses to avoid withdrawal symptoms
   d. The person uses to feel connected

7. This disorder's affect on adults was recognized by the DSM in the late 1980s. It is a neurodevelopmental disorder resulting in difficulty with movement, impulse control, and other issues. What is it?
   a. Autism spectrum disorder
   b. Asperger syndrome
   c. Cyclothymia
   d. Attention deficit hyperactivity syndrome

8. Which is the true statement?
   a. Bipolar disease is also called manic depression
   b. Bipolar disease only occurs in people with schizophrenia
   c. Bipolar disease always refers to the most extreme possible mood swings
   d. Bipolar disease is treated with antidepressants

9. Match the following:

a. Anorexia nervosa	__Bouts of overeating, followed by compensatory behavior
b. Bulimia nervosa	__Bouts of uncontrollable overeating that cannot be voluntarily controlled
c. Binge-eating disorder	__Habitual undereating to the point of self-starvation

10. Excoriation disorder, hair-pulling disorder, and hoarding are all considered subtypes of what condition?
    a. Obsessive-compulsive and related disorders
    b. Depression and related disorders
    c. Autism spectrum and related disorders
    d. Anxiety disorders and related disorders

11. Which condition requires that the patient is part of, or directly witnesses, an act of violence or destruction?
    a. Major depressive disorder
    b. Autism spectrum disorder
    c. Posttraumatic stress disorder
    d. General anxiety disorder

12. An occasional "lightning storm" of electrical impulses in the brain leads to involuntary motor activity. This describes…
    a. Narcolepsy
    b. Epilepsy
    c. Spastic cerebral palsy
    d. Complex regional pain syndrome

13. This condition usually affects an extremity. It involves a collection of signs and symptoms that include severe pain, and changes to the blood vessels, skin, and joints of the affected area. What is it?
  a. Dystonic cerebral palsy
  b. Spinal cord injury
  c. Meningitis
  d. Complex regional pain syndrome

14. A subdural hemorrhagic stroke involves…
  a. Bleeding in the arachnoid space
  b. A blood clot that traveled from the carotid artery
  c. A blood clot that traveled from the heart
  d. Bleeding in the cortex

15. The long-term consequences of this condition can include cognitive dysfunction, seizures, and changes in personality. What is it?
  a. Epilepsy
  b. Cerebral palsy
  c. Traumatic brain injury
  d. Trigeminal neuralgia

16. Which of the following conditions contraindicates massage to the face?
  a. Trigeminal neuralgia
  b. Bell palsy
  c. Blepharospasm
  d. Herpes zoster

17. Match the following:

a. Spina bifida	__Inner ear inflammation, usually connected to a viral infection
b. Cerebral palsy	__A birth defect in which the spinal cord may not be completely encased within the spine
c. Ménière syndrome	__A prenatal, birth, or early infancy injury leading to motor dysfunction and possible cognitive disability
d. Labyrinthitis	__A chronic inner ear condition with tinnitus, loss of hearing, and vertigo

18. This condition has features that include sleep disorders, central sensitization, and neurotransmitter imbalance. What is it?
  a. Myofascial pain syndrome
  b. Whiplash
  c. Fibromyalgia
  d. Complex regional pain syndrome

19. What is the typical trigger for tension-type headache?
  a. Musculoskeletal imbalance
  b. Food sensitivities
  c. Menstrual cycle
  d. Allergies

20. What is the typical trigger for migraine headache?
  a. Musculoskeletal imbalance
  b. Food sensitivities
  c. Overexercise
  d. Allergies

LEVEL 2: Application of Concepts

1. Your client has lateral amyotrophic sclerosis, in an early phase. Is it safe to work with him?
  a. Not unless you have a doctor's note
  b. No, because numbness contraindicates massage
  c. Yes, as long as you are extremely gentle
  d. Yes, as long as he can give clear feedback

2. Your client has Parkinson disease. What symptoms may massage be most likely to be able to address?
  a. Rigidity, tremor, sleeplessness
  b. Bradykinesia, dementia, micrographia
  c. Festinating gait, monotone speech, drooling
  d. All of the above

3. Your client had a bout of childhood viral encephalitis. What long-term repercussions is she most likely to have?
  a. Cognitive disability
  b. Blindness
  c. Hearing loss
  d. None of the above

4. Today you had a client recovering from shingles. What determines your risk of contracting this painful infection?
  a. Your history of exposure to herpes simplex
  b. Your history of exposure to herpes zoster
  c. How long you worked with your client
  d. Whether you touched any lesions on your client

5. Your client has been diagnosed with postpolio syndrome. She would like to stay active as long as possible. What is her best strategy?
   a. She should begin an exercise routine to build strength in weakened muscles
   b. She should focus on maintaining strength and supporting damaged muscles with efficient movement
   c. She should cut way back on exercise to preserve whatever muscle function she has left
   d. She should use massage therapy to bring blood and energy to underused muscles

6. Your client confides to you that she is terrified of being judged—so much so that coming for a massage feels like a major triumph. You observe that she is tight and needs reminding to breathe fully. With every comment, she apologizes for something that she thinks she's doing wrong. What condition is most likely to be present?
   a. Depression
   b. Social phobia
   c. General anxiety disorder
   d. Panic disorder

7. Your client has a hard time being quiet, and every topic he brings up is full of impending disaster, from his job that might be ending soon, to traffic, which almost made him miss his appointment, to climate change. What condition is probably present?
   a. Social phobia
   b. Panic disorder
   c. Posttraumatic stress disorder
   d. General anxiety disorder

8. The parent of a child on the autism spectrum made an appointment for his son. When they arrive, the 10-year-old boy is noncommunicative and doesn't make eye contact, but he is willing to get on the table. Your best strategy is to…
   a. Use firm, predictable pressure, to help with sensory integration
   b. Use light feathering strokes because ASD patients don't like touch
   c. Use reflexology on his hands and feet to avoid overtreatment
   d. Use craniosacral therapy, because this corrects ASD

9. Your client who has been using antidepressants for several months has decided that massage therapy is having such a positive impact that he can stop taking his medication. What is your best strategy?
   a. Congratulate him on successfully battling this difficult disorder
   b. Congratulate him on feeling better, and direct him to consult his doctor before changing his medication
   c. Refuse to work with him until he consults his doctor
   d. Recommend that he take his medication on alternating days to cut his dose in half before he stops altogether

10. You are midsession with a client who has a spinal cord injury. He experiences sudden flushing, accelerated heart rate, and sweating. What is your best choice?
   a. Call emergency medical services
   b. Be present with him as he processes his trauma
   c. Terminate the session, and reschedule when he is over his infection
   d. Change your technique to a modality that is less intense

11. Your client reports that she had a TIA 2 months ago. What area of the body must be treated with most caution?
   a. Suboccipital triangle
   b. Between the scapulae
   c. Anterior triangle of the neck
   d. Transverse process of C1

12. What is the main risk for a client with a vestibular balance disorder who wants to receive massage?
   a. The interaction of massage therapy with VBD medications can be dangerous
   b. People with VBD usually have an underlying condition that contraindicates massage
   c. The client may have dizziness or vertigo on lying down, rolling over, or getting up
   d. Massage therapy may overwhelm the vestibular activating system with too much stimulus

Note to educators: Due to space considerations, these review questions only address the most important material from Chapter 4. The Test Bank provides a much more comprehensive selection of questions, all of which are keyed to the relevant chapter objectives.

What Would *You* Do?

What happens now?

You are midsession with a client who has not reported any history of seizures, but he begins to contract and writhe; he is clearly having some kind of CNS episode. He is unresponsive to your voice, and his physical movements are becoming increasingly extreme. What happens now? Practice this with a classmate.

Falling asleep

Your client, whom you have seen for several years, has a flattering habit of falling asleep during his appointments. Lately though, you notice that his breathing during sleep is nonrhythmic, and sometimes he stops breathing altogether, followed by a loud snort. What is happening, and how will you talk to him about it that respects your role and scope of practice? Try this conversation with a partner.

Droopy face

Your client, who had to reschedule her appointment because she just had the flu, arrives for her session in a panic: one side of her face is drooping and she can't lift her lips to talk, or close her eye. She is eager for your input and for your massage, which she is sure will "fix her right up." Carefully analyze what you can safely do for her immediately and what recommendations you have for her before she visits again. Check your strategy with a partner to see if you came to similar conclusions.

Suggested Activities

1. For each condition covered in your curriculum, write down the following on a card:
   - A brief definition
   - Most common cause or contributing factor(s)
   - Major signs and symptoms
   - Risks and benefits of massage therapy
     - Variables that contribute to risks and benefits
     - Appropriate adaptations

   Use these as flash cards as you study.
2. For each condition covered in your curriculum, write one multiple-choice question. Share your questions with your classmates as you study together.
3. Quiz yourself using either the "labels off" feature in your enhanced e-book or the labeling exercise on thePoint® for Figures 4.1 and 4.2. Identify the following structures: Central neuron, Dorsal horn, Dorsal root ganglion, Endoneuron, Epineuron, Motor dendrite and cell body, Myelin, Neurilemma, Sensory dendrites, Sensory neuron, Stimulus, Ventral horn, Ventral nerve root, motor neuron.
4. Look up Sister Elizabeth Kenny and read about her revolutionary approach to treating polio. Given what you know about how this infection affects nerve and muscle tissue, describe why her strategy was successful.
5. Listen to Jill Bolte Taylor's TED talk: https://www.ted.com/speakers/jill_bolte_taylor. What insights does this give you about stroke and stroke recovery?

5

Circulatory System Conditions

Chapter 5 / Abbreviated Chapter Objectives

Having completed assignments and classroom time related to Chapter 5, the learner is expected to be able to...

- Identify definitions of the key terms in the introduction and those connected to the conditions covered in your curriculum.
- List and describe six general functions of the circulatory system.
- Name the chambers and dividing wall of the heart.
- Describe the three layers of blood vessels, identifying the main tissue type in each layer.
- Name the three types of blood vessels: those that carry blood away from the heart, those that carry blood toward the heart, and those that connect them.
- List the three types of blood cells or cell fragments, and describe their functions.
- Provide the following information for each condition covered in your curriculum:
  - Identify the definition of the condition.
  - List the most common causes or contributing factors to the condition.
  - List major signs and symptoms of the condition.
  - Identify possible risks and benefits of massage therapy, with:
    - Variables that contribute to risks and benefits
    - Appropriate adaptations for massage therapy

For detailed chapter objectives for each condition in this chapter, consult the student resource page at http://thePoint.lww.com/Werner6e. thePoint®

Introduction

Our cells are specialized and complex, each with an important function. Most of them are fixed: unable to move toward nutrition or away from wastes. They depend on the circulatory system for constant delivery of food and fuel and the carrying away of garbage. Suppose we needed hired help to get to the grocery store and to flush the toilets and take out the trash. What would happen if that service were interrupted? Very quickly, we would become overwhelmed by trash: unable to work normally, starving, and impeded at every step by our own wastes. That is the scenario behind many circulatory system disorders. Massage may promote circulatory activity, but under certain circumstances, it can also interrupt or interfere with this service: it is the therapist's job to determine which modalities are likely to be a help or a hindrance for clients with circulatory dysfunctions.

General Function: The Circulatory System

Diffusion, the random distribution of particles throughout an environment, is the main mechanism for the exchange of nutrients and wastes at the cellular level. Diffusion requires that substances be able to move freely: blood and lymph constitute the perfect medium for this process. An average adult contains about 23 L of combined blood and lymph. In every milliliter of it, particles flow, chemicals react, and life happens.

The circulatory system, through the medium of the blood, works to maintain **homeostasis**: the tendency to maintain a stable internal environment. It does this in a number of different ways:

- *Delivery of nutrients and oxygen*. The blood carries nutrients and oxygen to every cell in the body. If for some reason the blood can't reach a specific area, cells there starve and die. This is the situation with many disorders, including **stroke**, **heart attack**, **pulmonary embolism** (PE), renal infarction, and **decubitus ulcers**.
- *Removal of waste products*. While dropping off nutrients, the blood, along with lymph, picks up the waste products generated by metabolism. These include carbon dioxide and more noxious compounds that can cause problems if left in the tissues. Again, if blood and lymph supply to an area is limited, the affected cells can drown in their own waste products.
- *Temperature*. Superficial blood vessels dilate when it's hot, and they constrict when it's cold. Furthermore, blood prevents our most active places (the heart, the liver, working muscles) from overheating by distributing the extra warm blood throughout the body. In this way, the circulatory system helps to maintain a stable internal temperature.
- *Clotting*. Every time a rough place develops in the endothelium of a blood vessel, a complicated chain of chemical reactions results in the spinning of tiny fibers from plasma proteins. These nets catch red blood cells (RBCs) to plug any possible gaps. This is an absolutely critical, lifesaving mechanism. Unfortunately, in certain circumstances, this reaction causes more problems than it solves.
- *Protection from pathogens*. Without white blood cells, we would have no defense against the hordes of microorganisms that try to gain access to the body's precarious internal environment. This is discussed in more detail in the introduction to Chapter 6.
- *Chemical balance*. The body has a narrow margin of tolerance for variances in internal chemistry. A person can die if his or her blood gets even 15% too alkaline or too acidic. Happily, blood components, including RBCs, are supplied with enzymes and other buffers specifically designed to keep pH balance within the safety zone.

> **Homeostasis:** The tendency to maintain a stable internal environment.
>
> **Septum:** A wall between two chambers.
>
> **Atria:** The upper chambers of the heart.
>
> **Ventricle:** A cavity, in this case, the inferior chambers of the heart.

Structure and Function: The Heart

The heart is divided by the **septum** into left and right halves. The right half pumps blood to the lungs (the pulmonary circuit), and the left half pumps to the rest of the body (the systemic circuit), and in ideal circumstances, blood cannot pass directly from one side of the heart to the other (Figure 5.1). Each half of the heart is further divided into top and bottom. The small top chambers, where blood returning from the lungs and body enters, are called the **atria** (the singular form is **atrium** from the Latin for entrance hall), and the larger bottom chambers are the **ventricles** (from the Latin for belly). The two-part "lub-dup" of the heartbeat is the closing of the valves that separate the atria from the ventricles, and the ventricles from the arteries leaving the heart.

The cardiac muscle of the atria is much thinner and weaker than is that of the ventricles. This makes sense, because the atrial contraction has to push blood only a few centimeters downhill into the ventricles. The cardiac muscle of the ventricles is thicker and stronger than is that found in the atria, which is important, because the ventricular contraction pushes blood into the circulatory system—through

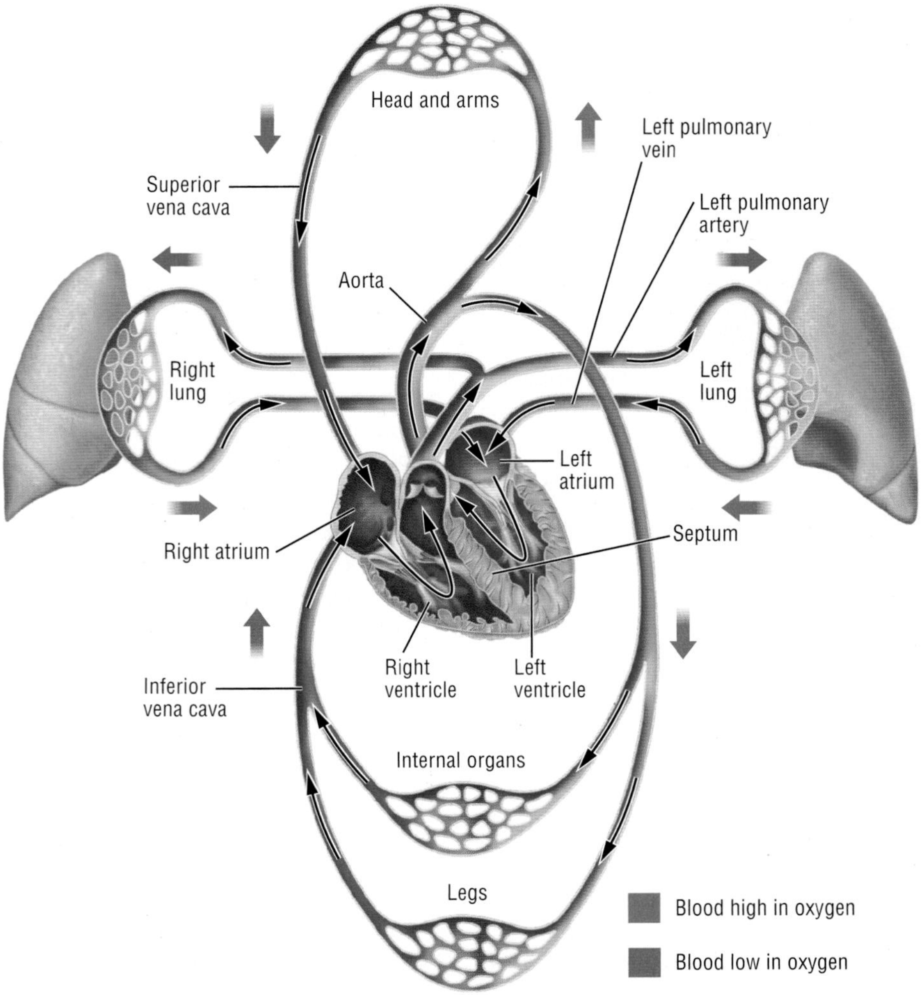

FIGURE 5.1 The pulmonary and systemic circuits

the pulmonary circuit to the lungs from the right ventricle and through the systemic circuit to the rest of the body from the left ventricle. The differences in the workload of various parts of the heart have great implications for the seriousness of heart attacks; the location of the damaged tissue determines how well the heart will function without it.

Structure and Function: Blood Vessels

The vessels leaving the heart are called arteries and arterioles; the vessels going toward the heart are called venules and veins; the vessels that connect them are called capillaries. Ideally, this should be a closed system. That is, although white blood cells are free to come and go through capillary walls, the RBCs should never be able to leave the 60,000 miles of continuous tubing that constitutes the circulatory system. If they do leak out, it means that the system has an injury, and a blood clot should be forming.

Arteries and veins share the basic properties of most of the tubes in the body. They have an internal layer of epithelium (it's called endothelium here because it's on the inside); this layer is called the **tunica intima**, or inside coat. The middle layer (**tunica media**) is made of smooth muscle, and the external layer of tough, protective connective tissue is called the **tunica externa**, or the **adventitia**. This combination of tissues makes these tubes strong, pliable, and stretchy (Figure 5.2).

Tunica intima: The endothelial, innermost layer of blood vessel walls.

Tunica media: The smooth muscle middle layer of blood vessel walls.

Tunica externa: The tough outermost layer of blood vessel walls.

Adventitia: The outermost connective tissue layer that covers organs and vessels.

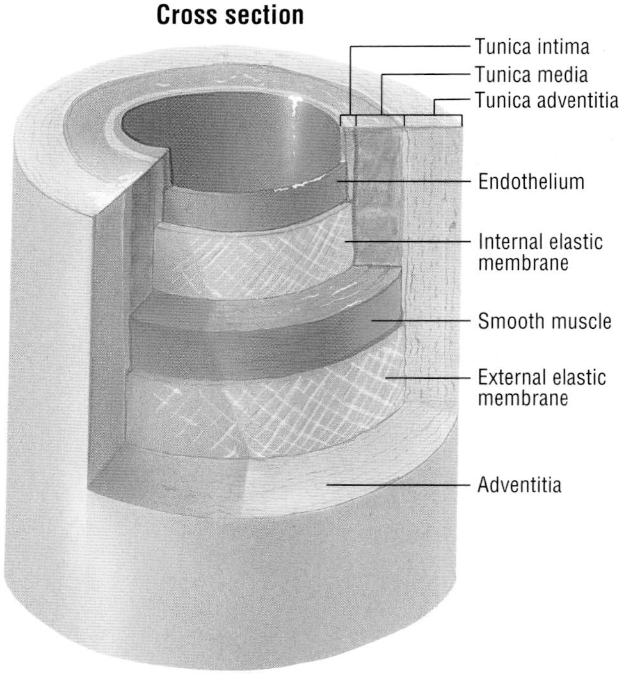

FIGURE 5.2 Arterial structure

Capillaries are delicate variations of basic tube construction. As the arteries divide into smaller arterioles, their outer layers get thinner and thinner. Finally, all that is left is one layer of simple squamous epithelium wrapped with smooth muscle cells: the capillaries. This construction is ideal for the passage of substances back and forth, because most diffusion happens readily through single-cell layers. But because capillaries lack the tougher muscle and connective tissue layers of the larger tubes, they are much more vulnerable to injury.

Blood cells and surrounding plasma leave the heart through the thick-walled arteries, crowd into arterioles, and line up one by one to squeeze through the capillaries. Once they've dumped their cargo of oxygen and picked up some carbon dioxide, they have more room; now they're in the venules. Again, the three-ply construction design is present, but with a difference. Much of the venous system operates against gravity. Blood flows upward in the legs, the arms, and the trunk, partly by indirect pressure exerted by the heart on the arterial system, but also with the help of **hydrostatic pressure** and muscular contraction. To help the blood move against gravity, small epithelial flaps called valves line the veins. Valves help to prevent venous backflow. The smooth muscle layer here is thinner and weaker than in the arteries, which have to cope with much higher pressure coming directly from the heart. Veins get wider, bigger, and stronger as they approach the heart, but they are never as strong as arteries.

When blood returns from the body to the heart (via the systemic circuit), it then goes to the lungs to be reoxygenated (via the pulmonary circuit). Each loop, from heart to destination and back again, takes about 60 seconds for a given blood cell to complete.

Structure and Function: The Blood

Red Blood Cells (Erythrocytes)

Almost all blood cells, red and white alike, are made in the red bone marrow. RBCs are created at the command of a hormone secreted by the kidneys called **erythropoietin** (EPO). They are in constant turnover, some being released into the bloodstream and others dying, at a rate of about 2 million every second. They constitute 98% of all blood cells. Their life span is about 4 months, and during that time, they do a single job: they deliver oxygen to the cells and carbon dioxide to the lungs. They are so devoted to this task that they give up their nuclei to make more room to carry their cargo.

Some disorders are related to a shortage of RBCs. An early sign is when too many immature erythrocytes (reticulocytes) are found in a blood sample: this suggests that the bone marrow is not keeping up with production needs.

RBCs are tiny; 1 mL of blood holds about 5 million of them. They are built around an iron-based molecule called **hemoglobin**. This molecule (250 million of them in each RBC) is extremely efficient at carrying oxygen and slightly less so at carrying carbon dioxide; most CO_2 is dissolved in plasma. Another characteristic feature of healthy RBCs is their shape: they are discs that are thinner in the middle than around the edges. They are smooth and flexible enough to bend and distort to get through the tiniest capillaries. If for some reason they are not round, smooth, and flexible, big problems ensue.

White Blood Cells (Leukocytes)

Leukocytes aren't really white; they're more or less translucent. Unlike RBCs, which are all identical, different classes of white blood cells fight off different types of invaders in

Hydrostatic pressure: The pressure exerted by a fluid due to the effects of gravity.

Erythropoietin: A hormone that stimulates the formation of red blood cells.

Hemoglobin: The protein in red blood cells that binds to oxygen.

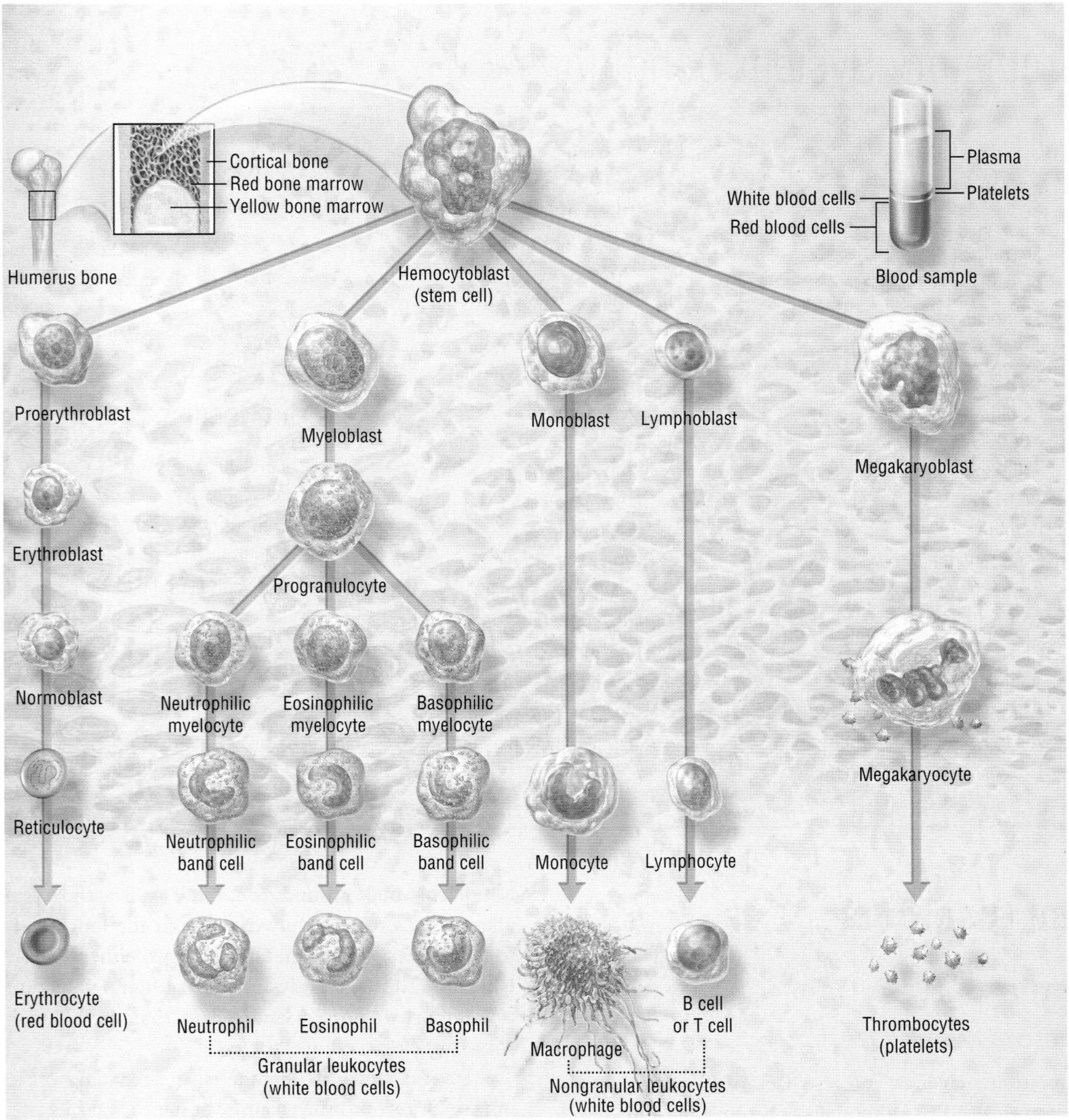

FIGURE 5.3 All blood cells are manufactured in cortical bone marrow

different stages of infection; this is discussed further in Chapter 6. White blood cells include neutrophils, basophils, eosinophils, monocytes, and lymphocytes.

Platelets (Thrombocytes)

Thrombocytes are not whole cells, but fragments of huge cells that are born in the red bone marrow, called megakaryocytes. Platelets are usually smooth, but when they are stimulated, they quickly become spiky and sticky. These cell fragments travel the system looking for leaks or rough places in the blood vessels. If they find one, they secrete chemicals that trigger tiny threads of **fibrin** to be woven from plasma proteins in the injured area. These fibers act as a net to catch passing RBCs, forming a crust on the skin or a clot (thrombus) internally.

All of these blood cells are manufactured in red bone marrow (Figure 5.3).

Fibrin: A protein that aids in blood clotting.

Circulatory System Conditions

Blood Disorders

- Anemia
  - Idiopathic anemia
  - Nutritional anemia
  - Hemorrhagic anemia
  - Hemolytic anemia
  - Aplastic anemia
  - Secondary anemia
- Embolism, thrombus
  - Pulmonary embolism
  - Arterial thrombus
  - Arterial embolism
- Hemophilia
  - Type A hemophilia
  - Type B hemophilia
  - von Willebrand disease
- Leukemia
  - Acute myeloid leukemia
  - Chronic myeloid leukemia
  - Acute lymphoid leukemia
  - Chronic lymphoid leukemia
- Myeloma
  - Multiple myeloma
  - Solitary myeloma
  - Extramedullary plastocytoma
- Sickle cell disease
- Thrombophlebitis, deep vein thrombosis

Vascular Disorders

- Aneurysm
  - Aortic aneurysm
  - Cerebral aneurysm
- Atherosclerosis
  - Coronary artery disease
  - Carotid artery disease
  - Peripheral artery disease
- Hypertension
  - Essential hypertension
  - Secondary hypertension
  - Malignant hypertension
- Raynaud syndrome
  - Raynaud disease
  - Raynaud phenomenon
- Varicose veins
  - Esophageal varices
  - Hemorrhoids
  - Telangiectasias
  - Varicoceles

Heart Conditions

- Heart attack
- Heart failure
  - Right-sided heart failure
  - Left-sided heart failure
  - Biventricular heart failure

Blood Disorders

Anemia

Definition: What Is It?

While the term "an-emia" suggests lack of blood, it actually means shortage of RBCs, or shortage of hemoglobin. Either way, oxygen-carrying capacity is limited. Anemia by itself is not a diagnosis; it is a description. The diagnosis is made when it is determined why a shortage of RBCs or hemoglobin has developed.

Demographics

Anemia can occur at all ages, depending on underlying conditions. It is estimated to affect about 3 million Americans, and it is seen in women of childbearing age twice as often as in others. Among seniors (those over 65 years of age), it is especially common, and some specialists recommend treating it as a freestanding entity within this group. Anemia is more common in women among people under 65 years of age, and more common in men for those over 65.

Etiology: What Happens?

RBCs are the most plentiful cell in the body, and healthy erythrocytes are packed full of hemoglobin. Hemoglobin, a molecule built around iron, binds well with oxygen. This allows RBCs to pick up oxygen from the lungs and deliver to the tissues. When anemia develops, either a shortage of RBCs or a shortage or dysfunction of hemoglobin interrupts this important process and means that the blood has lost some oxygen-carrying capacity.

Several kinds of anemia exist, depending on underlying conditions or other factors. Some of the most common varieties are discussed here. **Sickle cell disease (SCD)** is sometimes classified as a type of anemia, but it is found as a separate topic later in the chapter.

Types of Anemia

- *Idiopathic anemia*: This condition, which has no well-understood cause, may be due to poor nutritional uptake due to stress or to other factors.
- *Nutritional anemias*: These occur because the body is missing something vital in its diet. Iron deficiency may be the most common version (Figure 5.4), affecting women much more often than men because women need about twice as much iron, but take in fewer calories. Folic acid is a nutrient found in green leafy vegetables that is critical for the formation of RBCs. Because it is water soluble, folic acid can't be stored; a steady supply is necessary. Folic acid anemia is usually related to dietary insuffi-

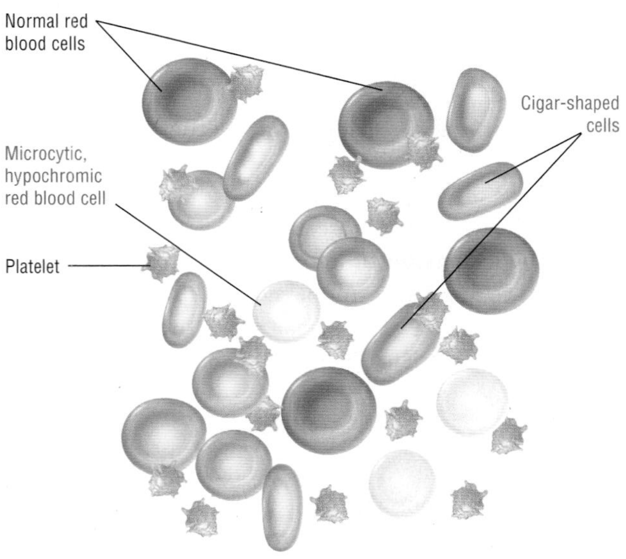

FIGURE 5.4 Iron deficiency anemia causes RBCs to become pale

ciency or malabsorption. Vitamin B_{12} is also necessary for RBC production. A B_{12} shortage or problems with uptake can lead to a serious complication called **pernicious anemia**. Because B_{12} is also critical to the maintenance of the central nervous system, a person with this deficiency experiences the slow onset of paralysis, loss of proprioception, and brain damage. People with untreated **celiac disease** can develop anemia related to poor absorption of iron, folic acid, and vitamin B_{12}. Anemia can also be the result of shortages of several other substances, notably copper and protein.

- *Hemorrhagic anemias*: These are brought about by blood loss. Often, the bleeding is a slow leak, but it can also be from trauma; this is acute hemorrhagic anemia. The most common causes are gastric or duodenal **ulcers**, chronic kidney problems, heavy menstruation, and large wounds.
- *Hemolytic anemias*: These are characterized by the premature destruction of healthy RBCs. In addition to the basic symptoms of anemia, **splenomegaly** and jaundice may be present. Another sign of hemolytic anemia is the presence of higher-than-normal numbers of **reticulocytes** in the blood.
- *Aplastic anemia*: In aplastic anemia, bone marrow activity is sluggish or nonexistent. The production of every kind of blood cell is slowed or suspended. Anemia develops with low RBC count, along with impaired immunity and circulatory and bleeding problems. Aplastic anemia can be caused by autoimmune attack against bone marrow, **renal failure**, folate deficiency, certain viral infections, exposure to radiation, and exposure to some environmental toxins, including lead and benzene.

  Myelodysplastic anemia is closely related to aplastic anemia, but in this case, the bone marrow makes multitudes of abnormal cells rather than being suppressed altogether. This can be a precancerous condition that indicates a risk of leukemia or myeloma.
- *Secondary anemias*: Anemia is a frequent complication of other disorders. Sometimes, a direct cause-and-effect relationship is obvious, and sometimes the association is a less clear. A partial list of the conditions that anemia frequently accompanies includes the following:
  - *Ulcers*. Gastric, duodenal, and colonic ulcers can all bleed internally. This may not be very obvious, but it results in a steady draining of RBCs, which can impair general oxygen uptake and energy levels. This is a type of hemorrhagic anemia, discussed earlier.
  - *Kidney disease*. When kidney capillaries are damaged, they can leak RBCs into the urine. The kidneys also secrete EPO, which stimulates RBC production. When the kidneys are not functioning well, EPO levels drop and RBC production goes down.
  - ***Hepatitis***. The liver contributes vital proteins to the blood, and it is responsible, with the spleen, for breaking down and recycling the iron from dead erythrocytes. If liver function is disrupted for any reason, the quality and amount of hemoglobin available to new RBCs may decline.
  - *Acute infection*. Anemia is sometimes an indicator that the body is under attack. It is a frequent follower of **pneumonia**, **tuberculosis**, or other infection. Anemia in these cases usually clears up spontaneously once the primary condition has been resolved.
  - ***Leukemia***, ***myeloma***, ***lymphoma***. In these conditions, masses of nonfunctional white blood cells are produced in bone marrow or in lymphatic tissues. These white blood cells essentially crowd out functional RBCs.

> **Pernicious anemia:** A condition in which the body does not produce enough red blood cells due to insufficient amounts of vitamin B_{12} (either due to inadequate consumption or because it is not properly absorbed).
>
> **Splenomegaly:** Enlargement of the spleen.
>
> **Reticulocytes:** Immature red blood cells.
>
> **Myelodysplastic anemia:** A form of anemia in which bone marrow manufactures abnormal cells. May be a precursor to myeloma or leukemia.

Signs and Symptoms

No matter what the cause of anemia is, some signs and symptoms are consistent. These include the following:

- *Fatigue*. Often, this is the first noticeable symptom of anemia. Less oxygen is available, so muscles tire sooner and stamina is compromised.

- *Pallor.* Pallor is present because of a reduced number of RBCs or a reduced amount of hemoglobin to carry the oxygen that gives the RBCs their color. Pallor is visible in the skin and in mucous membranes, gums, and nail beds. In dark-skinned people, pallor shows as an ashy-gray appearance to the skin.
- *Dyspnea, rapid breathing.* **Dyspnea** is a symptom of anemia because with less oxygen-carrying capacity, a person has to breathe more rapidly. Dizziness may accompany shortness of breath.
- *Rapid heartbeat.* Another term for this is **tachycardia**. This allows blood to travel faster through the body in an attempt to deliver adequate oxygen. The extra work of the heart may also be sensed as pounding in the ears.
- *Intolerance to cold.* Without adequate oxygen for rapid or sustained muscle contractions (i.e., shivering), cold becomes overwhelming very quickly.
- *Heart problems.* Aplastic anemia can cause arrhythmia, **cardiomegaly**, and heart failure as the circulatory system tries to cope with fewer blood cells of all types.

Treatment

Anemia is treated according to its cause. Anemia triggered by exposure to a specific substance is treated by removing the offending agent. Other interventions range from nutritional supplements to medications, transfusions, stem cell transplants, or other strategies to correct the underlying conditions.

Medications

- Oral or injected nutritional supplements for nutritional anemias
- Steroidal anti-inflammatories for autoimmune hemolytic anemias
- Synthetic EPO to boost RBC production

Massage Therapy Implications

RISKS	Anemia contraindicates massage when it accompanies other disorders that may be negatively affected. Specifically, if pernicious anemia has resulted in a decrease in sensation, or if anemia is due to acute infection, cancer, or other serious diseases, bodywork must be conducted with caution and as a part of an integrated health care strategy.
BENEFITS	Massage may help with the fatigue that anemia brings about, but it makes no lasting changes in blood cell production or nutrition. A client who manages anemia successfully can enjoy the same benefits from massage as does the rest of the population.

Embolism and Thrombus

Definition: What Are They?

An embolism is a traveling clot or collection of debris, and thrombus is a lodged clot (Figure 5.5). Thrombi and emboli that form on the arterial side of the systemic circuit are usually part of a wider cardiovascular disease (CVD) picture that includes **hypertension**, **atherosclerosis**, and a risk of **heart attack.** Thrombi that form on the venous side of the systemic circuit are discussed in detail in the **thrombophlebitis, deep vein thrombosis** (DVT) section of this chapter.

Etiology: What Happens?

Blood leaves the left ventricle of the heart via the aorta and goes to its destination through smaller and smaller vessels: arteries, arterioles, and finally capillaries. Nutrient-waste exchange happens at the capillary level, and then the vessels get bigger and bigger as they lead back toward the heart: from venules to veins to the vena cava. The same telescoping action happens in the pulmonary circuit: deoxygenated blood leaves the right ventricle through the huge pulmonary artery, and vessels going into the lungs get smaller and smaller. Oxygen and carbon dioxide are exchanged in capillaries in the lungs, and the freshly oxygenated blood goes back toward the heart through venules, veins, and finally the large pulmonary vein.

Platelets constantly flow through the whole system looking for rough spots in the endothelium, which indicate injury. If they find any disruption, they quickly develop spikes and stick to that spot. Then, they release the chemicals that cause blood proteins to weave fibrin, making a net to catch other blood cells: a clot is formed. Clots also form anywhere blood doesn't flow quickly; clotting factors thicken nonmoving blood, even without an injury to initiate the action. Tiny clots are constantly formed, especially on the venous side of the circuit, but they are dissolved by our naturally occurring **thrombolytics**. Sometimes, clot-forming mechanisms outwork clot-melting mechanisms, and then problems can follow.

The construction of the circulatory system does not allow clots to pass through capillaries; clots form in the larger vessels, they may break into fragments and travel, and then they are trapped by capillaries either on the arterial side of the systemic circuit or on the venous side. The damage that follows depends on the origin of the clot, its size, and where it finally gets stuck.

Dyspnea: Difficulty breathing.
Tachycardia: Rapid heartbeat.
Cardiomegaly: Abnormal enlargement of the heart.
Thrombolytic: Any substance that dissolves blood clots.

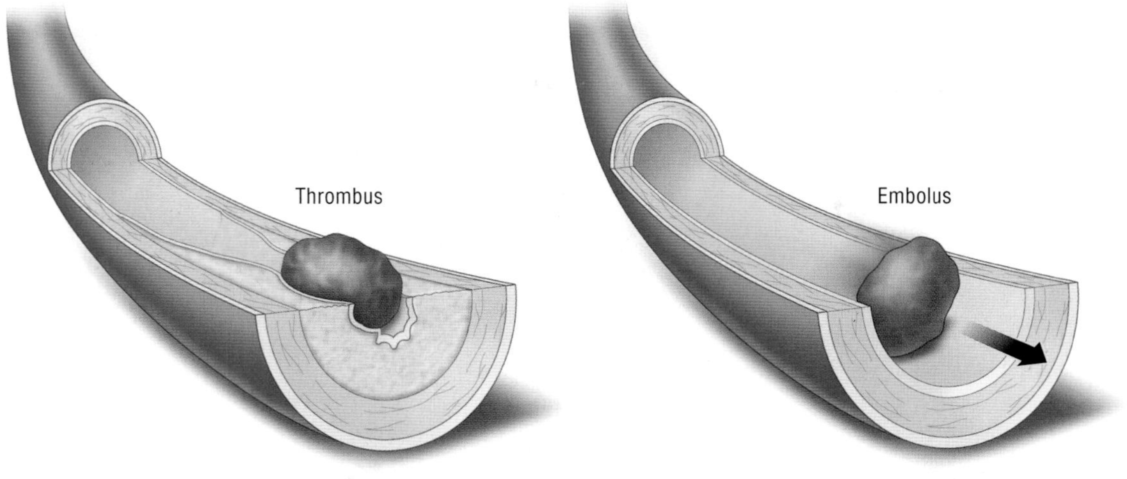

FIGURE 5.5 A thrombus is a lodged clot; an embolism is a moving piece of debris

Types of Thrombus and Embolism

- *Venous thrombosis*: This is discussed in detail in **thrombophlebitis**.
- *Pulmonary embolism*: Clots or debris anywhere on the venous side of the systemic circuit can only travel to the lungs (unless the heart has a structural defect called a **patent foramen ovale**, which allows blood to flow between the left and right sides). When a clot forms in a vein and some event—a sudden movement after prolonged immobility, for instance—knocks any debris loose, it travels toward the heart in increasingly large tubes. It goes through the right atrium and ventricle, enters the pulmonary artery, and ends up in the lungs (Figure 5.6). Most pulmonary emboli are fragments that lodge in multiple places in both lungs simultaneously. The extent of damage can vary from a temporary loss of a tiny bit of lung function to total circulatory collapse (Figure 5.7).

Risk factors for PE include other types of CVD, recent trauma, extended bed rest, and any kind of surgery: PE is a leading cause of death in hospitals. Women who are pregnant or who have recently given birth are at high risk for PE, as the weight of the uterus on the femoral vessels can obstruct blood flow, and hormonal changes associated with pregnancy and childbirth can also thicken the blood. Other risk factors include being overweight, smoking, and taking hormones for birth control or as hormone replacement therapy.

PE has some serous possible complications. A person with this history is at increased risk for another event.

Patent foramen ovale: A common defect in which an opening in the septum connects the left and right atria.

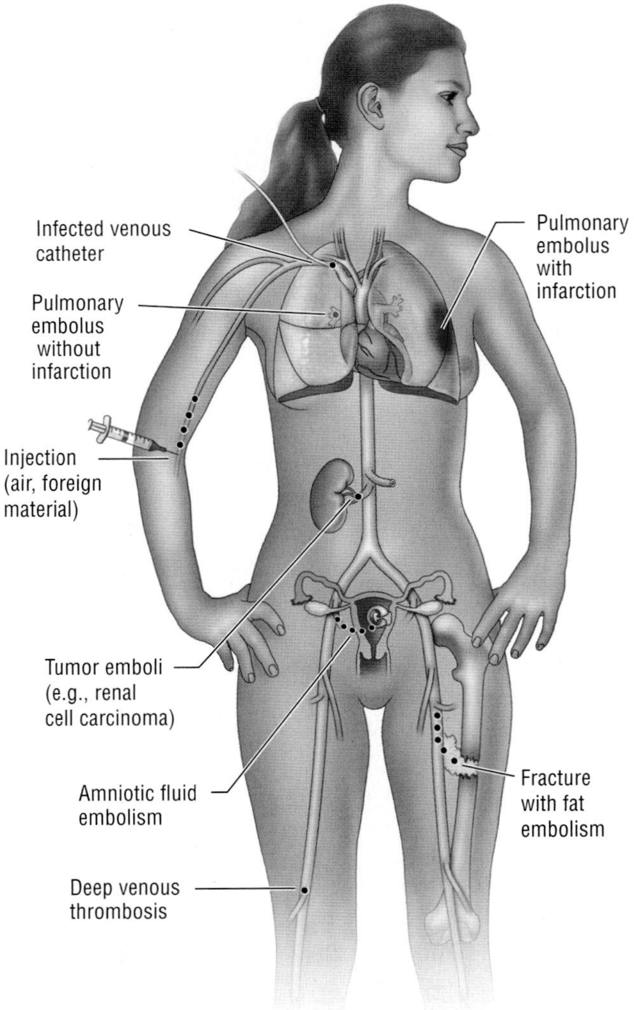

FIGURE 5.6 Sites of origin for pulmonary emboli

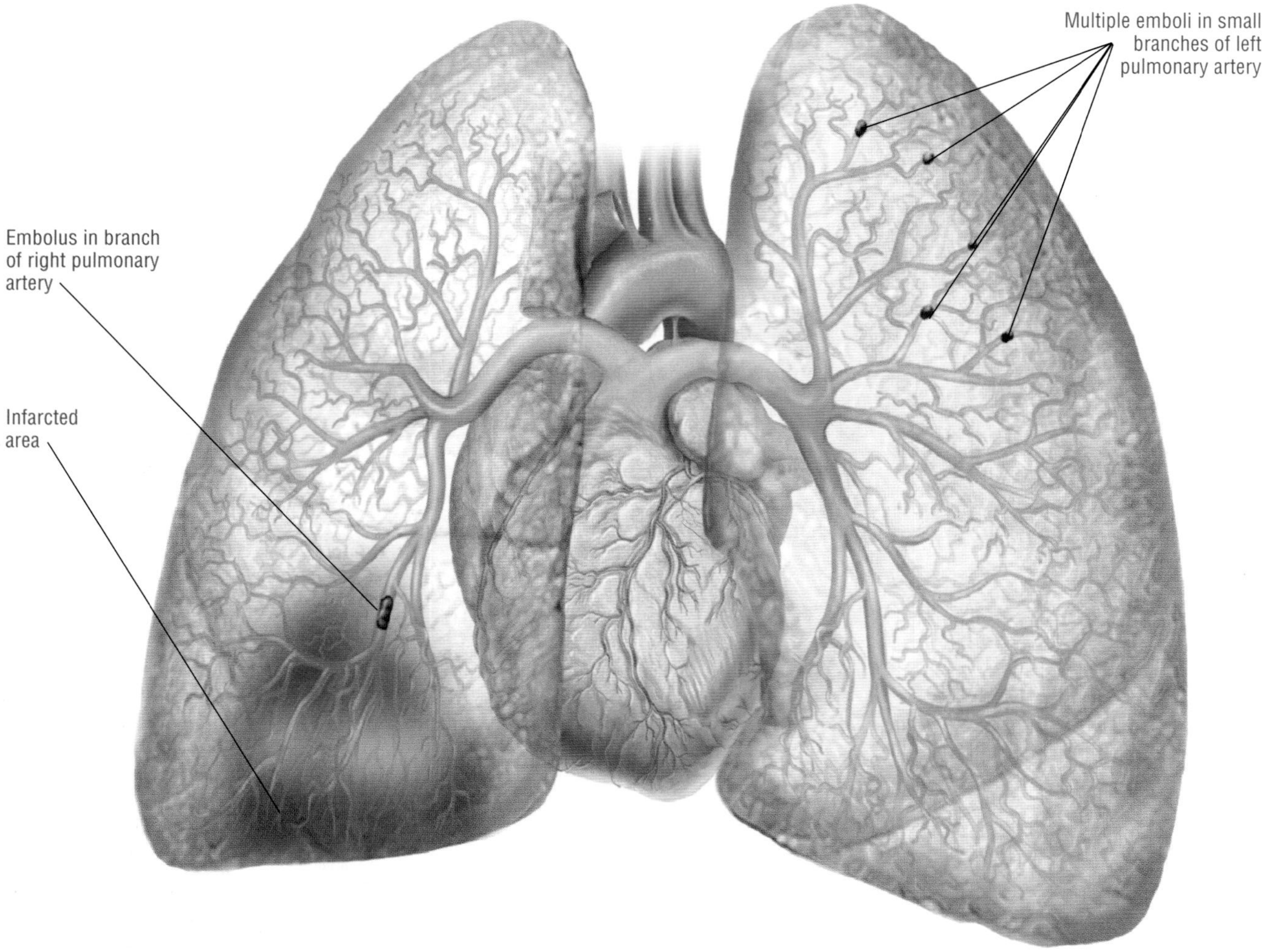

FIGURE 5.7 Pulmonary emboli can range from tiny to life threatening

Further, if a significant amount of lung function is lost, pulmonary hypertension and **right-sided heart failure** may develop as the heart tries to push blood through the damaged, restricted pulmonary circuit.

- *Arterial thrombus*: This is one of the many complications of **atherosclerosis**. Any roughness in the normally smooth artery or arteriole wall can trigger the production of a clot. Chronic inflammation, stress, and other factors can contribute to this as well. Clots can progressively grow to completely obstruct the **lumen** of the artery, or they can fragment to travel further along the system: this is an arterial embolism.
- *Arterial embolism*: Arterial emboli can originate as clots or plaques that form with atherosclerosis, or they can be related to atrial **fibrillation** or **rheumatic heart disease**. Emboli are often composed of clotted blood, but they can be any foreign object in the bloodstream such as a bit of plaque, a bone chip, an air bubble, or a clump of cancer cells. The brain, the arteries that supply the heart muscles, the kidneys, and the legs are the most common sites for arterial emboli to lodge (Figure 5.8). This is a common complication of invasive arterial surgical procedures.

Lumen: The space inside a tube, such as an artery or intestine.

Fibrillation: Rapid twitching of muscular fibrils.

Hemoptysis: Coughing up blood.

Signs and Symptoms

Many PE cases show no discernible signs or symptoms until after lung damage has occurred. Classic symptoms of PE include difficulty breathing, chest pains, and **hemoptysis**, but many people don't show this pattern. Other symptoms

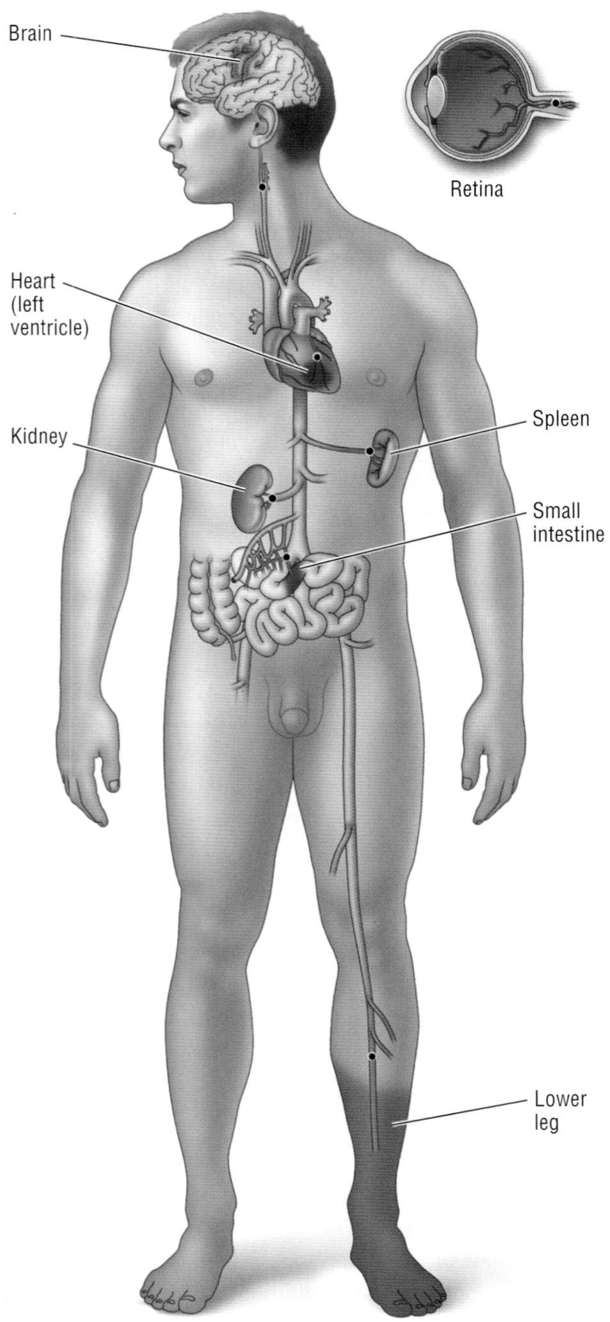

FIGURE 5.8 Arterial infarction sites

Infarction: The obstruction of blood supply to a tissue.

Venous thromboembolism (VTE): The combination of deep vein thrombosis and pulmonary embolism.

that may or may not be present are shortness of breath, lightheadedness, fainting, dizziness, rapid heartbeat, and sweating. Chest pain and chest wall tenderness along with back, shoulder, or abdominal pain are also possible.

Symptoms of arterial emboli in organs may be nonexistent until the affected tissue has significant damage: this is called an **infarction**. This is particularly dangerous in the kidneys, where many tiny clots can come to rest somewhere in the renal arteries, leading to **renal failure.** If clots lodge in the legs, however, symptoms are sharp pain followed by numbness, weakness, coldness, and blueness. Left untreated, this tissue may become necrotic in a matter of hours; immediate medical attention is necessary.

If the embolus lodges in the brain and the symptoms are short-lived, it is called a transient ischemic attack. A more serious brain embolism can cause an ischemic **stroke.** And finally, if debris lodges in a coronary artery, it's called a **heart attack**.

Treatment

The mainstay of treatment for thrombi or emboli is blood thinners, anticoagulants, and thrombolytics. A large clot lodged in the lung may be surgically extracted. When a thrombus in the lower extremity is threatening, a vena cava filter may be surgically implanted to prevent emboli from traveling to the lungs. Patients with damage from pulmonary emboli may supplement oxygen while their lungs heal. People at high risk for clots are counseled to stay well hydrated and sometimes to use compression stockings that assist in blood flow from the legs back to the abdomen (Sidebar 5.1).

Medications

- Blood thinners to reduce the production of new clots
- Anticoagulants to reduce the production of new clots
- Thrombolytics to help dissolve existing clots

SIDEBAR 5.1 DVT + PE = VTE

The link between DVT and PE is hard to overstate. When the two occur together (which probably happens more often than is officially recognized), the combined condition is called **venous thromboembolism** (VTE). The signs and symptoms for both DVT and PE can be subtle and easily missed: many people with DVT have a mild PE without realizing it, and for 25% of the people who die from PE, death is the first symptom ever recognized. VTE is considered an important public health issue, killing about 200,000 to 300,000 people each year.

Massage Therapy Implications

RISKS	The tendency to form clots is a caution for mechanical types of bodywork, both because of the risk of life-threatening emboli and because the medications to treat these disorders have bruising as a possible side effect. Whether that caution is for the whole body or local depends on how carefully the condition is being watched and treated and what kind of bodywork is being given.
BENEFITS	Nonmechanical forms of bodywork may be soothing and supportive for clients at risk of thrombus or embolism. It is important that they be under treatment, however. Clients who have a history of clotting issues but who have no lingering problems can enjoy the same benefits from massage as does the rest of the population.
RESEARCH	The interplay between massage therapy and thrombus or embolism is usually in the context of adverse events, or prevention of adverse events. Many massage therapists report counseling their clients to pursue a diagnosis when they present with symptoms of blood clots, and a few documented cases of embolism or thrombus that may have been disrupted by a massage treatment emphasize the need for caution in this context.[1–3] 1. Lim DC, Jayanthi HK, Money-Kyrle A, et al. Massaging the outcome: an unusual presentation of pulmonary embolism. *BMJ Case Reports* 2009;2009. http://www.ncbi.nlm.nih.gov/pmc/articles/PMC3029203/ 2. Crump C, Paluska SA. Venous thromboembolism following vigorous deep tissue massage. *The Physician and Sportsmedicine* 2010;38(4):136–139. http://www.ncbi.nlm.nih.gov/pubmed/21150153 3. Park H, Kim HJ, Cha MJ, et al. A case of cerebellar infarction caused by acute subclavian thrombus following minor trauma. *Yonsei Medical Journal* 2013;54(6):1538–1541. http://synapse.koreamed.org/DOIx.php?id=10.3349/ymj.2013.54.6.1538

Hemophilia

Definition: What Is It?

Hemophilia is a collection of genetic disorders characterized by the absence of some plasma proteins that are crucial in the clot-forming process.

The mutations that cause most forms of hemophilia are carried on the X chromosome, so males with hemophilia pass the chromosome along to their daughters, who become carriers. These female carriers pass the mutation on to about half of their sons. It is possible for a girl to have a typically male form of hemophilia, but she would need positive X chromosomes from both her father and mother, and this is very rare.

Demographics

About 20,000 people in the United States have hemophilia. Most of them are men, but one version of this condition is also seen in women. Over half of all patients have a severe form; about 25% have a moderate version, and 15% to 20% have a mild type of hemophilia.

Etiology: What Happens?

Thrombocytes constantly travel around the circulatory system looking for signs of damage. When they encounter any kind of rough spot inside a blood vessel, they stick to that spot and secrete a series of chemicals that cause a cascade of reactions in the blood plasma. Clotting factors from the liver work with thrombocyte secretions to weave nets of protein fibers called fibrin. These nets catch passing RBCs, forming a plug to limit the loss of blood through the damaged vessel. The plasma proteins that weave the fibrin nets have been identified as 12 distinct factors. Hemophilia occurs when a genetic mutation causes a deficiency in one or more of these clotting factors.

A person who is deficient in clotting factors has difficulty in forming a solid, long-lasting clot. Hemophiliacs don't bleed faster than average, but they do bleed longer. Hemophilia is rated as mild, moderate, or severe, depending on what percentage of normal levels of clotting factors the patient has. Severe hemophiliacs, who account for more than half of all hemophilia patients, have lower than 1% of normal levels of clotting factors.

Complications

While hemophilia is a manageable disease, it has serious potential complications. The leading cause of death for children with this condition is intracranial bleeding: even minor head trauma can cause major bleeding episodes in and around the brain, and this risk continues into adulthood. Bleeding into joint cavities is also a significant problem: unless clotting factors are administered quickly, the blood inside the joint may lead to an inflammatory response that damages cartilage and articulating bones. This condition is called **hemophilic arthritis**, and it occurs most often at the ankles, knees, and elbows.

Bleeding into muscles can cause pain and numbness as nerve endings are compressed. If the pressure is not quickly resolved, the muscle may develop a **compartment syndrome** or contracture, with a permanent loss of range of

> **Hemophilic arthritis:** Joint damage and inflammation, associated with hemophilia-related bleeding into joint cavities.

motion. The muscles most at risk for **hematomas** are in the calf, thigh, upper arm, and forearm. The psoas is also at risk for deep bleeds and resulting stiffness.

Contaminated blood products used to be another serious risk for people with hemophilia. This is no longer a major worry, but it is recommended that hemophiliacs and other people who regularly use blood products be vaccinated for hepatitis A and B.

Types of Hemophilia

- *Type A hemophilia*: This is the most common form of hemophilia, accounting for about 80% of all cases. It is characterized by a deficiency in clotting factor VIII. A rare version of this condition occurs when a mature person develops antibodies to factor VIII; this is called acquired hemophilia.
- *Type B hemophilia*: Also called Christmas disease, this is characterized by insufficient levels of factor IX. Hemophilia B accounts for about 15% of hemophilia cases.
- *von Willebrand disease*: Rather than a shortage of clotting factors from the liver, von Willebrand disease is a dysfunction of von Willebrand factor: a proclotting substance secreted by damaged endothelium. This substance normally helps platelets to clump together and helps factor VIII to do its work. Like type A or B hemophilia, von Willebrand disease is the result of a genetic mutation. Patients have bleeding problems that range from mild to severe, although the vast majority of cases are very mild and may go unrecognized. Unlike other forms of hemophilia, von Willebrand disease is not an X-linked disorder, so men and women are affected equally. It is the most common inherited bleeding disorder.

Signs and Symptoms

Hemophilia usually appears at birth, when the umbilical cord bleeds excessively, or in early childhood, as babies begin to engage in physical activities that involve minor bangs and bumps. These toddlers are subject to excessive bruising and bleeding with very mild irritation, and small scrapes and lesions tend to bleed for a long time.

As the person matures, he finds that he is prone to subcutaneous bleeding (bruising), intramuscular hemorrhaging (hematomas), nosebleeds (**epistaxis**), blood in the urine (**hematuria**), and severe joint pain brought about by bleeding in joint cavities. Bleeding episodes may follow minor trauma, or they may occur spontaneously.

Hematoma: A mass of clotted blood within an organ or tissue.

Epistaxis: Nosebleed.

Hematuria: Bloody urine.

Recombinant factors: Manufactured blood clotting proteins.

Treatment

Evidence shows that using prophylactic doses of clotting factor replacements leads to fewer bleeding episodes and better quality of life for hemophilia patients. Consequently, treatment strategies are shifting from treating bleeds as they come to trying to prevent them from happening, while living a normal, active life.

Progress in the production and packaging of clotting factors in a form that can be stored at home and self-administered as needed has radically changed the quality of life for patients with severe hemophilia. Instead of being dependent on whole blood transfusions or the use of blood products, **recombinant factors** allow patients to be independent enough to be able to work and travel.

People with mild hemophilia A can also treat themselves with an injected or inhaled form of the hormone desmopressin, which stimulates production of extra clotting factors in response to an injury.

In addition to managing bleeding, people with hemophilia are counseled to exercise (although they must obviously avoid contact sports) and to keep their weight under control; both of these can limit the risk of arthritis and muscle contracture.

Medications

- Prophylactic and as-needed recombinant clotting factors
- Concentrated clotting factors from donated blood
- Desmopressin to promote clotting factor production
- Antifibrinolytics to slow clot breakdown

Massage Therapy Implications

RISKS	Severe hemophilia contraindicates any rigorous bodywork or massage that might cause bruising or bleeding. If a client has this condition, it is wise to consult with his or her health care team to identify other risks.
BENEFITS	Gentle or light-touch massage is appropriate for clients with severe hemophilia, and this may be a potent way to help with the pain and stress of this complicated condition. For clients with milder forms of the disease, massage may be more rigorous, as long as it fits within their capacity for pressure without bruising.
RESEARCH	Massage therapy is mentioned in a review about treatment and prevention of hematomas for hemophiliac athletes,[1] but other scholarly articles generally recommend against massage therapy for this population. 1. Beyer R, Ingerslev J, Sorensen B. Muscle bleeds in professional athletes–diagnosis, classification, treatment and potential impact in patients with haemophilia. *Haemophilia* 2010;16(6):858–865. http://www.ncbi.nlm.nih.gov/pubmed/20491962

Leukemia

Definition: What Is It?

Leukemia, or "white blood," is a cancer that affects bone marrow function. Some overlap has been established between types of leukemia that affect lymphoid cells and lymphoma: cancer associated with lymph nodes. **Lymphoma** is discussed in Chapter 6.

Dozens of types of leukemia have been identified, but this discussion focuses on the four most common classifications. These types of leukemia have much in common, but each has some unique features that are examined under individual headings.

Demographics

About 15,000 people in the United States are diagnosed with acute myelogenous leukemia (AML) each year. Most are over 65 years old, but some children and teens are also susceptible. About 6,000 Americans are diagnosed with acute lymphocytic leukemia (ALL) each year; most of them are children or teens. Chronic myelogenous leukemia (CML) is found in about 6,000 people each year in this country; most are adults. And 16,000 people are diagnosed with chronic lymphocytic leukemia (CLL) each year; the vast majority of these are over 65 years old. Finally, about 6,000 people are diagnosed each year with one of several other rare forms of leukemia.

In all, this group of blood cancers is diagnosed about 49,000 times each year in the United States.

Etiology: What Happens?

Two types of stem cells, **myeloid** cells and **lymphoid** cells, manufacture most of our white blood cells in bone marrow. Leukocytes are classified as myeloid or lymphocytic, depending on their origin (refer to Figure 5.3 to review this information). Leukemia occurs when a mutation in the DNA of one or more stem cells in the bone marrow causes the production of multitudes of nonfunctioning leukocytes. These cells crowd out the functioning cells in the bone marrow and in the blood. Leukemia can be aggressive and quickly progressive, releasing immature cells into the circulatory system (acute), or it can be slowly progressive, leading to the release of mature but nonfunctioning cells (chronic). In either case, the mutated cells do not function as part of the immune system, and they live far longer than do normal cells, leading to dangerous accumulations of nonfunctioning cells that interfere with functioning cells.

Studies of cell lineage have revealed that the lymphocytic leukemias that affect T cells, B cells, and natural killer cells are essentially the same as associated forms of lymphoma; the only difference is in whether the targeted cells are stationary or circulating.

The genetic mutations seen with leukemia are usually acquired rather than inherited. Exposure to environmental toxins and radiation are cited most often as contributing factors. Electromagnetic fields are being studied as possible risk factors for leukemia, but results so far are inconclusive. Some forms of leukemia are linked to a congenital problem: Down syndrome and some other genetic anomalies can increase the risk for these diseases.

Untreated leukemia results in death from excessive bleeding or infection.

> **Myeloid:** Relating to bone marrow.
>
> **Lymphoid:** Producing or related to lymphocytes and antibodies.
>
> **Philadelphia chromosome:** A dysfunctional chromosome associated with the development of leukemia.

Types of Leukemia

- *Acute myelogenous leukemia* (AML): This is aggressive cancer of the myeloid cells that mainly affects people over 60 years old. The targeted immature cells are called blast cells, leading to the synonym acute myeloblastic leukemia. Other synonyms are acute myelocytic leukemia and acute granulocytic leukemia. The genetic damage that causes AML has been linked to certain environmental factors. High doses of radiation, chemotherapy for other types of cancer, and exposure to benzene all increase the risk of developing AML in later years. Unlike some other forms of leukemia, AML cells can congregate to form a tumor outside the bone marrow.
- *Chronic myelogenous leukemia* (CML): This is slowly progressive cancer of the myeloid cells. It is also called chronic granulocytic leukemia and chronic myeloid leukemia. CML has been traced to a specific dysfunctional chromosome, called the **Philadelphia chromosome**. It affects the production of myeloid cells, which include neutrophils, eosinophils, basophils, and monocytes. These faulty cells can interfere with and slow down normal immune system activity, but they do not usually bring it to a halt.

  CML patients often have abdominal pain and an enlarged spleen, as the cancerous cells congregate in this organ. Night sweats, unexpected weight loss, and a decreasing tolerance for warm temperatures are other signs and symptoms common to CML patients. CML occasionally changes its pattern and becomes more aggressive, in which case it is treated as AML.
- *Acute lymphocytic leukemia* (ALL): ALL is the type of leukemia found most often among children. Synonyms for ALL include acute lymphoid leukemia and acute lymphoblastic leukemia. It usually involves B cell production, although T cells may also be affected.

The proliferation of cells in a person with ALL is so overwhelming that all other bone marrow activity is suppressed, and immune system function is effectively crippled. Cancerous lymphocytes are released into the blood before they are fully mature. These lymphocytes may gather in lymph nodes, or they may cross into the central nervous system, where they can cause severe headaches, vomiting, and seizures.

- *Chronic lymphocytic leukemia* (CLL): This is a slowly progressive cancer of the lymphocytes. Although it can involve T cells or natural killer cells, most cases involve B-cell malignancies. These mutated cells can accumulate in bone marrow and lymph nodes. CLL is especially common among veterans of the Vietnam War who were exposed to Agent Orange.

  Sometimes, CLL is so stable and so nonthreatening that no treatment is recommended. If numbers of functioning blood cells drop to dangerous levels, chemotherapy may be recommended, along with radiation to shrink enlarged lymph nodes or other tissues.

Signs and Symptoms

Signs and symptoms of all types of leukemia point to bone marrow dysfunction. When the marrow is sabotaged by a genetic mutation that causes overproduction of nonfunctioning cells, functioning cells are produced in smaller numbers. A leading sign of leukemia is fatigue and low stamina due to **anemia:** low numbers of RBCs are available to deliver oxygen to working tissues. A person with leukemia bruises easily, and small cuts and abrasions may bleed for long periods. Unusual bleeding or bruising comes about because platelet production is suppressed (**thrombocytopenia**) and the person has limited ability to make blood clots. Finally, a person with leukemia is susceptible to chronic infections because they are lacking in white blood cells, especially neutrophils: a condition called **neutropenia**. This can manifest as skin infections like hangnails or pimples, respiratory infections like colds and flu, or chronic urinary tract infections. Whatever the infectious agent is, the person with leukemia has very limited resources to fight it off.

Thrombocytopenia: Low number of thrombocytes.

Neutropenia: A condition in which the body lacks sufficient neutrophils, leaving it susceptible to infection.

Refractory: Relapsed or recurring.

Autogenic transplant: A transplant using a person's own tissues.

Allogeneic transplant: A graft transplanted between genetically different individuals of the same species.

Other general symptoms include fever, headache, weight loss, abdominal pain, and enlarged lymph nodes.

Treatment

Leukemia treatment depends on what types of cells have been affected, how aggressive the disease is, and what kinds of treatments the patient has already had. Treatment usually begins with chemotherapy: administration of chemicals that are highly toxic to any cells that reproduce rapidly. Chemotherapy is usually administered in cycles of treatment followed by recovery. The goal is to suppress cancer cell growth so that the patient enters remission. Exactly which chemotherapy drugs are used and how they are administered depends on the type of cancer that is present.

If a person doesn't respond well to chemotherapy, or if the cancer keeps recurring (**refractory** leukemia), it is necessary to explore other treatment options. This can include adding radiation therapy or surgery, especially if cancerous cells have aggressively invaded a particular organ or location.

Bone marrow transplants with preserved marrow of the patient (**autogenic transplants**) or closely matched donors (**allogeneic transplants**) are useful for some leukemia cases, but the incidence of complications is high. It is also possible to harvest stem cells from the bloodstream, bone marrow, or umbilical cords of healthy people and to transplant these "cellular blanks" into leukemia patients so that they can make healthy, functioning blood cells.

New treatments for leukemia also include the use of biologic agents to slow the production of cancerous cells and the use of manufactured antibodies that are designed to identify and destroy cancer cells. One type of targeted therapy is especially useful for people who are positive for the Philadelphia chromosome; another is used for people with CLL.

The treatments for leukemia, especially the acute varieties, can take as hard a toll on the body as the disease itself. Chemotherapy introduces substances whose function is to kill off any rapidly reproducing cell. Unfortunately, this doesn't just mean cancer cells; it also means epithelial cells in the skin and the digestive tract and, ironically, healthy blood cells. The side effects of chemotherapy on epithelial tissues include development of ulcers in the mouth, nausea and diarrhea from gastrointestinal irritation, and hair loss as the epithelial cells in follicles are killed. One of the difficulties with digestive system disturbances is that if the patient can't eat well, the whole system becomes weaker and less able to cope with the stresses of both the disease and its treatment.

Medications

- Chemotherapeutic agents
- Biologic therapy agents, including interferon and monoclonal antibody therapy
- Drugs to mitigate side effects of cancer treatment, including blood cell growth factors to stimulate RBC production

Massage Therapy Implications

RISKS Leukemia and its treatments involve a high risk of bruising, bleeding, and infection. Any bodywork that increases these risks is of course not appropriate. A massage therapist should consult the client's health care team to assess the best timing for bodywork in the context of leukemia treatments.

BENEFITS The benefits that gentle bodywork can offer leukemia patients (reinforcing a parasympathetic state, improving sleep and appetite, reducing pain and anxiety) can be enjoyed with a minimum of risk if simple precautions are taken to allow for the client's fragility and medications. For more guidelines about massage in the context of cancer and cancer treatments, see Chapter 12.

RESEARCH A strong evidence base for massage therapy in the context of cancer has been accumulated. For leukemia specifically, massage has been seen to decrease some of the symptoms.[1] Another study found benefits from the relaxation effects of massage compared to aromatherapy and rest for blood cancer patients.[2]

1. Wesa KM, Cassileth BR. Is there a role for complementary therapy in the management of leukemia? *Expert Review of Anticancer Therapy* 2009;9(9):1241–1249. http://www.ncbi.nlm.nih.gov/pmc/articles/PMC2792198/
2. Stringer J, Swindell R, Dennis M. Massage in patients undergoing intensive chemotherapy reduces serum cortisol and prolactin. *Psycho-oncology* 2008;17(10):1024–1031. http://www.ncbi.nlm.nih.gov/pubmed/18300336

Myeloma

Definition: What Is It?

Myeloma (literally, "marrow tumor") is a blood cancer involving maturing B cells that are found in bone marrow.

Demographics:

Myeloma is almost exclusive to people over 50 years old. Estimates suggest that it is diagnosed about 22,000 times per year in the United States, leading to about 10,000 deaths. It is slightly more common among men than women, with a ratio of roughly 3:2. The average age at diagnosis is 68 years for men and 70 for women, but some cases develop in younger individuals. It is about twice as common among African Americans as it is among whites, and it is rare among those of Asian descent.

Etiology: What Happens?

Under normal circumstances, healthy bone marrow holds only a few maturing B cells. As soon as the new cells are ready, they normally migrate to lymph tissue, where they operate as **plasma cells**, producing antibodies. But when immature B cells undergo mutation and become cancerous, they rapidly proliferate into bone marrow tumors. These usually grow in the spine, pelvis, ribs, or skull, but occasionally tumors form elsewhere. These B-cell tumors are called **plastocytomas**.

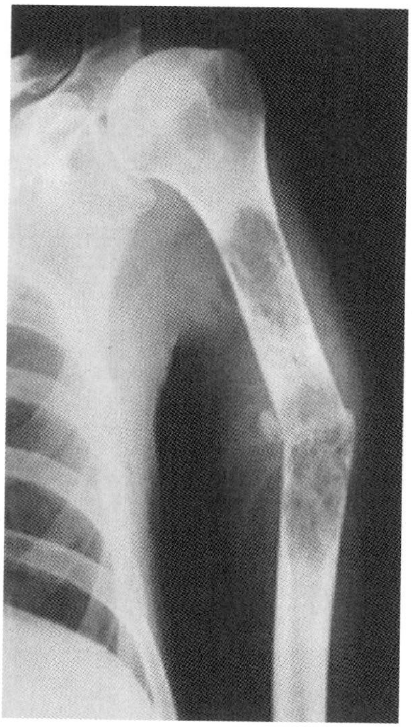

FIGURE 5.9 Multiple myeloma: two lesions in the arm of a 45-year-old man

Tumors inside bone marrow interfere with normal blood cell production, leading to the signs and symptoms of other blood cancers: **anemia**, poor clotting, and reduced resistance to infection. But myeloma cells also secrete cytokines that signal osteoclasts to dismantle bone tissue. This makes more room for the growing tumor, and it leads to pathologic thinning or spontaneous **fractures** in bone tissue (Figure 5.9).

Healthy B cells produce many types of functioning antibodies (also called **immunoglobulins**) that work in different ways to neutralize pathogens. Myeloma cells, on the other hand, produce massive numbers of nonfunctioning antibodies, called **monoclonal immunoglobulins**: monoclonal because they are all alike and immunoglobulins because they are technically anti-

Plasma cell: A B cell that produces a single type of antibody.

Plastocytoma: A tumor made of mutated immature B cells.

Immunoglobulin: An antibody.

Monoclonal immunoglobulins: Nonfunctioning antibodies produced by myeloma cells. Also called M proteins.

COMPARE & CONTRAST 5.1 Blood Cancers

Blood cancers are a confusing collection of conditions because they seem to overlap each other. Indeed, it has been found that some forms of leukemia are essentially the same as some forms of lymphoma, because they affect the same cells. The only difference is that when the cells circulate, it is called leukemia, and when cells are fixed inside lymph nodes, the disease is called lymphoma.

FEATURES	LEUKEMIA	MYELOMA	LYMPHOMA
Cells affected	Any white blood cell: myeloid (monocytes, neutrophils, basophils, eosinophils) or lymphoid (T cells, B cells, natural killer cells)	Nearly mature B cells in bone marrow only, although some cancerous cells may accumulate elsewhere	B cells, T cells natural killer cells, in lymph nodes or spleen
Earliest signs and symptoms	Anemia, thrombocytopenia, poor immune function	Bone pain from corroding tumors in marrow	Painless enlargement of lymph nodes, especially at the jaw, axilla, and groin

bodies, even though they don't offer any protective properties. Another name for monoclonal immunoglobulins is M proteins.

Normal antibodies are Y-shaped proteins, and they are too big to pass through the kidneys into the urinary system. M proteins have branches that sometimes break off during formation. These fragments are small enough to pass through the filters in the kidney to be excreted in the urine. The good news about this is that myeloma can be detected and to a certain extent tracked through urinalysis. The bad news is that if the disease is rapidly progressive, the kidneys can sustain extensive damage and even fail altogether.

Myeloma is seen on a spectrum of severity. A relatively common condition among mature people is called **monoclonal gammopathy of undetermined significance** (MGUS): this points to some dysfunctional B cells and the production of abnormal antibodies, but it does not always develop into aggressive disease. At the other end of the spectrum is aggressive, advanced, multiple, or extramedullary (outside the marrow) myeloma.

Myeloma seems particularly dependent on the environment where it grows and the secretion of the cytokines and other local chemicals that support its development. This line of inquiry may lead to more and better treatment options.

Monoclonal gammopathy of undetermined significance: A condition in which there are abnormal antibodies present in the blood.

Hypercalcemia: Abnormally high calcium levels.

Amyloidosis: A disease characterized by extracellular accumulation of amyloid proteins in various organs and tissues.

Types of Myeloma

- *Multiple myeloma*: This form produces tumors at several bone sites simultaneously. It is the most common form, accounting for 90% of myeloma diagnoses.
- *Solitary myeloma*: This is the development of a single myeloma tumor in the bone marrow.
- *Extramedullary plastocytoma*: This is the growth of myeloma tumors outside of bone tissue. These growths can develop in the skin, muscle, lungs, or other areas.

Signs and Symptoms

Myeloma can be silent in early stages; it is sometimes found during a routine medical examination. The earliest symptom for most people is pain, signs of spinal cord or nerve root compression, or **fractures** that occur as tumors corrode bone tissue and irritate nerves (Compare & Contrast 5.1). Other signs include **anemia**, frequent and persistent infections, kidney problems related to the excretion of fragmented M-proteins, **hypercalcemia** as bone tissue is dismantled, and the risk of **amyloidosis**: the accumulation of inflammatory proteins in the skin, tongue, or other organs like the heart or lungs, where they can do significant damage.

Treatment

Myeloma is often not responsive to treatment. If it is slow growing, and especially if the patient is elderly and in poor health, a period of watchful waiting is recommended to delay challenging procedures as long as possible. A combination of chemotherapy and bone marrow stem cell transplantation is usually suggested, but even with these intrusive interventions, the 5-year survival rate is relatively low.

Medications

- Chemotherapeutic agents
- Thalidomide and similar drugs to slow angiogenesis
- Corticosteroids, especially when amyloidosis occurs
- Bisphosphonates to promote healthy bone density
- Synthetic EPO to promote RBC production

Massage Therapy Implications

RISKS	Myeloma patients are very much at risk for spontaneous fractures at the affected bones and for renal failure. It is imperative that any bodywork in this context respect that possibility with adjustments in pressure, positioning, and any other adaptive demands. Cancer treatments carry their own set of complications and cautions for massage. As always in this context, it is wise to get special training and to work as part of a fully informed health care team. This is discussed in detail in Chapter 12.
BENEFITS	Gentle, noninvasive massage can be a helpful adjunct to care for a myeloma patient, through pain relief, anxiety reduction, improved sleep, and other benefits.

Sickle Cell Disease

Definition: What Is It?

Sickle cell disease (SCD) is an **autosomal recessive** genetic condition that results in production of abnormal hemoglobin, the protein that carries oxygen in RBCs. This causes the RBCs to collapse and lose their ability to pass easily through tiny capillaries.

Demographics

Blacks, Hispanics, and people from Italy, Greece, Turkey, and the Middle East are most likely to be carriers of the gene. SCD is estimated to affect between 70,000 and 100,000 people in the United States.

Etiology: What Happens?

The gene for SCD is recessive; this means if a person has only one copy of the gene, he or she has the sickle cell trait but not SCD. If two people who have the sickle cell trait have children together, each child has a 25% chance of inheriting a copy of the gene from each parent. This is the only way SCD is spread.

Being positive for the sickle cell trait carries no health consequences for the carrier. In fact may be beneficial if that person lives in an area where **malaria** is endemic—interestingly, those areas also happen to be the places where sickle cell genes are most common (Sidebar 5.2).

But having two copies of the sickle cell gene means that hemoglobin production is abnormal and many RBCs adopt a characteristic sickle shape (Figure 5.10). This prevents erythrocytes from squeezing through the smallest blood vessels and shortens their life span from about 4 months to about 10 days.

Some subtypes of SCD have been identified, depending on the exact nature of the genetic mutations, but their presentation and treatment options are all essentially the same.

Complications

SCD can lead to many serious and potentially life-shortening complications:

- *Sickle cell crises*: A sickle cell crisis occurs when sickle cells block a capillary, causing an infarction (Figure 5.11). This is often the first indicator of SCD in a young child.
- *Organ damage*: The spleen, as a collection site for dead and damaged RBCs, is often lost early in the disease process. Other organs that are frequently damaged include the liver, kidneys, and brain: even young children are vulnerable to ischemic **strokes**.
- *Infection*: The loss of spleen function makes an SCD patient vulnerable to serious and even life-threatening infections.

Autosomal recessive: Describing a condition that requires two copies of the gene in question to be present in order for the disease to develop.

SIDEBAR 5.2 Malaria and Sickle Cell Disease: A Close Connection

A person has SCD if he or she inherits a gene for it from both parents. If only one gene is present, a person has the sickle cell trait, but not the disease. This is a crucial distinction, because the sickle cell trait usually doesn't create any symptoms, although some people have mild anemia. But the presence of this single gene does limit the rupturing of erythrocytes during an attack of malaria. Sickle cell genes are mostly found in populations (and descendants of populations) from the Mediterranean, subtropical Africa, and Asia, otherwise called the malarial belt. Isn't it an amazing world?

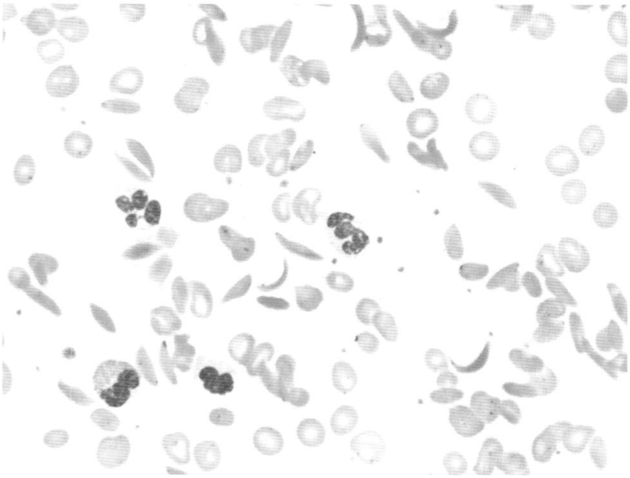

FIGURE 5.10 Sickle cell disease

Pneumonia is the leading cause of death among children with **SCD**.

- *Gallstones*: Accumulated bilirubin in the liver can concentrate into crystals that build up in the gallbladder.
- *Vision loss*: The accumulation of fragile RBCs in the arterioles that supply the retina can lead to blurred vision, hemorrhage, and blindness.
- *Acute chest syndrome*: Damaged cells accumulate in the lungs, leading to inflammation and pneumonia-like symptoms. This puts excessive strain on the right side of the heart and can lead to pulmonary hypertension and right-sided heart failure, in a situation called **acute chest syndrome**.
- *Others*: Other complications of SCD include delayed growth in children; chronic skin ulcers, usually at the lower legs; **avascular necrosis**; and priapism, a painful and long-lasting erection that occurs because the vessels that would allow blood to flow out are blocked with damaged RBCs.

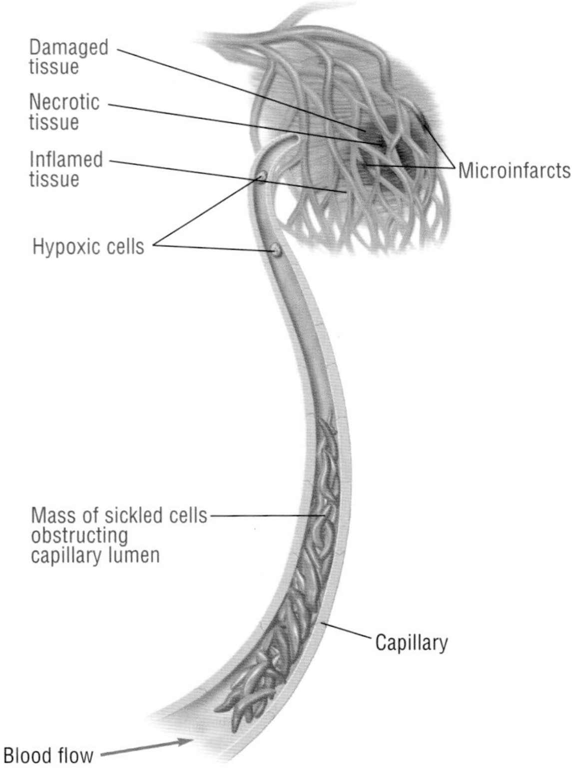

FIGURE 5.11 Sickle cell crisis

Signs and Symptoms

Having dysfunctional hemoglobin and brittle, fragile RBCs produces many consequences in the body. The symptoms of SCD include pain, fatigue, shortness of breath, and pallor related to **anemia**. **Jaundice** may develop as RBCs die and bilirubin accumulates in the liver and backs up into the bloodstream. Other symptoms are also complications, as already described.

Treatment

SCD is treated by trying to limit the severity and frequency of sickle cell crises. Mild episodes can be treated at home with over-the-counter pain medications and hot packs, but more severe attacks are often treated in the hospital with transfusions and intravenous opioid drugs. Stem cell transplantation that replaces faulty bone marrow may be curative, but it involves high-risk procedures that are not a good fit for every patient. A cancer drug called hydroxyurea slows sickling. It is now used with patients over 5 years of age.

Families with a child who has SCD often use many CIH strategies for pain management, and massage—often taught to a parent to give to a child—is a popular choice. Other nonpharmacologic interventions include acupressure and acupuncture, hydrotherapy, and TENS units.

The leading cause of death in children with SCD is pneumonia. This risk is managed with doses of prophylactic antibiotics until age 5, along with careful immunizations for flu, pneumonia, and other possible infections.

The life expectancy of a person with SCD has increased with better treatment options; today, a person with this condition can expect to live well into his or her 50s or later.

Medications

- Analgesics (nonprescription and prescription, including opioids) for pain management
- Prophylactic antibiotics in childhood for protection from infection
- Hydroxyurea, which slows sickling
- Supplements of folate to support healthy new RBC production

Acute chest syndrome: A complication of infection or a sickle cell blockage; can be life-threatening.

5 Circulatory System Conditions

Massage Therapy Implications

RISKS	Clients with SCD have severely compromised circulation, especially in the extremities. Any bodywork that demands circulatory adaptation may be simply too challenging for them to receive safely.
BENEFITS	Massage for the purpose of pain relief and anxiety reduction but without the intent of mechanically pushing fluids may be welcomed by SCD patients as a noninvasive way to deal with pain and to have a safe and positive physical experience.
RESEARCH	Massage therapy is often among the top choices of CIH therapies to manage the pain of SCD for adults and children.[1] A randomized controlled trial[2] found that children receiving massage from their parents (who had been trained by licensed massage therapists) had less depression, anxiety, and pain and higher levels of function. 1. Majumdar S, Thompson W, Ahmad N, et al. The use and effectiveness of complementary and alternative medicine for pain in sickle cell anemia. *Complementary Therapies in Clinical Practice* 2013;19(4):184–187. http://www.ncbi.nlm.nih.gov/pubmed/24199970 2. Lemanek KL, Ranalli M, Lukens C. A randomized controlled trial of massage therapy in children with sickle cell disease. *Journal of Pediatric Psychology* 2009;34(10):1091–1096. http://jpepsy.oxfordjournals.org/content/34/10/1091.long

Thrombophlebitis, Deep Vein Thrombosis

Definition: What Is It?

Thrombophlebitis and deep vein thrombosis (DVT) refer to veins that have become obstructed and possibly inflamed because of blood clots. These clots can form anywhere in the venous system, but they develop most often in the calves, thighs, and pelvis. Thrombophlebitis usually describes the presence of clots and inflammation in superficial leg veins (lesser and greater saphenous), while DVT is a similar problem in deeper leg veins, specifically the popliteal, femoral, and iliac veins.

Demographics

The annual incidence of thromboembolism in the United States is 1 to 2 cases per 1,000 individuals, leading to an estimated 300,000 to 600,000 cases each year. Signs of pulmonary embolism (PE) are present in 60% to 80% of DVT patients, even if clot is asymptomatic. Between 60,000 and 100,000 deaths each year are attributed to venous thromboembolism (VTE), which is the third leading cause of hospital deaths.

Etiology: What Happens?

Thrombophlebitis and DVT involve thrombi: stationary clots in the venous system, where, if they break loose, nothing stops them from traveling up the vena cava, through the right side of the heart, into the pulmonary artery, and finally to the lung, causing PE.

> **Hypercoagulability:** An excessive tendency to form blood clots.

Our ability to form blood clots is an important, lifesaving mechanism, but sometimes, we form clots faster than we can melt them. In the mid-1800s, a pioneer in pathology, Rudolf Virchow, first outlined three key factors in clot formation. The Virchow triad—injury to endothelium, **hypercoagulability**, and venous stasis, or slowed blood flow—is used today to describe the risk factors leading to the formation of blood clots in veins (Figure 5.12). Indeed, some specialists also apply the Virchow triad to assess the risk of clotting on the arterial side of the systemic circuit, finding that people who have a disorder on one side (DVT or thrombophlebitis) often have an increased risk for problems with the other (**arterial thrombosis or embolism**), and vice versa.

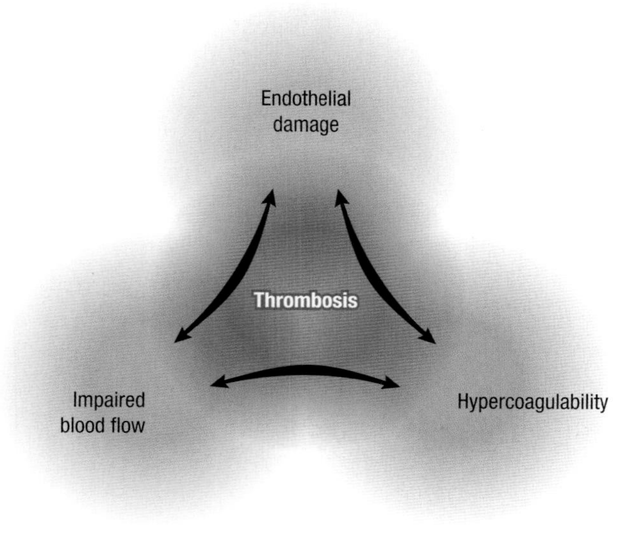

FIGURE 5.12 Virchow triad: contributing factors to blood clotting risk

CASE HISTORY 5.1 Deep Vein Thrombosis

Anne was a retired schoolteacher who spent her winters in Arizona and summers in the mountains of Colorado. In May, a week after she moved to her summer home, she took a bad fall over a curb and sustained a lateral plateau fracture to the tibia of her left leg, with which she had a history of **varicose veins** and phlebitis.

Her health maintenance organization was out of state, and it denied any treatment for conditions not considered life-threatening. For that reason, Anne, a mildly overweight moderate smoker, spent 3 days sitting in a chair all day at 10,000 feet of altitude (which thickens the blood, because less oxygen is in the air). She was unable to move except with the use of a walker. Her broken knee was never set or seen by an orthopedist.

By the third day, the swelling in the leg became so severely painful that she sought out a general practitioner in the Colorado town. He sent her to a local hospital for an ultrasound, which revealed a blood clot from her ankle to her groin. She immediately checked in, and began receiving anticoagulant medication.

ANNE, AGED 67: "It was just a broken knee!"

Four days later, she was sent home. Still basically immobile but taking anticoagulants, she returned to sitting in her chair with her leg elevated for 12 to 14 hours a day. On her second night home, she woke in the night with severe chest pains and shortness of breath. The emergency medical team took her back to the hospital, where it was revealed that she had thrown a large clot to the lung. At this point, her condition was too severe to be treated at a small rural hospital. After 2 days in the intensive care unit, she was transferred to a larger facility about 100 miles away, where a filter was inserted into her vena cava to prevent any further clots from reaching her lungs.

When she checked out of the second hospital, she was prescribed supplemental oxygen to compensate for the loss of lung function and the high altitude. She used an oxygen tank for several weeks, but began smoking again after that time. Now many years later, Anne is still active, but her breathing and stamina have never recovered.

Here are a few of the most common precipitators of thrombophlebitis or DVT:

- *Physical trauma*: Being kicked or hit in the leg can damage the delicate venous tissue, which is then prone to clot formation. Any fracture of bones in the leg can also increase risk (Case History 5.1).
- *Varicose veins*: Varicose veins involve damaged tissue and the risk of clot formation. The clots that form in superficial veins tend to embolize much less frequently than do those in deeper veins, but some people with varicose veins also develop DVT, either as a complication of treatment with a **sclerosing agent** or because the **perforator veins** allow clots from the superficial vessels to access the deeper ones.
- *Local infection*: This can cause an inflammatory reaction leading to clot formation. These infections are often related to surgical procedures involving catheters.
- *Physical restriction*: Too-tight socks or leg braces can cause the blood to thicken, even without damage to a vessel wall.

Sclerosing agent: A medicine injected into the blood vessels in order to shrink them.

Perforator veins: Veins that perforate the superficial fascia, connecting superficial veins to the deep ones into which they drain.

- *Immobility*: Sitting for long periods can contribute to DVT. This phenomenon has given rise to a layperson's term for this condition: "coach class syndrome."
- *Pregnancy and childbirth*: The weight of the fetus on femoral vessels slows blood return, and hormonal changes and stress can cause the blood to thicken.
- *Certain types of cancer*: Some cancers can lead to excessive clotting, either because of changes in the blood or because of irritation at the site of a catheter.
- *Surgery*: Thrombosis and subsequent PE are a leading cause of death following orthopedic surgery, especially for knee and hip **replacements**. Heart and any kind of pelvic surgery also hold high risks of thrombosis.
- *Hormone supplements*: High-estrogen birth control pills and hormone replacement therapy increase the risk of developing blood clots.
- *Other factors*: Cigarette smoking, **hypertension** and other cardiovascular diseases, paralysis, high altitude, and some genetic conditions lead to excessive coagulation in the blood.

Most blood clots causing DVT or thrombophlebitis form in the lower extremity, but they can develop elsewhere as a result of surgery or other trauma. Sudden movement or change in position is often the factor that causes part of a clot to fragment and travel to the lungs.

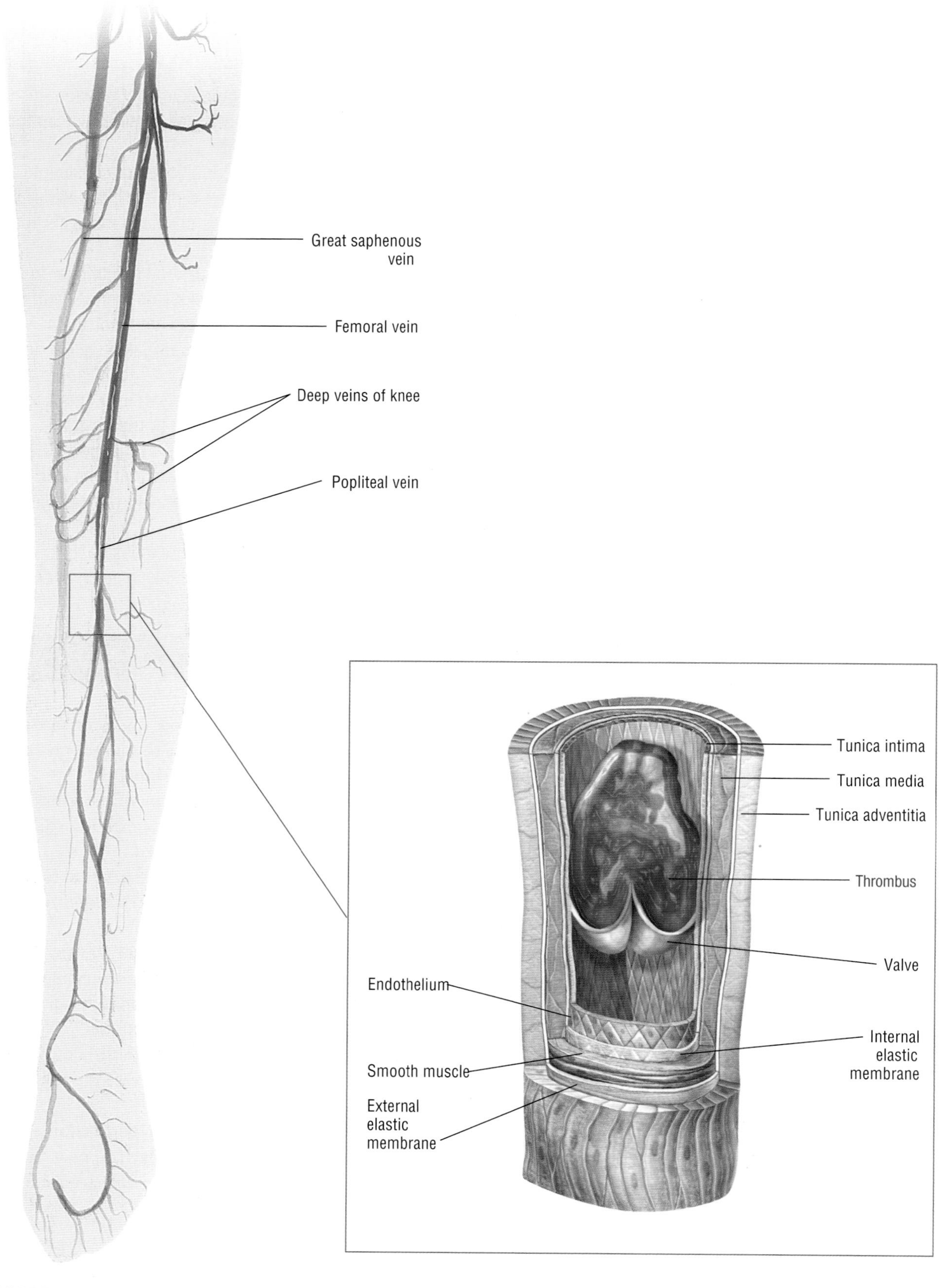

FIGURE 5.13 Deep vein thrombosis

One further twist occurs when a person has a defect in the cardiac septum. Many people have a small hole in the wall between the left and right sides of the heart, usually at the atrium. If clots from damaged veins that travel to the right side of the heart cross into the left side through this abnormal opening, they can go on through arteries to the brain as a **stroke**, to the cardiac muscle as a **heart attack**, or anywhere else as an **arterial embolism**.

Thrombophlebitis and DVT may do permanent damage to leg veins, including destruction of valves that assist with blood return to the heart. About 30% of all patients are at risk for **postthrombotic syndrome**, which can include permanent edema, pain, a feeling of heaviness in the affected leg, skin discoloration or ulcers, and very slow healing in the affected area.

Signs and Symptoms

Thrombophlebitis can show the major signs of **inflammation**: pain, heat, redness, and swelling. Sometimes, itchiness, a hard cord where the vein is affected, and edema with discoloration distal to the area are present (Figure 5.13). Thrombophlebitis that has become a chronic problem may result in poor blood flow to the skin, leading to flaking, discoloration, and **skin ulcers**. If it is caused by a local infection, fever and general illness may also be present.

DVT is considered the more dangerous of these two conditions because the clots in deeper veins can be big enough to do serious damage in the lungs. Unfortunately, not all DVT patients experience significant symptoms. When DVT does show signs, these include more swelling and edema than thrombophlebitis, because the clot inhibits more blood flow back to the heart. The backup forces extra fluid out of the capillaries and into the interstitial spaces, thus adding general edema to any swelling of the vein. The capillary exchange may become so sluggish that the edema pits, or leaves a dimple wherever it is touched.

> **Postthrombotic syndrome:** A combination of swelling, pain, and skin damage that sometimes follows DVT.
>
> **Pneumatic compression:** A technique in which venous circulation in a limb is mechanically increased through the use of intermittently inflated sleeves.

Treatment

The goals for a patient with thrombophlebitis or DVT are to stop clots from growing, to prevent clots from fragmenting and embolizing, and to prevent future clots from forming. The most common strategy is to supplement anticoagulants: drugs that prevent new clots from forming. Thrombolytics ("clot busters") are more powerful, but they have much more serious risks and are only used in the most extreme cases.

A bedridden patient may be given **pneumatic compression** to reduce the risk of thrombophlebitis or DVT. Support hose to prevent the accumulation of postoperative edema are also recommended.

High-risk patients may have a filter implanted in the vena cava to prevent clots from reaching the lungs. Surgery to remove a clot is sometimes performed, but other options are typically explored first.

Medications

- Aspirin (not well tolerated by some patients)
- Anticoagulants, including warfarin and heparin
  - Heparin is given through injection or intravenously; it is fast acting
  - Warfarin is taken orally for up to 6 months following an event
- Thrombolytics in extreme cases

Massage Therapy Implications

RISKS

A client with a diagnosed blood clot is not a candidate for any rigorous massage until that situation has completely stabilized. A client with signs of a blood clot (which can be simply deep unilateral calf pain) is likewise not a good candidate for circulatory massage until the source of the pain has been definitively determined not to be related to a blood clot. The risk, of course, is that a clot could fragment, embolize, and land in the lung.

Clients who are using anticoagulants are at significantly increased risk for bleeding and bruising. Any bodywork performed during this time must accommodate for those possibilities.

BENEFITS

A client who has successfully treated and recovered from thrombophlebitis or DVT can enjoy all the benefits from bodywork as does the rest of the population.

RESEARCH

The published research about massage therapy in the context of DVT mostly reports on adverse events. One paper dating from 1970[1] noted that DVT was often found postmortem in patients on bed rest after heart attack; deep calf massage was suggested as a preventive measure for such patients. This seems shocking by today's standards, but they had few reference sources at the time. This is a good example of how research builds and evolves in professional practice.

1. Bieri D, Heath J, Samios R. The effects of faradism under pressure on venous pressure. *The Australian Journal of Physiotherapy* 1970;16(4):159–160. http://www.ncbi.nlm.nih.gov/pubmed/25028255

Vascular Disorders

Aneurysm

Definition: What Is It?

An aneurysm is a permanent bulge in the wall of a blood vessel or the heart. They happen most often at the aorta (aortic aneurysm) and in the brain (cerebral aneurysm).

Demographics

Aneurysms are often silent, so accurate statistics are difficult to gather. It is estimated that 3 to 5 million Americans may have a cerebral aneurysm, but only 0.5% to 3% (about 30,000) will ever experience bleeding. Aortic aneurysms are highly correlated to age; most occur in people over 60 years old. Men are affected more often than women, with a ratio of about 3:1. Aneuryms cause some 15,000 deaths each year.

Etiology: What Happens?

The three-ply construction of the arteries includes the endothelial inside layer, the smooth muscle middle layer, and the tough connective tissue outer layer. Blood pressure in the aorta and the arteries that supply the brain is very high. If the walls of these vessels lose their elasticity, they can bulge wide with blood. This bulge is an aneurysm. As the aneurysm grows, the walls stretch and weaken, increasing the risk of rupture and death. Aneurysms are identified when the diameter of the affected section of the artery is more than 150% of normal.

Aneurysms happen most often in the thoracic or abdominal aorta and at the base of the brain. It is possible for multiple sites to develop simultaneously. The carotid arteries are occasional sites. Aneurysms sometimes develop in more distal vessels, but those cases are generally less threatening because the blood pressure drops with distance from the heart.

One complication of a major **heart attack** is an aneurysm in the left ventricle of the heart itself. The damage to myocardium reduces elasticity to the point that chronic pressure causes the whole wall of the ventricle to bulge. This is discussed further in the section on **heart failure**.

Several factors can contribute to the chances of developing an aneurysm:

- *Compromised smooth muscle.* Atherosclerotic plaques invade and weaken aortal muscle. Aortic aneurysms are a serious and common complication of **atherosclerosis** and **high blood pressure**.
- *Smoking.* The damage incurred to endothelium by carbon monoxide from cigarette smoke and a rise in blood pressure from nicotine makes smoking a leading risk factor for aortic aneurysm.
- *Congenitally weak arterial wall.* Sometimes, the tissue simply isn't strong enough to manage normal blood pressure, and with no warning, an aneurysm can rupture. Inherited connective tissue diseases such as **Marfan syndrome** and **Ehlers-Danlos syndrome** can contribute to this kind of event.
- *Inflammation.* A few diseases, such as polyarteritis nodosa and bacterial **endocarditis**, can cause inflammation and weakening of the arterial tissue.
- *Untreated* ***syphilis***. This can lead to damage in the aorta, sometimes decades after the initial infection.
- *Trauma.* Mechanical trauma, such as a car accident in which a person is injured by a steering wheel, may sometimes damage the outer layers of the aorta while leaving the inner one intact. This results in the characteristic bulging and stretching of the most delicate arterial tissue.

Complications

For the rare aneurysms that are not in the aorta or the brain, no serious complications may develop unless the aneurysm gets large enough to impede blood flow, which can lead to gangrene. But more typically, aneurysms press against nearby structures, which can interfere with function. If blood pools inside an aneurysm, clots may form and enter the bloodstream again. And of course, a rupture leads to hemorrhaging in the best case, and shock followed by circulatory collapse in the worst case. A ruptured cerebral aneurysm causes a **hemorrhagic stroke**; this is fatal about 50% of the time.

Types of Aneurysm

- *Saccular aneurysm.* These usually occur with thoracic or abdominal aortic aneurysms. The aortal wall bulges like a rounded sack, which throbs and pushes against neighboring organs and other structures.
- *Fusiform aneurysm.* This is a common type of aortic aneurysm; in this case, the bulge is less round and more tubular, as if the aorta were widened like a sausage for a few inches.
- *Berry aneurysm.* These small aneurysms are usually in the brain (Figure 5.14).
- *Dissecting aneurysm.* Also called false aneurysm, this is the least common and most painful type of aortic damage. The blood pressure actually splits the layers of the aorta between

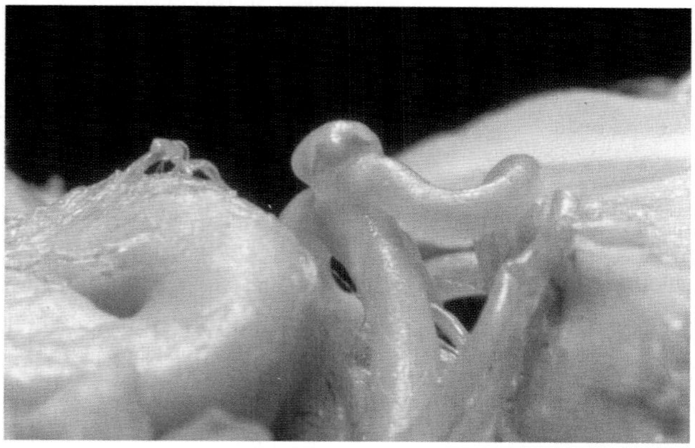

FIGURE 5.14 Berry aneurysm

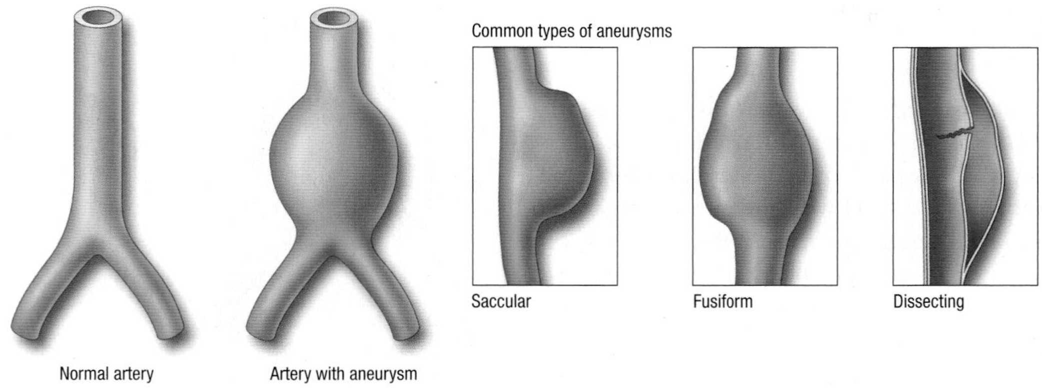

FIGURE 5.15 Varieties of aneurysms

the tunica intima and the tunica media. In some cases, this type of bulge can seal itself off when the blood trapped inside the split coagulates and solidifies. It is possible to have a dissecting aorta without an aneurysm (Figure 5.15).

Signs and Symptoms

Aneurysms can be difficult to identify early, because they often aren't painful until they become a medical emergency. With aortic aneurysms, the swelling might create some warning signals; this usually happens when the bulge is pressing on another organ. A pulsating mass may be palpable in the abdomen: this is pertinent for massage therapists doing abdominal work.

Thoracic aneurysms sometimes cause difficulty with swallowing, chest pain, hoarseness, and coughing that is not relieved with medication, because the protrusion presses on and irritates the larynx. Abdominal aneurysms sometimes show as a throbbing lump near the umbilicus, loss of appetite, weight loss, reduced urine output, and, if it's pushing against the spine, severe backache. Aneurysms in the brain may have no signs, but if they suddenly change, they may cause headache, numbness, weakness, or other symptoms, depending on what they press on.

Treatment

Aneurysms don't spontaneously retreat, because the pressure that causes them is unrelenting. They must be repaired, either with open surgery or with endovascular surgery. Open surgery involves clamping off the artery above and below the lesion and attaching either a replacement graft or a Dacron substitute to the two ends. This is usually successful, but it has to be done before a rupture. Endovascular surgery involves inserting a catheter through the femoral artery and threading it up to the aorta to insert a patch or stent at the aneurysm site. This is a much less invasive procedure with a lower risk of surgical complications.

NOTABLE CASES The first successful surgery for "triple A" (abdominal aortic aneurysm) happened in 1948. Just 1 year later, Albert Einstein underwent this radical new procedure, and he lived for another 6 years before dying at age 76 from aortic rupture.

Some aneurysms don't require immediate intervention. Many doctors recommend checking the size of small aneurysms by ultrasound every 6 months until the benefits of intervention outweigh the risks.

Medications

- Antihypertensives to reduce blood pressure
- Analgesics to manage pain and anxiety

Massage Therapy Implications

RISKS	Massage has been seen both to increase and decrease blood pressure. It causes superficial capillary dilation, which reroutes blood from elsewhere. It tends to shift functions toward a parasympathetic state, which may be positive for a person with an aneurysm, but all of these internal changes must be within that client's capacity for adaptation.
BENEFITS	A client with a stable aneurysm who is receiving medical care can receive massage that is within his or her capacity for adaptation. A good way to gauge this is to get an idea of the client's typical activities of daily living. A client who walks for a couple of miles a day has better adaptive capacity than does one who is totally bedridden, for instance.
OPTIONS	Modalities that focus on relaxation without emphasis on fluid movement are appropriate for aneurysm patients who can tolerate those challenges.

Atherosclerosis

Definition: What Is It?

Arteriosclerosis is hardening of the arteries from any cause. Atherosclerosis is a subtype of arteriosclerosis. It is a condition in which deposits of cholesterol, calcium, and other substances infiltrate and weaken layers of large- and medium-sized blood vessels, particularly the aorta and coronary arteries. It is compounded by local spasm and blood clots that form at the site of these deposits. These features contribute to occlusion of **lumen** of the arteries (Figure 5.16) and to the risk of forming and releasing blood clots on the arterial side of the systemic circuit: **arterial thrombus or embolism**.

Demographics

Coronary artery disease, in which the coronary arteries are the main location of the lesions, is estimated to affect about 16 million Americans. It is responsible for about 25% of all deaths in the United States each year: over 600,000.

Etiology: What Happens?

Development of atherosclerosis is a complex multifactorial process that varies according to gender, age, race, diet, and other factors. At this point, the most widely accepted idea of how atherosclerosis develops includes the following steps:

1. *Endothelial damage.* The tunica intima of arteries and other blood vessels is made of delicate epithelial tissue, and it is subject to a lot of abuse. A variety of things may hurl the first insult: constant **hypertension** in the aorta and arteries surrounding the heart, carbon monoxide from cigarette smoke, high levels of oxidized low-density lipoproteins (LDL) and triglycerides, or high blood sugar can begin endothelial erosion. Damage occurs most readily at branches or sharp curves in the arteries, where turbulence in blood flow most severely impacts endothelial health. At this point, LDLs may penetrate into the tunica intima.
2. *Monocytes arrive.* These small white blood cells are attracted to any site of damage in the body. The monocytes infiltrate the epithelial layer and become fixed macrophages, or big eaters. See animation at http://thePoint.lww.com/Werner6e. thePoint®
3. *Macrophages take up LDL.* LDLs are the "bad guys" of the cholesterol world. Their job is to escort usable cholesterol to the cells in the body. But when those cells don't need any more cholesterol, they stop accepting it. This leaves LDLs with nowhere to go. Macrophages in the tunica intima take up these light-colored packages of fat, which is why they are sometimes called foam cells at this stage. These foam cells merge to become large deposits of fat ("fatty streaks") in the tunica intima (see Sidebar 5.3).
4. *Foam cells infiltrate smooth muscle tissue.* Foam cells secrete growth factors; this causes the smooth muscle cells in the arterial wall to proliferate all around them. The grayish-white lumps of plaque are made of these extra muscle cells and cholesterol-filled macrophages. Foam cells also release enzymes that damage arterial walls and cause bleeding and clot formation.
5. *Platelets arrive.* Attracted by the changing texture of the arterial wall, platelets come and release their chemicals, which do three counterproductive things:
   a. Growth factors are secreted, and they reinforce the proliferation of new smooth muscle cells.
   b. Clots form, and they can further restrict the lumen of the artery.
   c. Vascular spasm occurs because the chemical that would normally prevent it can't penetrate through all

Arteriosclerosis: Hardening of the arteries.

Lumen: The space inside a tube, such as an artery or intestine.

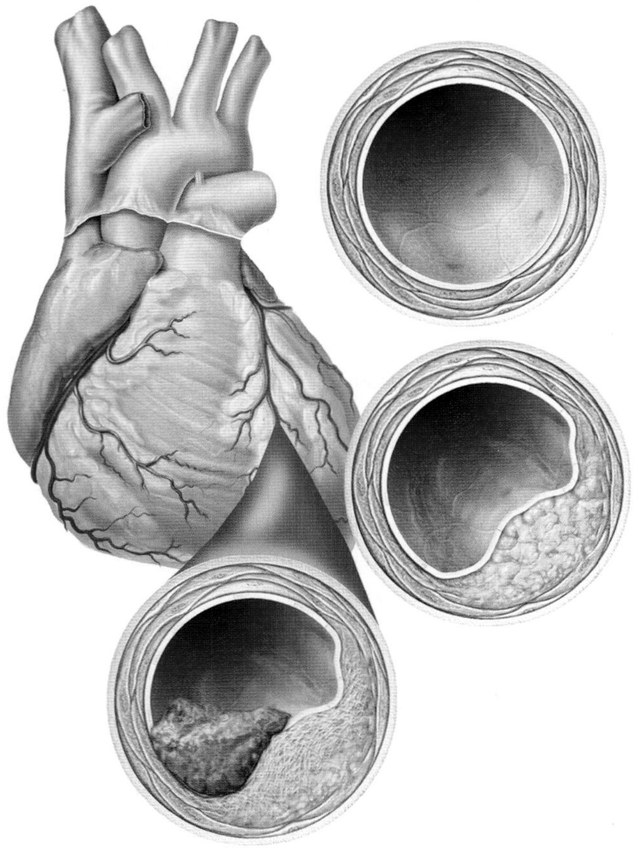

FIGURE 5.16 Progressive atherosclerosis of a coronary artery

SIDEBAR 5.3 A Brief Digression on Cholesterol

Cholesterol is a fatty substance produced in the liver and available in any animal product.

Cholesterol by itself has no access to the body's cells. Just as glucose must be escorted into cells by insulin, cholesterol must be escorted by lipoproteins, other chemicals also produced by the liver. When a cholesterol measurement is taken, it is actually the lipoproteins that are being counted.

Three varieties of lipoproteins are involved with the movement of cholesterol: **low-density lipoprotein** (LDL), **high-density lipoprotein** (HDL), and **triglyceride**. The LDLs ("bad cholesterol") deliver cholesterol to the body's cells. They are bad only when the body's cells have no more need for their cargo. At that point, the LDLs deposit the cholesterol in artery walls. The HDLs ("good cholesterol") are involved in reverse cholesterol transport. In this process, cholesterol is moved out of the arteries and back to the liver for metabolic processing. The third variety, triglycerides, are chemicals that help to convert fats and carbohydrates into energy for muscles. Elevated triglyceride levels contribute to plaque formation, so it is desirable to keep their numbers down.

When a person gets a cholesterol reading, it's useful to know not just what the overall levels are but in what ratios the carrier types occur. An ideal reading would find total levels below 200 mg/dL, with a relatively high proportion of HDLs (over 35 mg/dL) and lower numbers of LDLs and triglycerides (<130 mg/dL combined).

the plaque. This leads to a temporary lack of oxygen in the myocardium and the gripping chest pain called **angina pectoris**.

6. *Plaques form*. These are made of fat, and dead foam cells, with a fibrous cover made of smooth muscle cells and connective tissue proteins. This fibrous cap accepts deposits of calcium, which make the artery less flexible. Inside the plaque, clots form and tissue dies. Inflammation causes the fibrous cap to loosen, and the plaque ruptures. This releases the core of lipids, clots, and necrotic material into the blood.

Risk Factors

Risk factors for atherosclerosis can be divided into modifiable and nonmodifiable types.

Nonmodifiable Risk Factors

- *Heredity, genetics*: Heart disease certainly runs in families, but genetics are only one among many risk factors for atherosclerosis.
- *Gender*: While both men and women are affected by atherosclerosis, the average onset for men is typically around age 45, and for women, it is around age 55. This reflects the shift in hormones and blood chemistry that occurs after menopause.
- *Age*: The incidence of heart disease rises with age, but it is not a disease exclusively of the elderly.
- *Kidney disorders*: Atherosclerosis can sometimes lead to kidney problems. But if the kidney problems predate the circulatory ones, **high blood pressure** brought about by kidney failure can be a precipitator for atherosclerosis.

Low-density lipoprotein (LDL): A compound made up of both lipids and proteins, which is associated with an increased risk of cardiovascular disease.

High-density lipoprotein (HDL): A compound made up of both lipids and proteins, which is associated with a reduced risk of cardiovascular disease.

Triglyceride: A major component of natural fats and oils, containing glycerol and three fatty acids.

Angina pectoris: Severe chest pain.

Modifiable Risk Factors

- *Smoking*: Carbon monoxide from cigarette smoke is corrosive to endothelium. Furthermore, nicotine causes vasoconstriction and high blood pressure.
- *High cholesterol levels*: A predictable statistical link has been established between high cholesterol levels and the development of pathological atherosclerosis.
- *High blood pressure*: Chronic uncontrolled high blood pressure contributes to endothelial damage, which opens the door to the formation of plaques.
- *Sedentary lifestyle*: Regular moderate cardiovascular exercise, perhaps more than any other factor, can reduce the risk of atherosclerosis. It keeps arteries elastic and pliable; it reduces weight; it raises high-density lipoprotein (HDL) levels for the reduction of plaques; it reduces the risk of diabetes; and it lowers blood pressure.
- *Diabetes*: People with uncontrolled **diabetes** are especially susceptible to atherosclerosis because of the way their body metabolizes food. However, if the diabetes is controlled, the risk of atherosclerosis is much lower.
- ***Metabolic syndrome***: This is a collection of signs that indicate an increased risk for both heart disease and diabetes. It is discussed in Chapter 9.
- *Unrelieved mental stress and depression*: **Anxiety** and **depression** are mood disorders that have direct statistical correlation to atherosclerosis and other conditions that affect the circulatory system.

Other Risk Factors

Continued study into who develops atherosclerosis and what makes them different from the rest of the population has yielded some additional risk factors. It is unclear whether these are modifiable or not, and the exact relationship between these issues and heart disease is not thoroughly understood. However, identifying these issues early and controlling them may improve the outcome for many people.

- **C-reactive protein** is a liver enzyme secreted in the presence of a systemic inflammatory response. It is a dependable predictor for **heart attack**, **stroke**, and other conditions related to atherosclerosis, although the mechanism is not clearly understood. The connection between atherosclerosis and chronic inflammation may be at least partly explained by this phenomenon.
- **Homocysteine** is an amino acid in the blood. A small part of the population tends to have very high levels of homocysteine, which can contribute to endothelial damage. People with high levels are usually counseled to try to control this imbalance with folic acid and vitamins B_6 and B_{12}.
- Other risk factors that continue to be studied include **body mass index**, levels of fibrinogen, and subtypes of lipoproteins, some of which may be more involved with plaque formation than are others.

Types of Atherosclerosis

- *Carotid artery disease*: This is the formation of atherosclerotic plaque in the carotid artery where blood pressure is high and where, if a fragment breaks off, the only direction it can travel is into the brain where a transient ischemic attack or a **stroke** is the ultimate result (Figure 5.17).
- *Coronary artery disease*: This is atherosclerosis in the coronary arteries that supply the myocardium. Occlusion here, either from a clot that forms on-site or from a fragment that travels, can lead to the death of heart muscle. See "Myocardial Blood Flow" animation at http://thePoint.lww.com/Werner6e. thePoint®

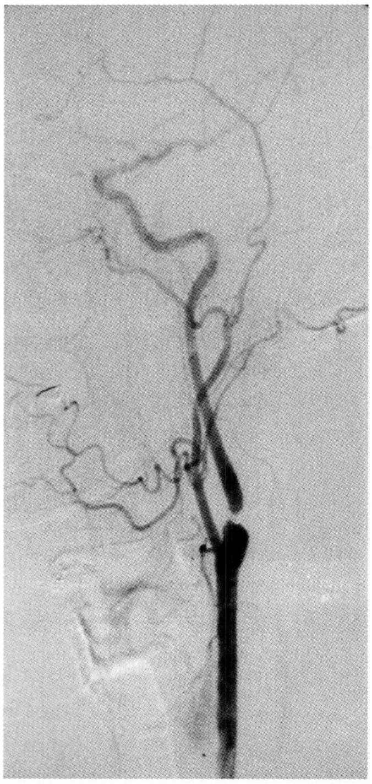

FIGURE 5.17 Carotid artery disease. Note the point of stenosis just past the bifurcation.

- *Peripheral artery disease*: This is the development of atherosclerosis away from the neck or heart. The abdomen or legs are the most frequent sites. If a clot builds or lodges in the renal artery, kidney damage occurs. In the legs, they can cause temporary pain and cramping (called **intermittent claudication**), **stasis dermatitis**, gangrene, and **skin ulcers** (Figure 5.18).

C-reactive protein: A liver enzyme secreted in the presence of inflammation. an excellent predictor of heart attack and stroke.

Homocysteine: An amino acid in the blood that contributes to endothelial injury.

Body mass index: A scale calculated using the ratio between a person's height and weight.

Intermittent claudication: Exercise-induced leg cramping caused by blocked arteries.

Complications

The complications of atherosclerosis are sometimes the first symptoms of the disease. Several of them are also topics discussed elsewhere in this chapter. They include but are not limited to these issues:

- *High blood pressure*. **Hypertension** is both a cause and a result of this disease; it contributes to the original damage to the tunica intima, and it is made worse when the arterial walls are too brittle to adjust to the constant changes in blood volume flowing through them.
- ***Aneurysm***. When the wall of an artery is rendered inelastic and defective, it can bulge and become thin, weak, and susceptible to rupture.
- *Arrhythmia*. Advanced atherosclerosis can contribute to the development of irregular or uncoordinated beating of the cardiac muscle as blood supply through the coronary arteries is periodically interrupted. Arrhythmia can cause

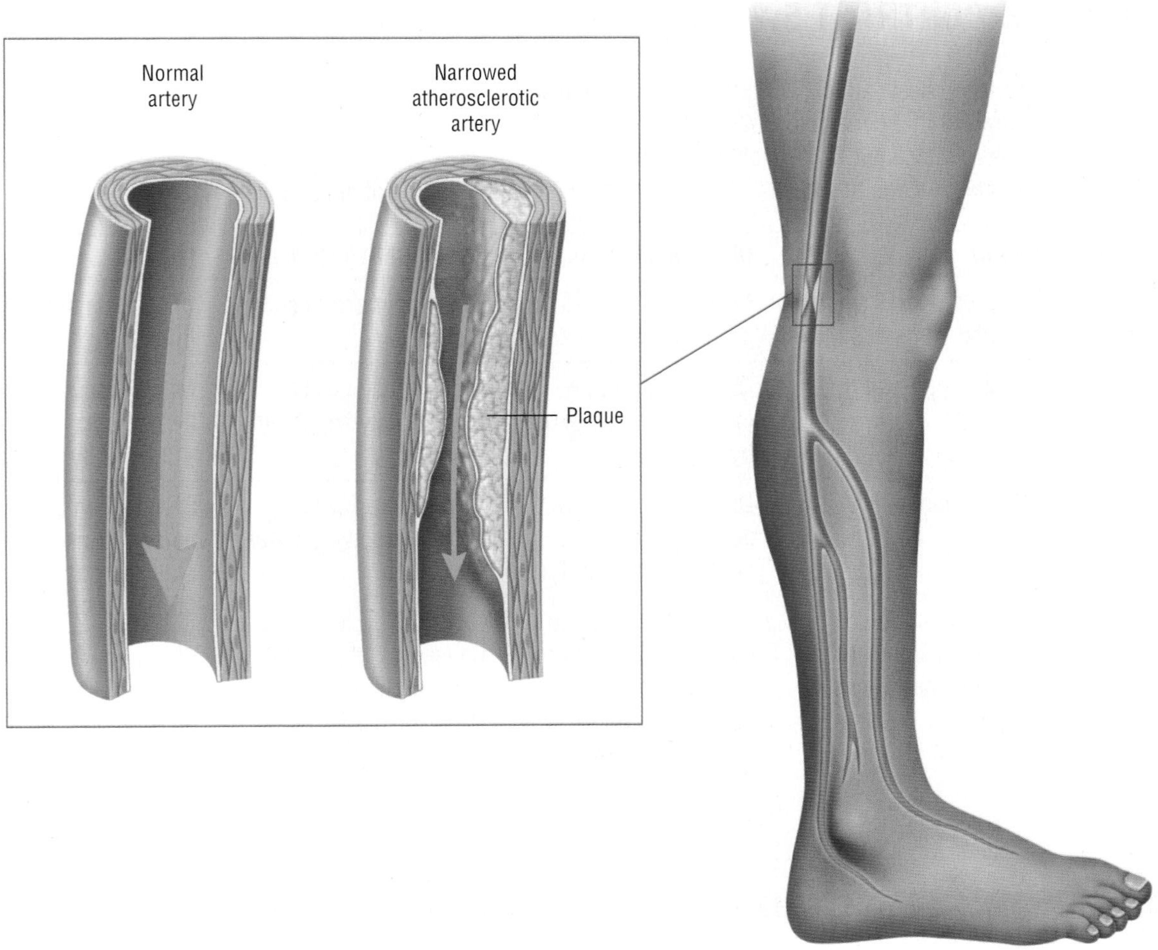

FIGURE 5.18 Peripheral artery disease

clots to form in the atria when the chamber doesn't empty completely. These clots can travel anywhere the aorta takes them.

- ***Thrombus or embolism***. Thrombi are the link between atherosclerosis and stroke or transient ischemic attack when they travel to the brain and between atherosclerosis and heart attack when they develop or lodge in the coronary arteries.
- *Angina pectoris*. The process of developing atherosclerotic plaques also creates a higher risk of short-term vascular spasm, which leads to heart and chest pain.
  - Stable angina pectoris means that chest pain is predictable with exercise or exertion and subsides during rest.
  - Unstable angina pectoris means that chest pain varies in intensity, is not associated with exercise, and is unpredictable. Unstable angina is related to the rupture of a plaque: it is associated with a high risk of heart attack (see Compare & Contrast 5.2).
- *Heart attack*. When rough plaques form on smooth artery walls, they attract thrombocytes. If a clot or fragment of plaque breaks off in the coronary artery, or if a plaque and clot completely occlude a section of the coronary artery, all of the myocardium that should have been supplied then dies. This is a myocardial infarction, or **heart attack**.

Signs and Symptoms

Until the damage has progressed to dangerous levels, atherosclerosis is completely silent, partly because the body doesn't depend on any single artery to do a job. Most areas have two or three

NOTABLE CASES Former President Bill Clinton underwent quadruple bypass surgery in 2004 to correct plaque accumulation associated with high cholesterol. While atherosclerosis is understood to be tied to a fatty diet, sedentary lifestyle, and smoking, evidence of it has been found in Egyptian mummies, who probably did not indulge in these modern temptations.

COMPARE & CONTRAST 5.2 Chest Pain, Chest Pain, Chest Pain

Not all chest pain means heart attack, although in a culture in which almost 25% of deaths are related to CVD, it seems logical to jump to that conclusion. What follows is a comparison of types of chest pain with some indications of what might be heart attack and what probably is not. However, heart attack symptoms are notoriously variable, and it is always a good idea to consult a health care professional when the source of chest pain is not clear.

FEATURES	ANGINA	HEART ATTACK	PULMONARY EMBOLISM	OTHERS
Duration	Chest pain lasts several minutes, subsides.	Chest pain progressively worsens.	Chest pain progressively worsens.	Chest pain subsides in <1 min.
Trigger	Usually triggered by activity	May or may not be immediately triggered by activity	May or may not be immediately triggered by activity	May or may not be immediately triggered by activity
Activity	Stops when activity stops	Doesn't stop when activity stops; continues to worsen	Doesn't stop when activity stops; continues to worsen	Stops when a person drinks water, changes position, or takes a deep breath
Causes	Caused by transient ischemia; heart muscle temporarily doesn't get enough oxygen to function.	Caused by permanent ischemia; blockage deprives cells of oxygen, and heart is irrevocably damaged.	Caused by blood clots in lung. Small clots may have little impact. Large clots may lead to pulmonary and circulatory collapse.	Caused by any number of factors, for example, musculoskeletal injury, gastroesophageal reflux

alternative vessels, or the body can generate new vessels that can be pressed into service if one of them is out of commission.

When signs of atherosclerosis begin to develop, they arise mainly from poor delivery of oxygen to the tissues. If the starved cells are in the heart, low stamina and shortness of breath are the earliest signs. Symptoms of atherosclerosis outside of the coronary arteries often take the shape of the previously discussed complications.

Angioplasty: A procedure for opening a blood vessel, usually by means of balloon dilation or the placement of a stent.

Endarterectomy: Excision of the diseased layers of an artery along with obstructing plaques.

Bypass surgery: A surgery in which a diseased blood vessel is bypassed by a grafted vessel in order to restore blood flow.

Restenosis: Recurring stenosis after corrective surgery.

Treatment

Treatment for atherosclerosis starts simply with adjustments in eating and exercise habits.

More advanced cases may require drugs and/or surgery. The drugs are generally designed to influence blood pressure, cholesterol levels, and platelet activity. Surgical intervention can include **angioplasty**, **endarterectomy**, or **bypass surgery**. Angioplasty is a procedure in which the artery may first be treated with a laser, which vaporizes plaques (laser angioplasty), and then a small balloon is inflated to widen the artery (balloon angioplasty). Unfortunately, the **restenosis** that occurs when the balloon is removed can be a dangerous complication of this procedure; new cells rapidly proliferate where the endothelium was scraped. In an endarterectomy, a tiny rotating drill is inserted into clogged arteries to shave off plaque, and the shavings are trapped and removed. This is sometimes used for carotid arteries when the risk of stroke is high. In bypass surgery, surgeons remove the damaged piece of artery and replace it, often with a graft from the internal mammary artery or a piece of saphenous vein. A single, double, triple, or however-many bypass refers to the number of sections of artery being replaced.

If a patient is not a good candidate for other interventions, or if the other approaches have failed, a procedure called percutaneous transmyocardial revascularization may be done. This procedure inserts a laser up through the femoral artery to the heart. The laser then creates tiny holes in the myocardium. This is intended to stimulate the growth of new blood vessels, improving circulation to the heart muscle and reducing angina.

Medications

- Cholesterol management drugs, including reductase inhibitors, fibric acid derivatives, and bile sequestering drugs
- Antihypertensive drugs, including beta-blockers, calcium channel blockers, and ACE inhibitors
- Anticoagulants, including aspirin
- Antianginal drugs, including nitroglycerin

Massage Therapy Implications

RISKS	Many people, perhaps the majority of adults in the United States, have a subclinical accumulation of plaque in major arteries (see Sidebar 5.4). Those with atherosclerosis severe enough to threaten other complications of heart disease (heart attack, heart failure, aneurysm, etc.) may not have the adaptive capacity to keep up with the challenges of rigorous circulatory massage. Choices must be made based on the client's resilience, his or her normal levels of activity, and what kinds of medications are used to control this condition.
BENEFITS	For a person with atherosclerosis who wants to support better health, careful massage along with dietary changes, exercise, and other self-care strategies can make a positive difference.
OPTIONS	While a person with any kind of heart disease may not be a good candidate for most types of massage, it is a wonderful feature of human construction that no major blood vessels run close to the surface on the upper back or between the scapulae. This means it is possible to give a wonderful massage, without having a profound or direct impact on the circulatory system. The main caution here is to remember that the anterior aspect of the trapezius muscle runs dangerously close to the carotid artery, and this is an endangerment site for carotid artery disease.

SIDEBAR 5.4 Heart Disease in the United States: Sobering Statistics

The statistics for all varieties of cardiovascular disease are not generally separated from each other, since most of these conditions have a circular relationship. A person is unlikely to have atherosclerosis without high blood pressure, for instance, and a person is unlikely to have a heart attack without the predisposing factor of atherosclerosis, even if it never produces any symptoms.

Statistics for CVD (this includes stroke, hypertension, heart failure, heart attack, angina, and congenital defects) in this country are sobering. These conditions collectively account for about 25% of all deaths each year. This is actually an improvement; not long ago, it was responsible for close to 40% of all deaths. Still, CVD is the leading cause of death for men and women. It kills more people each year than do the next four leading causes of death combined (cancer, chronic obstructive pulmonary disease, accidents, and diabetes).

1.5 million heart attacks occur each year, and half of them have no prior warning signs or symptoms. About 8 million heart attack survivors are alive today in the United States, and 80 million Americans live with more than one type of CVD.

About 33% of United States adults over 20 years of age have hypertension. Over 33 million adults over 20 years old have total serum cholesterol above 240 mg/dL, and more than 67% of United States adults are overweight.

Behaviors that limit the risk of heart disease have been identified to include not smoking, maintaining healthy weight, eating at least five servings of fruit and vegetables each day, and exercising for at least 30 minutes most days of the week. Other risk-lowering behaviors include having a diet that is low in trans fats, with a low glycemic load, high in fish oils, and high in folate. Studies consistently find that people for whom major risk factors are low in middle age have a greatly increased possibility of living to age 85 years or older without severe illness.

Hypertension

Definition: What Is It?

Hypertension is a technical term for high blood pressure. It is defined as blood pressure persistently elevated above 140 mm Hg systolic and/or 90 mm Hg diastolic.

Demographics

It is estimated that 67 to 76 million adults in the United States have high blood pressure, and of them, only about half manage it successfully. Another one in three adults has prehypertension. It is seen in men more often than women until women reach age 45; then it evens out and affects both genders equally. Age is a predisposing factor; about half of those over 60 years of age have high blood pressure. African Americans have higher hypertension rates than do other races in the United States, and higher risk of life-threatening complications.

Etiology: What Happens?

In hypertension, internal and external forces put excessive pressure on the arteries. Internal forces include any plaque or debris on arterial walls. The tightness of the artery also influences pressure. And external forces include water retention that presses in from the outside. When these forces add up, the artery is vulnerable to damage, and the interwoven picture of cardiovascular disease can begin.

A **sphygmomanometer** measures the pressure blood exerts against arterial walls at two moments: during contraction (**systole**) and relaxation (**diastole**). The blood pressure cuff converts the pressure in the arteries to millimeters of mercury.

The standard scale for hypertension in adults is based on how measurements correspond to the risk of developing **atherosclerosis**, **aneurysm**, **stroke**, **renal failure**, or **heart failure**. While a reading of 120/80 has traditionally been considered normal, the risk of secondary disease increases significantly when the systolic reading is consistently over 115 or when the diastolic reading is consistently over 75.

A person's blood pressure is based on the averages of two or more readings taken at each of two or more doctor visits, because blood pressure can change significantly from hour to hour. It's fairly common to see it shoot up from anxiety while a person is in a doctor's office; this is known as "white coat hypertension."

Blood pressure ratings are shown in Table 5.1. If a person is in two different levels for systolic and diastolic, he or she is labeled according to the higher stage.

Sphygmomanometer: An instrument for measuring blood pressure.

Systole: The phase of the heartbeat during which heart muscles contract, pushing blood out of the chambers.

Diastole: The phase of the heartbeat during which heart muscles relax, allowing the chambers to fill with blood.

TABLE 5.1 Blood Pressure Ratings

Category	Systolic BP (mm Hg)	Diastolic BP (mm Hg)
Optimal	<120	<80
Prehypertension	122–139	80–89
Hypertension		
Stage 1 (mild)	140–159	90–99
Stage 2 (moderate)	160+	100+

Complications

High blood pressure quietly and progressively erodes large- and medium-sized arteries, tearing up the endothelial lining and leading to a host of complications, including the following:

- *Edema*: High blood pressure forces fluid out of the capillaries at the nutrient-waste exchange sites. This adds to overall levels of interstitial fluid, causing edema. In a typically vicious circle, edema further raises blood pressure by putting external force on blood vessels.
- *Atherosclerosis*: Having blood pounding against arteries in an unceasing torrent simply wears out the walls, especially when the arteries have naturally lost some of their resiliency from age. As damage develops, the atherosclerotic process begins. This narrows arterial diameters, forcing blood pressure up.
- *Stroke*: Someone with hypertension is more likely to have a stroke than is someone who does not have hypertension. The stroke may be from an embolism, or it may be from ruptured arteries in the brain. Studies show that people whose blood pressure is in the high range of prehypertension have an almost 100% greater risk for stroke compared to those who do not have the condition.
- *Enlarged heart, heart failure*: Pushing against the narrowed arteries in the systemic circuit causes the left ventricle to grow considerably, but the coronary arteries do not

grow with it to handle the extra load. The muscle fibers of the heart also lose elasticity. Therefore, its contractions are weaker, because the muscle is not well supplied with blood and it can't contract fully. This can also cause angina. When the ventricles of the heart are so overtaxed that they simply cannot keep up with the workload, the patient risks heart failure.

- *Aneurysm*: This is the result of high blood pressure causing a bulge in the arteries.
- *Kidney disease*: This complication of high blood pressure demonstrates the circular relationship between hypertension and kidney dysfunction. If problems start with the circulatory system, hypertension causes atherosclerotic plaques to form in the renal arteries, which are subject to huge blood pressure. This causes changes in blood flow to the kidney, which impairs kidney function, leading to kidney damage, systemic edema, and yet more pressure exerted against vessel walls from that edema. If the problem starts in the kidneys, decreased kidney function causes fluid retention. This is often accompanied by extra release of **renin**. Excess renin results in vasoconstriction, water and salt retention, increased edema, increased blood volume, and high blood pressure.
- *Retinopathy*: Chronic high blood pressure can damage the blood vessels that supply the eyes, causing them to thicken and lose elasticity. Reduction of blood flow to eyes results in permanent visual distortion.

High blood pressure is the most important modifiable risk factor in the development of coronary artery disease, stroke, congestive heart failure, end-stage renal failure, and peripheral artery disease. To learn about the complications of this condition, see the animation "Hypertension" http://thePoint.lww.com. thePoint®

Types of Hypertension

- *Essential hypertension*: This is the focus of this discussion: it is not wholly dependent on some underlying factor. Essential hypertension accounts for about 95% of all diagnoses of high blood pressure.
- *Secondary hypertension*: This is a temporary complication of some other condition, such as pregnancy, kidney problems, adrenal tumor, or hormonal disorder.
- *Malignant hypertension*: This could be essential or secondary, but it involves diastolic pressure that rises very quickly, over a matter of weeks or months. It is extremely damaging to the circulatory system and a high risk for ischemic or hemorrhagic stroke. Left untreated, malignant hypertension is often fatal.

Renin: An enzyme produced by the kidneys that is involved in vasoconstriction and hypertension.

Signs and Symptoms

Hypertension, which is often called the silent killer, has few recognizable symptoms. When subtle signs are occasionally observed, they include shortness of breath after mild exercise; headaches or dizziness; swelling of the ankles, especially during the daytime; excessive sweating; anxiety; and occasional nosebleeds.

Treatment

Hypertension is a highly treatable condition, but because it has virtually no symptoms until it has progressed to very dangerous levels, it is frequently untreated or incompletely treated. Only about half of the people who treat their hypertension at all are successful at getting their blood pressure below 140/90.

Exercise and diet are the first strategies to manage this condition. The National Heart Lung and Blood Institute (NHLBI) has created the dietary approaches to stop hypertension (DASH) diet: it comprises high-fiber, low-fat foods that provide higher-than-average levels of calcium, magnesium, and potassium, while cutting sodium by about 20%. Following the DASH diet (which is useful for anyone, not just hypertension patients) has been found to be as effective as is treatment with any single type of blood pressure medication, without side effects or long-term health risks.

Exercise is also crucial for the development of healthy new blood vessels and for weight control. Losing even a small percentage of body weight for obese or overweight patients can have a profound effect on blood pressure and cardiovascular health.

Medication, if it's called for, includes diuretics, vasodilators, and beta-blockers, which decrease the force of ventricular contraction. Medicating high blood pressure can be challenging. Because the disease itself has no strong symptoms, and because the medicines often have mild but unpleasant side effects (including dizziness, insomnia, impotence, and others), it can be difficult for hypertension patients to be consistent with their medications. Most hypertension patients need two or more medications to successfully manage their condition.

Medications

- Diuretics for fluid management and kidney support
- Vasodilators (calcium channel blockers, ACE inhibitors, angiotensin receptor blockers) to reduce cardiac load
- Beta-blockers, alpha blockers to decrease the force of ventricular contraction

Massage Therapy Implications

RISKS	Clients with unmanaged or poorly managed hypertension may have complications that have cautions for massage, including kidney disease, atherosclerosis, and a risk of heart attack. All of these are concerns for massage therapists and bodywork practitioners. Further, clients who take medication for hypertension may feel dizzy or lethargic—this means they may need more time after a massage to make the transition back to full speed.
BENEFITS	Any client with mild or borderline hypertension who is encouraged to exercise is a good candidate for most kinds of bodywork. Clients with more advanced problems but who manage their hypertension successfully require some caution, but if they can exercise safely, they can probably also receive massage safely: judgments about massage must be made by comparing the challenges of bodywork with activities of daily living. Bodywork has been seen to have at least a short-term effect on blood pressure, but the overall stress-reducing effects may be more useful in the long run.
RESEARCH	A comparatively early study on massage therapy for hypertension found significant results with 10-minute sessions, three times a week.[1] Since then, many studies have considered the possibility. A systematic review[2] found weak evidence for massage therapy, but that was mainly because the research done so far has been of varying quality. The authors point out that massage with antihypertensive drugs appears to be more effective than the drugs alone. Similar conclusions were found in a systematic review limited to research on Tuina for hypertension.[3] One small study of Swedish massage[4] found that systolic and diastolic pressures decreased with treatment, as did markers for inflammatory chemicals associated with endothelial damage.[5] And one study compared types of massage, including Swedish, trigger point, and sports massage. They found that Swedish massage had the greatest impact on lowering hypertension.[6]

1. Olney CM. The effect of therapeutic back massage in hypertensive persons: a preliminary study. *Biological Research for Nursing* 2005;7(2):98–105. http://brn.sagepub.com/content/7/2/98
2. Xiong XJ, Li SJ, Zhang YQ. Massage therapy for essential hypertension: a systematic review. *Journal of Human Hypertension* 2014. http://www.ncbi.nlm.nih.gov/pubmed/24990417
3. Yang X, Zhao H, Wang J. Chinese massage (Tuina) for the treatment of essential hypertension: a systematic review and meta-analysis. *Complementary Therapies in Medicine* 2014;22(3):541–548. http://www.ncbi.nlm.nih.gov/pubmed/24906593
4. Supa'at I, Zakaria Z, Maskon O, et al. Effects of Swedish massage therapy on blood pressure, heart rate, and inflammatory markers in hypertensive women. *Evidence-Based Complementary and Alternative Medicine* 2013;2013:171852. http://www.ncbi.nlm.nih.gov/pubmed/24023571
5. Givi M. Durability of effect of massage therapy on blood pressure. *International Journal of Preventive Medicine* 2013;4(5): 511–516. http://www.ncbi.nlm.nih.gov/pmc/articles/PMC3733180/
6. Cambron JA, Dexheimer J, Coe P. Changes in blood pressure after various forms of therapeutic massage: a preliminary study. *Journal of Alternative and Complementary Medicine* 2006;12(1):65–70. http://www.ncbi.nlm.nih.gov/pubmed/16494570

Raynaud Syndrome

Definition: What Is It?

Raynaud syndrome is a condition involving the status of the arterioles in the hands and feet, although it can also affect the nose, ears, and lips. Primary Raynaud disease is a vasoconstriction disorder, while secondary Raynaud phenomenon is a complication of an underlying problem.

Demographics

Raynaud syndrome may affect 5% to 10% of the population. Most of those cases are the less serious form, Raynaud disease.

> **Vasospasm:** The sudden constriction of a blood vessel.

Many people with this condition have it so mildly that they don't seek medical intervention. Women are affected much more frequently than are men.

Etiology: What Happens?

Raynaud syndrome affects the arterioles in the extremities so that they develop **vasospasm**. It occurs in temporary episodes at first, but especially if it is a secondary complication, the vasoconstriction can become long-lasting. It can happen as a primary condition or as a symptom of an underlying disease.

Types of Raynaud Syndrome

- *Raynaud disease*: This is primary Raynaud syndrome; it occurs without an identified underlying pathology. It may be due to emotional stress, cold, or a mechanical irritation, such as operating machinery that influences blood vessel dilation. Raynaud disease generally has a slow onset, and

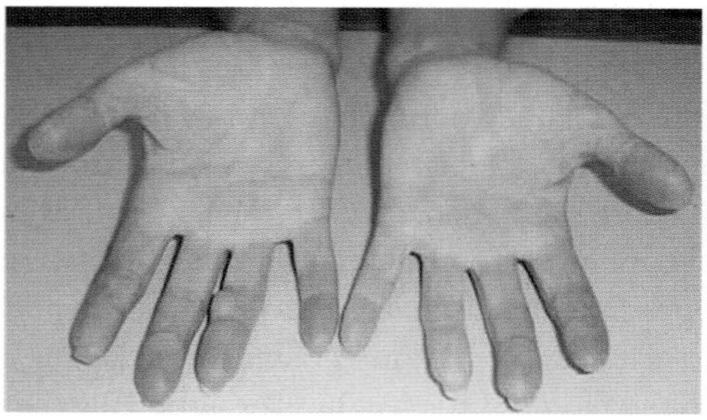

FIGURE 5.19 Raynaud syndrome

the attacks are less severe than when the symptoms occur as a secondary problem. If a person is prone to Raynaud disease, both the feet and hands tend to be affected.

- *Raynaud phenomenon*: This is a secondary reaction to an underlying condition. It generally has a much faster onset than does Raynaud disease, the age at onset is typically older, and the risk of serious complications is much higher. Raynaud phenomenon may develop before associated conditions are identified. Some conditions that are frequently seen with Raynaud phenomenon include the following:
  - Arterial diseases that involve occlusions, such as **diabetes**, **atherosclerosis**, and **Buerger disease**
  - Autoimmune connective tissue diseases, such as **scleroderma**, **lupus**, and **rheumatoid arthritis**
  - Sensitivity to some substances including beta-blockers, ergot compounds, and vinyl chloride
  - A history of tissue damage due to frostbite

Signs and Symptoms

Raynaud syndrome is usually bilateral. During an attack, patches of skin go through a characteristic cycle of colors: white as the blood is shunted away from the area (on dark-skinned people, the skin looks ashy gray); blue as the cells are starved for oxygen; and red as the attack subsides, the arterioles reopen, and the blood returns to the affected area (Figure 5.19). Some people only shift between blue and red; others show only pallor or blueness during an episode. It usually affects distal fingers and toes, not the thumb or the rest of the hand. Sometimes, only one or two digits are affected, and these may change from one episode to another.

While Raynaud disease episodes are typically short, attacks of Raynaud phenomenon can last anywhere from less than a minute to several hours. These can be so extreme and long-lasting that tissue may atrophy and ulcerations may develop. Arterioles in the nail beds can become thickened and distorted, the fingers may taper, and the skin can become thin, smooth, and shiny. Gangrene is a rare but possible complication for these extreme cases.

> **Buerger disease:** Inflammation of the intima of a blood vessel with thrombosis.
>
> **Sympathectomy:** A surgical procedure that destroys nerves in the sympathetic nervous system.

Treatment

Treatment depends on whether the patient has primary or secondary Raynaud syndrome. For primary Raynaud disease, a noninvasive approach is taken first. Quitting smoking, avoiding vasoconstrictors such as nicotine and caffeine, soaking in warm water, dressing appropriately for the weather, protecting the hands when working with cold or frozen foods, making sure that shoes aren't too tight, and even moving to a warmer climate are all suggested before more intrusive intervention is suggested. In addition, because primary Raynaud disease can be exacerbated by emotional upset, patients are often encouraged to find productive ways to manage stress. This can range from learning biofeedback techniques, to exercising regularly, to receiving massage therapy.

If results are unsatisfactory or if tissue damage from chronically impaired blood flow is a risk, the next step is medication to dilate the blood vessels.

Secondary Raynaud phenomenon often doesn't respond to medication. Surgery to interfere with sympathetic motor neuron stimulation of local capillaries may be conducted; this procedure, called a digital **sympathectomy**, is used only when no other options work, and it tends to be a temporary measure.

Medications

- Topical applications of prostaglandin analogues or nitroglycerin for vasodilation
- Calcium channel blockers, ACE inhibitors, for vasodilation
- Selective serotonin reuptake inhibitors for vasodilation

Massage Therapy Implications

RISKS	Raynaud phenomenon can be a symptom of lupus, scleroderma, or other serious problems that compromise the blood vessels. In this situation, whatever the underlying condition is must dictate the choices for bodywork. Clients with Raynaud disease may use vasodilating medications that have dizziness or lethargy as side effects. These clients may need adjustments in bodywork to deal with those changes.
BENEFITS	Raynaud disease indicates massage as long as the skin is intact and healthy and the medications that the client uses are accommodated.
OPTIONS	Many clients with Raynaud disease enjoy hydrotherapy applications, including warm baths or paraffin baths for the affected areas.

Varicose Veins

Definition: What Are They?

Varicose veins, named for the root word **varix**, are permanently distended, often twisted or ropy superficial veins. They occur when veins are not strong enough to keep up with a person's needs. This usually happens in the legs, where valves that support blood flow against gravity are compromised (Figure 5.20). As blood collects, the affected vein is stretched, distorted, and further weakened. Varicose veins are an early indicator of **chronic venous insufficiency**.

Demographics

Women are more vulnerable to varicose veins than are men for a variety of reasons, but anyone can develop them. About one-half of all people over 50 years old have varicose veins, and that percentage increases with age, especially for women. Being sedentary and overweight are also risk factors for varicosities.

Etiology: What Happens?

The veins in the legs are constructed in a way that helps to move blood from the toes all the way back to the heart. Small veins pick up the blood from the internal muscle capillaries. These veins tend to run on the superficial aspect of muscles. They feed into larger veins that perforate the muscle bellies and then join into the large deep veins that run under the muscles, close to the bones. When the leg muscles contract, the perforating veins are squeezed, sending their contents to the deep veins. When the leg muscles relax, the perforating veins draw in new blood from the smaller veins. The contraction and relaxation of the leg muscles (especially the soleus–"sump pump of the leg") is crucial to blood return. The valves inside the perforating veins and the deep veins ensure that blood does not collect in the smaller, weaker superficial veins.

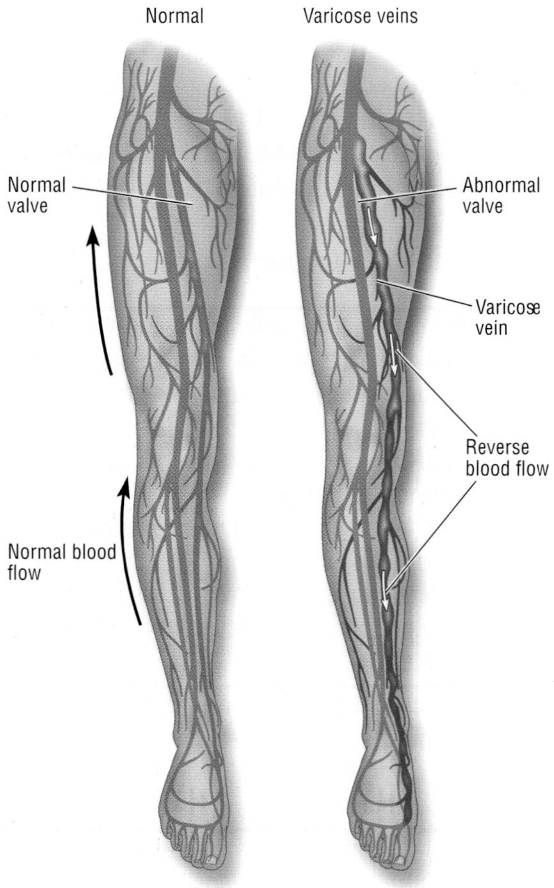

FIGURE 5.20 Varicose veins: note reverse blood flow

When valves in the superficial veins become weak, problems ensue. Weakness can develop because of simple wear and tear: being on one's feet for many hours a day, for instance, especially if the leg muscles are not allowed to fully contract and relax during that time. It could also be due to a mechanical obstruction to returning blood: knee socks that are too tight, a knee brace, or a fetus that presses on the femoral vein. Systemic problems from kidney or liver congestion have been seen to cause problems too. And finally, it could be simply congenitally weak veins or a structural anomaly at the junction between the great saphenous vein and the femoral vein.

Once a vein begins to widen, blood puts pressure on the inferior valves. Vascular incompetence ultimately causes the weakest superficial veins to become distorted, dilated, and twisted off their regular pathway. Deeper veins are protected from this process because they have the external support of muscle tissue.

Although varicosities are seldom more than annoying, they can create some unpleasant or even dangerous complications. Chronic venous insufficiency may result in varicose ulcers, which don't heal until circulation is restored. Skin irritation from poor circulation occasionally leads to a type of **dermatitis** that isn't resolved until the varicosity is relieved. Interruptions in blood flow increase the likelihood of night cramps. And slow-moving blood in a distended vein may coagulate, raising the possibility of clotting. Most clots that form in varicose veins are superficial and melt easily, however, so they are usually a lesser threat than are clots that form in deeper leg veins. Be aware, however, that the presence of grossly distended varicose veins may indicate an increased risk of DVT. This is true especially when the varicosities have a sudden onset or change in size and quality very rapidly.

Varices Dilated, distended veins. (singular: varix)

Chronic venous insufficiency: A condition in which the valves in the veins are weakened, resulting in edema as blood fails to return to the heart.

Types of Varicose Veins

In addition to the varicose veins that frequently develop in the legs, veins in other structures are vulnerable to distension and structural dysfunction.

- *Esophageal varices*: These are large, distended veins at the distal part of the esophagus. Esophageal varices are most common in people who struggle with advanced **cirrhosis** or other liver disease, or with **bulimia**. This situation carries a risk of dangerous internal bleeding. If it is determined that these varices are threatening, they may be surgically corrected
- *Hemorrhoids*: Technically speaking, hemorrhoids are clusters of vascular tissue around the anus. They can contain veins, capillaries, and small arterioles. Distended vessels can develop inside the rectum, where they are typically silent, or externally, where they can cause pain, itching, and bleeding with bowel movements. Hemorrhoids are usually associated with constipation and straining during bowel movements. If they are severely swollen or prolapsed, they can be surgically removed. Otherwise, they are typically treated by including more fiber and water in the diet and using soothing ointment.
- *Telangiectasias*: These are the very small permanently dilated capillaries and venules sometimes called spider veins. They can appear around the ankles, on the legs, or on the face. A new pattern of **telangiectasias** can sometimes indicate a deeper circulatory problem, but these phenomena are usually harmless (Figure 5.21).
- *Varicoceles*: These are dilated venous structures that supply the spermatic cord. They are often painless, but they can interfere with fertility and testosterone production. Varicoceles are treated by surgery.

Signs and Symptoms

Varicose veins look like lumpy bluish wandering lines on the skin of the legs (Figure 5.22). They are often visible on the back of the calf, where they affect the lesser saphenous vein, but more often, they affect the great saphenous vein, where they show anywhere from the ankle to the groin on the medial side. They may itch, throb, or cause cramping, especially when the person is tired.

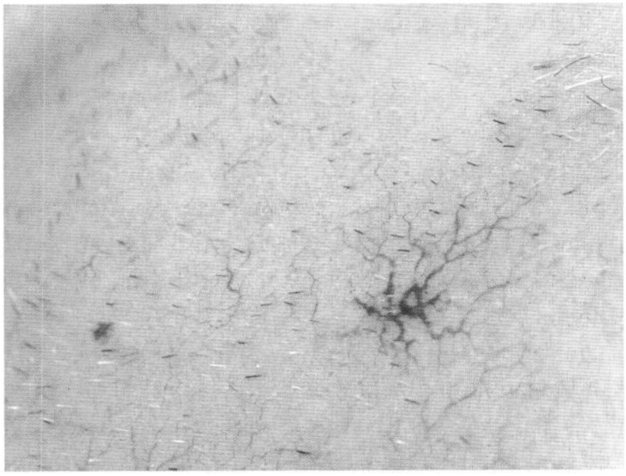

FIGURE 5.21 Harmless telangiectasias

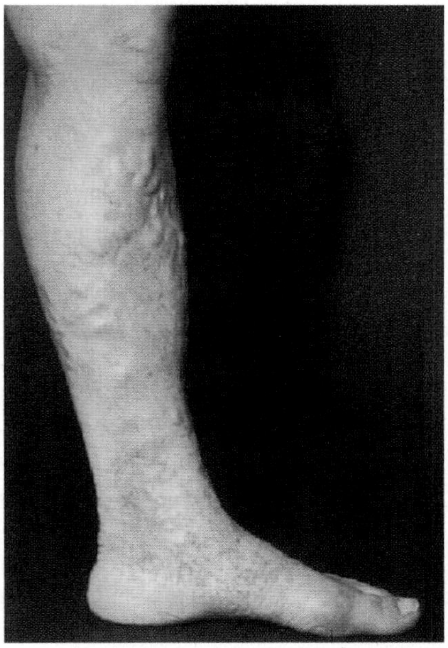

FIGURE 5.22 Varicose veins on medial side

Treatment

Support hose or elastic bandages can give extra help to damaged veins, and avoiding long periods of standing up without full contraction and relaxation of the muscles is often recommended. Clothes that constrict at the leg, the groin, or the waist should be avoided. Reclining with the feet slightly elevated also reduces symptoms.

Surgery for mild varicose veins is not generally recommended as a purely cosmetic intervention. However, varicose veins are a progressive condition; they don't usually spontaneously reverse, and if they are left untreated, their complications can be serious. Therefore, a certain number of patients eventually seek treatment for safety rather than cosmetic concerns.

Several strategies for reducing varicose veins have been developed. Vein stripping, ambulatory **phlebectomy** (ministripping), and sclerosing injections are all options, but using laser energy or radiofrequency through a catheter to large veins is usually successful with less risk of complications. In all of these treatments, the body's remarkable ability to generate new blood vessels quickly accommodates the closure or removal of the affected vein.

Telangiectasias: Small, permanently dilated blood vessels. Also called spider veins.

Phlebectomy: The surgical removal of a part of a vein.

Massage Therapy Implications

RISKS	If a client has very extreme distorted twisting varicose veins, and especially if his or her skin shows any signs of circulatory problems, this condition at least locally contraindicates massage. It is important to remember that people with varicose veins have an increased risk for DVT, so massage therapists must be aware of the signs and symptoms that can accompany this condition.
BENEFITS	While massage is unlikely to change the prognosis for varicose veins, if the skin is intact and healthy, then broad, gliding pressure is safe. Clients with varicose veins can enjoy the same benefits of bodywork as the rest of the population as long as locally affected areas are respected.
OPTIONS	If varicose veins are very mild, they can sometimes respond well to hydrotherapy. Alternating hot and cold application can provide exercise for the smooth muscle inside the superficial vein. This can be done in a massage setting, but clients can also do this for themselves at home.
RESEARCH	Little research has investigated the role of massage therapy in the context of venous insufficiency. One study compared standard massage to lymphatic drainage work for range of motion changes in the ankles of people with advanced varicose veins and ulcerations. The conclusion was that lymphatic drainage led to the greater improvement in range of motion.[1] 1. Pereira de Godoy JM, Braile DM, de Fatima Guerreiro Godoy M. Lymph drainage in patients with joint immobility due to chronic ulcerated lesions. *Phlebology* 2008;23(1):32–34. http://www.ncbi.nlm.nih.gov/pubmed/18361267

Heart Conditions

Heart Attack

Definition: What Is It?

A heart attack is a process that damages some portion of cardiac muscle tissue through ischemia, or lack of blood flow and oxygen supply (Figure 5.23). The starved cells do not grow back; they are replaced by inelastic, noncontractile scar tissue. The damaged area is referred to as an **infarct**. Another term for heart attack is myocardial infarction.

Demographics

Estimates of how many people have heart attacks and how many die as a result range widely. A well-accepted number is that about 1.5 million people have a heart attack in the United States each year, and 500,000 to 700,000 people die. Over 500,000 of those heart attacks are first-time heart incidents; the rest are repeat events. Heart attack is the leading cause of death for both men and women in this country.

Worldwide, heart attack and heart disease are leading causes of death in all industrialized countries and a rising cause of death in developing countries. This is not all bad news, however; while this statistic follows negative lifestyle changes that promote heart disease, it also reflects a decline in the mortality rate of infectious diseases.

> **Infarct:** An area of dead tissue resulting from lack of blood supply.

Etiology: What Happens?

A heart attack occurs when a portion of the cardiac muscle dies from lack of oxygen: an ischemic attack. Usually, it arises from **atherosclerosis** in the coronary artery. A plaque with adherent clots grows in place until it completely obstructs blood flow: a **thrombus**. It could also be from a loosened blood clot or a broken or ruptured piece of plaque that travels until it blocks the coronary artery: an **embolism**. Rarely, a heart attack may occur when a coronary artery goes into prolonged spasm; this is seen most often in cocaine or other drug overdose.

Risk factors for heart attack are similar to those for other cardiovascular diseases. They include age, gender (men with heart disease outnumber women until menopause, and then both genders are affected equally), family history of CVD, **diabetes, hypertension**, high cholesterol, obesity, lack of exercise, and stress.

Atherosclerotic plaques are important predisposing factors for heart attack risk. Older, harder plaques are relatively stable, but newer, softer plaques have a higher risk of rupturing to let go of clots or other debris that then block the coronary artery.

When a portion of the cardiac muscle is killed off by ischemic attack, the ability to contract with coordination and efficiency is badly damaged. If a heart attack is severe enough to trigger ventricular fibrillations, the risk of sudden death is very high.

The seriousness of a heart attack is determined by the size and location of the blockage, the length of time blood supply is deprived, and the metabolic needs of the cells that are affected. If it is relatively small and the affected area doesn't have to work especially hard, the heart attack is a mild one. But if the infarct is large enough to weaken the heart's

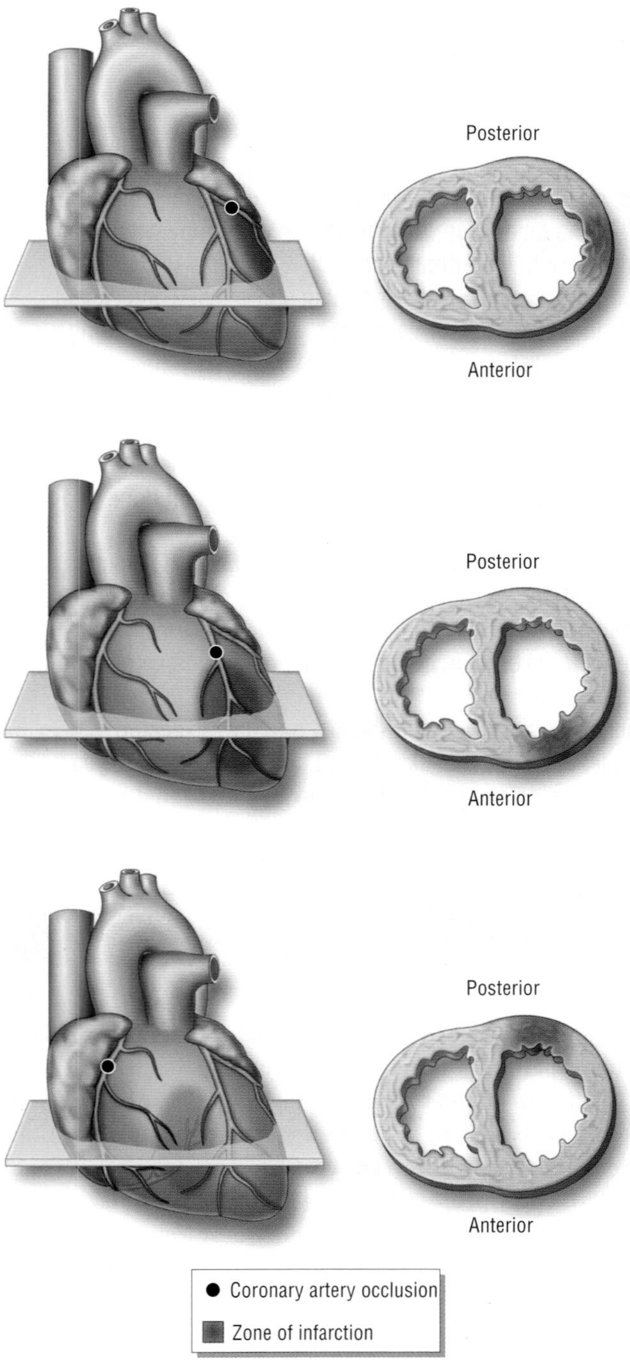

FIGURE 5.23 Myocardial infarctions

ability to contract, or if the damaged tissue involves the electrical conduction system for the heart, major intervention is necessary to save a life and create the possibility of recovery.

Complications

The chronology of heart problems is often circular rather than linear, which means that several heart attack complications are also heart attack contributors.

- *Atrial and ventricular fibrillations*: These are rapid, incomplete, weak attempts at contraction of the chambers. They occur most often if any part of the sinoatrial node, the heart's electrical pacemaker, has been damaged. These inefficient contractions allow blood to pool and thicken in the chambers of the heart and may contribute to the risk of embolism. Ventricular fibrillations, because they interfere with blood flow to the entire body, may result in death if they are not treated quickly.
- *Arrhythmia*: This is a potentially permanent consequence of losing some heart muscle function.
- *Embolism*: A heart attack can cause blood clots to form inside the chambers of the heart. Clots from the left side exit through the aorta and travel to wherever the bloodstream takes them; they can land in the brain, causing a **stroke**, or the renal arteries, where they can contribute to **renal failure**. Clots on the right side of the heart can raise the risk of PE.
- *Aneurysm*: Weakened cardiac tissue can create a bulge in the heart muscle itself similar to aortic **aneurysms**.
- *Heart failure*: In **heart failure**, the muscle is no longer strong enough to do its work. A heart with multiple patches of scar tissue is particularly vulnerable.
- *Shock*: In shock, the circulatory system swings reactively from a sympathetic to a parasympathetic state, opening the arteries to a maximum diameter in the process. The main danger with shock is loss of oxygen to the brain from radically decreased blood pressure.

NOTABLE CASES Former Vice President Dick Cheney is a survivor of five heart attacks and multiple surgeries and procedures. "Great Gatsby" writer F. Scott Fitzgerald succumbed to a heart attack in 1940 at age 44. Dancer, writer, and choreographer Bob Fosse died of a heart attack at age 60 in 1987. Heart attacks also shortened the lives of Grateful Dead musician Jerry Garcia, comedian John Candy, "Hitchhiker's Guide to the Universe" author Douglas Adams, "Sopranos" actor James Gandolfini, "Dragon Tattoo" series author Stieg Larsson, trumpet and cornet pioneer Louis Armstrong, and biologist Charles Darwin.

Signs and Symptoms

Heart attacks have a variety of signs and symptoms, some of which are extremely subtle and some of which are very severe (Case History 5.2). Some of the most common and dependable signs are these:

- Angina pectoris (literally, "chest pain"). This is one of the few early warning signs for the risk of heart attack. Not all people have this symptom, but those who do should pay close attention to it. Pain may spread to the shoulder, arm, neck, and jaw of the left side of the body. This is the referred pain pattern for the dermatome shared by the heart. Angina can be stable or unstable.
  - Stable angina is the simplest and most common form of angina. In this situation, the heart can get enough oxygen

CASE HISTORY 5.2 Heart Attack

BOB, AGE 49: The wake-up call.

After watching my mother go through heart disease and stent surgery, I began to seriously think about my own health. I talked to my doctor, and he set me up with a low-cost, on-site stress test that just used an exercise bike. He said if I could pass that, I'd be okay. I took it, and in the words of the technician, "My heart was not happy with what I was doing to it." So my doctor scheduled me with a cardiologist for a full treadmill test.

I didn't last long on the treadmill. When it was over, my blood pressure dropped and I had some really unpleasant symptoms, like dizziness, nausea, and a general feeling of crappiness. My doctor called my wife in from the waiting room, and with both of us together, he said, "My recommendation is to put you in the hospital now. We'll do an angiogram along with anything else that needs to be done."

I checked right in.

The next day, they found that the main section of the left coronary artery was 100% blocked. They had trouble pushing a wire through it, but when they got that done, they put in the balloon and then a titanium stent.

They also told me that they found evidence of a recent heart attack—one that was a fraction of an inch away from what they call a "widow maker." This was amazing to me, because I have no memory of any chest pains.

Three days after the angioplasty, I went home. They started my cardiac rehab right away. I have to exercise under supervision, next door to an emergency room. My doctors tell me if I ever let my heart rate get over 120 beats per minute, I run the risk of forming clots around the stent.

This episode was a real wake-up call for me. I'm the youngest man at my job and the last one they expected to have heart trouble. My identical twin went in for his own stress test and came back fine, but he was a couple of years later than me in developing his diabetes too, so he'll still have to keep an eye on it. I did some research about my situation, and I found that what I had—silent ischemia—is especially common in diabetic men over 40. I hope any man with type 2 diabetes over 40 or 45 will be sure to get his heart checked. You never know what you might find.

to perform regular tasks, but any extra effort, such as carrying something heavy or running up a flight of stairs, demands too much of the clogged coronary arteries. The result is moderate to severe, predictable chest pain that is relieved with rest and/or angina medication.

- Unstable angina can occur without unusual physical activity. It often appears in the night, with very extreme but short-lived chest pain. It is caused by vascular spasm at or near the site of atherosclerotic plaques or by plaques rupturing.

- Spreading pain, light-headedness, nausea, and sweating. These usually occur along with chest pain. When they occur without chest pain, they may still indicate a heart attack, but this is a less common presentation.
- Shortness of breath with or without chest pain; unexplained nausea, anxiety, or weakness; fainting; palpitations; and cold sweat.
- Stomach and abdominal pain.

A heart attack is a dynamic process. The critical blockage of the coronary artery may take place over several hours. This means that early intervention can preserve much of the myocardium. Survival rates for heart attacks are better than ever, because treatment is often instituted quickly. But if people ignore early warning signs and don't seek attention until symptoms have been present for many hours or even days, they experience much greater tissue loss.

It is important to point out that while heart attack symptoms can be severe, and heart attacks are part of a large and complex group of heart and circulatory problems, up to one-half of all the people who have a heart attack have no medical history of problems and no memory of warning symptoms.

Treatment

The first priorities with heart attack patients are to determine where the blockage is and to get rid of it as quickly as possible. This is done with clot-dissolving drugs, which can take effect in 90 minutes or less, and with immediate balloon angioplasty, which can open up most clogged arteries in about an hour. The technical term for this procedure is **percutaneous transluminal coronary angioplasty (PTCA)**. Other immediate-care options include the administration of oxygen and pain management with nitroglycerin and/or morphine.

Percutaneous transluminal coronary angioplasty (PTCA): A procedure in which a balloon is used to enlarge an artery.

Later care usually includes more clot dissolvers and nitroglycerin, which works to relax the smooth muscle tissue in the arteries. After the emergency has passed, a barrage of tests is conducted to determine the location and extent of damage to the cardiac muscle. These tests indicate one of three future courses of action: that the infarct was minor and requires no further medical intervention; that prescription anticoagulants are indicated; or that a serious and permanent narrowing of a coronary artery requires surgery to repair it. This surgery may be a more complete version of the angioplasty, or it may be coronary bypass surgery, in which damaged sections of the coronary artery are replaced with grafts of healthy vessels from elsewhere in the body.

Treatment in heart attack and heart surgery recovery must also embrace the lifestyle changes that will support a healthier future: eating sensibly, exercising regularly, controlling high blood pressure, and quitting smoking are the most important factors.

Some studies have indicated that taking aspirin regularly can decrease the chance of a repeat heart attack for people with a history of heart disease. This intervention is not risk free, however, so it should be undertaken with a doctor's oversight.

Medications

- Emergency care:
  - Aspirin for antiplatelet activity to prevent blockage from getting bigger
  - Analgesics
  - Nitroglycerin for smooth muscle relaxation
  - Thrombolytics and anticoagulants to lower blood clot risk
- Aftercare
  - Nitroglycerin
  - Anticoagulants, antiplatelet drugs
  - Cholesterol management drugs
  - Hypertension management drugs

Massage Therapy Implications

RISKS	The safety of massage for a heart attack survivor depends on how easily the client can withstand the changes in internal environment that this work will bring about. Anyone who is fragile or must exercise with great care may not be able to adapt to the changes that rigorous massage demands.
BENEFITS	Gentle, supportive bodywork of most kinds is appropriate for heart attack patients; this is an option that is now used in some hospital settings to help mitigate the pain and anxiety that goes along with heart disease surgery. A client with a history of heart attack but who is physically active can probably adapt to any changes that massage may bring about.

Heart Failure

Definition: What Is It?

Heart failure is a term for the progressive loss of cardiac function that accompanies age and a history of cardiovascular disease (CVD). It does not mean that the heart has stopped working altogether (that would be cardiac arrest); it simply means that the heart cannot keep up with the needs of the body.

Demographics

About 5.1 million people in the United States have heart failure, usually as a result of other CVDs, and over 500,000 new cases are identified each year. About half of people diagnosed with heart failure die within 5 years of diagnosis. This condition contributes to about 300,000 deaths each year. The prevalence of heart failure approximately doubles with each decade of life, but it also occurs in young people when it is connected to a congenital defect in heart function.

Etiology: What Happens?

A healthy heart pumps 2,000 gallons of blood each day. If resistance in the cardiovascular system increases (usually from **atherosclerosis**, **hypertension**, and other manifestations of CVD), the heart compensates in various ways. Any of these mechanisms works for short-term challenges, but over the long term, they add to the problem rather than helping to solve it.

In one compensation strategy, the heart muscle cells respond to chronic stress by growing larger. The ventricles appear to become bigger and thicker, allowing the heart to push harder against resistance in the pulmonary or systemic circuits. Ultimately however, this cardiac hypertrophy causes the ventricles to become stiff, so they no longer fill or contract normally.

Another compensation strategy is to secrete hormones, especially epinephrine and norepinephrine, which boost heart performance. This helps in the short term, but exacerbates long-term problems. Stress hormones make the heart work harder. Shifts in hormones also cause the body to retain salt and water. Both of these features compensate for weakness, but end up increasing blood pressure and adding to the workload of the overburdened heart.

In the long run, myocardium simply wears out and functions so inefficiently that blood flow to the rest of the body is inadequate for the most basic kinds of activities: climbing stairs, walking across a room, and even getting out of bed. Left untreated, the failed heart muscle goes into fibrillations, and the circulatory system collapses. To learn more, see "Congestive Heart Failure" animation, as well as the author's video "Heart Failure," at http://www.thePoint.lww.com/Werner6e. thePoint®

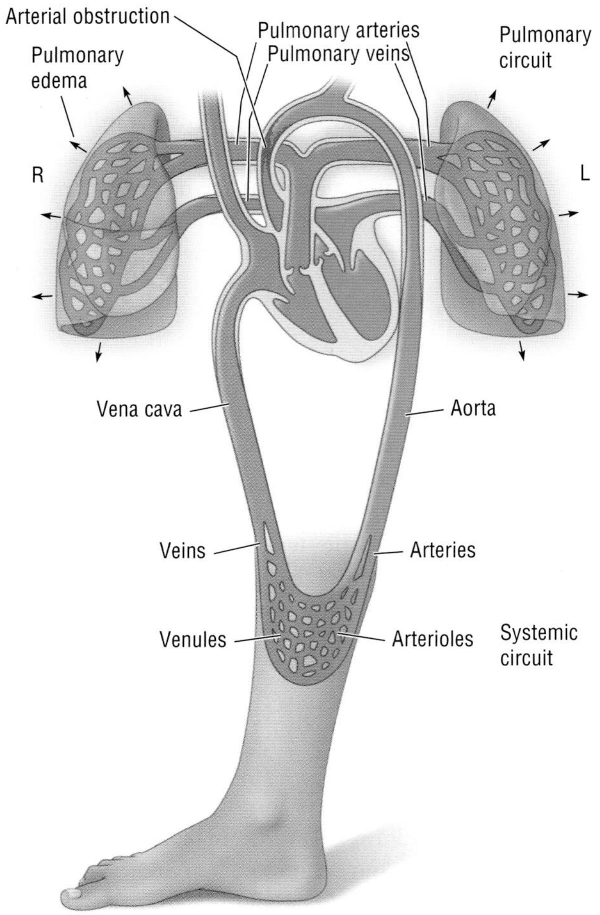

FIGURE 5.24 Left-sided heart failure: obstruction in the arteries leads to pulmonary edema

Most cases of heart failure are related to underlying CVD. A history of atherosclerosis or **heart attack** with resulting scar tissue in the heart muscle increases the risk of developing heart failure. High blood pressure, untreated **diabetes**, smoking, and alcohol and drug abuse can all be contributing factors as well. An especially potent setup for heart failure is any combination of these risk factors: uncontrolled high blood pressure along with smoking, for instance.

A smaller number of heart failure patients do not have a history of CVD but have sustained damage to the heart muscle for other reasons. Cardiomyopathy, valve diseases, infections of the valves or heart muscle, and congenital problems may all be factors in these cases.

> Cardiomyopathy: Disease of the heart muscle.
> Cor pulmonale: Enlargement of the right ventricle of the heart, often arising from lung disease.

Types of Heart Failure

- *Left-sided heart failure*: In this situation, the left ventricle is impaired, and blood backs up into the pulmonary circuit. This allows seepage of fluid back into the alveoli, causing pulmonary edema (Figure 5.24). Symptoms of left-sided heart failure include severe shortness of breath and stubborn coughing, perhaps with bloody sputum. Symptoms are worst when a person is active or lying down. One serious complication of this condition is the risk of **pneumonia** in the functionally impaired lungs.
- *Right-sided heart failure*: Also called cor pulmonale, this commonly results from pulmonary disease and high vascular resistance in the lungs—often as a complication of the pulmonary edema that accumulates with left-sided heart failure. Consequently, it becomes difficult for the right ventricle to pump blood through the pulmonary circuit, and the backup is felt through the rest of the body. Symptoms include severe edema, especially in the legs (Figure 5.25). Someone with this type of heart failure has ankles that look like they're spilling over the sides of her

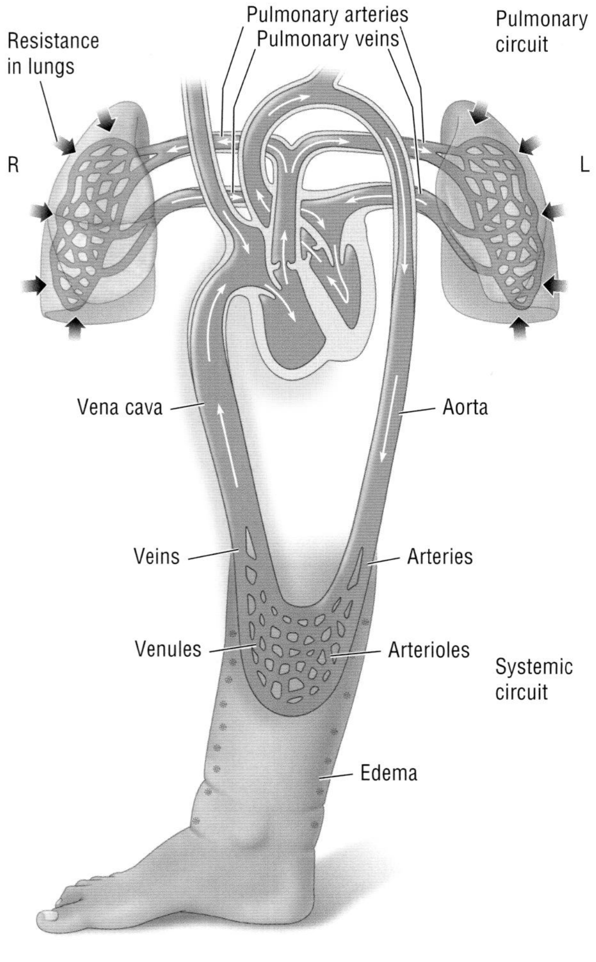

FIGURE 5.25 Right-sided heart failure (cor pulmonale): resistance in the lungs leads to a backup of fluid in the legs

shoes. If the patient is bedridden, the edema may occur in the abdomen or in the pelvis—wherever gravity is pulling most. Right-sided heart failure is also closely linked to enlarged liver and **renal failure**. As blood flow to the kidneys is reduced, the kidneys begin to retain water, which systemically increases blood pressure and makes the heart work even harder to push blood through narrow tubes.

- *Biventricular heart failure*: This is left- and right-sided failure simultaneously. It is the end stage of the disease, and if the patient doesn't respond to medications, he or she may be a candidate for a heart transplant or other surgery.

Signs and Symptoms

Signs of heart failure depend on which side of the heart is dysfunctional, as already described. Along with shortness of breath (often exacerbated by lying down), low stamina, and edema, heart failure patients may also have chronic chest pain; indigestion; arrhythmia; visibly distended veins in the neck; cold, sweaty skin; and restlessness.

Heart failure symptoms typically develop over a long period. If they have a sudden onset, they present a medical emergency.

Treatment

The treatment options for heart failure depend on how severe it is, and which side of the heart has been affected. Early interventions include rest, changes in diet (especially moving toward a low-sodium diet), and modifications in physical activity so that the heart can be exercised without being overly stressed.

If a patient doesn't respond well to these noninvasive treatment options, surgery may be considered. Surgery can range anywhere from repair to damaged valves, to wrapping a strong mesh bag around the heart, to a complete heart or heart and lung transplant.

Medications

- Anticoagulants to prevent excessive blood clotting
- Beta-blockers and ACE inhibitors to reduce the heart's workload
- Digitalis to slow and strengthen the heartbeat
- Diuretics to help shed excess fluid
- Statins to limit cholesterol levels

Massage Therapy Implications

RISKS

Most heart failure patients have a history of cardiovascular problems that contribute to their problems. Any massage that requires their ability to adapt to changing environments may be too challenging to receive safely. Accommodations must also be made for heart failure medications, many of which have dizziness and lethargy as side effects.

BENEFITS

Gentle bodywork that invites rather than imposes change may help to reduce blood pressure and perceived stress. This can be beneficial to heart failure patients in the short run, although it is unlikely to change their long-term prognosis.

RESEARCH

Jones et al.[1] found that foot reflexology treatment was safe for heart failure patients, but did not result in any measurable hemodynamic change in function. Another study of back massage found that recipients with heart failure reported reduced anxiety, and some had a reduction in systolic blood pressure,[2] but this study had no control group for comparison. Leduc et al.[3] investigated the safety of manual lymphatic drainage for lower limbs in patients with heart failure and found it to be a safe choice, with a decrease in limb girth and heart rate following treatment.

1. Jones J, Thomson P, Lauder W, et al. Reflexology has no immediate haemodynamic effect in patients with chronic heart failure: a double blind randomised controlled trial. *Complementary Therapies in Clinical Practice* 2013;19(3):133–138. http://www.ncbi.nlm.nih.gov/pubmed/23890459
2. Chen WL, Liu GJ, Yeh SH, et al. Effect of back massage intervention on anxiety, comfort, and physiologic responses in patients with congestive heart failure. *Journal of Alternative and Complementary Medicines* 2013;19(5):464–470. http://www.ncbi.nlm.nih.gov/pmc/articles/PMC3651680/
3. Leduc O, Crasset V, Leleu C, et al. Impact of manual lymphatic drainage on hemodynamic parameters in patients with heart failure and lower limb edema. *Lymphology* 2011;44(1):13–20. http://www.ncbi.nlm.nih.gov/pubmed/21667818

Explore and Apply

LEVEL 1: Receive and Respond

1. What is the best definition of anemia?
   a. Lack of blood
   b. Shortage of blood
   c. Lack of oxygen-carrying capacity
   d. Shortage of oxygen-carrying capacity

2. Match the following terms to their best descriptions:

a. Embolism	__A stationary clot that may grow in place
b. Thrombus	__Obstructs the lumen of medium- and large-sized arteries
c. Phlebitis	__A fragment of debris travels until it is lodged somewhere in the circulatory system
d. Plaque	__A vein is swollen and may be painful

3. What is true about hemophilia patients?
   a. They bleed faster than do other people
   b. They bleed longer than do other people
   c. They form larger clots than do other people
   d. They form smaller clots than do other people

4. Match the following terms to their best descriptions:

a. Hemophilia	__Clotting disorder that is not gender specific
b. Sickle cell disease	__Lack of clotting factors from the liver
c. Aplastic anemia	__A result of suppressed bone marrow function
d. von Willebrand disease	__A result of dysfunctional hemoglobin

5. Complications of untreated leukemia are most likely to involve…
   a. Infection and excessive bleeding
   b. Pulmonary embolism and circulatory collapse
   c. Myocardial infarction or heart failure
   d. Inflamed lymph nodes and tonsils

6. If a fragment breaks off a DVT, where will it most likely lodge?
   a. The brain
   b. The heart
   c. The lungs
   d. The kidneys

7. Match the following terms to their best descriptions:

a. Atherosclerosis	__A bulge in an arterial wall, usually in the aorta
b. Aneurysm	__Impaired oxygen-carrying capacity
c. Angina	__Pain related to lack of blood flow to supply myocardial cells
d. Anemia	__Development of arterial obstructions

8. Atherosclerosis is a frequent result of long-term, untreated…
   a. Varicose veins
   b. Angina
   c. Abdominal aortic aneurysm
   d. Hypertension

9. What is true about high blood pressure?
   a. It is often asymptomatic
   b. Most people treat it successfully
   c. It seriously impacts quality of life
   d. It often causes pulmonary embolism

10. Which blood vessels are most often affected by Raynaud syndrome?
    a. Capillaries in the fingertips
    b. Arterioles in the extremities
    c. Venules in the hands and feet
    d. Large- and medium-sized arteries throughout the body

11. Which of the following situations is usually present when atherosclerosis begins?
    a. Aneurysm
    b. Angina
    c. Hypertension
    d. Deep vein thrombosis

12. Which blood vessel is obstructed in a myocardial infarction?
    a. Carotid artery
    b. Coronary artery
    c. Cerebral artery
    d. Cephalic artery

13. What is the end result of a heart attack?
 a. Death
 b. Scarring
 c. Stroke
 d. Fibrillation

14. Which is most predictive of heart attack risk?
 a. Cholesterol level
 b. Blood pressure
 c. Stable angina
 d. Unstable angina

LEVEL 2: Application of Concepts

1. Your client reports that she had a pulmonary embolism 8 weeks ago. What medication is she likely to be using?
 a. Analgesics
 b. Anxiolytics
 c. Anticoagulants
 d. Antidepressants

2. Your client has sickle cell disease. Why is she likely to have poor immune function?
 a. This disease attacks functioning white blood cells
 b. This disease suppresses the production of white blood cells
 c. This disease often destroys the spleen
 d. This disease often destroys lymph nodes

3. Your client is undergoing treatment for multiple myeloma. What accommodation is he most likely to need?
 a. Extra care for infection control
 b. Positioning and pressure adjustments for fragile bones
 c. Working through the sheet to allow for his rash and itchiness
 d. Having extra coverings available, because these patients get cold easily

4. People with sickle cell disease are especially vulnerable to…
 a. Blocked blood vessels and infarctions
 b. Excessive bleeding
 c. Malaria
 d. Autoimmune disease

5. Your client reports that after playing soccer yesterday, her left calf feels sore and heavy, and she'd like you to work it out. You notice that it is warmer than the right calf, and it may also be bigger. Your best option is to…
 a. Continue the session but don't massage the left calf so that you don't disrupt a DVT
 b. Tell your client it's possible that she has a DVT and emphasize that she needs to have it checked right away, just in case
 c. Work deeply and specifically on the left calf to prevent the formation of a DVT
 d. Inform your client that she has a DVT and she needs to visit the ER as quickly as possible after her massage

6. Your new client is a 66-year-old woman. She comes to your office with an oxygen tank in tow. She huffs and puffs to climb the two stairs into your waiting room. Her legs are swollen, and her ankles overlap her shoes. What condition is probably present?
 a. Left-sided heart failure
 b. Right-sided heart failure
 c. Biventricular heart failure
 d. Ventricular fibrillation

Note to educators: Due to space considerations, these review questions only address the most important material from Chapter 8. The Test Bank provides a much more comprehensive selection of questions, all of which are keyed to the relevant chapter objectives.

What Would *You* Do?

Twin A

Your 50-year-old client had a heart attack 2 years ago. Afterwards, he took up bicycling to try to become more fit. He is a healthy weight, and he reports that he bikes about 100 miles a week, mostly on hills, in training for a big trip abroad next year. He wants to see if massage might help him train more efficiently. He takes a daily aspirin and medication to lower his cholesterol. What questions do you need to ask to be able to work safely with this client? What would a session with him look like? Role-play this conversation with a partner, and then switch roles, and refer to Twin B.

Twin B

Your 50-year-old client had a heart attack 2 years ago. He is about 30 pounds overweight and mostly sedentary, aside from golf most weekends. He has been prescribed drugs to manage

Explore and Apply (continued)

his blood pressure and cholesterol, but he confides that he is not always consistent about this. He has also been put on a drug to help with insulin uptake because he is borderline diabetic. He would like to take better care of his health, and he wonders if massage therapy might help him in this endeavor. What questions do you need to ask to be able to work safely with this client? What would his session look like? Role-play this conversation with a partner.

Can You Work Safely Here?

Mrs. Cortez, age 61, has been diagnosed with peripheral artery disease, hypertension, and high cholesterol. She has constant, sometime acutely severe pain in her legs. She would like to receive massage therapy for her leg pain, and she says her doctor thinks it's a good idea. Make a list of questions you need to ask to be able to work safely with her. Outline a treatment strategy that will maximize the benefits of massage while keeping her safe. Then, compare your strategy with a classmate's.

Massage Therapists are Role Models

Review the behaviors that limit the risk of heart disease, found in Sidebar 5.4. Being brutally honest, analyze how many of these you follow and where you have room for growth. What habits are on display for your clients to see? Discuss these with a partner, and strategize how you plan to be a role model for good health and heart disease prevention for your clients.

Suggested Activities

1. For each condition covered in your curriculum, write down the following on a card:
   - A brief definition
   - Most common cause or contributing factor(s)
   - Major signs and symptoms
   - Risks and benefits of massage therapy
     - Variables that contribute to risks and benefits
     - Appropriate adaptations

   Use these as flash cards as you study
2. For each condition covered in your curriculum, write one multiple choice question. Share your questions with your classmates as you study together.
3. Quiz yourself using either the "labels off" feature in your enhanced e-book or the labeling exercise on thePoint® for Figure 5.1. Identify the following structures: Aorta, Inferior vena cava, Left atrium, Left pulmonary artery, Left pulmonary vein, Left ventricle, Septum, Superior vena cava, Systemic circuit to the feet, and Systemic circuit to the head.
4. Quiz yourself using either the "labels off" feature in your enhanced e-book or the labeling exercise on thePoint® for Figure 5.2. Identify the following structures: Adventitia, Tunica intima, and Tunica media
5. Quiz yourself using either the "labels off" feature in your enhanced e-book or the labeling exercise on thePoint® for Figure 5.3. Identify the following structures: Point of origin for all blood cells, Platelets and their origin, B cells and T cells and their origin, Macrophages and their origin, Granular leukocytes and their origin, and Erythrocytes and their origin.
6. Use the student resources on thePoint® to find practice quiz questions and games.

6

Lymph and Immune System Conditions

CHAPTER 6 / Abbreviated Chapter Objectives

Having completed assignments and classroom time related to Chapter 6, the learner is expected to be able to ...

- Identify definitions of the key terms in the introduction and those connected to the conditions covered in your curriculum.
- Identify the source of interstitial fluid.
- Trace a droplet of interstitial fluid through both the lymphatic and circulatory systems.
- List five mechanisms for moving lymph through the lymphatic system.
- Explain the Starling equilibrium.
- Name the difference between specific and nonspecific immune system responses.
- Describe the function of an antibody.
- Define "allergy" and list three common allergens.
- Define "autoimmune disease" and list three common examples.
- Describe a type I hypersensitivity reaction.
- Describe a type IV hypersensitivity reaction.
- Provide the following information for each condition covered in your curriculum:
  - Identify the definition of the condition.
  - List the most common causes or contributing factors to the condition.
  - List major signs and symptoms of the condition.
  - Identify possible risks and benefits of massage therapy, with:
    - Variables that contribute to risks and benefits
    - Appropriate adaptations for massage therapy

For detailed chapter objectives for each condition in this chapter, consult the student resources page at <u>http://thePoint.lww.com/Werner6e</u>. thePoint®

Introduction

The lymphatic system is unlike any other organ system: its components are not even vaguely symmetrical, and it functions as a sort of subsystem to both the circulatory and immune systems. The conditions listed under this heading are influenced by either of the other two systems. Here is a brief overview of how the lymphatic system works.

Lymph System Structure

As blood travels away from the heart, it goes through progressively smaller tubes—the aorta branches into the arteries, which branch into arterioles, which finally divide into the very tiny and delicate capillaries. Blood leaves the heart under high speed and pressure; both speed and pressure fall as blood moves further into the body, away from the heart. Still, everything keeps moving at a good pace; a blood cell completes a loop through the systemic circuit about every 60 seconds.

The walls of the capillaries are made of one-cell-thick squamous epithelium, designed to allow diffusion of substances through the walls. Capillaries are so tiny that the red blood cells must line up one by one to pass through. This is the moment for the transfer of nutrients and wastes in the tissue cells. This is also where, having dropped off oxygen and picked up carbon dioxide, arterial blood becomes venous blood. And finally, this is the moment when some of the plasma from the arterial blood is squeezed out of the capillaries and into the tissues. In other words, this is the origin of interstitial fluid (Figure 6.1).

Interstitial fluid is absolutely vital. It is the medium in which all of the body's nutrients and wastes travel. But it must keep moving; if it stagnates, waste products or pathogens can accumulate and cause problems. Interstitial fluid keeps moving through the system by flowing into a different type of capillary: a lymphatic capillary. Lymphatic capillaries are similar to circulatory capillaries in construction, with one major difference: they are part of an open system. That means that interstitial fluid and small particles can flow into lymphatic capillaries at almost any point along the length of that capillary. By contrast, circulatory capillaries are closed to the extent that red blood cells are not able to come and go unless the vessel has been damaged.

When interstitial fluid is drawn into a lymphatic capillary, it is called lymph. Lymph is composed mainly of plasma that exited the bloodstream, loads of metabolic wastes that have been expelled by hardworking cells, and some chunks of particulate waste as well.

The new lymph is routed via the lymph capillaries to a series of cleaning stations called nodes, where the wastes are neutralized, and any small particles are filtered out. The nodes are also home to most of the body's specific immune response cells, so if any pathogens have been picked up and marked by macrophages in the lymph, this is where the specific immune response begins. The newly cleaned fluid reenters the circulatory system just above the right atrium of the heart, where the right and left thoracic ducts empty into the right and left subclavian veins, respectively.

Lymph System Function

Lymph flows through the lymphatic capillaries into bigger and bigger vessels, usually against the pull of gravity and without the aid of the heart's direct pumping action. Several processes help to move it along:

- Gravity helps to move lymph, if the limb is elevated.
- Muscle contractions push fluid through lymphatic vessels just as a hand squeezes toothpaste out of a tube. The larger lymphatic vessels also have smooth muscle tissue in their walls that contract rhythmically.
- Alternating hot and cold hydrotherapy applications can promote contractions in the smooth muscle tissue of lymphatic vessels to move fluid along.
- Deep breathing draws lymph up the thoracic duct during inhalation and squeezes forward out during exhalation.
- Massage with big mechanical manipulative movements like kneading and deep stroking can increase lymph flow, but small, extremely superficial movements can also cause fluid to be drawn into lymphatic capillaries. This is the mechanism employed with lymph drainage modalities.

If everything works well, fluid levels in the tissues are constant but not stagnant. The amount of fluid that leaves circulatory capillaries should be almost equal to the amount that re-enters circulatory capillaries, with about 10% left over to become interstitial fluid and then lymph. This is called the **Starling equilibrium**. But a backup anywhere in the system can result in major changes in fluid balance.

> **Starling equilibrium:** The principle that the amount of fluid squeezed out of circulatory capillaries should be almost equal to the amount being drawn into lymphatic capillaries.

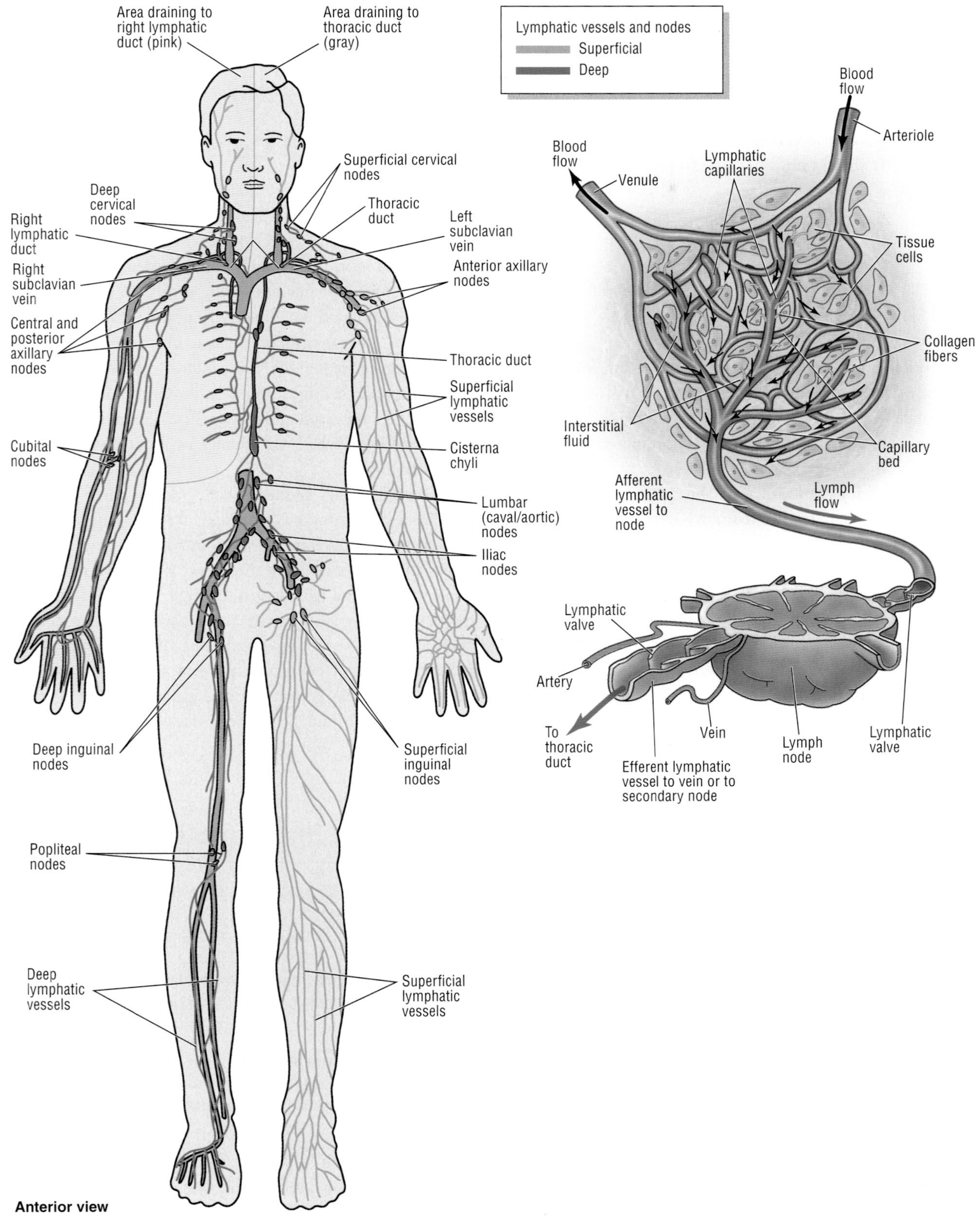

FIGURE 6.1 The lymphatic system and capillaries

If veins, lymph vessels, or nodes are blocked, then fluid can accumulate between tissue cells. The stagnant fluid quickly becomes a hindrance to diffusion and other chemical reactions, rather than the transfer medium it is designed to be. This is the problem with many of the diseases of the lymph system, and it is a serious concern for massage practitioners, who generally should not be trying to push fluid through a system that is already overtaxed.

Immune System Function

Unlike other organ systems, the immune system is not composed of a collection of organs performing a task for a coordinated total effort. Instead, it is a nebulous, complex collection of tissues, cells, and chemicals whose coordinated function is to keep the whole organism safe.

The primary function of the immune system is to distinguish what is self from what is nonself, and to eradicate anything that is nonself as quickly as possible. Immune system devices range from very general to highly specific in identifying exactly which antigens they attack (Sidebar 6.1). Some white cells attack anything; others simply ignore a pathogen if it's not their particular target. Most of our nonspecific immune devices, such as intact skin and the acidity of the gastric juices, are not discussed here. However, it is worthwhile to look at some of the specific immune machinery, because when it's working well, it's positively miraculous and when it's not working well or when it makes mistakes, things can go terribly wrong.

T Cells and B Cells

The two interlocking branches of the specific immune responses are cellular immunity (T cells) and humoral immunity (B cells). Neither of these extremely complicated systems can work at all unless their target pathogen is displayed by a nonspecific white blood cell. So that is the first step in fighting off an infection: a white blood cell must find, destroy, and display a piece of the microorganism in question. Fortunately, white blood cells are distributed generously all through the blood and interstitial fluid, and they are concentrated in the superficial fascia, lymph nodes, lungs, and liver, where the chance of meeting pathogens is especially high.

Consider the sequence of events when someone touches a contaminated doorknob and then wipes his or her eye: rhinovirus 14 has just been introduced into the body. A passing monocyte eats the virus. It displays that pathogen's marker, and it is drawn through lymphatic capillaries into a nearby lymph node. A T cell is waiting there. It is specially designed to recognize the flag of rhinovirus 14. The newly activated T cell gets very busy, replicating itself into several forms that go out into the bloodstream in search of more viruses to attack. In the process, the original T cell

SIDEBAR 6.1 Different White Blood Cells for Different Functions

White blood cells come in various sizes, classes, and strengths. Each type of leukocyte has a specific role in the immune system and inflammatory response. As researchers learn more about how these cells work and communicate with each other, we gain ability to influence their activities.

Neutrophils
Neutrophils are the smallest, fastest, and most common of the white blood cells. They are produced in bone marrow, and chemicals that leak from damaged cells stimulate their production in even greater numbers. Neutrophils typically have a short lifespan; they are the first to sacrifice themselves to disable potential invaders.

Monocytes
Monocytes begin as small white blood cells, but they have the power to change. When they are released into the bloodstream from the bone marrow, they circulate until they reach a target tissue. Then, they leave the circulatory system to infiltrate that tissue and grow into macrophages, "big eaters" that can devour pathogens and display bits of cell membrane that begin the specific immune response.

Monocytes and macrophages move slowly; they are usually involved in the subacute or chronic phases of inflammatory response.

Eosinophils and Basophils
These inflammatory agents are observed most often in the context of allergic reactions and responses against invading parasites.

Lymphocytes
Lymphocytes include B cells, T cells, and natural killer cells. These are manufactured in both bone marrow and lymphoid tissue, and are most often engaged in specific immune system responses to pathogens. These are the agents that allow us to develop immunity to infections.

stimulates its B-cell partner. This activated B-cell (now called a plasma cell) clones into hundreds of copies, and the new cells start producing out rhinovirus 14–specific antibodies at a mind-boggling pace: 2,000 antibodies per second. Antibodies are not alive. They are Y-shaped chemicals forged especially to lock onto their target pathogen and retire it. This can happen in any of several ways, depending on the pathogen and the antibodies involved. *To learn more, see the animation "Immune Response" available at* http://thePoint.lww.com/Werner6e. thePoint®

Back when the T cells and B cells were first becoming active, they each made a few copies of themselves that would outlive the infection and circulate through the body on the lookout for future attempts by the same pathogen to invade. These are memory cells, and thanks to them, people very seldom get sick with the same pathogen twice. If rhinovirus 14 gains access to the body again, an immune attack can mobilize against it and eradicate it so quickly that a person might never know he was even exposed.

Immune System Mistakes

The immune system is miraculous. Most of the time, T and B cells can somehow recognize their own special pathogen and launch exactly the right attack against it. But the immune system occasionally makes mistakes. Sometimes, it launches a full-scale attack, with an inflammatory response, antibody production, and collateral damage to nearby cells, against an antigen that's not dangerous: cat dander, oak pollen, or peanuts, for instance: this is called an allergic reaction. Allergies can range in severity from mildly annoying to life-threatening.

The other slip that the immune system can make is to mistake a part of the body for a dangerous pathogen. That is, it fails to distinguish self from nonself. Conditions involving this type of mistake are called autoimmune disorders. This group of diseases includes **multiple sclerosis**, **lupus**, **scleroderma**, **rheumatoid arthritis**, **myasthenia gravis**, and several other chronic, incurable problems that are discussed in this chapter. Both allergies and autoimmune dysfunction are sometimes discussed as **hypersensitivity reactions**.

Four types of hypersensitivity reactions have been classified. Because two of them can involve the skin and the other two can involve systemic disorders, it's useful for massage therapists to be familiar with them.

- *Type I hypersensitivity reactions*. These are an immediate reaction to an antigen or particle of nonself. In this situation, immunoglobulin E (IgE), a specific class of antibody, quickly sensitizes nearby mast cells to the presence of an "enemy," which may be a fragment of pollen, the proteins from peanuts or shellfish, or a droplet of bee venom. The alerted mast cells then release histamine and other chemicals that create dramatic changes in vascular permeability and that attract other white blood cells to the area. This inflammatory response produces the symptoms that are associated with typical allergic reactions: redness, swelling, itching, weepy eyes, and runny nose with hay fever; and nausea, vomiting, and diarrhea with certain food allergies.
- *Type II hypersensitivity reactions*. These are far less common than type I. They involve inflammatory cytotoxic (cell killing) reactions against a specific substance that may or may not belong to the body. Examples of type II reactions include hemolytic anemia, penicillin allergies, and reactions to the transfusion of mismatched blood.
- *Type III reactions*. These involve antibodies that bind with antigens, but the particles they form are too large to be phagocytized. These conglomerates, called **granulomas**, are eventually caught in the body's most delicate fluid filters: in the kidneys, the eyes, the brain, and the serous membranes surrounding the heart, lungs, and abdominal cavity. There they stimulate an aggressive response, which results in inflammation and damage to these very delicate structures. Examples of type III reactions include **systemic lupus erythematosus**, a specific type of kidney damage called glomerulonephritis, and possibly rheumatoid arthritis.
- *Type IV reactions*. These delayed reactions are cell mediated; they rely on T cells to stimulate an immune response to an irritant. **Contact dermatitis** is an example of a type IV hypersensitivity reaction. In this case, an inflammatory reaction appears on the skin after exposure to an irritating substance such as plant toxins, certain dyes, soaps, metals, or latex. This usually delayed reaction may occur 24 to 48 hours after an initial exposure.

To hear the author discuss autoimmunity and massage, view the video "Autoimmune Diseases" at http://thePoint.lww.com/Werner6e. thePoint®

Hypersensitivity reactions: Exaggerated responses to the stimulus of an agent.

Granuloma: A mass of granulation tissue formed in response to infection or a foreign substance.

Lymph and Immune System Conditions

Lymph System Conditions

- Edema
- Lymphangitis
- Lymphoma
  - Hodgkin lymphoma
  - Non-Hodgkin lymphoma
- Mononucleosis

Immune System Conditions

- Allergic reactions
  - Angioedema
  - Anaphylaxis
  - Multiple chemical sensitivity syndrome
- Chronic fatigue syndrome
- Fever
- HIV/AIDS

Autoimmune Disorders

- Ankylosing spondylitis
- Crohn disease
- Lupus
  - Drug-induced lupus
  - Neonatal lupus
  - Discoid Lupus
  - Systemic Lupus
  - Mixed connective tissue disease
- Multiple sclerosis
  - Benign MS
  - Relapse/remitting MS
  - Primary progressive MS
  - Secondary progressive MS
  - Progressive/relapsing MS
  - Malignant MS
- Psoriasis
  - Plaque psoriasis
  - Guttate psoriasis
  - Pustular psoriasis
  - Inverse psoriasis
  - Erythrodermic psoriasis
- Rheumatoid arthritis
  - Juvenile rheumatoid arthritis
- Scleroderma
  - Local scleroderma
    - Morphea scleroderma
    - Linear scleroderma
  - Systemic scleroderma
    - Limited systemic scleroderma
    - Diffuse scleroderma
    - Sine scleroderma
- Ulcerative colitis

Lymph System Conditions

Edema

Definition: What Is It?

Edema is accumulation of excessive fluid between cells. It may be a local or systemic problem, and it is usually associated with chemical imbalance, inflammation, or poor circulation.

Etiology: What Happens?

The Starling equilibrium states that the forces that cause fluid to leave blood capillaries should almost equal the forces that cause fluid to be reabsorbed by blood capillaries and that anything left over (which should be about 10%) should be processed by the lymph system. Lymph capillaries are perfectly designed to pick up excess interstitial fluid: each squamous cell is anchored to surrounding tissue by a collagen filament. When excess fluid accumulates in any area, these anchoring filaments pull back on the squamous cells, increasing that lymph capillary's ability to take in fluid. Sometimes, however, more fluid builds up in the tissues than the circulatory and lymph systems combined can take in; this is edema. Edema isn't generally noticeable until interstitial fluid volume is about 30% above normal.

Edema can have any of several causes; most of them are a combination of chemical and mechanical factors. Mechanical factors may involve a weakened heart, a dysfunctional liver, serious kidney problems, or an obstruction to venous or lymphatic return in the form of a blood clot or removed nodes. Even socks or knee braces that are too tight can cause distal edema. Chemical causes of edema usually have to do with accumulation of salts or proteins in the interstitial fluid, which causes the area to retain water. Other chemical factors include inflammatory responses to infection or allergens.

Systemic edema is usually indicative of an underlying condition that affects the heart, kidneys, or liver: all keystones for fluid movement. Localized edema is usually connected to a smaller-scale problem.

Lymphedema is different from simple edema; this is the result of damage to lymphatic structures and accumulation of proteins in the interstitial fluid. It is discussed in Chapter 12.

Signs and Symptoms

Edema varies in presentation according to the source, the duration, and the area that is affected. Tissue is often soft, puffy, or boggy. The area may be hot if the edema is related to a recent injury or infection, or cool if the edema is long standing and related to poor circulation.

When blood or lymphatic movement is chronically impaired, pitting edema may develop: a pit or dimple remains in the tissue for several minutes after it is gently compressed

(Figure 6.2). Tissue that is edematous because of chronic problems such as heart failure or lymph node loss may become indurated, or hardened.

Treatment

Edema is treated by addressing the underlying cause. This may mean treatment for something as complex as liver failure or as simple as a sprained ankle. Medications are likewise gauged to treat the contributing factors.

A person who experiences chronic or repeating edema may be counseled to follow a low-salt diet and to sit or recline with legs elevated whenever possible.

Medications

- Antihistamines for allergic reactions
- NSAIDs
- Steroidal anti-inflammatories
- Diuretics for heart, liver, or kidney dysfunction

Massage Therapy Implications

RISKS	Most types of edema contraindicate all but the lightest forms of bodywork because the delicate lymphatic capillaries are already working past capacity.
BENEFITS	Subacute or postacute musculoskeletal injuries may have long-term edema that hydrotherapy and massage can help to resolve safely.
OPTIONS	Lymphatic work from a trained practitioner is appropriate for edema in any stage that is not connected to an infection or other contraindicating condition.
RESEARCH	Techniques that focus on lymphatic movement are well supported in research and often recommended for appropriate edema-related situations, including postsurgery.[1,2] It is possible that muscle contractions may also be employed to help with edema, as in a study that compared proprioceptive neuromuscular facilitation to lymphatic massage.[3] 1. Warren AG, Janz BA, Borud LJ, et al. Evaluation and management of the fat leg syndrome. *Plastic and Reconstructive Surgery* 2007;119(1):9e–15e. http://www.ncbi.nlm.nih.gov/pubmed/17255648 2. Ebert JR, Joss B, Jardine B, et al. Randomized trial investigating the efficacy of manual lymphatic drainage to improve early outcome after total knee arthroplasty. *Archives of Physical Medicine and Rehabilitation* 2013;94(11):2103–2111. http://www.ncbi.nlm.nih.gov/pubmed/23810354 3. Hwang O, Ha K, Choi S. The effects of PNF techniques on lymphoma in the upper limbs. *Journal of Physical Therapy Science* 2013;25(7):839–841. http://www.ncbi.nlm.nih.gov/pmc/articles/PMC3820393/

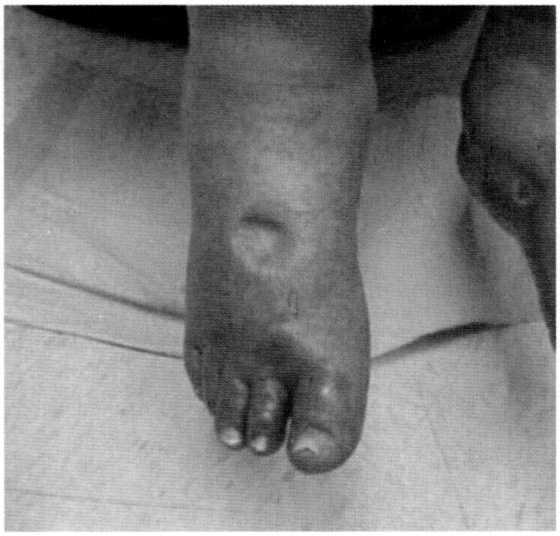

FIGURE 6.2 Severe pitting edema

Lymphangitis

Definition: What Is It?

Lymphangitis is an infection with inflammation in the **lymphangions**, or lymphatic capillaries. It is a particular risk for people with depressed immunity or poor circulation, because their white blood cell activity is sluggish. This allows any available bacteria the opportunity to establish a stronghold in the lymphatic system. Massage therapists are also at risk, because tiny lesions may be present on their hands. These are vulnerable to invasion by the bacteria that reside on the skin of even the healthiest clients.

Etiology: What Happens?

In lymphangitis, the lymph capillaries become infected, usually with one of the group A beta-hemolytic streptococci, although other pathogens, including staphylococcus, can also be the cause. This condition usually arises from a small injury on the skin. It can be a complication of **cellulitis** or of a viral or fungal infection such as **herpes simplex** or **athlete's foot**. People with **diabetes** or any condition that compromises immune system function are especially at risk.

When the pathogens gain entry, they set up an aggressive infection in the lymph vessel before macrophages or other white blood cells can stop them. Infections that invade the lymph nodes are called **lymphadenitis**. If even a few bacteria get past the filtering action of the lymph nodes, the

Lymphangion: A lymphatic vessel.

Lymphadenitis: Inflammation of one or more lymph nodes.

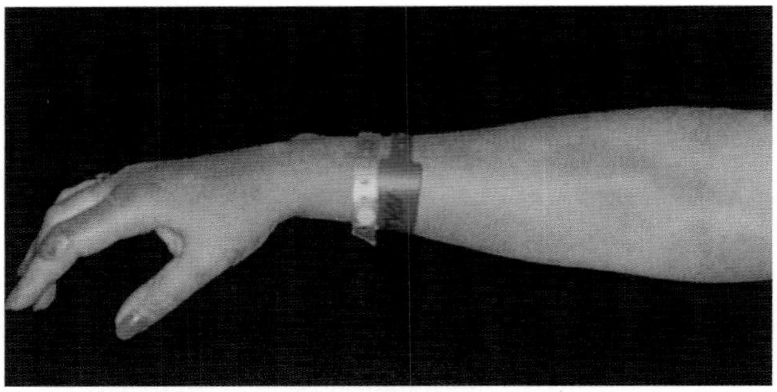

FIGURE 6.3 Lymphangitis

infection can enter the bloodstream at the right or left subclavian vein. Then, the situation is much more serious: the person has **septicemia**, or blood poisoning, which is potentially life-threatening. This is why, if lymphangitis is a possibility, medical intervention is advisable at the earliest possible opportunity.

Signs and Symptoms

Lymphangitis starts with signs of local infection: pain, heat, redness, and swelling, all focused around the initial site of infection. The infected lymph vessel may show a visible scarlet track running proximally from the portal of entry, which is usually some lesion in the skin such as a hangnail, an abrasion, or an insect bite (Figure 6.3).

If the infection is able to overwhelm the immune system response, it quickly moves deeper into the lymph system, leading to swollen nodes, fever, and a general feeling of misery. Blisters may develop along the line of infection. Depending on the virulence of the bacteria, extensive tissue damage may also occur to other tissues. This can happen surprisingly quickly; lymphangitis can become a systemic infection in a matter of hours.

Treatment

Lymphangitis is usually treated successfully with antibiotic therapy. Treatment must begin as soon as possible after the infection has been identified to avoid the risk of blood poisoning. Any abscesses may need to be drained.

Medications

- Antibiotics for bacterial infection
- Analgesics for pain
- Anti-inflammatories for inflammation

Septicemia: Blood poisoning.

Massage Therapy Implications

RISKS	A client with acute lymphangitis is unlikely to want to keep a massage appointment because he or she probably has a fever and general malaise along with throbbing pain and edema at the site of infection. This condition contraindicates massage locally because of the threat of communicable pathogens, and systemically because of the threat of complication to septicemia.
BENEFITS	A client who has fully recovered from lymphangitis can enjoy the same benefits from massage as the rest of the population.
OPTIONS	This condition can be an occupational hazard for massage therapists and bodywork practitioners whose hands may have open hangnails or other wounds that serve as a portal of entry. For this reason, it is important to keep as healthy as possible and to cover any compromised skin with a liquid bandage, a finger cot, or any another device that will prevent this risk.

Lymphoma

Definition: What Is It?

Lymphoma is a collective name for cancer that starts in the lymph nodes. Like **leukemia** and **myeloma**, lymphoma involves a mutation of the DNA in specific white blood cells. Some types of lymphoma affect the same cells as some types of lymphocytic leukemia, so the delineations between these cancer labels are no longer clear-cut.

Demographics

Non-Hodgkin lymphoma is a relatively common cancer in the United States. It is diagnosed in about 71,000 people and leads to about 19,000 deaths each year. This disease can occur in children, but 95% of patients are adults. Half of all patients are over 65 years old.

Hodgkin lymphoma is diagnosed about 10,000 times each year, leading to about 1,200 deaths.

Etiology: What Happens?

Lymphoma is cancer that originates in lymph tissues. It begins with a mutation of the DNA of the affected cells, usually some type of B cell (these account for about 80% of cases) or of T cells or natural killer cells. The mutated cells begin to replicate, producing massive numbers of nonfunctioning lymphocytes.

This causes the lymph tissues to enlarge, and it initiates the other symptoms associated with lymphoma, namely, **anemia**, night sweats, itchy skin, and fatigue, among others.

Mutated cells may travel through the lymphatic system to begin tumors elsewhere: this can occur in other lymph node regions or in the bones, the spleen, or the liver. In some cases, cells can gain access to the central nervous system and begin growing tumors there.

A statistical relationship exists between lymphoma and exposure to insecticides, herbicides, fertilizers, and black hair dye, but the direct cause-and-effect sequelae have not been established. Lymphoma risk is increased with some infections, including Epstein-Barr virus (EBV), **HIV**, **hepatitis** B and C, human T-cell lymphotropic virus (HTLV), and *Helicobacter pylori*—the bacterium linked with **peptic ulcers**. Other risk factors for lymphoma include the presence of autoimmune disease, using immunosuppressant drugs, and genetic predisposition.

The seriousness of lymphoma depends on what type of cell has mutated and how quickly it replicates. This disease is sometimes described by the behavior of its cells:

- Low-grade or indolent lymphoma grows slowly. It is often nonresponsive to treatment and may change to a more aggressive form later.
- Intermediate-grade lymphoma is aggressive, but responsive to treatment.
- High-grade lymphoma is aggressive and grows rapidly, but it may be resistant to treatment.

Types of Lymphoma

- *Hodgkin lymphoma (HL)*: This involves the mutation of B cells into large, malignant, multinucleate cells called **Reed-Sternberg cells**. It is seen most often in the submandibular nodes, but can also occur at the axillary and inguinal nodes. Eventually, the growths metastasize to organ tissues, particularly the liver or bone marrow. Several subtypes of HL have been identified, but their patterns of progression are similar. The process of metastasis tends to be predictable and organized, which distinguishes HL from NHL and which makes HL a very treatable form of cancer.
- *Non-Hodgkin lymphoma (NHL)*: This group comprises many subtypes of lymphoma that affect B cells, T cells, and natural killer cells. NHL is much more common than HL. It tends to be less predictable than Hodgkin lymphoma, and it can be harder to treat successfully.

Signs and Symptoms

The primary symptom of any kind of lymphoma is painless, nontender swelling of lymph nodes, especially in the neck, axilla, and inguinal area (Figure 6.4). Other symptoms include anemia, fatigue, weight loss, night sweats, itchy skin, and loss of appetite. These symptoms typically have a relatively fast onset and persist for 2 weeks or more. Indolent varieties of lymphoma may have symptoms that come and go; this is problematic, because it may cause a person to delay in getting an important diagnosis.

In later stages, lymphoma may show easy bruising and skin discoloration as platelet numbers drop, along with decreased resistance to **cold**, **flu**, or other infections; this reflects impaired immune system function.

Reed-Sternberg cells: Large transformed lymphocytes, indicative of Hodgkin disease.

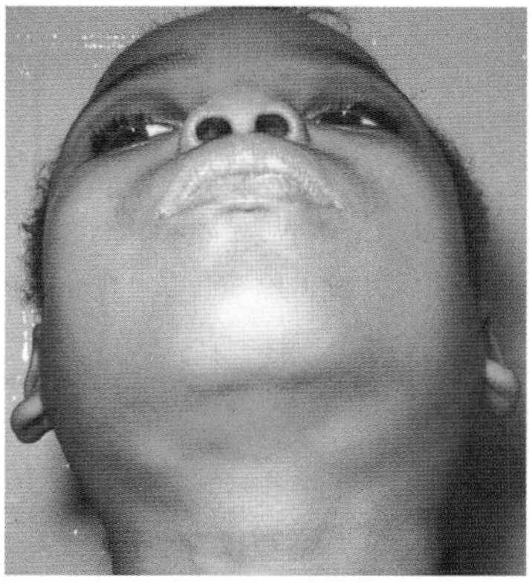

FIGURE 6.4 Hodgkin lymphoma: note the enlarged submandibular lymph nodes

NOTABLE CASES In 2009 cofounder of Microsoft Paul Allen was diagnosed with non-Hodgkin lymphoma, approximately 25 years after successful treatment for Hodgkin lymphoma. Jacqueline Kennedy Onassis was diagnosed with non-Hodgkin lymphoma in 1993 and died in 1994 at age 64. "Lucky Lindy" Charles Lindbergh, who first flew across the Atlantic in 1927, died of lymphoma at age 72 in 1974.

Treatment

Treatment choices for lymphoma depend on several factors, including exactly which type of cells are affected, the stage of the disease, and whether the stage is qualified by an A, B, E, or S finding (see Sidebar 6.2).

Chemotherapy and radiation are the usual choices, but some other options are finding success in dealing with lymphoma, including allogenic and autologous bone marrow transplants, stem cell transplants, and various types of biologic therapy involving radioactive antibodies, cancer vaccinations, and other strategies.

Medications

- Chemotherapeutic agents
- Medication to mitigate chemotherapy symptoms
- Biologic therapy agents

SIDEBAR 6.2 Staging Lymphoma

Lymphoma is staged by its degree of progression and by the microscopic appearance of the affected cells:

Stage I: The cancer is found in only one nodal region, or it has invaded only one nearby organ.

Stage II: Two or more nodal regions are affected, and they are on the same side of the diaphragm or multiple nodal regions along with one organ all on the same side of the diaphragm are affected.

Stage III: Nodes on both sides of the diaphragm are invaded, along with organ involvement; the spleen may or may not be affected.

Stage IV: The cancer is disseminated throughout the body, affecting nodes, organs, bone marrow, and/or the central nervous system.

Recurrent: Recurrent lymphoma is cancer that reappears after a full course of treatment.

In addition to a numerical stage, lymphoma is also described by letters A, B, E, and S:

A. There are no symptoms other than painless enlarged lymph nodes.
B. Fever, weight loss, and night sweats accompany enlarged lymph nodes.
E. Extranodal tumors are found.
S. Tumors are found in the spleen.

Massage Therapy Implications

RISKS	Lymphoma involves lymph nodes and possibly the spleen and other lymph tissues, so any bodywork that focuses on lymphatic or other fluid movement may be too demanding for patients to comfortably and safely receive.
BENEFITS	Massage can be a useful strategy to deal with the physical and emotional demands of dealing with both cancer and cancer treatments, as long as work is within a client's capacity to adapt and when bodywork is integrated into the rest of the treatment plan. See Chapter 12 for more detail. Clients who have fully recovered from lymphoma and who have no long-term complications can enjoy the same benefits from bodywork as the rest of the population.
RESEARCH	Massage for cancer patients has been well studied, and results consistently show that it is helpful, especially for pain and some of the mood-related aspects of this disease, especially anxiety and depression. One study compared therapeutic massage to individual meaning-centered psychotherapy for lymphoma patients and found that psychotherapy can help with some things, but the massaged group fared better on ratings for anxiety, depression, and hopelessness.[1] About 68% of long-term lymphoma survivors use CIH therapies, and massage is a popular choice for them.[2] 1. Breitbart W, Poppito S, Rosenfeld B, et al. Pilot randomized controlled trial of individual meaning-centered psychotherapy for patients with advanced cancer. *Journal of Clinical Oncology* 2012;30(12):1304–1309. http://www.ncbi.nlm.nih.gov/pmc/articles/PMC3646315/ 2. Habermann TM, Thompson CA, LaPlant BR, et al. Complementary and alternative medicine use among long-term lymphoma survivors: a pilot study. *American Journal of Hematology* 2009;84(12):795–798. http://www.ncbi.nlm.nih.gov/pmc/articles/PMC3154703/

Mononucleosis

Definition: What Is It?

Mononucleosis is a viral infection that begins in the salivary glands and throat and then moves into the lymphatic system. The causative agent in about 90% of all cases is the EBV, a member of the herpes family. Other pathogens that can cause mononucleosis include other members of Herpesviridae, specifically cytomegalovirus, **herpes zoster**, human herpesvirus 6 and 7, and others.

Demographics

EBV is extremely common in the United States, but not everyone who is exposed develops mononucleosis. It is estimated that about one-half of all American 5-year-olds have been exposed to the virus, and about 90% have been exposed by age 25.

The people most often diagnosed are young adults between 15 and 25 years old.

Etiology: What Happens?

EBV, the pathogen most often associated with mononucleosis, is fragile outside of a human host. While it may remain viable for a short time on a dish or suspended in a droplet of mucus in the air, the most dependable way to catch it is through direct saliva-to-saliva contact; this is why it is often called the "kissing disease."

Mononucleosis moves through the body in two stages. In the first stage, the virus invades cells in the epithelial tissue of the throat and salivary glands. It takes an unusually long time for the infection to get established; incubation can take up 4 to 6 weeks, during which time the patient is infectious but not strongly symptomatic. Once well established in the epithelial tissue of the throat, the virus moves on to infect B lymphocytes, which carry it to the lymph nodes, liver, and spleen.

As infected B cells proliferate, the body responds by producing high numbers of cytotoxic (killer) T cells. These T cells eventually establish control over the rogue B cells, and ultimately the virus becomes dormant in epithelial cells of the throat.

Once a person is infected with EBV, the virus follows the pattern of other herpes viruses: it is present forever, although usually dormant. It may intermittently reactivate, however. During these episodes, it is likely to be contagious but asymptomatic. This makes the spread of mononucleosis virtually impossible to control.

For most people, mononucleosis is an unpleasant but basically benign, self-limiting infection. It can significantly disrupt a person's life because it has such a powerful effect on stamina, resiliency, and general strength, but it is seldom life-threatening. A very small number of patients, however, do develop serious complications. These include infection of the central nervous system leading to **Bell palsy**, **seizures**, or **meningitis**; enlargement of the heart; temporary **anemia** and thrombocytopenia; and breathing problems when lymph nodes and tonsils get so inflamed that they block air passageways.

One fairly common complication of mononucleosis is a streptococcal infection of the throat ("strep throat"). It is important to be clear about what infection is causing which symptoms in this case, since while strep throat is easily treatable with antibiotics, mononucleosis is not. Further, the antibiotics used for strep throat can sometimes cause a rash in patients who also have mononucleosis.

Perhaps the greatest danger for most mononucleosis patients in the short run is the potential for damage to the spleen. This gland can become dangerously enlarged with lymphocytic activity. Since the spleen also breaks down and recycles dead red blood cells, it has a generous blood supply. If the enlarged organ should be injured by a fall or other trauma, it could rupture, which could lead to internal hemorrhage and rapid circulatory collapse. Persons recovering from mononucleosis are counseled to avoid contact sports for several weeks to reduce their risk of this kind of injury.

In the longer run, people who are infected with EBV carry the virus for a lifetime. If the host's immune system weakens and the EBV reactivates, it is possible for the proliferation of new B cells to change in character to become a type of Hodgkin or non-Hodgkin **lymphoma**.

Signs and Symptoms

Mononucleosis is notorious for presenting different symptoms in different patients. The younger a person is at exposure to EBV, the subtler the symptoms tend to be. Young children may go through exposure, infection, and recovery with no discernible symptoms at all.

In older patients, particularly adolescents and young adults, the signs and symptoms are more dependable. The prodromic stage, as the infection is becoming established but creates no strong symptoms, may be marked by general fatigue and malaise; the patient often does not feel well but may not feel sick, either. This may last anywhere from a few days to several weeks. Then as the infection becomes more aggressive, the leading triad of symptoms appears: fever of 102°F to 104°F (38.9°C to 40°C), an extremely sore throat, and lymph nodes that are swollen from the production of massive numbers of B cells and T cells. The cervical lymph nodes are usually affected most, but submandibular, axillary, and inguinal lymph nodes may also be palpably swollen and tender. Swelling around the throat can be severe enough to affect breathing.

Puffy, swollen eyelids are a common complaint among mononucleosis patients. **Splenomegaly** (enlargement of the spleen) occurs in about half of patients. Many also develop **hepatitis** and **jaundice**. Some mononucleosis patients develop a splotchy, measly rash, especially if they are taking amoxicillin or ampicillin, two penicillin-family antibiotics that are prescribed for strep throat.

Signs and symptoms of acute mononucleosis tend to last approximately 2 weeks before subsiding, but the whole infection is so wearing on the body that it can take several weeks or even months before a patient feels fully functional again.

Treatment

Although it is a viral infection, mononucleosis does not respond to antiviral medications. The typical approach is to treat the symptoms (acetaminophen to reduce fever and pain, rest, good nutrition, and generous hydration) and wait for it to be over. Patients may need to curtail activities to avoid exhaustion and avoid situations like contact sports that could put them at risk for damaging the spleen. A preventive vaccine for EBV is in development.

Medications

- Acetaminophen or ibuprofen for fever and muscle aches
- Steroidal anti-inflammatories for inflammation of the throat and tonsils

Splenomegaly: Enlargement of the spleen.

Massage Therapy Implications

RISKS	A client with fever, inflamed lymph nodes, and general malaise is not a good candidate for rigorous circulatory types of bodywork. Lymphatic congestion and fatigue may linger for weeks or even months after the acute phase, and these also require adaptation in bodywork choices.
BENEFITS	Work that supports healing properties without taxing the lymph or immune systems may be a valuable addition to the lengthy healing process for mononucleosis. A client with a history of this infection and no lingering weakness or illness can enjoy all the benefits from massage as the rest of the population.

Immune System Conditions

Allergic Reactions

Definition: What Are They?

Allergies are immune system reactions against stimuli that are not inherently hazardous. The immune system behaves as though an **allergen**, which could be oak pollen, cat dander, peanuts, or another essentially benign substance, were a potentially dangerous threat.

Demographics

Some experts estimate that 50 million Americans live with some kind of allergy, and that number continues to climb. It is hard to report how many people are affected by angioedema or anaphylaxis each year, but some estimates suggest that about 1,500 people die in this country each year from allergic reactions to food, penicillin, radiocontrast media, latex, and stings.

Etiology: What Happens?

Antibodies are the Y-shaped proteins manufactured by activated B cells against specific pathogens. Some classes of antibodies and some types of T cells are particularly reactive to noninfectious **antigens**, causing acute or chronic allergic symptoms. These hypersensitivity reactions have been classified into four distinct types. Details on types of hypersensitivity reactions are discussed in the introduction to this chapter.

Different types of allergies affect different parts of the population, depending on what substances people are exposed to and how often. The "hygiene hypothesis" suggests that rates of allergic rhinitis ("hay fever"), **asthma, eczema,** and some other allergies are on the rise in the United States because children are overprotected from exposure to allergens in early childhood, and this interferes with proper immune system development.

Alternatively, repeated exposure to some substances, especially latex, can lead to dangerous allergic reactions later in life. This is a particular problem for people with spina bifida or other medical problems that require frequent surgeries and for health care professionals who use latex gloves or latex-based equipment (e.g., catheters, syringes) on a regular basis. Allergies to latex are triggered by natural latex made from derivatives of rubber trees; synthetic latex does not appear to be a potent allergen.

Massage therapists frequently experience allergic reactions to lotions or oils, especially after long-term exposure.

Several conditions involving allergic reactions are discussed elsewhere in this book, in the chapter dedicated to the system that is most significantly affected. **Eczema** and **dermatitis** affect the skin, **asthma** and allergic **sinusitis** affect the respiratory system, and allergic **gastroenteritis** affects the digestive system. The rest of this section addresses three more general but extreme examples of hypersensitivity reactions: anaphylaxis, angioedema, and multiple chemical sensitivity syndrome.

> **Allergen:** A substance that elicits an allergic reaction.
>
> **Antigen:** A substance that provokes an immune response.

Types of Allergic Reactions

- *Anaphylaxis*: This is an acute, severe systemic allergic reaction leading to the release of massive amounts of histamine from previously sensitized mast cells. The result is a sudden drop in blood pressure (hypotension) and accumulation of fluid in the tissues (**edema**). If the reaction centers in the respiratory tract, it can dangerously interfere with breathing. Some of the most common triggers include antibiotics; blood products; the contrast medium used in diagnostic imaging; latex; venom of wasps, ants, and honeybees; and some foods, including peanuts and other nuts, soybeans, cow's milk, eggs, fish, and shellfish. The first exposure to a

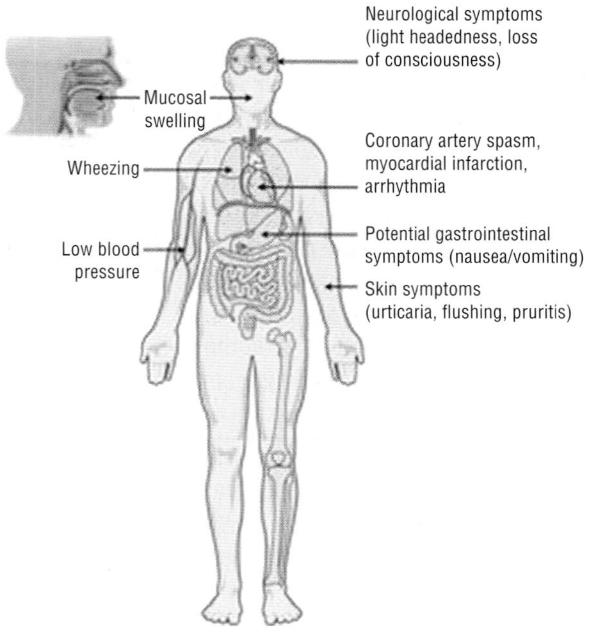

FIGURE 6.5 Anaphylaxis: Systemic symptoms

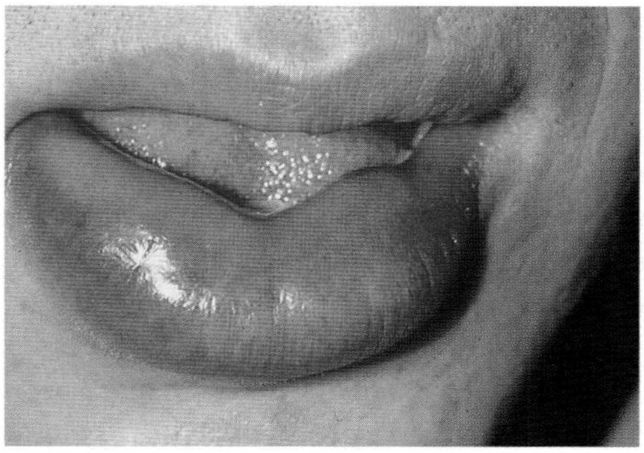

FIGURE 6.6 Angioedema: severe local swelling

trigger may not cause a significant allergic reaction, but repeated exposures lead to increased antibody activity, **complement** activation, and mast cell activity, all of which cause and prolong inflammation. Anaphylaxis is distinguished from angioedema because it occurs both at the site of exposure and systemically through the body (Figure 6.5).

- *Angioedema*: This is the rapid onset of localized swelling (Figure 6.6). The swelling can occur in the skin, genitals, extremities, or gastrointestinal tract. If it occurs in the tongue, larynx, or pharynx, angioedema can interrupt airflow, which is life-threatening. Allergens commonly associated with angioedema include peanuts or tree nuts, chocolate, fish, tomatoes, raw eggs, fresh berries, milk, and food preservatives. Medicines associated with this condition include aspirin, angiotensin-converting enzyme (ACE) inhibitors, and some other hypertension medications. Exposure to poison ivy, poison oak, or poison sumac can also create this kind of reaction (Sidebar 6.3).
- *Multiple chemical sensitivity syndrome* (MCSS): This is a condition in which a history of exposure to a trigger results in reactions that become increasingly severe. It is seen most often among people who have been exposed to chemical spills or other toxic crises. It affects multiple body systems, and as it progressively worsens, more and more triggers can cause reactions. Common allergens include cigarette smoke, perfume and cologne, diesel and gasoline exhaust, detergents, cleaners, varnish, shellac, and fumes from roadwork.

Complement: A group of proteins that work with antibodies during an immune response.

Urushiol: An oil that causes an allergic skin reaction in most people.

SIDEBAR 6.3 Poison Ivy, Poison Oak, and Poison Sumac

Poison ivy, poison oak, and poison sumac all have a chemical in their sap called **urushiol**. Urushiol causes a type IV delayed reaction on the skin involving inflammation, itchiness, and blisters. Up to 85% of the population has an allergic reaction to urushiol.

Poison ivy, poison oak, and poison sumac reactions occur in three ways: through direct contact with the sap, indirect contact with equipment or a pet that has been running through the woods, or through the air when plants are burned.

Many people are familiar with the signs of poison ivy: the rash is red, hot, and very itchy. It can appear to spread after the initial exposure, but this is often due to the fact that some areas of the skin tend to react more quickly than others. Blisters may form and crust over. The rash can take up to 10 days to heal fully. Poison sumac and poison oak produce the same symptoms because the allergen is the same chemical. Occasionally, a rash leads to a very extreme allergic reaction in the shape of angioedema or anaphylaxis; this is a risk especially when swelling takes place around the face or neck, where it can obstruct the airway.

Poison ivy and its relatives are of particular interest to massage therapists because they usually cause a delayed reaction: an exposed person may have no symptoms for 24 hours or more after contacting the plants, although the irritant is present on the skin until it is removed by bathing. This means if a client goes for a massage after a pleasant walk in the woods, it is possible for her therapist not only to spread the sap further on the client, but to spread the urushiol on her own body as well.

Signs and Symptoms

Typical respiratory allergies cause itchy eyes, nose, and throat, as seen in allergic sinusitis.

Anaphylaxis in the skin creates hives, itchiness, and flushing. Excessive edema can cause respiratory symptoms, including shortness of breath, coughing, and wheezing. A person may have so much swelling around the throat that swallowing becomes difficult; this is **dysphagia**. Gastrointestinal symptoms include nausea, vomiting, cramps, bloating, and diarrhea. In extreme circumstances, a person may have a slowed heart rate, hypotension, fainting, and shock. Anaphylaxis may take several hours to develop, and symptoms can appear to subside before returning in a more extreme form.

Signs of angioedema depend on where the inflammation takes place. The skin may be puffy and hot, although if it appears without hives, it may not be itchy. It is often asymmetrical, affecting only one part of the lip, for instance, or one side of the face. It has a rapid onset but usually resolves within 72 hours.

Symptoms of MCSS, while not life-threatening, can include headaches, joint pain, cognitive problems, muscle weakness, dizziness, and heat intolerance.

Treatment

Antihistamines are usually recommended to treat mild allergies. These block the release of histamine that triggers many allergy signs: itchy skin, runny nose, and irritated eyes.

Angioedema and anaphylaxis are on the more serious end of the allergic reaction spectrum, and they are typically treated in the short term with epinephrine and oxygen if breathing is impaired and steroidal anti-inflammatories after the crisis has passed. People at risk for anaphylactic reactions are taught how to avoid triggers and trained to keep medication, usually injectable epinephrine (an EpiPen), close at hand in case of emergency.

When a person has dangerous allergic reactions to insect stings, a long-term course of **desensitization** may be recommended; this process can reduce the risk of dangerous anaphylactic reactions.

Medications

- Antihistamines to block histamine activation sites
- Epinephrine for severe angioedema or anaphylaxis
- Steroidal anti-inflammatories

Dysphagia: Difficulty swallowing.

Desensitization: A therapy by which a person is introduced to gradually increasing amounts of an allergen in order to eliminate allergic reaction.

Massage Therapy Implications

RISKS A person with acute swelling, especially in a location that inhibits breathing, needs medical intervention more than massage. Practitioners must have hypoallergenic lubricants and be able to create a session room that is free from allergens like perfume and other heavy scents for clients who live with the possibility of severe allergic reactions.

A client with common respiratory allergies may be uncomfortable lying prone, as this puts pressure on the sinuses.

BENEFITS Chronic allergies can leave a person feeling exhausted. Massage that does not exacerbate symptoms can be a helpful restorative, as long as positioning and other environmental factors can be controlled for maximum comfort.

OPTIONS Any massage that works to reduce inflammation in the sinuses and throat may provide symptomatic relief from respiratory allergies.

RESEARCH Research points to the risk of developing contact dermatitis with prolonged exposure to some substances, especially essential oils; this is a caution for massage therapists than for their clients.[1-3] Angioedema and anaphylaxis, on the other hand, do not tend to be issues in massage therapy settings.

1. Lakshmi C. Allergic contact dermatitis (type IV hypersensitivity) and type I hypersensitivity following aromatherapy with Ayurvedic oils (Dhanwantharam Thailam, Eladi coconut oil) presenting as generalized erythema and pruritus with flexural eczema. *Indian Journal of Dermatology* 2014;59(3):283–286. http://www.ncbi.nlm.nih.gov/pmc/articles/PMC4037951/
2. Trattner A, David M, Lazarov A. Occupational contact dermatitis due to essential oils. *Contact Dermatitis* 2008;58(5):282–284. http://www.ncbi.nlm.nih.gov/pubmed/18416758
3. Crawford GH, Katz KA, Ellis E, et al. Use of aromatherapy products and increased risk of hand dermatitis in massage therapists. *Archives of Dermatology* 2004;140(8):991–996. http://www.ncbi.nlm.nih.gov/pubmed/15313817

Chronic Fatigue Syndrome

Definition: What Is It?

Chronic fatigue syndrome (CFS) is a collection of signs and symptoms that affect multiple systems in the body. It varies in severity from mildly limiting to completely debilitating.

CFS was named in 1988 by scientists at the Centers for Disease Control, and its definition continues to evolve. The name is vague on purpose because this disease affects different people in very different ways. Nonetheless, some people feel this title trivializes their condition, and CFS is therefore also called chronic fatigue immune dysfunction syndrome (CFIDS). In Europe and

Canada, a condition called **myalgic encephalomyelitis** (ME) is sometimes referred to as a synonym for CFS.

Demographics

Estimates for the incidence of CFS vary widely. The Centers for Disease Control suggest that it has been diagnosed in about 1 million Americans, but many more may meet or come close to meeting the diagnostic criteria.

Etiology: What Happens?

The etiology of CFS is not well understood. It seems clear that it arises from a combination of factors that may or may not involve infectious agents, mentally or emotionally stressful events, neuroendocrine dysfunction, and other factors.

For many years, the leading theory was that a person was infected with a common virus (probably Epstein-Barr, the herpesvirus that causes most cases of **mononucleosis**) and then the body simply continued to behave as though the infection were acute long after the danger had passed. Although blood studies of patients with CFS often show some immune system abnormalities (levels of the inflammatory cytokines and some antibodies are high, while natural killer cell levels tend to be unusually low), it now seems clear that not all CFS cases begin with mononucleosis.

Other pathogenic exposures have been implicated in CFS, specifically mycoplasma, some enteroviruses and retroviruses, *Chlamydophila pneumoniae*, and other infectious agents. No single pathogen has been found to be present in most CFS patients, however, and most people who have been exposed to these agents do not develop CFS symptoms.

The more we learn about CFS, the clearer it becomes that this is probably a multifactoral disorder, with input from many different sources, including viruses and other pathogens, abnormalities in the hypothalamus-pituitary-adrenal axis, an overreactive immune system, and depression or other psychiatric or emotional factors. The net result in the central nervous system is a dysfunctional HPA axis, disturbed sleep cycles, and imbalances in dopamine, serotonin, epinephrine, and norepinephrine.

Interestingly, the cortisol levels in people with CFS tend to be lower than normal. This suggests some level of adrenal depletion rather than freedom from low-grade stress, and the absence of normal cortisol (a power anti-inflammatory) means that **allergies** tend to be very extreme for CFS patients.

Signs and Symptoms

Fatigue is the central symptom of CFS. The fatigue is unrelenting and not restored by sleep or rest. The basic diagnostic criterion for CFS includes unrelenting fatigue that persists for a minimum of 6 months, the fatigue is severe enough to interfere with work and daily activities, and at least four of the following are also present at the same time:

- Poor short-term memory, poor concentration, and mental fogginess
- Changes in sleep quantity and quality
- Muscle aches
- Headache in a new pattern
- Tender lymph nodes, especially in the neck and axilla
- Joint paint with no inflammation
- Recurring sore throat
- Postexertional pain, out of proportion to the amount of exercise

Of these, poor memory and concentration, along with significant postexertional pain, are the most consistent nonfatigue CFS symptoms. Patients may also report extreme allergies, abdominal bloating, nausea, diarrhea, cramping, chest pain, irregular heartbeat, coughing, dizziness, fainting, dry eyes and mouth, weight loss, jaw pain, morning stiffness, night sweats, and psychological problems related to living with chronic illness, especially depression, and/or anxiety.

This list of symptoms points to an important feature of CFS: it closely resembles two other chronic stress-related conditions, **fibromyalgia** and **irritable bowel syndrome**, and it frequently occurs along with them. In fact, so much overlap exists between these conditions that many people with aspects of all three disorders are simply diagnosed with whatever syndrome's primary features appear first: irritable bowel syndrome for gastrointestinal discomfort, fibromyalgia syndrome for predominant muscle and joint pain, or CFS if the leading symptom is unrelenting fatigue. Other common comorbidities include **multiple chemical sensitivity syndrome**, **interstitial cystitis**, and **temporomandibular syndrome**.

> **NOTABLE CASES** It is thought that Florence Nightingale, who was a pioneer in modern nursing practices during the Crimean War, had CFS. Author Laura Hillenbrand (*Seabiscuit: An American Legend*) is an active spokesperson for patients with this condition.

One of the most difficult issues for CFS patients is that symptoms are variable and unpredictable. They may come and go with no connection to activity or other triggers. When a person enters a period of remission, the tendency to overexert can then put them back into an exhausted state.

Treatment

The primary treatment for CFS is making lifestyle choices that support the body as fully as possible. This means managing stress (any stimulus—emotional or physical—that requires the body

> **Myalgic encephalomyelitis:** Another name for chronic fatigue syndrome.

to adapt to a change) as well as possible. It also means avoiding stimulants (caffeine, sugar) and depressants (alcohol) and exercising consistently and gently, so as not to exacerbate symptoms.

An important part of treatment for CFS patients is education; the more they learn about their condition, the better equipped they are to handle its challenges. Some evidence indicates that cognitive-behavioral therapy can be effective as CFS patients seek coping skills to live with this condition.

Medical intervention may include low-dose antidepressants, but many experts suggest that these drugs are not particularly effective for CFS patients. Other medications are geared toward symptomatic treatment.

Research shows that CFS patients do best with a multipronged approach to treatment that encompasses cognitive-behavioral therapy, exercise, and self-care (which can include massage) along with standard medical care.

Medications

- NSAIDs for muscle and joint pain
- Anxiolytics
- Antiallergy medication to control allergic symptoms

Massage Therapy Implications

RISKS	CFS patients tend to have low stamina and may not welcome a rigorous, long, demanding massage that could leave them more fatigued than after their treatment than before.
BENEFITS	Evidence suggests that massage can help with pain, sleep, and perceived anxiety: all issues for CFS patients. Gentle massage is a safe and appropriate choice for clients with this condition. More rigorous bodywork can be helpful with clients who have improved resilience.
RESEARCH	A systematic review of complementary and integrative health therapies for CFS found positive outcomes for massage therapy.[1] Jones et al.[2] found that people with CFS and other fatiguing pathologies are willing users of CIH—especially body-based therapies like massage and chiropractic—so it is important for people in this field to be educated about CFS. 1. Alraek T, Lee MS, Choi TY, et al. Complementary and alternative medicine for patients with chronic fatigue syndrome: a systematic review. *BMC Complementary and Alternative Medicine* 2011;11:87. http://www.ncbi.nlm.nih.gov/pmc/articles/PMC3201900/ 2. Jones JF, Maloney EM, Boneva RS, et al. Complementary and alternative medical therapy utilization by people with chronic fatiguing illnesses in the United States. *BMC Complementary and Alternative Medicine* 2007;7(12). http://www.ncbi.nlm.nih.gov/pmc/articles/PMC1878505/

Fever

Definition: What Is It?

Fever, also called **pyrexia**, is an abnormally high body temperature. It is usually brought about by bacterial or viral infection, but sometimes it is triggered by other types of tissue damage. Exactly when fever is identified is a bit of a moving target: most people vary in internal temperature by a degree Fahrenheit or more throughout the day. Fever is a controlled change in temperature, which distinguishes it from other types of **hyperthermia** (Sidebar 6.4).

Etiology: What Happens?

Several steps are involved in the development of an infection-based fever:

1. A person is infected with some microorganism, such as bacteria, viruses, or fungi.
2. White blood cells find and eat those invaders.
3. Some pieces of the bacterial cell membranes are displayed by the macrophages. They stimulate other white blood cells to secrete **interleukin-1** and other proinflammatory cytokines.
4. Interleukin-1 circulates through the system, including the brain. It causes a series of chemical reactions involving prostaglandins that tell the hypothalamus to reset the body's thermostat to a higher level. In this situation, interleukin-1 is acting as a **pyrogen**, a fever starter.
5. Orders from the hypothalamus ripple through the body, setting up the muscular and glandular responses that raise the core temperature. These responses include shivering, constriction of superficial capillaries, and increased metabolism.

The characteristic shivering and chills that go along with a rising fever are part of the mechanism to increase the core temperature: this is called the chill phase. Once that goal has been met, the shivering stops, but processes keep working to maintain the increased temperature until the stimulating chemicals have been removed. This peak is called the crisis of the fever. When the crisis has passed, the body's cooling mechanisms, sweating and capillary dilation, take over: the flush phase. At this point, the worst is over, and the fever is broken.

Pyrexia: Fever.
Hyperthermia: Abnormally high body temperature.
Interleukin-1: A protein that raises body temperature.
Pyrogen: A fever-inducing agent.

SIDEBAR 6.4 Types of Hyperthermia

Fever is a systemic rise in body temperature that is carefully controlled by the hypothalamus. It has the advantages of speeding up immune system activity while slowing and starving infectious agents. Fever is an extraordinarily efficient mechanism to fight infection.

Sometimes, however, a person's core temperature rises without hypothalamic control. This generally occurs when a person generates more heat than he or she can release. In this case, the body temperature continues to rise until external factors work to cool off the person. If environmental factors don't allow this to happen, the person is at risk for brain damage or death.

The three levels of hyperthermia are heat cramps, heat exhaustion, and heat stroke. They are most commonly seen in people who are physically very active in warm, humid environments. Massage therapists who work at summertime sporting events can expect to see any of these manifestations of hyperthermia. A fourth condition, malignant hyperthermia, is a genetic condition that may be triggered by exposure to anesthesia.

- *Heat cramps*: Muscle cramping is a frequent result of the dehydration that accompanies excessive heat production. The body sweats in an attempt to lower its temperature, and the result is a deficit in interstitial fluid. This makes it more difficult for the calcium ions that stimulate muscle contractions to be reabsorbed into their storage containers. The consequence is that muscle contractions are sustained and uncontrolled. Fortunately, massage along with rehydration is an excellent way to move fluid back into the muscle bellies and stimulate the chemical and neurological reactions that reduce the spasm.
- *Heat exhaustion*: Heat exhaustion occurs when muscular activity generates more heat than a person can release. It is marked by excessive sweating, headache, vasodilation, and dehydration. Excessive sweating may lead to low blood pressure, light-headedness, and fainting. Fast hydration is the best recourse for this situation.
- *Heat stroke*: Heat stroke is the final stage of hyperthermia. In this condition, body temperature rises to dangerous levels (~104°F, or 40°C, for adults). Prolonged dehydration may lead to lack of sweating and circulatory shock from loss of water and electrolytes. The person may become confused or delirious. Heat stroke can be fatal if the core temperature is not quickly but carefully reduced to safe levels.
- *Malignant hyperthermia*: This is not an activity-related problem, but rather a genetic anomaly that allows the body temperature to rise to dangerous, even fatal, levels with a minimum of muscular work. It is sometimes seen as part of an allergic reaction to anesthesia. Many people don't know they are at risk for this disorder until they have a dangerous episode.

Pathogenic invasion is the causative factor of most but not all fevers. Severe injury can upset the hypothalamic thermostat, as can poison, certain cancers, and some autoimmune diseases.

This culture has a strange and troubling discomfort with discomfort. Often, people would rather hide a symptom than feel it and figure out what it's trying to tell them. This is true particularly with fever, which can be disagreeable and inconvenient. In rare cases, it can get high enough to do some serious damage, but most of the time fever is a sign that the body is working in the most efficient possible way to get rid of invading pathogens. Some of those mechanisms include the following:

- Interleukin-1 and other cytokines not only help to reset the body's thermostat, they also stimulate T-cell production. Increased T-cell production stimulates B cells and the production of antibodies.
- Interferon, a powerful antiviral agent, becomes much more active in the presence of fever.
- Increased temperature limits iron secretion from the liver and spleen, slowing bacterial and viral activity.
- Increased temperature raises the heart rate (10 beats per minute per degree), which in turn increases the distribution of white blood cells throughout the body.
- Increased temperature increases cell wall permeability and speeds chemical reactions. This promotes faster recovery for damaged tissues.

Fever occasionally presents a danger, particularly when the temperature rises over 104°F (40°C) for adults; this is called **hyperpyrexia**. The most common complications are dehydration (from prolonged sweating), **acidosis**, and brain damage. Death from fever occurs somewhere around 112°F to 114°F (44.4°C to 44.5°C) for adults. If a fever comes down too fast, it can quickly dilate blood vessels. This can lead to circulatory shock, which can be dangerous, especially to older patients.

Hyperpyrexia: Dangerously high fever.

Acidosis: The state of having abnormally acidic body fluids or tissues.

Signs and Symptoms

The primary sign of fever is self-evident: it is a body temperature that is higher than normal. It is important to remember that many individuals have a "normal" temperature that is not exactly 98.6°F, and also our temperature varies throughout the day, so small fluctuations without other symptoms like headache or malaise may not be significant. Other symptoms include the chills and shivering that go with raising internal temperature and the flushing and sweating that go along with lowering it.

Treatment

Generally, fever is identified when an undertongue thermometer registers 101°F (38.3°C) or more. That said, anyone with a persistent fever below that target should investigate it with a primary health care provider.

Experts don't agree about the best time to treat simple fevers in adults. Suppressing symptoms may prolong an infection, and allowing a person to go back to work or school puts them in contact with other people who may subsequently become infected. On the other hand, fevers are uncomfortable and inconvenient, and it is natural to want to interrupt their course.

Medications

- Aspirin, ibuprofen, or acetaminophen to interrupt hypothalamic control of internal temperature
- Note: aspirin is NOT appropriate for use with children

Massage Therapy Implications

RISKS	Fever systemically contraindicates most types of bodywork for the dual reason that the client is already challenged, and the practitioner shouldn't run the risk of exposure to a contagious condition.
BENEFITS	Gentle bodywork may help a client with a fever feel better, although it may have no impact on the fever itself. Any client who has fully recovered from a condition involving fever can enjoy the same benefits from bodywork as the rest of the population.

HIV/AIDS

Definition: What Is It?

AIDS (acquired immune deficiency syndrome) was first recognized as a specific disease in the United States in 1983. The causative virus, HIV (human immunodeficiency virus), attacks various agents of the immune system with disastrous results.

Demographics

The World Health Organization estimates that in 2013 a total of 35 million people in the world were living with HIV. About 2.1 million people developed new infections, and of those, 240,000 were in children under 15 years old. We lost 1.5 million people to AIDS in 2013.

In the United States, 1.3 million people are HIV positive, although up to 14% may be unaware of their status. About 50,000 new infections are diagnosed, and some 35,000 people progress from being HIV positive to having AIDS each year. Roughly 14,000 deaths in the United States each year are attributed to HIV infection.

HIV/AIDS impacts many more men than women in this country. Almost 80% of infections are in men, and of those, most are related to male-to-male sexual contact. Heterosexual contact and injected drug use account for the majority of infections among women.

Etiology: What Happens?

HIV enters the body by way of body fluids: blood (including transfusions and on shared needles), semen, vaginal secretions, and breast milk are the most efficient carriers of the virus.

HIV can attach to cells in mucosal epithelium to gain entry to the body. Any other sexually transmitted infection, such as **syphilis**, genital **herpes**, **chlamydia**, or **gonorrhea**, can significantly increase the risk of transmitting the virus. Once in the tissue, the virus invades a target cell through a molecular portal of entry on the membrane called CD4, along with coreceptor sites, which vary. Monocytes, macrophages, T cells, stem cells for blood, fibroblasts, and several cells found in the central nervous system all have this molecular doorway, so these are called CD4+ cells. HIV often invades circulating monocytes and macrophages and uses these hosts as transport to concentrations of CD4+ cells in the bone marrow, lymph nodes, spleen, tonsils, adenoids, and central nervous system.

These targets are significant for a couple of reasons. First, when the virus pools in macrophages before moving up in the immune system hierarchy, its presence does not immediately trigger the production of antibodies, which makes it difficult to identify early in a blood test. Second, consider the consequences of a virus that targets immune system cells: the entire immune system collapses and leaves the body vulnerable to a wide array of opportunistic diseases.

SIDEBAR 6.5 A Virus Primer

Viruses consist of a protein coat of variable complexity wrapped around a core of DNA or RNA. Outside a host cell, viruses have no metabolic functions and cannot replicate. Inside a host cell, the virus reprograms the functions of that cell to replicate more viruses. In other words, the host cell becomes a virus factory. When the factory is full of inventory, it either seeps virions (viral particles) from its membrane, or it ruptures, releasing hordes of new viruses in search of other hosts. Enormous amounts of damage occur with any viral infection, not just to the cells attacked by the virus, but to the cells the body sacrifices to fight back.

Most viruses cause short-term acute infections that spread easily. The coughing and sneezing seen with respiratory tract infections such as cold and flu are remarkably efficient distributors of virus. Likewise, the diarrhea that occurs with intestinal infections is an effective way to spread virus through fecal contamination. The immune system response to these viruses is severe and usually successful; most infections are curtailed, and the viruses are expelled in short order.

A few viruses, however, cause long-term chronic infections instead of short-term acute illness. Hepatitis B and C, herpesviruses, and HIV are notorious among these. For a virus to live in a body for a long time, it must be able to hide from immune system cells to escape attack and destruction. It is precisely the ability of HIV to hide from typical immune system activity that makes it so difficult to fight. In addition to being good hiders, chronic infectious viruses have been seen to produce decoy particles that draw antibody attack away from themselves and to secrete fake cytokines, chemical messengers that confuse and slow down immune system response.

As we learn more about how chronic infectious viruses pool in hidden reservoirs in the body, our ability to fight back will improve. We may someday be able to eradicate these hidden invaders permanently.

HIV can move from one CD4+ cell to another, and it can pool in the core of lymph nodes, where it eventually causes the cells to degenerate and the lymph node to lose all function. HIV has also been found in astrocytes and microglial cells in the central nervous system. This breaks down the **blood-brain barrier**, so accumulations of wastes in the brain can lead to neurological symptoms.

HIV is composed of RNA rather than DNA, which holds the blueprints for our own cells. (See Sidebar 6.5.) Once inside a CD4+ cell, this retrovirus uses the enzyme **transcriptase** to convert its RNA to DNA in order to replicate (Figure 6.7). In the process, the virus is often minutely altered—just enough to make it resistant to identification or treatment. Ultimately, the virus replicates so much that the infected CD4+ cells die through membrane rupture or **apoptosis**.

Blood-brain-barrier: A highly selective filter formed by endothelial cells and astrocytes to prevent the passage of material from the blood directly into the central nervous system.

Transcriptase: An enzyme that converts RNA to DNA.

Apoptosis: Programmed cell death.

Titer: A measurement of concentration (as in the concentration of a virus in the blood).

Progression

Each stage of HIV/AIDS is associated with decreasing numbers of active CD4+ cells and increased viral **titers** (counts of virus). The typical pattern looks like this:

- *Phase 1.* A person is infected with HIV. The virus pools in white blood cells and doesn't elicit an immune response. Consequently, tests are negative, and no symptoms are present, but the person can transmit the disease because the viral load is high. This incubation phase can last a year or more, although the average is 3 weeks to 6 months in sexually transmitted cases.
- *Phase 2.* In the acute primary phase, HIV infection antibodies become detectable in blood tests. Many people have fatigue, swollen glands, fever, weight loss, headaches, drowsiness, and confusion within several weeks of exposure. These signs and symptoms usually last about 2 weeks and are often mistaken for flu or mononucleosis.
- *Phase 3.* No signs, symptoms, or opportunistic diseases are obvious. Although immune system cells are being destroyed in lymphatic tissue, the body is able to produce some antibodies against the virus. It is during this phase that medical intervention inhibits viral replication and prolongs life expectancy. The length of the asymptomatic phase without treatment varies widely, lasting anywhere from 1 to 20 years or more, with a median of 10 years.

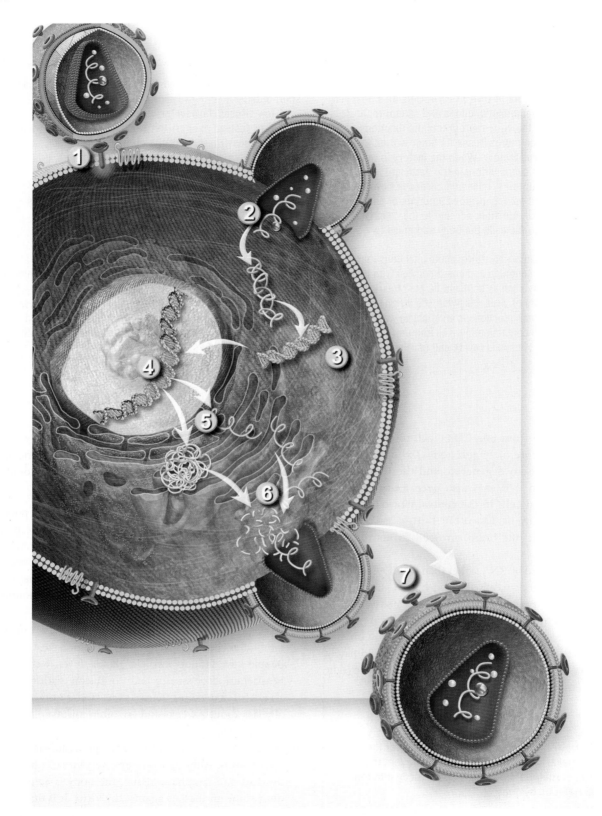

FIGURE 6.7 HIV/AIDS. *1.* The virus attaches to a CD4 site on a target cell. *2.* RNA enters the cytoplasm. *3.* RNA uses transcriptase to become DNA. *4.* The virus reprograms the cell's function in the nucleus. *5.* The cell now manufactures many copies of HIV RNA, along with its protein coats. *6.* Viruses are manufactured in the cell. *7.* Newly formed viruses leave to find new targets.

- *Phase 4.* Signs and symptoms of opportunistic diseases or AIDS-related cancers become apparent and eventually debilitating. A normal T-cell count is 800 to 1,000 cells per milliliter of blood. AIDS is diagnosed when these levels drop to 200 cells per milliliter or below, and indicator diseases begin to develop.

HIV Resistance

Some HIV/AIDS research has focused on the variables that determine how long an infected person can stay healthy. Some people who are infected with HIV never develop symptoms or develop them much more slowly than most people. These "long-term nonprogressors" can provide important clues to ways the virus may be fought once infection has been established. It seems clear that most long-term nonprogressors or very slow progressors have a combination of factors working in their favor. Three main variables have been identified:

- *Host resistance.* Some HIV patients have a genetic mutation in their immune system that produces few receptor sites on their macrophages and T cells for the virus to latch on to. It takes more exposure over a longer time to establish an infection in these people, because the chance for a successful invasion is much lower.
- *Immune system response.* When most cells are invaded by a virus, they display a fragment of that virus on their membrane. This serves as a signal to immune system agents that the cell is compromised and should be destroyed. HIV is capable of slowing down this display reaction or of hiding from it altogether by mimicking normal cell membranes. If the efficiency of the display mechanism is improved, immune system response is more aggressive.
- *Virulence of the virus.* Sometimes HIV is partially weakened by medication or an immune system response, but remains transmittable to another person. Infection with a weakened virus generally means the new host is better able to control it. Relative virulence of individual viruses is difficult to measure, however.

Communicability

HIV is spread from one person to another through the exchange of intimate fluids. These include blood (as from contaminated blood products, shared needles, or maternal-fetal circulation), semen, vaginal secretions, and breast milk. HIV does not accumulate in concentrations high enough to cause infection in other body fluids, such as sweat, saliva, or tears. The virus quickly falls apart outside a human host, so it is not considered to be transmissible through contaminated surfaces or insect vectors such as mosquitoes, ticks, or bedbugs.

Complications

When HIV has virtually disabled normal immune function, the body is incapable of fending off attacks from pathogens that are not threatening to healthy people. A group of formerly obscure diseases are now so closely associated with AIDS; they are called indicator diseases. Here are some of the most common and serious ones:

- *Pneumocystis carinii pneumonia.* This is a fungal infection of the lungs. It is now also called *Pneumocystis jirovecii*.
- *Cytomegalovirus.* This member of the herpes family can cause retinitis and blindness, colitis, pneumonia, and infection of the adrenal glands.
- *Kaposi sarcoma.* This is a type of skin cancer (Figure 6.8) related to infection with human herpesvirus 8. Kaposi sarcoma is much more common in men with AIDS than in women.
- *Non-Hodgkin lymphomas.* HIV has been found to specifically initiate cancer cell replication with a variety of **lymphomas**. They tend to be aggressive, they frequently metastasize to the central nervous system, and they are highly resistant to treatment.

Other opportunistic indicator diseases include toxoplasmosis, a protozoan that can cause **encephalitis** or **pneumonia**; **candidiasis**; and Cryptococcus neoformans, a fungal infection that can cause meningitis and pneumonia.

In addition to these indicator diseases, people with AIDS are highly susceptible to gastrointestinal disturbances, **herpes simplex, meningitis, shingles, cervical cancer, hepatitis C,** and many other conditions. When **tuberculosis** occurs simultaneously with HIV, the risk of having tuberculosis become an active, contagious condition rises with each year of coinfection.

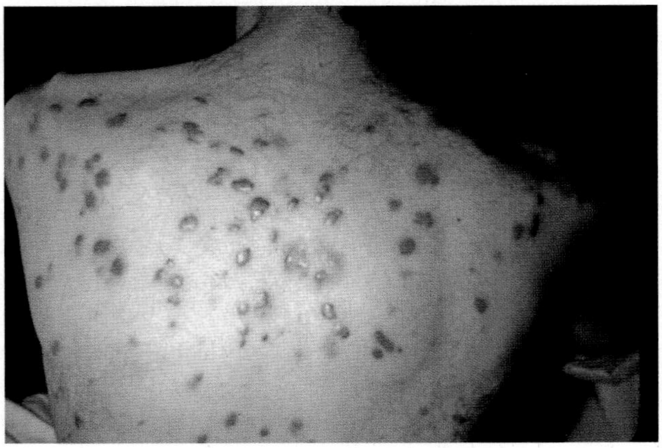

FIGURE 6.8 Kaposi sarcoma

It is important to point out that while it is difficult to catch HIV from an infected person without some kind of intimate contact, it might not be difficult to catch some of the contagious complications of AIDS. Tuberculosis, herpes, and other infections don't discriminate between HIV-positive and other persons.

Signs and Symptoms

Signs and symptoms of HIV depend on the stage of infection; these are described earlier in this section.

Prevention

Until recently, the only way to prevent the spread of HIV was to avoid all high-risk behaviors. Good education in this strategy has led to a plateau in the number of new diagnoses, but more is needed, especially for those in relationships with people who are HIV positive. A protocol called preexposure prophylaxis (PrEP) uses specific antiretroviral drugs in a single daily pill that radically reduces the risk of HIV transmission: the rate of infection for people who consistently use the medication is 92% lower than for those who do not. This strategy is not risk-free, however, and needs to be used along with other interventions like safe sex practices and regular testing for best results.

NOTABLE CASES The list of important and influential people lost to AIDS is too long to attempt. Perhaps the first "big name" to go public with this disease was actor Rock Hudson, but he was only one of thousands, including actor Tony Perkins ("Psycho") and tennis grand slam winner Arthur Ashe. Basketball legend Magic Johnson may be the public figure with the longest history of being both healthy and HIV positive; he was diagnosed in 1991 and continues to be an activist for AIDS prevention and accessibility of treatment.

Treatment

One of the things that makes finding a cure for AIDS so difficult is that when it reproduces, the virus can minutely change—just enough to make it resistant to drugs as well as to immune system activation. The solution to that problem has been to combine various drugs to anticipate the mutations of the virus. This has been highly successful in laboratory settings, but these drug combinations are often prohibitively toxic to the actual patients. Another challenge is the spread of drug-resistant forms of the virus to people who have never been treated. Not surprisingly, this is a bigger issue in the United States, Australia, and Western Europe than in the rest of the world, where antiretroviral therapy is harder to access.

The most successful AIDS treatments so far have involved using multiple strategies to interrupt viral replication. The use of highly active antiretroviral therapy (**HAART**) has been seen to slow progression in many patients, but it can't eradicate the virus. Although the goal of eliminating the virus from an infected person is still a long way off, studies of patients who manage to control their infection efficiently continue to point the way to better treatment options, and the life expectancy for a person with HIV today (who can afford to treat it) is better than it has ever been.

The biggest controversy in HIV treatment currently is deciding when it is best to initiate antiviral therapy. It is clear that drugs prolong the lives of AIDS patients, but they are also highly toxic and have many serious side effects, including low blood cell count, **peripheral neuropathy**, **pancreatitis**, insulin resistance, chronic diarrhea, liver inflammation, **kidney stones**, and many others. One of the most visible side effects of HIV medication is **lipodystrophy**: fat in the cheeks and the buttocks degenerates, but fat in the upper back, breasts, and around the belly accumulates. Furthermore, many AIDS patients live in isolation, and they are more likely than most to be depressed and/or substance abusers, which increases the risk of their not taking their medication according to prescription: this gives rise to ever more resistant strains of the virus.

Treatment recommendations vary. If HIV is identified during the primary phase of flu-like symptoms, some research predicts the best prognosis if therapy is started right away. Health care workers who get needlesticks with a risk of contamination are treated immediately to reduce the risk that the virus can take hold. But if the virus isn't identified until the person is asymptomatic, many experts recommend holding off on aggressive treatment until CD4+ levels drop to below a specific threshold.

Medications

- Antiretroviral drugs

HAART: Highly active antiretroviral therapy. A combination of at least three drugs used to suppress HIV.

Lipodystrophy: The abnormal redistribution of fat in the body.

Massage Therapy Implications

RISKS	It is possible (although not typical) for a person who is HIV positive to have an opportunistic disease that is potentially contagious through casual contact. This is obviously a caution for massage therapists working with HIV-positive clients, but in most cases, the person most at risk for getting sick when an AIDS patient receives massage is not the therapist; it's the client. Therefore, care must be taken that the practitioner does not carry active pathogens that may put a client with AIDS at risk. Some side effects of ART include problems that contraindicate some types of massage, like nausea and vomiting, rashes, pancreatitis, and heart problems.
BENEFITS	Asymptomatic HIV indicates massage. Some studies indicate that massage boosts immune system activity and efficiency for clients who are HIV positive. Further, stress management techniques appear to promote the production of healthy lymphocytes in HIV-positive persons. Clients with advanced AIDS can also benefit from massage that is specifically adjusted to meet their special needs. Bodywork can be a wonderful treatment option and an important source of support and comfort for people who are often rejected, ignored, or actively persecuted by society. Some side effects of HAART can be successfully addressed by massage therapy, including constipation, peripheral neuropathy, fatigue, and insomnia.
RESEARCH	A substantial amount of research has been done about massage therapy for people with HIV/AIDS or to address some of the issues peripheral to the disease. Depression is a frequent complication that can interfere with good self-care. Poland et al.[1] found that massage therapy (compared to two-handed touch with no massage or no intervention) led to significantly reduced symptoms. Several studies suggest that in addition to promoting parasympathetic response, massage may also boost immune system activity.[2] 1. Poland RE, Gertsik L, Favreau JT, et al. Open-label, randomized, parallel-group controlled clinical trial of massage for treatment of depression in HIV-infected subjects. *Journal of Alternative and Complementary Medicine (New York, N.Y.)* 2013;19(4):334–340. http://www.ncbi.nlm.nih.gov/pmc/articles/PMC3627430/ 2. Hillier SL, Louw Q, Morris L, et al. Massage therapy for people with HIV/AIDS. *Cochrane Database of Systematic Reviews* 2010;(1):CD007502. http://www.ncbi.nlm.nih.gov/pubmed/20091636

Autoimmune Disorders

Ankylosing Spondylitis

Definition: What Is It?

Ankylosing spondylitis (AS) is spinal inflammation (spondylitis) leading to stiff joints (ankylosis). In this condition, the joints between and around vertebrae can become permanently fused. AS is a progressive inflammatory arthritis of the spine. It is sometimes called rheumatoid spondylitis.

Demographics

Unlike most autoimmune diseases, AS affects males more often than females; the ratio is about 3:1, depending on age. This may be misleading, however, because symptoms are often less severe in women, and diagnoses may be missed. Most diagnoses are made between ages 20 and 40. It is estimated that about 500,000 Americans currently live with AS, but up to 2.7 million people live with associated spondyloarthropathies (see Sidebar 6.6.)

Etiology: What Happens?

Ankylosing spondylitis is generally recognized as an autoimmune disease, but the blood of people with AS shows no sign of the **antinuclear antibodies** (ANA) that are typical of other autoimmune diseases. For this reason, it is classified as a **seronegative spondyloarthropathy**. Other seronegative

> **Antinuclear antibodies:** Antibodies produced by the immune system that attack the body's own cells.
>
> **Seronegative spondyloarthropathy:** An autoimmune disease of the vertebral column that does not result in antinuclear antibodies in the blood.

6 Lymph and Immune System Conditions

SIDEBAR 6.6 The Spondyloarthritis Family

Ankylosing spondylitis is an autoimmune condition that involves progressive inflammation and damage of the spine and other tissues. It is the most common of a whole group of autoimmune conditions, known collectively as spondyloarthritis. The primary feature that all of these conditions share is enthesitis: inflammation and damage where bones connect to other tissues.

Other diseases in this group include psoriatic arthritis, a common complication of psoriasis; arthritis associated with inflammatory bowel disease; juvenile spondyloarthritis; reactive arthritis (formerly known as Reiter syndrome); and undifferentiated spondyloarthritis.

The guidelines for massage therapy in the context of spondyloarthritis in general follow the same principles as those for ankylosing spondylitis: do what is possible to reduce inflammation, and focus on increasing and preserving range of motion.

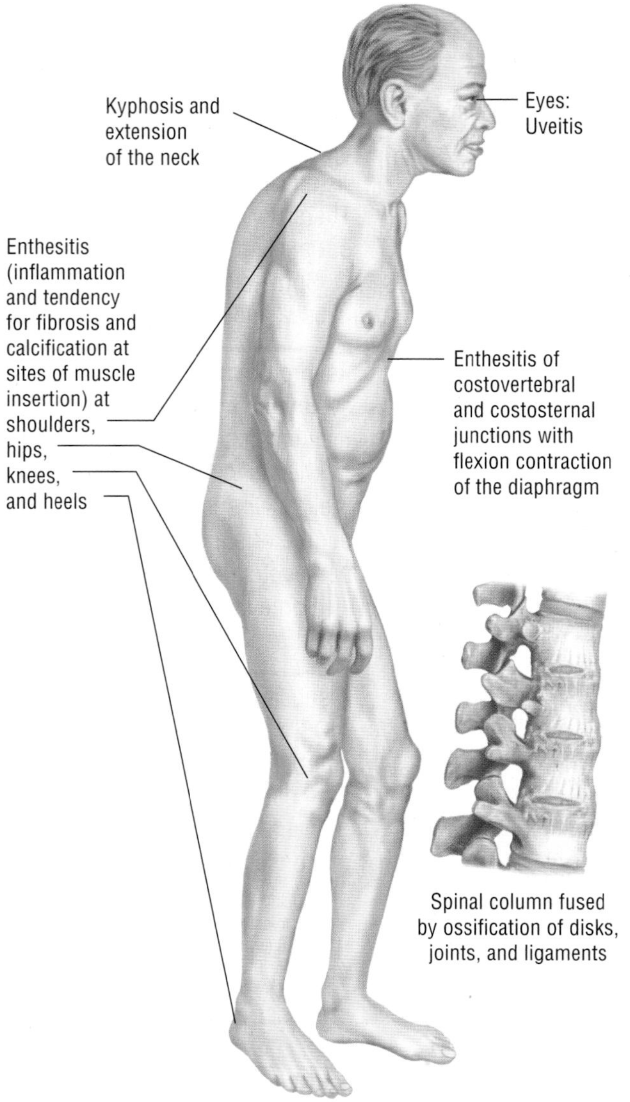

FIGURE 6.9 Ankylosing spondylitis

autoimmune diseases include inflammatory bowel disease (**Crohn disease** and **ulcerative colitis**), **psoriasis**, and psoriatic arthritis. Interestingly, these conditions are frequently seen in people with AS or in the family members of AS patients. A specific gene (HLA-B27) has been identified with an increased risk for AS, but it is not a definitive marker.

AS typically begins with chronic inflammation at the sacroiliac joint on one or both sides. Inflammation affects points of connection between bone and ligament or tendon, in a condition called **enthesitis**. Cartilaginous discs ossify, and bony deformation leads to the squaring of vertebral bodies. These fusions are called **syndesmophytes**, and this process leads to a distinctive "bamboo spine" appearance. Although it is usually limited to intervertebral and costal joints, the heels, hips, shoulders, toes, and sternoclavicular joints may be affected too.

The pattern of inflammation and damage proceeds up the spine, leaving in its wake a trail of injured vertebrae that may eventually fuse sometimes with a flattened lumbar curve and an exaggerated thoracic curve. If the progression reaches all the way up to the neck, the cervical vertebrae may fuse with the head in a permanently flexed position as well. Fusions may also occur at the vertebrocostal joints, resulting in a locked rib cage and difficulty breathing (Figure 6.9).

AS carries a high risk of **osteoporosis** and vertebral **fracture**. Poor support from damaged ligaments means a greater chance of peripheral nerve pressure or cauda equina syndrome.

Loss of lung capacity is an important complication of AS. Fusions at the costovertebral joints interfere with lung capacity, which results in constant shortness of breath, low stamina, and reduced resistance to **pneumonia**. Further, rib rigidity and limited lung capacity may contribute to right-sided **heart failure**.

Enthesitis: Inflammation of sites where ligaments or tendons meet bone.

Syndesmophytes: A bone spur attached to a ligament.

Inflammation outside of joints may affect the eyes, heart, aorta, prostate, gastrointestinal tract, and kidneys.

Signs and Symptoms

AS usually starts as chronic low back pain. Often, pain is felt in the buttocks, sometimes all the way down into the heels, which can sometimes lead to a misdiagnosis of **disc disease**. The spine and hips feel stiff and immobile. Unlike more typical low back pain, AS is usually much worse in the morning or after rest; it improves with activity.

AS has flare and remission stages. During flare episodes, a general feeling of fatigue, illness, and a slight fever may be present. The eyes may become dry, red, and uncomfortable; this is called **iritis**. Pain and stiffness gradually spread up the spine. When the inflammation subsides, the fever and acute pain are resolved, but stiffness and pain may continue to be present. Usually, the disease is limited to the low back, but it can progress to the neck or other joints in the body: hips and shoulders are most often affected.

Treatment

The first option for dealing with AS (which has no known cause and therefore no cure) is exercise. Physical therapy is recommended to preserve the suppleness of the spine and the strength of the paraspinals without aggravating the condition. Maintaining correct posture is the primary goal, since the vertebrae tend to fuse in a flexed position.

If exercise alone doesn't help, painkillers and anti-inflammatories are usually prescribed. **Disease-modifying antirheumatic drugs** (DMARDs) might be recommended. In very extreme cases, surgery may be suggested: an **osteotomy** is a procedure that fuses joints in a straightened position. If the knees, shoulders, or hips have been impaired, **joint replacement surgery** may also be suggested.

Medications

- Analgesics
- NSAIDs
- Oral and injected steroidal anti-inflammatories
- DMARDs to alter immune system activity
- Biologic agents to alter immune system activity

Iritis: Inflammation of the iris of the eye.

Disease-modifying antirheumatic drugs (DMARDs): Agents that apparently alter the course and progression of rheumatoid arthritis, rather than simply suppressing inflammation and pain.

Osteotomy: The surgical cutting of bone.

Inflammatory bowel disease: An umbrella term encompassing both Crohn disease and ulcerative colitis.

Massage Therapy Implications

RISKS	Ankylosing spondylitis is a progressive, inflammatory condition that spreads up the spine and affects other tissues as well. For these reasons, massage or bodywork during periods of flare must be gauged not to promote inflammation of any kind.
BENEFITS	Between flares, massage for pain and relaxation can be helpful not only to preserve function but to deal with the stress that inevitably accompanies a chronic, painful, progressive disease.
OPTIONS	Careful range of motion, proprioceptive work, and massage that focuses on deep breathing may be especially helpful for AS patients who place a high priority on preserving freedom of movement for as long as possible.
RESEARCH	Not much research has been done on AS and massage therapy, but a pioneering case report[1] demonstrated less stiffness and improved range of motion with one client after seven sessions.

1. Chunco R. The effects of massage on pain, stiffness, and fatigue levels associated with ankylosing spondylitis: a case study. *International Journal of Therapeutic Massage and Bodywork* 2011;4(1):12–17. http://www.ncbi.nlm.nih.gov/pmc/articles/PMC3088527/

Crohn Disease

Definition: What Is It?

Crohn disease is a progressive inflammatory disorder that can affect any part of the GI tract, from the mouth to the anus. Advanced cases may also involve tissues outside the digestive system.

Crohn disease and **ulcerative colitis** are often described together under the umbrella term **inflammatory bowel disease**, but they have some important differences. Although Crohn disease can and often does affect the large intestine, it also affects the upper GI tract; this is not seen with ulcerative colitis. For more information on how these two conditions are alike and different, see Compare & Contrast 6.1.

Demographics

Crohn disease is diagnosed most often in young adults, ages 13 to 30. Whites and especially Ashkenazi Jews are affected more than other ethnic or racial groups, but that trend is beginning to change. It is estimated that about 1.4 million Americans have some form of inflammatory bowel disease. Some estimate that Crohn disease accounts for roughly one-half of that; others say that ulcerative colitis is more common.

COMPARE & CONTRAST 6.1 Crohn Disease and Ulcerative colitis

Crohn disease and ulcerative colitis are two conditions linked under the description inflammatory bowel disease, or IBD. This may create the impression that these two disorders are slightly different manifestations of the same problem, but they are significantly different in etiology, progression, and long-term prognosis. Although differentiating between these conditions has little impact on a massage therapist's decision, it may have big impact on the life of the client.

CHARACTERISTICS	CROHN DISEASE	ULCERATIVE COLITIS
Area affected	Often begins in ileum but can spread to colon or to rest of small intestine	Almost always begins in rectum May spread up colon but never to small intestine
Pattern of progression	Unpredictable, disconnected patches may appear anywhere along GI tract.	Contiguous lesions
Depth of lesions	Ulcers may burrow through mucosa, into muscular or serous wall of GI tract. Perforation fairly common	Ulcers penetrate only mucosa or submucosa of colon; seldom perforate
Complications	Can lead to liver problems, skin and mouth ulcers, eye inflammation, peritonitis, bladder infections, and colorectal cancer	Significantly raises risk of colorectal cancer; other complications: liver inflammation, arthritis, skin rash, anemia
Surgery	Surgery can remove affected areas, but disease often continues to attack healthy tissue; surgery often must be repeated.	Surgery to remove affected area is curative.

It is clear that these diseases occur most frequently in highly developed urban areas compared to rural ones, and they are more common north of the equator than south of it. IBD in general and Crohn disease in particular are becoming more common, as urbanization affects more of the globe.

Etiology: What Happens?

Crohn disease involves the development of inflamed areas in the large and small intestine. Many cases begin in the distal portion of the small intestine, the ileum, but this progressive disease can affect upper regions of the GI tract as well as the colon and the anus.

Crohn disease is an idiopathic disease. It is considered to be a multifactoral problem, with aspects of pathologic invasion, genetic predisposition, immune system dysfunction, environmental influences, and dietary triggers. A dysfunctional inflammatory response against bacteria in the gut is part of the picture, but it is unclear whether that response is the cause or the result of the disease.

Some experts consider that the limited exposure to intestinal pathogens that comes with being part of an urbanized culture may lead to weaknesses in the immune response of susceptible people. Then, when they are exposed to a trigger, the immune system overreacts. This is similar to the "hygiene hypothesis" that is applied to **allergies** and other hypersensitivity reactions. This point of view is supported by research that shows that certain common rural parasites appear to prevent the development of Crohn disease in animal models.

One of the distinguishing features of Crohn disease is that the areas it affects are not contiguous; the inflamed regions appear in an unpredictable patchwork anywhere in the GI tract. Eventually, these ulcers can cause accumulations of scar tissue that cause stenosis of the intestines, or they can stimulate the development of abnormal connecting tubes from the colon to other hollow organs (the bladder, uterus, other loops of intestine) or to the surface of the skin (Figure 6.10). These tubes are called **fistulas**, and they allow fecal material to exit the GI tract.

Fistula: An abnormal opening between two hollow organs or between a hollow organ and the outside of the body.

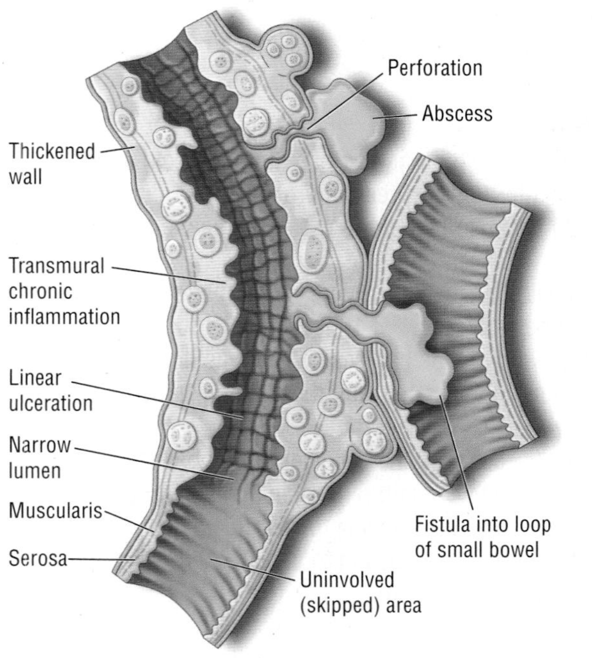

FIGURE 6.10 Crohn disease with chronic inflammation, ulcerations, perforation, abscess, and fistula

Crohn disease disrupts normal digestion in several ways. Inflammation in the intestines interferes with absorption; this means a patient is at risk for serious malnutrition, **gallstones**, and a specific type of **kidney stone**. When Crohn disease occurs in young children, it can lead to stunted growth and delayed development. This disease can also cause bowel obstruction, at first by swelling and spasm, and eventually by scar tissue strictures. Deep ulcers may bleed into the GI tract or perforate, leading to **peritonitis**. Adhesions can form between layers of the peritoneum. Abscesses can form in the GI tract or around the anus. If fistulas into the bladder form, leaking fecal material can cause serious **urinary tract infections** that can also invade the kidneys. Chronic irritation to epithelial cells in the GI tract also increases the risk of **colon cancer**.

Crohn disease is linked to problems outside the GI tract as well. It is associated with inflammation of the spine, as discussed in Sidebar 6.6. It can cause inflammation at the bile duct, leading to **cirrhosis**, **jaundice**, and gallstones. Poor nutrient absorption leads to **osteoporosis**. It can lead to acute inflammation affecting the liver, eyes, and joints. It can cause ulcers called aphthae in the mouth and lesions on the skin as well; these open sores most often appear around the ankles and lower legs.

> **Aphthae:** A small ulcer on a mucous membrane, especially the mouth (singular, aphtha).
>
> **Aminosalicylates:** A type of medicines used to treat inflammatory bowel disease.

Signs and Symptoms

Crohn disease occurs in periods of flare and remission. During periods of remission, a patient may have no symptoms at all, but during a flare, the most common symptoms include abdominal pain, especially at the distal end of the ileum in the lower right quadrant, along with cramping, diarrhea (often with blood), and bloating. Weight loss, fever, joint pain, small ulcers in the mouth and throat, and lesions on the skin may also accompany acute flares. Many Crohn disease patients also have severe pain around the anus, along with anal fissures and abscesses.

> **NOTABLE CASES** In 1956, just 9 months after a major heart attack, President Dwight D. Eisenhower had an emergency ileotransverse colostomy. The 30 cm of removed tissue showed signs of Crohn disease. He was back at his desk 5 days after his surgery.

Treatment

The damage to the whole length of the digestive system that Crohn disease can cause is serious, so it is usually treated aggressively. Treatment during flares usually begins with a class of drugs called aminosalicylates: these quell inflammation and immune system activity in the GI tract. Antibiotics may be necessary for abscesses or infections. Steroidal anti-inflammatories and other immune modifiers are used if other drugs are unsuccessful. Most Crohn disease patients eventually have surgery to remove affected sections of intestine or open blockages, but this is not curative; new patches of inflamed tissue may arise in other places, requiring further surgery.

Crohn disease patients have to be extraordinarily careful about their diet, especially during flares. High-fiber, bulky foods can exacerbate symptoms and create obstructions if scar tissue has narrowed the passageway. Sometimes a high-calorie liquid diet is recommended during these episodes. In extreme cases, the patient may take in all nutrients intravenously to give the whole system a break from the stress of digesting food (Case History 6.1).

Medications

- Aminosalicylates to by mouth, enema, or suppository to suppress inflammation in the GI tract
- Antibiotics as needed
- Oral, injected, or topical steroidal anti-inflammatories to limit inflammation and scarring
- Immune-modifying drugs to interfere with immune system response

CASE HISTORY 6.1 Crohn Disease

Karen was diagnosed with Crohn disease when she was a young adult, but she has had stomach pain as long as she can remember. "When I was a kid, my mother literally had to hold my head and put food in my mouth. She wasn't being mean; it's just what the doctors told her to do because I wouldn't eat. All I knew was food hurt."

Karen's doctor was convinced that there was nothing wrong with her. "It's all in your head," he told her. The Thanksgiving she was 22, she collapsed on a trip to California. She had a fever of 105°F. She had formed an abscess on her intestine, and the infection had invaded her bloodstream: she had sepsis and was hospitalized in Los Angeles for a week. After the attack subsided, she had her first colonoscopy, and the evidence of Crohn disease was clear.

After her diagnosis, Karen tried two medications to control the disease, but one gave her severe headaches, and another, a sulfa drug, caused some breathing problems. Fortunately, she went into remission and had no problems for several years. Then in 1995, she developed severe stomach pain with diarrhea. Unable to absorb adequate nutrition from food, she developed bone pain, and her hair began to fall out. At this time, she began treating her disease with stronger medication.

KAREN, AGED 41: "All I knew was, food hurt."

Karen's first surgery was conducted in 1997. Her small intestine was resected where a stricture had obstructed it; a fistula was repaired, adhesions between abdominal organs were released, and her appendix was taken out. She had remarkable relief after this, but it was short-lived. "Most Crohn disease patients go about 4 years between surgeries; I go more like 2 years."

Karen's Crohn disease involves a tendency to build up scar tissue in the small intestine, leading to strictures, fistulas, and obstruction. She took infliximab (Remicade) to control symptoms, but several months ago, it seemed to stop working. She finds that prednisone controls most of her symptoms, but she can use it only for about 6 weeks before developing serious side effects.

One of Karen's challenges is monitoring the progress of her disease. A colonoscopy goes only to the ileocecal valve, and a barium swallow shows problems only in the esophagus and stomach; Karen's problems are between the two points. She tried to use a new technology, a tiny camera in a pill-sized capsule, called a capsule endoscopy, that takes hundreds of pictures as it travels through the GI tract, but the camera got caught at an intestinal stricture, and she needed surgery to have it removed.

When she is in remission, Karen finds she doesn't have to be especially careful about her diet, but she doesn't tolerate caffeine well. When her disease is active, she has to avoid any roughage; she needs a low-fiber diet. She takes vitamins to make up for some lost absorption in her small intestine.

Karen works out 4 days a week in a gym, which she says is very helpful for managing her stress. A massage therapist visits her office once a month. She enjoys this, but she reports that when her disease is active, she has a hard time receiving massage: "Obstructive pain is intense! The intestines are twisting and turning, trying to shove the stuff through. I get terrible spasms in my back, and the therapist says the muscles in my back are stiff as a board."

Karen had five surgeries between 1997 and 2006, and she says she now recognizes the symptoms of another stricture forming, just 6 months since her last surgery. She gets along well with her doctor, who she calls GI Joe, and she enjoys interaction with other Crohn disease patients. She is happy to "share my agonies" with anyone who asks, and she does so with laughter and good will. "You have to laugh," she says. "What else are you gonna do?"

Massage Therapy Implications

RISKS	During a Crohn disease flare, a person may not be at ease with some positions on the table, and rigorous bodywork may be too challenging to be comfortable. Further, the medications that Crohn disease clients take may carry some cautions for massage therapists.
BENEFITS	When Crohn disease is in remission, massage can be supportive and safe choice. Intrusive abdominal work should probably be avoided, but any strategy that can establish a parasympathetic state can support efficient digestion.
OPTIONS	Extremely gentle work or simply holding on the abdomen can help the body to "organize" its responses to stimuli. This can be especially important to help incorporate this problematic area for a client who struggles with digestive discomfort.

Lupus

Definition: What Is It?

Lupus is an autoimmune disease in which various types of tissues are attacked by the immune system. Lupus can be mild, but has the potential to be life-threatening. In extreme cases, this disorder can attack the heart, the lungs, the kidneys, and the brain, with devastating results.

Demographics

Like many autoimmune disorders, many more women are affected by lupus than men; in this case, the ratio is about 9:1. Most people are affected between the ages of 15 and 44. Lupus in its mild and serious forms is estimated to affect about 1.5 million people in the United States. People of color have a higher incidence, along with earlier onset and more severe complications than whites.

Etiology: What Happens?

Lupus is a condition with a wide range of presentations, but the common factor is immune system attacks against a variety of tissue types throughout the body. These attacks often begin in small blood vessels, which can cause inflammation, clotting, and nutrition supply problems to all the tissues downstream of the damage.

The precise cause or causes of lupus are unknown; it seems to be a combination of racial and genetic predisposition, hormones, and environmental exposures. A genetic link is clearly a factor, but a child of a parent with lupus has only a small risk of developing the disease. Further, when one identical twin develops lupus, the other twin may not. This indicates that although a genetic susceptibility may be inherited, other factors must also contribute to the development of the disease. Another indicator that genetics is not the primary issue is that while lupus in the United States and the United Kingdom has the highest incidence among black women, lupus is very rare among women in Western or Central Africa.

Environmental contributors may include exposure to certain viruses, ultraviolet light, certain medications, and high levels of estrogen. Women with lupus often report a change in symptoms with their menstrual cycle, and estrogen replacement therapy that is employed to reduce the risk of osteoporosis can increase the risk of lupus for some women.

> **Malar, or malar rash:** A rash of the cheeks, often associated with lupus or erysipelas. Also known as a "butterfly rash.

Types of Lupus

- *Drug-induced lupus*: This is brought on by some prescribed medications for high blood pressure, heart arrhythmia, psychosis, and epilepsy. These symptoms resolve when the medications are discontinued.
- *Neonatal lupus*: This occurs when a mother with lupus or another autoimmune disease transfers antibodies to a newborn baby. The baby develops a skin rash, liver problems, or a low blood count for a few weeks or months until the antibodies are no longer active. At that time, the symptoms disappear, usually with no long-term consequences.
- *Discoid lupus erythematosus (DLE)*: This is a chronic skin disease. It can involve small scaly red patches with sharp margins that don't itch, or the characteristic butterfly or **malar** rash of redness over the nose and cheeks (Figures 6.11 and 6.12). The skin can become very thin and delicate, or

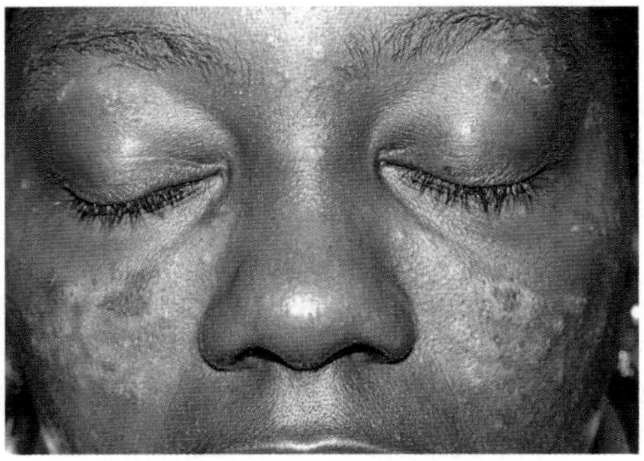

FIGURE 6.11 Discoid rash

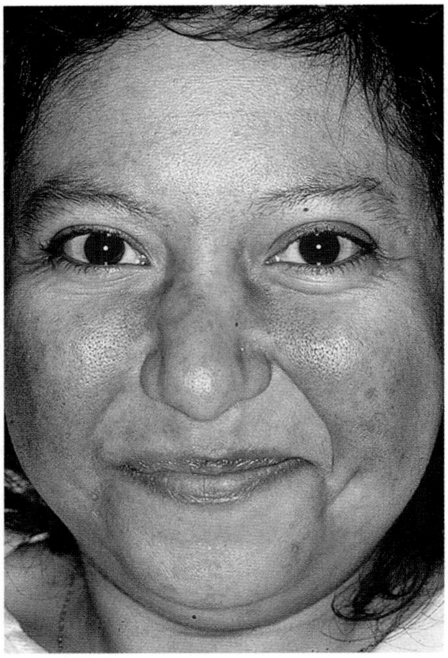

FIGURE 6.12 Malar rash

lesions may become permanently discolored and thickened. DLE is sometimes described as a subset of skin disorders called **subacute cutaneous lupus**. A small number of people with DLE go on to develop systemic lupus erythematosus.
- *Systemic lupus erythematosus (SLE)*: This is caused by antibody attacks against a variety of tissues throughout the body. This can result in **arthritis**, **renal failure**, **thrombosis**, psychosis, **headaches**, **seizures**, **coronary artery disease**, **carditis**, and **pleurisy**. SLE can usually be controlled, but at this time it cannot be cured. SLE sometimes begins as DLE, but not always.
- *Mixed connective tissue disease*: About 10% of people diagnosed with lupus have it simultaneously with other autoimmune diseases, especially **scleroderma**, **rheumatoid arthritis**, polymyositis, and dermatomyositis. Rheumatoid arthritis and lupus occur together so often that a new name has been coined for this situation: **rhupus**. This combination of conditions is sometimes called mixed connective tissue disease.

Signs and Symptoms

Lupus can look like a lot of different diseases. While it does have some markers in the blood that can help to identify it, those markers are sometimes present in people without lupus, so they can't be used as a definitive diagnosis. Along with blood markers, lupus usually involves four or more of the following, not necessarily simultaneously:

- Debilitating fatigue
- Mental confusion, cognitive dysfunction, and short-term memory loss
- **Alopecia**
- Malar rash
- Discoid skin rash that can cause permanent scarring
- Photosensitivity
- Mucous membrane ulcers, particularly in the mouth, nose, or throat
- Arthritis in more than two joints, specifically in the hands or feet (not in the spine)
- Pleurisy and/or pericarditis
- Kidney problems: blood or protein in the urine
- Brain irritation: headaches, seizures, or psychosis
- Blood count abnormalities: low red blood cell count, white blood cell count, or platelet count
- Immunologic disorders: special antibodies and/or lupus anticoagulants are present in the blood
- Antinuclear antibodies in the blood

Lupus flares are exacerbated by certain kinds of stimuli. Excessive exposure to ultraviolet light, emotional stress, injury, infection, or trauma can be triggers. Pregnancy is a trigger for some women, while for others it may suppress flares. Someone who has lupus must identify the stimuli that are particularly potent for her and avoid them carefully.

One of the challenges in identifying lupus is that symptoms fluctuate and may change entirely over time.

Lupus can affect virtually every system in the body (Figure 6.13). Because some of the features of this disease make profound changes in health, it is worth looking at how SLE affects several systems.

Subacute cutaneous lupus: A type of cutaneous lupus that is between chronic and acute in nature.

Rhupus: Term for the common combination of rheumatoid arthritis and lupus.

Alopecia: Baldness. Can refer to body and facial hair as well as hair on the head.

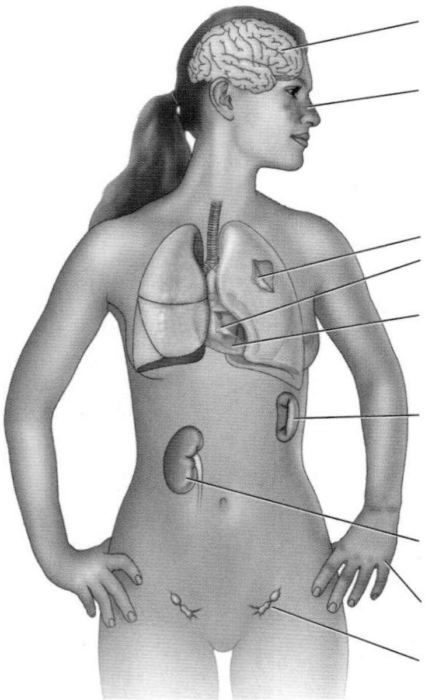

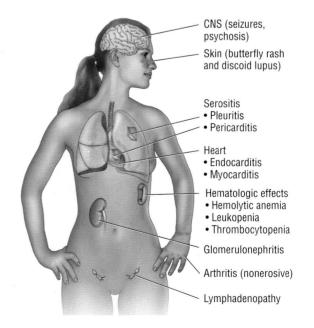

FIGURE 6.13 Lupus: systemic effects

- *Integumentary system.* The characteristic rashes seen with lupus have already been described. These rashes may be exacerbated by sunlight in a condition called **photosensitivity**. Lupus can also cause ulcers in the mucous membranes, particularly in the nose, throat, and mouth. When SLE causes superficial blood vessels to become inflamed, symptoms may appear on the skin in the shape of telangiectasias ("spider veins"), welts, red lines, and painful bumps.
- *Musculoskeletal system.* Most people with lupus eventually develop painful, swollen, but nonerosive arthritis. Joint pain usually occurs asymmetrically at the hands or knees, but seldom in the spine. Nonspecific muscle pain is another common symptom, and many lupus patients also meet the diagnostic criteria for **fibromyalgia**.
- *Nervous system.* Nervous system complications can range from extreme **headaches** to psychosis (including paranoia and hallucinations) to **fever** or **seizures**, depending on which part of the brain is adversely affected by blood vessel inflammation. When the clotting disorders that may accompany this disorder occur in the brain, the result is a transient ischemic attack or **stroke**.
- *Cardiovascular system.* Lupus can lead to inflammation of major blood vessels, opening the door to rapidly progressive **atherosclerosis** and the risk of **heart attack**, even in young people. Lupus is also associated with slow clot formation and slow clot dissolving. This problem can lead to **thrombophlebitis** or **pulmonary embolism**. In addition to blood vessel damage, lupus inflames the serous membranes of the heart, leading to arrhythmia and severe chest pain. **Anemia** is a frequent complication of long-term inflammation and bone marrow suppression. **Thrombocytopenia** may occur when lupus antibodies have attacked thrombocytes. Finally, **Raynaud phenomenon** is a sign of **vasculitis**.
- *Respiratory system.* A common complication of lupus is pleurisy, or inflammation and fluid accumulation in the serous membranes that line the lungs. This causes pain on inhalation and restricted movement of the lungs. If enough resistance in the lungs develops, a lupus patient may be at risk for pulmonary hypertension and right-sided **heart failure**.

Photosensitivity: Abnormal sensitivity to light.

Thrombocytopenia: Decreased number of thrombocytes.

Vasculitis: Inflammation of a blood or lymphatic vessel.

Glomerulonephritis: Acute kidney inflammation.

Osteonecrosis: Death of bone tissue on a macroscopic scale.

- *Urinary system.* Tissue damage in the kidneys leads to a specific type of **glomerulonephritis**. Kidney damage can accumulate without symptoms until the kidneys are on the brink of renal failure.
- *Reproductive system.* The clotting disorder associated with lupus can make it difficult to carry a child to term. Repeated spontaneous miscarriages are sometimes the first sign of the disease that will lead to a diagnosis. Pregnant women with lupus face special challenges, as some of the medications that control symptoms are not safe for the baby.

Treatment

The treatment emphasis for lupus is to promote remission, to limit or prevent tissue damage, and to improve the quality of life of the patient. If the case is not very severe, it may be managed with nonsteroidal anti-inflammatories. These drugs are inexpensive and easily accessible, and they are often effective against inflammation. Unfortunately, they are also associated with chronic stomach irritation, and long-term use can irritate and damage the kidneys—a special point of concern for lupus patients.

Steroidal anti-inflammatories (especially prednisone) are sometimes prescribed for short-term use, especially during flares. These are very powerful anti-inflammatories, but they are also associated with many dangerous side effects, including mood changes, weight gain, liver damage, bone thinning, and **osteonecrosis**, especially in the hips and shoulders.

Antimalarial drugs have found success in treating some of the symptoms of lupus, especially skin rashes and ulcers of mucous membranes, and reducing the needed dose of corticosteroids. Some antimalarial drugs cause changes in eye function, so an ophthalmologist must closely monitor their use.

NOTABLE CASES Singer Michael Jackson was diagnosed with lupus shortly after his signature album *Thriller* was released. Singer Seal carries the facial scars from the malar rash associated with discoid lupus. Musicians Toni Braxton and Paula Abdul have the condition, as did southern Gothic writer Flannery O'Connor.

In very severe cases, immunosuppressant drugs may be recommended. This of course leaves the patient vulnerable to secondary infections.

Other treatment options for lupus depend on the presenting symptoms. Acute rashes may be treated with topical steroid creams or ointments. If a patient has blood-clotting problems, anticoagulants may be administered. It is a high priority to treat lupus symptoms quickly as they arise; early intervention can reduce the amount of damage that accrues during flares and keep the body functioning at normal levels during periods of remission.

Medications

- NSAIDs for low-grade pain and inflammation
- Steroidal anti-inflammatory during flare
- Antimalarial drugs for skin rashes
- Immunosuppressant drugs
- Drugs for symptomatic and side effect treatment: steroid cream, anticoagulants, bisphosphonates for osteoporosis, etc.

Massage Therapy Implications

RISKS	Active flares of lupus involve inflammation that can damage the skin, heart, lungs, and kidneys and cause painful swelling at joints. Rigorous massage during these acute episodes may exacerbate symptoms and put undue stress on an inflamed cardiovascular system.
BENEFITS	Gentle and reflexive massage may be soothing during flares, and more rigorous massage during remission (within tolerance of course) may help to deal with pain and stiffness, allowing the client with lupus to be more active when it is possible.

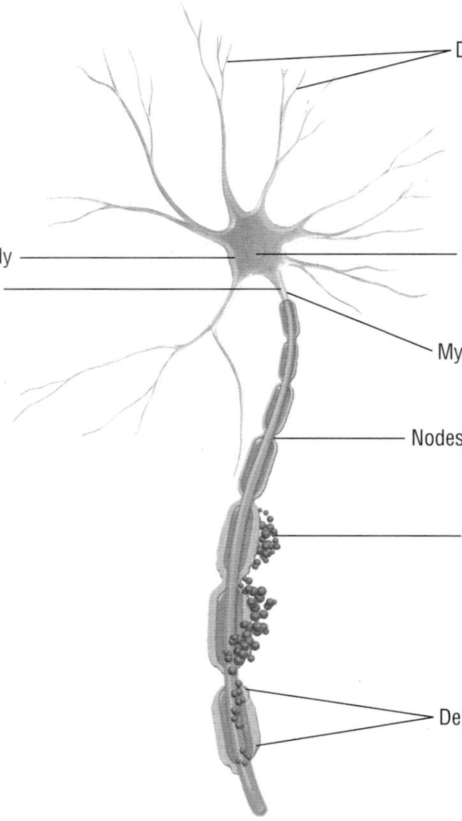

FIGURE 6.14 Myelin destruction with multiple sclerosis

Multiple Sclerosis

Definition: What Is It?

Multiple sclerosis (MS) is a condition characterized by inflammation and degeneration of myelin sheaths in the spinal cord and brain. It is an autoimmune disease, but the triggering pathogens or other stimuli appear to vary.

Demographics

MS is estimated to affect about 400,000 Americans and 2.3 million people worldwide. Women outnumber men by about 2–3:1, depending on the age at diagnosis. Although the progression of this condition is highly variable, about half of all patients need assistance to walk within 15 years of diagnosis. It is usually found in young adulthood, but about 10% of all cases involve a pediatric version that targets children.

The numbers of MS diagnoses are rising, but that may be because diagnostic testing has improved and it is being found earlier.

Etiology: What Happens?

The word sclerosis means hardened scar or plaque. In multiple sclerosis, T cells, B cells, antibodies, and destructive cytokines attack and destroy myelin in patchy areas of the CNS. Oligodendrocytes, the myelin-producing cells in the CNS, multiply and attempt to repair the damage, but eventually they fail.

As attacks progress, normal myelin is replaced with scar tissue plaques. Electrical impulses are either slowed or completely obstructed. If flares are persistent and repetitive, the damage may penetrate to affect the neuron itself (Figure 6.14). In this case, lost function is more likely to be permanent. The result is loss of motor control, cognitive changes, paralysis, pain, and numbness.

MS, like many autoimmune diseases, often works in cycles of inflammatory flares followed by periods of remission. During flares, the myelin is under attack and is replaced by scar tissue. During remission, inflammation subsides, and some myelin regenerates. In this way, MS patients may lose some neurological function during flares but regain some or all of it during remission.

It seems clear that a genetic predisposition raises the risk of developing MS, but this appears to be a relatively small factor. The population-wide risk of developing MS is less than 1%. People with a first-degree relative who has the disease carry a risk of 1% to 3%. If one identical twin has the disease, the other twin has 25% to 30% chance of developing MS.

Further, epidemiologists have examined why the incidence of MS appears to increase with distance from the equator. The key factor here appears to be the availability of vitamin D: this nutrient, which is manufactured with the stimulus of exposure to sunlight, decreases proinflammatory cytokines. People with high vitamin D levels appear to have a lower-than-average risk of developing MS. The issue appears to be connected to where a person spends the majority of their adult life; if she is born in the tropics, but moved to the extreme northern or southern hemisphere by age 15, the risk of her developing MS is the same as for the rest of the population for that area.

This collection of information indicates that MS is probably an autoimmune disease to which some people are genetically predisposed, but that requires some combination of environmental triggers to initiate the disease process.

Types of Multiple Sclerosis

- *Benign MS*: This version of MS involves one episode, followed by virtually no progression.
- *Relapse/remitting MS*: This is the most common form of MS, involving cycles between flare and remission. While some recovery of the myelin sheath can occur during remission, ultimately some level of damage is usually permanent. RRMS affects about 87% of MS patients.
- *Primary progressive MS*: This version involves a chronic, low-grade progression that is not marked by periods of acute flare or remission.
- *Secondary progressive MS*: In this version, cycles of flare and remission occur, but recovery during remission is only partial. The patient experiences a progressive loss of function.
- *Progressive/relapsing MS*: This form involves a slow but steady decline, marked by periods of extreme flare.
- *Malignant MS*: This rare form involves a fast and relentless decline, leading to disability and death within weeks or months of diagnosis.

SIDEBAR 6.7 Diagnosing Multiple Sclerosis

MS is notoriously difficult to diagnose, because the signs that appear on tests (including various types of MRIs and a spinal tap to look for fragments of damaged myelin) often don't correspond to the severity of symptoms.

The medical convention is to describe a person's disease as possible, probable, or definite MS. To achieve a conclusive diagnosis, a patient must have these findings:

- Objective evidence of at least two episodes. (This can be determined through MRI, examination of cerebrospinal fluid, or evoked potential tests that show the speed of nerve transmission in the brain.)
- Episodes of flare that are separated by at least a month and by location of affected function.
- No other explanation for symptoms that can be found.

Several conditions can produce MS-like symptoms. Part of a thorough diagnosis is ruling out the following:

Lyme disease	HIV/AIDS	Scleroderma
Vascular problems in the brain	Disc disease	Lupus
CNS tumors	Fibromyalgia	Encephalitis
B12 or folic acid deficiency		

Signs and Symptoms

This disease is sometimes called "the great imitator" because its initial symptoms can look like a variety of other diseases, depending on which areas of nerve tissue have been affected (Sidebar 6.7). The order with which symptoms appear also varies greatly from one person to the next. Some of the most dependable signs and symptoms are as follows:

- *Weakness*. The onset of this problem may be gradual or sudden. It comes about because the loss of myelin makes nerve transmission slow.
- *Spasm*. This can take the form of chronic muscle stiffness or of active acute cramping.
- *Changes in sensation*. MS patients often report numbness or **paresthesia** in various parts of the body. These sensations may last for hours or days at a time.
- *Optic neuritis*. Attacks on the myelin of the optic nerve result in extreme eye pain coupled with progressive loss of function. Vision may be minimally impaired (for instance, some people have red-green color distortions), or it may be fully lost until the episode has passed. Most MS patients recover full or close to full vision when they go into remission.
- *Urologic dysfunction*. MS patients may find it difficult to urinate, or they may be incontinent.
- *Sexual dysfunction*. Difficulty maintaining an erection for men or having an orgasm in women are sometimes early signs of this disease.
- *Difficulty walking*. This problem can be a product of several factors, including muscle stiffness, numbness, dizziness, balance problems, and loss of coordination.
- *Loss of cognitive function*. A frequently overlooked issue for many MS patients is a change in mental ability. Short-term memory and the ability to learn and perform complex tasks are often challenged. A small percentage of MS patients undergo severe changes in cognitive skills that results in dementia.

Paresthesia: An abnormal sensation, such as burning, prickling, tickling, or tingling.

NOTABLE CASES Actress Teri Garr is a powerful spokesperson for the MS community. Prolific writer Joan Didion, the late comedian Richard Pryor, talk show host Montel Williams, and the late Mouseketeer Annette Funicello are other recognizable names with this condition.

  - *Depression*. This is a complication of many chronic progressive diseases, especially in situations as unpredictable as those of MS.
  - *Digestive disturbances*. Many MS patients have severe digestive disturbances (nausea, diarrhea, constipation) that vary greatly from day to day.
  - *Sensitivity to heat*. Many MS patients find that warm temperatures, especially rapid changes from cool to warm, trigger painful spasms.
- *Fatigue*. Perhaps the most common symptom for MS patients is debilitating fatigue, which is particularly exacerbated by heat. The fatigue may be a result of slower or impaired nerve transmission (requiring fewer muscle fibers to work harder), muscle spasm, and other factors.

Treatment

The mainstay of current MS treatment is a class of drugs called DMAMS: disease-modifying agents for MS. These include several types of interferons, which can shorten the periods of flare and prolong periods between episodes, and methotrexate and similar drugs, which slow cell growth and quell immune system activity. Steroidal anti-inflammatories are also used, but it is important to point out that all of these medications carry strong side effects, some of which can be life-threatening.

Other medications are used to control symptoms like fatigue, constipation, bladder control, cognitive difficulties, and other problems.

Nonpharmacological options for people living with MS include careful exercise and physical or occupational therapy designed to maintain strength and function as long as possible. Eating well and getting adequate amounts of high-quality sleep are important for maintaining health and prolonging remissions. Stress management techniques, including massage, are often recommended for the same reasons (Case History 6.2).

Medications

- Immunomodulators, including injected glatiramer acetate, interferons, methotrexate, and others
- Steroidal anti-inflammatories
- Medication for symptomatic control
  - Anticholinergics for bladder control
  - Laxatives for constipation
  - Amantadine for fatigue
  - Analgesics for pain
  - Antidepressants as necessary

Massage Therapy Implications

RISKS	Massage that is too deep or two fast can sometimes stimulate painful and uncontrolled muscle spasms, even for clients who are in remission. Areas of numbness call for special caution, since clients can't rate their comfort with pressure. Sudden changes in environment, including pressure, temperature (especially heat), and other variables, appear to be difficult for many MS patients to process.
BENEFITS	Massage may help MS patients to sleep better, to manage stress and depression, and thereby to reduce the frequency of flares.
OPTIONS	Some MS patients experience weakness or spasm in the extremities. Massage can be used to slow or minimize this, as long as sensation is present.
RESEARCH	Massage therapy for MS has a substantial body of evidence in research literature, but much of it shows a null result for specific functional goals, with a positive result for pain, quality of life, mood, and self-efficacy. Researchers suggest that the reduction of stress perception helps the patient cope more positively with his or her challenges.[1,2] One study found that a specific type of massage at the injection site helps MS patients tolerate the treatment with fewer side effects from the injections.[3] Abdominal massage for people with MS can help with constipation.[4,5]

1. Schroeder B, Doig J, Premkumar K. The effects of massage therapy on multiple sclerosis patients' quality of life and leg function. *Evidence Based Complementary and Alternative Medicine* 2014;2014:640916. http://www.hindawi.com/journals/ecam/2014/640916/
2. Finch P, Bessonnette S. A pragmatic investigation into the effects of massage therapy on the self efficacy of multiple sclerosis clients. *Journal of Bodywork and Movement Therapies* 2014;18(1):11–16. http://www.ncbi.nlm.nih.gov/pubmed/24411144
3. Marquez-Rebollo C, Vergara-Carrasco L, Diaz-Navarro R, et al. Benefit of endermology on indurations and panniculitis/lipoatrophy during relapsing-remitting multiple sclerosis long-term treatment with glatiramer acetate. *Advances in Therapy* 2014;31(8):904–914. http://www.ncbi.nlm.nih.gov/pubmed/25047757
4. Coggrave M, Norton C, Cody JD. Management of faecal incontinence and constipation in adults with central neurological diseases. *Cochrane Database of Systemic Reviews* 2014;(1):CD002115. http://www.ncbi.nlm.nih.gov/pubmed/24420006
5. McClurg D, Hagen S, Hawkins S, et al. Abdominal massage for the alleviation of constipation symptoms in people with multiple sclerosis: a randomized controlled feasibility study. *Multiple Sclerosis (Houndmills, Basingstoke, England)* 2011;17(2):223–233. http://www.ncbi.nlm.nih.gov/pubmed/20940182

CASE HISTORY 6.2 Multiple Sclerosis

About a year and a half ago, we had just moved into a new house and my youngest child had just started school. For the first time in 15 years, I was looking forward to having some time, to getting on with my life. Then, there was a pain in my left heel that felt like a stone bruise. We were just back from a long vacation, so I thought it was from too much walking. Two weeks later, my foot went numb, and it traveled up my leg to my knee. It began affecting my right leg too. Then, there was numbness and tingling in my left hand. It felt like I had just had a shot of Novocain, it was that kind of tingling.

My doctor sent me to a neurologist who checked me out and watched me walk. Then while I was sitting there, he went out into the hall with another doctor and they started speaking in medical jargon that I couldn't understand; it made me really nervous. When he came back, he asked me, "Will you come in for a spinal tap?"

"Why?"

"There are some things we want to check out."

"What do you think I have?"

"I think you have MS."

"Excuse me?"

I never dreamed it would be something like this.

TRICIA, AGE 36: "It takes all the courage I can muster just to stand up in the morning."

They started me on intravenous steroids. The next morning, I got up after a bad night, and for the first time in 2 months, I could walk normally. I was so excited; I woke my family and called my mom on the phone. But by the end of that morning, I was already beginning to feel tired.

The head of the department was prepared to tell my family I had progressive MS, and I could be dead in a matter of weeks. I finally decided that I needed to be home; I needed to be with my family, so I checked out even though they didn't want me to.

I continued physical therapy at a local clinic. At first, they would have me sit in a warm pool with jets of water after I exercised, and I would go home feeling so drained and worn out; it was awful. Finally, they adjusted that part of it, and I did better.

Today, I still don't have much sensation below my knees. It takes all the courage I can muster just to stand up in the morning. I never know what kind of day I'll have, whether I'll be able to walk without a cane and whether I'll be tied to the house because my digestive system is unpredictable. I have terrible headaches that begin on the lower half of one side of my face and go up into my ear. I have days when I can't eat at all. I've had episodes of dizziness and double vision. I'm not on steroids now, but I take an antidepressant for the headaches. We're still struggling to find the right dose. My greatest fear, even more than being in a wheelchair, is that I will lose bladder or bowel control or go blind.

But my doctor says my scenario is good. It's been a year and a half without any exacerbations, and he says I'm in remission. The only thing that's worse is my headaches, which are more painful and happen more often.

I think everything depends on your attitude. A major thing for me is to feel needed. If I have a purpose, I feel better. I have five wonderful children and a husband who loves me. My doctor thought I was going to die, and here I am in remission. I just feel so lucky to be here.

Psoriasis

Definition: What Is It?

Psoriasis is a chronic skin disease in which cells, which normally replicate every 28 to 32 days, are replaced every 3 to 4 days. Instead of sloughing off, they accumulate into itchy, scaly plaques on the skin, usually on the trunk, elbows, and knees. Most specialists now classify psoriasis as an autoimmune disease.

Demographics

Estimates on the prevalence of psoriasis in the United States range from 2% to 3%, suggesting that close to a million Americans could be living with this condition in one phase or another. It appears to affect men and women about equally.

Etiology: What Happens?

Normal skin cells are produced at the stratum basale and then move toward the surface as new ranks are formed

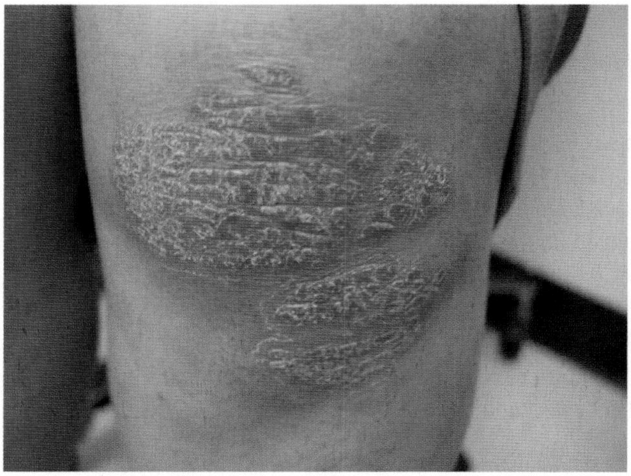

FIGURE 6.15 Plaque psoriasis, mild

underneath. The process from birth to exfoliation typically takes 28 to 30 days. When a person has psoriasis, however, changes in function cause skin cells to replicate faster, and they don't slough off as readily.

Like many autoimmune conditions, psoriasis appears to be related to a combination of genetic predisposition, immune system dysfunction, and environmental exposures.

The genetic patterns seen with this condition have to do with a tendency to produce abnormally high levels of pro-inflammatory chemicals. Interestingly, this anomaly is also associated with insulin resistance, and the overlap between psoriasis and **metabolic syndrome** is high enough that people diagnosed with psoriasis are often counseled to test for heart disease and diabetes as well.

The immune system dysfunction seen with psoriasis is based on the presence of T cells that can stimulate inflammation and new capillary growth in the epidermis. This discovery has opened the door to new treatment options that interfere with these T cells' activities.

Environmental triggers for psoriasis flares are fairly predictable. Emotional stress ranks high on this list, and because the disease and its treatment are both extremely challenging, this can become a self-fulfilling prophecy. Other triggers include viral and bacterial infections, reactions to medications, weather (especially dry cold winter air), and skin injuries. A psoriasis flare that develops 10 to 14 days after a minor skin wound is so predictable that this has a name: **Koebner phenomenon**. Smoking and hormonal fluctuations are also risk factors for psoriasis flares.

Types of Psoriasis

- *Plaque psoriasis*: This is by far the most common presentation, affecting about 80% of all psoriasis patients. It involves small to large lesions (Figures 6.15 and 6.16) in a symmetrical distribution that itch and flake. Plaque psoriasis sometimes progresses to a more severe form.
- *Guttate psoriasis*: This is often triggered by a viral or bacterial infection. It involves multiple round shallow lesions that are small and regular ("guttate" comes from the Latin for "drop," as in raindrop) (Figure 6.17).
- *Pustular psoriasis*: This involves small pus-filled noninfectious blisters. These can appear anywhere, but palms and soles are especially vulnerable. It can be quite serious because the risk of secondary infection is high (Figure 6.18).
- *Inverse psoriasis*: This condition appears at skin folds. The skin is red and shiny and vulnerable to secondary yeast or fungal infection.
- *Erythrodermic psoriasis*: This serious condition is often triggered by sun exposure or topical steroidal anti-inflammatory use or cessation. It can involve extensive damage, infection, and fluid loss and may become a medical emergency (Figure 6.19).

> **Koebner phenomenon:** Heightened susceptibility to the effects of trauma and chemical exposure.

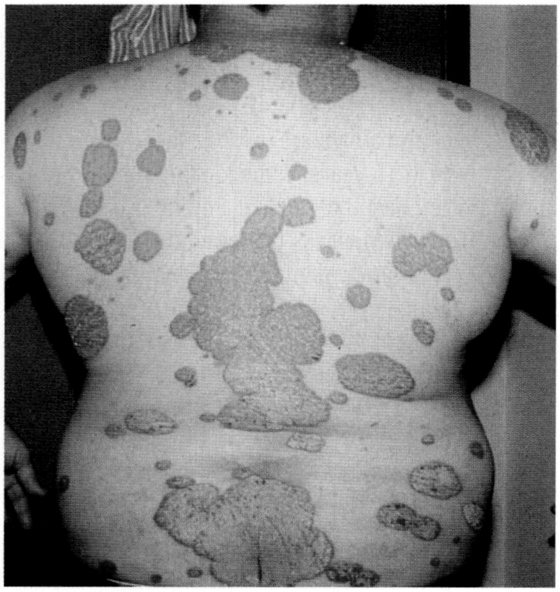

FIGURE 6.16 Plaque psoriasis, severe

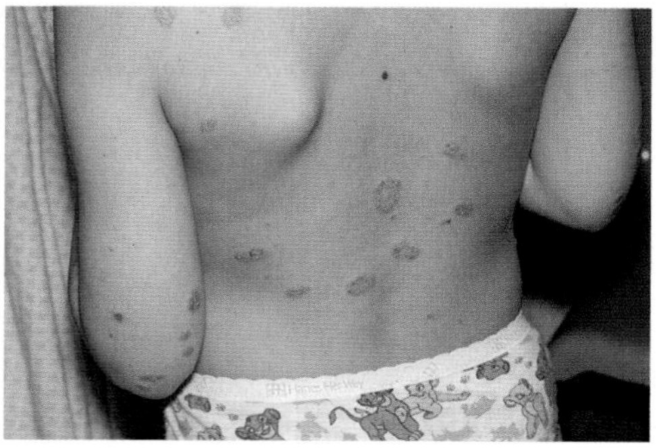

FIGURE 6.17 Guttate psoriasis

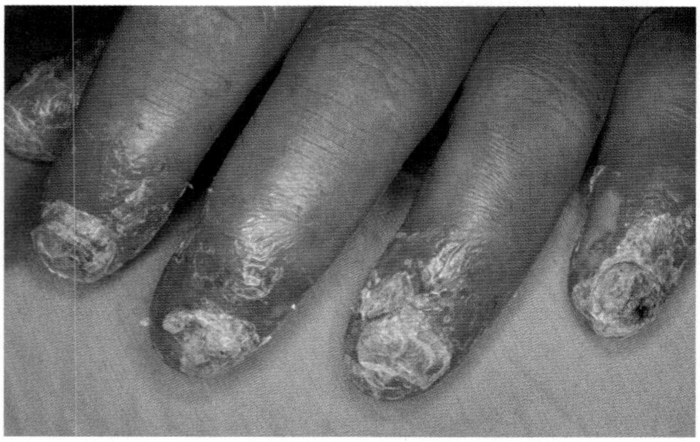

FIGURE 6.18 Pustular psoriasis with onycholysis

Signs and Symptoms

Signs and symptoms of psoriasis vary with the type. They often run in cycles of flare and remission. The lesions tend to have well-defined edges, and if they have been present for a prolonged time, they may be covered with a silvery flaky scale. Small lesions close together may converge into larger ones.

Most psoriasis lesions develop on the trunk, scalp, elbows, or knees, but they can be found on the palms, soles, and under nails, where lesions can destroy the whole nail: this is called **onycholysis**. More rarely, it can develop in skin folds, inside the mouth, or on the genitals.

Complications

Psoriasis is rarely life-threatening, but because it can be at least temporarily uncomfortable and disfiguring, it can certainly interfere with quality of life. Additionally, 10% to 30% of patients develop joint pain in an associated condition called psoriatic arthritis. This situation is complex and has several subtypes, but in many ways, it resembles **rheumatoid arthritis** in the extremities, and **ankylosing spondylitis** at the spine, and can be addressed by bodywork practitioners in the same way.

Treatment

Psoriasis has no permanent cure, and treatment options tend to be only temporarily successful or carry potentially dangerous side effects. Consequently, a person with a moderate to severe case may need to alternate his or her treatments on a regular cycle. To complicate things further, some treatment options react negatively with others, so this is a situation that requires careful oversight.

Psoriasis treatment typically begins with topical applications and then careful doses of UV radiation. If these are unsuccessful, then biologic therapies that impact immune system function might be applied. A limited amount of research into psoriasis and herbal remedies has been conducted. Topical applications of capsaicin and aloe vera tested well. Oral doses of dong quai and milk thistle also showed some good responses, but these carry a risk of negative interactions with other medications.

NOTABLE CASES Five-time Pro Bowl football player Mark Gastineau, musicians Art Garfunkel and Tom Waits, and "the Beaver" Jerry Mathers are all psoriasis patients.

Medications

- Topical applications of soothing lotion or medicated creams, including steroidal anti-inflammatories, retinoids, or coal tar extract
- Vitamin D analog cream (calcipotriene): Note, this is not vitamin D, and rubbing vitamin D on lesions is ineffective
- Injections of steroidal anti-inflammatories directly into plaques to help dissolve them
- PUVA: This is the use of psoralen (a systemic drug that heightens photosensitivity) along with UV radiation
- Biologics to alter immune system activity

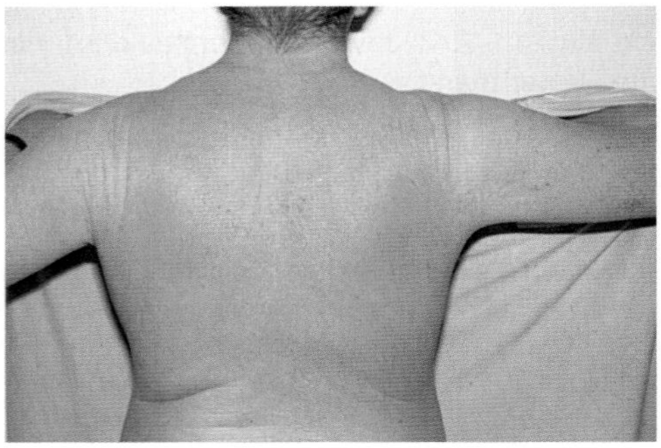

FIGURE 6.19 Erythrodermic psoriasis

Massage Therapy Implications

RISKS	Massage may make itchy lesions itchier. Of course, any open lesion is a possible portal of entry for infectious agents. Otherwise, psoriasis carries no specific contraindications for massage.
BENEFITS	Massage can be a welcome experience for people who have trouble with their skin. Stress is seen to be a significant trigger, and massage may help to modulate that. Because this condition isn't contagious and doesn't spread through touching, massage anywhere the skin is intact and not irritated is safe and appropriate.
OPTIONS	Choose a hypoallergenic lubricant for clients with psoriasis.

Onycholysis: Loosening of the nails.

Rheumatoid Arthritis

Definition: What Is It?

Rheumatoid arthritis is an autoimmune condition in which the synovial membranes of various joints are attacked by immune system cells. Unlike other forms of arthritis, rheumatoid arthritis can also involve inflammation of tissues outside the musculoskeletal system.

Demographics

This disease affects about 3.1 million people or about 1% of all Americans. Like many autoimmune diseases, women are affected more often than men; in this situation, the ratio is about 3:1.

Etiology: What Happens?

Rheumatoid arthritis is an autoimmune disease in which the immune system attacks the synovial membranes of certain joints, but other areas (blood vessels, serous membranes, the skin, eyes, lungs, liver, and heart) may also be affected.

When a synovial membrane is under immune system attack, all of the signs of inflammation develop: heat, pain, redness, swelling, and loss of function. Studies of joint tissues show that B cells, T cells, antibodies, and many proinflammatory chemicals are present during a flare. In response, the synovial membrane thickens and swells. Fluid accumulates inside the joint capsule, which causes pressure and pain. The inflamed tissues release enzymes that erode cartilage and bone; tendons and ligaments may also be affected. This causes the telltale deformation of the joint capsules and gnarled appearance of rheumatoid arthritis (Figure 6.20).

Synovial membranes are just one of the types of tissue that may be attacked. Other possibilities include:

- The **sclera** of the eyes may develop rheumatic nodules.
- The salivary glands and tear ducts may be dysfunctional in a condition called **Sjögren syndrome**.
- Attacks on the serous lining of the lungs may lead to pleuritis, which makes breathing painful and increases vulnerability to lung infection.
- The heart or pericardial sac may develop **carditis** or **pericarditis**.
- An attack on the liver may lead to **hepatitis**.
- Blood vessels can be targeted with vasculitis. This complication carries another set of risks: **Raynaud syndrome**, skin ulcers, bleeding intestinal **ulcers**, and internal hemorrhaging.
- Other immune system attack can trigger **bursitis** and **anemia**, especially when onset of the disease occurs in childhood.

Advanced structural damage brings a different set of complications. Deformed and bone-damaged joints may dislocate or collapse, rendering them useless. The tendons that cross over distorted joints sometimes become so stretched that they rupture. If the disease is at the C1 to C2 joint and the joint collapses, the resultant injury to the spinal column may result in problems with sphincter control or paralysis.

Types of Rheumatoid Arthritis

- *Juvenile rheumatoid arthritis (JRA).* JRA is a group of chronic arthritic conditions that affect children. Three main subtypes have been identified: **pauciarticular JRA**, **polyarticular JRA**, and **systemic JRA**, sometimes called "**Still disease**." The treatment goals for JRA are to help the patient live as normal a life as possible using diet, exercise, and pain management strategies along with drugs.

Signs and Symptoms

Symptoms of rheumatoid arthritis vary considerably at the onset of the disease. Most patients have a period of weeks or

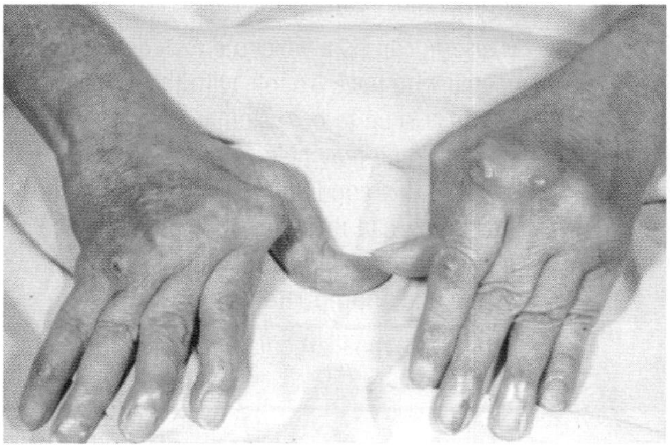

FIGURE 6.20 Rheumatoid arthritis with joint deformation

Sclera: The white, outer layer of the eye.

Sjögren syndrome: An autoimmune disorder in which the glands that produce tears and saliva are destroyed.

Pauciarticular JRA: Juvenile rheumatoid arthritis affecting fewer than five joints.

Polyarticular JRA: Juvenile rheumatoid arthritis affecting five or more joints.

Systemic JRA, Still disease: The most serious type of juvenile rheumatoid arthritis, affecting at least one joint as well as causing inflammation in various internal organs.

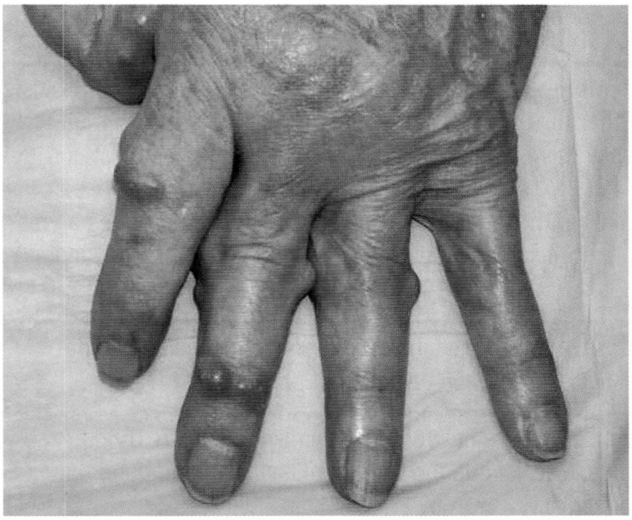

FIGURE 6.21 Rheumatic nodules

months with a general feeling of illness: lack of energy, lack of appetite, low-grade fever, and vague muscle pain, which gradually becomes sharp, specific joint pain. A few patients have a sudden onset with joint pain alone. **Rheumatic nodules** on and around the fingers, elbows, and other pressure-bearing areas are also common indicators of the disease (Figure 6.21).

In the acute stage of RA, the targeted joints are red, hot, painful, and stiff, although they improve considerably with heat and moderate amounts of movement and stretching. The joints rheumatoid arthritis most often attacks are the knuckles in hands and toes. It frequently develops in the ankles and wrists; knees are less common. One of the most serious places to get it is in the neck, where it can lead to dangerous instability. It generally affects the body bilaterally, although it is sometimes worse on one side than the other.

Like many autoimmune diseases, rheumatoid arthritis appears in cycles of flare followed by periods of remission. Some patients have only a few flares in their life and are never affected again. Moderate cases involve cycles of flare and remission up to several times a year. Severe rheumatoid arthritis involves chronic inflammation that never fully subsides.

Rheumatic nodules: Lumps under the skin that occur near joints affected with rheumatoid arthritis.

Complications

One of the often underaddressed comorbidities with RA is **osteoporosis**. This condition is a possible complication of RA because the medications sometimes result in bone loss, but also because reduced movement and weightbearing stress leads to bone loss, as does the simple fact of being a mature female: the group affected by RA more than any other. The overlap between RA and osteoporosis means that the risk of unstable joints is accompanied by the risk of bones that easily fracture and heal slowly.

NOTABLE CASES French impressionist painter Renoir struggled with rheumatoid arthritis and used to paint from a wheelchair with a brush jammed into his twisted fingers. Actress Kathleen Turner is an outspoken advocate for rheumatoid arthritis research and treatment.

Treatment

It is a high priority to correctly diagnose RA as quickly as possible, because delaying treatment, even for just a few months, increases the risk of permanent joint damage. The goals of treatment are to reduce pain, to limit inflammation, to halt joint damage, and to improve function. Medications that help to achieve these goals include DMARDs, biologic agents, steroids, NSAIDs, and analgesics. Most of these have serious potential side effects, and some are extremely expensive, so working out a drug strategy is an important part of RA treatment.

Nonmedical intervention for rheumatoid arthritis can include adjustments to diet, exercise, and stress reduction techniques, including massage. Splints, orthotics, canes, or other devices that make it easier to get through the day may become necessary.

Surgery can be a successful option for rheumatoid arthritis patients, if the disease has affected joints that can be easily treated. Joint fusion or replacement is sometimes an option, along with surgery to rebuild damaged or ruptured tendons and to remove portions of affected synovial membranes.

Medications

- NSAIDs, including COX-2 inhibitors
- Analgesics
- Steroidal anti-inflammatories
- DMARDs, including gold salts, antimalarial medications, methotrexate, and others
- Biologic agents, including tumor necrosis factor alpha inhibitors, IL-1 inhibitors, and others

Massage Therapy Implications

RISKS	In its acute (flare) phase, rheumatoid arthritis is an inflammatory condition that affects not just joints, but possibly the entire body. Rigorous massage during this phase is not appropriate, but gentle, soothing work may help ease this experience. Many patients appreciate heat and gentle manipulation of painful joints. Be aware that the medications a client with RA takes may also have impact decisions about bodywork: analgesics and anti-inflammatories alter tissue responses. Other drugs may depress immune system responses.
BENEFITS	Massage can be effective for pain, stress, and muscle tension. All of these benefits can be specifically applied for RA patients, especially between episodes of flare.
OPTIONS	Painless passive range of motion exercises can be helpful for RA patients who are trying to maintain flexibility at their affected joints. Special attention to the muscles and tendons that cross the painful joints may also be effective.
RESEARCH	One recent study compared light pressure to moderate pressure massage for RA patients and found that those who received moderate pressure massage to the arm and shoulder reported less pain and greater grip strength than the light pressure group.[1] A case report on a client with RA and digestive difficulties found that sustained myofascial release helped with both RA pain and GI function.[2] 1. Field T, Diego M, Delgado J, et al. Rheumatoid arthritis in upper limbs benefits from moderate pressure massage therapy. *Complementary Therapies in Clinical Practice* 2013;19(2):101–103. http://www.ncbi.nlm.nih.gov/pubmed/23561068 2. Cubick EE, Quezada VY, Schumer AD, et al. Sustained release myofascial release as treatment for a patient with complications of rheumatoid arthritis and collagenous colitis: a case report. *International Journal of Therapeutic Massage and Bodywork* 2011;4(3):1–9. http://www.ncbi.nlm.nih.gov/pmc/articles/PMC3184472/

Scleroderma

Definition: What Is It?

Scleroderma is an autoimmune disease in which inflammation stimulates fibroblasts in small blood vessels to produce abnormal amounts of collagen. This frequently occurs in the skin, hence the name: sclero (Greek for hard) and derma (Greek for skin) or "hard skin." But other tissues and organs may also be affected.

Demographics

Scleroderma affects about 300,000 people in the United States. As with other autoimmune diseases, women are affected more often than men, at a ratio of about 3 or 4 to 1. Unlike most other autoimmune diseases, scleroderma affects children as well as adults.

Etiology: What Happens?

Scleroderma is the result of an immune system attack against the lining of small blood vessels: the arterioles, capillaries, and venules. Damage to these tiny vessels causes local edema and stimulates nearby fibroblasts to spin out huge amounts of type I and III collagen, the basis for scar tissue. Eventually, the edema subsides, but the scar tissue deposits remain hard and unyielding for years at a time.

The cause of scleroderma is unknown, but several contributing factors have been identified. Abnormal immune responses and chronic inflammation stimulate the fibroblasts to produce excessive collagen. Other factors include exposure to chemicals, including silica, vinyl chloride, epoxy resins, uranium, and aromatic hydrocarbons. Organic solvents and viral infections (especially with cytomegalovirus or human herpesvirus 5) may also be environmental triggers.

Types of Scleroderma

- *Local scleroderma.* In this form of scleroderma, the areas of damage are limited to the skin. The initial edema may last for several weeks or months, the thickening of the skin may accumulate over a course of about 3 years, and then the symptoms gradually stabilize or even reverse. Local scleroderma is often discussed in two forms:
  - *Morphea scleroderma.* **Morphea** scleroderma takes the shape of discrete oval patches that develop on the trunk, face, or extremities. The lesions first appear as areas where the skin seems dry and thick. Eventually, they become pale in the center and purplish around the edges.
  - *Linear scleroderma.* This appears as a discolored line or band on a leg or arm or over the forehead. In this location, it may be called "coup de sabre" because it resembles a sword-fight scar (Figure 6.22).

Morphea: A localized form of scleroderma.

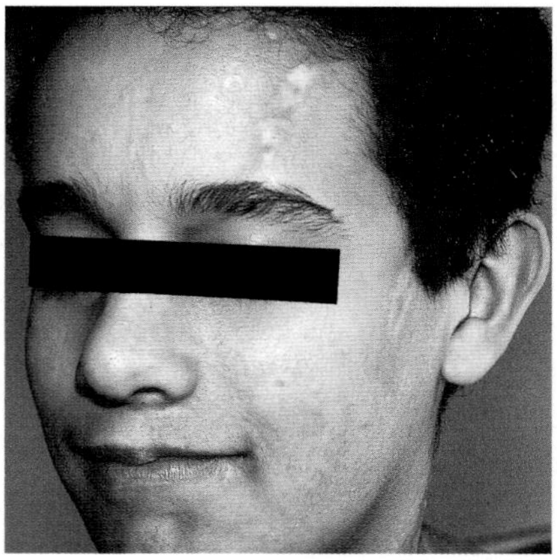

FIGURE 6.22 Scleroderma: coup de sabre lesion

- *Systemic scleroderma.* This has a slow onset that begins as CREST syndrome (described below), but may eventually infiltrate internal organs. Tissues most at risk are in the digestive tract, the heart and circulatory system, the kidneys, the lungs, and various parts of the musculoskeletal system, especially synovial membranes in joints and around tendons. This disease may stabilize and even reverse itself, but it can also be fatal. Systemic scleroderma is also called "systemic sclerosis." It occurs in three major subtypes.
  - *Limited systemic scleroderma.* This version begins with CREST syndrome, and it is only slowly progressive.
  - *Diffuse scleroderma.* This has a more sudden onset and earlier involvement of internal organs.
  - *Sine scleroderma.* **Sine scleroderma** doesn't involve the skin at all; it only involves internal organs.

Signs and Symptoms

Scleroderma can produce a variety of symptoms, depending on which blood vessels are under attack. The term **CREST syndrome** has been coined as a mnemonic for the most common scleroderma symptoms:

- C: **Calcinosis** refers to accumulation of calcium deposits in the skin, especially in the fingers.

> **Sine scleroderma:** An unusual form of systemic scleroderma with significant organ involvement and minimal affect on the skin.
>
> **CREST syndrome:** A mnemonic for the most common scleroderma symptoms: calcinosis, Raynaud phenomenon, esophageal motility disorders, sclerodactyly, and telangiectasia.
>
> **Calcinonsis:** Calcium deposits in the skin or any soft tissue.
>
> **Sclerodactyly:** Stiffness of the skin of the fingers.
>
> **Microstomia:** Literally, "small mouth". Scleroderma can limit the range of motion allowed for opening the oral aperture.

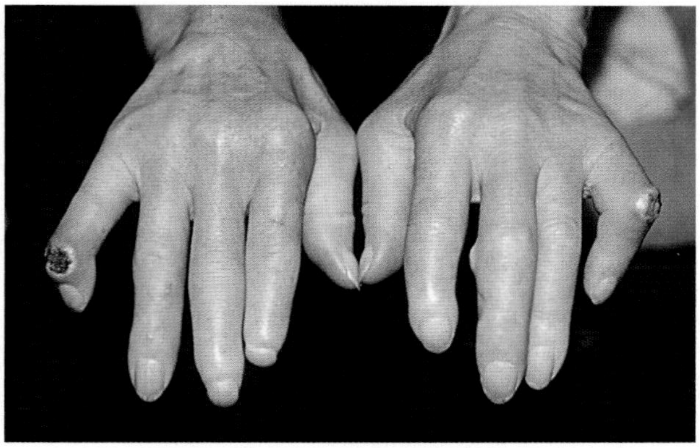

FIGURE 6.23 Scleroderma: sclerodactyly

- R: **Raynaud phenomenon** is a result of impaired circulation and vascular spasm in the hands.
- E: Esophageal dysmotility refers to sluggishness of the digestive tract and chronic gastric reflux.
- S: **Sclerodactyly** is a result of the accumulation of tight, shiny scar tissue in the hands (Figure 6.23).
- T: Telangiectasia is a discoloration of the skin caused by permanently stretched and damaged capillaries. It is also known as "spider veins."

Other symptoms of scleroderma include tight, hardened skin, usually on the hands or face; skin ulcers in which circulation prevents normal nutrition for healthy cells; changes in pigmentation; and hair loss in the affected patches. Muscles may become weak, while tendons and tendinous sheaths become painful and swollen. **Trigeminal neuralgia** and **carpal tunnel syndrome** may develop as a result of nerve entrapment. **Sjögren syndrome** may also be a part of the picture. Lungs may accumulate edema or fibrosis where blood vessels are under attack, opening the door to pneumonia. Heart pain, arrhythmia, and **heart failure** may develop as the heart tries to push blood through a system that cannot accommodate it. And kidneys, working under high blood pressure and with damaged arterioles, may fail.

Complications

Complications of the most serious forms of scleroderma range from mild to serious and potentially life-threatening. While the skin tightens visibly on the hands, a less visible result is tightening in the face, leading to difficulties with opening the mouth (**microstomia**). This makes eating, speaking, and oral care problematic. Blood clots may lead to **embolism** or **thrombus. Renal failure**, pulmonary fibrosis, and **heart failure** are all possible for people with systemic diffuse scleroderma. Pulmonary hypertension is a major predictor of mortality in patients with scleroderma.

Treatment

Treatment for this condition is directed at managing the symptoms and complications of the disease. In addition, immune system modifiers are increasingly effective. Physical or occupational therapies are employed to maintain flexibility in the hands and face. Patients are usually advised to avoid smoking, cold conditions, and spicy foods to minimize symptoms.

Medications

- Immune system modifiers to suppress immune system overactivity
- Steroidal anti-inflammatories (with the caution that these may stress the kidneys)
- Calcium channel blockers for Raynaud phenomenon
- ACE inhibitors for kidney function
- Diuretics for kidney function
- Antacids and proton pump inhibitors for gastric reflux
- NSAIDs for muscle and joint pain

Massage Therapy Implications

RISKS	Because scleroderma can involve permanent damage to blood vessels as well as skin lesions, lung, and kidney problems, any kind of massage must be done with some caution. Decisions must be based on the resilience of the client; this can be a moving target that changes from one day to the next. Be aware that some medications—especially anti-inflammatories and blood pressure drugs—used to control scleroderma may have side effects that impact decisions about bodywork.
BENEFITS	Any bodywork that can be done to restore parasympathetic balance without over challenging a damaged circulatory system could prove beneficial for scleroderma patients.
RESEARCH	Lymphatic drainage of the arm has been used to improve hand function for some scleroderma patients.[1] Massage therapy, along with exercise and other interventions, was also shown to be a promising strategy for joint motion, skin compliance, hand function, and quality of life.[2] 1. Bongi SM, Del Rosso A, Passalacqua M, et al. Manual lymph drainage improving upper extremity edema and hand function in patients with systemic sclerosis in edematous phase. *Arthritis Care and Research* 2011;63(8):1134–1141. http://www.ncbi.nlm.nih.gov/pubmed/21523925 2. Poole JL. Musculoskeletal rehabilitation in the person with scleroderma. *Current Opinion in Rheumatology* 2010;22(2):205–212. http://www.ncbi.nlm.nih.gov/pubmed/21523925

Ulcerative Colitis

Definition: What Is It?

Ulcerative colitis is a disease involving inflammation and shallow ulcers in the colon (Figure 6.24). Ulcerative colitis and Crohn disease are sometimes referred to collectively as inflammatory bowel disease. The inflammation with ulcerative colitis is limited to the large intestine, however, which distinguishes it from **Crohn disease**. For more information on the connections between Crohn disease and ulcerative colitis, see Compare & Contrast 6.1.

Demographics

About 1 million people in the United States are affected with ulcerative colitis. Women slightly outnumber men, but not by a wide margin. Whites are affected more than other ethnic or racial groups. UC is far more common in the Western world than anywhere else; its prevalence is low in Asia and the Far East.

Etiology: What Happens?

The initial cause of ulcerative colitis is a subject of some debate, although most specialists agree that it is an autoimmune disease with some genetic factors and possibly triggered by an abnormal response to colon-dwelling bacteria. It almost always begins in the rectum when immune system cells attack the most superficial layer of the colon. The resulting inflammation kills tissue and results in the formation of shallow ulcers: open sores that may never fully heal. Colon function is extremely limited,

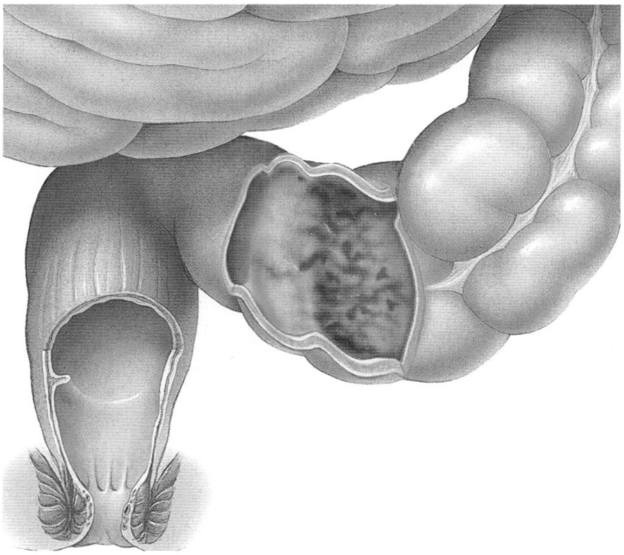

FIGURE 6.24 Ulcerative colitis

and the patient has chronic bloody diarrhea. The sores may become infected, leading to the release of blood and pus in the stools.

Ulcerative colitis is classified by what part or parts of the colon are affected. Disease that is limited to the rectum is called ulcerative **proctitis**; **proctosigmoiditis** describes progression to the sigmoid colon. Left-sided colitis involves the descending colon, and **pancolitis** describes inflammation of the entire colon. The most extreme and dangerous form of ulcerative colitis is **fulminant** colitis. In this condition, the whole colon is acutely inflamed and ulcerated, and the risk of life-threatening complications from a condition called **toxic megacolon** is high.

About half of all ulcerative colitis patients have it in a mild form that doesn't become threatening. Patients with ulcerative colitis that involves the whole colon are at significantly more risk for developing **colorectal cancer** than the general population. This risk goes up significantly 8 to 10 years after diagnosis of ulcerative colitis. For this reason, surgery to remove the affected part of the colon is frequently recommended.

Signs and Symptoms

Symptoms of ulcerative colitis depend largely on how much of the bowel is affected: the greater the extent of inflammation, the worse the symptoms tend to be. Symptoms run in cycles of flare and remission. During flares, the primary symptom is painful chronic diarrhea with blood and pus in the stools. Abdominal cramping, **tenesmus**, loss of appetite, and mild fever may also occur during acute episodes.

Between acute episodes, the ulcerative colitis patient may have only minimal abdominal pain but must be careful to avoid any triggers of abdominal cramping or discomfort.

Proctitis: Ulcerative colitis that is present only in the rectum or anus.

Proctosigmoiditis: Ulcerative colitis that is present in both the rectum and the sigmoid colon.

Pancolitis: Inflammation of the entire colon.

Fulminant: Sudden and severe.

Toxic megacolon: Acute non-obstructive dilation of the colon.

Tenesmus: A constant or recurring feeling of needing to have a bowel movement, regardless of the actual contents of the colon.

Cholangitis: Inflammation of the bile ducts.

Uveitis: Inflammation of the uvea of the eye.

Colostomy: A procedure in which an artificial opening is created between the skin of the abdomen and the colon.

Complications

Like most autoimmune diseases, ulcerative colitis affects tissues outside its primary area. A person with UC may also have inflammation of the liver or gallbladder ducts (**cholangitis**), **osteoporosis** from poor nutritional absorption, **anemia** from blood loss, and **kidney stones** from the disruption in electrolyte balance and chronic dehydration that accompanies long-term diarrhea. **Uveitis**, or inflammation of structures in the eye, may result in permanent vision loss if it is not treated. Some skin lesions are also associated with ulcerative colitis; these may occur in connection with flares or may outlive a flare to be a chronic infection. Ulcerative colitis is also associated with the spondyloarthropathies discussed in Sidebar 6.6.

Treatment

Treatment options for ulcerative colitis begin with aminosalicylates: a class of medications that lessen the severity of flareups and prolong periods of remission. If these don't control the inflammation satisfactorily, corticosteroids may be prescribed for short periods. Immunosuppressive drugs and, surprisingly, nicotine patches have also been found to improve symptoms.

If these options are not satisfactory, or if inflammation of the colon has progressed to a dangerous degree, surgery is the only permanent solution. Several surgical options have been developed; all of them involve the removal of the bowel. External **colostomy** bags, internal colostomy bags, and the joining of the small intestine to the muscles of the rectum are options for replacing the main functions of the colon.

Medications

- Oral, suppository, or enema application of aminosalicylates to control inflammation and immune system response
- Oral or injected corticosteroids to suppress inflammation
- Immune-modifying drugs to alter immune system response

Massage Therapy Implications

RISKS	Ulcerative colitis in a flared stage contraindicates local intrusive massage. Even during remission, it's important to remember that the colon sustains permanent damage; consequently, deep abdominal work must be done with caution. Clients who use colostomy bags may require some special positioning adjustments in order to receive massage comfortably.
BENEFITS	A client with ulcerative colitis that is in remission can receive any massage that is well tolerated, although of course abdominal work must be done with care. A client who has fully recovered from ulcerative colitis surgery can enjoy all the benefits from massage as the rest of the population, with adjustments for a colostomy bag.
OPTIONS	Clients with ulcerative colitis or other conditions that cause digestive discomfort can especially benefit from reflexive work or gentle holding that focuses on the abdomen in order to help incorporate this painful and problem-laden part of the body into the whole.
RESEARCH	While little research has been done on what massage therapy can do for people with UC specifically, we do know that many inflammatory bowel disease patients pursue complementary and integrative health care therapies along with conventional medicine and that massage therapy is a leading choice among them.[1] 1. Rawsthorne P, Clara I, Graff LA, et al. The Manitoba Inflammatory Bowel Disease Cohort Study: a prospective longitudinal evaluation of the use of complementary and alternative medicine services and products. *Gut* 2012;61(4):521–527. http://www.ncbi.nlm.nih.gov/pubmed/21836028

Explore and Apply

LEVEL 1: Receive and Respond

1. What is the source of interstitial fluid?
   a. Lymph nodes
   b. Mast cells
   c. Thoracic duct
   d. Circulatory capillaries

2. Which of the following is a mechanism to help move lymph through the thoracic duct?
   a. Deep breathing
   b. Healthy digestion
   c. Hydrostatic pressure
   d. Osmotic pressure

3. Which pathogen usually causes mononucleosis?
   a. *Streptococcus aureus*
   b. Herpes simplex virus
   c. Epstein-Barr virus
   d. Mycobacterium tuberculosis

4. Which is the best description of angioedema?
   a. Acute, severe systemic reaction leading to hypotension and systemic edema
   b. Rapid onset of localized swelling; can be fatal if it interrupts airflow
   c. Red, swollen, itching eyes, runny nose
   d. Nausea, vomiting, diarrhea in reaction to a food allergen

5. What term is sometimes used as a synonym for chronic fatigue syndrome?
   a. Multiple chemical sensitivity syndrome
   b. Fibromyalgia syndrome
   c. Myalgic encephalomyelitis
   d. Central sensitization syndrome

6. What are the three phases of a fever (in correct order)?
   a. Chill, crisis, flush
   b. Crisis, chill, flush
   c. Flush, chill, crisis
   d. Crisis, flush, chill

7. Which is the list of body fluids most capable of carrying HIV to a new host?
   a. Saliva, breast milk, semen
   b. Blood, sweat, tears
   c. Semen, sweat, blood
   d. Semen, blood, breast milk

8. Match the following terms to their best descriptions:

a. Ankylosing spondylitis	—Inflammatory arthritis at several joints, skin rash, high risk of renal failure
b. Rheumatoid arthritis	—Progressive inflammation of the spine, high risk of pneumonia, heart failure
c. Scleroderma	—Stiff fingers and face; CREST syndrome
d. Lupus	—Affects synovial joints, but may also involve nodules on the sclera of the eye and Sjögren syndrome

9. Inflammatory bowel disease comprises…
   a. Irritable bowel syndrome, fibromyalgia, chronic fatigue syndrome
   b. Ulcerative colitis, Crohn disease
   c. Crohn disease, celiac disease, rheumatoid arthritis
   d. Lupus, ulcerative colitis

10. Which of the following is true for both Crohn disease and ulcerative colitis?
    a. Increased risk of colorectal cancer
    b. Involves only the upper GI tract
    c. Involves only the lower GI tract
    d. Surgery is curative

Explore and Apply (continued)

LEVEL 2: Application of Concepts

1. When the Starling equilibrium is overwhelmed, the resulting situation is probably...
   a. Infection
   b. Edema
   c. Hypersensitivity
   d. Autoimmunity

2. Why are massage therapists especially vulnerable to lymphangitis? What precautions can be taken to keep this risk to a minimum?

3. Your 30-year-old client had Hodgkin lymphoma 4 years ago, but is now declared to be cancer-free. What accommodations are necessary for this client?
   a. The same as for any client without a history of cancer
   b. A gentle massage that doesn't overtax this person's impaired lymph system
   c. Precautions for positioning because of the risk of brittle bones
   d. Gloves for the therapist to avoid exposure to chemotherapeutic drugs

4. Your client has chronic fatigue syndrome. Besides fatigue, what symptoms are probably foremost for her?
   a. Sensitivity to cold
   b. Sluggish digestion
   c. Poor memory and concentration
   d. Chronic muscle stiffness

5. What happens in phase 3 of HIV infection?
   a. Indicator diseases develop
   b. The immune system keeps up with viral progression
   c. Symptoms that look like flu or mono develop
   d. T-cell counts drop below 200 per cubic mL of blood

6. The functional changes seen with multiple sclerosis become permanent when...
   a. Both CNS and PNS structures are attacked
   b. All the oligodendrocytes are destroyed
   c. Inflammation affects the axons
   d. Antibodies attack neuron cell bodies

7. Your client has advanced plaque psoriasis in a flared state. What is your best strategy?
   a. Reschedule the appointment for a time when she is no longer contagious
   b. Use a hypoallergenic lotion and work in a way that doesn't exacerbate itchiness
   c. Recommend that she change her medication, because it clearly doesn't work
   d. Work normally but wear gloves to avoid spreading the rash

Note to educators: Due to space considerations, these review questions only skim over the most important material from Chapter 8. The Test Bank provides a much more comprehensive selection of questions, all of which are keyed to the relevant chapter objectives.

What Would *You* Do?

"I've Never Heard of That One..."

Your client tells you she has been diagnosed with enteropathy-type intestinal T-cell lymphoma. How will you determine the safety of massage therapy? Where will you look for information? Make a list of resources (books, websites, etc.) where you will gather this information. Then, make a list of potential risks and benefits for massage therapy.

Is Massage a Good Choice for People with Autoimmune Diseases?

Some research suggests that massage therapy can promote immune system activity. If that is the case, could it have a negative effect for a client who lives with an autoimmune disease like lupus or scleroderma? Choose a partner and discuss how you plan to address this question. What will you do if a client wants a specific answer?

Suggested Activities

1. For each condition covered in your curriculum, write down the following on a card:
   - A brief definition
   - Most common cause or contributing factor(s)
   - Major signs and symptoms
   - Risks and benefits of massage therapy
     - Variables that contribute to risks and benefits
     - Appropriate adaptations

   Use these as flash cards as you study.
2. For each condition covered in your curriculum, write one multiple-choice question. Share your questions with your classmates as you study together.
3. Quiz yourself using either the "labels off" feature in your enhanced e-book or the labeling exercise on thePoint® for Figure 6.1. Identify the following structures: Afferent lymph vessel, Capillary bed, Efferent lymph vessel, Lymphatic capillaries, Right lymphatic duct, Superficial cervical nodes, Superficial inguinal nodes, Thoracic duct (inferior), Thoracic duct (superior), Tissue cells.
4. Use the student resources on thePoint® to find practice quiz questions and games.

7

Respiratory System Conditions

Chapter 7 / Abbreviated Chapter Objectives

Having completed assignments and classroom time related to Chapter 7, the learner is expected to be able to…

- Identify definitions of the key terms in the introduction and those connected to the conditions covered in your curriculum.
- List the six structures of the respiratory system in order from proximal to distal.
- Describe the basic mechanisms of efficient respiration.
- Identify where in the lungs gaseous exchange takes place.
- Explain why it is important for cilia to move the mucus blanket.
- List three muscles involved in inhalation.
- Name the structures most responsible for successful passive exhalation.
- Provide the following information for each condition covered in your curriculum:
  - Identify the definition of the condition.
  - List the most common causes or contributing factors to the condition.
  - List major signs and symptoms of the condition.
  - Identify possible risks and benefits of massage therapy with:
    - Variables that contribute to risks and benefits.
    - Appropriate adaptations for massage therapy.

For detailed chapter objectives for each condition in this chapter, consult the student resources page at <u>http://thePoint.lww.com/Werner6e</u>. thePoint®

INTRODUCTION

Respiratory System Structure

The easiest way to discuss the structure of the respiratory system is to follow a particle of air through it (Figure 7.1). Take a deep breath. Air drawn in through the nose encounters mucous membranes. Various types of mucous membranes line any cavity in the body that communicates with the outside world: specifically the respiratory, digestive, reproductive, and urinary systems. In the respiratory system, the mucous membranes start inside the nose and mouth, and they line the sinuses and throat all the way down into the small tubes in the lungs. The wet, sticky mucous membranes in the respiratory system are responsible for warming, moistening, and filtering the air that passes by.

Once past the nose and mouth, air enters first the pharynx, then the larynx, the trachea, and the left and right bronchi. The bronchi are asymmetrical. The right bronchus is bigger, wider, and straighter leading into the three lobes of the right lung. The left bronchus is smaller in diameter, and it curves off to the side to reach the two lobes of the left lung. This is significant if a foreign object is inhaled into the lungs; it almost always follows the path of least resistance to the right side.

The bronchi divide into the bronchioles, which then separate out 23 times until they terminate in microscopic

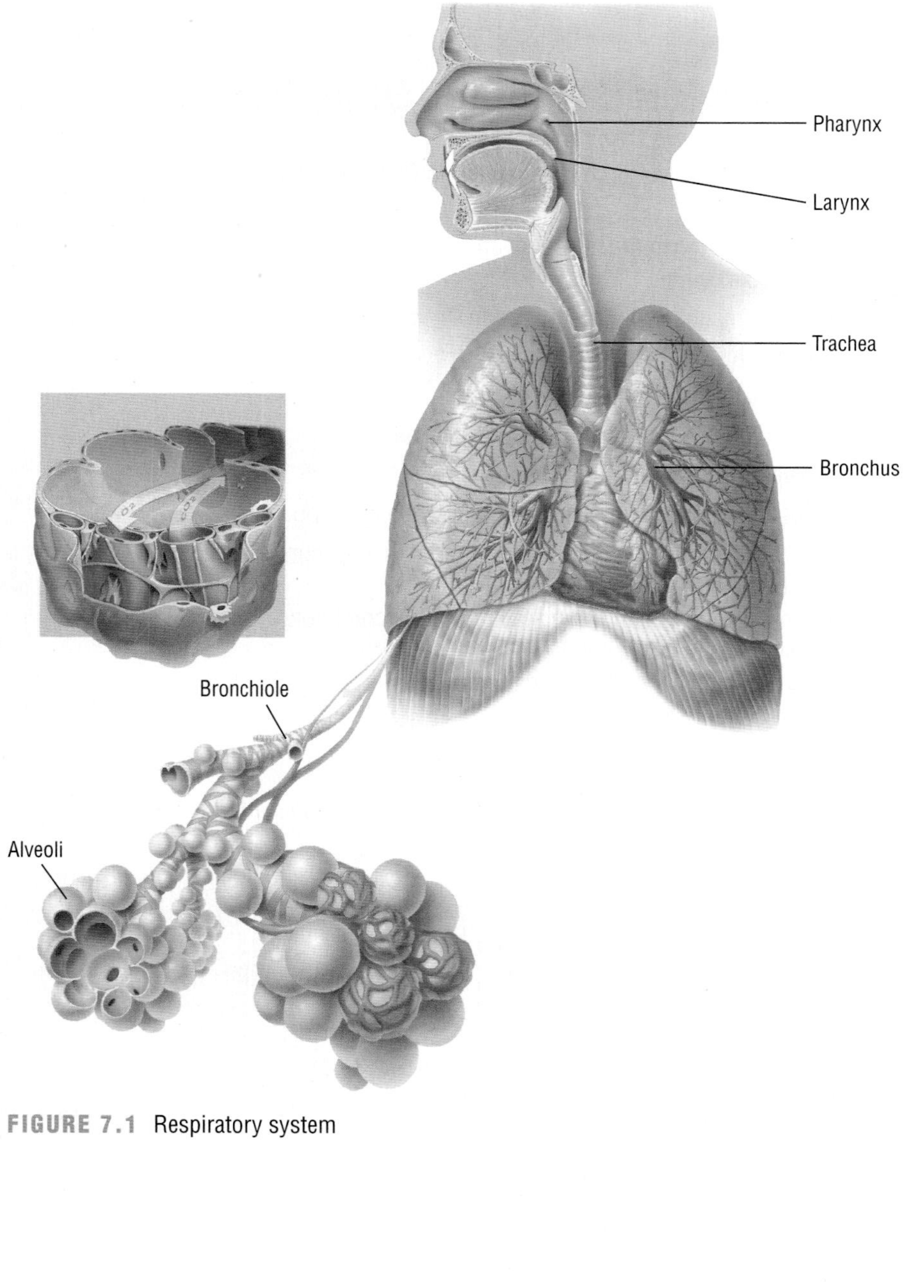

FIGURE 7.1 Respiratory system

alveoli. These grape-shaped clusters of epithelial bubbles are like tiny balloons, each one surrounded by blood capillaries. Gaseous exchange occurs through the permeable surfaces of the alveoli and the capillaries. If the alveoli are impaired or not functioning correctly, the body cannot make an efficient trade of fresh air for used air. *An explanation of this process is in the animation "Asthma," available at* http://thePoint.lww.com/Werner6e. thePoint®

The structure of the lungs themselves is well suited for fighting off infection. Each lung has two or three separate lobes (two on the left and three on the right), and each of those lobes has smaller separate segments called lobules. These isolated segments make it difficult for pathogens to infect the whole structure. All of the tubes are lined with mucous membrane, which traps pathogens and other particles. Then the cilia in the tract help move the **mucus blanket** toward the mouth and nose for expulsion. Smooth muscle tissue lines all of the tubes down to the smallest bronchi; when an irritant is trapped in these tubes, a healthy cough reflex quickly moves it out of the body.

Alveoli: Small cavities or sockets. Specifically, the tiny air sacs in the lungs where the exchange of gases takes place. (Singular: alveolus)

Mucus blanket: The mucus covering of the respiratory epithelium.

Respiratory System Function

Air cycles through the lungs 12 to 20 times per minute. The lungs themselves do not have any muscle tissue to expand or contract; they are simply limp-walled sacs that inflate or deflate according to the air pressure inside and outside of them. A change in air pressure is brought about by a change in the shape of the thoracic cavity. If the cavity is made larger, the air pressure inside the lungs is low until air rushes in to equalize it. In other words, the act of inhaling is simply filling a vacuum. When the pressure inside and outside the lungs is about equal, we relax our inhaling muscles, and air eases out again: exhalation.

The muscles involved in inhalation are the diaphragm, which lowers the "floor" of the thoracic cavity during contraction; the external intercostals and serratus posterior, which expand the "walls" of the thoracic cavity, and the scalenes, which lift the "roof." When they work together, the size of this hollow space enlarges, and air rushes in to fill it.

Exhalation is mostly a passive process; elastic connective tissue fibers in the lungs pull them back to their original size, so relaxed exhalation does not involve muscular activity unless a person invests effort to remove air from the lungs. In that situation, the internal intercostals and transversus abdominus are the main players.

The efficiency of this mechanism is astonishing. Even though oxygen–carbon dioxide exchange is only partial with each breath (a typical inhalation contains roughly 21% oxygen, while a typical exhalation still contains about 16% oxygen), the respiratory system supplies the entire body with enough oxygen to function with minimal effort: a healthy person invests only 5% of resting calories in the act of breathing.

Respiratory System Conditions

Infectious Respiratory Disorders

- Acute bronchitis
- Common cold
- Influenza
  - Seasonal flu
  - H5N1 Avian flu
  - H1N1 Swine flu
- Pneumonia
  - Bronchopneumonia
  - Lobar pneumonia
  - Double pneumonia
  - Community-acquired pneumonia
  - Nosocomial (hospital-acquired) pneumonia
  - Aspiration pneumonia
- Sinusitis
  - Noninfectious sinusitis (Hayfever)
  - Infectious sinusitis
- Tuberculosis
  - Drug susceptible tuberculosis
  - Multidrug resistant tuberculosis
  - Extensively drug resistant tuberculosis

Chronic Obstructive Pulmonary Diseases

- Chronic bronchitis
- Emphysema

Other Respiratory Disorders

- Asthma
  - Bronchial asthma
  - Exercise-induced asthma
  - Silent asthma
  - Cough variant asthma
- Cystic fibrosis
- Laryngeal cancer
- Lung cancer
  - Small cell lung cancer
  - Nonsmall cell lung cancer
  - Other types of lung cancer

Infectious Respiratory Disorders

Acute Bronchitis

Definition: What Is It?

Acute bronchitis, sometimes called "chest cold," is a self-limiting inflammation of the respiratory tract, specifically of the bronchial tree. It is usually a complication of the **common cold** or **flu**. Acute bronchitis typically resolves within 10 days to several weeks of onset. This helps to distinguish it from **chronic bronchitis**, which is an irreversible condition with a very different etiology and prognosis.

Demographics

About 10 million adults develop acute bronchitis each year, mostly in the fall and winter. It is among the most common reasons people visit a doctor, but it occurs less frequently than cold (66 million cases per year) or flu (91 million cases per year).

Etiology: What Happens?

When the bronchi are irritated or infected by any kind of pathogen, an inflammatory response ensues. The tubes swell, the cilia are damaged, excessive mucus is produced, and the result is coughing and wheezing as air moves through passageways that are obstructed with swelling and excessive sticky secretions. Most cases of acute bronchitis are complications of a cold or flu in which the viruses simply move from the upper respiratory system to the bronchial tubes. Other causative agents include a variety of bacteria and fungi. Noninfectious irritants, like fumes, air pollutants, and other contaminants can create an environment where pathogens can thrive. Chronic reflux from the esophagus can also irritate the bronchi; acute bronchitis can be a complication of **gastroesophageal reflux disorder**.

An important feature of acute bronchitis is that it is self-limiting and results in no permanent changes to the bronchi, cilia, or mucous membranes. This distinguishes acute bronchitis from chronic bronchitis (Compare & Contrast 7.1).

Signs and Symptoms

The primary sign of acute bronchitis is a persistent cough. It often starts dry, but within a few days becomes productive. **Sputum** may be clear or opaque. Wheezing, nasal congestion, headache, low fever, muscle aches, chest pain, and fatigue may also be present. Most of the symptoms of acute bronchitis subside within about 10 days of onset, but the cough may persist for several weeks while the delicate lining of the bronchial tubes heals.

If fever persists or exceeds 101°F (38.3°C), or if the sputum becomes greenish, yellow, or blood streaked, the possibility of **pneumonia** must be considered. This is a more serious condition that usually needs medical intervention.

> **Sputum:** Mucus and other material that is coughed up from the respiratory tract.

Treatment

The best treatment options for most cases of acute bronchitis include rest, fluids, and warm, humid air to liquefy mucus and aid in its expulsion. Antibiotics are not effective in most cases of acute bronchitis, but they may be appropriate when the causative agent has been identified as bacterial. Many experts agree that antibiotics are often over-prescribed for acute bronchitis patients, however.

Bronchodilators and cough suppressants may help to manage some of the symptoms of acute bronchitis, but they do not eradicate the infection, and research suggests that they do little to shorten the duration of the cough.

Medications

- NSAIDs for general discomfort and fever reduction
- Cough suppressants
- Bronchodilators
- Antibiotics if necessary

Massage Therapy Implications

RISKS	Any massage that demands a significant adaptive response should be delayed until the acute phase of a bronchial infection has passed. At any point during acute bronchitis accommodations may have to be made for a client who is uncomfortable lying flat on a table.
BENEFITS	Gentle, nondemanding bodywork may be appropriate for someone with acute bronchitis, as long as precautions are taken to protect the therapist from infection. When the client is in recovery, massage may be helpful for improving fatigue.
OPTIONS	Within client tolerance, focus on the breathing muscles may improve efficiency of breathing function.

COMPARE & CONTRAST 7.1 Acute Bronchitis, Chronic Bronchitis, or Bronchiectasis: Which Is Which?

The lungs are particularly vulnerable to infection, stationed as they are at the receiving end of everything that enters the body through the nose. They have some structural features that make it easy to isolate sites of infection, and they are well stocked with immune system cells to fight off incoming invaders, but they are susceptible to a variety of disorders that can cause both short-term and long-term damage. Three lung problems have similarities and differences that make it useful to examine them side-by-side:

- *Acute bronchitis* often accompanies upper respiratory infections or flu. This is a viral attack directly on the bronchi, although it can also complicate into a bacterial infection.
- *Chronic bronchitis* involves long-term irritation to the bronchial lining, all the way down to the terminal bronchioles. This irritation can cause the lining to become permanently thick with excessive mucus production that can make it difficult to breathe. Chronic bronchitis raises the risk for lung infections, but it doesn't start with a pathogenic invasion.
- ***Bronchiectasis*** is a disorder brought about by repeated lung infections that cause structural changes to the bronchial tubes; they become permanently widened. When the bronchi become unable to move mucus out of the body, it pools in the lungs, creating a risk of further infection and more structural damage.

If a lung disorder is present, it is useful for the massage therapist to have a clear idea of the situation so that the client may be made as comfortable as possible on the table and so that the risk of spreading infection is minimized.

CHARACTERISTICS	ACUTE BRONCHITIS	CHRONIC BRONCHITIS	BRONCHIECTASIS
Cause	Viral attack on lungs; often accompanies cold or flu.	Long-term lung irritation, for example, cigarette smoke, pollution, particles in air.	History of multiple lung infections, including acute bronchitis, pneumonia.
Symptoms	Productive cough with clear sputum (colored sputum: suspect secondary bacterial infection); fever, aches, pains.	Productive cough with clear sputum (colored sputum: suspect secondary bacterial infection). Excessive mucus production, frequent throat clearing. Susceptibility to lung infections. Wheezing, shortness of breath, cyanosis.	Frequent cough with green or yellow sputum, especially when lying down.
Prognosis	If basically healthy, full recovery with no long-term problems.	If irritation to lungs halts, may not progress but is not reversible. If it progresses, may develop into emphysema, right-sided heart failure, respiratory failure.	Patient must avoid lung irritants and possibility of further lung infections, which may further damage bronchi.
Implications for massage	Should not receive rigorous massage until infection resolves.	May receive massage if positioned on table so as not to exacerbate symptoms. Essential to rule out possibility of circulatory stress.	May receive massage if positioned on table so as not to exacerbate symptoms.

Common Cold

Definition: What Is It?

The common cold is an infection of the upper respiratory tract brought about by any of hundreds of viruses.

Over the course of a lifetime people are exposed to multitudes of different cold viruses. They get sick, they establish immunity to that particular pathogen, and they move on to the next infection. Much of this happens in childhood, so by adulthood people have encountered most of what they are likely to see, and the frequency of infections generally subsides. But no single infectious agent causes the so-called common cold, so no effective single vaccine against common cold may ever be developed.

Demographics

About 66 million colds affect adults each year. Adults have an average of 2 to 3 colds per year. Children, who are still building their collection of immunities, usually have 6 to 10 colds per year.

Interestingly, only humans, chimpanzees, and other higher primates get colds. By contrast, many mammals and birds are vulnerable to flu viruses.

Etiology: What Happens?

Human sinuses are constructed with a great deal of surface area. This promotes the conditioning of air—heating, filtering, and moistening it—before it gets into the more delicate lungs. Cilia that line the nasal sinuses keep mucus constantly in movement, but the passageway by which it can leave the sinuses is about 3 mm, or the diameter of a pencil lead. It is not surprising then that when the sinuses are inflamed or extra mucus is produced that we get a "stuffy" or congested sinus passage.

The common cold, also known as an upper respiratory tract infection (URTI), **coryza**, or viral rhinitis, is caused by any of hundreds of viruses. Rhinoviruses cause approximately half of colds; this group has about 110 subtypes and is most active in autumn and spring. Other pathogens include coronaviruses (these are the group that also cause **severe acute respiratory syndrome**, or SARS), adenoviruses, and respiratory syncytial virus. Most of these viral infections are low grade and not dangerous, but some can cause very severe infections, especially in infants and young children.

The viruses that cause the common cold enter the nose, where the temperature is about 91°F (32.8°C), a perfect growth environment. The cilia in the mucous membrane carry the viruses to the back of the throat, where they have access to their target cells in the lymphoid tissue of the adenoids. When a virus gains access to its target, it infiltrates that cell and takes over its processes until the cell literally bursts with new viruses. Cold viruses act fast: the incubation period between being exposed and developing symptoms can be as short as 12 hours.

While the damage that cold viruses cause is substantial, it pales in comparison with the damage caused by the immune system when it is fighting off a cold virus. Signals released by infected cells trigger an aggressive response, which cause the area to be flooded with inflammatory chemicals and aggressive immune systems cells. It is the immune system response to a viral threat that causes most of the discomfort associated with common cold symptoms.

Coryza: Inflammation of the mucous membrane of the nose.

Severe acute respiratory syndrome: A highly contagious respiratory illness caused by a type of coronavirus.

Anosmia: Total or partial absence of the sense of smell.

Cold viruses can stay viable for several hours outside the body, depending on the local environment. The viruses are airborne after an infected person coughs or sneezes, but they are even more readily spread when someone gets a virus on the hand, and it finds access to the body through a portal of entry: the mouth, the eyes, or the nose. Picking up a virus from a light switch, a doorknob, a keyboard, or a piece of money, and then rubbing the nose is a very efficient way to spread the disease.

The best way to prevent the spread of colds and other infectious diseases is by frequently washing the hands, focusing on the cuticles and nails, using soap or detergent and scrubbing for 20 to 30 seconds before rinsing. Using paper tissues and disposing of them carefully, avoiding contact with people who are sick, and employing good judgment about sleep, diet, and exercise can also help to prevent the spread of colds.

Colds are seldom dangerous, except when they complicate into a secondary infection. The compromised integrity of the membranes and the accumulations of mucus, a perfect growth medium, leave the body vulnerable to secondary infections that can include ear infection, laryngitis, **acute bronchitis**, **sinusitis**, and **pneumonia**. People with **asthma** or chronic obstructive pulmonary disease (**chronic bronchitis** and/or **emphysema**) also frequently find that colds exacerbate their respiratory symptoms.

Signs and Symptoms

The symptoms of a cold are probably familiar to everyone: stuffy, runny nose, sneezing, sore throat, dry coughing, headache, and a mild fever. Symptoms generally last less than 2 weeks, although the cough may linger for 3 weeks or more.

Treatment

Because colds are viral infections, antibiotics are useless in this context. Getting extra rest, drinking lots of fluids, and isolating oneself from family, classmates, and coworkers who could get infected are all high priorities. Using a humidifier may relieve some of the irritation to mucous membranes, although some types of humidifiers can be breeding grounds for fungi or bacteria, so it is important to keep them scrupulously clean.

Over-the-counter drugs can relieve the symptoms of a cold, but they do not reduce recovery time. In fact, by inhibiting the ways a body fights off infection (reducing fever, drying up the sinuses), over-the-counter drugs may actually increase the amount of time the infection is present in the body.

Medications

- NSAIDs for fever and pain
- Cough suppressants
- Decongestants
- Zinc lozenges (note: zinc nasal sprays have been associated with a risk of permanent **anosmia**—loss of the sense of smell)

Massage Therapy Implications

RISKS Anecdotal reports suggest that clients who receive a rigorous circulatory massage while a cold or flu infection is taking hold may get sicker than if they had delayed. By contrast, clients who receive massage while in recovery from a respiratory tract infection often find that their symptoms are temporarily exacerbated, and then their recovery is shortened. No research has been published on this issue, however.

Rigorous massage that demands an adaptive response is best delayed until the acute phase of a cold has passed. Cold viruses are contagious through casual contact, so therapists must also take precautions on behalf of their own health. Massage during recovery may be safe, but clients may be uncomfortable being prone for prolonged periods, as this puts pressure on the sinuses.

BENEFITS Gentle work may be soothing and effective to promote good sleep at any stage of a cold. Someone who is recovering from a cold may especially appreciate what massage can do to help clear the sinuses. A client who has fully recovered from a cold can enjoy the same benefits from bodywork as the rest of the population.

Influenza

Definition: What Is It?

Influenza or flu is a viral infection of the respiratory tract. Seasonal flu is usually a relatively benign, self-limiting infection, but it can become life-threatening if an aggressive virus invades a vulnerable patient. A flu infection with a particularly virulent virus, or in a person with limited immune resources, can be a deadly situation.

Demographics

It is estimated that the flu affects anywhere from 5% to 20% of the United States population each year. Flu and its complications hospitalize 200,000 people, and kill an average of 23,000 to 36,000 Americans each year, although some years that number approaches 50,000.

Etiology: What Happens?

Flu viruses work in the usual way of infectious agents: they gain access to the body, usually by inhalation or touch from a contaminated surface that carries the virus to a portal of entry: the nose, mouth, or eye. Then the viruses invade their primary targets: mucus-producing cells that line the respiratory tract.

Once the infection is established, the immune system response causes most of the extreme symptoms. White blood cells attack infected cells, causing sore throat and coughing. They also release the chemicals that stimulate fever. It can take 2 or 3 days for symptoms to appear, but the person is shedding virus in oral and mucous secretions during that time. The peak of communicability is usually around day 4 of the infection. The person continues to shed virus throughout the acute and subacute stages.

Three classes of flu virus have been identified. The type A viruses are the most virulent, responsible for major epidemics that can claim millions of lives (Sidebar 7.1). Type A viruses

SIDEBAR 7.1 We Are All under the Influence: The History of Flu

Symptoms of the infectious disease now called flu have been documented since the 5th century BCE. It was observed in those early days of medicine that this disorder could spread throughout a population, but symptoms sometimes wouldn't appear for a few days after exposure, and it continued to spread for several days after all symptoms were gone among the original patients. Because its course seemed so mysterious, it was assumed to be controlled by the influence of the planets and stars. In the early 1500s, the Italian term for influence (influenza) became the common name for this disorder.

The first recorded pandemic of flu virus is known from records from Europe from 1580. The 20th century saw three pandemics of flu infections and a strong threat of a fourth. So far the 21st century has seen one pandemic.

- 1918 to 1921. The "Spanish Lady" was a flu virus that in the course of 3 years killed half a million people in the United States and more than 30 to 40 million people worldwide. It is credited with helping to end WWI because so many soldiers were lost to this pandemic: most of the deaths were in people 15 to 35 years old.
- 1957. Asian flu: 70,000 deaths in the United States, 1 to 2 million worldwide.
- 1968. Hong Kong flu: 34,000 deaths in the United States, about 1 million worldwide.
- 1997. In Hong Kong a new flu virus was identified that was directly communicable from birds to people. It infected 18 people and killed 6, but if it had escaped Hong Kong, it could have killed millions more. It was controlled by an aggressive public health effort that ended in the slaughter of all of Hong Kong's domestic poultry to limit the spread of the virus. The flu that appeared in 1997 is the same virus (H5N1) that is now called "bird flu"; it is closely related to the virus that caused the "Spanish Lady" pandemic of 1918.
- 2009. An alarming outbreak of "swine flu" (H1N1) began in April, and by June it was labeled a pandemic. It was especially virulent among adults under 65—a population that is not usually threatened by flu infections. It killed 12,000 Americans in 2009, but coverage for H1N1 in subsequent flu vaccines has made it a much less threatening infection.

mutate quickly and so can cause repeated infections in the same person. Type B flu viruses can also spread, but they are not as aggressive or widely spread as type A viruses. Type C flu viruses are not associated with epidemics, and they are relatively stable. They create much less severe symptoms than the other types.

Type A flu viruses are remarkably adaptable. They can infect several species besides humans, including birds, pigs, ferrets, seals, whales, and horses. It appears that when flu passes from one species to another, it undergoes some minor changes to its enzymes that allow it to invade its new host. In some cases, it may move directly from animals to humans without mutation. Type A flu viruses also have the ability to mutate as they develop resistance to attack. This makes it impossible for a person to establish permanent immunity, because each time we are exposed, the pathogen is different.

Type A viruses are labeled according to the presence of certain proteins, called **hemagglutinin** and **neuraminidase**, on their outer coat. Researchers have identified 15 subtypes of hemagglutinin and 9 subtypes of neuraminidase, and individual strains of virus are named for the subtypes they carry. For instance, the most common forms of human flu are H2N2 and H3N1.

Flu can become life-threatening because it can allow the possibility of an opportunistic secondary infection in the shape of **pneumonia** or **acute bronchitis**. This is a particular danger for high-risk populations: those under 2 to 5 years old; those over 65 years old; smokers; diabetics; and people who are immunosuppressed, living in long-term care facilities, or affected by chronic lung or heart problems.

Types of Influenza

- *Seasonal flu*: This is the most common form of flu, and it can involve several different subtypes of type A viruses. It is most active from fall through early spring.
- *H5N1* (Avian flu): Also called "bird flu," this is a variety that passes from wild water birds (swans, geese, ducks) to domestic poultry with devastating results. In rare cases, it has passed from birds to humans (typically when people are working or living with infected poultry), and very rarely from person to person. Since 2003 only about 630 people have been diagnosed with bird flu worldwide with 375 deaths. This strain is extremely virulent with a high mortality rate among humans, so it is being watched closely. If it mutates with a more communicable form of seasonal flu, the results could be very dangerous.
- *H1N1* (Swine flu): This variety was recognized in a fast-moving international outbreak in 2009. H1N1 is unique among flu viruses in that it appears to target people under 65 years old with very extreme and sometimes fatal consequences.

> **Hemagglutinin:** A type of protein that causes agglutination of red blood cells. Found on the outer coating of influenza and other antigens.
>
> **Neuraminidase:** A protein found on the outer surface of influenza viruses.
>
> **Neti pot:** A container used to administer nasal flushing in order to clear the sinuses.
>
> **Neuraminidase inhibitors:** A class of antiviral drugs that targets influenza.

Signs and Symptoms

Flu symptoms can range from subtle to fatal within hours or days. For most common infections, the symptoms look like a bad cold: respiratory irritation with runny nose and dry cough, sore throat, headache, chills, and a long-lasting high fever (see Figure 7.2). While not all flu patients develop a fever, it is not unusual for flu-related fever to go over 102°F (38.9°C) in adults, and it may last for 3 days or more. Most flu infections cause symptoms that affect more than the upper respiratory tract, however. Many patients have aching muscles and joints, and debilitating fatigue. For more information on how flu differs from the **common cold**, see Compare & Contrast 7.2.

One area that flu viruses generally don't attack is the gastrointestinal (GI) tract. What is commonly referred to as "stomach flu" is far more likely to be infection with Norovirus or a case of food poisoning. Flu infections can involve vomiting and diarrhea, but this is related to systemic stress and inflammation rather than a specific attack in the GI tract.

Flu symptoms usually appear about 3 days after exposure to the virus, and they may persist for up to 2 weeks. If they persist longer than that, or if the coughing begins to produce a lot of streaked or opaque phlegm, it may be that the original viral infection has complicated to a secondary infection of the lungs: pneumonia.

Treatment

As a viral infection, flu is unaffected by antibiotics. Good-sense measures include rest and liquids. Over-the-counter drugs may abate the symptoms but do not speed healing. They can be useful, however, if the symptoms are preventing a person from getting the sleep necessary to heal. **Neti pots** and other nasal rinsing devices help some people, but it is important to keep this equipment scrupulously clean, or these devices may serve to spread infections instead of helping to treat them.

A group of antiviral drugs called **neuraminidase inhibitors**, includes the name brands Tamiflu and Relenza. These need to be started within 48 hours of symptom onset, but they can shorten the duration of a flu infection, reduce the severity of symptoms, and decrease the risk of complications.

Every year the Food and Drug Administration distributes a vaccine to fight a combination of type A and type B viruses. These vaccines are formulated about 9 months ahead of flu season. Because viruses mutate quickly, flu vaccines must be updated every year. The Centers for Disease Control and Prevention recommend flu vaccines for most people, but especially for high-risk populations,

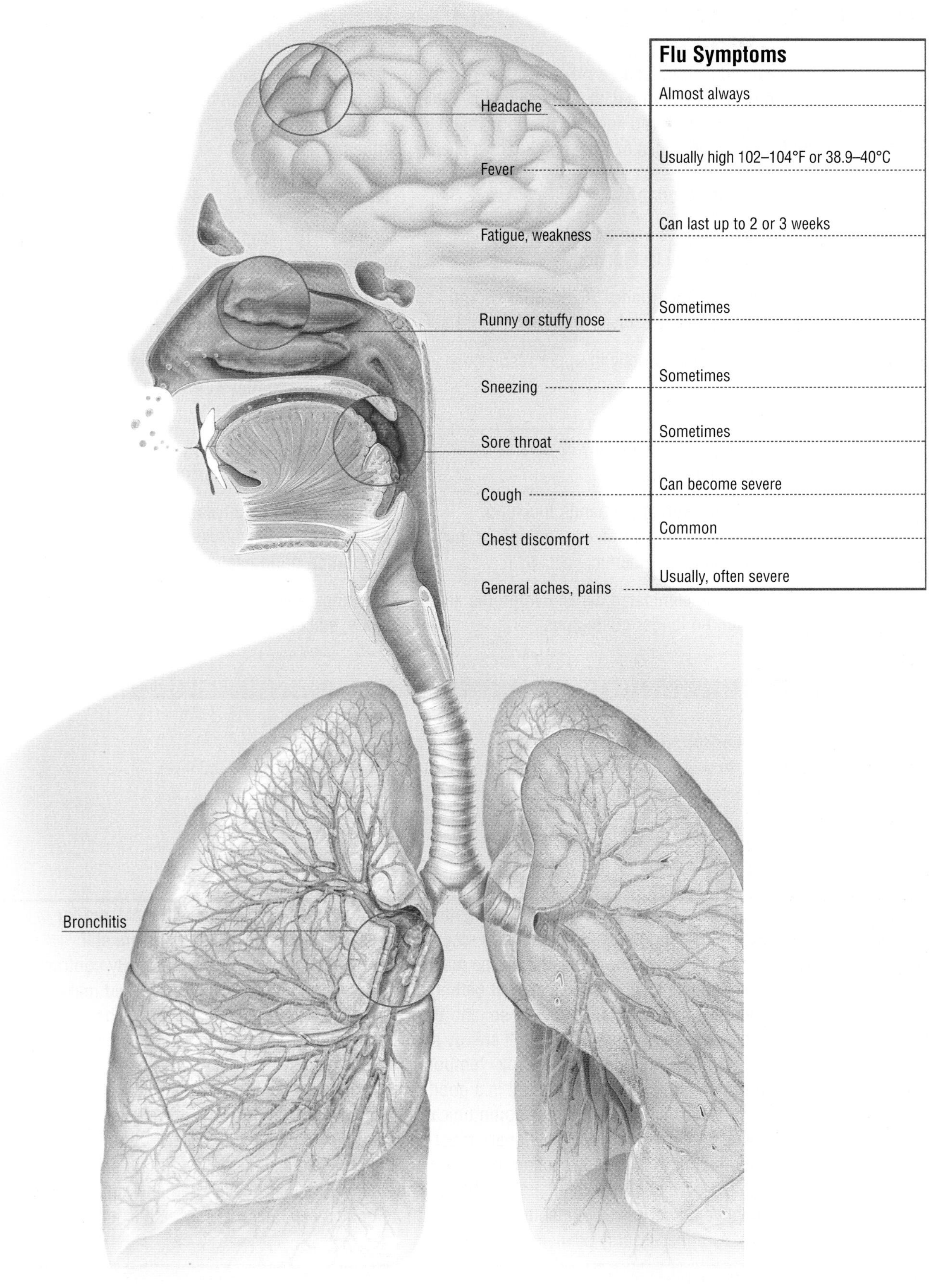
Flu Symptoms
Headache
Almost always
Fever
Usually high 102–104°F or 38.9–40°C
Fatigue, weakness
Can last up to 2 or 3 weeks
Runny or stuffy nose
Sometimes
Sneezing
Sometimes
Sore throat
Sometimes
Cough
Can become severe
Chest discomfort
Common
General aches, pains
Usually, often severe
Bronchitis

FIGURE 7.2 Symptoms of flu

COMPARE & CONTRAST 7.2 Is It a Cold? Is It the Flu? Does It Matter?

Colds and flu are both caused by viral attacks on cells in the respiratory tract. They have similar symptoms, and they carry similar cautions about working with clients who have these infections. Still, flu can be much worse than a cold. Flu is more contagious, and it can linger in the body much longer, and it can occasionally be life-threatening. Therefore, it's useful to have a clear idea of which pathogen a client is battling.

PRESENTATION	COMMON COLD	INFLUENZA
Duration	Usually less than a week, although the cough may last longer.	Could be 10 days or more.
Fever	Usually low (under 102°F, 38.9°C) and short-term (resolves within 48 hours).	Usually high (over 102°F, 38.9°C) and long-term (may persist for 3 days or more).
Location	Symptoms strictly in upper respiratory tract.	Possible systemic muscle and joint pain, inflamed lymph nodes, irritated GI tract, debilitating fatigue.
Complications	Complications usually involve sinus or ear infection.	Complications affect the lower respiratory tract as bronchitis or pneumonia.
Communicability	Usually spread by hands touching contaminated surfaces. Contagious, but not usually epidemic.	Usually spread by inhalation of airborne virus. Often highly virulent; may infect high proportion of population.
Resolution	Quickly eliminated; when symptoms are over, no longer contagious.	May linger several days after symptoms abate, still communicable.

including those who are immunosuppressed and who have chronic respiratory illnesses: these are people for whom a flu infection is most likely to complicate to life-threatening pneumonia.

Medications

- NSAIDs for general malaise and fever
- Antivirals
- Neuraminidase inhibitors

Massage Therapy Implications

RISKS

A lot of anecdotal evidence has been gathered about massage for clients with cold and flu. Experience suggests that if a person receives a massage while these infections are still becoming established, then he or she may be more extremely ill than otherwise. By contrast, many people have experienced that getting a massage after a cold or flu has peaked makes them feel sick again for a day or so, and then the rest of their recovery appears to be shortened: they come back to full energy and vitality quickly. For this reason, it is important to inform clients that massage may temporarily exacerbate symptoms so they can make an informed choice about whether it is a good time for them to receive bodywork.

Influenza viruses are highly communicable through airborne droplets as well as by way of contaminated surfaces. Practitioners must be aware that working with clients who have flu puts them at risk for contracting this infection. Clients in an acute stage of flu are engaged in fighting off an aggressive infection. While gentle bodywork that doesn't demand an extensive adaptive response may be soothing and promote good sleep, any more intrusive bodywork may be unnecessarily challenging.

BENEFITS

Gentle, nondemanding bodywork during an acute phase of flu may be highly relaxing, as long as the practitioner takes appropriate precautions. After the acute phase has passed, massage to promote good sleep and rebounded energy may be useful.

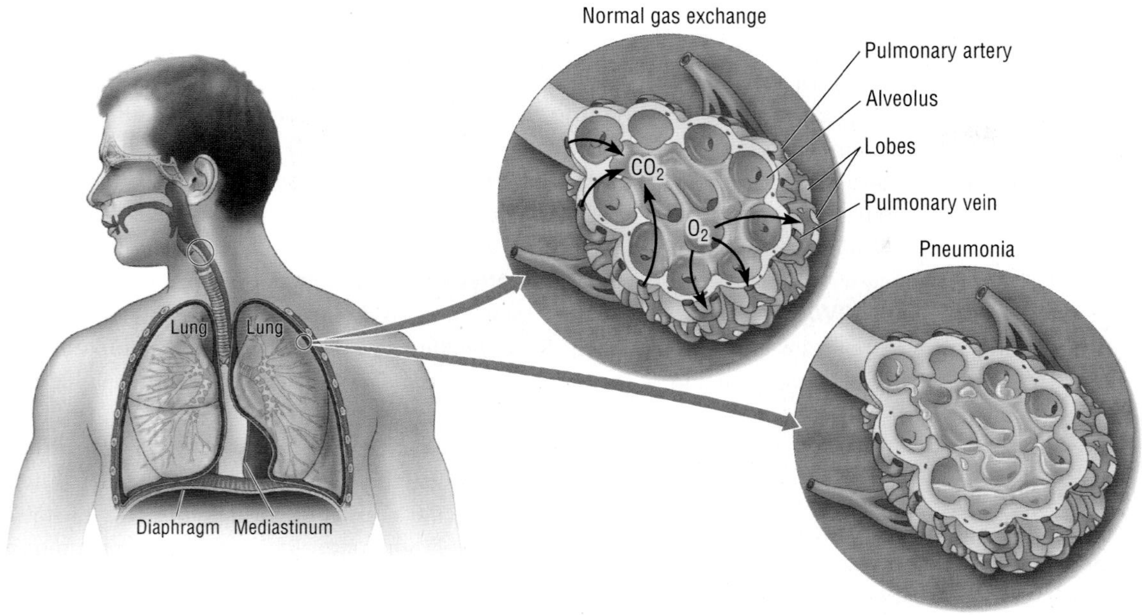

FIGURE 7.3 Pneumonia: the alveoli fill with mucus and gaseous exchange cannot take place

Pneumonia

Definition: What Is It?

Pneumonia is a general term for inflammation of the lungs, usually due to an infectious agent. The severity of pneumonia ranges from being not much worse than a bad cold to being a cause of death within 24 hours.

Demographics

Because it is an opportunistic infection that takes advantage of weak immune systems, pneumonia is the leading cause of death by infectious disease in the United States. It accounts for about 1.1 million hospital stays each year; each one is an average of 5 days. Pneumonia is responsible for about 52,000 deaths each year, most of them in people over 65 years old.

Etiology: What Happens?

The alveoli are the tiny hollow balloons with walls made of squamous epithelium found at the very end of the bronchioles in the lungs. A net of tiny capillaries from the pulmonary circuit surrounds each alveolus: this is the site of oxygen-carbon dioxide exchange. In an infectious agent enters these tiny structures, the alveoli fill with dead white blood cells, mucus, and fluid seeping back from the capillaries (Figure 7.3). Eventually, the normal diffusion of gases is impossible. Abscesses may form, and capillary damage may occur, allowing bleeding into the alveoli and eventually into the sputum.

In extreme infections, the pleurae may be affected as well as the lung tissue. Scar tissue can develop between layers, leading to pain and limited movement with each breath; this is called **pleurisy**. Alternatively, the pleural fluid itself can host infection in a condition called **empyema**.

Several infectious agents can cause pneumonia, and more than one type of pathogen may be present at a time: a fact that sometimes makes diagnosis and treatment of this condition a challenge.

- *Viruses*. Viral infections account for about half of pneumonia cases. Influenza and **respiratory syncytial virus** are the most common culprits. Other viruses include cytomegalovirus, herpes simplex, and adenovirus. The incubation period of viral pneumonia is 1 to 3 days. Viral pneumonia tends to be short-lived and not serious. It appears most frequently in children.
- *Bacteria*. Varieties of staphylococci and streptococci often live harmlessly in the nose and throat, but when resistance is low, they may invade the lower respiratory tract to set up an infection in the lungs. The toxins released by the bacteria initiate an inflammatory response, leading to edema in the alveoli and a reduced ability to draw oxygen into the system. This kind of infection usually responds well to antibiotics. *Streptococcus pneumoniae*, also called pneumococcus, is the most common form of bacterial pneumonia. Another infection is caused by *Legionella pneumoniae*, named for the Legionnaires' convention where it was first identified in 1977. Chlamydia (a different pathogen from the chlamydia that causes sexually transmitted infections) and tuberculosis bacilli can also cause bacterial pneumonia.
- *Mycoplasma*. Often described as tiny bacteria, mycoplasma are the smallest free-living infectious agents ever found. The incubation period for mycoplasma pneumonia is 1 to 4 weeks, and

Empyema: Pus in a body cavity.

Respiratory syncytial virus (RSV): A common virus that causes colds in healthy adults, but can be serious in infants and the immunocompromised.

7 Respiratory System Conditions

because it tends not to be as severe as bacterial or viral types of infection, it is sometimes called "walking pneumonia" or "atypical pneumonia." Fortunately, like bacterial pneumonia, mycoplasma pneumonia responds well to antibiotics.

- *Fungi.* Some fungi that are endemic to certain areas of the United States are associated with pneumonia.
- *Pneumocystis carinii. Pneumocystis carinii*, also called pneumocystis jiroveci, is subtype of fungus that causes an infection almost exclusively associated with immunosuppressed patients, such as those with **HIV/AIDS**; people receiving chemotherapy for cancer or immunosuppressive drugs to prevent the rejection of organ transplants; and those who don't have a functioning spleen.

Considering the delicacy of the epithelium in the lungs, it is amazing that if a pneumonia infection is short-lived, it is completely reversible. The body can liquefy and absorb the consolidated matter in affected alveoli, and it can reabsorb the fluid from any inflamed part of the lung. A basically healthy patient who gets appropriate treatment can expect to recover fully within 2 weeks. Untreated pneumonia, however, has a high mortality rate. It can also complicate into **meningitis**, respiratory failure, and bacteremia (the presence of bacteria in the blood, a type of blood poisoning); these situations are nearly always fatal.

In long-standing cases with accumulation of **pulmonary fibrosis** and scar tissue, permanent damage to the elasticity of the epithelial tissue may occur, or the freedom with which the lungs move in the pleural cavity may be compromised. This can raise the risk of future infections.

When people develop pneumonia as a complication of an underlying disorder, this infection can be life-threatening. Secondary pneumonia is an opportunistic disease. It is often the final complication of other serious conditions, even noninfectious ones. People who have had a **stroke**, **heart failure**, **alcoholism**, or **cancer** die of pneumonia more often than any other disease. People who are bedridden or paralyzed are susceptible too, because their cough reflex is often impaired; they cannot expel mucus easily. Having a preexisting respiratory problem such as **flu**, **chronic bronchitis**, **emphysema**, or **asthma** is an open invitation. And finally, being immunosuppressed because of tissue transplant, **AIDS**, **sickle cell disease**, steroid use, **leukemia**, or cytotoxic drug use makes a person particularly vulnerable to pneumonia.

Many cases of pneumonia could be prevented through appropriate vaccine use. The annual flu vaccine, if it is effective against the circulating viruses, prevents flu infections from complicating into viral or bacterial pneumonia. Pneumovax, a vaccine against pneumococcus, is also available. This vaccine is recommended for high-risk patients and for people who live or work in long-term care facilities or hospitals.

Types of Pneumonia by Location

- *Bronchopneumonia*: This starts as a bronchial inflammation and spreads into the lungs. It appears in a patchy pattern all over the lungs, not segregated to a specific area.
- *Lobar pneumonia*: This is restricted to one lobe of the lungs. Eventually, the whole lobe may be affected (Figure 7.4).
- *Double pneumonia*: This affects both lungs. It can be bacterial or viral.

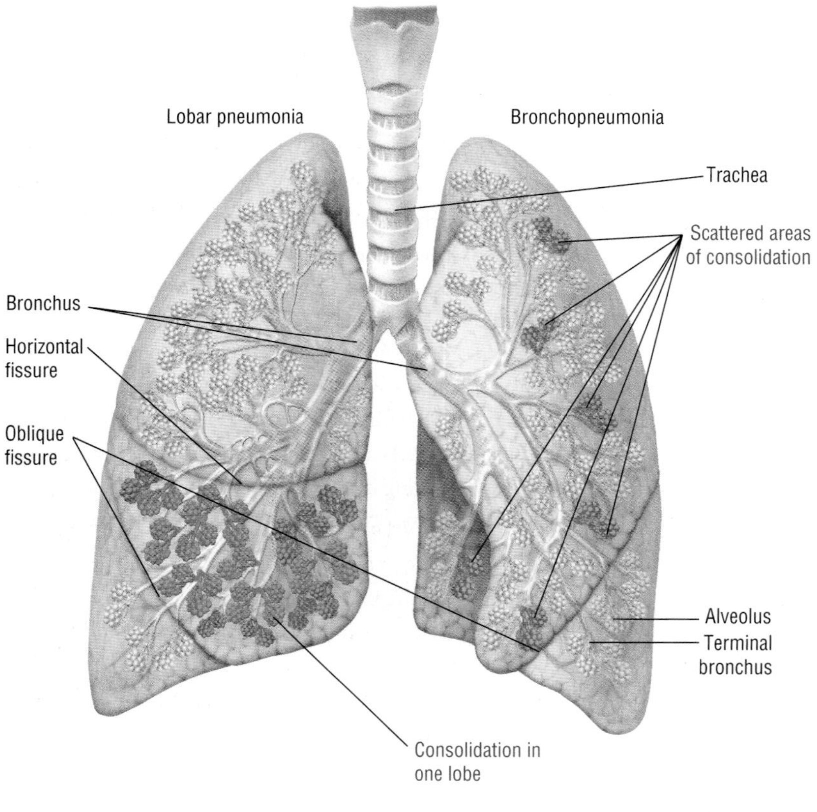

FIGURE 7.4 Lobar pneumonia is confined to one area; bronchopneumonia is in patchy areas all over the lung

Types of Pneumonia by Source of Infection

- *Community-acquired pneumonia*: This is the most common form. It is usually a bacterial infection or a complication of flu.
- **Nosocomial** *or hospital-acquired pneumonia*: This is an infection in that develops within 48 hours of being in a hospital or other healthcare setting.
- *Aspiration pneumonia*: This is an infection brought about when a person accidently inhales food, liquid, or other substances into the lungs. It is a particular risk for anyone with swallowing difficulties or with a weakened cough reflex.

Signs and Symptoms

Signs and symptoms of pneumonia vary widely depending on the causative factor and how much of the lung is affected. They include coughing, very high fever, chills, sweating, delirium, chest pains, **cyanosis**, thick and colored sputum, shortness of breath, muscle aches and pains, and pleurisy.

Pneumonia can have a sudden or gradual onset. Very often it follows the same course as flu, but instead of getting better, the respiratory symptoms get rapidly worse and are accompanied by fever up to 104°F (40°C).

Treatment

Treatment depends entirely on what type of pneumonia is present. Bacterial and mycoplasma pneumonias generally respond well to antibiotics, but these do not apply for viral infections. Cough suppressants are generally discouraged because they interfere with the ability to move contaminated mucus.

Symptomatic relief and supportive therapy include breathing humidified air, drinking ample fluids, and supplementing oxygen, if necessary. If damage to the pleurae is extensive, surgery to drain the pleural space may be conducted.

Medications

- Antibiotics if necessary
- Antiviral medication if necessary
- NSAIDs for fever reduction and general malaise

Nosocomial: A hospital-acquired infection.

Cyanosis: A bluish coloration of the skin and mucous membranes due to insufficient oxygenation.

Rhinitis: Inflammation of the nasal mucous membrane.

Massage Therapy Implications

RISKS	Pneumonia is a serious and complicated condition that frequently accompanies other serious disorders. A client with this condition should not be challenged by rigorous massage. Gentle, reflexive work may be supportive, as long as the therapist is safe from the risk of infection.
BENEFITS	When the acute phase of pneumonia has passed, massage can be helpful for a person is undergoing a long and slow recovery. A person who has fully recovered from pneumonia can enjoy all the benefits from bodywork as the rest of the population.
OPTIONS	Although today this is typically done by machine, manual percussion on the chest to loosen mucus can be helpful for a person recovering from pneumonia.

Sinusitis

Definition: What Is It?

Sinusitis, as the name implies, is a condition in which the mucous membranes that line the sinuses become inflamed and swollen. It can be due to infectious or noninfectious causes. The difference between sinusitis and **rhinitis** is that the sinuses encompass more than the nose, so rhinitis could be seen as a subset of sinusitis.

Demographics

It is estimated that 37 million Americans or more develop sinusitis each year. These numbers are increasing, possibly from increased indoors and outdoors pollution, and more antibiotic resistance.

Etiology: What Happens?

Sinuses are hollow areas lateral to, above, and behind the nose (Figure 7.5). They provide resonance for the voice, and they lighten the weight of the head. The mucous membranes lining sinuses are provided with cilia, tiny hairs that move the mucus along so that trapped pathogens and particulate matter can be expelled or swallowed and destroyed instead of reaching the lower respiratory system.

When the cilia break down or are paralyzed, often as a result of viral infection or environmental irritants, pathogen-laden mucus lingers over delicate epithelial cells, and stimulating an inflammatory response. Soon the hollow

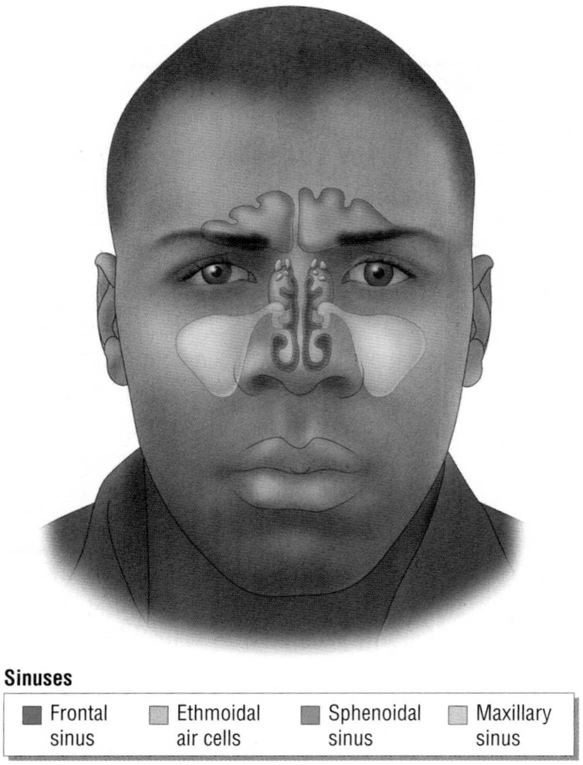

FIGURE 7.5 Location of sinuses

areas fill with sticky, pus-filled mucus that cannot drain. This forms an ideal growth medium for bacteria that normally colonize the sinuses.

Alternatively, the cilia may remain intact and highly functional, but the mucous membranes are stimulated to respond to oak pollen or other allergens as if they were life-threatening pathogens. Inflammation ensues with the production of huge amounts of thin, runny mucus; puffy, itchy eyes; and all of the symptoms associated with allergic rhinitis or hay fever. This can also provide a hospitable environment for local bacteria, so a person with hay fever has a significantly higher than normal risk of intermittent sinus infections.

Many different factors can cause inflamed sinuses, including the following:

- *Viruses and bacteria*. The most common types of sinusitis begin as viral infections such as **cold** or **flu**. Then when defense mechanisms are low, the bacteria that normally colonize the skin and mucous membranes take advantage, and begin to multiply. The bacteria most commonly associated with these infections are *Streptococcus pneumonia*, *Haemophilus influenza*, or *Moraxalla catarrhis*.
- *Fungi and bacteria*. Some people with chronic sinusitis have significant amounts of fungal growth in their sinuses. These micro-organisms can trigger an immune system response that causes all the symptoms of sinusitis. This is a problem particularly for persons with **diabetes**, **HIV/AIDS**, or other immunosuppressive disorders.
- *Structural problems*. A deviated septum or the growth of nasal polyps can obstruct the flow of mucus out of the sinuses. Structural anomalies in the shape of the facial bones can also block drainage. This is not an infection to begin with, but mucus held back from normal flow is an inviting growth medium for bacteria, so what begins as a simple structural anomaly can become a true infection.
- *Environmental irritants*. Exposure to cigarette smoke (first- or second-hand), indoors and outdoors pollutants, cocaine, or other irritants can destroy cilia and increase the risk of infection.
- *Other conditions*. Acute or chronic sinusitis is frequently seen with other conditions. Severe dental **caries** raises the risk of sinusitis, probably from the availability of local bacteria. **Asthma** is closely associated with sinusitis, as both conditions have to do with excessive mucus production and a hyperreactive inflammatory response.

Types of Sinusitis

- *Noninfectious sinusitis*: Also called allergic rhinitis or hay fever, this causes inflammation of the sinus membranes without underlying infection. Hay fever is often distinguished from infectious sinusitis by the lack of congestion and by the quality of the nasal discharge. It tends to be thin and runny, rather than thick and sticky. People with hay fever do have inflamed sinuses however, which puts them at risk for secondary infections.
- *Infectious sinusitis*: This is a pathogenic invasion followed by an inflammatory response that creates a vicious circle: the body creates excessive mucus to help remove infectious agents, but the inflamed tissues make drainage of that mucus (which can harbor bacteria and other pathogens) difficult or impossible. Sinus infections are often complications of respiratory tract infections like colds or flu.

Signs and Symptoms

Signs and symptoms of sinusitis vary according to the cause of the inflammation and which sinuses are involved. Severe **headache** is a key feature, especially upon waking. Bending over makes it much worse, because that position increases pressure on already stressed membranes. The affected area may be extremely painful to the touch, and swelling or puffiness around the eyes or cheeks may be visible. Fever and chills may accompany an acute bacterial infection. Sore throat, coughing (caused by postnasal drip), and congestion or runny nose may appear with any type of sinus irritation, along with bad breath and possible ear pain. And regardless of whether it is infectious or allergic, people with sinusitis

Caries: Severe decay of tooth or bone.

are likely to experience fatigue and general malaise because the body is fighting hard to cast off an invader.

The mucus expressed with a sinus infection is likely to be streaked or opaque, in shades that range from pale green to yellow to brown. It tends to be thick and sticky. The mucus expressed with hay fever, on the other hand, tends to be thin, runny, and clear.

The duration of an episode of sinusitis depends on what causes it and how it is treated. Nasal inflammation associated with seasonal allergies may persist for weeks or months at a time, while infections may resolve within 2 weeks if antibiotics are effective.

Treatment

Treatment for sinusitis begins with self-help measures: staying in humid air or breathing steam to help moisturize and liquefy clogged mucus is an important step. Increasing daily water intake and reducing the use of alcohol, caffeine, and other diuretics may also help to soften and loosen thick, sticky mucus. Many experts recommend using a saline wash to rinse the sinuses regularly with a Neti pot or other device; the Centers for Disease Control and Prevention have developed some guidelines to reduce the risk of contamination and nasal irritation: keeping the instrument clean is vital, but even more so is the preparation of the water. Safe-to-drink tap water may harbor pathogens that can survive in the sinuses, so it is important to use sterile water. Using air filters to remove irritating particles from the air can also help.

Drugs prescribed for this disorder begin with antibiotics if the infection is bacterial. Sinuses are difficult to access, and the bacteria associated with most cases of sinusitis tend to be drug resistant, so this condition often requires a long-term course of specialized antibiotics.

Decongestants are sometimes recommended to shrink the mucous membranes, but these are only appropriate for short-term use because they can create a significant rebound effect when usage is stopped. Corticosteroids in nasal spray form can reduce swelling, but they can take several weeks to become effective.

In very extreme cases surgery is recommended. This involves inserting a tube through the nose and enlarging sinus passages, removing polyps, repairing a deviated septum, and doing anything else that may assist the mucus to drain freely. Using tiny balloons on catheters (**balloon sinusotomy**) tends to have fewer risks than traditional endoscopy, and it can also be used with children, unlike some other interventions.

> **Balloon sinusotomy:** A procedure in which a balloon is inflated inside the sinuses in order to restructure them without extensive scarring.

Medications

- Antibiotics if necessary, along with acidophilus to reduce the risk of yeast infections
- Mucolytics to help dissolve mucus
- Antihistamines
- Antifungal medication if necessary
- Decongestants and antihistamines
- Steroidal anti-inflammatories by nasal spray

Massage Therapy Implications

RISKS	Acute sinus infections, especially with fever, headache, and general malaise, contraindicate any bodywork that might exacerbate symptoms. While gentle work away from the face is unlikely to make this problem worse, a person running a fever is better off delaying rigorous massage until this crisis has been resolved. Clients with an acute infection are also likely to be uncomfortable lying flat on the table, prone, or supine.
BENEFITS	Clients who have inflamed sinuses that are not due to infection may derive benefits from bodywork, as long as they are comfortable on the table. Gentle and lymphatic work on and around the face may help the sinuses to drain, which can help to relieve symptoms.
OPTIONS	Therapists trained in lymphatic work find that this approach is often particularly successful for allergic sinusitis.

Tuberculosis

Definition: What Is It?

"Tubercle" means bump, as in the greater tubercle of the humerus. Tuberculosis (TB) is a disease involving pus- and bacteria-filled bumps, usually in the lungs but sometimes in other locations as well.

Demographics

The World Health Organization reports that almost 9 million people develop the active form of TB disease each year, and it causes about 1.5 million deaths. It is estimated that a new TB exposure happens roughly one time every second.

In the United States TB rates are going down. About 15 million Americans have been exposed, but in 2012, the Centers for Disease Control and Prevention reported just under 10,000 cases of active TB; this is the lowest number of active TB cases in this country since 1953, when record-keeping began. Distribution of TB in the United States is

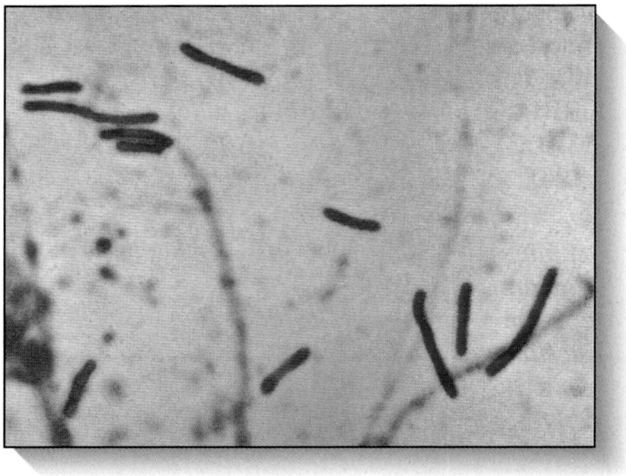

FIGURE 7.6 *Mycobacterium tuberculosis*: rod-shaped bacteria from a sputum sample

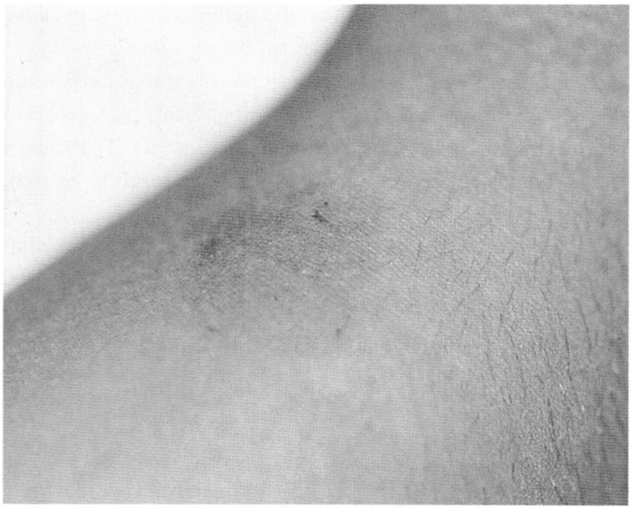

FIGURE 7.7 To check a patient for immunity to tuberculous, a Mantoux test is performed. Purified protein derivative, made from the bacteria, is injected intradermally. Then, 48 to 72 hours after the injection, an indurated inflamed area shows a positive sign.

not demographically even. It occurs in highest numbers among recent immigrants (63% of reported cases are among people who were born outside the United States), Native Americans, people of color, people with limited access to health care, and people in prisons or homeless shelters. TB is responsible for about 500 deaths in the United States each year.

Etiology: What Happens?

Tuberculosis is an airborne disease caused by *Mycobacterium tuberculosis* (see Figure 7.6). This is a bacterium with a waxy coat that allows it to survive outside of a host. When a person with an active infection coughs or sneezes, thousands of infective droplets are released into the air. The tiny bacteria, protected from drying out by their waxy covering, drift in the air until another host comes along and takes a deep breath.

Tuberculosis moves in the body in two phases:

- *Primary phase: TB exposure.* A person inhales some bacteria that travel all the way to the alveoli, where they are engulfed by macrophages. Their waxy coating makes them resistant to the macrophages' digestive enzymes. Instead, the bacteria slowly build up whole colonies inside the alveoli. Unable to expel these invaders, the body builds a protective fibrous wall around the site of infection: a tubercle. Tubercles are usually found in the lungs, but if some of the bacteria seep out into the bloodstream or lymph system, the same process happens elsewhere. Kidneys, the spine, and the central nervous system are the most common other locations for extrapulmonary tuberculosis.

  A single, tiny cyst in the lung is where TB stops for most people. This is TB exposure, but not the active disease; it is also called a **latent infection**. Within 10 to 12 weeks T-cells are activated, and a specific immune response ensues. The body is prepared to react to another contact with the bacillus, which is the mechanism behind the Mantoux skin test that looks for past exposure (see Figure 7.7). The inhaled bacteria remain contained inside their tidy fibrous package. They may stay there forever unless something happens to set them free: this is usually a depression in immune system function. A person with a latent infection cannot spread that infection to others.
- *Secondary phase: active disease.* Between 5% and 10% of the people exposed to TB eventually develop the active disease. This usually happens within the first year after exposure, but it can be decades later. The bacteria escape and spread into other areas in the lungs or wherever else in the body they may be stationed. The body attempts to surround the new sites with bigger and bigger fibrous capsules, which can cause permanent scarring. **Pleurisy**, the scarring and sticking of the pleurae, is a frequent complication of active TB. Inside the capsules, the bacteria destroy cells, and the tissue is necrotic or dead (Figure 7.8).

New tubercles eventually erode enough lung tissue to impede function. A cough begins, and gradually produces bloody sputum; this phlegm actually contains detached

NOTABLE CASES The list of historical and current public figures with tuberculosis is impressive indeed. It includes King Tutankhamen; writers John Keats, Emily Bronte, Fyodor Dostoevsky, and Robert Louis Stevenson; artist Paul Gaugin; First Lady Eleanor Roosevelt, former President of South Africa, and Nobel Peace Prize winner Nelson Mandela.

Latent infection: A condition in which a pathogen is present in a person but is dormant, causing no symptoms.

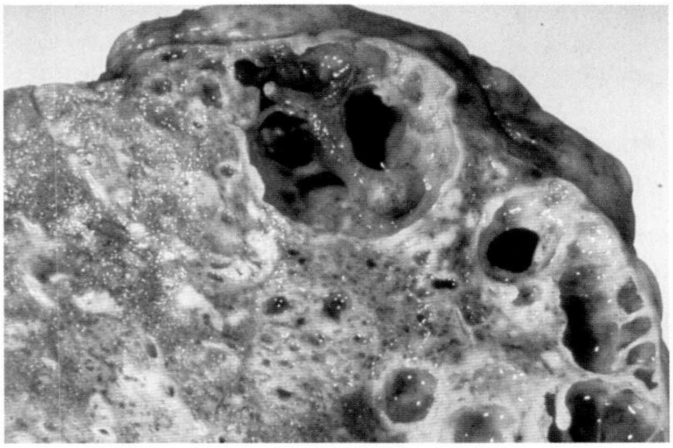

FIGURE 7.8 Cavitations with tuberculosis

pieces of the bacteria-infested tubercles, which is why active TB is contagious. If several of the tubercles join together, their necrotic centers can cause a large **cavitation** in the lung. Surrounding blood vessels may hemorrhage into the cavity leading to coughing up blood or hemoptysis. Similar lesions can develop in the kidneys if the tubercles form there. Infections in the bones tend to weaken bone structure and destroy articular cartilage.

The major risk factor for TB infection is exposure to someone with active disease. Travelers to parts of the world where TB is most common are at risk, as are people who spend time with immigrants from those areas, hospital workers, or residents of close living quarters where the disease may be rampant, such as prisons, nursing homes, and homeless shelters.

Once a person has been exposed to TB, the question is whether he or she will develop an active infection. Several variables that influence this process have been identified, including HIV status, socioeconomic standing, the use of injected illegal drugs, alcoholism, the presence of other immunosuppressive diseases or medications, age, and a history of not completing TB medication.

Coinfection with **HIV** is a major risk factor for TB making the transition from lesions to active disease. The risk that latent TB will become active increases each year that a person carries both infections. Studies suggest that about 20% of the people in the United States who have TB are also HIV-positive. Furthermore, having HIV and TB simultaneously can interfere with an accurate TB skin test, because a damaged immune system may not produce an adequate response to the purified test sample.

Types of Tuberculosis

- *Drug-susceptible tuberculosis*. This is the most common type of tuberculosis that is the main focus for this discussion. It is sensitive to first-line antibiotics, and the prognosis for a fully treated patient is excellent.

Cavitation: The formation of pits or holes.

- *Multidrug resistant tuberculosis (MDR-TB)*. This is a mutation that occurs when a patient does not fully treat drug-susceptible tuberculosis. The bacteria are resistant to all first-line antibiotics, so it requires much more expensive treatment with drugs that may have dangerous side effects. A person with active MDR-TB in an active form spreads this mutation of the bacteria to others. Seventy-two cases of MDR-TB were reported in the United States in 2012.
- *Extensively drug resistant tuberculosis (XDR-TB)*. This strain of TB is resistant to most antibiotics, so its treatment is limited to less effective drugs. Between 1993 and 2011, 63 cases of XDR-TB were been identified in the United States. It is most common in the former Soviet Union, parts of Asia, and among HIV-positive populations in South Africa.

Signs and Symptoms

The primary phase of TB is so benign a person may never know about the exposure; the symptoms, if any develop at all, are the same as for a mild flu. But the active disease shows much more severe symptoms. They include fever, sweating, weight loss, and exhaustion. Chest pain and shortness of breath are common. A stubborn cough that starts dry and becomes productive of bloody or pus-filled phlegm is a cardinal sign. Other symptoms arise if other organs have been infected as well: bone pain, blood in the urine, or central nervous system symptoms, for instance.

Treatment

In the old days, wealthy TB patients were sent to sanitaria, where it was hoped that sunlight, rest, and good food would enable them to outlive their infection. Many modern day spas and resorts began their lives as TB sanitaria. Fresh air, rest, and good nutrition are still good ideas, but they work even better when they are combined with the right antibiotics (See sidebar 7.2).

Anyone who has drug-susceptible TB, whether the infection is latent or active, can successfully treat it, including people who are HIV-positive. People identified with latent TB who are high risk for active disease are recommended to treat it with a single medication called isoniazid (INH) for 9 months. Alternatively, they could use a combination of INH and another drug called rifampin (RIF) for a shorter time. People with active TB need INH or RIF along with several other medications for 6 to 9 months in order to prevent mutation to a drug resistant form. Common side effects include sensitivity to sunlight, and yellow or orange tears, sweat, and saliva. More serious side effects include liver damage, neuropathy, joint pain, dizziness, tinnitus, and other problems. These are most likely to develop if a person takes TB medication while consuming alcohol.

Drug resistant forms of TB may need 2 years or more of multipronged antibiotic therapy.

SIDEBAR 7.2 A Tuberculosis Vaccine?

A vaccine against tuberculosis has been developed and is in use in some countries, but because of some inherit difficulties, it is not used in the United States. It is called the BCG, or bacille Calmette-Guérin, vaccine.

BCG vaccine can reduce the risk of contracting TB, but it comes with some problems. It is most effective for infants and young children; it is only sporadically effective for adults, and because it initiates an immune response to TB, a person vaccinated with BCG shows positive on all TB tests. This means that if the vaccine fails and a person is truly infected, the infection is difficult to identify while it is still latent.

Work on a more effective TB vaccine is under way. This, along with better means of delivering drugs, working with governments to educate patients and doctors, and many public outreach programs to limit the spread of TB around the globe, may eventually mean that this disease will be a thing of the past.

Medications

- Antibiotics: one for latent TB or up to four for active or MDR-TB.

Massage Therapy Implications

RISKS	Tuberculosis is contagious through indirect casual contact. For this reason, active untreated disease contraindicates massage. Clients treating TB may have side effects that impact massage choices.
BENEFITS	A client who is treating TB and who has received clearance risk of communicability can receive massage safely. A client who tests positive for TB exposure, but who has no active disease can also enjoy all the benefits from bodywork as the rest of the population, as long as drug side effects don't interfere with nerve, liver, or kidney function.

Chronic Obstructive Pulmonary Disorders

Chronic Bronchitis

Definition: What Is It?

Chronic bronchitis is part of a group of the closely connected lung problems called **chronic obstructive pulmonary disease (COPD)**. Chronic bronchitis, as its name implies, is long-term irritation of the bronchi and bronchioles, which may occur with or without infection. It is a progressive disorder that may be halted or slowed but not reversed. It often occurs simultaneously or as a predecessor to **emphysema**.

Demographics

COPD is the fourth leading cause of death in the United States. Statistics on COPD often don't separate chronic bronchitis from emphysema, as the two conditions are essentially on a sequential arc. Approximately 32 million Americans have been diagnosed with COPD. It is an age-related condition, much more common among those over 65 years old than among younger people. Men with COPD slightly outnumber women, but that ratio has been approaching equal for many years.

Chronic obstructive pulmonary disease (COPD): A progressive respiratory disease characterized by difficulty breathing.

Etiology: What Happens?

The act of breathing is a deceptively simple process. The muscles of inhalation lift and separate the ribs, which creates a vacuum in the thoracic cavity. Air rushes in to fill the empty space. When tissues are stretched, the impulse to inhale stops, and elastin fibers embedded in the lungs and all the membranes of the thorax essentially snap the rib cage back to its original shape. The lungs themselves do not dilate or contract; they are passively filled by muscles contracting to expand the rib cage, or emptied by the action of elastin fibers.

Chronic bronchitis is the result of long-term irritation to bronchial tubes. When the delicate lining of the respiratory tract is chronically insulted with cigarettes (first-hand, second-hand, or sidestream smoke), air pollutants, industrial chemicals, or other contaminants, an inflammatory response follows. Attacks against the bronchial lining destroy elastin fibers and cause overgrowth of mucus-producing cells, excessive production of mucus, and increased resistance to the movement of air in and out of the lungs (Figure 7.9). Eventually, the damage to the bronchioles is permanent; chronic bronchitis is an irreversible progressive disorder.

While exposure to tobacco smoke and other air pollutants is listed as the leading risk factor for developing chronic bronchitis, hyperreactivity in the bronchi is a close second.

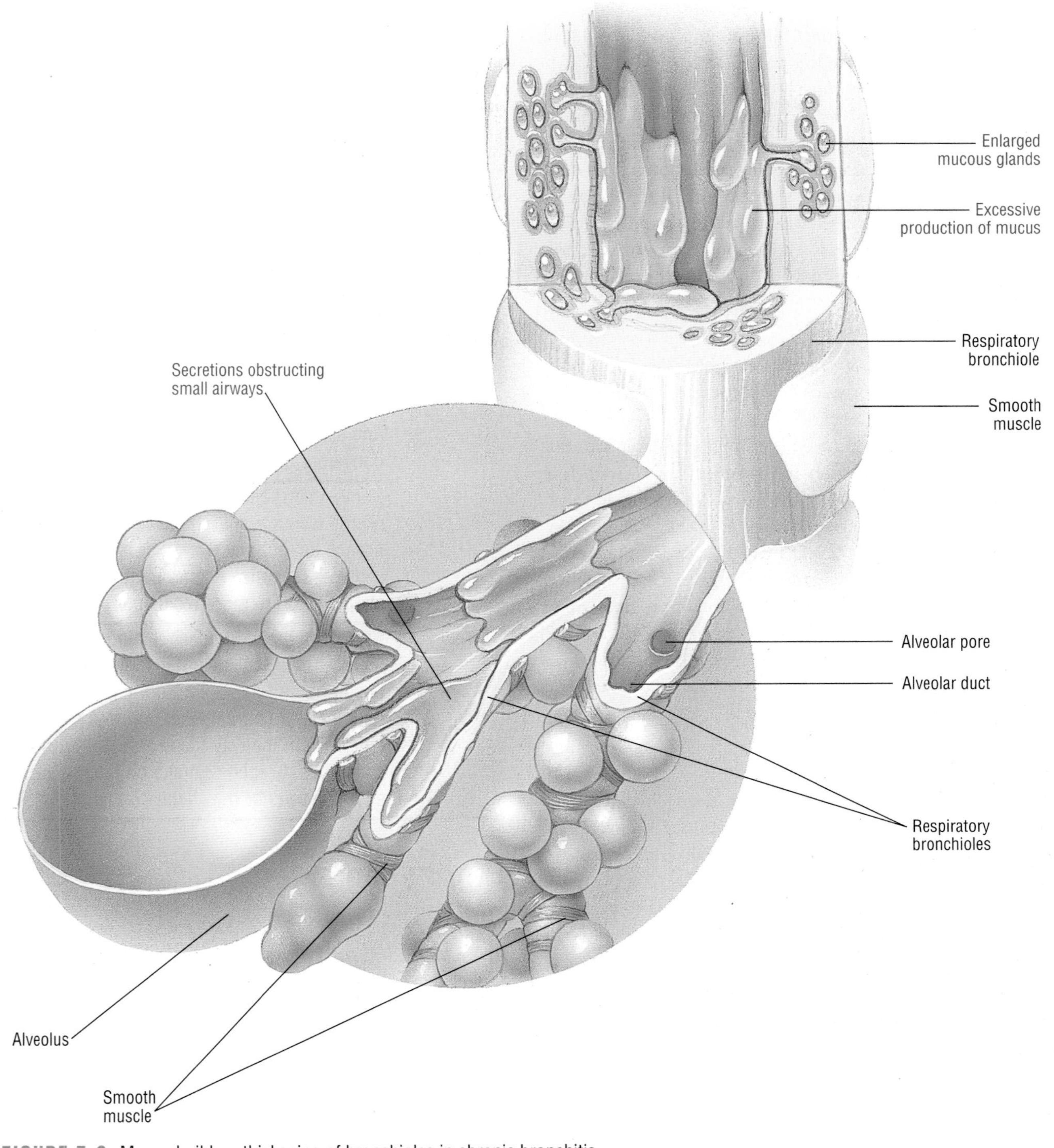

FIGURE 7.9 Mucus buildup, thickening of bronchioles in chronic bronchitis

These points to a very important priority for **asthma** patients to control their condition carefully.

As elastin breaks down, the act of exhalation becomes more difficult. At the same time, resistance in the airways means that less oxygen enters the body with each breath. The heart has to work harder to push enough blood into the lungs to supply the body with fuel. Further, red blood cell production may increase in an effort to provide more access to any oxygen that can seep into the capillaries. The blood may become thicker with excess erythrocytes (**polycythemia**), so the heart has to work even harder to push it through the pulmonary circuit. As oxygen levels in the blood drop, acidosis develops; this contributes to vasoconstriction in the

Polycythemia: An abnormally high number of red cells in the blood.

pulmonary arteries and worsens **pulmonary hypertension**. Eventually, **right-sided heart failure** may develop and lead to edema, especially in the legs and ankles.

Complications of chronic bronchitis are serious. Bronchi that are chronically inflamed and producing a lot of mucus are highly to viral or bacterial infection. A person with chronic bronchitis can develop life-threatening **pneumonia** from **cold** or **flu** viruses much more easily than the general population. In addition, the risk of right-sided heart failure is significant. This serious prognosis is the reason it is important to stop the progression of chronic bronchitis as soon as it can be recognized.

Signs and Symptoms

Signs and symptoms of chronic bronchitis develop slowly, often taking months or years before they are severe enough to attract attention. The process usually begins with a mild cough, perhaps following a typical flu or cold infection. But the cough lingers long after the infection has cleared. It is present most days for 3 months or more, producing thick, clear sputum. This pattern occurs for at least 2 years in a row.

Patients may have to clear their throat very often, especially in the morning; this reflects the excessive production of mucus in the lungs. Shortness of breath progresses and people become highly vulnerable to respiratory infections.

Later in the process, chronic bronchitis patients may develop signs of oxygen deprivation, including cyanosis and eventually edema related to right-sided heart failure.

Treatment

People with chronic bronchitis are especially susceptible to viral and bacterial infections of the respiratory tract. If a bacterial infection arises, aggressive treatment with antibiotics may be recommended to prevent life-threatening pneumonia. Chronic bronchitis patients are encouraged to be vaccinated against pneumococcus pneumonia and to get yearly flu shots for the same reason.

Other than preventing secondary infections, treatment for chronic bronchitis focuses on halting the progression of the damage and keeping the patient as comfortable as possible. Quitting smoking, if that is an issue, is the single most important step a chronic bronchitis patient can take. Patients are advised to avoid polluted air and known triggers of bronchial spasm. Oxygen may be provided in a medical emergency, but most chronic bronchitis patients don't need to supplement oxygen on a regular basis.

Balancing short-acting bronchodilators with longer-acting anti-inflammatories is often a successful strategy to manage this irreversible condition. Ultimately, a combination of medication, education, and careful exercise to rehabilitate underused tissues may slow or even stop the progression of chronic bronchitis.

Medications

- Bronchodilators to clear the airways.
- Inhaled and oral corticosteroids to control inflammation.
- Expectorants to assist in the clearing of mucus.
- Antibiotics as necessary to fight bacterial infection.

Massage Therapy Implications

RISKS	Chronic bronchitis patients may be uncomfortable lying flat on a table. Further, clients with chronic bronchitis are especially prone to respiratory infections that can rapidly become life-threatening. Any client in this situation should delay bodywork until the infection has resolved.
BENEFITS	Gentle massage can be supportive for clients who are quite frail with chronic bronchitis, but any work that requires an adaptive response should be reserved for people who are more resilient.
OPTIONS	Bodywork that addresses the intercostal muscles, the scalenes, the serratus posterior, and the diaphragm—all within tolerance, of course—can improve the efficiency in the way these muscles work, which has profound impact on fatigue and energy levels for the client.

Emphysema

Definition: What Is It?

The name emphysema means "blown up" (as in inflated, not exploded); this describes what happens to the alveoli as part of this disease process. Emphysema, along with chronic bronchitis, involves irreversible destruction of structures in the respiratory system. The collective name for **chronic bronchitis** and emphysema is COPD: chronic obstructive pulmonary disease. Because chronic bronchitis and emphysema are so often seen together, some specialists do not delineate between these two diseases.

Demographics

COPD is the third leading cause of death in the United States, and it is involved in about 125,000 deaths per year. For more on COPD statistics, see Sidebar 7.3.

Etiology: What Happens?

During a normal breathing cycle, muscles contract to increase the size of the thoracic cavity, and air rushes in to fill the vacuum. When those muscles relax, elastin in the epithelium of

Pulmonary hypertension: Abnormally high blood pressure in the arteries of the lungs.

SIDEBAR 7.3 Statistics on Chronic Obstructive Pulmonary Disease

It can be difficult to separate statistics for emphysema and chronic bronchitis, the two main conditions that make up the group called COPD, because many people have both conditions and many more have them in silent stages that aren't identified until their lungs have accrued extensive damage. About 13 million people in the United States have been diagnosed with COPD, but about 24 million adults have signs of impaired lung function, so COPD may be underdiagnosed. This disease spectrum costs the United States about $50 billion a year in direct healthcare expenses and indirect morbidity and mortality expenses.

The single greatest contributing factor to COPD is cigarette smoking; smoking causes 80% or more of COPD deaths. Men with COPD outnumbered women for many years, but for the last several years, mortality rate has been higher for women than men.

COPD kills (usually with overwhelming infection and respiratory failure) about 134,000 people every year, making it the third leading cause of death in the United States.

the lungs and elsewhere pulls the thoracic cavity back to its original size. In this way, exhalation is mainly a passive process that doesn't require muscular contraction. To forcibly expel extra air from the lungs (this is called **expiratory reserve volume**), the internal intercostals and transversus abdominus contract to compress the abdomen and thoracic cavity.

Normal, healthy lungs can be compared to a new balloon: filled with air it is stretched tight, and when it is released, the elastic walls force air out. If we want that to happen faster or more completely, we can squeeze the balloon from the outside. But when the balloon gets old and stretched out, it doesn't snap back to its original size. Its elastic walls don't compress well, and air can linger inside and become stale. This is essentially what happens to the alveoli in emphysema.

The lungs have 300 million alveoli that provide sites for oxygen-carbon dioxide exchange. Each one forms a tiny cup with its own circulatory capillary to allow the exchange of oxygen and carbon dioxide. All healthy alveoli are coated with **alpha-1 antitrypsin**, a protein that protects elastin from breaking down. Long-term exposure to cigarette smoke or other pollutants overcomes the protective abilities of alpha-1 antitrypsin, resulting in destruction of the alveolar elastin fibers. The alveoli lose their recoil ability, and they fill up with mucus, which interferes with their ability to exchange oxygen and carbon dioxide. Instead of emptying and filling with every breath, they only partially empty or stay altogether full. This usually begins in a small area, but if the irritation continues, inflammatory chemicals secreted by damaged cells can cause structural damage throughout the lung. The alveolar walls eventually break down and merge with each other forming larger sacs called **bullae** (Figure 7.10). These sacs have less volume and less surface area for gaseous exchange than the uninjured alveoli did, and they lack the elasticity and capacity for rebound that healthy alveoli have.

As the alveoli fuse and surface area for gaseous exchange is lost, the emphysema patient has to work much harder to move air in and out of the lungs. A person with healthy lungs expends about 5% of resting energy in the effort of breathing. A person with advanced emphysema puts closer to 50% of resting energy into this job and must do this every minute, 24 hours a day. For this reason, both eating and sleeping become extremely challenging for emphysema patients.

When alveoli lose function, gaseous exchange is impaired, leading to reduced oxygen levels in the blood or **hypoxia**. This is not only toxic to brain cells, but it triggers several vicious circles that affect respiration and cardiovascular function. Hypoxia causes the epithelial walls of the alveoli to thicken into tough fibrous connective tissue, which allows even less diffusion than before. As breathing becomes more difficult, respiration rate slows. This leads to even higher concentrations of carbon dioxide in the blood: hypoxia is exacerbated. The blood vessels supplying the damaged alveoli also sustain damage, and hypoxia can cause vascular spasm, so it becomes harder to pump blood through the pulmonary artery.

In addition to cardiovascular challenges, emphysema patients lose much of their ability to resist secondary infection, so they are extremely vulnerable to **influenza** and **pneumonia**. Another complication occurs if the bullae rupture; this allows air into the pleural space (which is supposed to be completely closed) and ends in total lung collapse or **pneumothorax**; and finally, the stress to the circulatory system is very great. The right ventricle, trying to pump blood through the partially collapsed pulmonary circuit, enlarges and eventually develops **right-sided heart failure** or cor pulmonale. The risk of blood clots forming in the circuit is also high, which results in **pulmonary embolism**. Eventually,

Expiratory reserve volume: The amount of air that can still be expelled from the lungs after a normal exhalation.

Alpha-1 antitrypsin: A protein that protects alveoli.

Bulla: A lesion in the lungs where alveoli join in cavities of 1 cm or larger.

Hypoxia: Abnormally low oxygen levels in the body.

Pneumothorax: The presence of air or gas in the pleural cavity.

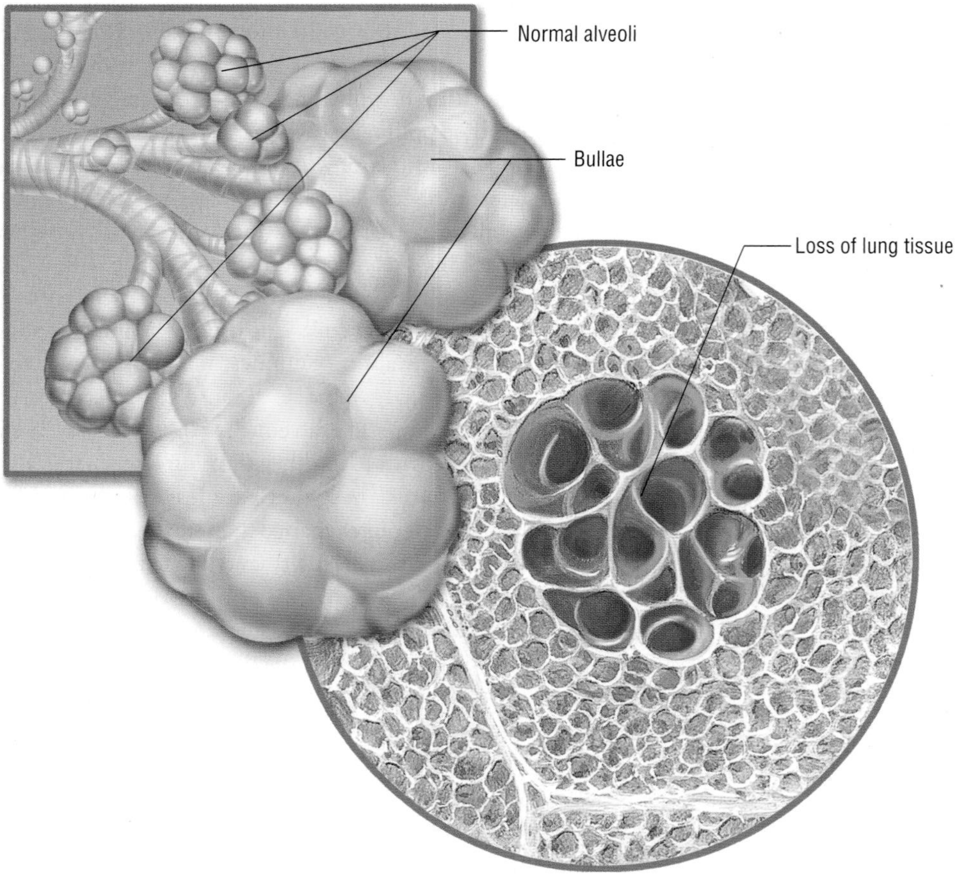

FIGURE 7.10 Emphysema with bullae and loss of alveolar surface area

an untreated emphysema patient undergoes respiratory and circulatory collapse.

The leading cause of the damage seen with both chronic bronchitis and emphysema is exposure to cigarette smoke, although genetic predisposition also clearly plays a role. A small percentage of emphysema patients have an inherited condition in which they are deficient in alpha-1 antitrypsin, so the elastin in their lungs tends to break down early, regardless of whether they smoke.

Signs and Symptoms

It can take many years for emphysema to advance to a stage where symptoms demand that a person seeks medical help. Because it usually affects people over 65 years old, early symptoms are often assumed to be normal signs of aging. These include pain with breathing, shortness of breath, a dry cough, and wheezing. Weight loss often occurs, as a person who must exert so much energy in breathing has little interest in eating. **Rales**, a characteristic bubbling, rasping sound of air moving through a narrowed passage, may occur. Exhalation is a labored, and the patient may develop a habit of pushing air out through pursed lips. This is an attempt to push against increasing back-pressure in the lungs. Because the lungs no longer deflate normally with each breath, the diaphragm becomes permanently flattened. The emphysema patient often develops "barrel chest"; that is, the intercostals lock into a position that holds the rib cage out as wide as possible.

NOTABLE CASES A short list of influential people whose lives were shortened by COPD includes poet T.S. Eliot, talk show host Johnny Carson, the original "Frankenstein" Boris Karloff, founder of Alcoholics Anonymous Bill Wilson, iconic American painter Norman Rockwell, and "Mr. Spock," Leonard Nimoy.

Treatment

Emphysema is irreversible. If it is found and treated early, further progression can be slowed or stopped. But once the alveoli have begun to break down, they don't recover. The first course of action is to remove any irritating stimulus; usually this is cigarette smoke.

Medication for emphysema can dilate the bronchi and take pressure off the alveoli, remove mucus and edema from the lungs, and ward off potential lung infections. Emphysema

Rales: An abnormal rattling sound when breathing.

CASE HISTORY 7.1 Emphysema

Roberta started smoking in 1947 and quit in 1984. In the mid-1980s she noticed that she was frequently short of breath, she had low energy, and she had consistent headaches on rising each morning. She was unable to walk far or fast. In an effort to catch her breath she hyperventilated easily, which only made matters worse. She had a lot of stress and frustration because breathing was so difficult and she could no longer accomplish the things she wanted to do.

Roberta's primary care physician diagnosed COPD and chronic bronchitis. She also saw a pulmonary specialist who diagnosed emphysema. This finding was based on a number of tests, including chest radiography, spirometry, an analysis of arterial blood gases, and measurement of the air volume she was able to expel.

ROBERTA F, AGE 68:
"Emphysema makes it hard for Roberta to do anything... every daily routine has to be altered."

Emphysema makes it hard for Roberta to do anything. The activities of daily living are difficult, and every daily routine has to be altered to accommodate the disease. Stairs and hills are especially challenging. Emphysema dulls the thinking by depriving the brain of oxygen. It reduces appetite, and the lack of oxygen reduces the benefit from what food is eaten. It also strains the heart, because the heart has to work harder to push more blood, which contains less oxygen, through the body.

Roberta also has osteoporosis. This condition, in combination with her breathing difficulties, has significantly altered her posture. Her shoulders rise to her ears as she attempts to get more air, and her chest is compressed because of her spine.

Another aspect of Roberta's experience with emphysema is how it has seriously affected her resistance to disease. In June 1997 she had a bad cold, which put her in the hospital for 4 days.

In January 1998 Roberta contracted pneumonia, which was confirmed by chest radiography. She was in the hospital for 5 days. The pneumonia cleared up with antibiotics, and she returned home.

Roberta is now feeling improved. She still supplements oxygen, and her daily activities have become a little easier. She tries to keep up with her exercises, eat properly, and reduce stress. She also attends Better Breathing Club meetings sponsored by the American Lung Association to keep up with new information about techniques to deal with her disease, and she sees her pulmonary specialist regularly.

Author's note: Roberta passed away from pneumonia in 2002. Many thanks to her and her family for generously sharing her story.

and other COPD patients are strongly urged to be vaccinated against pneumococcus pneumonia and to get a yearly flu shot, because they are at higher risk for serious lung infections than the general population (Case History 7.1).

Oxygen supplementation may be recommended during sleep or following exercise.

Lung volume reduction surgery removes only damaged portions of the lung. This increases thoracic capacity for the diaphragm to work and improves circulation. Lung transplants are a last-ditch option that has been successful for some patients: emphysema is the leading reason for lung transplants.

Medications

- Nicotine patches or gum to aid in quitting smoking
- Short-acting and long-acting bronchodilators to reduce airway resistance
- Inhaled and oral corticosteroids to manage inflammation.
- Mucolytics and expectorants to help clear the lungs of mucus
- Antibiotics as necessary

Massage Therapy Implications

RISKS	The major risks for working with a client with emphysema include the possibility of cardiovascular problems, difficulty lying flat, and secondary respiratory infection. These can be accommodated with adjustments to positioning and modality choices.
BENEFITS	Gentle massage (with respect for the possibility of respiratory infection) is appropriate for emphysema patients, who often feel debilitating fatigue. More specific work on muscles of the chest, shoulders, and neck can be beneficial, if the client can tolerate it.
OPTIONS	Massage that focuses on the muscles of inspiration and expiration can be especially helpful for COPD patients and anyone who has breathing difficulties. Reducing the effort that it takes to breathe can allow patients to feel energized and less fatigued.

Other Respiratory Disorders

Asthma

Definition: What Is It?

Asthma is a chronic disorder of the airways that interferes with breathing. It may be triggered by external factors such as allergens or pollutants, but it is also linked to internal factors such as emotional stress. Asthma is both more common and more serious in African-Americans than among other races. This could be a genetic factor, but may also reflect more exposure to pollutants and disparities in access to health care.

Demographics

About 24 to 26 million people in the United States have been diagnosed with asthma; more than 7 million of them are children. Asthma is estimated to lead to 2 million emergency room visits, and 15,000 deaths in this country each year.

Etiology: What Happens?

All bronchioles are sensitive to foreign debris, but asthmatics' bronchioles are extremely irritable and hyperreactive. Furthermore, the bronchial tubes of a person with asthma appear to be in a state of ongoing inflammation, always poised to begin an attack. When they encounter a trigger, the irritated membranes lining these tubes swell and secrete extra mucus (Figure 7.11). Some small passageways may become completely obstructed by mucous plugs during an attack. People with asthma find it very difficult to breathe, especially to exhale, during an episode; this is called respiratory distress.

To see how this condition works, view the animation "Asthma," available at http://thePoint.lww.com/Werner6e. thePoint®

Pet-related allergens, cigarette smoke, dust mites, and cockroach wastes have been found to be especially potent asthma triggers. The high rate of asthma among young children supports the "hygiene hypothesis": infants and toddlers, especially in industrialized countries, are generally more protected from immune system challenges than those of previous generations. This appears to set up the immune system to be more reactive to potential allergens. Among adults, **gastroesophageal reflux disorder** (GERD), sensitivity to aspirin, and some occupational exposures have also been seen to exacerbate asthma.

NOTABLE CASES Many elite athletes report that they live with asthma. Among them are the following Olympic medalists: Greg Lougainis (diving), Tom Dolan (swimming), Bill Koch (cross-country skiing), and Jackie Joyner-Kersee (track and field).

Asthma is typically rated by severity and pattern. These labels help to determine the best balance of treatment options to control symptoms.

- Mild, intermittent asthma means that episodes occur less than twice a week, and between episodes breathing is normal. This variety may have little impact on activity.
- Mild, persistent asthma means that episodes occur more often than twice a week, up to once a day. Nighttime episodes might happen once a month. Frequency and severity may affect activities.
- Moderate, persistent asthma is characterized by episodes every day and nighttime attacks at least once a week.
- Severe, persistent asthma means that attacks occur most days and nights, and activity is severely limited.

Types of Asthma

- *Bronchial asthma.* This is a typical form with tight bronchioles and excessive mucus production and wheezing during episodes.
- *Exercise-induced asthma.* Sometimes called exercise-induced bronchoconstriction, this version occurs with physical exertion, although symptoms are sometimes delayed for several hours. It is probably a multifactoral problem, but the central issue may be that hard-working athletes might not be able to adequately warm, filter, and moisten the air they take into their lungs, leading to a higher risk of irritation.
- *Silent asthma.* In this situation, no symptoms warn of an impending episode, but then the patient suddenly is dangerously short of breath.
- *Cough variant asthma.* This form shows coughing alone as its primary symptom. It is frequently worst in the middle of the night.

Signs and Symptoms

Symptoms of asthma include dyspnea (shortness of breath), wheezing, and coughing that may or may not be productive. While inhaling is not difficult, exhaling is extremely limited: the bronchioles are constricted, so the alveoli don't empty easily. Even with deep inhalation, oxygen levels drop because the stale air in the lungs cannot be replaced; hyperinflation of the lungs is the result. *To hear the sounds of normal and asthmatic breathing, see the animation "Breathing Sounds" available at* http://thePoint.lww.com/Werner6e. thePoint®

If the symptoms are extreme and prolonged, the asthmatic person may start to feel panicky. This may add sweating, increased heart rate, and anxiety to the list of symptoms. In emergencies the lips and face may take on a bluish cast when access to oxygen is severely restricted.

Asthma attacks are sporadic, lasting anywhere from a few minutes to a few days, but between attacks the lungs are normal. Eventually, however some airway remodeling may

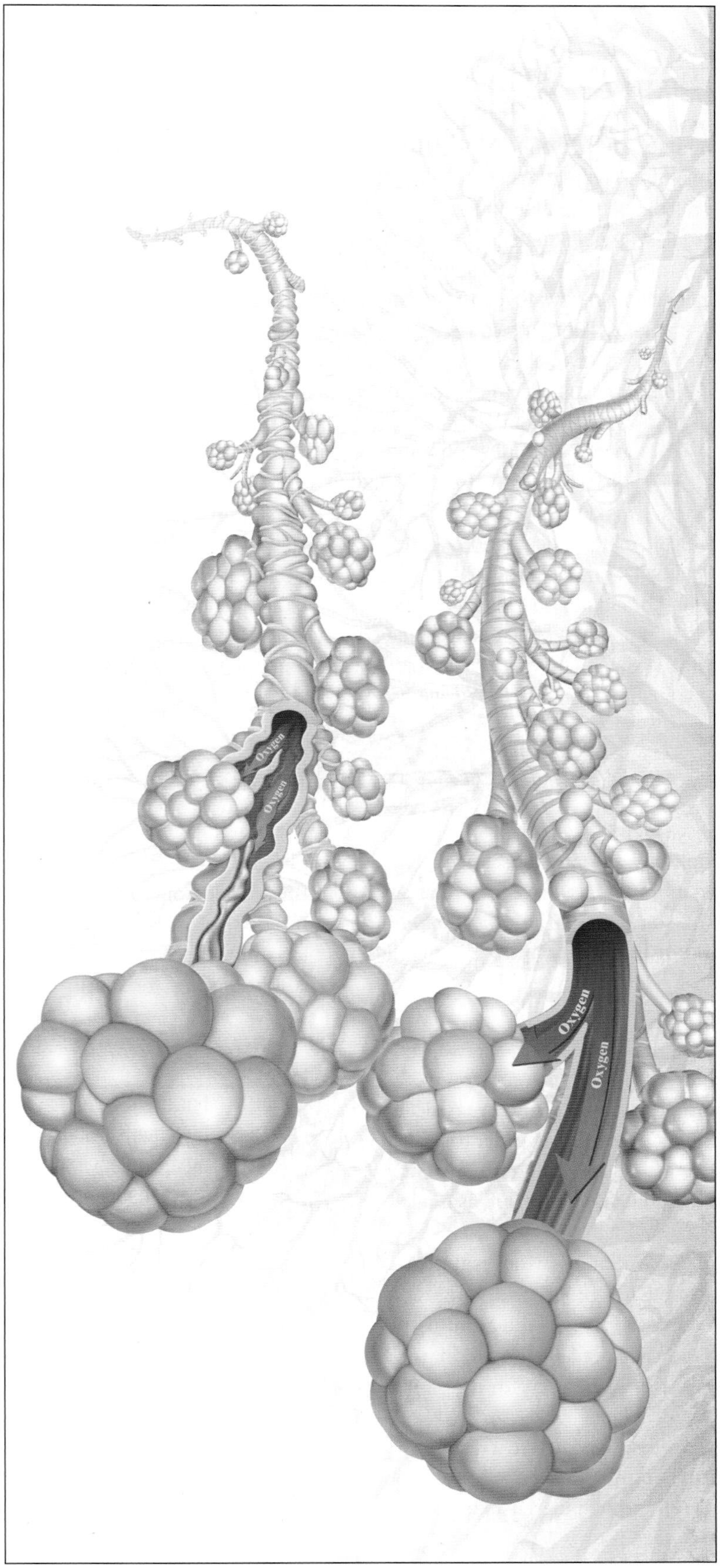

FIGURE 7.11 Asthma: constricted bronchioles, inflammation, and excessive mucus

CASE HISTORY 7.2 Asthma

RICHARD L., AGE 52: "Do you have any pets?"

I didn't contract asthma until I was 22, after I got back from Vietnam. I was living in Los Angeles, and I got real bad bronchitis. I was diagnosed then with just a common smog problem.

Then I moved to Corvallis, Oregon, and ran into the Willamette Valley crud: they have pollination 10 months of the year there. I saw an allergist who gave me skin tests, and I came up positive to 95% of the things he tested me for. I realized it wasn't just the smog; I had a lung problem.

When I moved to Seattle, I wound up with an asthma specialist who's been really good for me. I've had a few bouts here; one time a cold put me in the hospital for about a week.

I've been doing massage since the 1960s but just recently went to school and got licensed. I'm really sensitive to perfumes, and massage school students are 90% female, so I'd always choose where to sit away from anyone wearing perfume. But I never thought about massage oils until we got into it. I knew to stay away from oils and lotions that are scented at all. When I got a massage with almond oil I noticed my skin would turn really red, but it wasn't until someone worked on my chest and back that I noticed about an hour later my breathing was affected.

Asthma affects my life in all kinds of ways. My lung capacity is only about 65% of normal. I like to go listen to music, but the venues where the good bands play are always too smoky. I have to stay away from flower shops. It was almost impossible to go into a mall because you have to walk past the perfume counter to get through the big department stores. Asthma really limits my social life too. When someone asks us over to dinner, our first question has to be, "Do you have any pets? You do? Sorry, we can't."

become evident. Hypertrophy of smooth muscle cells and fibrosis of the epithelial membranes can leave a permanent mark of asthma affects, and some people with asthma are at increased risk to develop **chronic bronchitis**: part of the COPD picture.

Treatment

Treatment for asthma begins with limiting exposure to the stimuli that are known to trigger attacks. Drugs are typically prescribed to manage this chronic disorder, in order to reduce the risk of acute attacks. Patients are also taught to recognize the warning signs of an attack so it can be treated as quickly as possible.

Medical intervention is available in several forms with two basic goals: immediate relief and long-term control. Short-term intervention involves the administration of beta-agonist inhalers that act as bronchodilators. Inhaled or orally taken steroids can be used for long-term control.

When asthma attacks are directly related to a respiratory allergy, patients are often advised to take allergy medication and to consider immunotherapy to help desensitize the system to a particular allergen (Case History 7.2).

To learn more how you can support your clients with asthma, see the author's video "Asthma and the Massage Room Environment" available at http://thePoint.lww.com/Werner6e. thePoint®

Medications

- Bronchodilators to reduce airway resistance.
- Inhaled or oral corticosteroids as long-term anti-inflammatories.
- Antihistamines for allergy control.

Massage Therapy Implications

RISKS	For clients who have asthma and other hypersensitivity situations, it is important to create an environment that is as free from allergens as possible. This means avoiding any heavy scents, essential oils that are irritating, and lubricants that are not hypoallergenic. Clients with asthma may use medication that demands adaptation for massage.
BENEFITS	Massage can be soothing for a person who lives in anxiety about being able to draw a deep breath, and it can help make profound changes in the ease with which breathing happens.
OPTIONS	Specific attention to the muscles of inhalation and exhalation (intercostals, scalenes, serratus posterior, and diaphragm) can make a dramatic difference in the resting tension and overall efficiency of these muscles.

Cystic Fibrosis

Definition: What Is It?

Cystic fibrosis (CF) is an autosomal recessive genetic disorder. This means that a person must inherit one faulty gene from each parent to develop this condition. It affects exocrine glands, causing the production of thick, viscous secretions. The digestive, integumentary, and reproductive system glands are all involved with this disease, but the greatest impact is on the respiratory system.

Demographics

CF is the most common life-limiting genetic disorder among whites in the United States. It is estimated that about 10 million Americans carry the CF gene, although many don't know. About 30,000 people in this country have CF at any given time, and 1,000 to 2,500 babies are born with this disease each year.

Before the 1950s, the life expectancy for a person with CF was under 10 years. Today, the median life expectancy is 37.4 years, and getting higher with the development of new treatment options. Men tend to live longer with this disease than women. Improved life expectancy has given rise to what is essentially a new population of patients: adults with CF who have different complications and challenges than children.

Etiology: What Happens?

Several hundred slightly different mutations can lead to CF, but the net result is that the **transmembrane conductance regulator gene** is altered so that cell membranes in secreting tissues can't conduct chloride. This changes how these cells use water, and leads to abnormally thick, sticky secretions in many exocrine glands but most particularly in the respiratory tract, digestive tract, skin, and reproductive tract (Figure 7.12).

- *Respiratory system.* CF usually has its most profound effects on the respiratory system. The changes in mucous membrane function cause mucus in the respiratory tract to become thick, gluey, and difficult to dislodge. This provides an inviting environment for bacteria. Because of the genetic dysfunction, immune system action against pathogens reinforces the inflammatory response, which causes more damage and supports, rather than suppresses infection. A variety of bacterial agents may create chronic infection, but the one that is the most difficult to eradicate is *Pseudomonas aeruginosa*.

  Other respiratory system changes include the growth of nasal polyps and the development of chronic rhinitis. Ultimately, congestion in the lungs can impair blood circulation to the lungs and lead to the possibility of **right-sided heart failure**.
- *Digestive system.* Digestive system dysfunction can affect both the GI tract and the accessory organs. A warning sign for CF is a baby born with an intestinal obstruction; this happens because the mucus in the small and large intestines doesn't move well. Poor absorption in the small intestine also leads to greasy, bulky stools and failure to thrive. Limited access to vitamins and minerals can cause important deficiencies.

  Adults with CF are vulnerable to **osteoporosis** because of poor absorption. CF can interfere with the normal production of bile and drainage of bile into the small intestine, leading to an enlarged spleen, **gallstones**, portal hypertension, liver congestion, or **cirrhosis**. Poor secretion of bicarbonate and digestive enzymes from the pancreas can lead to **diabetes** and **peptic ulcers** in the duodenum and pancreatitis.
- *Integumentary system.* CF affects sweat glands in the skin, leading to abnormally thick, salty perspiration, and the risk of heat stroke and salt depletion, especially in infants.
- *Reproductive system.* Almost all men with CF are sterile. This occurs because the epididymis cannot secrete normally, or because the vas deferens doesn't form completely. Women with CF often have normal reproductive systems and can have successful pregnancies.

> **Transmembrane conductance regulator gene:** A gene that is responsible for proteins that conduct chloride in and out of cells. Mutation is associated with cystic fibrosis.
>
> **Clubbing:** A deformity of the fingers and fingernails that is associated with several lung and heart conditions.

Signs and Symptoms

Signs and symptoms of CF vary by the system that is affected most severely. Respiratory symptoms are most common. They include a dry or productive cough, shortness of breath, wheezing, chest pain, cyanosis, hemoptysis, and **clubbing** of fingers, which occurs with long-term oxygen deprivation in the extremities.

Signs and symptoms of other affected systems are discussed in the Etiology section.

Treatment

CF is not curable; treatment options focus on symptoms and complications. Devices to help break up congestion in the lungs, along with breathing exercises to maintain and improve function, are often suggested. Taking food in easily digestible forms, supplementing vitamins and enzymes, and exercising to increase or maintain lung function are recommended for people who are not fighting acute infection or intestinal blockages.

Bronchodilators, mucolytics, antibiotics to fight infection, and anti-inflammatories are typical medical interventions for CF

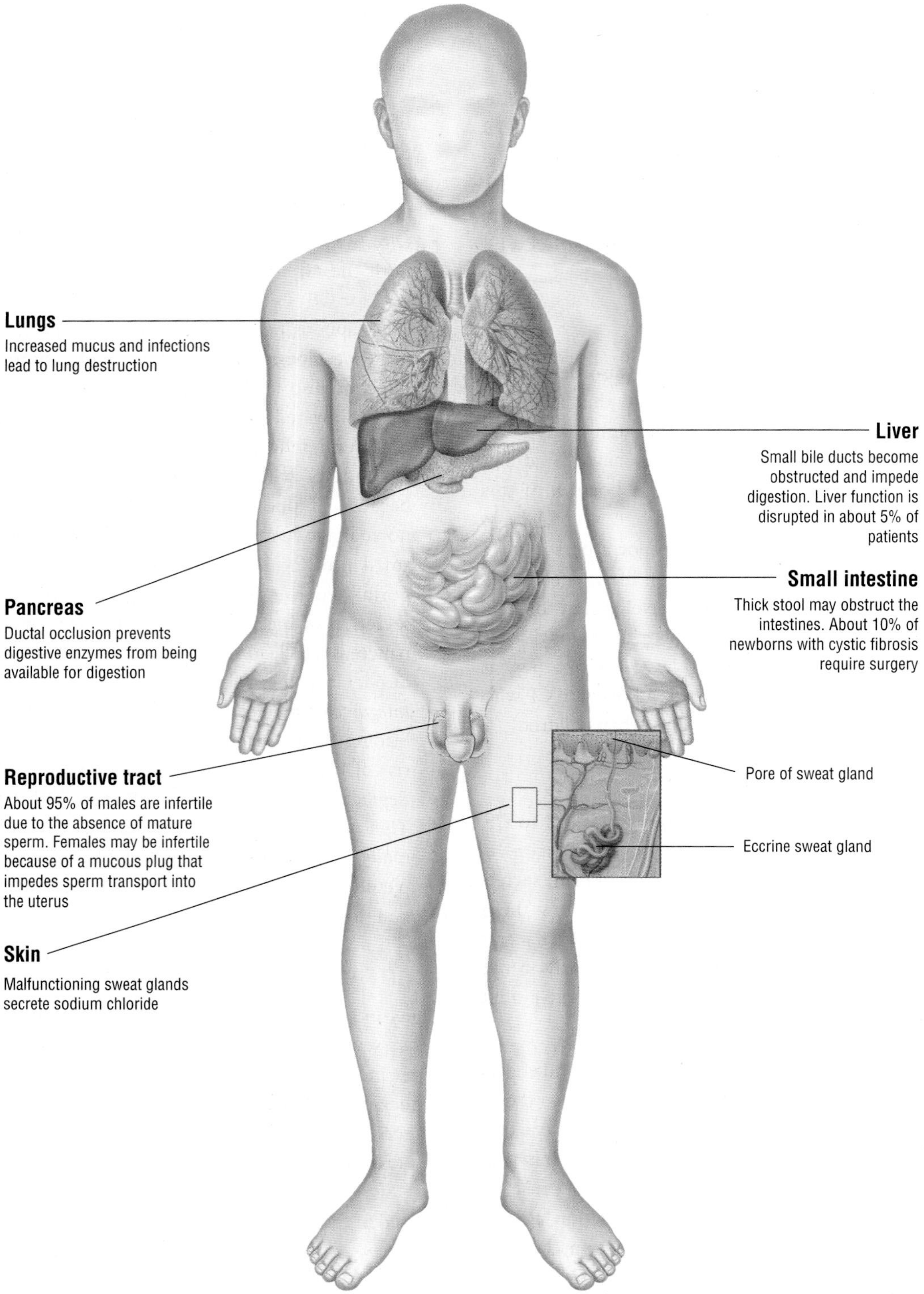
Lungs
Increased mucus and infections lead to lung destruction
Liver
Small bile ducts become obstructed and impede digestion. Liver function is disrupted in about 5% of patients
Small intestine
Thick stool may obstruct the intestines. About 10% of newborns with cystic fibrosis require surgery
Pancreas
Ductal occlusion prevents digestive enzymes from being available for digestion
Reproductive tract
About 95% of males are infertile due to the absence of mature sperm. Females may be infertile because of a mucous plug that impedes sperm transport into the uterus
Pore of sweat gland
Eccrine sweat gland
Skin
Malfunctioning sweat glands secrete sodium chloride

FIGURE 7.12 Systemic changes in cystic fibrosis

patients. Patients with advanced cases may be candidates for lung transplants, although this procedure has a high rejection rate.

In addition to treating all the issues related directly to CF, patients must also manage their complications. This means drugs to manage ulcers, osteoporosis, diabetes, and others may be on their medications list.

Medications

- Inhaled bronchodilators to reduce resistance in airways
- Inhaled mucolytics and saline to help dissolve mucus
- Inhaled and oral antibiotics as needed for bacterial respiratory infection
- Anti-inflammatories

Massage Therapy Implications

RISKS	The primary risk for working with a client who has CF is respiratory infection: either the client may be ill or the therapist may be inadvertently carrying pathogens that put a client at risk.
BENEFITS	Many children and adults with CF undergo intense physiotherapy to dislodge deposits of mucus in the lungs, and when no acute infection is present, they are recommended to exercise within tolerance to build stamina and strength. Massage is probably safe and appropriate under these circumstances as long as the therapist works with the rest of the health care team, is healthy, and doesn't share any virulent pathogens with the client. Adults with CF are prone to other secondary issues, namely anxiety and/or depression as they struggle to manage this disease. Massage therapy may be a helpful intervention in this situation, with caution for the significant chance of osteoporosis, diabetes, and other complications.
RESEARCH	An Australian study[1] found that a single treatment of massage and mobilization techniques reduced pain and improved the ease of breathing for adults with CF. An earlier systematic review[2] concluded that preliminary evidence supports massage therapy for children with CF, specifically for reducing pain, improving health outcomes, and improving the quality of life for the children and their families. 1. Lee A, Holdsworth M, Holland A, et al. The immediate effect of musculoskeletal physiotherapy techniques and massage on pain and ease of breathing in adults with cystic fibrosis. *Journal of Cystic Fibrosis* 2009;8(1):79–81. http://www.cysticfibrosisjournal.com/article/S1569-1993(08)00111-2/pdf 2. Huth MM, Zink KA, Van Horn NR. The effects of massage therapy in improving outcomes for youth with cystic fibrosis: an evidence review. *Pediatric Nursing* 2005;31(4):328–332. http://www.ncbi.nlm.nih.gov/pubmed/16229132

Laryngeal Cancer

Definition: What Is It?

Laryngeal cancer is the development of malignant growths on and around the larynx.

Demographics

Laryngeal cancer is a relatively common disease, diagnosed about 12,000 times a year in the United States, and leading to about 3,600 deaths. It usually affects mature people, often with a history of tobacco use. Men are affected more than women at a ratio of about 4:1.

The incidence of laryngeal and other throat cancers has been rising among young people, largely because it can be a complication of exposure to human papilloma viruses; these are the same viruses that cause **genital warts** and may lead to **cervical cancer**.

Etiology: What Happens?

The larynx is the portion of the throat where the division of the digestive and respiratory tracts occurs. This 2-inch long and 2-inch wide structure is often discussed as three subparts: the **supraglottis**, which connects to the pharynx; the **glottis**, which holds the vocal cords, and the **subglottis**, which connects the larynx to the trachea. A small flap called the **epiglottis** forms a protective shield over the respiratory tract to prevent the aspiration of liquids or solids into the lungs.

A healthy larynx is vital for speech, swallowing, protection of the respiratory tract, and breath control. When the larynx is compromised any of these functions may be impaired, and the risk for a life-threatening lung infection from aspirated material is very high (Figure 7.13).

The larynx is vulnerable to several types of growths, including polyps, nodules, and tumors. When tumors are cancerous they almost always begin in the squamous cell lining of the glottis, and may spread from there through the throat to the tongue, and into other structures of the neck, including the cervical lymph nodes. Metastasis to the lungs is common for this form of cancer.

A specific cause for laryngeal cancer has not been identified. Rather, as with many types of cancer, risk factors appear to accumulate to increase the possibility that a person will develop this disease. The main risk factors for laryngeal cancer include using tobacco of any kind,

Supraglottis: The upper part of the larynx.

Glottis: The vocal cords and the slit between them. Part of the larynx.

Subglottis: The lower portion of the larynx that connects it to the trachea.

Epiglottis: The flap of tissue that covers the windpipe during swallowing.

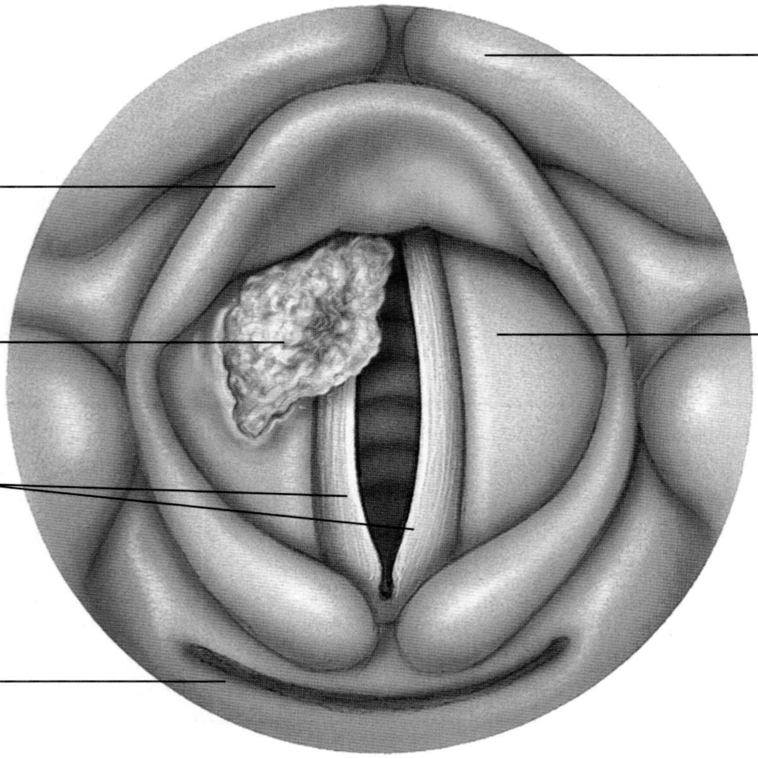

FIGURE 7.13 Laryngeal cancer affecting the true and false vocal cords

and drinking excessive alcohol, and these two habits tend to potentiate each other, that is, the risk associated with drinking *and* smoking is greater than for the risks of each behavior accrued separately. Other risk factors include age, gender, exposure to human papilloma virus, poor dental hygiene, a diet poor in vitamin A and beta-carotene, a history of **gastroesophageal reflux disorder**, a history of radiation to the neck for other reasons, and a history of exposure to nickel, sulfuric acid, or asbestos.

Signs and Symptoms

Early signs and symptoms of laryngeal cancer may be subtle. They typically include a chronic cough, hoarseness, sore throat, and a feeling of something being "stuck" in the back of the throat. Bad breath, problems breathing, and ear ache are also frequently reported. Later in the process a person with laryngeal cancer may have blood in their sputum and unintentional weight loss.

Treatment

Laryngeal cancer is treated aggressively, but the larynx performs such vital functions that oncologists consider preserving the best function possible as a high priority. Consequently, radiation and chemotherapy, which spare the larynx, are often pursued before surgery to remove cancerous tissue. Surgical procedures also emphasize preserving the best possible function, so that the risk of future problems with speech or accidental aspiration of solids or liquids into the trachea can be minimized (See sidebar 7.4).

Medications

- Chemotherapeutic drugs
- Analgesics following surgery

Massage Therapy Implications

RISKS	As with other cancers, risks for working with laryngeal cancer patients center more on the treatments than on the cancer itself. Radiation, chemotherapy, and surgery must all be accommodated with modality choices.
BENEFITS	Massage can reduces anxiety and depression, improves appetite and sleep, and generally adds to the quality of life for a person with laryngeal or other types of cancer.
OPTIONS	Laryngeal cancer patients may have a temporary stoma placed in their neck; this is vulnerable to disruption and contamination. More information about massage in the context of cancer patients is found in Chapter 12.

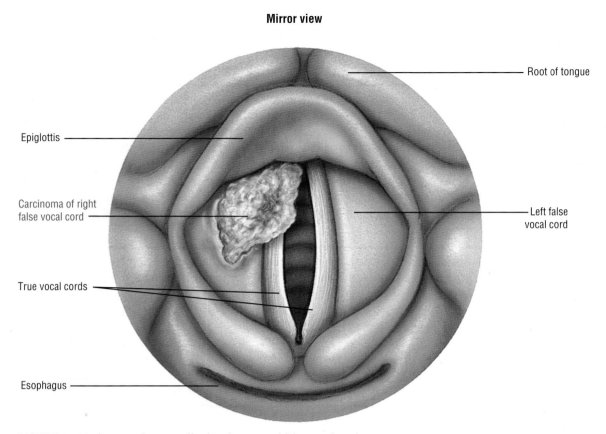

SIDEBAR 7.4 Staging Laryngeal Cancer

Laryngeal cancer staging identifies three major factors to predict the prognosis and to determine the best treatment options:

- The number of subsites on the larynx where the cancer is found.
- The mobility or fixedness of the vocal cords.
- The presence of metastases to the cervical lymph nodes and beyond.

(T) Tumor assessment

Tx	Tumor cannot be assessed.
T0	No evidence of primary tumor in situ.
T1	One subsite affected; vocal cords are mobile.
T2	Invasion into nearby tissues; vocal cord mobility is mildly impaired.
T3	Invasion into nearby tissues, vocal cords are fixed.
T4	Invasion throughout larynx, local cartilage, and soft tissues of the anterior neck.

(N) Node assessment

Nx	Node involvement cannot be assessed.
N0	No node involvement.
N1	One node is invaded with a growth <3 cm.
N2	One node is invaded with a growth 3 to 6 cm, or Multiple nodes on the same side with growths <6 cm, or Multiple nodes on both sides with growths <6 cm.
N3	Any growths in nodes >6 cm.

Laryngeal subsites are identified as the supraglottis, the glottis, and the subglottis.

Here is a simplified version of the laryngeal cancer staging protocol, first in the TNM format, and then translated into the stages 0 to IV format:

(M) Metastasis

Mx	Metastasis cannot be assessed.
M0	No distant metastasis is found.
M1	Distant metastasis is found.

Stages 0 to IV

Stage 0	TIS, N0, M0
Stage I	T1, N0, M0
Stage II	T2, N0, M0
Stage III	T3, N0, M0, or T1-3, N1, M0
Stage IVa	T4, N0, M0, or T4, N1, M0, or T-any, N2, M0
Stage IVb	T4, N-any, M0, or T-any, N3, M0
Stage IVc	T-any, N-any, M1

Lung Cancer

Definition: What Is It?

Lung cancer is the growth of malignant cells in the lungs. These cells eventually form tumors, but because they have extremely easy access to both the circulatory and lymph systems, they are capable of spreading to other tissues (metastasizing) before tumors are detectable.

Lung cancer is an example of epithelial cancer that tends to grow where tissue is vulnerable to repeated irritation and damage.

Demographics

It is estimated that about 224,000 people are diagnosed and 159,000 people in the United States die of lung cancer each year. It is the leading cause of death by cancer, killing more people each year than breast, prostate, and colorectal cancers combined.

About 380,000 lung cancer patients are alive in the United States today. At just under 17%, the 5-year survival rate is lower for lung cancer than for most other types of cancer. The survival rate is better when the cancer is found before it spreads outside the lungs, but this happens in only 15% of all cases.

Etiology: What Happens?

Lung cancer occurs in epithelial cells that are chronically irritated by environmental contaminants. Although cigarette, pipe, and cigar smoke are responsible for 85% to 90% of cases of lung cancer, other causes have also been identified, including exposure to **radon**, asbestos, uranium, arsenic, and air pollution. These are all much more potent carcinogens when they are paired with smoking.

When the epithelial cells that line the respiratory tract have a long history of exposure to highly toxic substances, their orderly pattern of replication and repair is eventually disrupted. Abnormal cells accumulate in uncontrolled and disorganized patches. A rich supply of blood and lymph vessels allows mutated cells to travel out of their immediate area

Radon: A radioactive gas.

7 Respiratory System Conditions

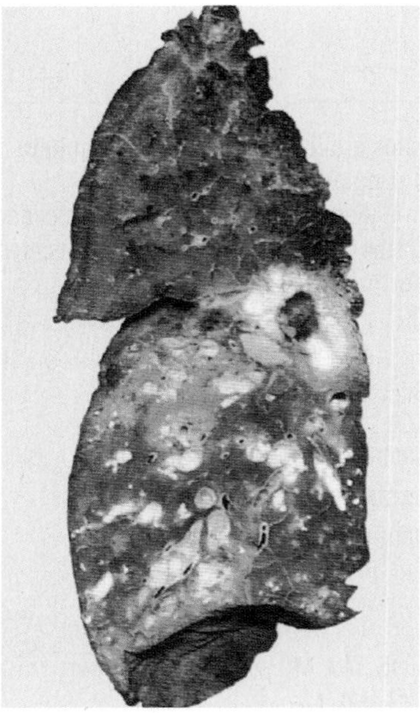

FIGURE 7.14 Lung cancer

before a detectable tumor appears; this is why lung cancer is seldom found before metastasis (see Figure 7.14).

The lymph nodes around the lungs and in the mediastinum are often the first site of metastasis for lung cancer. From there the cells have access to distant places in the body. The liver, bone tissue, adrenal glands, and brain are frequently invaded.

NOTABLE CASES The list of influential lives that have been cut short by lung cancer is too long to contemplate. Among them are musician George Harrison; water lilies painter Claude Monet, singer Rosemary Clooney, animator and innovator Walt Disney, actor and director Paul Newman, and Dana Reeve ("Superman" Christopher Reeve's wife), who never smoked.

The most obvious risk factor for lung cancer is smoking. Cigarette smoke contains multiple known carcinogens, and the tar in cigarettes holds the damaging chemicals close to the delicate linings of the lungs. In addition to airborne toxins, lung cancer is a risk for people who have had radiation to the chest for **breast cancer** or other treatments; or a history of **tuberculosis**, **chronic obstructive pulmonary disease**, or severe **pneumonia**.

Every year thousands of people who were never smokers die of lung cancer. These cases are often linked to second-hand or sidestream smoke or other risk factors, but the potential for inherited predisposition is now being actively pursued through genetic research. This may eventually yield ways to identify people at particularly high risk for lung cancer, along with ways to identify it early and treat it more successfully.

Types of Lung Cancer

- *Small cell lung cancer.* This is also called "oat cell" carcinoma. It accounts for 20% of lung cancers. Small cell lung cancer grows fast, spreads quickly, and is rarely operable.
- *Nonsmall cell lung cancer.* This includes several types of cancers depending on which cells they affect first. Nonsmall cell carcinomas account for about 85% of lung cancers. They include squamous cell carcinoma, adenocarcinoma, large cell carcinoma, etc. Most of these grow more slowly than small cell carcinoma, but the symptoms they produce are so subtle that diagnosis doesn't usually happen until long after the cancer has spread beyond its original area.
- *Other types of lung malignancies.* Small cell and nonsmall cell lung cancers account for most types of lung cancer, but a few cases of other types are identified as well. These include carcinoid tumors, adenoid cystic carcinoma, sarcomas, etc. **Mesothelioma** is a type of cancer that arises in the pleural sac that surrounds the lung; this is closely associated with asbestos exposure.

Signs and Symptoms

One of the most challenging problems with lung cancer is that it is extremely difficult to identify early. The growth of abnormal cells in alveoli, bronchial linings, or mucous membranes stimulates virtually no changes in function or sensation. A persistent smoker's cough is one early sign, along with bloodstained phlegm, chronic chest pain, wheezing, and possibly shortness of breath. None of these symptoms seems cause for alarm, since a smoker or someone who works with irritating chemicals often has them regardless of the health of their respiratory tract cells.

It is a bit of a mystery that a healthy lung imbued with a full complement of immune system cells, which protect us against practically every possible inhaled antigen, does not launch a similar attack against the growth of cancer tissue. It turns out that one of the features of lung tumor cells, at least in nonsmall cell lung cancer, is that they attract increased numbers of T-regulatory cells: the ones that tell the rest of the immune system to stand down because the attack is over. This is part of the mechanism that allows tumors to grow silently in their early stages.

Later signs of lung cancer may be more revealing. If a tumor grows near the apex of the lung, it may put mechanical pressure on the brachial plexus, leading to symptoms that mimic **thoracic outlet syndrome**. A tumor that presses on the superior vena cava may cause facial swelling and dilated blood vessels in the neck and face; this is called **superior vena cava syndrome**. If a tumor protrudes

Mesothelioma: Cancer of the mesothelium.

Superior vena cava syndrome: A condition caused by compression of the superior vena cava, usually by a tumor.

SIDEBAR 7.5 Staging Lung Cancer

The staging protocol for lung cancer depends on whether the diagnosis is for small cell or nonsmall cell lung cancer. It is important to stage any kind of cancer accurately to choose the best possible treatment options. Patients may also choose to volunteer for clinical trials to add to the body of knowledge about best options according to stage.

Small cell lung cancer, because it is so aggressive and is usually inoperable, is described as being either limited or extensive. Limited small cell lung cancer means that it is found in only one lung and local lymph nodes; extensive small cell lung cancer means that it is found in both lungs, multiple nodes, and in distant areas as well.

Nonsmall cell lung cancer comes in several forms, but they are similar in presentation and treatment protocols, so they are all staged together using a combination of the TNM and stages 0 to IV classifications. These staging protocols are described in detail in Chapter 12. Here is a simplified version of nonsmall cell lung cancer staging:

TUMOR (T)	NODE (N)	METASTASIS (M)
Tx: positive findings on tests; no lesion found.	N0: no nodes involved.	M0: no metastasis found.
Tis: cancer in situ, limited to endothelial cells.	N1: some nodes involved near affected lung.	M1: distant metastasis found.
T1: tumor <3 cm in diameter.	N2: nodes in mediastinum on side of affected lung.	
T2: tumor is 3 to 7 cm in diameter; may involve pleura or bronchi.	N3: Nodes on opposite side of involved thorax.	
T3: tumor >7 cm, extensions into nearby structures.		
T4: tumor invasion of mediastinal structures.		

These delineations are then translated into stages 0 to IV in this way:

STAGE	TUMOR	NODE	METASTASIS
IA	T1	N0	M0
IB	T2	N0	M0
IIA	T1–T2	N1	M0
IIIA	T1–3	N1–2	M0
IIIB	T1–4	N1–3	M0
IV	T-any	N-any	M1

on the esophagus or larynx, a person may have chronic hoarseness. Tumors that press on the phrenic nerve can paralyze the diaphragm.

Treatment

Treatment for lung cancer depends on what kind of cancer is growing and how far it has progressed (See sidebar 7.5). For the lucky few who find nonsmall cell lung cancer while it is still local, surgery followed by radiation may be adequate. The surgery could involve the removal of a small section of lung tissue (a wedge resection), the removal of an entire lobe (a **lobectomy**), or even the removal of an entire lung (a **pneumonectomy**).

Small cell carcinoma grows so fast and spreads so quickly that it is generally treated with radiation and chemotherapy alone; surgery usually has no chance of containing the growth. While this can be successful in the short run, most small cell lung cancer patients have a recurrence within 2 years, and the cancer tends to become unresponsive to treatment.

Targeted therapies for lung cancer include the use of biologically engineered antibodies that deliver drugs or radiation to cancer cells; drugs that interfere with angiogenesis; drugs that inhibit cancer cell growth factors; drugs that make cancer cells sensitive to light; and a cancer "vaccine" that essentially introduces a substance that makes immune system cells more sensitive to cancer cells. All of

Lobectomy: The surgical removal of a lobe of an organ.

Pneumonectomy: The surgical removal of a lung.

these are still in experimental use, and they all carry serious potential side effects, but they may eventually be both more effective and less risky than traditional cancer treatments.

Medications

- Chemotherapeutic agents to kill fast-growing cells
- Targeted therapies to
  - Deliver treatment to cancer cells
  - Interfere with angiogenesis
  - Suppress local growth factors
  - Use light to kill cancer cells
  - Stimulate immune system responses against cancer cells
- Medication to lessen the side effects of chemotherapy

Massage Therapy Implications

RISKS	A person with lung cancer may be undergoing extremely aggressive treatment to manage this disease; chemotherapy, radiation, and surgery all have specific cautions for massage. Alternatively, he or she may be at the end of life and seeking strictly palliative care, in which case bodywork must be adjusted for frailty, the risk of problems with bones or major organs, and any medical equipment that can be disrupted.
BENEFITS	Massage can be a supportive strategy for a person going through a challenging time. It can help with insomnia, pain, fatigue, anxiety, and depression—all of which can make both the cancer and the side effects of medication seem worse.
OPTIONS	Details about massage in the context of cancer are covered in Chapter 12.
RESEARCH	An overview of several complementary and integrative health care therapies for patients with lung cancer[1] suggests that massage therapy, among other interventions, can be a useful supportive measure for these populations, so it is useful for conventional medical practitioners to be familiar with our work. 1. Deng GE, Rausch SM, Jones LW, et al. Complementary therapies and integrative medicine in lung cancer: diagnosis and management of lung cancer, 3rd ed: American College of Chest Physicians evidence-based clinical practice guidelines. *Chest* 2013;143(5 suppl):e420S–e436S. http://www.ncbi.nlm.nih.gov/pubmed/23649450

Explore and Apply

LEVEL 1: Receive and Respond

1. When a healthy person is at rest, he invests ___ of his energy in the act of respiration.
   a. 5%
   b. 10%
   c. 50%
   d. 2%

2. The process of normal expiration happens because of...
   a. The contraction of specific thoracic muscles
   b. Gravity
   c. The resilience of elastin fibers in lung tissue
   d. Hydrostatic pressure

3. What is the typical etiology of acute bronchitis?
   a. It is a complication of cold or flu
   b. It is a result of long-term damage to the bronchi
   c. It is an allergic reaction with inflammation and excessive mucus production
   d. It is related to the development of scar tissue between the pleural layers

4. Who is most prone to "catch cold"?
   a. Elders
   b. Young children
   c. Middle-aged people
   d. All ages have equal risk

5. What is the best description of flu?
   a. An infection of the lungs leading to scarring and the potential for permanent dysfunction, the leading cause of death by infection
   b. A benign respiratory infection involving about a week of congestion and fever
   c. A lung disease that causes the alveoli to fuse and sometimes to rupture
   d. A potentially dangerous infection that kills up to 50,000 people in the United States each year

6. Match the condition to the best description

a. Pneumonia	— Part of chronic obstructive pulmonary disease
b. Sinusitis	— A contagious bacterial infection of the lungs
c. Emphysema	— Inflammation of mucous membranes from bacteria, viruses, or fungi
d. Tuberculosis	— Infection that blocks gaseous exchange in the alveoli

7. What is a consequence of not taking tuberculosis drugs as prescribed?
   a. The infection can come back and become chronic
   b. The drugs become toxic when they expire
   c. The infection can mutate to cause cancer
   d. The bacteria can mutate into a stronger pathogen

8. What two factors are associated with asthma?
   a. Antibiotic resistance and chronic infection
   b. Degeneration of elastin and alveolar dysfunction
   c. Inflammation of bronchioles and excess mucus production
   d. Poor gaseous exchange and inefficient inhalation

9. Which glands are affected by cystic fibrosis?
   a. Endocrine
   b. Exocrine
   c. Epithelial
   d. Endothelial

10. Physicians recommend chemotherapy and radiation for laryngeal cancer rather than surgery because...
    a. It is usually at stage IV at diagnosis
    b. Preserving the larynx is important to future health
    c. Laryngeal surgery is prohibitively risky
    d. Surgery may spread the disease to other parts of the body

11. What is true about lung cancer?
    a. It has usually spread beyond the lungs when it is diagnosed
    b. It usually spreads before tumors develop
    c. It is usually found by accident during tests for some other reason
    d. It may be self-limiting

Explore and Apply (continued)

LEVEL 2: Application of Concepts

1. If elastin in the lung tissue breaks down, what is an expected consequence?
   a. It takes more effort to inhale
   b. It takes more effort to exhale
   c. Oxygen and carbon dioxide no longer cross over
   d. Alveoli fill with fluid

2. With what you now know about oxygen content of the air and exhaled breath, explain why rescue breathing works. Would it work if we absorbed all available oxygen from the air into our bloodstream? Why or why not?

3. Your client has allergic sinusitis. What accommodation will probably help her be most comfortable?
   a. She should spend most of the session face-down so her sinuses can drain
   b. Avoid long periods of prone work so she doesn't have pressure on her sinuses
   c. Use eucalyptus oil to help clear her sinuses
   d. Reschedule the massage for after her symptoms have passed

4. Your client has asthma. What are some things you can do to promote her comfort in the session room?
   a. Use essential oils in your massage lubricant designed for respiratory soothing
   b. Burn incense to rid the room of the last client's perfume
   c. Prepare for her cold feet with extra blankets
   d. Avoid any scents or stimulants that might trigger an attack

5. Your client reports that he has no symptoms, but he had a positive TB skin test. This means that…
   a. He has TB exposure but not TB disease; he is not contagious
   b. He is contagious; you need to reschedule until after he completes antibiotic treatment
   c. He is only contagious if he sneezes or coughs near you
   d. He needs extensive work on his chest to loosen mucus in his lungs

6. Reread the section on chronic bronchitis. Then, without referring to the text, describe how chronic hypoxia can become a vicious cycle.

Note to educators: Due to space considerations, these review questions only skim over the most important material from Chapter 8. The Test Bank provides a much more comprehensive selection of questions, all of which are keyed to the relevant learning objectives.

What Would *You* Do?

"I REALLY Want a Massage!"

You volunteer at a low-income health clinic in a large city. One day your client for chair massage has a heavy, phlegmy cough, and she is running a slight fever. She says she has been this way for a month. She has really been looking forward to her massage—this is they only access she has. Role-play a conversation with a partner to come to a conclusion about a massage for this client, then switch roles and do it again.

Is This within Your Skillset?

Your new 80-year-old client has emphysema and osteoporosis. The shape of her thorax further limits her ability to breathe. She would like to see if you could help her with this breathing and her debilitating fatigue. Design a treatment plan that respects her conditions. Anticipate challenges like table positioning, the frailty of her ribs, and the fact that she is likely to have cardiovascular problems as well.

Explore and Apply (continued)

Suggested Activities

1. For each condition covered in your curriculum, write down the following on a card:
   - a brief definition
   - most common cause or contributing factor(s)
   - major signs and symptoms
   - risks and benefits of massage therapy
     - variables that contribute to risks and benefits
     - appropriate adaptations

   Use these as flash cards as you study.

2. For each condition covered in your curriculum, write one multiple choice question. Share your questions with your classmates as you study together.

3. Quiz yourself using either the "labels off" feature in your enhanced ebook, or the labeling exercise on thePoint® for Figure 7.1. Identify the following structures: Alveoli, Bronchi, Bronchioles, Larynx, Pharynx, and Trachea.

4. Use the student resources on thePoint® to find practice quiz questions and games.

8

Digestive System Conditions

CHAPTER 8 / Abbreviated Chapter Objectives

Having completed assignments and classroom time related to Chapter 8, the learner is expected to be able to…

- Identify definitions of the key terms in the introduction and those connected to the conditions covered in your curriculum.
- Name the sections of the gastrointestinal (GI) tract listing at least four structures in correct order.
- Identify the structure that separates the esophagus from the stomach.
- Identify the structure that separates the stomach from the small intestine.
- Identify the structure that separates the small intestine from the large intestine.
- Describe the chemical environment inside the stomach.
- Describe the internal surface of the small intestine.
- Identify the portal vein and describe its function.
- List three accessory organs.
- Describe how stress can lead to digestive discomfort.
- Explain why persistent digestive system discomfort should be pursued with a primary care provider.
- Provide the following information for each condition covered in your curriculum:
  - Identify the definition of the condition.
  - List the most common causes or contributing factors to the condition.
  - List major signs and symptoms of the condition.
  - Identify possible risks and benefits of massage therapy with:
    - Variables that contribute to risks and benefits.
    - Appropriate adaptations for massage therapy.

For detailed chapter objectives for each condition in this chapter, consult the student resources page at http://thePoint.lww.com/Werner6e. thePoint®

Structure and Function of the Digestive Tract

The best way to review how the digestive tract works when it is healthy is to follow a piece of food through the system (Figure 8.1).

When our teeth grind up a morsel of food, it is broken into small pieces so that the digestive enzymes in saliva and the rest of the gastrointestinal (GI) tract have access to available nutrients. The food moves from the mouth down the esophagus, through the **lower esophageal sphincter**, and into a wide place in the tube: the stomach. Here, it is further pulverized by powerful muscular contractions and exposed to more acidic chemicals. When the former food, now referred to as **chyme**, moves through the pyloric valve into the small intestine, the gallbladder and pancreas add their secretions. By now the barrage of digestive enzymes has reduced the meal into its most primitive building blocks: sugars, fats, and proteins.

The small intestine loops and twirls around the abdomen, secured by sheets of connective tissue membrane called the **mesentery**, a part of the **peritoneum**. It is lubricated on the outside by other layers of the peritoneum, which allow it to move freely as a person twists, squirms, and changes positions. The inside of a healthy small intestine looks like velvet or velour, with millions of tiny **villi**, each one supplied with blood and lymph capillaries for the absorption of nutrients and fats. This is where amino acids and glucose enter the bloodstream, and fats are drawn into the lymph system. Rhythmic waves of smooth muscle contraction called **peristalsis** gently ease the chyme along the tube until at the distal end of the small intestine, and the leftovers pass through the **ileocecal valve**, the entryway to the colon.

The colon, or large intestine, is a much shorter and wider section of tubing than the small intestine. It differs also in the absence of villi, and the presence of anchoring bands of connective tissue that bind the colon down at the four flexures or corners of the abdomen. A healthy colon has segments called **haustra**. Water is squeezed out of the fecal matter in the colon, and reabsorbed back into the body. This is also the site of vitamin K synthesis. The colon functions like a trash compactor; everything left of a meal that makes it this far is condensed and excreted.

Lower esophageal sphincter: The bundle of muscles surrounding the passage from the esophagus to the stomach.

Chyme: Partially digested food in the stomach or small intestine.

Mesentery: A fold of tissue that anchors the intestines and other abdominal organs to the posterior abdominal wall.

Peritoneum: The membrane that lines the abdominal cavity.

Villi: Finger-like projections that increase the surface area of the small intestine, which in turn increases nutrient absorption.

Peristalsis: The wave-like contractions of the intestines that move their contents forward.

Ileocecal valve: The passage from the small intestine to the large intestine.

Haustra: The small pouches of the colon. (Singular: haustrum.)

Glycogen: The form in which the body stores carbohydrates.

Structure and Function of the Accessory Organs

The continuous tube that winds from mouth to anus is only one part of the digestive system; the accessory organs contribute to the process of turning food into energy or building blocks as well. These organs include the liver, gallbladder, and pancreas, each of which produce or release chemicals into the digestive tract. Here is a brief review of each of these organs.

The Liver

The liver is an organ of immense complexity with literally hundreds of functions. This organ has an amazing ability to regenerate; hepatocytes are remarkably adaptable. Livers that have been partially removed can recover full functional size soon after surgery, and small pieces of liver that have been transplanted into other hosts can grow to full function within a similar short period. The liver also has twice the blood supply of most other organs; between the hepatic artery delivering oxygen and the portal vein delivering fresh products of digestion from the GI tract, it's no wonder that this organ is hot and dark red.

The liver is the largest organ in the body. It is the destination of the portal system detour, receiving almost all of the vitamins, amino acids, and glucose that are extracted from the small intestine. By storing glucose as **glycogen**

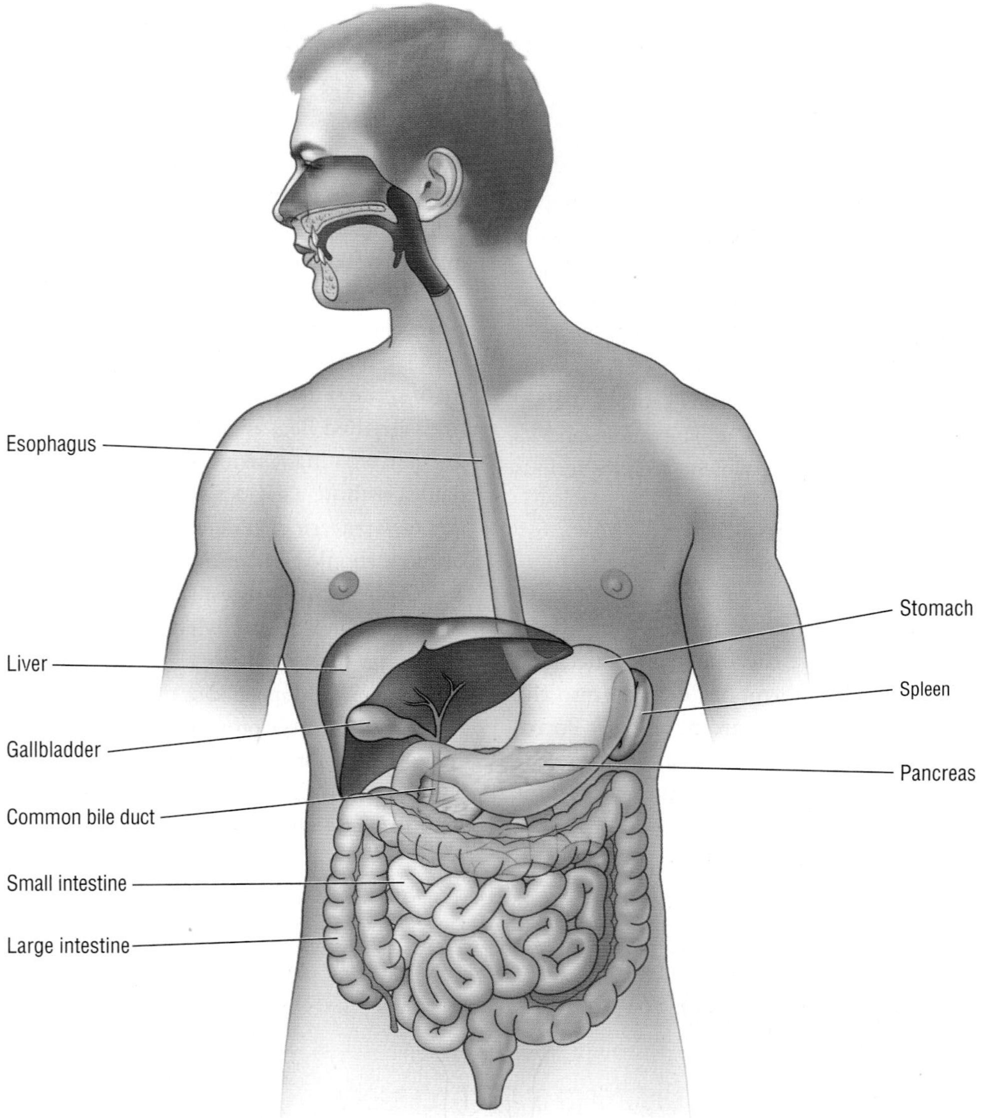

FIGURE 8.1 Digestive system overview

until it is called for, the liver also acts as a sugar buffer, preventing the radical swings in blood glucose levels that would happen without an intermediate stop for sugar. The liver synthesizes many of the enzymes that support cellular activity, as well as the blood proteins that regulate intracellular fluid levels and blood clotting.

Kupffer cells: Phagocytes (cell-eating cells) found in the liver.

Heme: The nonprotein part of hemoglobin that contains iron.

Bilirubin: A dark bile pigment formed from the hemoglobin of dead red blood cells.

Detoxification functions of the liver are well known. The liver alters many drugs into forms that are less toxic than the original, or that can be excreted. A functioning liver prevents many substances, including alcohol, from reaching toxic levels in the bloodstream. It also processes the wastes generated by protein digestion, changing them to uric acid to be excreted by the kidneys.

In addition to these functions, **Kupffer cells** are constantly watching for any pathogens that they can eradicate. Finally, the liver helps to recycle the **heme** from dead red blood cells into **bilirubin**, a major component of bile, which is vital for the digestion of fats. The liver produces up to three cups of bile each day. Bile leaves the liver via the cystic duct and enters the gallbladder.

The Gallbladder

The gallbladder is a small green sac that hangs off the liver about halfway along the right costal angle. Its function is fairly simple: it receives bile from the liver, stores it, and concentrates it. The gallbladder can hold up to one cup of bile at a time. On hormonal command, it releases the bile into the duodenum via the common bile duct. There the bile helps to emulsify fats, that is, separate them into tiny separated globules to make them easier to digest. The gallbladder and its ducts are susceptible to dysfunction, which can have serious repercussions.

The Pancreas

The pancreas is both an exocrine gland releasing digestive juices into the intestine via the pancreatic duct, and an endocrine gland, releasing hormones directly into the bloodstream. Its exocrine secretions are potentially corrosive. Any blockage in the pancreatic duct can lead to very serious tissue damage, as the pancreas is quite capable of digesting itself.

Digestive System Problems and Massage

Most of the digestive system problems that respond well to massage are related to autonomic imbalance; when a person is under stress, digestion is a low priority. If this state of affairs goes on for a long time, problems inevitably develop. The most common disorders of this type are spastic or flaccid constipation, indigestion, and gas.

The first concern, however, is to eliminate the possibility of more serious conditions that contraindicate circulatory massage. Red flags include severe local pain, bloody stools, anemia, bloating, and fever; any of these along with digestive pain constitute a good reason to visit the doctor. In addition, any new pattern of milder digestive pain persists for 2 weeks or more should be investigated.

Problems in the digestive system are impossible to pin down without diagnostic tests, which are outside the scope of practice of massage therapy. Massage should not be performed when the client has any unexplained or undiagnosed pain. Any temporary relief that a massage provides may delay the client getting medical assistance for a serious and acute illness. Although spastic constipation is not inherently dangerous, colon cancer is—and massage therapists are not equipped to tell the difference.

Digestive System Conditions

Disorders of the Upper Gastrointestinal Tract

- Celiac disease
- Esophageal cancer
- Gastroenteritis
- Gastroesophageal reflux disorder
- Peptic ulcers
- Stomach cancer

Disorders of the Large Intestine

- Colorectal cancer
- Diverticular disease
- Irritable bowel syndrome
  - IBS-D
  - IBS-C
  - IBS-M
  - IBS-A

Disorders of the Accessory Organs

- Cirrhosis
- Gallstones
- Hepatitis
  - Hepatitis A
  - Hepatitis B
  - Hepatitis C
  - Other forms of hepatitis
- Liver cancer
- Pancreatic cancer
  - Adenocarcinoma of the pancreas
  - Neuroendocrine tumors of the pancreas
- Pancreatitis
  - Acute pancreatitis
  - Chronic pancreatitis

Other Digestive System Conditions

- Candidiasis
  - Mucocutaneous candidiasis
  - Vulvovaginitis
  - Invasive candidiasis
  - Others

Disorders of the Upper Gastrointestinal Tract

Celiac Disease

Definition: What Is It?

Celiac disease is a condition in which the intestinal villi are flattened or destroyed altogether as part of a reaction in the presence of gluten, a group of proteins present in many types of grains. It is also known as celiac sprue, nontropical sprue, or gluten-sensitive enteropathy.

Demographics

Best estimates suggest that celiac disease occurs in about 0.7% of the United States population (about 2 million people), although the majority of people with this condition are undiagnosed. It is significantly more common in non-Hispanic whites than among any other races. Some evidence suggests that the prevalence of celiac disease is substantially higher than it was in the 1950s.

Etiology: What Happens?

Gluten is an umbrella name for a group of proteins found in many grains, including wheat, rye, barley, spelt, and others. When a person without celiac disease consumes gluten, digestive enzymes break it down into small chains of amino acids that are absorbed into the intestinal villi. When celiac disease is present, gluten is broken into its component pieces, including a long chain of amino acids called gliadin, but gliadin resists enzyme action to break it up any further. For reasons that are not completely clear, gliadin is absorbed into the villi of people with celiac disease, where it triggers a mild or severe inflammatory response.

Eventually, repeated inflammatory attacks on intestinal villi cause them to degenerate, lie flat, or disappear altogether (Figure 8.2). The person then loses access to absorbable nutrition not only from sources of gluten, but from other sources as well. Glucose from dairy products is often particularly difficult to digest, which leads to symptoms of lactose intolerance, although the problem is not with the lactose itself but with the villi that are meant to absorb it. Fats become similarly unavailable, and they pass through the digestive system to be expelled in the stools. Poor uptake leads to signs of malabsorption and malnutrition, although the diet of a person with celiac disease may be identical to that of an average person.

Celiac disease is at least partly related to immune system hyperactivity, and it frequently occurs concurrently with autoimmune disorders, including type 1 **diabetes**, **hypothyroidism**, **hyperthyroidism**, **lupus**, **rheumatoid arthritis**, and **Sjogren syndrome**. A genetic link in celiac disease is easy to trace, since the incidence within families is significantly higher than in the general population. Age at onset varies significantly, however. Some people develop symptoms in early childhood, and others develop symptoms after a significant stressful trigger in adulthood, such as surgery, childbirth, or trauma. Still others may go throughout life with symptoms so mild, they are ignored or misdiagnosed as other GI disorders.

Some people with celiac disease don't have significant GI symptoms, but they develop a painful, itchy rash called dermatitis herpetiformis. It usually clears when gluten is eliminated from the diet.

> **Celiac sprue:** Chronic inflammation and atrophy of the mucosa of the small intestine related to an allergy to gluten. Also called celiac disease.
>
> **Gluten-sensitive enteropathy:** Another name for celiac disease.
>
> **Gliadin:** A class of proteins found in gluten.
>
> **Malabsorption:** Impaired absorption of nutrients by the small intestine.
>
> **Dermatitis herpetiformis:** A chronic condition characterized by a rash of extremely itchy blisters.
>
> **Osteomalacia:** A condition characterized by the progressive softening of bones.

Complications

Complications of celiac disease have to do with poor uptake of nutrients. Young children with celiac disease have delayed growth and development, and many never reach their projected height. Poor uptake of iron and vitamins leads to **anemia**, folic acid deficiency, and a high risk of miscarriage or neural tube defects in a growing fetus. Poor uptake of calcium leads to osteomalacia in children or **osteoporosis** in adults. Muscle weakness, chronic spasm, and joint pain may develop. Behavioral changes, irritability, **peripheral neuropathy**, and a risk of seizures can be linked to a vitamin B_{12} deficiency.

Constant irritation and inflammation of the GI tract also raises the risk of adenocarcinoma or **lymphoma** in the small intestine. Non-Hodgkin lymphoma is a significant cause of death for persons whose celiac disease is never identified.

Signs and Symptoms

Signs and symptoms of celiac disease typically center on malabsorption of nutrients and malnutrition. While some patients have pain or discomfort in the GI tract, many others have only the results of poor vitamin and nutrient uptake. Symptoms may be determined by the section of the small intestine that is most affected. Damage to the duodenum, for instance, results in different nutritional deficiencies from those of damage to the jejunum.

GI symptoms include gas, bloating, and diarrhea. Stools are often high-volume, pale, and foul-smelling, as they contain much of the fat and other material that would normally have been absorbed in the small intestines. It can be difficult to differentiate between symptoms of celiac disease and

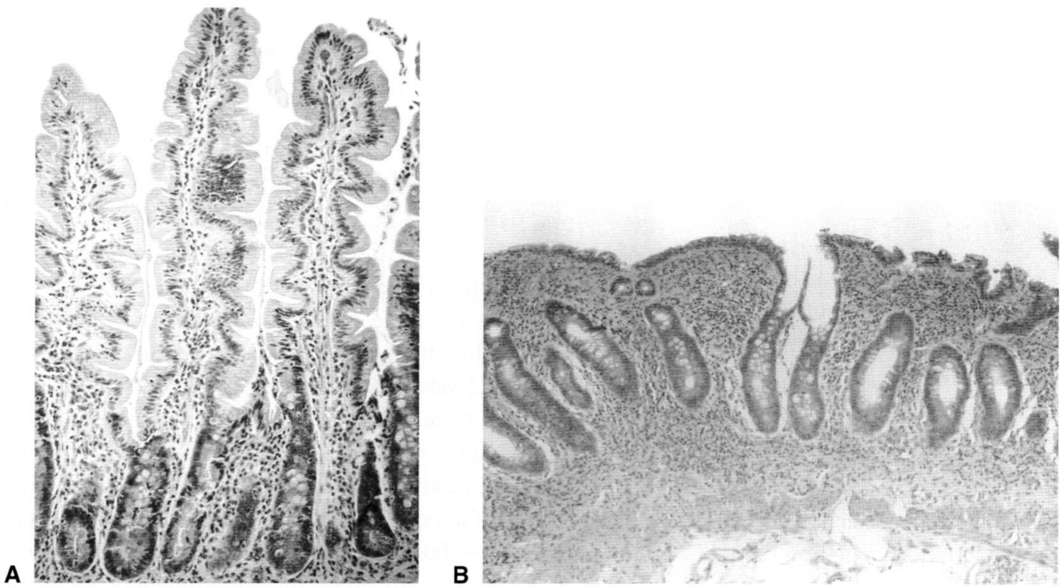

FIGURE 8.2 **A:** Normal villi. **B:** Villi are missing and large lymphocytes are present, indicating an inflammatory response in the mucosal layer.

those of **irritable bowel syndrome (IBS)**. Furthermore, these conditions can occur simultaneously. It is useful to have a full clinical picture however, because each of them responds to a different treatment strategy.

Other symptoms include weight loss (or failure to gain weight in children), anemia, irritability, **depression**, behavior changes, muscle **cramps** and weakness, poor stamina, tooth discoloration, and **dermatitis**. **Seizures**, migraine **headaches**, tingling in hands and feet, missed menstrual periods, repeated miscarriage, and joint pain are other possible symptoms (Sidebar 8.1).

Treatment

No reliable treatment exists for celiac disease, except to avoid gluten in any form. Gluten is present in many grains, including wheat, rye, barley, spelt, triticale, and kamut. Many (but not all) people with celiac disease are also sensitive to oats, although whether this grain actually contains gluten or is frequently contaminated with it is somewhat questionable. Gluten is also used in many other products, including vitamins and other pills, cosmetics (especially lipstick), and as a thickener in many processed foods.

Gluten is not present in corn, quinoa, potatoes, beans, nuts, rice, or soy; flour made from these foods can frequently be substituted to help comprise a gluten-free diet. Other gluten-free foods include fruits, vegetables, and meats. It is possible to have a varied and well-balanced gluten-free diet, but eating processed foods or at restaurants may be problematic.

The majority of celiac disease patients who avoid all sources of gluten for months or years can heal completely, and achieve the complete rebuilding of their intestinal villi. However, this reconstruction can easily be undone if

SIDEBAR 8.1 Gluten Sensitivity ≠ Celiac Disease

Some people report that they have some sensitivity reactions to food with gluten, although their standard tests for celiac disease are negative. Many people make a connection to gluten and intestinal discomfort without going through testing or elimination diets at all—essentially self-diagnosing with gluten sensitivity. This trend has led to a certain level of skepticism inside and outside the medical community. Claims of gluten sensitivity have given rise to a whole field of "gluten-free" food lines, and many consumers have jumped on the bandwagon, perhaps assuming that gluten-free food must be healthier than conventional food.

This is a fallacy of course. Gluten-free bread or crackers or cookies have the same number of calories as conventional ones. They can have the same problems with processed foods as other packaged products from hidden sugar to hydrogenated fats to preservatives. The only thing they lack is a particular protein that breaks down in a particular way in the small intestine.

That said, nonceliac gluten sensitivity is a recognized pathology leading to abdominal pain, diarrhea, and many other symptoms. Is this truly a sensitivity to gluten? Or is it related to other as-yet-undetermined factors? It doesn't really matter for massage therapists. But because many clients consider us a source of accurate information about their health, it is important to be able to share accurate information about the relative healthiness of gluten-free foods.

gluten-rich foods are consumed; a person with celiac disease must commit to a lifelong dietary adjustment.

Medications

- Short-term steroidal anti-inflammatories if restricting gluten does not improve symptoms quickly enough.
- Vitamin and mineral supplements as necessary.
- Topical medication for dermatitis herpetiformis.

Massage Therapy Implications

RISKS	Any relief that follows massage may cause a client to delay getting an important diagnosis, so therapists need to support clients in pursuing nagging digestive symptoms. Abdominal work for a client with diagnosed celiac disease must be conducted conservatively and with ample client feedback for comfort. The characteristic rash that many celiac disease patients have locally contraindicates massage.
BENEFITS	A client who has been diagnosed with celiac disease and manages it successfully can enjoy all the benefits of bodywork as the rest of the population.
OPTIONS	Most experts agree that gluten and gliadin cannot be absorbed through the skin. Nonetheless, some patients find that using hair or skin products with wheat in them causes celiac symptoms. It may be that a different allergic reaction is being triggered. Because celiac disease patients may have other hypersensitivity reactions, it is a good idea to use hypoallergenic oil or lotion for clients with this condition.

Esophageal Cancer

Definition: What Is It?

Esophageal cancer is the development of malignant cells in the esophagus. It typically appears in either of two forms: cancer that grows in the thoracic or proximal area of the esophagus, which is a type of squamous cell carcinoma, or cancer that grows at the distal end, a type of **adenocarcinoma**.

> **Adenocarcinoma:** A malignant tumor of glandular epithelial cells.
>
> **Barrett esophagus:** A condition in which normal esophageal tissue is replaced by tissue similar to intestinal lining.

Demographics

Worldwide, squamous cell esophageal cancer (often related to smoking) is quite common. In the United States, adenocarcinoma (related to reflux) is the most common form of esophageal cancer, and it is one of the few types of cancer with an increasing rather than decreasing incidence.

About 18,000 diagnoses of esophageal cancer are made in the United States annually: 12,000 with adenocarcinoma and 6,000 with squamous cell cancer. The mortality rate for this cancer is high; about 15,000 people die of this disease each year. Men are much more vulnerable to this disease than women with a ratio of about 4:1.

Etiology: What Happens?

The esophagus is a tube about 10-inch long running from the throat to the lower esophageal sphincter that opens into the stomach. It is composed of four main layers of tissue: the mucous membrane that lines the tube; the submucosa that provides blood and lymph support for the active mucus-producing cells; the muscularis that provides strong wave-like contractions to move a food bolus from the throat into the stomach; and the adventitia is a connective tissue outer layer. The esophagus does not have a serous membrane covering.

When malignant cells grow in the upper or middle sections of the esophagus, they tend to appear in squamous epithelial cells of the mucous membrane; this is called squamous cell carcinoma of the esophagus. This condition is closely related to smoking or alcohol use, and smoking in combination with alcohol use increases the risk of malignancies by a large margin.

When esophageal cancer originates at the distal end of the tube, close to the lower esophageal sphincter, it is a glandular cancer. A condition called **Barrett esophagus** is a complication of **gastroesophageal reflux disease** (GERD), and it is considered a precancerous state for adenocarcinoma. Barrett esophagus is the result of exposure to a chronic, repeated barrage of gastric juices from reflux that causes cells of the esophageal mucosa to mutate. This raises the risk of malignancy so significantly that many physicians recommend surgery or other interventions before cancer is confirmed.

Malignant cells from esophageal cancer can invade other tissues in several ways. Because the esophagus has no serous membrane cover, any tumor that penetrates through all four layers of the esophagus can spread easily to nearby structures. The trachea, diaphragm, aorta, vena cava, and laryngeal nerve are most susceptible (Figure 8.3). Because the esophageal submucosa has a generous supply of lymphatic capillaries, lymphatic spread of the disease is also a risk. The lymph system can carry malignant cells to nearby nodes and other tissues, including the lungs, liver, and bones. Esophageal cancer can also spread through the bloodstream, although this appears to happen more rarely than other routes for metastasis.

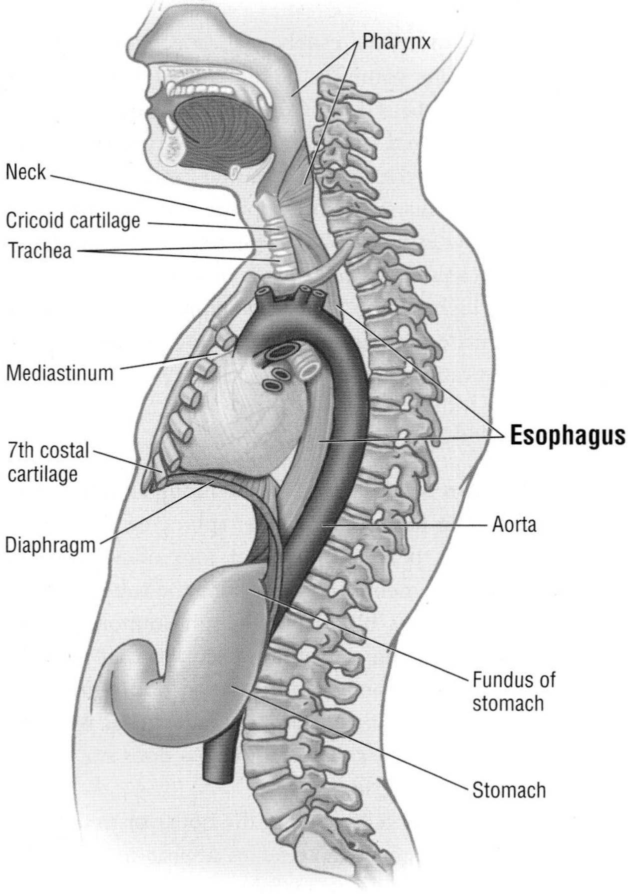

FIGURE 8.3 If esophageal cancer penetrates through the wall of the esophagus, it can spread to several other structures through direct contact

Smoking and alcohol use increase the chance of developing upper esophageal cancer, and GERD increases the risk of lower esophageal cancer. Other risk factors include obesity (this may contribute to GERD), a history of any other head or neck cancer, exposure to toxic substances (i.e., ingesting lye or other poisons), exposure to human papillomavirus in the throat, and a lifetime habit of drinking extremely hot beverages. Worldwide studies also reveal that a shortage of vitamins A, B, and C, beta-carotene, and selenium are common among esophageal cancer patients. Interestingly, having a *Helicobacter pylori* infection—a major contributor to **peptic ulcers**—turns out to be associated with a reduced risk for Barrett esophagus and esophageal cancer. Some researchers suggest that reduced acid output in the stomach is the reason.

Signs and Symptoms

Early signs and symptoms of esophageal cancer are practically nonexistent, which is why this disease has such a high mortality rate; it is often undetected until a tumor is large enough to create a mechanical obstruction, and metastasis to other nearby organs and/or lymph nodes has already occurred.

The symptoms that most often cause people to go to the doctor include dysphagia, a feeling of food or liquid "getting stuck" on its way to the stomach, pain with swallowing, and unplanned weight loss. A chronic cough, with or without blood, may also occur. Hoarseness may be related to mechanical irritation of the trachea or to damage at the laryngeal nerve. Hiccups may indicate damage to the phrenic nerve.

Other signs suggest that the cancer has spread or that complications have developed. Deep pain indicates possible metastasis to bones. Fever and lung infection may be connected to a tracheo-esophageal fistula, which allows materials into the respiratory tract that shouldn't be there.

Treatment

Treatment for esophageal cancer could include surgery, chemotherapy, radiation therapy, or photodynamic therapy, in which specially designed drugs are absorbed into cancerous cells, and exposure to a laser destroys them. Surgery may be conducted to remove the affected section of the esophagus, or simply to create a more functional passageway. Radiation may be externally or internally applied. Chemotherapy is not generally successful by itself, but may be used as part of a larger treatment strategy.

Treatment options are determined by the stage of cancer at diagnosis. Staging protocols are provided in Sidebar 8.2.

Recovery from treatment for esophageal cancer is often problematic, since good nutrition is essential to heal from such invasive procedures, and eating is often very difficult.

Medications

- Chemotherapeutic agents
- Photodynamic therapy

Massage Therapy Implications

RISKS	As with other cancers, massage for esophageal cancer patients must be adjusted according to the client's general resilience and the treatment options (along with commensurate side-effects) that are in use. This client may have a reduced ability to tolerate rigorous massage, so bodywork must be carefully accommodated.
BENEFITS	Massage for cancer patients has been seen to improve sleep and appetite, reduce depression and anxiety, and help with pain. All of these can benefit esophageal cancer patients with appropriate accommodations. More information on massage in the context of cancer appears in Chapter 12.

SIDEBAR 8.2 Staging Esophageal Cancer

The staging of esophageal cancer is determined by how deeply the esophagus has been penetrated by cancer cells, and by whether lymph nodes have been affected or metastasis has developed. Esophageal cancer is staged using both the TNM (tumor, node, and metastasis) technique and numerical staging from 0 to IV. Here is a somewhat simplified version of esophageal cancer staging.

TUMOR (T)	NODE (N)	METASTASIS (M)
T is: cancer in situ, limited to superficial mucosa: dysplasia.	N0: no nodes involved.	M0: no metastasis found.
T1: mucosa and/or submucosa invaded.	N1: 1–2 nearby nodes involved.	M1a: distant lymph nodes involved.
T2: muscularis invaded.	N2: metastasis in 3–6 regional nodes.	M1b: distant organs involved.
T3: adventitia invaded.	N3: metastasis in 7 or more regional nodes.	
T4: nearby structures invaded.		

HISTOLOGIC GRADE (G)	
Gx	Grade cannot be assessed.
G1	Cells are well-differentiated.
G2	Cells are moderately differentiated.
G3	Cells are poorly differentiated.
G4	Cells are undifferentiated.

These delineations are then translated into stages 0 to IV in this way:

STAGE	TUMOR	NODE	METASTASIS	GRADE
0	T is	N0	M0	1x
IA, B	T1	N0	M0	1–3
IIA, B	T2–3	N0-1	M0	1–3
III	T3–4	N any	M0	Any
IVA, B	T any	N any	M1a,b	Any

Gastroenteritis

Definition: What Is It?

Gastroenteritis is inflammation of the GI tract, usually the stomach or small intestine. By convention, gastroenteritis is usually discussed as a result of an infection with bacteria, viruses, or parasites. Noninfectious problems can also cause inflammation of the GI tract, however; and it can sometimes be difficult to identify the cause of a person's symptoms.

Demographics

Norovirus is the most common cause of acute gastroenteritis in the United States. It causes about 20 million illnesses and contributes to up to 800 deaths each year. It is not possible to develop immunity to norovirus, so one individual can be infected multiple times.

Bacterial gastroenteritis is likewise common, although the causative agents may be different between children and adults. One bacterial infection, *Clostridium difficile*, is often associated with hospital and nursing home stays. Its incidence has more than tripled since 2000.

Gastroenteritis is a condition with a high mortality rate among vulnerable populations. Worldwide it is a leading cause of death for infants and young children. In the United States, it is associated with about 17,000 deaths each year, mostly among people over 65.

Etiology: What Happens?

The symptoms of gastroenteritis are caused by damage to the intestines that can occur in a variety of ways. Some pathogens produce toxins that injure the intestinal mucosa. Others directly invade mucosal cells to destroy them. When peristalsis is slowed or delayed, which can occur with **diabetes** and some other diseases, pathogens that would normally be expelled can linger and overpower protective mechanisms so that gastroenteritis becomes a complication of another disease.

When the GI tract is damaged or inflamed, absorption of nutrients and water is severely limited. Both water and valuable electrolytes are lost through diarrhea and vomiting.

Gastroenteritis can have several causes:

- *Viruses.* The most common cause of GI inflammation among adults in the United States is Norwalk virus (one of a group called noroviruses). Among children, rotavirus infections are most common. Any of the **hepatitis** viruses can cause GI inflammation, as can any member of the enterovirus family. Viral gastroenteritis is highly communicable and can reach epidemic levels.
- *Bacteria.* Common bacterial pathogens include *Salmonella, Shigella, Campylobacter,* and several varieties of *Escherichia coli.* Bacterial gastroenteritis is usually spread through improperly stored or prepared food or contaminated water or ice. "Traveler's diarrhea" is almost always from *E. coli* or *Campylobacter jejuni. Helicobacter pylori,* the pathogen associated with **peptic ulcers** is a common source of gastroenteritis. One increasingly common bacterial infection of the GI tract is caused by *C. difficile* (C-diff). It is particularly dangerous, because C-diff produces toxins that can seriously damage the wall of the colon. It is sometimes called necrotizing colitis or pseudomembranous colitis. C-diff is resistant to many antibiotics, and is seen frequently in hospital patients.
- *Parasites.* Microscopic animal parasites can invade the GI tract, causing typical symptoms of gastroenteritis. Among the most common are *Giardia, Cryptosporidium,* and *Entamoeba histolytica.*
- *Others.* Other causes of gastroenteritis include fungal infections (i.e., candidiasis), toxins (i.e., poisonous mushrooms or shellfish, or seafood from red tide areas), dietary problems (i.e., food allergies), medications (i.e., antibiotics or magnesium-containing laxatives or antacids), and other conditions that interfere with absorption or cause inflammation. These include **celiac disease, appendicitis, Crohn disease, ulcerative colitis,** and **diverticulitis.** And weakness at the **pyloric valve** may allow contents of the duodenum to back up into the stomach, causing local irritation. This is called bile reflux.

NOTABLE CASES Twelfth United States President Zachary Taylor died on July 9, 1850 at age 65. He had experienced 4 days of intense cramping, nausea, vomiting, diarrhea, and dehydration. These symptoms followed his eating a lot of cherries and cold milk as a part of July 4th celebrations. It is theorized that he died of cholera, a deadly form of bacterial gastroenteritis that he contracted either through contaminated cherries or milk. President Taylor had been in office for only 16 months. He was succeeded by Millard Fillmore.

Pathogenic forms of gastroenteritis are highly communicable. They can spread through an environment via oral-fecal contamination, or via contaminated water or ice. Food prepared on contaminated surfaces can carry viruses or bacteria. For these reasons, travelers to places where gastroenteritis is common are advised to use only bottled water for drinking and brushing teeth, and to avoid raw fruits and vegetables that may have been rinsed in contaminated water.

The most serious complication of gastroenteritis is dehydration from the massive fluid and mineral loss that goes along with diarrhea and vomiting. The loss of critical fluid and electrolytes can be fatal; gastroenteritis is a leading cause of death in many developing nations. In the United States, the people most at risk for this extreme reaction are infants, immunocompromised persons, and elders, whose systems are not capable of coping with this extreme change in internal environment. Signs of dangerously progressed dehydration include sunken eyes, lack of urination or very dark urine, and skin tenting: when the skin is pinched it does not immediately go back to its original position.

Some gastroenteritis factors can cause other problems as well. *Campylobacter* has been linked with **Guillain-Barré syndrome**, and *Salmonella* can complicate into **meningitis** or blood poisoning. Some forms of *E. coli* are highly toxic and can lead to **renal failure**.

Most cases of gastroenteritis resolve within 2 or 3 days without medical intervention. If symptoms persist longer than 2 to 3 weeks, it is no longer considered an acute infection, but a chronic condition. This leads medical professionals to look for an underlying condition such as food allergy, **IBS**, diverticulitis, Crohn disease, ulcerative colitis, **hepatitis**, or **HIV/AIDS**.

Signs and Symptoms

Different causative factors of gastroenteritis can lead to varying signs and symptoms, but the basic trio of intestinal inflammation includes nausea, vomiting, and

Pyloric valve: The ring of muscle at the passage from the stomach to the small intestine. Also called the pyloric sphincter.

diarrhea. These are appropriate responses to infection, as they are efficient methods of clearing out the GI tract, but several of these diseases are spread through oral-fecal contamination, so hygiene is critical when dealing with these symptoms.

Other signs that may develop with gastroenteritis include bloating, cramps, gas, and mucus or blood in the stools.

Treatment

Gastroenteritis is much easier to prevent than to treat. When it occurs in large outbreaks, it is often due to a specific source of contamination: a shipment of tainted vegetables, a contaminated well, or shellfish harvested from polluted water. Since foodstuffs are now shipped quickly all over large areas, it is a constant public health challenge to track down the source of infection and to limit its spread among the rest of the population.

Gastroenteritis is usually an acute, self-limiting condition, and is generally treated with rest, fluid, and electrolyte replacement. Viruses do not respond to antibiotics, and antibiotics for bacterial infections of the GI tract are problematic, because they may make intestinal inflammation worse. The use of anti-diarrhea medications is often discouraged, because they interfere with the process of shedding pathogens, and so may prolong the infection.

Treatment focuses on preventing dehydration. If taking fluids by mouth aggravates vomiting, it may be necessary to use intravenous fluid replacement in a hospital setting.

Medications

- An oral vaccine for rotavirus is available.
- Antibiotics, if tolerated, for bacterial infection.
- Antiemetics to control vomiting.

Massage Therapy Implications

RISKS	Acute gastroenteritis contraindicates massage mainly because the client is unlikely to be comfortable. Pathogenic infections may also be communicable if surfaces are contaminated.
BENEFITS	If a client has digestive system irritation that is unrelated to infection, cancer, or other dangerous causes, bodywork could be helpful in promoting a parasympathetic state that can improve function and comfort.

Gastroesophageal Reflux Disease

Definition: What Is It?

Gastroesophageal reflux disease (GERD) is a condition involving damage to the epithelial lining of the esophagus, when it is chronically exposed to digestive juices from the stomach. It is usually associated with a weakness at the lower esophageal sphincter, but several other factors may contribute as well.

Demographics

Many people experience some gastric reflux at some point; up to 40% of the United States population (including infants and children) have this condition from time to time. A smaller percentage, about 10%, have it more than once a week. The frequency of GERD symptoms may be a predictor for its complications.

Etiology: What Happens?

Most cases of GERD are connected to some combination of four problems: the lower esophageal sphincter is too relaxed; the lower esophageal sphincter doesn't allow appropriate clearing of foods from the esophagus into the stomach; the **esophageal hiatus** in the diaphragm has trapped a portion of the stomach; or the stomach is slow to empty, adding to backpressure at the lower esophageal sphincter.

Any one of these problems allows stomach contents, including highly corrosive hydrochloric acid (and occasionally bile and pancreatic enzymes that have backed up from a weak pyloric valve), to enter the esophagus, which lacks the thick layer of mucus that protects the stomach from acid exposure (Figure 8.4).

Risk factors for GERD include pregnancy, obesity, smoking, a diet high in fatty or spicy foods, caffeine and alcohol use, and connective tissue disease like **lupus** or **scleroderma**. A hiatal **hernia**, which is an enlargement of the opening in the diaphragm where the esophagus passes through the stomach, may catch and irritate the superior part of the stomach. Most people with hiatal hernias have GERD, although not all GERD patients have hiatal hernias. Some diseases, including **diabetes**, **peptic ulcers**, and **spinal cord injuries**, cause reduced peristalsis and sluggish movement of substances through the GI tract. When stomach contents linger too long, the accumulation of pressure and gastric juices can cause them to put backpressure on the esophagus.

Esophageal hiatus: The opening in the diaphragm through which the esophagus passes.

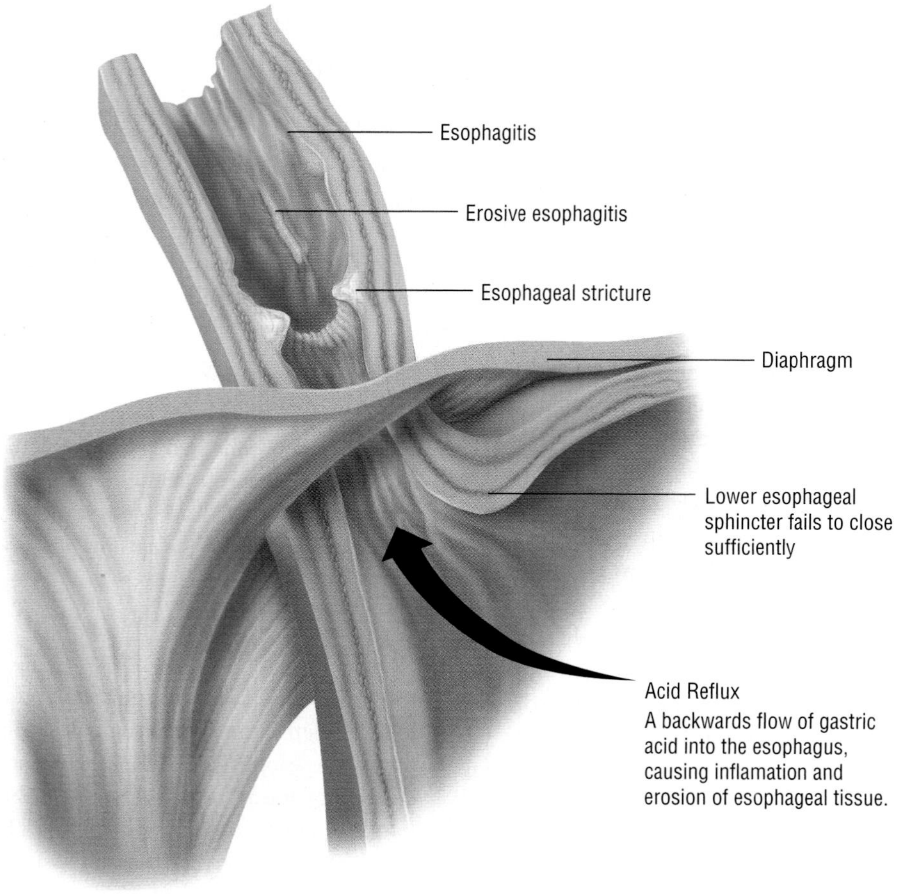
Esophagitis
Erosive esophagitis
Esophageal stricture
Diaphragm
Lower esophageal sphincter fails to close sufficiently
Acid Reflux
A backwards flow of gastric acid into the esophagus, causing inflamation and erosion of esophageal tissue.

FIGURE 8.4 Gastroesophageal reflux disorder: backsplash from the stomach enters the esophagus

Complications

Chronic irritation of the esophageal lining can cause several reactions:

- *Respiratory injury*. This may occur if gastric secretions reach up to the larynx where these substances can be aspirated into the lungs. GERD may be a risk factor for laryngeal cancer.
- *Decay of tooth enamel*. This may develop as acidic juices are increasingly present in the mouth.
- *Esophageal ulcers*. These lesions may become infected, or they may bleed into the GI tract.
- *Stricture*. The esophageal wall thickens with scar tissue in response to irritation. Strictures may make it difficult to swallow normally.
- *Barrett esophagus*. This is a pathological change in the normal esophageal cells; they mutate into cells that resemble the stomach lining. Barrett esophagus has been identified as a precancerous condition, opening the door to adenocarcinoma, an increasingly common and dangerous type of **esophageal cancer**.

Signs and Symptoms

Signs and symptoms of GERD are produced mainly by the action of gastric juice on the delicate esophageal lining. A bitter taste, a feeling like some food has been regurgitated, gas, indigestion, bloating, and pain in the chest behind the sternum are common symptoms. The pain of GERD can be mistaken for **heart attack** or angina. Symptoms are reliably aggravated by bending over or lying down.

Other GERD symptoms that occur less frequently include trouble swallowing, along with coughing, wheezing, and hemoptysis, if ulcers in the esophagus have eroded into a blood vessel.

Treatment

Treatment for GERD falls into two categories: management and repair. Managing GERD so that it doesn't progress includes strategies like losing weight; eating smaller portions; not lying down within 2 hours after a meal; avoiding caffeine, alcohol, and nicotine; raising the bed about 6 inches at the head; loosening clothing that puts pressure around the waist; and putting a heating pad on the stomach when it is painful. Foods that are associated with reflux include chocolate, coffee, peppermint, fatty or spicy foods, tomato products, and alcoholic beverages. Research suggests that traditional and electroacupuncture can be helpful for symptom management as well.

Medications for GERD can work in a variety of ways. Antacids neutralize stomach acid, but over-the-counter brands may also cause the stomach to expand with gas and putting more pressure on the esophageal valve. Other medications can block receptors in the stomach that stimulate acid production, increase stomach motility to assist in sluggish movement, and block the release of hydrogen ions that contribute to the stomach's acidic environment.

Surgery usually focuses on strengthening the esophageal sphincter and taking pressure off the stomach. If the esophagus is limited by the development of a scar tissue stricture, this may be dilated. A portion of the stomach may be wrapped around the sphincter to give it external support in a procedure called a **fundoplication**. And if a hiatal hernia puts pressure on the stomach, surgery may be performed to correct it.

Medications

- Antacids to reduce the acidic environment in the stomach.
- H2 blockers to reduce histamine activity and acid production.
- Proton pump inhibitors to reduce acid production.
- Coating agents to protect tissues from acid.
- Promotility agents to promote peristalsis and tighten the lower esophageal valve.

Massage Therapy Implications

RISKS	It is important to work with GERD patients in a way that does not exacerbate their symptoms. This may mean not working with them lying flat on a table, or scheduling massage appointments for at least a couple of hours after their last meal.
BENEFITS	Clients who successfully treat this condition can enjoy the same benefits of massage as the rest of the population, although work around the superior aspect of the abdomen should probably be conservative.
OPTIONS	Clients with GERD may accept massage most comfortably if they can sit in a recliner or a massage chair.
RESEARCH	The main body of research about massage therapy for GERD symptoms has been done with infants and their parents. Not surprisingly, it was found that an infant having GERD is disruptive to parent-child interactions, and that teaching caregivers to give massage to the infant can have a positive effect on that bond.[1] 1. Neu M, Schmiege SJ, Pan Z, et al. Interactions during feeding with mothers and their infants with symptoms of gastroesophageal reflux. *Journal of Alternative and Complementary Medicine* 2014;20(6):493–499. http://www.ncbi.nlm.nih.gov/pubmed/24742255

Peptic Ulcers

Definition: What Are They?

An ulcer is the result of progressive tissue damage due to constant irritation or some impediment to the healing process. Cells in the lesion die, and a crater erodes into deep layers of tissue. An ulcer is a perpetually open sore, and an invitation to infection. This section focuses on peptic ulcers of the inner surfaces of the stomach and duodenum, but an ulcer has the same properties, whether it is in the GI tract or on the skin.

Demographics

Peptic ulcers affect about 4.5 million people in the United States each year, and approximately 10% of all people have some signs of a duodenal ulcer at some point.

Helicobacter pylori is a factor in many ulcers, but a person can be infected with *H. pylori* and never develop a peptic ulcer. *Helicobacter pylori* is probably present in 20% of all Americans under 40, and in 50% of those over 60-year old.

Etiology: What Happens?

Ulcers in the esophagus, stomach, or small intestine are called peptic ulcers, named for **pepsin**, the protein-digesting enzyme that contributes to their development (Figure 8.5).

Until fairly recently, ulcers have been assumed to be caused by too much stress and/or spicy or acidic food. Ulcer patients have historically been counseled to eat bland food, to drink lots of milk, and to avoid getting upset or overly excited. Many found that their ulcers eventually subsided, but would recur later; they were essentially a lifelong condition. A more current understanding of these lesions show that they are multifactorial condition involving fluctuations in stress, bacterial infection, and some medications.

Stress and Ulcers

The link between stress and ulcers is a significant factor, but the incidence of ulcers across the population doesn't follow demographics that are associated with high-stress situations, so variables in individual stress coping mechanisms evidently influence this process.

The normal environment inside a stomach has some features that can be classified as aggressive and others that are defensive. Aggressive features include the production of

Fundoplication: Suture of the fundus of the stomach around the esophagus to prevent reflux with hiatal hernia.

Pepsin: The main digestive enzyme in the stomach.

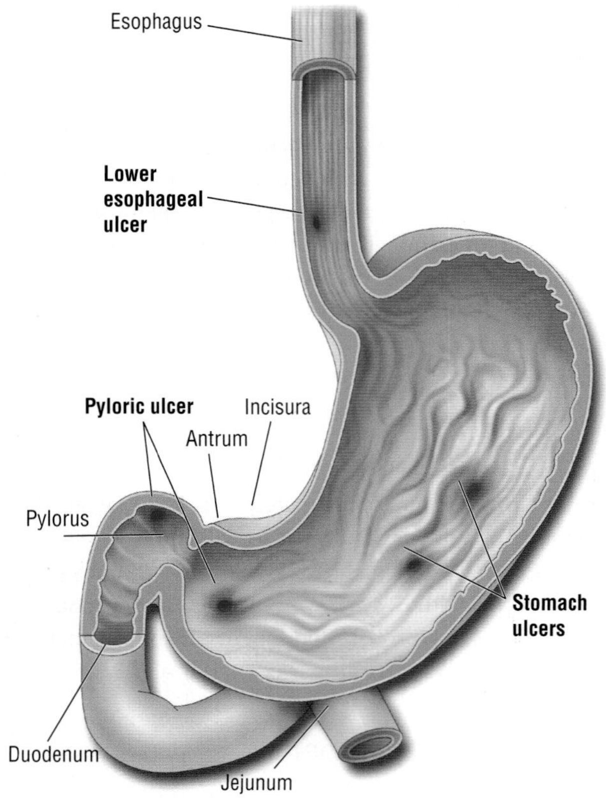

FIGURE 8.5 Sites of peptic ulcers

hydrochloric acid and pepsin, which help to digest proteins. Defensive features include a generous blood supply to the stomach wall, which serves to help damaged cells regenerate quickly, and supports rapid mucus production. Mucus protects the stomach wall from acid and pepsin. The acid is then neutralized in the first section of the small intestine by bicarbonate from the pancreas. These aggressive and defensive mechanisms work best when they keep each other in balance.

Recall that when a person is in a sympathetic state, blood supply to the whole digestive tract is suppressed, and stomach activity is suspended. Lack of blood flow means that mucus production is slowed, but so is acid and pepsin production: the two mechanisms stay in balance. But when stress is lifted and a person shifts back into a relaxed, parasympathetic state, stomach secretions are stimulated again. The problem is that the stomach produces acid and pepsin much faster than it rebuilds a delicate mucus lining. This imbalance between aggressive and defensive features leaves the stomach wall vulnerable to damage. In other words, ulcers seem to be more related to the fluctuations in stress than to the perception of stress alone.

> **NOTABLE CASES** Iconic Irish writer James Joyce (*Ulysses*, *The Dubliners*) died of complications related to a perforated ulcer at age 59. English writer Rudyard Kipling (*The Jungle Book*, *Gunga Din*) lost his life at age 70 to a perforated duodenal ulcer. And "Bird" jazz saxophone pioneer Charlie Parker was officially said to have died of a bleeding ulcer at age 34, but the recent heart attack, cirrhosis, and pneumonia that were all present at the same time might also have contributed.

Helicobacter pylori and Ulcers

In 1984, a remarkable discovery revealed an unexpected phenomenon: a bacterium that can survive and thrive in the highly acidic environment of the stomach. This bacterium, *H. pylori*, is found in many biopsies of ulcers. It is an unusual bacterium, shaped like a bacillus (it can be rod-shaped), but it also has spiral flagella (Figure 8.6). Identification of *H. pylori* led to the conclusion that imbalances in GI tract chemistry can initiate tissue damage to the mucosa, but bacterial infection makes the ulcer a long-term chronic problem. (For more information on *H. pylori*, see Sidebar 8.3.)

Anti-inflammatories and Ulcers

The use of nonsteroidal anti-inflammatory drugs (NSAIDs) for everything from headaches to back pain to heart disease and stroke prevention has led to significant disruption

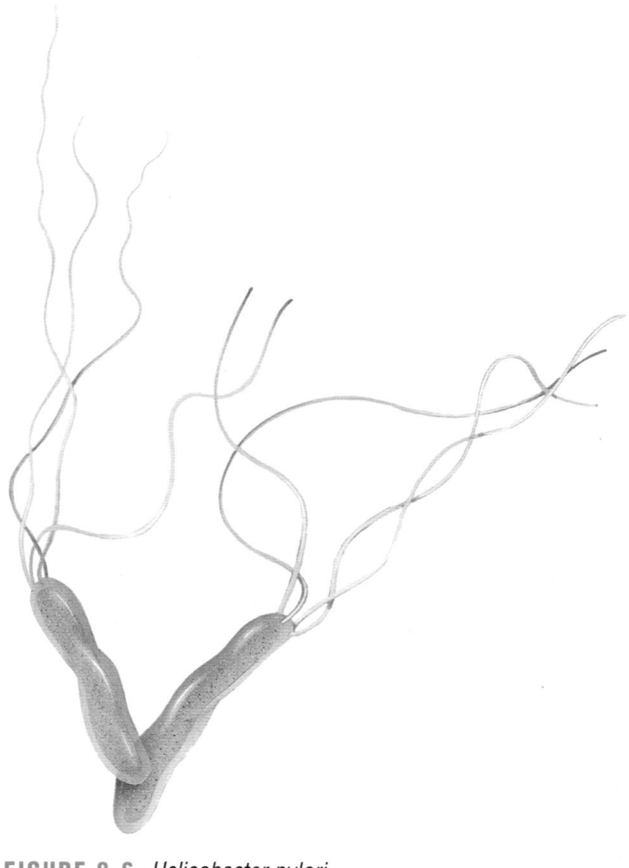

FIGURE 8.6 *Helicobacter pylori*

SIDEBAR 8.3 What is *Helicobacter pylori*?

Helicobacter pylori is a bacterium that is admirably designed to withstand and even thrive in the corrosively acidic environment of the stomach. The bacterium has several anatomical features that allow it to infect the mucous membranes of the stomach and duodenal wall.

Until 1984, it was never even considered that a bacterium could survive in the digestive tract. When pioneer researchers Barry Marshall and Robin Warren proposed the possibility and a scientific meeting, they were all but laughed offstage. But biopsies of lesions consistently revealed the presence of *H. pylori*. And when ulcer patients found that combining appropriate antibiotics with other acid-limiting medications led to a permanent cure for their ulcers—something that was unheard of at the time—the approach to treating this common condition completely changed. In 1994, the National Institutes of Health issued a statement that it was clear that *H. pylori* does indeed cause most peptic ulcers, and is also a contributing factor to stomach cancer and lymphoma.

What is *H. pylori*, and where does it come from? Little is well understood about this pathogen. It is a short, **microaerophilic gram-negative bacillus** with spiraling flagella. It is sensitive to common antibiotics such as tetracycline and amoxicillin.

The discovery of *H. pylori* and its role in peptic ulcers has raised as many questions as it has answered:

- How is the bacterium communicated? No one knows, but most researchers believe it is through oral-fecal contamination or through salivary contact.
- How can it be prevented? It is impossible to prevent the spread of *H. pylori* without knowing how it gets from one person to another.
- If it is sensitive to common antibiotics, why isn't it eradicated when a person takes amoxicillin or tetracycline for something else? Antibiotics for *H. pylori* seem to work only when an ulcer has formed or when the infected person has acute gastritis from bacterial irritation.
- Does the presence of *H. pylori* contribute to general indigestion? It is unclear, but taking antibiotics for indigestion definitely doesn't clear up an *H. pylori* infection or relieve symptoms of **dyspepsia**.
- What diseases are associated with *H. pylori*? This bacterium has been definitively associated with an assortment of serious conditions, including chronic active gastritis, stomach cancer, peptic ulcers, and lymphoma that begins in the stomach.

of stomach function for many patients. Aspirin, ibuprofen, and naproxen sodium all inhibit the **cyclooxygenase-1 pathway**, so they impede the production of prostaglandins that would otherwise stimulate blood flow and healthy mucus production. Interestingly, these medications also inhibit the production of bicarbonate in the pancreas, which should neutralize stomach acid. This means the duodenum is especially vulnerable to corrosion.

Complications of ulcers can be serious. When they erode into capillaries, cumulative slow bleeding into the GI tract can lead to **anemia**. If the damaged blood vessel is a larger arteriole or artery, untreated hemorrhaging can lead quickly to shock and death. Ulcers can also perforate, or eat all the way through the organ wall, releasing bacteria and partially digested food into the peritoneal space, leading to **peritonitis**. Perforation happens more often with duodenal than stomach ulcers. Ulcers can create a combination of scar tissue and inflammation that causes the pyloric valve to spasm. If this is not quickly resolved, surgery can be required to reopen the digestive tract. Finally, having a peptic ulcer significantly raises the risk of developing **stomach cancer**. Although stomach cancer is on the decline in the United States, it is still the second leading type of cancer worldwide. Another type of cancer, mucosal-associated lymphoid-type **lymphoma**, is also associated with *H. pylori* and a history of peptic ulcers.

Helicobacter pylori and the use of NSAIDs (or a combination of the two) account for the majority of peptic ulcers, but about 20% of diagnosed ulcers may be related to entirely other factors. These idiopathic peptic ulcers are the subject of active study.

Microaerophilic: Describing a type of bacteria that requires very little oxygen to live.

Gram-negative bacillus: One of a class of bacteria that can be identified by the way in which they do not retain violet coloring when using a gram stain.

Cyclooxygenase-1 pathway (COX-1 pathway): The sequence of events that leads to an inflammatory process.

Dyspepsia: Indigestion.

Signs and Symptoms

The primary symptom of peptic ulcers is a gnawing, burning pain in the chest or abdomen that can last anywhere from 30 minutes to 3 hours. When the pain occurs in relation to eating varies greatly from one person to another, and it can depend on the location of the ulcer. Pain is generally relieved by antacids or eating more food.

Other signs of ulcers can include nausea, vomiting, loss of appetite, and bleeding into the GI tract.

Treatment

Treatment for most ulcers includes antibiotics for the *H. pylori*; **bismuth** that protects the delicate stomach lining; and several medications that limit histamine release (H2 blockers) or acid production (proton pump inhibitors). When the treatment regimen is carefully followed, ulcers may be permanently healed.

Ulcers caused by the use of NSAIDs do not respond to antibiotic therapy. The only way to limit them is to suspend the use of the medications that damage the stomach lining. That said, some people need NSAID therapy for specific conditions. It is now recognized that if any trace of *H. pylori* is eradicated in these patients before they begin their antibiotic therapy, their risk of bleeding ulcers is diminished.

Ulcers that don't heal satisfactorily or that continue to bleed, perforate, or cause strictures may be surgically corrected, either by removing damaged sections of the stomach, or by severing the appropriate branch of the vagus nerve to limit acid secretion.

Medications

- Antibiotics for *H. pylori*
- Bismuth to protect the stomach lining
- H2 blockers to limit histamine release in the stomach
- Proton pump inhibitors to limit acidity in the stomach

Massage Therapy Implications

RISKS	Because massage stimulates a parasympathetic press response, which can promote digestive activity, a person with ulcers may be most comfortable timing their massage appointments around their eating schedule for the least discomfort. If lying flat on a table exacerbates symptoms, massage may be better offered in a reclining chair or on a massage chair.
BENEFITS	While massage has no direct impact on peptic ulcers, the general parasympathetic response that it brings about can be helpful for a person with ulcers.
RESEARCH	Some preliminary evidence suggests that deep reflex muscular massage along with exercise may elicit an immune system response that promotes peptic ulcer relief, but if that work has ever been replicated or built upon, it is not readily available.[1] 1. Aksenova AM, Teslenko OI, Boganskaia OA. Changes in the immune status of peptic ulcer patients after combined treatment including deep massage. *Vopr Kurortol Fizioter Lech Fiz Kult* 1999;(2):19–20. http://www.ncbi.nlm.nih.gov/pubmed/24742255

Stomach Cancer

Definition: What Is It?

Stomach cancer is the development of malignant tumors in the stomach that can block the passage of food through the digestive system, and can spread to other organs either through direct contact or through blood and lymph flow.

Demographics

About 21,000 people are diagnosed, and some 11,000 die each year in this country from stomach cancer.

Worldwide, stomach cancer is the second leading cause of death by cancer. It is more common in men than in women, it usually affects people over 60-year old, and it is associated with tobacco smoking, a history of stomach surgery, obesity, and a diet high in salted, smoked, or pickled foods.

Etiology: What Happens?

Although several types of cancer have been observed to grow from stomach cells, most stomach cancers are adenocarcinomas, involving mutations of glandular cells (Figure 8.7). It is not always clear what triggers these mutations, but a comparison of eating habits and the history of both refrigeration and antibiotic use yields some clues.

Stomach cancer rates in the United States began to decline in the 1930s, about the time that refrigeration became accessible for most Americans. The average diet shifted away from smoked, pickled, and salted foods, and toward more fresh meats and fresh, canned, or frozen vegetables. In countries where stomach cancer is very prominent, the consumption of salted, smoked, or pickled foods is significantly higher than it is in the United States.

> **NOTABLE CASES** Actor John Wayne survived lung cancer in 1964, but succumbed to stomach cancer in 1979. Everybody's favorite neighbor Fred Rogers died of stomach cancer at age 74. At the opposite end of the personality spectrum, Napoleon Bonaparte's death may have been due to stomach cancer, although some speculate that he may have been the victim of arsenic poisoning.

Most stomach cancer patients test positive for *H. pylori*. This bacterium, which is associated with **peptic ulcers**, converts the **nitrates** and **nitrites** in high-risk foods (mainly

> **Bismuth:** A chemical element sometimes used in the treatment of ulcers.
>
> **Nitrate:** A common preservative in meats. Contains one more oxygen than nitrites.
>
> **Nitrite:** A salt or ester of nitrous acid, commonly used as a preservative.

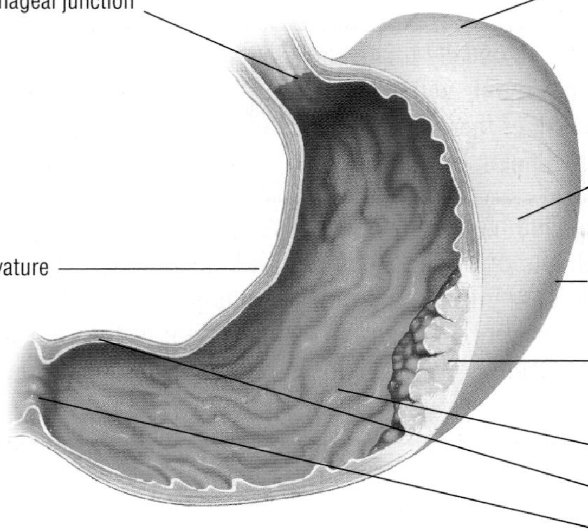

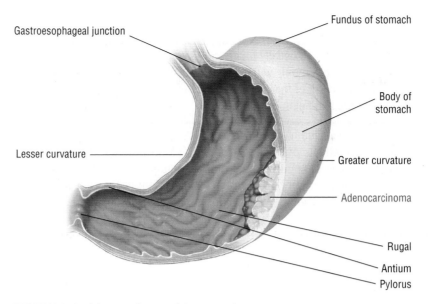

FIGURE 8.7 Adenocarcinoma of the stomach

cured meats) into carcinogens. Infection rates of this not well-understood bacterium are low in the United States, compared with many other countries.

When the environment in the stomach is insufficiently acidic, ingested materials don't break down properly and many become carcinogenic. Any situation that impedes the production of gastric digestive secretions increases the risk of stomach cancer. This can include a history of *H. pylori* infection, atrophic gastritis (long-term inflammation that destroys acid-producing cells), stomach surgery, **pernicious anemia**, and other factors.

At its most complex, the stomach wall has five distinct layers: the mucosa, the submucosa, the muscularis, the visceral layer of the peritoneum, and the parietal layer of the peritoneum. In some areas, however, the serous membranes don't separate the stomach from adjacent organs.

As the mucosal layer of the stomach wall is assaulted with chronic exposure to carcinogens, tiny changes in the glandular cells may develop. These precancerous changes are virtually silent, and are almost never detected. Malignant cells eventually grow into tumors large enough to obstruct the passage of food through the digestive tract, or they can invade and perforate the muscular layer and the serous membranes, allowing them to contact and then spread to nearby abdominal organs. It can also use the circulatory and lymph systems to metastasize. By the time stomach cancer is detected, it has usually moved through the portal vein to the liver or into the lymph system.

Adenocarcinomas account for 90% to 95% of stomach cancer diagnoses. Other types of cancers in the stomach include a type of non-Hodgkin **lymphoma**, **carcinoid tumors** that arise from hormone-producing cells, and **stromal tumors** that can occur anywhere in the GI tract.

Signs and Symptoms

Signs and symptoms of stomach cancer are mostly related to the sensation of having an obstruction in the digestive tract. They include a feeling of fullness after only a little food, vague abdominal pain above the navel, unintentional weight loss, heartburn and other **ulcer** symptoms, nausea and vomiting, and the development of **ascites**: the accumulation of excessive fluid in the peritoneal space. Tumors may bleed slightly, leading to small amounts of blood in the stool and possible anemia.

Treatment

Staging protocols for stomach cancer are discussed in Sidebar 8.4. This condition is treated with a combination of chemotherapy, externally applied radiation therapy, and surgery. Many patients undergo a course of chemotherapy both before and after surgery to improve the odds of success.

Medications

- Chemotherapeutic agents to limit neoplastic cell growth.
- Biologic therapies, including monoclonal antibodies to target cancer cells.

Carcinoid tumors: A rare kind of cancer found in the digestive tract.

Stromal tumor: A tumor that arises from the connective tissue stroma rather than epithelium.

Ascites: The accumulation of fluid in the peritoneal cavity.

Massage Therapy Implications

RISKS	Stomach cancer is usually treated very aggressively, which means clients with this condition will be dealing not only with cancer, but with the challenges of surgeries, chemotherapy, and radiation. All of these require adjustments in bodywork, but with care, massage can be appropriate and helpful.
BENEFITS	Because massage has been seen to ease pain, anxiety, depression, sleeplessness, and other side-effects of cancer treatment, it has some well-defined benefits to offer stomach cancer patients. Any treatment must be gauged according to the resilience of the client, and the cautions connected to the advancement of the cancer and treatment strategies that are being used. For more information on massage in the context of cancer, see Chapter 12.

SIDEBAR 8.4 Staging Stomach Cancer

Stomach cancer is staged using a combination of the TNM (tumor, node, and metastasis) and numerical (0 to IV) protocols.

TUMOR RATINGS	NODE RATINGS	METASTASIS RATINGS
Tx: tumor can't be assessed.	Nx: nodal involvement can't be assessed.	Mx: metastasis can't be assessed.
T0: no evidence of primary tumor.	N 0: no nodal involvement.	M0: no metastasis.
T is: in situ cancer, affecting mucosa only.	N1: 1–2 nearby nodes invaded.	M1: distant metastasis.
T1: affects submucosal layer.	N2: 3–6 nearby nodes invaded.	
T2: affects muscularis.	N3a: 7–15 nearby nodes invaded.	
T3: affects subserosa.	N 3b: > 16 nearby nodes invaded.	
T4: whole serosa affected; adjacent organs may be involved.		

These ratings are then discussed as stages in this way:

STAGE	TUMOR	NODE	METASTASIS
0	T is	N0	M0
IA	T1	N0	M0
IB	T1–2	N0–1	M0
IIA	T1–3	N0–2	M0
IIB	T1–4	N0–3	M0
IIIA	T2–4	N1–3	M0
IIIB	T3–4a or b	N0–3	M0
IIIC	T4a or b	N2–3	M0
IV	T any	N any	M1

Disorders of the Large Intestine

Colorectal Cancer

Definition: What Is It?

Colorectal cancer is the development of tumors anywhere in the large intestine from the ascending right side to the rectum. Although the two conditions are linked, malignant colon or rectal cancer is not the same thing as the presence of **adenomas** or colon **polyps**.

Demographics

Colorectal cancer is a relatively common form of cancer in this country, diagnosed about 147,000 times per year (94,000 colon cancer and 53,000 rectal cancer), and leading to about 50,000 deaths. It is the third leading cause of death by cancer in the United States. Colorectal cancer diagnoses are in decline, perhaps because of better prevention habits. Colorectal cancer deaths have also been declining, thanks to widely used screening that leads to early and successful treatment.

Colorectal cancer occurs about equally in men and women, and it is almost always in people over 50-year old, although African Americans have a higher-than-average risk of developing colorectal cancer before age 50. If it is found early, it is highly treatable. Over 1 million Americans are colorectal cancer survivors.

Etiology: What Happens?

The colon or large bowel is the last and widest section of the digestive tract. In this 6-foot long tube, the remnants of food are compacted, water is reabsorbed, and feces are stored in the rectum until they are expelled. The inner lining of the colon is composed of epithelium, which as has been seen in other discussions of cancer, is particularly susceptible to uncontrolled cell growth.

Most colon cancers begin with the development of adenomas, small polyps in the bowel. Minor chromosome damage is believed to cause the formation of these polyps. The cells in the mucosa of the colon multiply in a disordered and disorganized way, and produce small pile ups of excess tissue (Figures 8.8 and 8.9). But if the polyps are present for a long period, two things happen: **oncogenes** are activated and **tumor suppressor genes** are

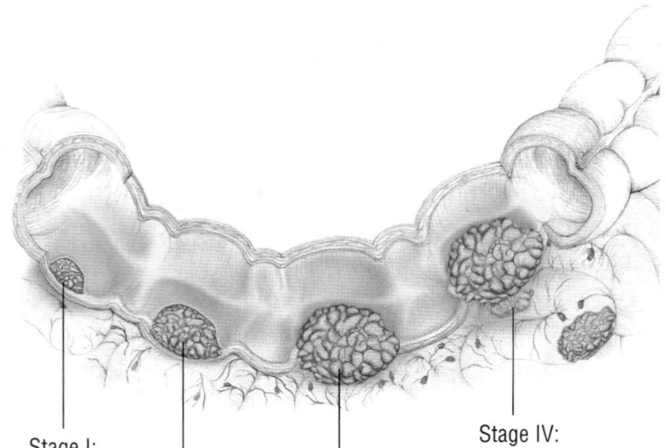
Stage I:
Submucosa
is invaded
Stage II:
Muscularis
is invaded
Stage III:
Serous membranes
are penetrated,
lymph nodes
involved
Stage IV:
Tumor invades,
adheres to other
structures

FIGURE 8.8 Colorectal cancer from left to right: in situ; invasion of colon wall; invasion of colon wall with substantial growth into colon lumen; growth, invasion of wall, and metastasis through lymph and direct contact

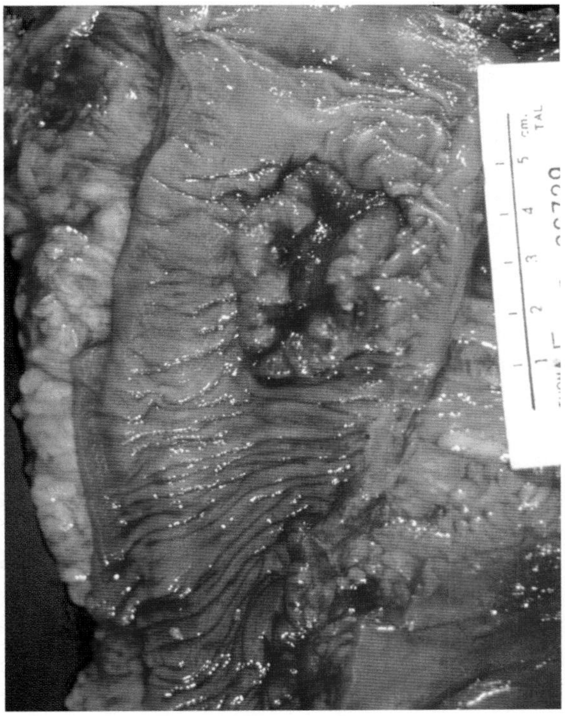

FIGURE 8.9 Colorectal cancer tumor

Adenoma: A benign tumor of glandular epithelial cells.

Polyp: An abnormal growth that projects from a mucous membrane.

Oncogene: Any of a family of genes that normally code for proteins related to cell growth, but which can encourage the development of cancer if mutated or abnormally activated.

Tumor suppressor gene: A gene that suppresses or protects against cancer. Also called an antioncogene.

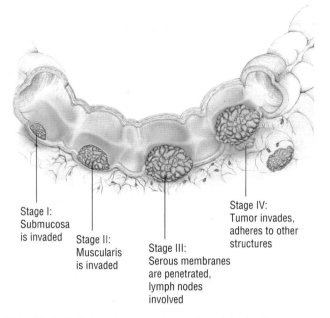

suppressed. The net result is that cells on the surface of the colon mucosa continue to replicate, and don't die off. They can invade the deeper layers of the bowel and even erode all the way through it to reach out to other pelvic organs. They can obstruct the movement of fecal matter through the GI tract; and they can metastasize through the lymph system to other places in the body, notably, the brain, liver, and lungs.

It is not clear why common colon polyps, which occur in up to 50% of older Americans, become malignant. One theory is that high-fat foods linger in the colon longer than other types of food, and some of their byproducts are carcinogenic. This theory also suggests that diets that are high in fiber help material to move through the colon faster and more completely, "scrubbing" the bowel walls of damaging or irritating materials.

> **NOTABLE CASES** The list of notable personalities with colon or rectal cancer is extremely varied, ranging from the French composer Claude Debussy, to the original Cat Woman Eartha Kitt, to the United States President Ronald Reagan, and to the "Peanuts" creator Charles Schulz. Football coach Vince Lombardi and early science fiction writer H.P. Lovecraft were also colon cancer patients.

Research into the influence of diet and colon cancer is sometimes contradictory. General associations can be made between a high-fat, low-fiber diet, and an increased risk of colorectal cancer, but when it comes to individual cases, other variables appear to influence the development of polyps and cancer, so diet is just one factor among many.

As with many diseases, the risk factors for developing colorectal cancer include some that can be controlled and others that can't. Risk factors for colorectal cancer include the following:

- *Obesity, sedentary lifestyle.* People who are obese have a relatively high chance of developing colon cancer. People who get little exercise are also prone to this disease; regular exercise has been shown to be protective against colorectal cancer.
- *Genetics.* **Familial adenomatous polyposis** and **hereditary nonpolyposis colorectal cancer syndrome** are genetic conditions that predispose some people to the development of colorectal cancer. Although people with these genetic profiles have a 90% to 100% chance of developing the disease, they constitute only a small percentage of colorectal cancer patients.
- *Inflammatory bowel disease.* **Ulcerative colitis** and **Crohn disease** are very closely connected with colon cancer. The younger a person is when diagnosed with either of these problems, the greater the chances of eventually developing colon cancer. The risk is so high that for some people preventive surgery to remove the whole colon is suggested before the cancer has a chance to develop.
- *Age.* The chances of having colon cancer rise with age; 90% of colon cancer patients are over 50 years of age.

Signs and Symptoms

Like many other types of cancer, colon cancer often doesn't show distinctive symptoms until it has progressed to a dangerous stage. Symptoms vary according to where tumors grow. Cancer in the spacious ascending colon is often first manifested as unexplained **anemia**: tumors can bleed slowly but continuously into the colon, making less iron, and therefore less oxygen, available to body cells. Iron deficiency anemia, especially among men and postmenopausal women, is a warning sign for colon cancer.

Growths in the more constricted descending colon are experienced as constipation or narrowed stools. Other signs of colon cancer that a person may or may not be aware of include blood in the stools (sometimes it is obvious and bright red, sometimes it occurs in invisible, microscopic amounts), lower abdominal pain, a feeling that bowel movements are incomplete, and unintentional weight loss.

Treatment

Treatment for colorectal cancer depends on the stage at which it is identified. Staging protocols are discussed in Sidebar 8.5. Treatment typically involves a combination of surgery, internally or externally applied radiation, chemotherapy, and using **monoclonal antibodies** and other biologic therapies to attack cancer cells. For information about colorectal cancer prevention, see Sidebar 8.6.

Medications

- Chemotherapeutic agents to slow the growth of cancer cells.
- Biologic therapies, specifically monoclonal antibodies that target cancer cells.

> **Familial adenomatous polyposis:** Genetic condition characterized by the presence of numerous polyps, which can become cancerous.
>
> **Hereditary nonpolyposis colorectal cancer syndrome:** A genetic condition that causes a predisposition to colorectal cancer. Also called Lynch syndrome.
>
> **Monoclonal antibodies:** A type of antibodies that are made by identical cells that are clones of one parent cell. They attach to one specific epitope, making them useful in targeting cancer cells without harming surrounding tissues.

SIDEBAR 8.5 Staging Colorectal Cancer

The TNM classification system identifies the progress of tumors, lymph node involvement, and the extent of metastasis. Here is a simplified version of the TNM system for colorectal cancer:

TUMOR	NODE	METASTASIS
Tx: can't be assessed	Nx: can't be assessed	Mx: can't be assessed
T0: no evidence of tumor	N0: no nodal involvement	M0: no distant metastasis
T IS: in situ tumor (affects mucosa only)	N1: 1–3 nearby nodes involved	M1a: distant metastasis to one organ or site
T1: submucosa invaded	N2: ≥4 nearby nodes involved	M1b: metastases to more than one site
T2: muscularis invaded		
T3: subserosa invaded		
T4a: tumor penetrates through visceral serosa		
T4: tumor invades or adheres to other organs and structures		

The TNM classifications are then applied to a numerical staging system as follows:

STAGE	TUMOR	NODE	METASTASIS
0	T is	N0	M0
I	T1–T2	N0	M0
IIA	T3	N0	M0
IIB	T4	N0	M0
IIIA	T1–T2	N1–N2	M0
IIIB	T3–T4	N1–N2	M0
IIIC	T any	N2	M0
IVA	Any	Any	M1a
IVB	Any	Any	M1b

SIDEBAR 8.6 Colorectal Cancer Prevention

While it has been difficult to prove specific diet and lifestyle causes of colorectal cancer, protective mechanisms have been somewhat easier to identify. The following habits are associated with a lower-than-average risk of developing this disease:

- Eat at least five servings of fruits and vegetables every day; choose whole-grains for starches
- Reduce most fats in the diet, especially saturated fats
- Get recommended vitamins and minerals, particularly calcium, magnesium, vitamin B_6, and folate
- Limit alcohol consumption to two drinks a day for men and one per day for women
- Don't smoke
- Be physically active and maintain a healthy weight

Massage Therapy Implications

RISKS	Colorectal cancer patients may undergo any combination of surgery, radiation, chemotherapy, and other treatment strategies, all of which require some adaptation on the part of a massage therapist or bodywork practitioner.
BENEFITS	Massage can be an important and useful addition to colorectal cancer treatment, as long as the challenges of treatment are respected. For more information about massage in the context of cancer, see Chapter 12.
OPTIONS	Some massage therapists may be nervous about working with a client who uses a colostomy bag. Because these devices take many forms, it is best simply to consult with the client about how to make him or her most comfortable. Be aware that massage oil or lotion may dissolve the adhesive on the bag.
RESEARCH	A study from Thailand[1] used Thai massage and aromatherapy to look for impact on immune system function and other outcomes for colorectal cancer patients undergoing chemotherapy, as compared to standard care. They found that the massaged patients had more active lymphocytes, and that their pain and stress were significantly lower than those in the usual care group. 1. Khiewkhern S, Promthet S, Sukprasert A, et al. Effectiveness of aromatherapy with light thai massage for cellular immunity improvement in colorectal cancer patients receiving chemotherapy. *Asian Pacific Journal of Cancer Prevention* 2013;14(6): 3903–3907. http://www.ncbi.nlm.nih.gov/pubmed/23886205

Diverticular Disease

Definition: What Is It?

Diverticular disease is a condition of the small intestine or colon in which the mucosal and submucosal layers of the GI tract bulge through the outer muscular layer to form a sac or **diverticulum**. It happens most often in the descending section or sigmoid bend of the colon. The presence of these bulges is called diverticulosis. If they become infected, this is called diverticulitis.

Demographics

Diverticular disease is most common in countries where diets are based on animal fats and processed grains. Interestingly, it was first documented in the early 1900s, just when new technology had been developed to remove the bran from wheat and the American diet shifted to rely heavily on low-fiber white flour. Up to half of the United States population aged 60 to 80, may have diverticular disease, and two-thirds or more of people over 85-year old. Not everyone develops infections, so this condition is often silent.

> **Diverticulum:** An abnormal bulging out of the intestine. (Plural: diverticula.)
>
> **Fecalith:** A hard, rock-like mass of feces in the intestine.

Etiology: What Happens?

Diverticular disease is a multifactoral condition involving a combination of inefficient colon motility, changes in the strength of the colon wall, and the lack of sufficient dietary fiber.

Contractions of the large intestine are very strong, but without adequate bulk supplied by soluble and insoluble fiber, internal pressure between areas of contraction causes colon walls to bulge. This is especially problematic if the collagen matrix of the muscularis is impaired (as with **Marfan syndrome** or **Ehlers-Danlos syndrome**) or weakened by age. In this situation, the mucosa and submucosa of the colon can herniate through the outer muscular layer to form small sacs or diverticula. These sacs may fill with fecal matter and bacteria, and the potential for infection or diverticulitis is high (Figure 8.10). Material that accumulates inside the pouches can harden, becoming a **fecalith**.

Most diverticula form in the sigmoid flexure or descending colon, but they have been found throughout the GI tract, all the way up to the esophagus. The more diverticula a person has, the more likely he or she is to develop diverticulitis.

Complications of diverticulitis are rare, but they can be serious enough to become life threatening very quickly. They can include the following:

- *Bleeding*. Sometimes capillaries get stretched over the dome of the protrusion, and they may tear open and bleed into the colon. This is a specific situation called diverticular bleeding.
- *Abscess*. Infected diverticula may have tiny tears that allow contents to leak out. If this is small, an abscess develops.

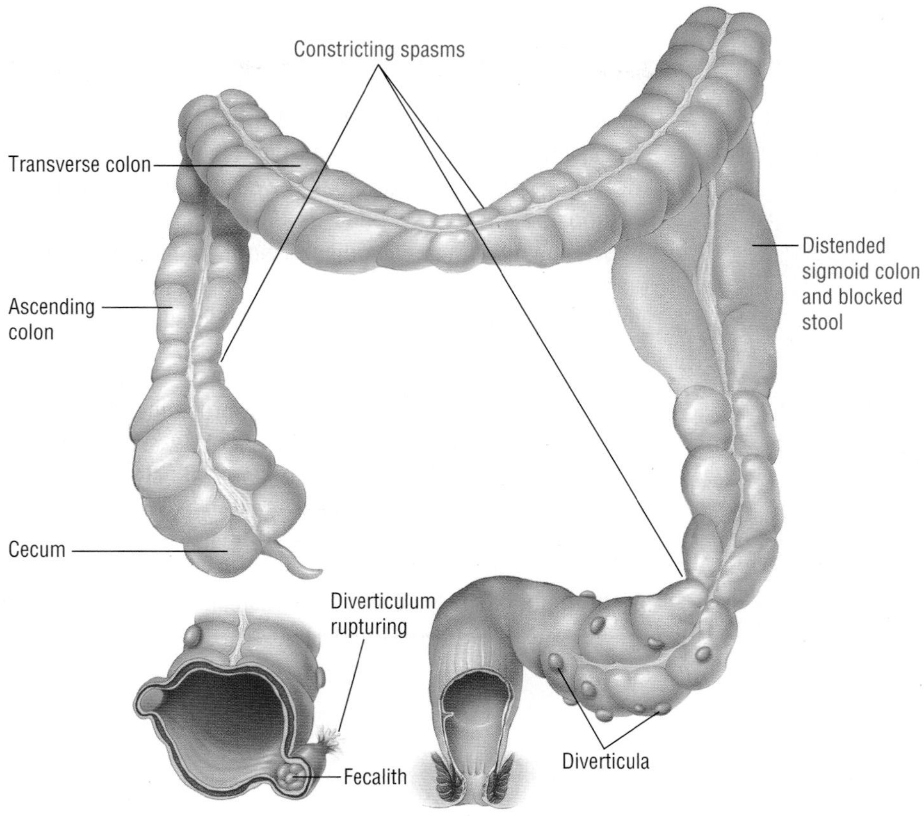

FIGURE 8.10 Diverticular disease

If an abscess ruptures, its contents may be released into the peritoneum, causing **peritonitis**.

- *Perforation and rupture.* Diverticula may tear open and release their contents into the peritoneum leading to peritonitis.
- *Blockage.* The accumulation of scar tissue where diverticula have formed may block the colon.
- *Fistula.* In the areas that have been damaged by long-term inflammation and scarring, small passageways or fistulas may develop between hollow organs, allowing the passage of fecal matter into spaces where it doesn't belong. In this situation, the colon may connect with the urinary bladder, small intestine, or uterus.

Signs and Symptoms

Symptoms of diverticulosis may be nonexistent. When infection is present however, symptoms include bloating, nausea, fever, cramping, and severe pain, usually on the lower left side of the abdomen. Diarrhea and or constipation may also occur. Symptoms of diverticulitis often have a sudden onset and become rapidly worse, but some people have several days of mild discomfort before severe infection sets in.

Treatment

Diverticular disease is more easily prevented than corrected. Daily fiber intake is recommended to be 25 to 30 g/d, along with 64 ounces of fluid. Without healthy amounts of soluble and insoluble fiber to create bulk in the colon, the smooth muscle has to work hard to compact fecal material and even harder to expel it from the body. The fact that vegetarians and people whose diets are built on whole grains, fruits, and vegetables seldom develop diverticular disease is an indication that healthy levels of dietary fiber might reduce the risk of developing this problem.

Treatment for diverticulosis isn't usually necessary. Although the diverticula are not reversible, further growths can be prevented with changes toward a higher-fiber diet and exercise.

Treatment for diverticulitis starts with antibiotics and a clear liquid diet for several days. If substantial tissue damage has occurred, including a bowel obstruction, uncontrolled bleeding, perforation, large abscesses, or fistulas, surgery may be performed. Depending on the seriousness of the condition, surgery may involve a simple resection of the colon, removing the infected or damaged area, or it may require a temporary or permanent colostomy.

Medications

- Antibiotics when infection is present
- Analgesics as necessary
- Anti-inflammatories as necessary
- Antispasmodics to decrease internal colon pressure

Massage Therapy Implications

RISKS	It is important to realize that the signs and symptoms of diverticular disease can be similar to those of simple digestive upset. If massage temporarily eases these symptoms, it may delay the client in getting a very important diagnosis. Consequently, if symptoms include a fever, or if they persist for more than 2 weeks, it is important to advise clients to pursue a formal diagnosis. When a client has been diagnosed with diverticular disease, care must be taken with abdominal work, because the colon is structurally compromised. During flares of acute inflammation (diverticulitis), it is best to delay any intrusive bodywork until the infection has passed.
BENEFITS	Massage or bodywork is unlikely to improve the prognosis for a person with diverticular disease, but as long as care is taken not to exacerbate symptoms, bodywork may be a helpful strategy to deal with anxiety and abdominal pain.
OPTIONS	Because abdominal pain can be a chronic problem for people with diverticular disease, any gentle work on the belly: clockwise stroking or even simple touch through a sheet can help to incorporate this problematic area back into the whole person.

Irritable Bowel Syndrome

Definition: What Is It?

Irritable bowel syndrome (IBS) is a condition involving digestive system dysfunction without major structural changes. It has also been known as spastic colon, irritable colon, mucus colitis, and functional bowel syndrome.

It is considered a biopsychosocial disorder, involving aspects of basic health processes as they relate to mood and stress management.

Demographics

IBS may affect as much as 10% of the U.S. population, although the majority of people with symptoms may not seek medical attention. Women in the United States are more likely than men to have this condition, with a ratio of 2 to 3:1. Symptoms often begin in childhood, although the syndrome is usually identified in adults.

Etiology: What Happens?

In a normal colon, fecal matter is squeezed and compacted, while water and salts are reabsorbed into the bloodstream. Strong contractions move the formed stools into the rectum, where they are stored until another wave of contractions moves them out of the body altogether. The shorter the transit time for material to move through the colon, the less water is reabsorbed; this leads to watery stools or diarrhea. The longer the transit time, the more water is absorbed, and stools become extremely dense and compacted: constipation. Diarrhea and constipation are both factors in IBS.

The development of IBS symptoms is related to three main factors: hypersensitivity in the intestines, problems with motility or organized peristalsis, and psychosocial factors like **depression** or **anxiety** that often accompany IBS and tend to make symptoms worse (Figure 8.11).

While this syndrome is usually discussed as a digestive system disorder, it is also connected to a dysfunction of the **brain-gut axis**, that is, the link of continuous feedback between GI tract sensation and motor response from the central nervous system. Many people with IBS also have other smooth muscle tissue dysfunction. IBS frequently appears simultaneously with **chronic fatigue syndrome** and **fibromyalgia**: two chronic conditions that both have important central nervous system components.

One subset of IBS patients develops long-term symptoms after having an acute infection of the gut. Tissue studies of these patients reveal the possibility of low-grade inflammation, which may indicate the presence of infection. This is significant finding, as it suggests treatment options that are not successful with other IBS patients.

Brain-gut axis: The ongoing process of biochemical interaction between the gastrointestinal tract and the nervous system.

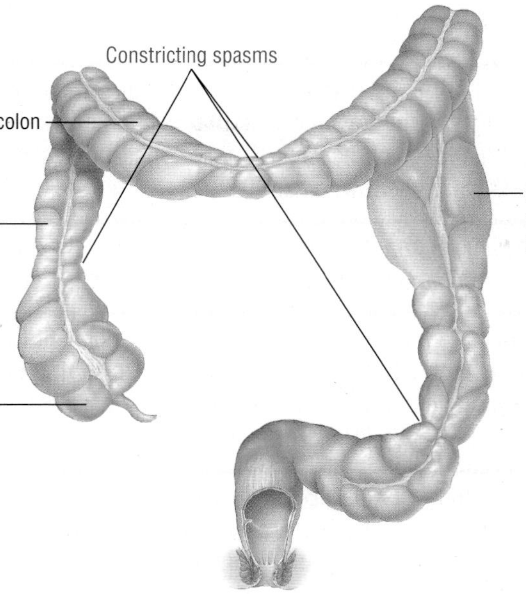

FIGURE 8.11 Irritable bowel syndrome can lead to constipation, diarrhea, or both

Types of Irritable Bowel Syndrome

- *IBS-D*. This describes IBS, in which the primary symptom is a chronic diarrhea.
- *IBS-C*. This describes IBS, in which the primary symptom is chronic constipation.
- *IBS-M*. In this version, a person can experience both diarrhea and constipation within a short time span; "m" is for "mixed."
- *IBS-A*. This describes alternating IBS, in which symptoms fluctuate between diarrhea and constipation.

Signs and Symptoms

Symptoms of IBS can range from occasionally inconvenient to severely debilitating, but it is not a life-threatening disease. It can mimic several serious digestive system conditions, however. In particular, **diverticulitis**, **colorectal cancer**, **ulcerative colitis**, and **Crohn disease** must be eliminated as possibilities. This can be problematic, because IBS and inflammatory bowel disease can be comorbid.

An internationally recognized symptomatic profile for IBS identifies leading symptoms as recurrent abdominal pain at least 3 days every month, pain with defecation, changes in stool frequency, and changes in stool appearance. Other symptoms can include gas, bloating, headaches, and general malaise.

The changes brought about by IBS are purely functional; no structural anomalies like scar tissue, ulcers, polyps, or tumors develop because of this disorder. For this reason, if a person with IBS develops a fever, has blood in the stool, develops **anemia**, or has unintended weight loss. IBS is not the cause and these new symptoms should be reported to a physician.

Treatment

Treatment for IBS depends on the individual. The first recourse is to consider dietary and stress factors. Nicotine, caffeine, alcohol, the artificial sweetener sorbitol, and dairy products have been found to be particularly irritating, but no particular food or drink is a definitive trigger for IBS attacks for all patients. Some doctors recommend fiber supplementation; the addition of bulk to the diet can fill the colon more completely and help to limit spasm.

Complementary treatments for IBS have found some success. Some herbs, peppermint, and the use of probiotics to restore normal intestinal bacteria have shown success with some patients.

Medications

- Antispasmodics to limit colon hyperreactivity
- Fecal binders for diarrhea
- Bulking agents
- Laxatives for constipation
- Antidiarrheals as necessary
- Antacids to limit digestive discomfort
- Antidepressants/anti-anxiety medications for stress management
- Antibiotics if low-grade bacterial infection is confirmed

Massage Therapy Implications

RISKS	Some clients with IBS are extremely self-conscious about passing gas during a massage appointment. This, or nervousness about touch in general, may make it difficult for a person to enjoy the experience of massage. If these challenges can be addressed, massage has no particular risks for a client who has IBS.
BENEFITS	Because massage is an effective way to address anxiety and stress, clients with IBS welcome touch may find this a powerful tool to help manage their condition.
OPTIONS	The key factor for someone who has IBS to derive benefit from massage is for them to be able to relax and not worry about passing gas. To address this issue for all her nervous clients, I know one massage therapist who has a plaque up on her wall that states "It's not a good massage until somebody farts."
RESEARCH	Some evidence suggests that IBS and associated disorders share a CNS feature in the lack of endocannabinoid uptake sites. Massage therapy and some other interventions have been seen to improve this uptake for relief of some symptoms.[1] Other research supports the use of massage therapy for fibromyalgia, and IBS is often a part of that picture. 1. McPartland JM, Guy GW, Di Marzo V. Care and feeding of the endocannabinoid system: a systematic review of potential clinical interventions that upregulate the endocannabinoid system. *PLoS One* 2014:9(3);e89566. http://www.ncbi.nlm.nih.gov/pmc/articles/PMC3951193/

Disorders of the Accessory Organs

Cirrhosis

Definition: What Is It?

The word cirrhosis, from the Greek "kirrhos," means "yellow condition," referring to the jaundice that can develop as a complication of this condition. Cirrhosis is a result of long-term liver damage. It describes the crowding out and replacement of healthy liver cells with nonfunctioning scar tissue. This interferes with virtually every function of the liver with potentially fatal repercussions.

Demographics

Cirrhosis leads to about 35,000 deaths each year; it is the ninth leading cause of death in the United States. **Hepatitis C** and **alcoholism** have been the leading causes of cirrhosis, but the long-term effects of fatty liver disease are expected to have a big impact on cirrhosis statistics in the near future. Given that nonalcoholic fatty liver disease is present in up to 40% of the general population, and that this is likely to progress to cirrhosis in many cases; this is essentially inevitable.

Hepatocyte: An active liver cell.

Etiology: What Happens?

The liver is composed of highly organized layers of epithelial **hepatocytes**: cells that produce a myriad of vital chemicals vital for metabolism and survival. The liver produces bile, which helps to metabolize fats, and other enzymes that metabolize proteins and carbohydrates. Clotting factors, proteins that maintain the proper balance of tissue fluid, and the cells that help filter and neutralize toxins and hormones are all produced in the liver.

Under normal circumstances, the liver has great powers of regeneration. But chronic long-term irritation or infection may suppress the growth of healthy, organized cells. Instead, collagen and other components of extracellular matrix proliferate. Healthy cells are crowded into abnormal nodules leading to a knobby, "hobnailed liver" appearance (Figure 8.12),

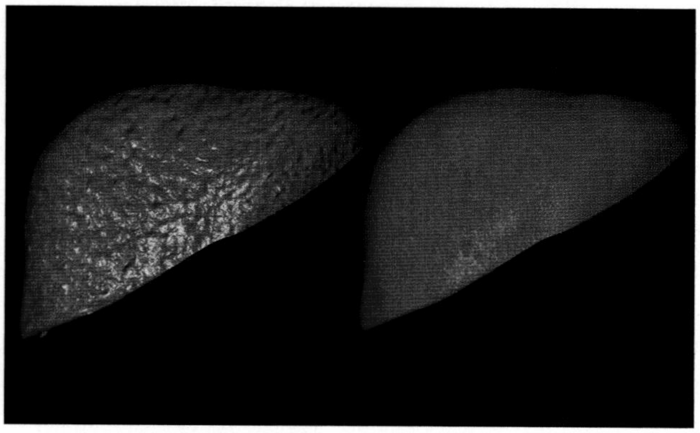

FIGURE 8.12 Cirrhotic liver compared to normal liver

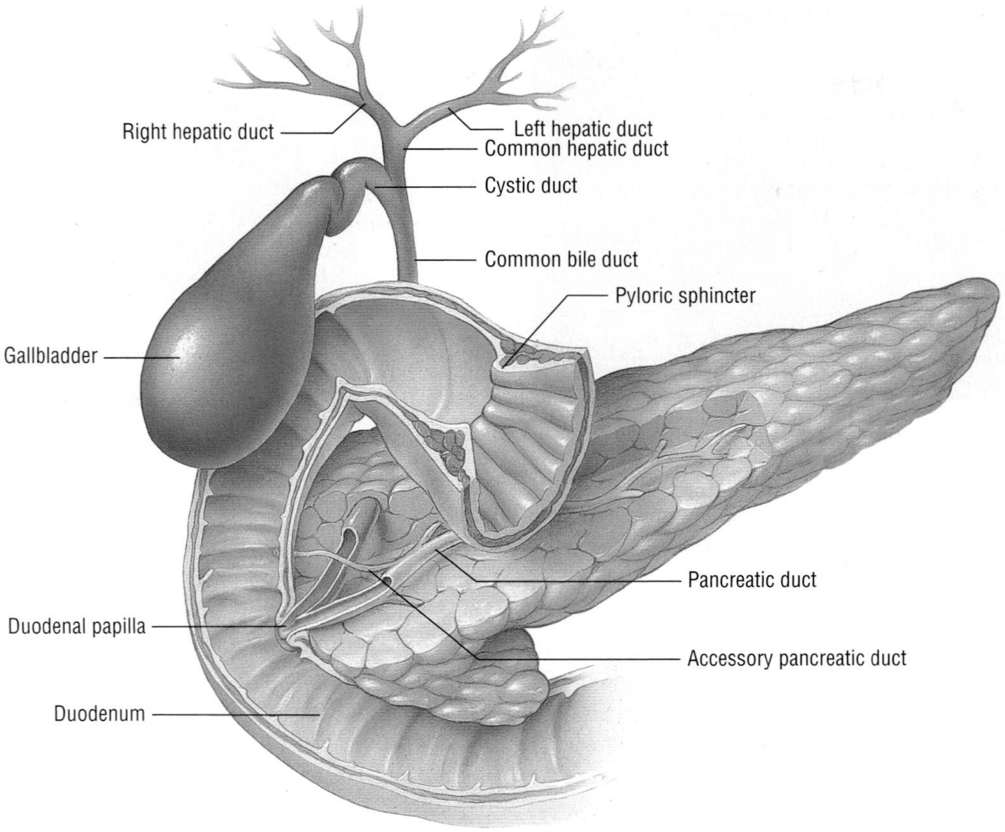

FIGURE 8.13 Cirrhosis: gallbladder and duct system: any blockage can cause back-ups and damage to the liver

and the tiny channels that are meant to direct the flow of bile and other fluids to the appropriate vessels become blocked.

Traditionally, alcoholism has been the leading cause of cirrhosis in the United States. Now, hepatitis C probably causes cirrhosis at least as often as long-term alcohol abuse. Cirrhosis can also arise from types B and D, drug-related, and autoimmune hepatitis. **Nonalcoholic fatty liver disease** (NAFLD) is also a significant contributor to cirrhosis: this is a complication of obesity, **type 2 diabetes**, and high triglycerides. NAFLD progresses to another condition, **nonalcoholic steatohepatitis** (NASH) in some adults. Steatohepatitis is inflammation of fatty tissue in the liver. Chronic inflammation then leads to the formation of excessive connective tissue—the hallmark of cirrhosis.

Other causes for cirrhosis include any factor that can obstruct the complicated bile duct system (Figure 8.13), including **gallstones**, **pancreatic cancer**, and congenital malformation of the bile duct system. Long-term exposure to environmental toxins can contribute to cirrhosis, as can congestive **heart failure** and some congenital diseases. It is important to bear in mind that most people with cirrhosis have multiple factors that may contribute to this disease: hepatitis B along with obesity, for instance, substantially increases the risk of developing cirrhosis.

One very rare form of cirrhosis is related to a genetic defect and it occurs exclusively in infants of Ojibway-Cree descent.

Nonalcoholic fatty liver disease: A condition, often asymptomatic, characterized by fatty deposits in the liver of a person who consumes little to no alcohol.

Nonalcoholic steatohepatitis (NASH): Inflammation of fatty tissue in the liver.

Portal hypertension: Elevated pressure in the hepatic portal due to damaged liver tissue.

Complications

As the liver progressively loses function, many complications arise, many of which are linked to **portal hypertension**. In this situation, the liver becomes so congested that it cannot freely accept blood delivered from the digestive and accessory organs, and pressure accumulates in the portal system veins. Other complications arise as the liver simply no longer produces enough vital blood components or inadequately filters and neutralizes hormones and toxic materials. Complications of cirrhosis include the following:

- *Splenomegaly*. The spleen enlarges because it can't drain through the portal vein. The danger with splenomegaly is that when fluid backs up in this organ, the risk of rupture and internal hemorrhage is high.

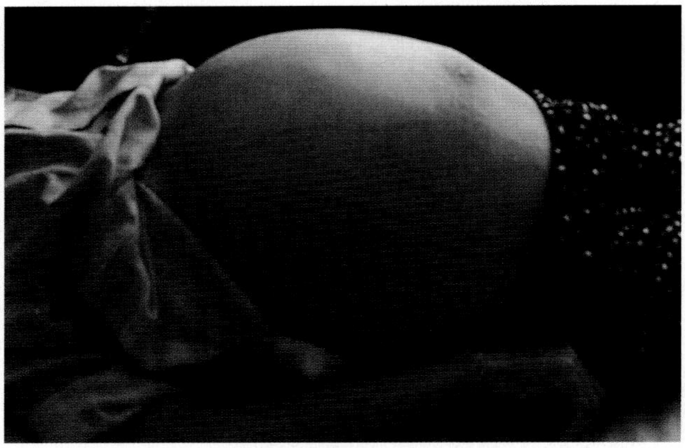

FIGURE 8.14 Cirrhosis-related ascites

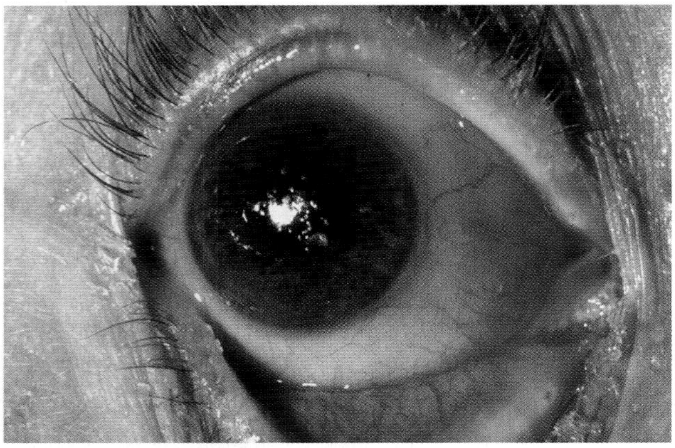

FIGURE 8.15 Cirrhosis can cause jaundice and the yellowing of the sclera

- *Ascites*. When pressure in the portal system increases, plasma seeps out of the veins and lymphatic vessels into the peritoneal space, causing the abdominal distension known as **ascites** (Figure 8.14). The bacteria that normally inhabit the GI tract may seep out to set up an infection in this fluid, causing spontaneous bacterial **peritonitis**, a potentially life-threatening infection. Ascites in the peritoneum can also seep across the diaphragm to cause **pleural effusion**.
- *Internal varices*. Pressure in abdominal veins grows as fluid backs up through the system. This can lead to internal venous distensions and varicosities, especially in the esophagus and stomach. Internal varicose veins can hemorrhage during vomiting, leading to bloody vomit, internal bleeding, shock, or death.
- *Bleeding, bruising*. When the liver no longer produces adequate clotting factors, the ability to heal from minor injury is severely impaired. Cirrhosis patients may bruise extensively and bleed for abnormally long periods.
- *Osteoporosis*. The liver helps to process vitamin D. Without this function, it is impossible to absorb adequate calcium from the diet, so **osteoporosis** is likely to develop.
- *Muscle wasting*. When the enzymes that aid in protein metabolism are in short supply, a cirrhosis patient may undergo progressive atrophy of the skeletal muscles.
- ***Jaundice***. **Bilirubin** is produced in the spleen, and it is meant to be recycled in the liver to be a component of bile. When cirrhosis interferes with this process, water-soluble components of bilirubin accumulate in the bloodstream. Bilirubin is strongly pigmented, and it can add a yellowish tint to the skin and the sclera of the eye. It can also cause rashes and itching, as some people have an extreme reaction to this unfamiliar chemical in their skin (Figure 8.15).
- *Systemic edema*. One of the critical proteins for maintaining fluid balance in the body, **albumin**, is significantly lowered in advanced cirrhosis. Without albumin, the body cannot maintain proper fluid levels, and **edema** accumulates systemically in all interstitial spaces.
- *Hormone disruption*. The liver of men with cirrhosis no longer inactivates their normal low levels of estrogen; feminizing characteristics such as breast development, loss of chest hair, impotence, and atrophy of the testicles soon follow. For women, hormonal changes include the cessation of periods, infertility, and the growth of body hair. Both men and women with cirrhosis can expect a decreased sex drive.
- *Encephalopathy*. **Encephalopathy** is a consequence of advanced cirrhosis; it is a signal that the liver's detoxifying agents are out of commission. Furthermore, the blood-brain barrier, which usually keeps the central nervous system safe from low levels of metabolic byproducts, becomes much less effective with cirrhosis. Wastes accumulate in the blood, cross into the CNS, and eventually cause brain damage. Symptoms include somnolence, confusion, tremors, hallucinations, even coma, and death.
- *Kidney failure*. Advanced cirrhosis can impair blood flow to the kidneys, resulting in kidney failure. **Hepatorenal syndrome** is an emergency that requires a liver transplant for survival.

NOTABLE CASES Cirrhosis and its complications was the cause of death for many influential people, including musician and songwriter Billie Holiday, who died at age 44, novelist Jack Kerouac (age 47), statesman Daniel Webster (age 70), and short story writer and master of the surprise ending, O. Henry (age 48).

Ascites: The accumulation of fluid in the peritoneal cavity.

Pleural effusion: The accumulation of fluid in the pleural cavity.

Bilirubin: A dark bile pigment formed from the hemoglobin of dead red blood cells.

Albumin: A protein found in blood.

Encephalopathy: A disease affecting brain function.

Hepatorenal syndrome: Renal failure in a person with liver disease.

- *Liver failure, end-stage liver disease.* The progressive loss of liver function can lead to a failure of the liver to keep up with daily needs. A person with end-stage liver disease is a candidate for a liver transplant.
- *Liver cancer.* Chronic inflammation in the liver increases the risk of cellular mutation and **liver cancer**.

Signs and Symptoms

The liver readily compensates for slowly progressive losses in function. Consequently, by the time symptoms are observable without blood tests, cirrhosis is likely to be advanced. Early symptoms are vague and can be attributed to any number of other common disorders. They include nausea, vomiting, weight loss, and the development of red or itchy patches on the skin. Later symptoms are usually identified by the complications discussed above.

Treatment

The prognosis for someone in the early stages of cirrhosis caused by alcoholism or drug abuse is excellent, if the damage can be stopped. Medication is sometimes administered to counteract the complications of this disease: diuretics for edema, antacids for intestinal discomfort, and **levulose** to bind with ammonia so that it can be excreted. Vitamins and minerals are recommended to guard against malnutrition. Cirrhosis due to hepatitis is treated with interferon as an antiviral measure. Steroids for inflammation due to autoimmune hepatitis are occasionally prescribed. Surgical repair of internal varicosities may be necessary, and if the kidneys are impaired, **hemodialysis** can assist in their function until the crisis has passed.

When these interventions are inadequate, a liver transplant is considered. In this country about 15,000 liver transplants are conducted each year. The liver regenerates so readily that a person can give about 60% of a healthy organ, and both the donor and recipient can have healthy functioning livers within a few months.

Levulose: A sugar found in many fruits. Also called fructose.

Hemodialysis: A medical procedure in which blood is purified outside of the body, used when the kidneys cannot perform this function normally. Commonly called dialysis.

Cholecyst: Another name for the gallbladder.

Cholelithiasis: The presence of a gallstone in the gallbladder or bile ducts.

Cholecystitis: Inflammation of the gallbladder.

Choledocholithiasis: The presence of a gallstone in the common bile duct.

Cholangitis: Inflammation of the bile duct.

Medications

- Diuretics for water retention.
- Beta blockers for portal hypertension.
- Antacids for digestive discomfort.
- Levulose to help eradicate ammonia.
- Steroidal anti-inflammatories for autoimmune problems.
- Interferon for chronic viral hepatitis.

Massage Therapy Implications

RISKS	Complications of cirrhosis can damage the skin, interfere with blood clotting, promote blood toxicity, and generally impair function of several systems. Clients with advanced cirrhosis do not have the adaptive capacity to manage rigorous massage or bodywork.
BENEFITS	Gentle work that invites calm and reduces anxiety can be helpful for any person with a complicated disease. If a client is encouraged to exercise to promote recovery of muscles, massage may fit into this context as well.

To see some of the physical effects of end-stage liver disease (one of the complications of cirrhosis), see the video "Physical Examination of End Stage Liver Disease" at http://thePoint.Lww.com/Werner6e. thePoint®

Gallstones

Definition: What Are They?

Gallstones are concentrated deposits of bile salts or pigments in the gallbladder. The technical term for gallbladder is **cholecyst**, because it is a cyst (holding tank) that collects, among other things, cholesterol. The formation of tiny crystals or stones in the gallbladder is called **cholelithiasis** ("lith" means stone). Inflammation of the gallbladder from a stuck stone or other cause is called **cholecystitis**. When stones become lodged in the common bile duct, the condition is called **choledocholithiasis**. Inflammation of any of the ducts in the biliary system (the exocrine ducts of the liver, gallbladder, and pancreas) is called **cholangitis**.

Demographics

It is estimated that in this country some 20% of people over 65 have gallstones, and this condition is diagnosed about a million times each year. Gallstone surgery happens about 500,000 times each year.

While many people consider gallstones to be an inconvenience, they can be very serious. They lead to about 7,000 deaths each year through surgical complications, pancreatitis, and gallbladder cancer, which can be an outcome of chronic gallbladder disease.

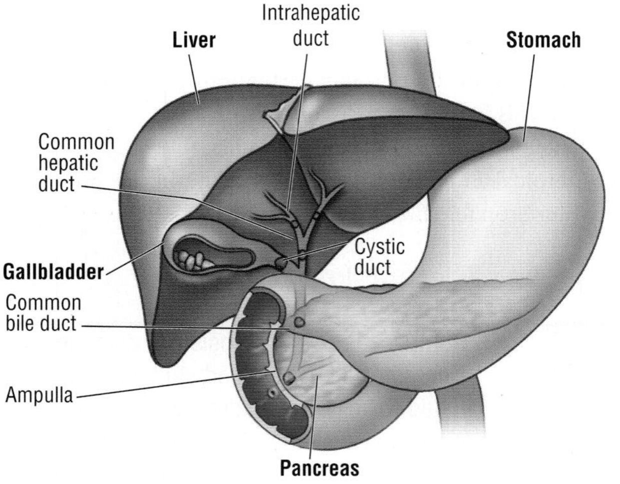

FIGURE 8.16 Gallstones in ducts

Women are far more prone to developing gallstones than men. Depending on age, they outnumber men by about two to one.

Etiology: What Happens?

Bile is produced in the liver and delivered to the gallbladder through the hepatic duct and the cystic duct (Figure 8.16). When a person eats a high-fat meal, hormonal commands cause the gallbladder to release its contents into the cystic duct. The bile flows into the common bile duct, and then into the small intestine. Pancreatic secretions also use the common bile duct for access to the small intestine.

The purpose of bile is to hold particles of fat in tiny, discrete pieces, so that they can be absorbed into the **lacteals**; this is emulsification. Without bile, fat particles tend to stick together in indigestible clumps, which reduce access to important fat-soluble vitamins and nutrients.

Bile is primarily made up of water, **bile salts**, bilirubin from recycled red blood cells, and cholesterol, which is filtered out of the bloodstream by the liver. When either cholesterol or bilirubin occurs in higher-than-normal concentrations in bile, they can precipitate out of the liquid to become tiny granules called "bile sludge," or larger stones (Figure 8.17).

A relatively small percentage of gallstones (10% to 20%) are made of bilirubin, the coloring agent for feces. Bilirubin stones are also called "pigment stones." These are usually a sign of some type of blood dysfunction that causes the premature destruction of red blood cells, resulting in abnormally

> **Lacteals:** Lymphatic vessels of the small intestine, through which fats are absorbed.
>
> **Bile salts:** Salts created from bile acid, which serve to assist in the digestion of fats.
>
> **Bariatric surgery:** Stomach surgery used to induce weight loss.

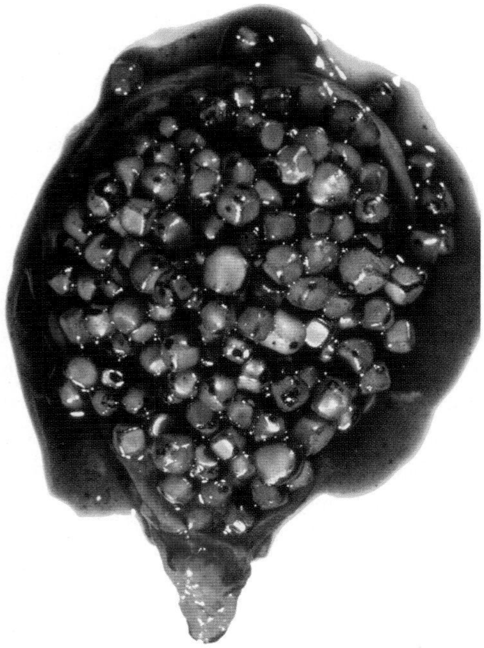

FIGURE 8.17 Gallstones

high levels of bilirubin in the blood and in the liver. Gallstones that occur in children are most likely to be some form of pigment stone.

Most gallstones (80% to 90%) are composed of cholesterol. Several factors can increase the risk of developing cholesterol stones, including the following:

- *Obesity*. This increases the amount of cholesterol manufactured by the liver and stored in the gallbladder.
- *Estrogen*. This tends to increase the amount of cholesterol in bile while decreasing gallbladder activity, which allows the cholesterol to crystallize. Estrogen levels may be related to pregnancy, birth control pills, or hormone replacement therapy.
- *Race*. Native Americans and Mexican Americans have the highest incidence of gallstones of any specific racial groups.
- *Gender*. Women age 16 to 60 with gallstones outnumber men by about two to one.
- *Cholesterol-lowering drugs*. Drugs that are designed to lower blood cholesterol help to concentrate cholesterol in the gallbladder, increasing the risk of forming stones.
- *Diabetes*. This causes high levels of triglycerides, which raises the risk for gallstones.
- *Rapid weight loss*. This causes the liver to metabolize fat for fuel, resulting in higher levels of cholesterol in the bile. Gallstones are a common complication of **bariatric surgery**.
- *Fasting*. This reduces gallbladder emptying, so bile becomes concentrated and cholesterol precipitates out into stones.
- *History of gallstones*. People who have had gallstones in the past are more likely than the general population to develop them again.

- *Other diseases.* People with **Crohn disease**, **cirrhosis**, and **diabetes** have a higher incidence of gallstones, although the mechanisms for this are not clear.

Gallstones in themselves are not usually a serious threat, but they can create unpleasant or even life-threatening complications. The most obvious is an obstruction of the cystic or hepatic duct, which can lead to jaundice or acute pancreatitis. The pooling of stagnant bile can also lead to cholecystitis. It is possible for an infected gallbladder to rupture, releasing its contents and causing abscesses or **peritonitis** And a person with chronic gallbladder irritation has an increased risk of developing fibrosis and gallbladder cancer.

Signs and Symptoms

Most people who have gallstones never know, because symptoms are typically generated only when a stone becomes lodged in the hepatic duct, the cystic duct, or in the common bile duct. If this happens, it causes extreme local pain called **biliary colic**, which may last for hours, build to a peak, and then gradually subside when the stone moves out of the duct and into either the gallbladder or the duodenum. The pain may be intense enough to induce nausea and vomiting. If the stone is immovably stuck, the patient may require hospitalization to have it surgically removed.

The gallbladder refers pain between the scapulae and over the right shoulder. Although most patients have pain in the upper right quadrant of the abdomen, some feel it primarily in the upper back (where even the most gifted massage won't relieve it).

Treatment

Laparoscopic **cholecystectomy** is the most common intervention to deal with gallstones. The whole gallbladder is removed in this procedure.

Another surgical option uses a scope on a thin tube that is inserted through the mouth, down the esophagus, through the stomach, and into the small intestine and biliary duct system. This scope may be used as a diagnostic tool, but in some cases a device can be attached to the scope to remove or dislodge gallstones.

If the gallstones are determined to be small and cholesterol-based, a long-term dosage of chemicals that can dissolve stones may be recommended. This can also be a preventive measure for people undergoing rapid weight loss, as seen with bariatric surgery.

Biliary colic: Acute pain associated with the impaction of a gallstone in the cystic duct.

Cholecystectomy: The surgical removal of the gallbladder.

SIDEBAR 8.7 Lose the Gallbladder, Keep the Fat

Bile, manufactured in the liver and stored in the gallbladder, suspends consumed fats in tiny pieces so the body can absorb and digest them in the small intestine. A person who loses her gallbladder has less access to incoming fat, so she absorbs less fat from her diet.

Why, then, do gallbladder surgery patients not lose a lot of weight after surgery? It seems like gallbladder removal would be a popular form of elective surgery!

It turns out that to burn fat that is stored in the body's lipid cells, we must consume the kinds of fats that will help to soften those lipid cells' membranes. When a person loses her gallbladder—and access to incoming nutrition in the form of fats—it actually becomes harder to lose weight, because the body much more tenaciously retains whatever fat is in the lipid cells. Since obesity is a leading contributor to the formation of gallstones, losing one's gallbladder makes it doubly hard to resolve problems with being overweight.

A person whose gallbladder has been removed can still produce bile, but it is dripped into the duodenum in a steady stream rather than being saved for high-fat meals. It is rare, but possible, for this steady stream of bile to crystalize in the bile duct; in other words, gallstones may form without a gallbladder. However, the more common concern in this situation is that the patient may lose some access to important fat-soluble vitamins. Fortunately, digestive supplements can aid in the emulsification of fats (Sidebar 8.7).

Medications

- Analgesics for acute gallbladder attacks.
- Ursodeoxycholic acid or chenodeoxycholic acid for 6 to 18 months to dissolve small cholesterol-based gallstones.

Massage Therapy Implications

RISKS	Acute biliary colic (a gallbladder attack) contraindicates massage until the problem has been addressed. When gallstones have been identified but no symptoms are present, the right costal angle is a local caution.
BENEFITS	A client with a history of gallstones but no current symptoms, or someone who has had uncomplicated gallbladder surgery, can enjoy the same benefits of massage as the rest of the population.

Hepatitis

Definition: What Is It?

Hepatitis means inflamed liver. It can be caused by drug reactions, inflammation related to fatty deposits, autoimmune disease, or exposure to certain toxins, but it is most often one of a variety of viral infections that can mildly or severely impair liver function. Seven types of viral hepatitis have been identified to date: hepatitis A through G. Hepatitis A, B, and C cause about 90% of viral liver infection in the United States; they are the primary focus of this discussion.

To hear the author discuss the different types of hepatitis and implications for massage, go to http://thePoint.lww.com/Werner6e. thePoint®

Demographics

Various forms of liver inflammation are common in the United States. Up to 30% of all adults have been exposed to hepatitis A, although they may have no memory of an infection. It is estimated that up to 1.4 million people have hepatitis B, although many of them don't know. About 3.2 million Americans carry hepatitis C, a form of liver infection that has a very high risk of long-term liver disease. Hepatitis C is the most common blood-borne infection in the United States.

Liver inflammation can occur without a viral infection: nonviral liver inflammation due to fatty liver (NASH or nonalcoholic steatohepatitis) affects 2% to 5% of people in this country.

Etiology: What Happens?

Hepatitis A, B, and C all are viral attacks against liver cells. Each type of virus is unique, however. Exposure to one type of hepatitis does not impart immunity to any other type of hepatitis.

Once a hepatitis virus gains access to the body, it attacks liver cells and stimulates an immune system response. Viral hepatitis can be identified and diagnosed by the presence of antibodies in the blood, and also by the presence of enzymes that indicate liver damage.

NOTABLE CASES Hepatitis C has affected a number of notable personalities. Musician Lou Reed died in 2013 of complications related to the infection. David Crosby and Gregg Allman are liver transplant recipients; Allman is an active hepatitis C awareness spokesperson. Natalie Cole and Steven Tyler have both been treated successfully for this infection.

Viral hepatitis of any kind may be described in four basic phases:

- *Phase 1.* New infection and viral replication. During this phase, the virus attacks cells in the liver, but the liver compensates for the damage, so no symptoms develop. Blood tests for indicator enzymes or antibodies are positive.
- *Phase 2.* Prodromal stage. Symptoms develop in this stage. Food aversion, nausea, vomiting, and malaise are the most common complaints.
- *Phase 3.* Icteric stage. At this point the signs of **jaundice** develop, including **icterus**, pale stools, dark urine, and **hepatomegaly**.
- *Phase 4.* Convalescence. During this time the liver heals, jaundice resolves, enzymes return to normal levels, and health is restored.

For information about communicability, prognosis, and prevention for various types of viral hepatitis, see Compare & Contrast 8.1.

Types of Hepatitis

- *Hepatitis A.* This used to be called infectious hepatitis. It is usually spread through oral-fecal contamination, but it can be spread less efficiently through contact with intimate fluids. It is a short, acute infection (relative to other types of hepatitis), and it usually causes no long-lasting damage. One exposure creates lifelong immunity. Hepatitis A virus (HAV) incubates for 2 to 6 weeks after exposure before symptoms appear, but it is highly contagious during this period. Once symptoms develop, the virus is present for another 2 to 3 weeks, although a person may not feel fully restored to health for up to 6 months.
- *Hepatitis B.* Hepatitis B virus (HBV) is spread through contact with intimate fluids: blood, semen, breast milk, or vaginal secretions. It causes long-term infections with subtle symptoms. In this case, the virus itself is not responsible for most liver injury; chronic inflammation is the cause of most of the damage. HBV incubates for 2 to 6 months before symptoms develop, but it is communicable during this time. Most adults who are exposed to hepatitis B recover fully within 15 months. However, most infants who contract the disease from their mothers, about half of children infected between age 1 and 5, and about 5% of exposed adults develop chronic infections. These individuals are long-term carriers of the virus, and their risk of developing other liver diseases—especially **liver cancer**—is higher than that of the general population. On a global basis, it is possible to see elevated numbers of deaths related to liver cancer in areas where hepatitis B is especially common.

Unlike many pathogens, HBV is sturdy outside of a host, and is communicable through indirect blood-to-blood contact with a contaminated surface. Furthermore, it occurs in high concentrations, so limited exposure can cause an infection. For this reason, it is especially important to sterilize any

Icterus: Abnormal yellowing of the skin and eyes. Also called jaundice.

Hepatomegaly: Abnormal enlargement of the liver.

COMPARE & CONTRAST 8.1 The ABCs of Hepatitis

The three most common types of hepatitis seen in developed countries are caused by viruses that, while they are unrelated to each other, share a common target: hepatocytes. For this reason, they create a similar symptomatic picture, but with varying severity. This chart compares other important features of these viruses, namely communicability, prognosis, and the availability of a preventive vaccine.

	COMMUNICABILITY	PROGNOSIS	VACCINE AVAILABLE?
Hepatitis A	HAV concentrates in the feces of an infected person; therefore, it is most easily transmitted through oral-fecal contact, often by way of contaminated food or water. Hepatitis A is the reason for "employees must wash hands before returning to work" signs in restaurant bathrooms. Raw or undercooked shellfish grown in contaminated water can spread the disease to humans. Hepatitis A can also be shared through sexual activity, but this does not appear to an efficient method of communication.	Hepatitis A usually develops over several weeks, spontaneously resolves, and does not cause long-term complications.	Yes; one vaccine is sufficient.
Hepatitis B	HBV occurs in high concentration in the blood, and is viable outside a host for many hours or days. It is communicable through exposure to intimate fluids, but doesn't necessarily require direct contact. Sharing a tattoo needle, body piercing equipment, an intravenous needle, or even a razor or a toothbrush with a person who has hepatitis B is a potent mechanism for communicating the virus from host to another. Infants born to mothers with hepatitis B are at very high risk for chronic liver disease unless they are treated immediately.	Hepatitis B infections can be long-lasting and silent, requiring treatment for many months before the virus is eradicated. About 5% of hepatitis B patients are long-term carriers, and resistant to treatment. Untreated hepatitis B patients and long-term carriers experience chronic liver inflammation. This can lead to the development of varicose veins on the stomach and esophagus, which may rupture and bleed. Liver failure, cirrhosis, and liver cancer are other possible complications.	Yes; a series of three vaccines over a period of 6 months needs to be repeated about every 20 years.
Hepatitis C	Hepatitis C is most communicable through blood-to-blood contact (i.e., accidental needle sticks in healthcare settings, transfusions, shared needles, tattoo or piercing equipment, or sexual activity with damage to mucous membranes). It does not appear to be easily communicable without direct contact, but some cases develop from sexual contact, indirect blood contact (e.g., sharing a razor or toothbrush), or unknown sources of exposure.	Only about 25% of hepatitis C patients recover spontaneously. Of those with chronic hepatitis C, many are at risk for chronic liver disease, including cirrhosis, liver failure, and liver cancer. The presence of other illnesses, specifically HIV, hepatitis B, or alcoholism, raises the risk of complications from long-term hepatitis C infections.	No vaccine is available for hepatitis C.

To hear the author speak more on hepatitis A, B, and C, go to http://thePoint.lww.com/Werner6e. thePoint®

CASE HISTORY 8.1 Hepatitis C: "I feel totally worthless. It sucks."

RANDY, AGE 64

I spent a lot of time in Southeast Asia—Vietnam and afterwards. I was probably infected with hepatitis C when I was in the military.

In the late 80s I felt healthy. I was a musician and a music producer. I was into playing, engineering, stage-managing. I was on the road a lot. And it was the culture—I indulged in drugs, especially cocaine.

Then I was told I had "hep non-A, non-B."

It was all a guessing game to figure out how it happened or what to do. Everyone contradicts everyone else. Eventually, you have to go by what you trust. I ended up using some herbal remedies and supplements. I stopped drinking, and reduced stress, and things seemed to be okay. I got married, had kids, and got away from big crowds. I had learned building as another way to earn a living.

But my energy levels just got worse and worse. That was my big indicator.

It can get to where I can only work 3 or 4 hours a day. My desire to do things—to go fishing, to play music—are gone. Some days nothing matters. It impacts my home, my relationships. I feel totally worthless. It sucks.

I never treated my hep C with interferon—it turns out that the type of virus coming out of Southeast Asia had a really poor response to that. I am hoping to start a new treatment protocol this year. I feel like hep C has taken more than my energy. It's taken my personality—my whole psyche. I hope I can get some of that back.

instruments that come in contact with human blood: tattoo needles, body piercing equipment, acupuncture needles, and professional medical and dental tools all fall into this category. Further, sharing household items that might contact blood, such as razors or toothbrushes, must be avoided.

- *Hepatitis C.* Before the viruses D, E, F, and G were discovered, hepatitis virus C (HCV) was called "hepatitis non-A and non-B."

  Hepatitis C is carried by more than 4 million Americans, and of those, about three-quarters have it as a chronic infection; those individuals are at high risk for **cirrhosis**, liver failure, or **liver cancer**. Anywhere from 1% to 5% of those long-term carriers will probably die from complications related to this infection.

  HCV is unique in that it damages the liver so slowly that symptoms may not develop until decades after exposure (see Case History 8.1). The individual can spread the virus during that period, however.
- *Other forms of hepatitis.* Liver inflammation may be caused by other viruses. Hepatitis D is a form that can only exist alongside hepatitis B. Types E–G are rare pathogens that are uncommon in the United States. Two members of the herpes family, Epstein-Barr virus and cytomegalovirus have also been seen to cause liver inflammation.

Nonviral hepatitis is an occasional reaction to certain medications or an autoimmune attack launched against hepatocytes. Autoimmune hepatitis frequently accompanies other autoimmune diseases, including **type 1 diabetes**, **Graves disease**, and **ulcerative colitis**. Nonalcoholic fatty liver disease is a rising cause of liver inflammation. This condition is a precursor to NASH or nonalcoholic steatohepatitis: inflammation of fatty deposits in the liver that lead to scarring and a high risk of **cirrhosis**.

Signs and Symptoms

The severity of hepatitis symptoms varies widely from one person to another depending on the phase of the infection, the general health of the patient, and the type of virus involved. The basic picture of hepatitis symptoms includes general malaise, weakness, fever, nausea, food aversion, and sometimes jaundice. Hepatitis A typically presents the most extreme symptoms for the shortest time; hepatitis B and C tend to be much subtler, developing symptoms only when so much liver function has been lost that it can no longer compensate for the damage. Blood tests for antibodies or liver enzymes can indicate infection long before symptoms suggest an illness. A person infected with any type of hepatitis who has other form of liver disease is at risk for a much more serious case than someone who begins with a healthy liver.

Treatment

Hepatitis A is typically treated with a shot of **immunoglobulin** (usually equine antibodies) to begin fighting the

Immunoglobulin: A protein that helps the immune system recognize and attack foreign objects. Also called antibodies.

virus while the patient establishes an immune response. Hepatitis B and C are treated with antiviral agents, rest, good nutrition, and patience during a long recovery period. New antiviral medications are always in development for hepatitis B and C; the prognosis for people with these infections is generally positive, if they can tolerate the treatment.

The side-effects from antiviral treatments can be severe, including fatigue, headache, fever, nausea, rashes, weight loss, and depression. These can be severe enough to interfere with a patient's ability to take medication as directed, thus allowing the infection to progress. Massage is sometimes recommended as a coping strategy for this challenge.

If significant liver function is lost due to hepatitis C, a liver transplant may be recommended; this is the leading reason for liver transplants in the United States.

Medications

- For hepatitis A: immunoglobulin injection to boost active antibodies while the patient establishes an immune response.
- For hepatitis B and C: any combination of lamivudine, ribovirin, interferon, or other antiviral agents.

Massage Therapy Implications

RISKS	Acute hepatitis carries a risk of several serious complications, including jaundice, cirrhosis, and liver failure. Any bodywork that puts an extra adaptive stress on the body may be overwhelming rather than supportive during this time. Further, some types of hepatitis are communicable via indirect contact with body fluids; this presents a risk to the therapists as well as the client.
BENEFITS	Massage that is within the capacity of a client to adapt can be appropriate for client with hepatitis that is not acute. While it probably won't have a profound impact on the progress of the disease, it can improve the quality of life for a person dealing with a very challenging situation. Carefully administered massage may also help hepatitis patients better tolerate the side-effects of medication. Clients who have fully recovered from any type of hepatitis can enjoy the same benefits from bodywork as the rest of the population.

Liver Cancer

Definition: What Is It?

Primary liver cancer, also called hepatocellular carcinoma, is cancer that originates in the liver. This is distinguished from secondary liver cancer, or metastatic liver disease, which is a result of cancer that originates elsewhere and spreads to the liver.

Demographics

Liver cancer is diagnosed about 33,000 people each year, and leads to about 23,000 deaths. It is the fastest-growing cause of cancer death in this country, with diagnostic rates that have more than doubled in the past 20 years. This is probably because of rising NAFLD, and the long-term influence of both hepatitis B and C on an aging population. In other parts of the world, especially in developing countries, liver cancer is a leading cause of mortality.

In this country, liver cancer is typically diagnosed in mature people; the average age at diagnosis is 65 years. It is found in men more often than women.

Etiology: What Happens?

Liver cancer develops when hepatocytes replicate uncontrollably. A history of slow-acting viral infection, alcoholism, and long-term inflammation along with cirrhosis are all contributing factors to rampant cellular activity. This is true especially when any combination of these factors affects a single person.

Liver cancer tumors may develop singly, or they may occur in several disconnected areas throughout the left and right lobes. They tend to be highly invested with blood vessels, which raises the risk for distant metastasis (usually to the lungs) before signs and symptoms lead to a diagnosis. Interestingly, most liver cancer tumors are supplied by the hepatic artery, while the rest of the liver's tissues are supplied mostly by the portal vein. This means medication can be administered via the portal artery with minimal damage to nontumor cells.

Several risk factors for liver cancer have been identified. They are especially potent when they appear in combination.

- *Hepatitis B infection.* This virus has specifically been seen to cause, not just appear frequently with, a specific type of liver cancer. Genetic material from **HBV** can be found in the malignant cells of liver cancer. Hepatitis B is an especially high risk for liver cancer when the infection was contracted in infancy or childhood.
- *Hepatitis C infection.* The relationship between **HCV** and liver cancer is not completely understood; some research indicates that the virus may actually cause the cancer, while other studies suggest that liver cancer develops indirectly through the chronic inflammation associated with hepatitis C. Regardless, about 5% to 10% of people diagnosed with hepatitis C eventually develop liver cancer. Because HCV infects over 3 million people in the United States, liver cancer rates are expected to keep rising for the next several years.

- *Alcoholism.* **Alcohol abuse**, especially in combination with hepatitis B or C, greatly raises the risk of liver cancer. Ironically, it appears that it is the cessation of alcohol use that triggers the cellular mutation: when a person stops drinking and the liver begins to regenerate, cells are more likely to become malignant.
- *Hemochromatosis.* This is a genetic blood disorder, involving the production of too many red blood cells. Persons with untreated **hemochromatosis** are at high risk for **cirrhosis**, which may then progress to liver cancer.
- *Nonalcoholic fatty liver disease (NFALD).* NFALD can lead to NASH, which leads to cirrhosis. This is a relatively new risk factor for liver cancer, but it is an important one in a country where two-thirds of the adult population is overweight.
- *Cirrhosis.* This condition, the result of long-term liver damage with scarring, develops in the presence of chronic viral infection, alcoholism, toxic exposure, or other circumstances. It is possible, but unusual, for liver cancer to develop without cirrhosis.
- *Aflatoxin B1.* This is a chemical from a mold called *Aspergillus flavus* that grows on peanuts and grains stored in hot, humid conditions. **Aflatoxin B1** is an extremely potent carcinogen responsible for many liver cancer cases in Asia and sub-Saharan Africa.

Signs and Symptoms

Tumors in the liver can interfere with normal function, but because hepatitis and/or cirrhosis are often also present, these early signs are easily missed or ignored. The most commonly reported signs and symptoms of liver cancer include vague abdominal pain that becomes increasingly intense, unintended weight loss and food aversion, muscle wasting, ascites (which may obscure signs of weight loss), fever, an abdominal mass, and if the bile duct is blocked, **jaundice**. Blood tests may reveal signs of liver dysfunction. One specific substance, **alpha fetoprotein**, is often present in the blood when liver cancer is present. Other blood tests may show unusual hormonal activity, as cancerous cells sometimes secrete hormones.

NOTABLE CASES Liver cancer was the cause of death for composer Johannes Brahms, musicians Ray Charles and John Coltrane, baseball great Mickey Mantle, and dancer/actor/director Gregory Hines.

Hemochromatosis: A genetic disorder characterized by the over absorption of iron.

Aflatoxin B1: A toxin produced by some strains of *Aspergillus flavus* that causes cancer in some animals.

Alpha-fetoprotein: A protein produced by a fetus. Levels can be measured to detect neural tube defects before birth.

Treatment

Even when liver cancer is caught in its earliest recognizable stages, survival for more than 5 years is rare. Staging protocols for liver cancer are discussed in Sidebar 8.8. Most survivors of liver cancer surgery have a recurrence within several months, unless they are lucky enough to receive a new liver in a transplant surgery before metastasis occurs. This cancer is aggressive and difficult to control, and most patients have serious underlying liver disease that makes them poor candidates for many types of surgery. Furthermore, liver cancer tends not to respond well to chemotherapy or radiation. Consequently, a number of treatment options have been developed that try to control the growth of the cancer without invasive surgery. These include techniques to burn or freeze tumors through laparoscopic or percutaneous instruments; injections of ethanol to destroy tumor cells; and the use of drugs or implements to block the blood vessels that supply tumors. No single treatment option shows outstanding promise for a long-term cure, however.

Surgery typically entails a resection of the liver (removing the portion or portions in which tumors are present) or liver transplant. The fact that many liver cancer patients have a long history of cirrhosis and/or hepatitis makes both resections and transplant surgeries difficult.

Medications

- Chemotherapy administered by catheter to sections of the liver to kill off targeted cells.
- Oral anti-angiogenic agents to inhibit the growth of blood vessels supplying tumors.
- Injections of ethanol to destroy tumor cells.
- Medication to manage liver cancer complications, including pain, encephalopathy, and ascites.

Massage Therapy Implications

RISKS	Liver cancer often involves aggressive therapies including various types of surgery and surgical devices, which require adaptation in bodywork choices. For more information about massage in the context of cancer, see Chapter 12.
BENEFITS	Treatment for liver cancer is a highly stressful process, and patients are often encouraged to use whatever stress management mechanisms might suit them; careful, highly informed massage therapy could be applied in this context. Because liver cancer is often terminal, massage therapy may be welcomed as a way to provide comfort, pain relief, and other benefits at the end of life.

SIDEBAR 8.8 Staging Liver Cancer

Staging protocols for liver cancer have several variations. The typical TNM classification with numerical groupings follows this pattern:

TUMOR (T)	NODE (N)	METASTASIS (M)
T1: One tumor, no vascularization. T2: One tumor with vascularization or multiple tumors <5 cm. T3: Multiple tumors >5 cm or one tumor involving portal vein or hepatic artery. T4: Multiple tumors with direct invasion of adjacent organs and/or perforation of visceral peritoneum.	N0: no nodes involved. N1: regional nodes involved.	M0: no metastasis found. M1: tumors found outside the liver.

These delineations are then translated into stages I to IV in this way:

STAGE	TUMOR	NODE	METASTASIS
I	T1	N0	M0
II	T2	N0	M0
IIIA	T3	N0	M0
IIIB	T4	N0	M0
IIIC	Any	N1	M0
IV	T any	N any	M1

Liver cancer staging may be discussed in stages 0 through IV, as other cancers are, but it is also discussed in terms of best treatment options.

- *Localized resectable cancer.* This indicates that a single tumor smaller than 2 cm without signs of spreading to blood or lymph vessels has been found. The tumor can be fully removed surgically.
- *Localized unresectable cancer.* This means that although metastasis is not obvious, the liver is too damaged by cirrhosis or other factors to make surgery safe.
- *Advanced cancer.* This indicates that distant metastasis has occurred, and while chemotherapy and radiation may slow the progress, the cancer is probably not curable.
- *Recurrent cancer.* This is cancer that returns after previous treatments.

Pancreatic Cancer

Definition: What Is It?

Pancreatic cancer begins as mutation of certain genes that trigger uncontrolled growth of cells in the pancreas. It usually occurs in the exocrine ducts of this gland, but occasionally it is found in the hormone-producing cells.

Demographics

Pancreatic cancer is aggressive, metastasizes easily, and is difficult to detect in early stages; consequently, it is the fourth leading cause of death from cancer in this country. About 46,000 people are diagnosed and about 39,000 deaths are attributed to pancreatic cancer each year.

Etiology: What Happens?

The pancreas is a small, spongy gland behind the stomach. It produces digestive enzymes that collect in an extensive duct system, and eventually enter the duodenum by way of the common bile duct. It also manufactures insulin and other hormones for maintenance of blood sugar levels.

Pancreatic cancer comes about when mutations of cells lead to the growth of invasive, aggressive, and life-threatening tumors. When these tumors arise in the exocrine ducts, they are **adenocarcinomas**. When they grow in the islet cells, they are **neuroendocrine tumors**. In either case, the tumors tend to grow quickly and easily invade nearby tissues simply by spreading out. The duodenum, stomach, and peritoneal wall are often affected by these local extensions. When cells invade the abdominal lymph system or large blood vessels, the liver is often the first site of metastasis.

Exact causes or triggers of pancreatic cancer have not been identified, but a number of risk factors have been seen to increase the chance that pancreatic cells may mutate. The primary risk factors for pancreatic cancer include the following:

NOTABLE CASES Pancreatic cancer has shortened the lives of many notable personalities, including musician Dizzy Gillespie, opera singer Luciano Pavarotti, actors Michael Landon and Patrick Swayze, and Apple Computer co-founder Steve Jobs. As of this writing one well-known pancreatic cancer survivor is Supreme Court Justice Ruth Bader Ginsburg.

- Age (most diagnoses are among people 60 to 80 years old).
- Race (it occurs slightly more frequently among African Americans).
- A history of smoking (this may be responsible for up to 30% of genetic mutations).
- A history of **type 2 diabetes**.
- Chronic **pancreatitis**, especially when due to alcohol abuse.
- Obesity and diet (high in animal fats, red meat and processed meat; low in fresh fruits and vegetables).
- Inherited characteristics, including a family history of pancreatitis, or a genetic predisposition to **colorectal cancer**, **breast cancer**, or **melanoma**.

Types of Pancreatic Cancer

- *Adenocarcinoma of the pancreas*. This is cancer of the exocrine ducts. It affects the secretion of digestive enzymes, sometimes by blocking the pancreatic duct. Pancreatic adenocarcinoma is the most common form of pancreatic cancer, causing about 96% of all cases.
- *Neuroendocrine tumors of the pancreas*. This is cancer of the endocrine cells of the pancreas, specifically the islet cells that produce insulin and other hormones. A problem with these cells leads to difficulties with regulating blood glucose.

Adenocarcinoma: A malignant tumor of glandular epithelial tissue.

Neuroendocrine tumor: Tumors of tissues of the endocrine and neurological systems, which can be either benign or malignant.

Pruritis: Itchiness.

Signs and Symptoms

Early pancreatic cancer creates such subtle symptoms that people rarely consult their doctor about them: abdominal discomfort, mid-back pain, loss of appetite, and unintended weight loss typically occur for 2 months or more before most people seek a diagnosis.

If a tumor obstructs the common bile duct, **jaundice** may develop, sometimes with **pruritis**. Other late-stage signs of include difficulty with digestion, ascites, and enlargement of the liver and spleen. If the cancer affects the endocrine cells, difficulty with the regulation of blood glucose may arise.

Treatment

Because pancreatic cancer is so difficult to identify in early stages, the majority of patients have local or distant metastasis when they are diagnosed. Staging protocols for pancreatic cancer are discussed in Sidebar 8.9. A small percentage of patients are good candidates for resection, and, not surprisingly, they have a better prognosis than others. Nonetheless, surgery for this condition is invasive and often requires removing not only parts of the pancreas but also the gallbladder, part of the stomach, and some of the small intestine. The chance of recurrence after surgery is very high.

If it is determined that a person has inoperable cancer, various combinations of chemotherapy, targeted therapy, and radiation therapy may be used to slow the tumors' growth and prolong life. In some cases, the combination of chemotherapy and radiation can reduce a growth to the point that it can be surgically excised, or these interventions can add to the postsurgical life expectancy of the patient.

Biologic or targeted therapies to use immune system agents to attack specific cancer cells are in development for pancreatic cancer, but they have not yet reached mainstream application. The promise for these therapies, which may eventually be highly customizable to each patient, is rich.

Surgery may be performed to relieve some of the symptoms of pancreatic cancer. This may include bypassing the exocrine ducts, inserting a stent to keep ducts open, or damaging the local nerves to reduce pain.

Ultimately, the treatment options for pancreatic cancer probably include hospice care for a dying person. At this point, any appropriate comfort measures are welcome.

SIDEBAR 8.9 Staging Pancreatic Cancer

Staging for pancreatic cancer follows the pattern for TNM classification and numerical assignments, but it can be difficult to evaluate the extent of lymph node involvement without surgery. Consequently, the true extent of the cancer progression may not be known before treatment options are chosen. Staging is as follows:

TUMOR (T)	NODE (N)	METASTASIS (M)
T1: only pancreas involved; tumor <2 cm.	N0: no nodes involved.	M0: no metastasis found.
T2: only pancreas involved; tumor >2 cm.	N1: regional nodes involved.	M1: tumors outside pancreas.
T3: cancer has spread but not invaded large blood vessels.		
T4: cancer has spread and invaded large blood vessels.		

These delineations are then translated into stages I to IV in this way:

STAGE	TUMOR	NODE	METASTASIS
IA	T1	N0	M0
IB	T2	N0	M0
IIA	T3	N0	M0
IIB	T1-3	N any	M0
III	T4	N any	M0
IV	T any	N any	M1

Because it can be difficult to assess pancreatic cancer without surgery, many experts simply discuss it in terms of possible treatment options:

- *Potentially resectable* means a growth is isolated to a particular area that is accessible through surgery for removal. Life expectancy is much better, if it is caught while operable.
- *Locally advanced* means tumors reach out and invade local tissues such as the stomach, liver, and peritoneum. This often happens before distant metastasis.
- *Metastatic cancer* means that tumors have invaded the lymph system and may be growing far from their site of origin.

Medications

- Chemotherapy to kill fast-growing cells.
- Biologic or targeted therapy to kill cancer cells.
- Narcotic analgesics, sometimes with antidepressants and antiemetics to address pain and side-effects of treatment.

Massage Therapy Implications

RISKS	Pancreatic cancer patients are likely to be fragile, in pain, and facing the end of life. Any bodywork offered in this context must be given with the utmost sensitivity and care. For more on massage and cancer, see Chapter 12.
BENEFITS	Appropriate massage can help with pain, anxiety, depression, and general quality of life for a person who dealing with this often-terminal disease.

Pancreatitis

Definition: What Is It?

Pancreatitis is inflammation of the pancreas. Acute pancreatitis can be triggered by alcohol binging, **gallstones**, toxic exposures, blunt trauma, or other factors; chronic pancreatitis is usually related to long-term **alcohol abuse**.

Demographics

About 274,000 patients are admitted to the hospital for treatment of acute pancreatitis in this country each year, and this disorder has a mortality rate of about 5% (about 13,700 deaths per year). It affects more men than women, and African Americans are affected far more often than other races. Chronic pancreatitis is less common; it leads to about 122,000 doctor visits and 56,000 hospitalizations each year.

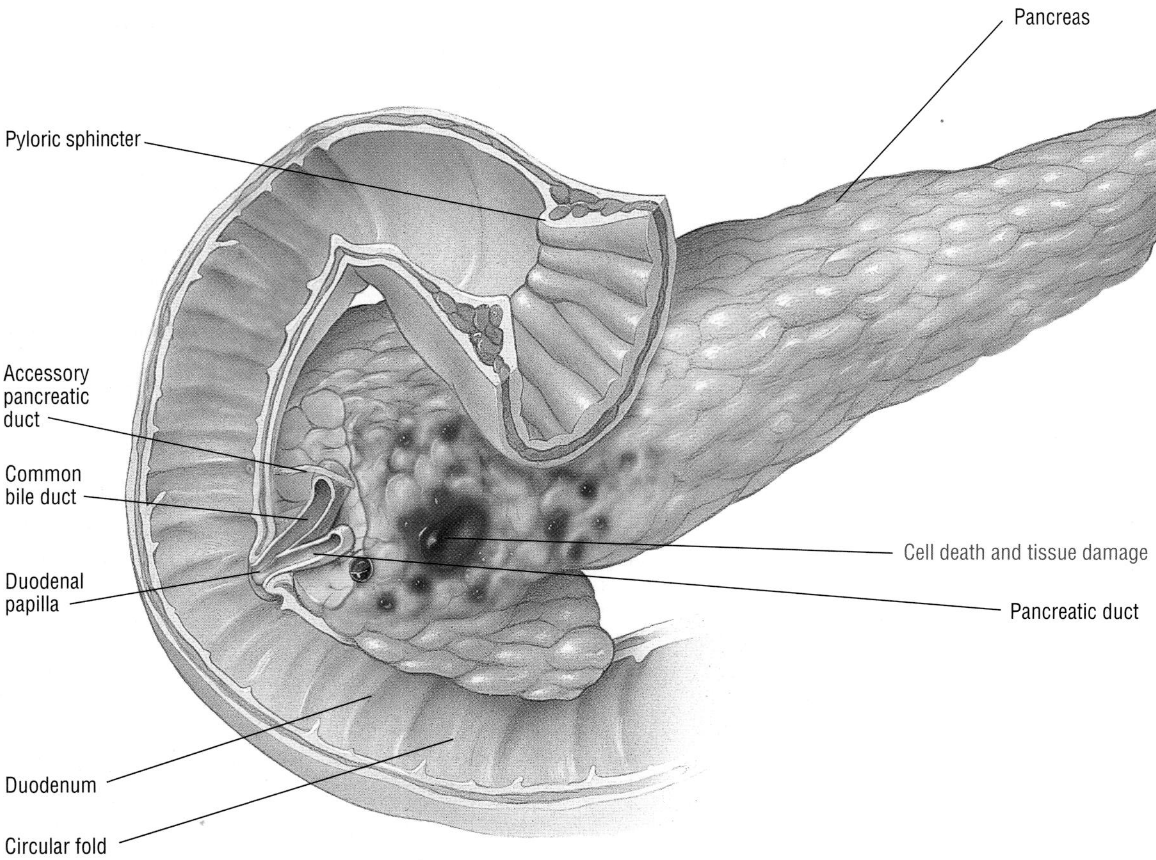

FIGURE 8.18 Acute pancreatitis

Etiology: What Happens?

The pancreas manufactures both endocrine and exocrine secretions. Its exocrine products are produced in **acinar** cells. They include bicarbonate to neutralize material exiting the highly acidic stomach, and digestive enzymes that break down carbohydrates, proteins, and fats into absorbable particles. If the ducts in the pancreas are blocked, or if the gland develops cysts or abscesses, these functions are lost, and the secretions may even destroy the pancreas tissue itself; this is called **autodigestion**.

Types of Pancreatitis

- *Acute pancreatitis*. This is a sudden onset of symptoms related to a blockage of the pancreatic ducts, so that corrosive secretions are trapped within the gland (Figure 8.18). This can be brought about by **gallstones** lodged in the common bile duct, alcohol use, blunt trauma to the abdomen, a congenital malformation of the pancreas, **cystic fibrosis**, or other problems. Acute pancreatitis is usually short-lived with a full recovery, if intervention happens quickly. But when it is severe, cysts, abscesses, necrosis, and the release of dangerous toxins into the bloodstream can occur. The results may include circulatory shock, **renal failure**, or **adult respiratory distress syndrome**.
- *Chronic pancreatitis*. In this situation, long-term wear and tear leads to permanent, irreversible damage to the delicate epithelial tissue of the gland. Chronic pancreatitis is almost always related to alcohol abuse. **Ethanol** can cause digestive enzymes to be released prematurely, damaging the gland, promoting fibrosis and scarring, and forming protein plugs that may calcify to become pancreatic stones. Long-term alcohol abuse is the most common cause of chronic pancreatitis, but other causes include inherited problems like cystic fibrosis, congenital anomalies in how the pancreas is formed, autoimmune dysfunction, and gallstones.

Signs and Symptoms

Dull upper abdominal pain is the leading symptom of acute and chronic pancreatitis. With acute pancreatitis the pain has

Acinar: Describing a raspberry-shaped cluster of cells that produces a secretion.

Autodigestion: A process in which cells are digested by enzymes produced within them.

Adult respiratory distress syndrome (ARDS): An acute condition characterized by widespread inflammation of the lungs.

Ethanol: Ethyl alcohol.

a sudden onset. It may appear with nausea, diarrhea, vomiting, fever, and rapid pulse.

In chronic pancreatitis, the pain may be episodic, lasting for many hours and then subsiding until the next attack. Episodes get closer together until the pain is severe and unremitting. Pancreatic pain often refers into the back, which is an issue of concern for massage therapists, of course.

Other symptoms suggest the loss of pancreatic enzymes and hormones: unintended weight loss, malabsorption of nutrients and steatorrhea, difficulties with the regulation of blood glucose, and the possibility of **jaundice**, if the obstruction of the pancreatic duct also affects the common bile duct.

Treatment

Pancreatitis is treated according to the cause. Many patients undergo a few days of taking no food by mouth to allow the organ to heal. Surgery is often part of a treatment plan. If the pancreatitis is related to gallstones, these are removed so the ducts can flow freely. If abscesses form, these are drained or removed. If tissue has died because of autodigestion, that is also removed. The pancreatic duct may be surgically reopened or a stent may be inserted. Digestive enzymes may be taken orally to relieve the pancreas of the work of producing them. Finally, if the pain from chronic pancreatitis is unresponsive to any other interventions, surgery may be performed to sever the sensory nerves from the gland.

Medications

- Antibiotics if necessary
- Analgesics for pain management
- Supplementary digestive enzymes if necessary

Massage Therapy Implications

RISKS	Pancreatitis, which is rare but potentially dangerous, can refer pain to the midback, which may push clients toward seeking massage rather than medical care; this is a situation where undiagnosed abdominal pain is a good reason to visit a doctor with persistent symptoms.
BENEFITS	Clients who are appropriately treating pancreatitis can receive any massage that fits within their capacity for adaptation, and those who have fully recovered can enjoy all the benefits that bodywork offers the general population.

Other Digestive System Conditions

Candidiasis

Definition: What Is It?

Candida albicans is one type of about 20 yeast-like fungi that inhabit the digestive tract, often from the mouth to the anus (Figure 8.19). They usually live in balance with other flora and fauna of the GI tract. Under certain circumstances that balance is upset and *Candida* replicates too easily leading to a variety of problems. This condition of having levels of *Candida* become abnormally predominant is called candidiasis.

Demographics

Candida fungi are present in about 60% of all healthy people.

Oral candidiasis is fairly common among infants and immunosuppressed people, and rare among the general population. People with **diabetes**, those who use dentures, or those who use long-term corticosteroids are at increased risk for active *Candida* infections of the mouth and throat.

Candida that affects the genital tract of women is very common; up to 75% of all women report having at least one yeast infection at some point.

Invasive candidiasis is a situation where the yeast becomes aggressive and can lead to fungal infection of the bloodstream. It is rare in people who are basically healthy, but in hospital settings it is the fourth most common bloodstream infection in the United States, affecting some 25,000

Steatorrhea: Abnormal amounts of fat in the feces resulting from poor absorption of fats in the intestines.

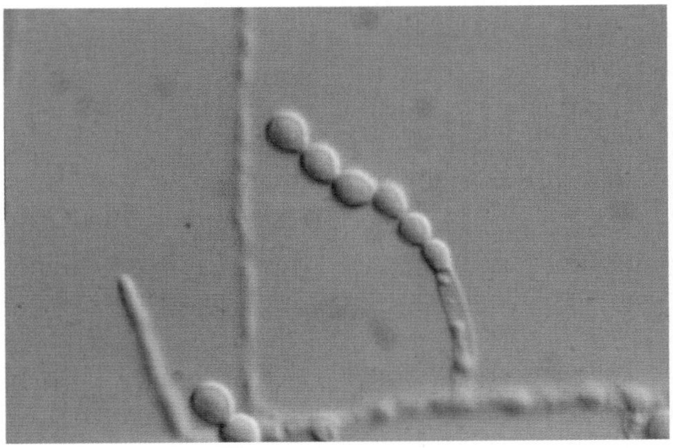

FIGURE 8.19 *Candida albicans*

people each year. Underweight premature infants are also at risk for invasive candidiasis.

Etiology: What Happens?

Under normal circumstances, a balanced environment of flora (plant-like organisms) and fauna (animal-like organisms) peacefully coexist in the GI tract. The flora keep the fauna from replicating too much, and the fauna do likewise for the flora. These organisms live in balance with each other, and in **symbiosis** with the human digestive system: a mutually beneficial relationship with their human hosts.

When a disruption in the balance of the GI tract occurs, either plants or animals can dominate. When bacteria are suppressed, *Candida* in the GI tract converts from benign, helpful yeast-like organisms to more aggressive fungi. In the absence of balancing bacteria, the fungi have more opportunity to reproduce and spread. Because *Candida* is already present, the exact delineation between colonization and infestation is not always clear. Opinions vary about how extensive a *Candida* colonization has to be before it causes symptoms or becomes a problem (Sidebar 8.10).

Often the trigger for intestinal imbalance is use of antibiotics. These medications, designed to kill harmful bacteria, may also kill beneficial bacteria. This is why many healthcare providers recommend supplementing lactobacilli along with antibiotic prescriptions. Other well-accepted causes of candidiasis include immunosuppression as seen with **HIV/AIDS** patients, and people undergoing treatment for cancer, genetic immune system dysfunctions, thymus tumors, and hormonal imbalances.

SIDEBAR 8.10 It's Candidiasis, But Is It a Problem?

Two schools of thought dominate the discussion of candidiasis. The more conservative allopathic approach generally assumes that the overgrowth of *Candida* isn't a problem until very severe symptoms occur, which may involve the skin, mucous membranes, or invasive candidiasis, a systemic infection of the blood.

Many naturopathic and holistic practitioners propose that milder overgrowths of *Candida* can also cause many chronic, low-grade symptoms. The fungi may grow and spread throughout the intestines, sinking root-like structures into the walls. They produce waste products that can be irritating to the host. Invasion of the intestinal wall may also allow other substances to enter the bloodstream, where immune system responses launched against incompletely digested material may be extreme. Between losing access to nutrition because the fungi get it first, dealing with yeasts' metabolic wastes, and immune system responses against digestive contents, a person with chronic, low-grade candidiasis may develop a number of persistent, subtle, or severe symptoms.

Practitioners who deal with candidiasis as a contributor to many other chronic disorders often report success when helping their patients change their diet and lifestyle in ways that restore balance to intestinal flora and fauna. This clinical evidence has yet to be reproduced in a formal research setting however, which leads to resistance to the acceptance of candidiasis as a common, chronic disorder responsible for symptoms that range from fatigue to menstrual pain to food allergies.

Types of Candidiasis

- *Mucocutaneous candidiasis*. This describes yeast infections that appear in the mouth or on the skin. **Thrush** is one form that is commonly seen in infants and immunosuppressed people. This type of infestation can cause painful fissures to develop around the mouth (**angular cheilitis**), and ulcers to erupt in the digestive tract. *Candida* can also colonize fingernails and toenails. Other skin signs include **intertrigo** (colonies in skin folds around the groin, axillae, and breasts) and the diaper rash and jock itch that appear when yeasts from the GI tract colonize the external skin around the anus.
- *Vulvovaginitis*. This is the development of candidiasis in and around the vagina. It is a common infection for women. It can cause itching and burning at the vagina, painful intercourse, and characteristic cottage cheese-like, yeasty-smelling vaginal discharge.
- *Invasive candidiasis*. Also called candemia, this is *Candida* that has invaded the bloodstream. It is most often seen in hospital settings, among patients who are in an intensive care unit, who have a central venous catheter, or who had weakened immune systems. Invasive candemia can lead to organ failure.
- *Others*. Rarer types of candidiasis can affect the bladder, penis, urinary tract, and kidneys.

Symbiosis: A mutually beneficial relationship between two organisms.

Thrush: *Candida* infection of the mouth.

Angular cheilitis: A condition characterized by inflammation and cracking at the corners of the mouth.

Intertrigo: Inflammation of the skin in and around folds.

Signs and Symptoms

Candidiasis can show a variety of signs and symptoms depending on the severity of the condition, its location, and the underlying health of the affected person. Symptoms range from patchy, painless white lesions in the mouth (thrush) to yeasty vaginal discharge (vulvovaginitis), and can include variations like skin lesions, chemical sensitivities, and headaches on the mild end, to drug-resistant fever, chills, and organ failure on the severe end of the spectrum.

Treatment

Various topical or oral antifungal medications may be recommended for severe versions of candidiasis.

For subtler versions of this condition, reestablishing internal flora to balance out the fungi is a high priority. This requires dietary changes that essentially rule out simple carbohydrates, sweet things, fermented foods, and many processed foods. Some clinicians suggest that most people would feel more energetic and less sluggish with a dietary change of this sort, so whether an overabundance of yeasts has been addressed or not may be moot.

Medications

- Topical antifungal medication for cutaneous or vaginal candidiasis.
- Oral antifungal medications:
  - The "-azole" group to block essential materials in the yeast cell wall. These are used with caution, as some of these drugs have been associated with severe liver damage.
  - The polyene group including nystatin or amphotericin B for more resistant infestations.

Massage Therapy Implications

RISKS	Extreme cutaneous candidiasis is usually seen in the context of significant immune system impairment, which carries its own cautions for massage therapy.
BENEFITS	Mild candidiasis has no risks for massage, and clients with this condition can enjoy the same benefits from bodywork as the rest of the population. The use of essential oils to treat *Candida* of the skin should be done only be trained providers for whom it is within the scope of practice.

Explore and Apply

LEVEL 1: Receive and Respond

1. What triggers an inflammatory response in people with celiac disease?
   a. Gluten
   b. Gliadin
   c. Glucose
   d. Glycogen

2. Esophageal cancer at the proximal end of the esophagus is usually connected to…
   a. Reflux
   b. Obesity
   c. Smoking
   d. Genetics

3. Most people with a hiatal hernia also have…
   a. Barrett esophagus
   b. Gallstone
   c. Obesity
   d. GERD

4. Gastric cancer is most closely associated with …
   a. Eating a lot of salted, pickled, or smoked foods
   b. Eating fresh vegetables that have been contaminated with pathogens
   c. Smoking combined with excessive alcohol consumption
   d. Chronic irritation from GERD

5. Which condition involves NO structural changes to the GI tract?
   a. Inflammatory bowel disease
   b. Irritable bowel syndrome
   c. Gastroesophageal reflux disease
   d. Diverticular disease

6. What is the most common symptom of gallstones?
   a. Nothing
   b. Biliary colic
   c. Right upper quadrant pain
   d. Scapular pain

7. Indicate which type of viral hepatitis goes with the following descriptors:

Only 25% recover spontaneously	(C)
About one-third of the United States population has been exposed	(A)
Could be spread through touching toothbrushes	(B)
About 5% of infected adults are at risk for long-term liver disease	(B)
Least long-term consequences	(A)
No vaccine has yet been developed	(C)

8. Liver cancer is almost always seen along with…
   a. Splenomegaly
   b. Gallstones
   c. Hepatitis A
   d. Cirrhosis

9. Chronic pancreatitis is usually related to…
   a. Alcohol abuse
   b. Autoimmune disease
   c. Diabetes mellitus
   d. High fat diet

10. Candidiasis is a reflection of the overgrowth of…
    a. Bacteria
    b. Fungi
    c. Viruses
    d. Prions

LEVEL 2: Application of Concepts

1. Your client has persistent low-grade abdominal pain and a change in bowel habits in a new pattern. Massage relieves symptoms for a day or 2, but then they return. What is the most appropriate course of action?
   a. Tell him to begin an elimination diet to determine his food sensitivities
   b. Tell him to stop consuming dairy products, as his symptoms point to lactose intolerance
   c. Tell him to consult a primary care provider in case something serious is happening
   d. Tell him to wear looser clothing and to avoid caffeine, chocolate, and spicy food

2. Your client had extreme gastroenteritis 2 days ago, but is beginning to feel better. What is the best advice for her recovery?
   a. Rest and drink fluids to prevent dehydration
   b. Get a rigorous massage to help clear any lingering infection
   c. Resume activities as normal to avoid deconditioning
   d. Get vaccinated to avoid another bout of stomach flu

3. Write a paragraph describing the difference (if any) between heartburn and gastroesophageal reflux disorder. Elucidate the complications that GERD can involve.

4. Which is the most accurate statement about peptic ulcers?
   a. They only occur in the stomach,
   b. They are related to fluctuations between stress and relief,
   c. They are caused by prolonged stress,
   d. They are the result of a lifetime diet of spicy and fatty food,

5. Your client has a colostomy bag after having had colorectal cancer 6 years ago. He is physically active, but his left hip and hamstrings are giving him problems. What is your best strategy?
   a. Work normally, making whatever adjustments he needs for his comfort,
   b. Refuse to work with him without a doctor's note,
   c. Ask him to remove his bag during your session,
   d. Do only light massage to avoid the risk of disturbing remaining cancer cells,

6. What is the leading symptom of diverticulosis?
   a. None; this condition is silent
   b. Bloating, gas, nausea
   c. Alternating diarrhea and constipation
   d. Fever, abdominal pain, headache

7. Your new client reports abdominal discomfort, frequent headache, general puffiness, tremor, and itchy patches on the skin. How can you accommodate for her needs?
   a. This client needs deep abdominal work for improved digestive function,
   b. This client needs to detoxify before receiving massage,
   c. This client needs gentle massage to avoid overwhelming a delicate system,
   d. This client needs to avoid massage therapy altogether,

8. Your very large client informs you that he is not really overweight: he has been diagnosed with ascites. What organ is most likely to be dysfunctional?
   a. Spleen
   b. Gallbladder
   c. Liver
   d. Stomach

9. How can having gallstones lead to death?
   a. Fragments of a stone may embolize and lodge in a coronary or cerebral artery.
   b. Gallstones are sharp and they can cause massive internal bleeding, if they scrape the interior hepatic duct.
   c. A severe immune reaction to a gallstone can lead to anaphylaxis and shock.
   d. A gallstone may block the pancreatic duct leading to acute pancreatitis and death.

Note to educators: Due to space considerations, these review questions only skim over the most important material from Chapter 8. The Test Bank provides a much more comprehensive selection of questions, all of which are keyed to the relevant chapter objectives.

What Would *You* Do?

Two High-Risk Clients

You have two clients booked for the morning. The first is a 55-year-old man in ill health; he is coinfected with hepatitis B and hepatitis C. He is in treatment, which is why he wants to see you; the antiviral medications are making him very uncomfortable. Your second client is a woman in her 40s, who is 6-weeks pregnant, after many years of trying. She is coming for a relaxation massage, because she is so nervous about losing this baby. Consider whether you have any specific concerns about this line-up of clients. What (if any) special actions might you take in this situation? Would you inform the pregnant client about the previous client? Would you exercise any extra cleaning precautions? Why or why not?

Nonspecific Symptoms

Regarding the client in question no. 7 who reports abdominal discomfort, frequent headache, general puffiness, tremor, and itchy patches on the skin: what suggestions do you have for his continued care? Role-play a conversation with a partner in which the client asks for advice, and the massage therapist must stay within scope of practice in responding. For the purposes of this exercise, the client has no easy access to a primary care physician, and is distrustful of the medical system in general.

Explore and Apply (continued)

Suggested Activities

1. For each condition covered in your curriculum, write down the following on a card:
   - A brief definition
   - Most common cause or contributing factor(s)
   - Major signs and symptoms
   - Risks and benefits of massage therapy
     - Variables that contribute to risks and benefits
     - Appropriate adaptations

   Use these as flash cards as you study.
2. For each condition covered in your curriculum, write one multiple choice question. Share your questions with your classmates as you study together.
3. Quiz yourself using either the "labels off" feature in your enhanced ebook, or the labeling exercise on thePoint® for Figure 8.1. Identify the following organs: Esophagus, Stomach, Small intestine, Large intestine, Liver, Gallbladder, Pancreas, Spleen.
4. Using the "Diseases of the Digestive System" labeling exercise on thePoint® identify the following lesions: Peptic ulcer (stomach), Peptic ulcer (duodenum), Gallstones, Polyps, Acute pancreatitis, Colorectal tumor, Hobnailed liver (cirrhosis), Stomach cancer tumor, Esophageal cancer, Barrett esophagus, Diverticulum.
5. Use the student resources on thePoint® to find practice quiz questions and games.

9

Endocrine System Conditions

CHAPTER 9 / Abbreviated Chapter Objectives

Having completed assignments and classroom time related to Chapter 9, the learner is expected to be able to…

- Identify definitions of the key terms in the introduction and those connected to the conditions covered in your curriculum.
- Identify the single structure that controls most endocrine system function.
- Describe an example of an endocrine system negative feedback loop.
- Identify the functions of the following hormones:
  - Calcitonin/parathyroid hormone
  - Glucagon/ insulin
  - Cortisone and epinephrine
  - Thyroxine and triiodothyronine.
- Provide the following information for each condition covered in your curriculum:
  - Identify the definition of the condition
  - List the most common causes or contributing factors to the condition
  - List major signs and symptoms of the condition
  - Identify possible risks and benefits of massage therapy, with:
    - Variables that contribute to risks and benefits
    - Appropriate adaptations for massage therapy

For detailed chapter objectives for each condition in this chapter, consult the student resource page at http://thePoint.lww.com/Werner6e. thePoint®

Endocrine System Introduction

The endocrine system is a collection of glands that secrete hormones: chemicals that relay messages instructing other glands and tissues in the body to function in a variety of ways (Figure 9.1). Where the autonomic nervous system exerts electrical control over homeostatic body functions, the endocrine system exerts chemical control. Interestingly, the control center for both systems is the same structure, the hypothalamus.

The hypothalamus is a nondescript mass of tissue deep in the brain. It has a generous blood supply, which allows it to monitor functions of the body. The hypothalamus is primarily responsible for maintaining homeostasis, or a stable internal environment. It does so through electrical transmission to the brainstem to manage heart rate, blood pressure, temperature, and other functions and also through electrical and chemical transmission to the pituitary gland, which then sends out signals to the targeted tissues. Sometimes, the hypothalamus sends its own hormones to be released into the blood by the pituitary gland by way of a stalk called the **infundibulum**. While the pituitary is sometimes called the "master gland" of the endocrine system, the hypothalamus controls the pituitary by determining what to secrete and when to secrete it.

Chemicals released by the hypothalamus and pituitary travel to their target glands through the circulatory system. They stimulate those glands to release their hormones. When those secretions reach appropriate levels in the blood,

Infundibulum: The hollow structure that connects the hypothalamus to the posterior pituitary gland.

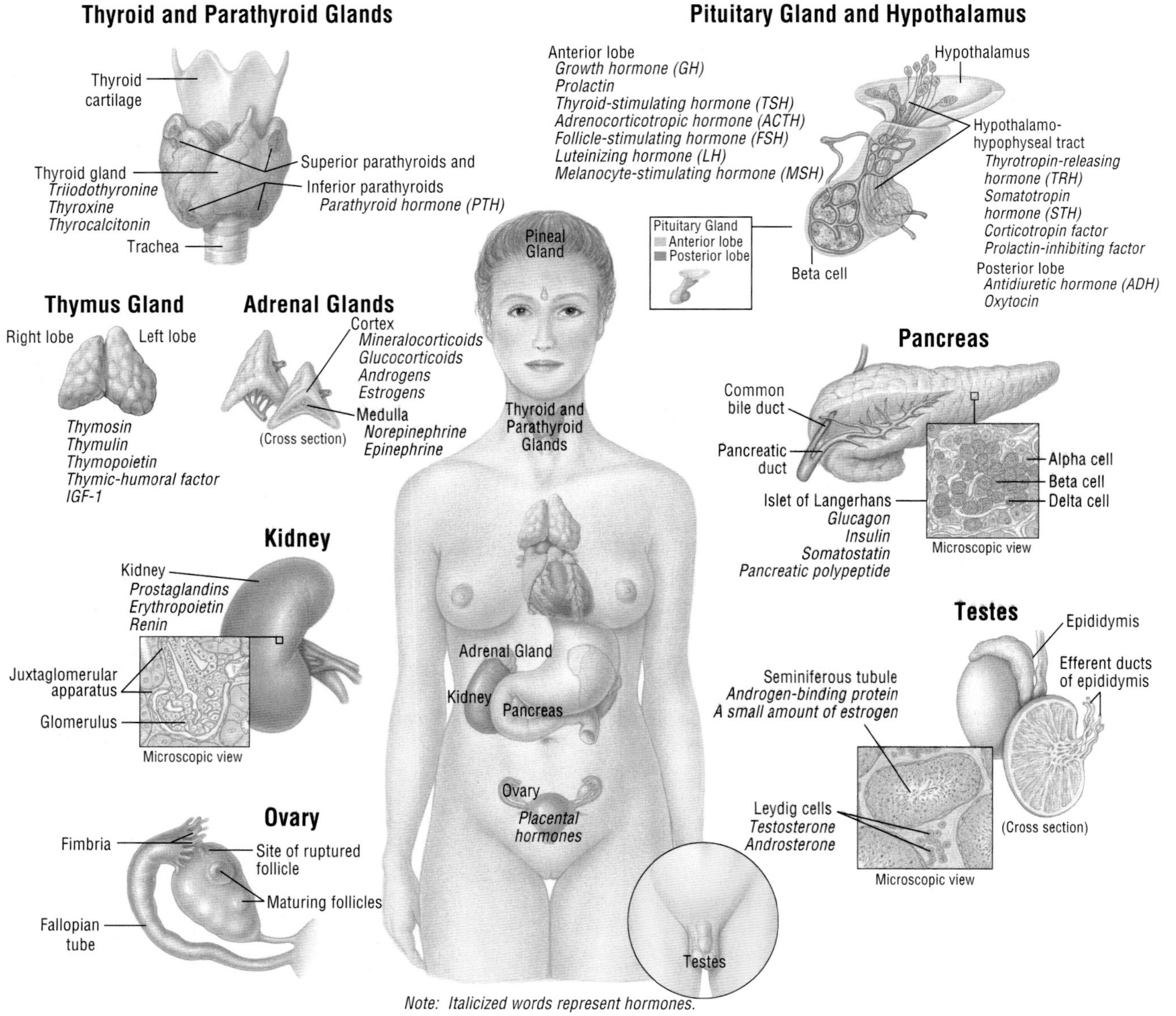

FIGURE 9.1 Major organs of the endocrine system

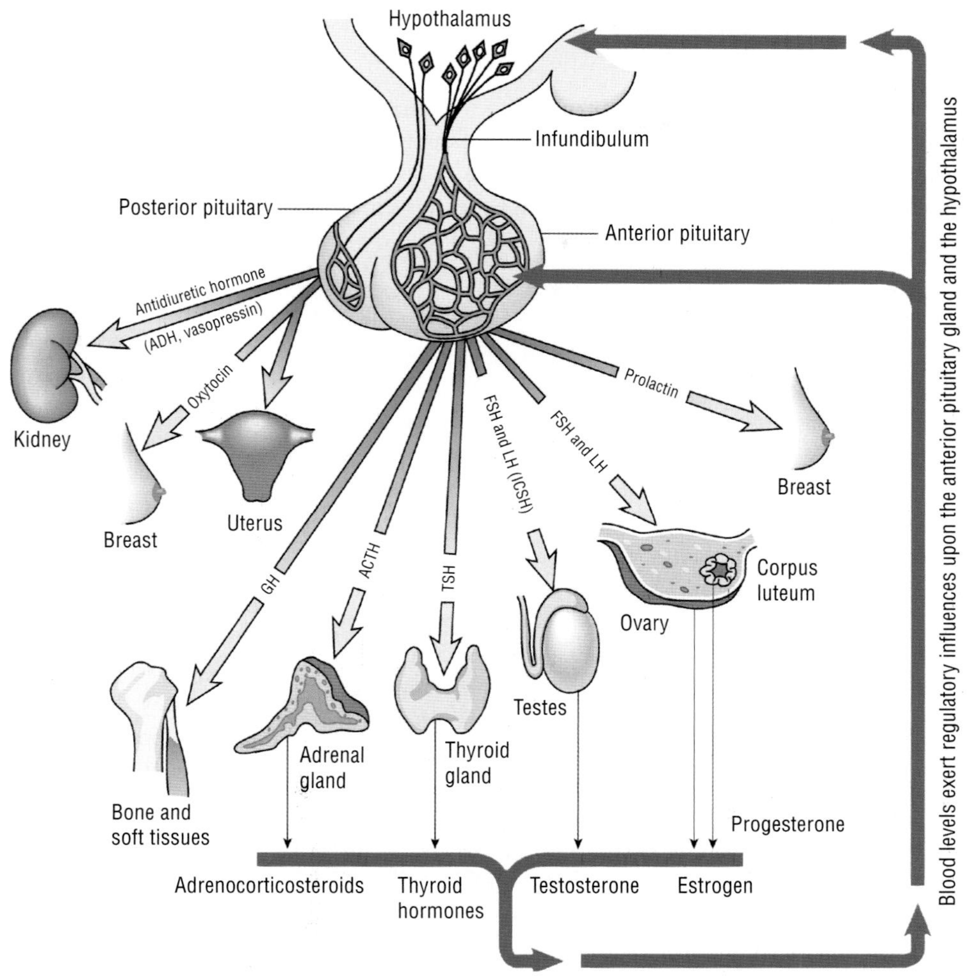

FIGURE 9.2 The hypothalamus and pituitary gland control several other endocrine glands in a negative feedback loop

the hypothalamus and pituitary stop sending out signals; most endocrine regulation is operated via this **negative feedback loop** (Figure 9.2).

The cycle of hormone stimulation and suppression usually works best when it occurs in gentle, rhythmic fluctuation. For example, when a person's blood sugar gets low, two things happen: he perceives that he is hungry and his pancreas secretes glucagon, a hormone that stimulates the liver to release stored glucose. He eats, his digestive tract absorbs sugar from his meal, and his blood sugar rises. This stimulates the pancreas to release insulin to carry the sugar out of the blood and into cells, lowering blood sugar. When levels are low enough, the person gets hungry, beginning the cycle again. The blood sugar-insulin cycle takes place several times a day; it takes only a few hours to move from one state to another. Another endocrine cycle, the circadian rhythm, moves on a roughly 24-hour rotation. The menstrual cycle also depends on regular fluctuations, but this one lasts about 4 weeks. Other cycles, specifically those related to stress and perceived threat, depend on external circumstances to determine their frequency and duration.

> **Negative feedback loop:** A process in which a response reduces the stimulus causing it.
>
> **Peptides:** A compound made up of two or more amino acids.
>
> **Amines:** A category of organic compounds found in the body.
>
> **Steroids:** A group of chemical compounds that includes some types of hormones.

Endocrine system glands secrete dozens of chemicals, each of which has specific target tissues and functions. Endocrine effects may also be determined by the frequency with which they are released into the bloodstream and the balance between each hormone and its antagonists.

Hormones fall into three chemical classes:

- **Peptides** are the most common type of hormones. Growth hormone, erythropoietin (EPO), and parathyroid hormone are peptide hormones.
- **Amines** are derived from a specific amino acid, tyrosine. Adrenaline and thyroxine are examples of amine hormones.
- **Steroids** are lipids. Cortisol and testosterone are steroid hormones.

Major Hormones

It is useful for massage therapists to be able to recognize the names of most hormones and their actions, since this is a key feature of physiology. But a few hormones are so strongly implicated in basic health issues that massage therapists may benefit from more than just passing familiarity:

- Growth hormone, also called **somatotropin**, is released from the pituitary gland and stimulates conversion of fuel into new cells. Infants, children, and teenagers secrete massive amounts of growth hormone; adults secrete less. When a person has finished growing, the primary purpose of growth hormone is to stimulate regeneration and repair of damaged tissue, in other words healing. Growth hormone is secreted primarily in stage IV sleep. **Sleep disorders** can lead to a shortage of this important chemical.
- Epinephrine, also called adrenaline, is a steroid hormone. It comes from the adrenal gland medulla, along with a very similar hormone, noradrenaline. It is associated with short-term, high-grade stress and acts to reinforce the reactions initiated by the sympathetic nervous system. An inefficient connection between the pituitary gland and the adrenal glands can cause a sluggish stress response system.
- Cortisol, another steroid hormone, is one of a group of **glucocorticoids** secreted by the adrenal cortex. It is the hormone secreted under long-term, low-grade stress. Cortisol is important for several reasons: it is a very powerful anti-inflammatory and is sometimes used systemically or locally in a synthetic form for that purpose. It also suppresses immune system response to disease and infection. It can damage connective tissues, so people with systemically high levels of cortisol are prone to musculoskeletal injury and **osteoporosis**. Cortisol in the saliva, blood, or urine is sometimes used as a marker for perceived stress.
- Aldosterone is a major **mineralocorticoid**. Mineralocorticoids are other adrenal cortex secretions; these help to regulate electrolyte balance and control fluid retention.
- Insulin and glucagon work together to regulate blood glucose (BG): insulin decreases BG, and glucagon increases it. Both are manufactured and released by the pancreas.
- Thyroid hormones are secreted by the thyroid gland in two molecular forms, triiodothyronine (T3) and thyroxine (T4). These hormones stimulate the metabolism of fuel into energy. Thyroid pathologies have to do with overproduction or underproduction of these hormones.

> **Somatotropin:** Another term for growth hormone.
>
> **Glucocorticoid:** A category of hormones with anti-inflammatory effects.
>
> **Mineralocorticoid:** One of the steroids from the adrenal cortex that influence salt metabolism.

- Calcitonin, another thyroid secretion, stimulates osteoblasts to extract calcium from the blood and add to bone density. In other words, it decreases blood calcium.
- Parathyroid hormone comes from the tiny parathyroid glands located deep in the thyroid gland. It is the antagonist of calcitonin, stimulating osteoclast activity and pulling calcium off the bones to raise blood calcium.
- Testosterone, estrogens, and progesterone are steroid hormones released mainly by the gonads (testicles for men, ovaries for women). They have to do with secondary sexual characteristics, menstrual cycles, maintaining pregnancy, and a host of other issues. Supplements of anabolic steroids can increase muscle mass; this is why they are sometimes employed by athletes, often with dangerous results. The negative feedback loops in these hormone relationships seem to be especially precarious, possibly because environmental exposures to various types of steroids (in medications, dairy products, meat, plastics, pesticides, and other environmental sources) unbalance the scales.
- Other hormones have less implication for massage, but a big impact on how well the body works. One is EPO, secreted by the kidneys. EPO stimulates the production of red blood cells. It can be artificially supplemented to increase RBC count and the oxygen-carrying capacity of the blood, but this may also increase the risk of blood clots. Thymosin is a hormone from the thymus; it is involved with the maturation of T cells. Melatonin comes from the pineal gland and helps to regulate wake-sleep cycles. Prostaglandins are hormones produced by almost any kind of cell for local action. Prostaglandins produce a myriad of effects in the body, including smooth muscle contraction and increased pain sensitivity.

Endocrine glands release their secretions (usually under direction of the pituitary-hypothalamus unit) directly into the blood. This distinguishes them from exocrine glands, which send their secretions into ducts for release into specific local areas. The hormones circulate systemically through the body and attach to specific receptor sites on their target tissues. Then, they stimulate the target cells or tissues to perform some function, such as making red blood cells (EPO from the kidneys acting on stem cells in the bone marrow) or pulling calcium off the bones (parathyroid hormone acting on osteoclasts).

Most endocrine system disorders have to do with imbalances in hormone production. Autoimmune attacks or tumors may stimulate or suppress certain glands, leading to problems with the negative feedback loop. When too much or too little of any hormone is present in the blood, symptoms can be felt throughout the body. Other endocrine disruptions occur when circulating hormone levels are normal but target tissues have developed resistance to their action.

Explore how the endocrine system works by watching the author's video "HPA Axis" at http://thePoint.lww.com/Werner6e. thePoint®

Endocrine System Conditions

- Diabetes mellitus
  - Type 1 diabetes mellitus
  - Type 2 diabetes mellitus
  - Prediabetes
  - Double diabetes
  - Other types of diabetes
- Hyperthyroidism
  - Graves disease
  - Multinodular goiter
  - Thyroiditis
  - Toxic adenoma
- Hypothyroidism
  - Hashimoto thyroiditis
  - Congenital hypothyroidism
  - Idiopathic hypothyroidism
  - Iodine deficiency hypothyroidism
  - Secondary hypothyroidism
  - Other types of hypothyroidism
- Metabolic syndrome
- Thyroid cancer
  - Papillary thyroid cancer
  - Follicular thyroid cancer
    - Hurthle cell cancer
  - Medullary thyroid cancer
  - Anaplastic thyroid cancer
  - Thyroid lymphoma

Endocrine System Conditions

Diabetes Mellitus

Definition: What Is It?

The word "diabetes" comes from the Greek for "siphon" or to "pass through," referring to the tendency for diabetics to urinate very frequently. "Mellitus" is from Latin for "sweetened with honey." Diabetes mellitus essentially means sweet pee.

Diabetes is not a single disease, but rather a group of related disorders that all result in **hyperglycemia**. Two main varieties, type 1 and type 2 diabetes, are examined in this section, with a brief look at others. Type 1 and 2 diabetes account for about 98% of diabetes diagnoses.

The animation "Diabetes Mellitus" provides a brief overview of this condition; visit http://thePoint.lww.com/Werner6e. thePoint®

Demographics

Estimates vary, but most resources suggest that about 29 million Americans have type 2 diabetes (i.e., 9.3%), although about 8 million people don't know it yet. About 1.6 million people are diagnosed with diabetes each year. Researchers credit an aging population along with higher numbers of obese young people and sedentary lifestyles for these alarming figures.

Type 1 diabetes is less common than type 2. It is estimated that about 1 million Americans live with type 1 diabetes, and it is diagnosed about 16,000 times per year in young people.

Diabetes costs $245 billion in direct and indirect health care expenses each year, making it one of the most expensive diseases seen in the United States.

Etiology: What Happens?

Many cells, especially those in muscles, do best when they can use glucose for fuel. Glucose is an efficient energy source, and the leftovers of this "burn" are easy to process; they are carbon dioxide and water. But glucose does not have direct access to the cells that need it. Insulin, a hormone produced by **beta cells** in the pancreas, is required to escort glucose across cell membranes. Insulin also aids in the removal of fat from the blood into lipid storage cells. Diabetes develops when insulin is in short supply, or because insulin receptor sites have developed resistance, or both. Consequently, hungry muscle cells must resort first to stored fat reserves and then to proteins for fuel sources, while glucose and fats accumulate dangerously in the bloodstream (see Sidebar 9.1 for more information on insulin resistance).

Type 1 diabetes is an autoimmune disease connected to genetic background and childhood exposure to agents that might stimulate an immune system mistake and an attack on insulin-producing cells.

By contrast, type 2 diabetes is more likely to be related to genetic predisposition along with diet and lifestyle factors that are more controllable. Risk factors for type 2 diabetes include being over 45 years old (although it is often diagnosed among younger people); being 20% or more over healthy weight; having a family history of diabetes; having a racial predisposition for diabetes (i.e., being Native American, Hispanic, a Pacific Islander, Asian American, or African American); and having problems with glucose tolerance, **hypertension**, **gestational diabetes**, or **polycystic ovarian syndrome**.

A close look at diabetes rates and eating habits reveals that the fewer animal products that are consumed, the lower the risk of developing type 2 diabetes. The converse is also true: the more animal products in the diet, the higher the

Hyperglycemia: Abnormally high blood sugar levels.

Beta cell: A type of cell, located in the islets of Langerhans in the pancreas, which produces insulin.

SIDEBAR 9.1 Insulin Resistance: Silent and Dangerous

Insulin resistance is a condition in which a given concentration of insulin does not have the expected effect on cellular uptake of BG. It is typically related to decreased numbers of insulin receptors on cell membranes, often in conjunction with postreceptor problems inside the cell. Blood sugar levels climb, stimulating the production of more insulin. In this way, hyperglycemia and **hyperinsulinemia** (the presence of excessive insulin in the blood) occur simultaneously. This situation, along with excessive release of glucose from the liver, opens the door to type 2 diabetes mellitus.

Insulin resistance is also considered a contributing factor for another disorder, **metabolic syndrome**, which is associated with a dangerously increased risk of many forms of heart disease.

Insulin resistance is directly connected to overloaded abdominal fat cells. These fat cells are metabolically different from subcutaneous fat cells; they produce many chemicals that have adverse effects on body functions. Losing 5% or more of overall fat storage can reduce the risk of insulin resistance and its associated diseases.

Insulin resistance itself is often a silent disorder. Some patients develop a skin discoloration called **acanthosis nigricans**, velvety brown patches that appear around the skin folds, especially at the axilla. It is thought that excessive insulin interacts with skin cells to produce this sign. Episodes of hypoglycemia occasionally affect people with insulin resistance; this indicates that antibodies have destroyed damaged insulin receptor sites, temporarily causing a sudden uptake of BG.

Insulin resistance may be identified by testing BG and/or insulin after fasting, when levels should be low. Other experts suggest that a glucose tolerance test, which measures glucose in the blood 2 hours after a patient ingests 75 mg of sugar, is more indicative of the early stages of this disorder.

risk of developing insulin resistance and/or diabetes. This is a consistent finding, even when other issues like sedentariness, physical activity, and age are factored in. It is not clear how eating animal products leads to diabetes, but most experts consider it to be a connection between ingesting saturated fats and developing changes in cell membranes: cell membranes must be sensitive to insulin in order to lower blood sugar. When they develop resistance, a person may secrete a normal amount of insulin, but still have diabetes.

Complications

Complications of diabetes are potentially serious, and they are often the first signs of the disease that cause a person to seek medical intervention.

- *Cardiovascular disease.* Diabetics are especially prone to cardiovascular disease, because high BG and insulin resistance lead to chemical changes that damage endothelium, leading to **atherosclerosis** throughout the circulatory system. Diabetes more than doubles the risk of **stroke**, **hypertension**, and **aneurysm**, and cardiovascular disease is the leading cause of death for people with diabetes.
- *Edema.* **Edema** develops in the extremities because of sluggish blood return. It can also give rise to **stasis dermatitis**. Kidney damage may also contribute to systemic edema.
- *Ulcers, gangrene, and amputations.* When the body's blood vessels are caked with plaque, even minor skin lesions don't heal well. Ingrown toenails, blisters, or pressure spots on the feet can become life-threatening for diabetics: the tissue either dies of starvation or is infected with pathogens that are impossible to fight off, forming characteristic diabetic ulcers, usually on the feet (Figure 9.3). Diabetes is the leading cause of nontraumatic foot and leg **amputations** in this country, leading to about 73,000 surgeries each year.
- *Kidney disease.* Renal vessels are especially vulnerable to atherosclerosis, because they are one of the first diversions from the descending aorta. Excessive BG, which acts as a powerful diuretic, is also hard on the kidneys, causing reduced formation of **glomerular filtrate** and a thickening

Hyperinsulinemia: Abnormally high levels of insulin in the blood.

Acanthosis nigricans: A condition characterized by the formation of velvety brown or black patches on the skin, usually around creases and folds.

Glomerular filtrate: The liquid pushed from the glomerulus into the Bowman capsule.

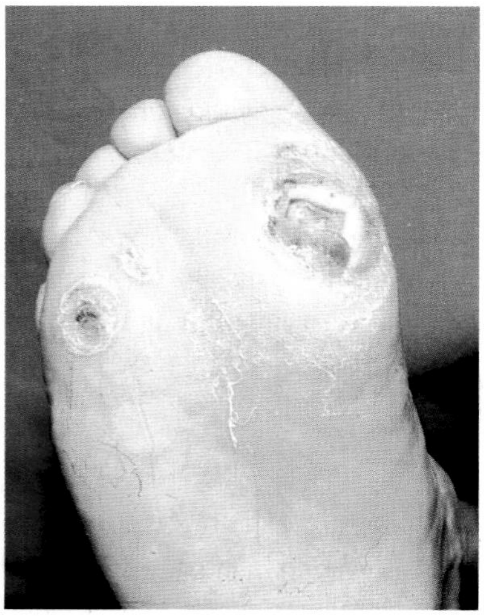

FIGURE 9.3 Diabetic ulcers: notice multiple lesions

of the basement membrane in the Bowman capsule. Consequently, diabetes is the leading cause of end-stage **renal failure** and of the need for kidney transplants.

- *Impaired vision.* The capillaries of the eyes of diabetic patients can become abnormally thickened, depriving eye cells of nutrition. Diseased capillaries leak blood and proteins into the retina. Microaneurysms can form, and these also cut off circulation. All of these factors contribute to diabetic retinopathy. Excessive glucose also binds with proteins in the lens, causing first cataracts, then blindness. Almost 5 million people have serious vision impairment due to diabetes in this country; it is the leading cause of new blindness among people 20 to 74 years old.
- *Neuropathy.* Lack of capillary circulation and excessive sugar in the blood both contribute to nerve damage. Symptoms of **peripheral neuropathy** include tingling or pain and eventual numbness. Neuropathy of the autonomic motor system—especially at the vagus nerve—can lead to an inability to maintain postural blood pressure, delayed or inefficient emptying of the stomach, diarrhea, constipation, and sexual impotency for both genders. One especially dangerous consequence of neuropathy is hypoglycemia insensitivity, a loss in the ability to sense when blood sugar is too low.
- *Others.* Diabetes affects every body system in some way. It is linked to **urinary tract infections**, **candidiasis**, birth defects, a mold infection of the nose and sinuses called mucormycosis, aggressive ear infections that can invade the cranial bones (malignant otitis externa), and higher-than-normal rates of gingivitis and tooth loss.

Types of Diabetes Mellitus

- *Type 1 diabetes mellitus.* Type 1 diabetes, formerly known as insulin-dependent diabetes mellitus (IDDM), is an autoimmune disorder. It can be brought about by a number of factors, including exposure to certain drugs and chemicals or as a complication of some kinds of infections. Immune system cells of people with type 1 diabetes attack the beta cells in the pancreas where insulin is produced. The destruction of these cells leads to a lifelong deficiency in insulin. People who have type 1 diabetes are also at increased risk for other autoimmune endocrine conditions, including **Hashimoto thyroiditis**, **Graves disease**, and **Addison disease**.

  Type 1 diabetes usually shows symptoms before age 30, but one variety, called latent autoimmune diabetes in adults (LADA), may not be identified until later. Type 1 diabetes is the rarer and more serious of the two basic types of diabetes. It accounts for 5% to 10% of diabetes in this country.
- *Type 2 diabetes mellitus.* This variety is used to be called non–insulin-dependent diabetes mellitus (NIDDM), but since many patients do end up supplementing insulin, that name is no longer accurate. The exact cause of type 2 diabetes is probably a combination of prodiabetes behaviors along with genetic predisposition.

  Type 2 diabetes can be controllable with diet, exercise, and possibly some antidiabetes drugs, depending on how far advanced it is when treatment begins, but many patients eventually benefit from supplementing insulin.
- *Prediabetes.* In this case, BG levels are consistently higher than normal, but not up to diabetes diagnostic criteria. Up to 79 million Americans—35% of all adults—may be living in this state, and many will progress to develop type 2 disease.
- *Double diabetes.* This is a situation in which a person has type 1 diabetes, but also develops the insulin resistance seen with type 2 diabetes.
- *Other types of diabetes.* Other types of diabetes include gestational diabetes and secondary diabetes. Gestational diabetes occurs when a woman develops a transient case during pregnancy. This condition can cause birth defects in the child as well as changing fetal metabolism, which results in very high birth weights and a high incidence of cesarean sections. Women who have gestational diabetes and their babies also have an increased risk of developing type 2 diabetes later in life. This is discussed further in the section on pregnancy in Chapter 11.

  Secondary diabetes may develop with damage or trauma to the pancreas or as a symptom of some other endocrine disorder, such as **acromegaly** or **Cushing syndrome**. And **diabetes insipidus** is a dysfunction of the pituitary gland and insufficient production of antidiuretic hormone (ADH).

> Bowman capsule: The beginning segment of a nephron, which surrounds the glomerulus.
>
> Retinopathy: Noninflammatory degenerative disease of the retina of the eye.
>
> Hypoglycemia insensitivity: Loss of the ability to sense when one's blood sugar is low.
>
> Mucormycosis: A fungal infection of the sinuses.
>
> Gingivitis: Inflammation of the gums.
>
> Antidiuretic hormone: (ADH) A hormone that encourages water retention and increased blood pressure. Also called vasopressin.
>
> Polyuria: Excessive urination.
>
> Polydipsia: Excessive thirst.
>
> Polyphagia: Excessive eating.

Signs and Symptoms

Three defining "polys" are common to all types of diabetes. Polyuria, or frequent urination, results from elevated blood sugar, which acts as a diuretic; it pulls water from the cells in the body, and excess water is expelled in the urine. Polydipsia means excessive thirst, which accompanies the loss of water with polyuria. Polyphagia refers to increased appetite, since diabetics must get most of their energy from fats and proteins instead of carbohydrates, which provide the fuel that is easiest to burn. Other symptoms of diabetes include fatigue, weight loss, nausea, and vomiting.

Very often, signs of diabetes are missed until the disease has damaged other organs. It is estimated that an average adult diagnosed with diabetes has probably had the disease for 4 to 7 years by the time it is identified.

Diabetic Emergencies

People with diabetes are vulnerable to two classes of medical emergencies, both of which can be fatal if not treated promptly.

- *Ketoacidosis*. This is a critical shortage of insulin and lack of glucose in the cells in type 1 diabetics; people with type 2 diabetes don't have this problem. The body partially metabolizes fats for fuel, and the acidic byproduct of that metabolism (**ketones**) dangerously changes the pH balance of the blood. **Ketoacidosis** is identifiable by a characteristic sweet or fruity odor to the breath. Diabetics can test themselves for ketoacidosis with test strips that look for signs of ketones in the urine. Ketoacidosis can be brought on by stress, infection, or trauma and can lead to shock, coma, and death. An analogous condition in type 2 diabetics is **hyperosmolality**. This causes a change in the pH of the blood, which can lead to shock, coma, and death.
- *Insulin shock*. This is an emergency at the other end of the scale. In this case, too much insulin is circulating, either because too much has been administered or because a skipped meal, sudden exertion, stress, infection, or trauma has resulted in the consumption of all available blood sugar. The consequence of having too much available insulin is a dangerously low blood sugar level, or hypoglycemia. Symptoms of insulin shock include dizziness, confusion, weakness, and tremors. It too can lead to coma and death if not treated (with sugar tablets, juice, milk, candy, or nondiet soda to replace blood sugar) quickly.

NOTABLE CASES The list of influential people with diabetes is long and varied. It includes Rania Al-Abdullah (Queen of Jordan), Anwar Sadat (President of Egypt), and Mike Huckabee (American politician). Johnny Cash had it, and as of this writing, B.B. King is still going strong with his diabetes. McDonald's founder Ray Kroc had diabetes, along with actors Tom Hanks, Halle Berry, James Cagney, and Mary Tyler Moore. Writers Ernest Hemingway and H.G. Wells had this disease, and so did inventor and innovator Thomas Edison.

Ketones: A potentially toxic byproduct of metabolism

Ketoacidosis: A dangerous metabolic state characterized by high blood acidity (acidosis), which occurs when the body, unable to break down sugars, instead uses fats, releasing an acidic byproduct called ketones

Hyperosmolality: Increased concentration of a solution

Hyperlipidemia: Abnormally high levels of fats in the blood

Treatment

Before the development of insulin in 1921, the diagnosis of diabetes was a death knell. Most people lived only a few years after the disease was identified. Now, diabetes is a highly treatable disease, although not all diagnosed people treat it aggressively enough to prevent complications.

The goals for diabetes treatment are to improve insulin production in the pancreas when possible, to inhibit the release of glucose from the liver, to increase the sensitivity of target cells to insulin, and to decrease the absorption of carbohydrates in the small intestines. In addition to these measures, special care of eyes and feet can reduce the risk of blindness and amputations associated with the disease.

Type 1 diabetes is treated primarily with various forms of insulin. This can be delivered by injection; with an insulin pen, which delivers a measured dose under the skin without a hypodermic needle; or with insulin pumps, which feed a steady drip into the body through a plastic tube.

Type 2 diabetes is first addressed with changes in diet and exercise, but many patients are eventually treated with drugs that influence how insulin is used and insulin supplementation (see Sidebar 9.2 for more about managing BG).

Diabetes is the leading cause for nontraumatic amputation in the United States, and it is an ongoing struggle to try to reduce these surgeries. For small bone infections in the foot, some research suggests that antibiotics lead to about the same outcomes as surgery, but leaves the foot intact. This may influence the amputation statistics related to this disease.

Many diabetic patients eventually develop renal insufficiency; their kidneys simply cannot keep up with their needs. Hemodialysis is a treatment in which the blood is routed through a filtering machine that removes excess water and waste products before returning the blood to the body. Dialysis of any kind is often a stopgap measure while a person waits for a kidney to become available for transplant.

Medications

- Fast-acting and slow-acting insulin by injection, inhalation, pen, or pump (insulin cannot be administered orally) to reduce blood sugar for type 1 and some type 2 diabetes
- Medications including metformin to stimulate insulin release and insulin uptake
- Medications to address **hyperlipidemia**
- Antihypertensives, especially angiotensin converting enzyme inhibitors and angiotensin II receptor blockers
- Medications to address other complications of diabetes

Massage Therapy Implications

RISKS	The risks of massage for a person with advanced or poorly managed diabetes are complex. Cardiovascular disease, kidney disease, skin ulcerations and neuropathy comprise a short list of common complications that alter bodywork choices. Injection sites or insulin pump attachment sites are local contraindications. In addition, timing bodywork choices around insulin doses is preferable, to avoid triggering a hypoglycemic episode.
BENEFITS	An active client who has healthy, responsive tissue well-controlled diabetes can enjoy the same benefits from bodywork as the rest of the population.
OPTIONS	Because massage has been seen to drop blood sugar, it is a good idea to try to schedule massage or bodywork sessions when levels are most stable: in the middle of a cycle, rather than just after or just before administering insulin. It is also wise to ask a diabetic client ahead of time how he or she would want to handle a hypoglycemic episode. Some people keep sugar tablets with them; others prefer milk, juice, or other options.
RESEARCH	People with diabetes are often enthusiastic users of complementary and integrative health care modalities, especially massage therapy, so conventional providers are encouraged to be familiar with these interventions.[1] Further, the finding that many people with diabetes and other chronic diseases seek complementary and alternative medicine points to a need for evidence-based practice education for CAM providers.[2] A Swedish study[3] found that light massage compared to relaxation exercises led to some significant changes in diabetes biomarkers; this was especially true for the women in the study. Some research supports the theory that massage therapy temporarily lowers BG, but the duration of effect has not been well established.[4] Connective tissue massage on the lower leg was studied to see its effects on peripheral artery disease; it successfully improved local arterial pressure and oxygen saturation, and some effects lingered for several months, compared to the control group.[5]

1. Canaway R, Manderson L, Oldenburg B. Perceptions of benefit of complementary therapy use among people with diabetes and cardiovascular disease. *Forsch Komplementmed* 2014;21(1):25–33. http://www.ncbi.nlm.nih.gov/pubmed/24603627
2. Hawk C, Ndetan H, Evans MW, Jr. Potential role of complementary and alternative health care providers in chronic disease prevention and health promotion: an analysis of National Health Interview Survey data. *Preventive Medicine* 2012;54(1):18–22. http://www.ncbi.nlm.nih.gov/pubmed/21777609
3. Wandell PE, Arnlov J, Nixon Andreasson A, et al. Effects of tactile massage on metabolic biomarkers in patients with type 2 diabetes. *Diabetes & Metabolism* 2013;39(5):411–417. http://www.ncbi.nlm.nih.gov/pubmed/23642641
4. Sajedi F, Kashaninia Z, Hoseinzadeh S, et al. How effective is Swedish massage on blood glucose level in children with diabetes mellitus? *Acta Medica Iranica* 2011;49(9):592–597. http://acta.tums.ac.ir/index.php/acta/article/view/4400
5. Castro-Sanchez AM, Moreno-Lorenzo C, Mataran-Penarrocha GA, et al. Connective tissue reflex massage for type 2 diabetic patients with peripheral arterial disease: randomized controlled trial. *Evidence- Based Complementary and Alternative Medicine* 2011;2011:804321. http://www.hindawi.com/journals/ecam/2011/804321/

SIDEBAR 9.2 Managing Diabetes: Blood Glucose Highs and Lows

Keeping blood glucose within a limited range of variation can be a complicated undertaking. Normal fasting blood sugar (a measurement that is taken before eating in the morning) is 110 mg/dL of blood or less. Diabetes is diagnosed when fasting levels rise over 126 mg/dL for 2 or more consecutive days.

Another test, called the hemoglobin A1c test, measures how much sugar sticks to the hemoglobin in circulating erythrocytes. This is often considered a better long-term test, since it reflects general blood sugar levels for 3 months or more, instead of in increments of several hours. A normal reading is 4% to 5.9%; diabetes is diagnosed when A1c tests show 8% or more glucose.

The opposite problem with blood sugar can also be a problem for people with diabetes. Hypoglycemia can develop quickly if the schedule of eating and medication is disrupted in such a way that insulin levels are high, but not enough sugar is entering the bloodstream from the intestines. Hypoglycemia is recognized when circulating levels of glucose dip below 70 mg/dL.

Signs and symptoms of hypoglycemia include confusion and dizziness, feeling shaky, alterations in vision and hearing, hunger, headache, and irritability. Pale skin, racing pulse, sweating and weakness are also possible. Hypoglycemia can be dangerous; it can lead to loss of consciousness and coma. More often it simply calls for some easily absorbable simple sugar, in a hurry. Many people with diabetes will have a favorite option for this: sugar tablets, a gel tube, fruit juice, or hard candies are common options.

Hypoglycemia can develop occasionally in people who don't have diabetes, but it is typically a serious, ongoing problem only for those with a history of liver, kidney or pancreatic diseases, who have been through stomach surgery, or who have other metabolic problems.

Because massage therapy has been seen to lead to lower blood sugar levels, it is important to inform clients who have diabetes of this phenomenon, and to have a plan ahead of time in case a diabetic client feels unsteady after a session.

CASE HISTORY 9.1 Type 2 Diabetes

MAUREEN, AGE 43
"A do-it-yourself project."

Maureen had gestational diabetes while pregnant with two of her three children. At age 42, she began having chronic yeast infections, unintentional weight loss, blurred vision, and unusual thirst. When she went for her annual checkup, she was not happy but also not surprised to be diagnosed with type 2 diabetes.

At first, Maureen was intimidated by the glucose testing equipment she had to use, and she was terrified by the long-term complications that often develop with diabetes. But as she did more research, she came to the conclusion that diabetes is very much a do-it-yourself project. She found that proper control can be achieved through exercise, good nutrition, mindfulness of her glucose levels, and stress reduction.

She tests her blood frequently and sees immediate relationships between her glucose levels and how much stress she's going through and how much exercise she gets. Since her diagnosis, Maureen's diabetes medication has been cut in half, and she is able to maintain reasonable glucose levels by being proactive about her health. Although she is still upset about her disease, she is thankful that she was diagnosed early enough to take control of her situation and change it for the better.

Hyperthyroidism

Definition: What Is It?

Hyperthyroidism is a condition in which the thyroid gland produces excessive amounts of hormones that stimulate metabolism of fuel into energy. It falls under a larger heading of **thyrotoxicosis**, which describes any situation in which too much thyroid hormone is present in the blood (see Sidebar 9.3).

Demographics

Hyperthyroidism is a common disorder, affecting about 1% of the United States population at some time in their lives. This condition can affect young children, elders, and everyone in between, but Graves disease is most common among 20 to 40 year olds, while toxic multinodular goiter is most common among people of 60 years and older.

SIDEBAR 9.3 Thyrotoxicosis and Hyperthyroidism Semantics

Hyperthyroidism is a condition in which the thyroid gland is overactive and produces too much hormone, but it is not the only situation in which T3 and T4 can flood the system. **Thyrotoxicosis** describes any situation in which too much thyroid hormone is present. This includes hyperthyroidism, but also includes some forms of thyroiditis (which leads to stored hormones being released), oversupplementation of replacement hormones, active thyroid cells elsewhere in the body (in metastatic **thyroid cancer** tumors or dermoid cysts, for instance), and the consumption of too much iodine, which can happen with some kinds of medications, cough syrups, or seaweed.

Etiology: What Happens?

Hyperthyroidism is usually caused by one of three things: an autoimmune attack against the thyroid gland that causes it to secrete excessive amounts of metabolic hormones, a nodule or group of nodules that become hyperactive for unknown reasons, or inflammation of the whole thyroid. In all of these cases, the body is flooded with thyroid hormones that serve to speed up the metabolic rate, including heart rate, respiration, and digestion. It is associated with dangerously irregular heartbeat and an increased risk of stroke, especially for young patients.

Under normal circumstances, secretions of thyroid-stimulating hormone (TSH) from the pituitary control thyroid activity. When hyperthyroidism is well established, circulating levels of TSH drop significantly, but the thyroid still produces too much of its hormones T3 (triiodothyronine) and T4 (thyroxine). The result is that the conversion of fuel into energy increases by 60% to 100%, and many body systems are affected (see Figure 9.4).

In addition to affecting the thyroid and associated hormones, hyperthyroidism can cause problems in several other tissues. **Osteoporosis** is a special risk, because normally, the thyroid and parathyroid glands work together to secrete hormones that maintain bone density. When hyperthyroidism alters the balance between these antagonistic hormones, bone tissue is dismantled faster than it is reconstructed.

Eyes are affected in a couple of ways by hyperthyroidism. One fairly common condition is elevation of eyelids in a way

Thyrotoxicosis: Excessive levels of thyroid hormone.

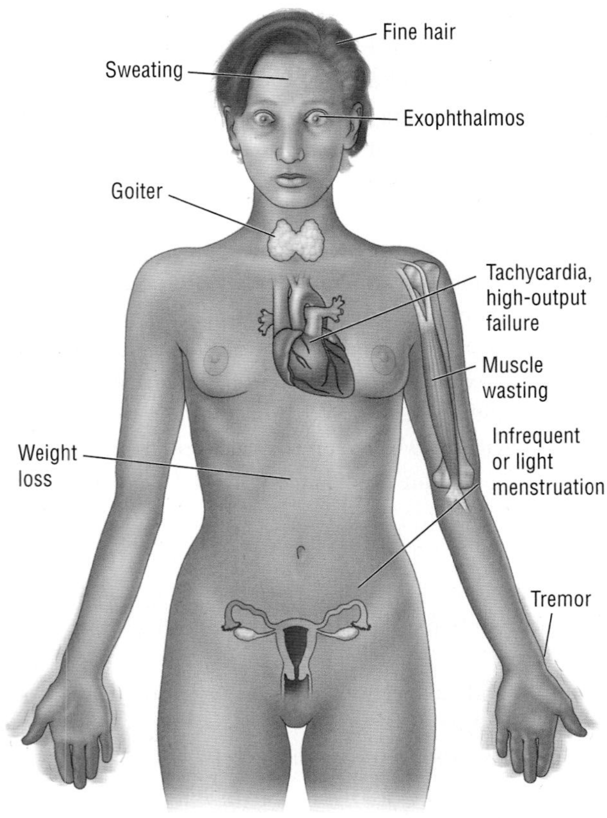

FIGURE 9.4 Hyperthyroidism

that makes the eyes seem to bulge. Protrusion of the eyes is known as **exophthalmos** or **proptosis** (Figure 9.3). Another eye problem is a rare disorder called **Graves ophthalmopathy**. This causes the eyeball to protrude beyond its protective orbit, because tissues behind it swell. The front surface of the eye can dry out, causing light sensitivity, double vision, decreased freedom of movement within the orbit, pain, and excessive tearing.

Some hyperthyroidism disease patients develop raised red patches of skin on their shins, feet, or elsewhere. These rashes, called **pretibial myxedema**, are caused by deposition of **mucopolysaccharides** in the dermis. They are generally not painful or dangerous. Another fairly rare complication is thyroid **acropachy**: the skin around the fingernails becomes swollen but is not typically painful.

In addition to eye and skin problems, some hyperthyroidism patients have occasional episodes of dangerously high metabolism called thyroid storms. In these episodes, symptoms suddenly become acute and may include rapid heartbeat, fever without infection, intolerance to heat, nausea, confusion, agitation, and finally shock. Thyroid storms are medical emergencies and require immediate intervention to slow the heart and bring down the fever.

Hyperthyroidism during **pregnancy** can lead to problems for both mother and baby if it is not controlled. Miscarriage, preeclampsia, and preterm delivery are all associated with hyperthyroidism during pregnancy. Finally, long-term hyperthyroidism can lead to dangerous changes in arterial and cardiac tissues. The ventricles become thickened, raising the risk for pulmonary edema and **heart failure**, and the heartbeat may be vulnerable to atrial fibrillations.

Exophthalmos: Abnormal bulging of the eyes. Also called eye proptosis.

Proptosis: Abnormal bulging of the eyes or other body parts.

Graves ophthalmopathy: Bulging of the eyes caused by increased water content in the eye tissues. Often associated with hyperthyroidism.

Pretibial myxedema: A rash that occurs in the tibial region, specifically associated with hyperthyroidism.

Mucopolysaccharides: Long chains of sugars, commonly found in mucus. Often called glycosaminoglycans.

Acropachy: A condition characterized by clubbing and swelling of the ends of the fingers and toes.

Types of Hyperthyroidism

- *Graves disease*. This is autoimmune hyperthyroidism, the most common form of this condition. In this situation, antibodies called thyroid-stimulating immunoglobulins attack the thyroid gland, causing it to grow and to secrete excessive levels of thyroid hormones, especially thyroxine. While genetics clearly plays a major part in the development of Graves disease, its onset often seems to be connected to a stressful trigger. Other risk factors for developing this disorder include exposure to x-rays of the neck and having taken antiviral medications such as interferon or interleukin. Graves disease often occurs along with other autoimmune conditions (see Sidebar 9.4).

NOTABLE CASES Marty Feldman (Igor in the movie *Young Frankenstein*) built a comic career out of the exophthalmos that was a complication of his hyperthyroidism. Former President and First Lady George and Barbara Bush both have hyperthyroidism (as did their dog). Sprinter Gail Devers did not let hyperthyroidism interfere with her athletic goals: after treatment for her condition, she won multiple track and field Olympic and World Champion medals.

- *Multinodular goiter*. The accumulation of small, nonfunctioning thyroid nodules is not unusual, but they sometimes become active, leading to excessive hormone production or mechanical impingement on the trachea or esophagus.
- *Thyroiditis*. This is inflammation of the thyroid leading to temporary hyperactivity. It is sometimes due to a viral infection, but may also be a complication of childbirth.

SIDEBAR 9.4 Graves Disease and Autoimmune Polyglandular Syndrome: Why Have Just One?

A strong genetic link has been established in Graves disease; if one person has this disorder, it is likely that some kind of thyroid dysfunction will be present in some other first- or second-degree relative. In some families, Graves disease shows as one of several problems that are known collectively as **autoimmune polyglandular syndrome**. Related conditions in this syndrome include **type 1 diabetes, systemic lupus erythematosus, pernicious anemia**, and others.

- *Toxic adenoma*. This is the development of a benign tumor or thyroid nodule, and it is related to chronic iodine deficiency. Because iodine is a key ingredient in thyroid secretions, a shortage of this mineral can be dangerous. Table salt is supplemented with iodine, so most Americans don't have to deal with iodine deficiency.

Signs and Symptoms

Signs and symptoms of hyperthyroidism are mostly related to the excessive secretion of thyroid hormones. They include anxiety, irritability, insomnia, rapid heartbeat, tremor, increased perspiration, sensitivity to heat, frequent bowel movements, and unintentional weight loss. Skeletal muscles, especially in the upper arms and thighs, often become weak in a condition called **thyrotoxic myopathy**. Other symptoms may include light flow during menstrual periods, dry skin and brittle nails, and problems specifically with the skin and eyes. Many hyperthyroidism patients develop a **goiter**: the thyroid becomes enlarged enough to create a visible painless swelling in the neck.

Treatment

Hyperthyroidism can be treated in a number of ways, depending on the underlying causes and the severity of the symptoms. Most treatment options eventually lead to **hypothyroidism**, which is treatable and much less threatening than hyperthyroidism.

Radioactive iodine is often used as a diagnostic tool to track iodine uptake, but it can also be used to kill off hyperactive thyroid cells. Some medications prevent the thyroid from producing too much T4, or they reduce its effect. These medications may be used to prepare a patient for surgery or radioactive iodine treatment, but they are occasionally successful by themselves. Beta blockers may be recommended to reduce heart rate and palpitations. Patients who can't take antithyroid drugs or radioactive iodine may consider a **thyroidectomy**. This is a risky procedure, however, because the parathyroids, which control calcium metabolism, are often damaged in the process, along with the vocal cords and laryngeal nerves.

Autoimmune polyglandular syndrome: A descriptor for a group of conditions that frequently appear together or within families, including Graves disease, type I diabetes, systemic lupus erythematosus, and others.

Thyrotoxic myopathy: A neuromuscular disorder connected to hyperthyroidism that involves weakness, the breakdown of muscle tissue, and intolerance to heat.

Goiter: An enlarged thyroid gland that can be seen as a swelling in the neck.

Thyroidectomy: Surgical removal of the thyroid gland.

Medications

- Radioactive iodine to identify and kill off overactive thyroid tissue
- Antithyroid medications to interfere with thyroid hormone production
- Beta blockers for symptomatic relief

Massage Therapy Implications

RISKS	If a client has skin damage as part of his or her hyperthyroidism, massage may be a local caution. Otherwise, massage carries no specific risks for this condition.
BENEFITS	If a client's skin is healthy and intact, massage may be able to offer temporary relief from the frenetic pace of life that many people with hyperthyroidism experience, even though long-lasting changes to thyroid function are not a realistic expectation.
RESEARCH	No strong research to date supports massage therapy as a way to deal with the hormonal imbalances of hyperthyroidism, but it is possible that practitioners trained in lymphatic drainage work may be able to help with the inflammation seen with pretibial myxedema. Further, it is clear that a client with a goiter is not a good candidate for deep specific work at the anterior neck; one case study marks the development of thyrotoxicosis after such a treatment[1].

1. Tachi J, Amino N, Miyai K. Massage therapy on neck: a contributing factor for destructive thyrotoxicosis? *Thyroidology* 1990;2(1):25–27. http://www.ncbi.nlm.nih.gov/pubmed/1715747

Hypothyroidism

Definition: What Is It?

Hypothyroidism is a condition in which circulating levels of thyroid hormones are abnormally low. This interferes with the body's ability to generate energy from fuel.

Demographics

Estimates suggest that almost 4% of the US population meet the criteria for subclinical hypothyroidism, although many may not know. It is more common in women than in men, especially among women who were small at birth and had a low **body mass index** (BMI) during childhood.

This condition can be seen at any age, but it is much more common among those who are 60 years old and older: it is estimated to affect about 6% of women and 2.4% of men in this age range.

Etiology: What Happens?

The thyroid gland produces thyroid hormone in two forms, T3 (triiodothyronine) in small amounts and T4 (thyroxine) in larger amounts. It does this under the direction of the hypothalamus and the pituitary gland, which releases TSH. The liver and other tissues convert T4 to T3, which is more usable by the body. When adequate amounts of T3 and T4 are circulating in the blood, the pituitary gland reduces its secretions of TSH. This is the negative feedback loop that keeps thyroid and pituitary secretions in balance.

The purpose of thyroid hormones is to stimulate the conversion of fuel (oxygen and calories) into energy or work. In hypothyroidism, inadequate amounts of T3 and T4 are produced, so any available fuel in the form of calories is simply stored and not used. In a typical early case of hypothyroidism, the pituitary gland releases lots of TSH, and whatever T4 is secreted by the thyroid is converted to T3 immediately. Consequently, at this stage, TSH levels are high, T4 levels are significantly low, but T3 levels are close to normal. In later stages, TSH remains high, but both T3 and T4 levels drop.

Whatever causes the thyroid to release less T3 and T4, the net result is that a person has difficulty turning fuel into energy. Changes in thyroxine-sensitive cells lead to decreased contractility of the heart muscle, heart enlargement, low cardiac output, and high levels of low-density lipoproteins (the **atherosclerosis**-promoting form of cholesterol). Heart disease and **diabetes** are common overlaps for hypothyroidism. Other consequences include slow gastrointestinal activity (gastric stasis), delayed puberty, menstrual changes, and infertility.

Body mass index (BMI): A weight to height ratio, used to screen for under- and overweight relative to height.

Hypothalamus-pituitary-thyroid axis: The interrelationship between the hypothalamus, the pituitary gland, and the thyroid gland and the hormones they each secrete, which serve to modify the activity of the others.

Myxedema coma: A profound loss of consciousness resulting from low levels of thyroid hormone in the body.

Types of Hypothyroidism

- *Hashimoto thyroiditis*. This is an autoimmune attack against the thyroid gland that results in suppression of thyroid secretions.
- *Congenital hypothyroidism*. This describes a birth defect in which the thyroid is smaller than normal, or missing altogether. In this country, it is mostly seen in premature babies, but in areas where iodine deficiency is a problem, it is a common occurrence.
- *Idiopathic hypothyroidism*. Some cases of hypothyroidism don't seem to be related to any specific underlying disorder but simply arise without known cause. Because many patients exhibit the signs and symptoms of hypothyroidism without strongly indicative blood test confirmation, the identification and treatment of hypothyroidism for these patients is controversial. Another term for this situation is subclinical hypothyroidism.
- *Iodine deficiency hypothyroidism*. Worldwide, this is the most common cause of hypothyroidism. In the United States, it is rare, largely because of the use of iodized salt and other supplemented foods.
- *Secondary hypothyroidism*. Most **hyperthyroidism** patients who use radioactive iodine or surgery to suppress thyroid activity eventually develop hypothyroidism.
- *Other types of hypothyroidism*. Thyroid suppression can be a side effect of some medications (especially the lithium-based drugs used for **bipolar disease**), a tumor or brain injury that interferes with the **hypothalamus-pituitary-thyroid axis**, exposure to radiation, or a transient complication of childbirth.

NOTABLE CASES Singer Linda Ronstadt and talk show icon Oprah Winfrey both struggle with hypothyroidism.

Signs and Symptoms

Signs and symptoms of hypothyroidism are often subtle but steadily progressive (Figure 9.4). A person who cannot convert fuel into energy is likely to gain weight, feel fatigued and depressed, and have a sluggish digestive system with chronic constipation. Heart rate and basal temperature drop, and reflexes may become slow. A patient may have poor tolerance of cold, and her skin may be puffy but dry. Fluid retention in the extremities raises the risk of carpal tunnel syndrome and other nerve entrapment syndromes. Her hair becomes brittle and may even break off or fall out. For some reason, this is especially common at the lateral aspect of the eyebrows. Menstrual periods tend to be heavy and long lasting. Some hypothyroidism patients develop goiter, a painless enlargement of the thyroid (Figure 9.5).

Very severe or untreated cases may cause a person to become so cold and drowsy that she becomes unconscious. This is called **myxedema coma**, and it is a rare but dangerous complication of hypothyroidism, especially among elderly patients (Figure 9.6).

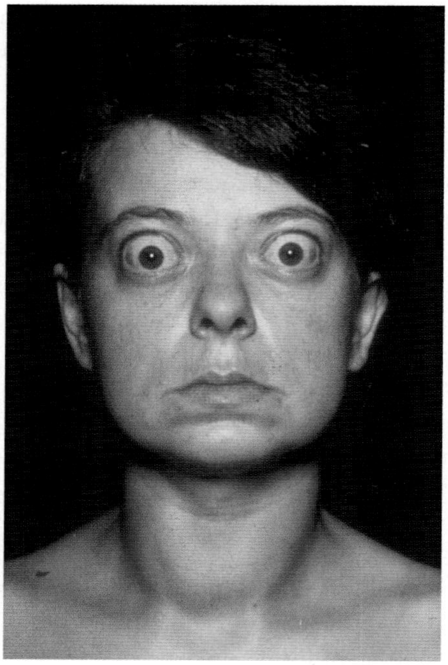

FIGURE 9.5 Hyperthyroidism: goiter and exophthalmos

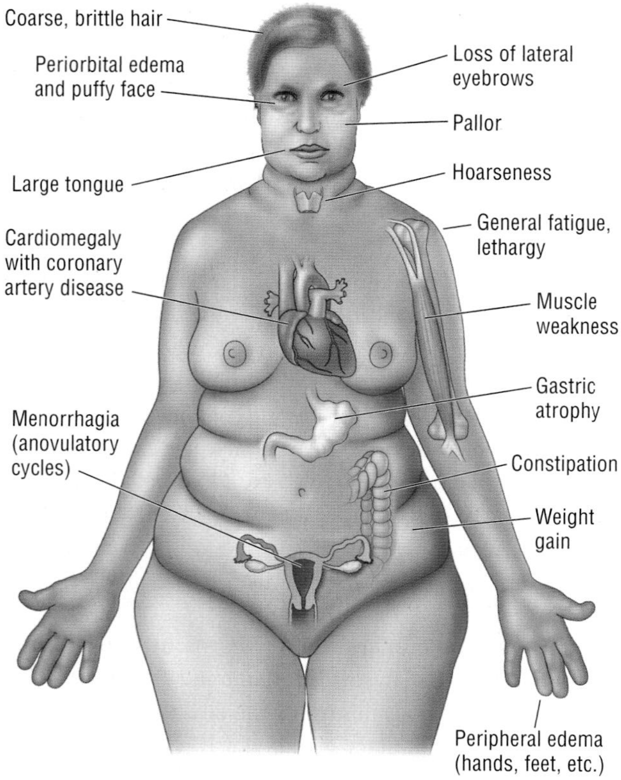

FIGURE 9.6 Hypothyroidism

Treatment

Identifying the need to treat hypothyroidism can sometimes be a challenge. The symptoms of this condition are often vague; it can resemble **depression**, **fibromyalgia**, **chronic fatigue syndrome**, and several other chronic conditions. Also, whether standard scales of "normal" blood tests are accurate for all patients is controversial; subclinical hypothyroidism doesn't fit the typical tests, but can respond well to treatment. Further, it is important to work toward normal thyroid secretion levels, because hypothyroidism can contribute to heart disease. For these reasons, the identification and treatment of mild cases of hypothyroidism may vary from one professional to another (see Sidebar 9.5).

It is especially important for pregnant women to be tested for thyroid function. Pregnancy can hide some symptoms of hypothyroidism, which can create serious repercussions for the unborn child. Most newborns are tested for thyroid function as a matter of course; early intervention in the rare cases when thyroid function is subnormal can prevent stunted growth and mental disability.

The usual treatment for hypothyroidism is to supplement thyroid hormones, usually in the form of synthetic T4, which most people can metabolize into adequate amounts of T3. While many people find relief with this treatment, others must

SIDEBAR 9.5 Hypothyroidism Testing

Hypothyroidism is diagnosed primarily through the measurement of TSH, the hormone secreted by the pituitary gland that tells the thyroid to release T3 and T4. If TSH is high but T3 and T4 are normal or low, it is a sign that the thyroid is not able to answer the demands of the pituitary. The only exception to this rule is when a pituitary tumor interferes with the normal secretion of TSH, and that is quite rare.

Levels of TSH are rated in terms of milliunits per liter (mu/L) and graded in this way:

A TSH test may be accompanied by a test for free T3 and T4 and/or a test for the presence of antithyroid antibodies, which could indicate an immune system attack on the thyroid, Hashimoto thyroiditis.

HYPERTHYROIDISM	NORMAL RANGE OF TSH	SUBCLINICAL RANGE OF HYPOTHYROIDISM	HYPOTHYROIDISM
0.0–0.4	0.4–4.0	4.0–10.0	10.0+

explore other options to find the right supplement for both T3 and T4. This can be in the form of synthetic versions of these hormones or as desiccated porcine or bovine glands. Using animal products for hormone replacement is challenging, though, because the potency from one batch to another can vary greatly.

It is important to remember that hypothyroidism can be a progressive disease, and the appropriate dosage may change over time.

Medications

- Synthetic T4 (levothyroxine)
- Synthetic T3
- Desiccated animal gland (Armour)

Massage Therapy Implications

RISKS	Persons with hypothyroidism are at increased risk for cardiovascular complications, and that informs some choices about massage. However, this situation is so prevalent in the American population that it is safe to assume that most mature clients live with some degree of cardiovascular disease.
BENEFITS	Massage won't necessarily improve thyroid activity, but it may help to ameliorate some of the fatigue and depression that often accompanies this condition.

Metabolic Syndrome

Definition: What Is It?

Metabolic syndrome is not a freestanding disease. Instead, it is a group of problems that, when seen in combinations, have been identified as indicators for a high risk of developing type 2 diabetes and cardiovascular disease.

Demographics

Estimates of the incidence of metabolic syndrome vary widely, but most agree that about 30% to 35% of adult Americans would fit the diagnostic criteria for this condition, although many do not know it. The risk for this condition increases with age, but even more directly with increasing BMI.

Etiology: What Happens?

Metabolic syndrome is identified as a cluster of five main features, including high triglycerides, low high-density lipoproteins (the "good" cholesterol), **hypertension**, central obesity (fat retention in the **omentum** more than in superficial fascia), and high fasting BG levels. Other possible features in metabolic syndrome include a high risk of blood clotting, high levels of **C-reactive protein** and other indicators of inflammation, and **polycystic ovary disease** in women.

These factors are not particularly alarming when they appear individually, but in combination, they set the stage for a high risk of **type 2 diabetes, atherosclerosis, heart attack, heart failure,** and **stroke**. Nonalcoholic fatty liver disease, early cognitive decline, and an increased risk for some kinds of cancers are also associated with metabolic syndrome.

The primary risk factors for metabolic syndrome are obesity and insulin resistance. Further, obesity tends to cause insulin resistance, and insulin resistance can cause obesity, forming a vicious circle. This is complicated by the fact that fat cells in the omentum are metabolically more active than those in subcutaneous fat, and they can produce proclotting and proinflammatory secretions. Both of these raise the risk for cardiovascular problems.

Signs and Symptoms

Metabolic syndrome typically appears as central obesity (much of the body weight is carried around the abdomen in an "apple" rather than a "pear" shape), along with disruptions in cholesterol, hypertension, and higher-than-normal BG. The point at which this is associated with risk varies by racial profile; Asian Americans are at risk for the consequences of metabolic syndrome with a smaller abdominal measurement than other races. Outside of excessive body weight however, metabolic syndrome does not typically have noticeable signs; its other components are silent.

Metabolic syndrome is identified when three of these five risk factors are simultaneously present:

- High fasting BG (over 100 mg/dL after 9 hours of fasting) or needing medication to manage BG
- Abdominal obesity: a waist measurement of over 88 cm (35 inches) for women or over 102 cm (40 inches) for men; for Asian Americans, the risk begins at 80 cm (32 inches) for women and 90 cm (35 inches) for men
- Elevated triglyceride levels (>140 mg/dL for men, > 150 mg/dL for women)
- Low levels of high-density lipoproteins (<40 mg/dL for men, <50 mg/dL for women)
- Hypertension (systolic blood pressure >130 mm Hg, diastolic >85 mm Hg)

Having blood chemistry that shows a propensity for clotting and long-term inflammation also appears on metabolic syndrome criteria lists, but without specific measures.

Omentum: An apron-like layer of fatty tissue that hangs down over the abdominal organs.

C-reactive protein: A protein found in the blood, high levels of which are indicative of inflammation in the body.

Treatment

Treatment for metabolic syndrome is often divided into short-term and long-term goals. Short-term goals include lowering BG and correcting cholesterol levels with diet, exercise, and medical intervention.

Long-term goals include increasing physical activity and losing weight. Reducing body weight by 5% to 7% (this is only 10 to 14 lb for a 200-lb person) reduces the risk of complications by about 60%, and exercise improves insulin action and decreases BG. Limiting alcohol use and quitting smoking are other important steps.

Medications

- Metformin or other insulin-regulating medication
- Antihypertensive medications, with respect for the ones that exacerbate insulin resistance
- Cholesterol-lowering drugs to manage hyperlipidemia
- Low-dose aspirin as needed for antiplatelet activity

Massage Therapy Implications

RISKS	The safety of massage for clients with metabolic syndrome depends on their resilience and ability to adapt to homeostatic challenge. A person at high risk for cardiovascular disease or diabetes may have more trouble with rigorous massage than someone with a milder version of this condition.
BENEFITS	While massage alone is unlikely to have a profound impact on metabolic syndrome, along with diet and exercise, it can be a part of a supportive change in lifestyle practices that can reduce the risk of this condition becoming a more serious problem.

Thyroid Cancer

Definition: What Is It?

Thyroid cancer is any type of cancer that originates in the thyroid gland. Most varieties of thyroid cancer are slow growing and easily treatable, but some forms are more aggressive.

Demographics

About 23,500 people are diagnosed with thyroid cancer in this country each year. Most of them are over 40 years old. Women outnumber men with this condition by about 3:1.

Etiology: What Happens?

The thyroid gland is composed of two main types of epithelial cells: follicular cells, which normally produce T3 and T4, and parafollicular cells, also called C cells, which produce calcitonin, a hormone that pulls calcium out of the blood to increase bone density.

Cancer develops when DNA in thyroid cells is damaged and cell growth becomes uncontrolled and disorganized. Thyroid cancer is often related to a history of radiation exposure. People who were treated with radiation for **acne**, tonsillitis, or an enlarged thymus are at increased risk for this disease. Similarly, people exposed to radioactive fallout from nuclear testing or nuclear reactor accidents have a higher-than-normal risk for thyroid cancer; this is one of the long-term repercussions of the Chernobyl nuclear accident in 1986. Radiation from standard neck or dental radiography is not associated with an increased risk of thyroid cancer.

Other forms of thyroid cancer are related to inherited genetic characteristics. Children of people with the genetic mutation for thyroid cancer have a 50% chance of developing the disease themselves. Inherited forms of thyroid cancer tend to be more aggressive and harder to treat than other forms, so when this condition is discovered, all family members, especially children, are recommended for genetic testing.

It is important to delineate between thyroid cancer and thyroid nodules. Nodules on this gland are fairly common and usually completely benign (Figure 9.7).

Types of Thyroid Cancer

- *Papillary thyroid cancer.* This is the most common type of thyroid cancer, accounting for about 85% of all diagnoses. Papillary cells look like fern leaves, with many tiny extensions; they arise from follicular cells. This type of cancer usually stays local, and while it may intrude on local lymph nodes, it is usually stable and doesn't tend to grow or invade other tissues. In rare cases, it does metastasize through the lymph system to the bones or the lungs.
- *Follicular thyroid cancer.* This form of thyroid cancer also arises from follicular cells. It is less common than papillary thyroid cancer, accounting for about 9% of thyroid cancer diagnoses. Follicular thyroid cancer is more likely to metastasize than papillary thyroid cancer, particularly if it is diagnosed in someone over 50 years old.
  - Hurthle cell carcinoma is a subtype of follicular thyroid cancer. It tends to have a poor prognosis because it is harder to find early and less responsive to treatment than other forms of thyroid cancer.
- *Medullary thyroid cancer.* This form of cancer arises from C cells that normally produce calcitonin. It is rare but it can be aggressive. It is often related to a group of identified genetic mutations.
- *Anaplastic thyroid cancer.* Also called undifferentiated thyroid cancer, anaplastic thyroid cancer is highly aggressive, metastasizing easily to the **mediastinal** lymph nodes, trachea, lungs, and bones. It originates from benign or low-grade thyroid tumors and usually affects people over 60 years old.

Mediastinal: Relating to the mediastinum, the space in the chest containing all of the thoracic organs except the lungs

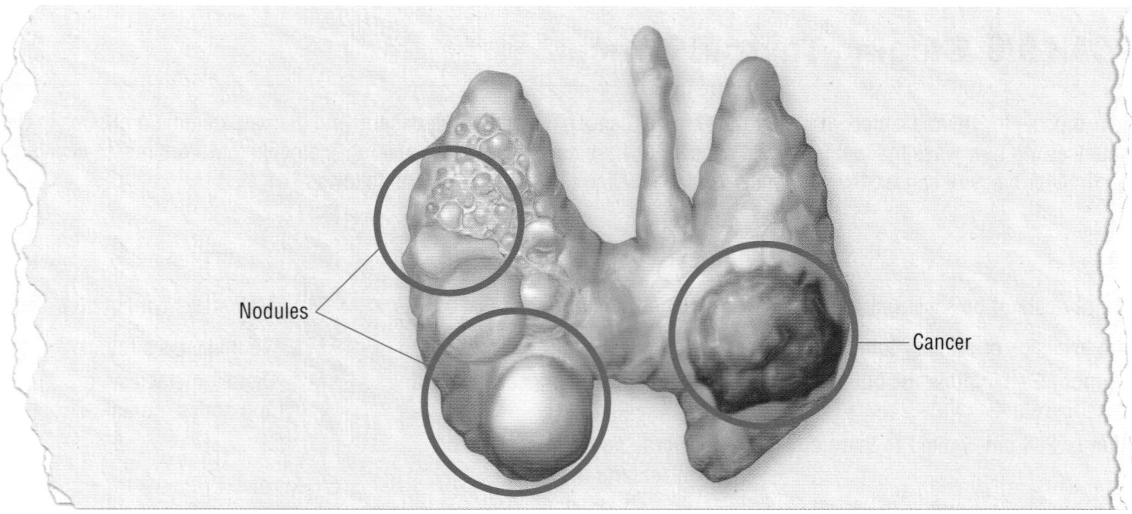

FIGURE 9.7 Thyroid nodules and cancer

- *Thyroid lymphoma*. Lymphocytes in the thyroid gland are also vulnerable to DNA mutation. This is most likely to happen along with **hypothyroidism** in the form of Hashimoto thyroiditis.

Signs and Symptoms

Nonaggressive forms of thyroid cancer may be silent, especially in early stages. Later symptoms include painless enlargement in the throat. This may press on the esophagus or trachea, leading to problems with breathing, coughing, hoarseness, and difficulty with swallowing.

Later stages of aggressive thyroid cancers may include tumors in the lungs or on bones; symptoms may be related to these complications.

Treatment

Most cases of thyroid cancer are successfully treated with surgery to remove part or all of the thyroid gland. Thyroid hormones must be supplemented after this procedure. Lymph nodes in the neck are often dissected to look for signs of metastasis.

Surgery may be followed with doses of radioactive iodine or external beams of radiation at tumor sites. This regimen is successful for most cases of thyroid cancer, even if it recurs after surgery.

Aggressive forms of thyroid cancer are typically treated with radioactive iodine and other forms of chemotherapy, but not surgery, since the chance of getting all of the cancer cells is negligible.

Thyroid cancer has a fairly common recurrence rate, so many experts are working on ways to identify the factors that predict recurrence for the best possible outcomes.

Staging protocols for thyroid cancer are discussed in Sidebar 9.6.

NOTABLE CASES Film critic Roger Ebert had radiation treatment for an ear infection when he was young, and later, he developed papillary thyroid cancer. His multiple surgeries led to the loss of his voice, but did not keep him from being actively involved in his profession. He died at age 70 in 2013. Other thyroid cancer patients have included Supreme Court justice William Rehnquist and prolific science fiction author Isaac Asimov. Singer Rod Stewart is a thyroid cancer survivor.

Medications

- Chemotherapeutic agents
- Radioactive iodine
- Thyroid hormones to stabilize blood levels and to inhibit the secretion of TSH

Massage Therapy Implications

RISKS	As with other types of cancer, massage for thyroid cancer is based on the treatment options and the general resilience of the patient. One special caution for this population is that someone undergoing treatment with radioactive iodine must be kept in isolation until the treatment is complete. This means massage must be delayed as well. For more information about massage in the context of cancer, see Chapter 12.
BENEFITS	Because massage can offer relief of pain, anxiety, depression, and other problems that accompany cancer treatment, it can be helpful for someone with living with this disease, as long as the challenges presented by the cancer and its treatments are respected.

SIDEBAR 9.6 Staging Thyroid Cancer

Staging protocols for thyroid cancer are tied to the type of cancer, the age of the patient, and the best treatment options in the circumstances. As new ways to identify thyroid cancer early are developed, these staging protocols may continue to evolve.

As with other types of cancer, thyroid cancer is staged using the TNM system, as follows:

TUMOR (T)	NODE (N)	METASTASIS (M)
T X: Tumor cannot be assessed	N X: Nodes cannot be assessed	M X: Metastasis cannot be assessed
T 0: No evidence of primary tumor	N 0: No nodes involved	M 0: No metastasis found
T 1: Tumor <2 cm, within the boundaries of the thyroid	N 1a: Some nodes in neck involved	M 1: Distant metastasis to lymph nodes, organs, or bones
T 2: Tumor 2–4 cm, limited to thyroid	N 1b: Some nodes in neck and mediastinum involved	
T 3: The tumor is >4 cm; or the tumor has invaded nearby tissue.		
T 4a: Tumor any size; has invaded anterior neck tissues		
T 4b: Tumor any size; has invaded posterior neck, spine, or large blood vessels		

These delineations are translated into stages I to IV in this way:

For papillary or follicular thyroid cancer in patients under 45 years old:

Stage I	any T, any N, M0
Stage II	any T, any N, M1

For anaplastic thyroid cancer

Stage IVa	T4a, any N, M0
Stage IVb	T4b, any N, M0
Stage IVc	any T, any N, M1

For papillary or follicular thyroid cancer in patients over 45 years old:

Stage I	T1, N0, M0
Stage II	T2, N0, M0
Stage III	T1–3, N0–N1a, M0
Stage IVa	T1–4a, N0–1b, M0
Stage IVb	T4b, any N, M0
Stage IVc	any T, any N, M1

Explore and Apply

LEVEL 1: Receive and Respond

2. The pituitary gland is often called the "master gland," but it is under the control of which other structure?
   a. Thymus
   b. Thalamus
   c. Hypothalamus
   d. Thyroid

3. What is an antagonist to parathyroid hormone?
   a. Calcitonin
   b. Thyronine
   c. Somatotropin
   d. Cortisol

4. This condition can cause blindness, renal failure, amputation, stroke, and heart attack. What is it?
   a. Hyperthyroidism
   b. Metabolic syndrome
   c. Diabetes
   d. Hypothyroidism

5. What is a medical emergency associated with hyperthyroidism?
   a. Ketoacidosis
   b. Thyroid storm
   c. Pretibial myxedema
   d. Hyperosmolality

6. Which is a collection of signs that suggest an increased risk of diabetes or heart disease?
   a. Hypothyroidism
   b. Hyperthyroidism
   c. Hypoglycemia
   d. Metabolic syndrome

7. Match the following terms to their best definitions

a. An undetermined condition leading to decreased thyroid hormone production	__Graves disease
b. An autoimmune condition leading to increased thyroid hormone condition	__Metabolic syndrome
c. An autoimmune condition leading to decreased pancreatic secretions	__Double diabetes
d. A combination of impaired insulin production and insulin resistance	__Idiopathic hypothyroidism
e. A combination of factors leading to diabetes and/or heart disease	__Type 1 diabetes

LEVEL 2: Practical Application

1. Your client who has diabetes has enjoyed a long, late afternoon massage. As she gets ready to leave, you notice that she seems a little dizzy and disoriented. What is your best strategy?
   a. Take her to the hospital immediately.
   b. Offer her something sweet: juice, candy, or milk.
   c. Apply an ice pack to her neck.
   d. Offer her some protein: nuts, jerky, or peanut butter.

2. Your client is a 32-year-old woman. She is thin, and although it is winter, she is dressed in a T-shirt and shorts, and she complains that she is too hot. She has a hard time relaxing on the table. What condition might be present?
   a. Hypothyroidism
   b. Hyperthyroidism
   c. Thyroid cancer
   d. Iodine deficiency

3. Compare Graves disease to Hashimoto thyroiditis. What do they have in common? How are they different?

4. Your client is a 71-year-old woman. She is overweight, and she complains of having no "get up and go." She is cold in your 75° session room. You notice that her hair and skin are very dry. What condition might be present?
   a. Hypothyroidism
   b. Hyperthyroidism
   c. Thyroid cancer
   d. Diabetes

5. Your 35-year-old client is a survivor of thyroid cancer. Her surgery was 5 years ago, and her last chemotherapy treatment was 4 years ago. What accommodations does she need for this situation?
   a. She needs doctor's note affirming that she is cancer-free.
   b. Avoid working prone so that her neck is not compressed.
   c. The same accommodations that you make for any healthy client.
   d. Very light work to avoid disrupting latent tumor cells elsewhere in the body.

Note to educators: Due to space considerations, these review questions only address the most important material from Chapter 9. The Test Bank provides a much more comprehensive selection of questions, all of which are keyed to the relevant chapter objectives.

What Would *You* Do?

The Diabetic Twins

You have two clients: identical twin brothers who are 42. Both have type 2 diabetes, but the similarities stop there. One twin manages his condition with careful monitoring, exercise, diet, and medication. The other is less diligent. He is overweight, he's had one heart attack, and his eyesight is going. Outline a treatment strategy for each client, with a list of goals and potential cautions or complications for each.

A Frightened Thyroid Cancer Patient

Your client is a young woman anticipating treatment for thyroid cancer. She will be undergoing treatment with radioactive iodine. She is eager to receive massage during this process. What questions do you need to have answered in order to work safely? How will you explain your choices to her?

Suggested Activities

1. For each condition covered in your curriculum, write down the following on a card:
   - A brief definition
   - Most common cause or contributing factor(s)
   - Major signs and symptoms
   - Risks and benefits of massage therapy
     - Variables that contribute to risks and benefits
     - Appropriate adaptations

   Use these as flash cards as you study
2. For each condition covered in your curriculum, write one multiple choice question. Share your questions with your classmates as you study together.
3. Quiz yourself using either the "labels off" feature in your enhanced ebook or the labeling exercise on thePoint® for Figure 9.1. Identify the sources of the following hormones: Insulin, Testosterone, Thyroxine, Erythropoietin, Epinephrine, Aldosterone, Glucagon, Adrenaline, Thymosin, Growth hormone, Cortisol, Calcitonin.
4. Use the student resources on thePoint® to find practice quiz questions and games.

10

Urinary System Conditions

CHAPTER 10 / Abbreviated Chapter Objectives

Having completed assignments and classroom time related to Chapter 10, the learner is expected to be able to…

- Identify definitions of the key terms in the introduction and those connected to the conditions covered in your curriculum.
- Label the parts of the urinary system.
- Identify the structures involved in the first exchange of fluid between the circulatory system and the urinary system.
- Name the basic structural unit of the kidney.
- Describe how the kidneys contribute to normal blood counts.
- Describe the relationship between normal blood pressure and healthy kidney function and between hypertension and kidney damage.
- Provide the following information for each condition covered in your curriculum:
  - Identify the definition of the condition.
  - List the most common causes or contributing factors to the condition.
  - List major signs and symptoms of the condition.
  - Identify possible risks and benefits of massage therapy, with:
    - Variables that contribute to risks and benefits
    - Appropriate adaptations for massage therapy

For detailed chapter objectives for each condition in this chapter, consult the student resource page at http://thePoint.lww.com/Werner6e. thePoint®

Urinary System Introduction

The urinary system is a relatively small system composed of the kidneys, ureters, bladder, and urethra (Figure 10.1).

The huge renal artery comes directly off the abdominal aorta and enters the kidneys. It rapidly decreases in diameter and splits up to form thousands of capillaries, terminating in tiny knots called **glomeruli**. Each of these is surrounded by a **Bowman capsule**, the entry point to the **nephron**. Blood pressure forces fluid from the glomeruli into the Bowman capsule. Nephrons and circulatory capillaries exchange water and waste products as they intertwine along the **loop of Henle** (Figure 10.2). By the time fluid enters the collecting tubules, any water, electrolytes, or other material the body needs has been reabsorbed, so that only waste products are left. This fluid is urine. The collecting tubules pour their contents into the renal pelvis, the renal pelvis empties into the ureters, they lead to the urinary bladder, and urine is excreted from the bladder through the urethra.

To view an animation of the kidney process, see "Renal Function" at http://thePoint.lww.com. thePoint®.

The kidneys have another function that is not directly involved in the removal of waste products from the blood. **Erythropoietin** (EPO), a hormone that stimulates red blood cell production, is produced in the kidneys. Damage to these delicate organs can therefore sometimes be identified by changes in red blood cell count and **anemia**.

The kidneys are constructed primarily of epithelial tissue, which makes them vulnerable to injury. When the kidneys have been damaged, red blood cells leak from capillaries into the nephrons. This shows as **hematuria**. It is evidence of trauma, infection, or another possibly dangerous condition in the kidneys.

Filtration, the movement of substances through a membrane by external mechanical pressure (in this case the blood

Glomerulus: The tiny knot of capillaries at the end of a kidney tubule.

Bowman capsule: The beginning segment of a nephron, which surrounds the glomerulus.

Nephron: A functional unit of the kidney.

Loop of Henle: The U-shaped loop of tubule in the nephron of a kidney.

Erythropoietin: A hormone produced by the kidneys that stimulates the production of red blood cells.

Hematuria: The presence of blood in the urine.

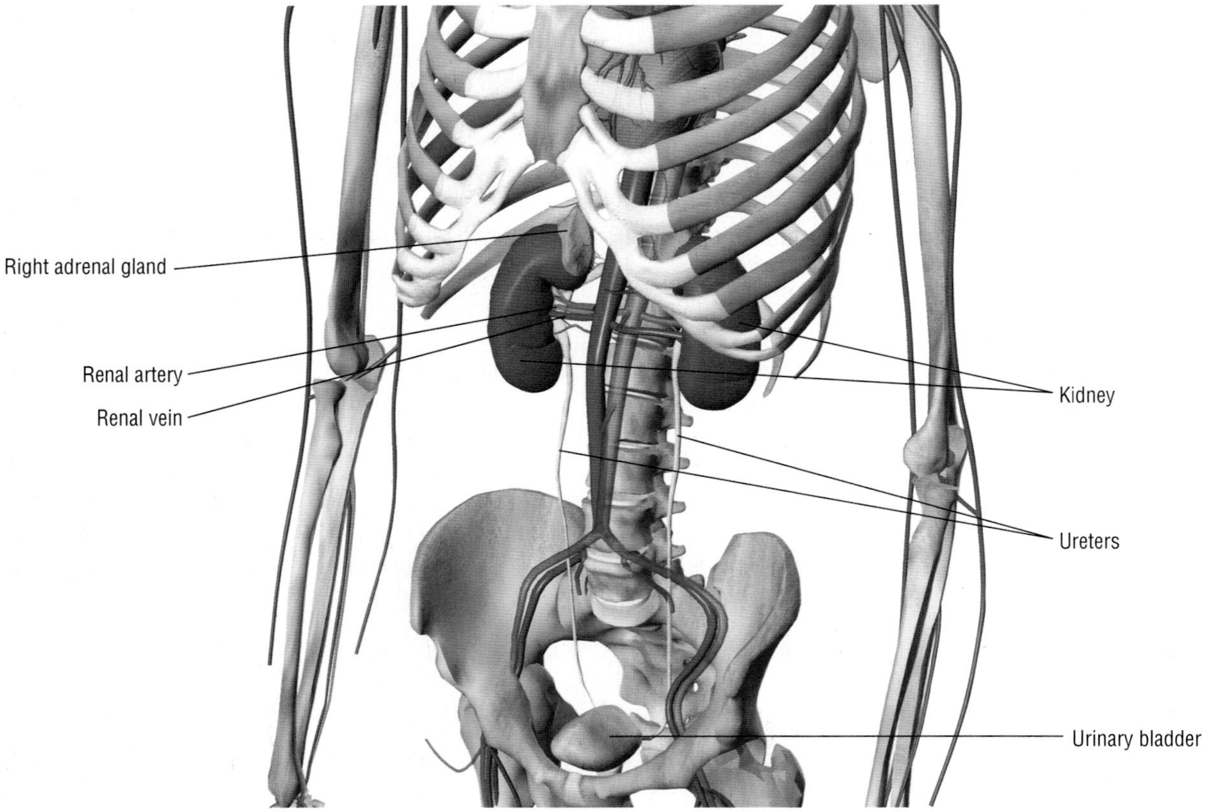

FIGURE 10.1 Urinary system overview

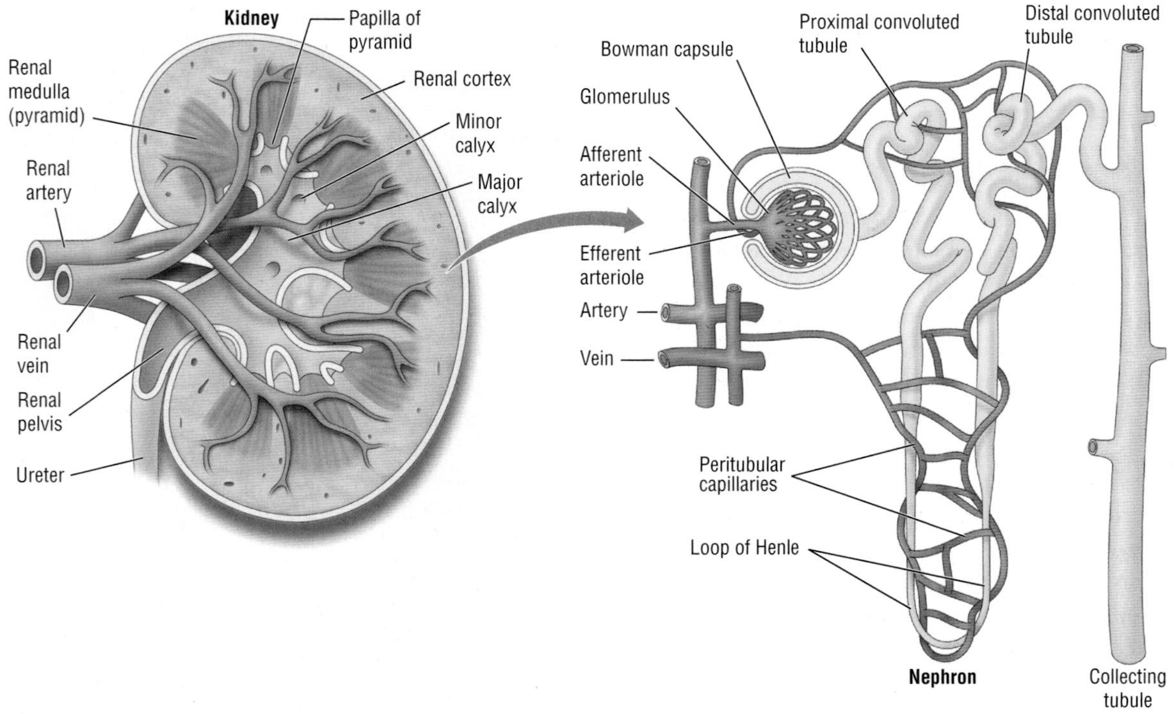

FIGURE 10.2 Kidney function

pressure), is the mechanism that initially pushes waste-filled plasma into the kidneys. The speed with which this happens is called the **glomerular filtration rate**, or GFR. Normal GFR is 120 mL/min: this adds up to 180 L of fluid moving through the kidneys each day! (Of course, most of the glomerular filtrate is reabsorbed into circulatory capillaries and put back into the bloodstream.)

> **Glomerular filtration rate:** The rate at which blood passes through the glomeruli of the kidneys.
>
> **Positive feedback loop:** A process in which a stimulus prompts a response, which in turn amplifies the stimulus, heightening the response.

It is clear then, how closely blood pressure and kidney health are interrelated. If blood pressure is consistently too high, the kidneys sustain damage and become less efficient. At the same time, if the kidneys are not functioning adequately, the body accumulates excessive fluid, which raises blood pressure. This **positive feedback loop** is a recurring theme in kidney dysfunction etiology.

Urinary System Conditions

Kidney Disorders

- Kidney stones
  - Calcium stones
  - Struvite stones
  - Uric acid stones
  - Cystine stones
  - Other stones
- Polycystic kidney disease
- Pyelonephritis
  - Acute pyelonephritis
  - Chronic pyelonephritis
  - Emphysematous pyelonephritis
- Renal cancer
  - Renal cell carcinoma
  - Transitional cell carcinoma
  - Wilms tumor
- Renal failure
  - Acute renal failure
  - Chronic renal failure

Bladder and Urinary Tract Disorders

- Bladder cancer
  - Transitional cell carcinoma
  - Squamous cell carcinoma
  - Other types of bladder cancer
- Interstitial cystitis
- Urinary tract infection

Kidney Disorders

Kidney Stones

Definition: What Is It?

Also called renal calculi or **nephrolithiases**, kidney stones are crystals that sometimes develop in the renal pelvis. The size of kidney stones varies widely, depending on how long they have been developing and what they are made of. Most stones range between the size of grains of sand to about 1 inch in diameter. Some stones are much larger, growing into the cortex of the kidney, forming a staghorn calculus (Figure 10.3).

Small stones may pass through the urinary tract with no symptoms, but larger ones may get stuck in the ureters. The technical name for stones in this location is **ureterolithiases**.

Kidney stones usually form in the absence of adequate fluids. Thus, they are most common in hot environments, where people tend to lose more liquid through sweat than they replace. Peak months for the diagnosis of kidney stones in the United States are June through August, for the same reason.

Demographics

About 10% of all Americans will have a kidney stone at some point. These crystals are the cause of about half a million emergency room visits and 2 million outpatient visits each year. Most stones occur in White or Asian men between 20 and 50 years old, but men of other ages and races, along with women and children, can have them too.

Within the United States, the highest number of kidney stones occur in the southeastern region, which has given rise to the term "the stone belt" for that part of the country.

Etiology: What Happens?

Tiny crystals often form in the kidneys and cause no problems or symptoms; these are called **nidi**. But if a sizable stone moves into the urethra, then pressure may build up behind it. This makes the affected kidney swell, causing the characteristic grabbing pain associated with kidney stones.

Most kidney stones that are big enough to cause problems are excruciatingly painful but eventually pass into the bladder and out in the urine without causing long-lasting damage to the urinary system. Occasionally, however, a stone grows large enough to seriously disrupt kidney function. This may lead to **chronic** or acute **renal failure**.

> **Nephrolithiasis:** A crystalline mass found in the kidneys or ureters. Also called a kidney stone.
>
> **Ureterolithiasis:** A kidney stone that is lodged in a ureter.
>
> **Nidus, nidi:** A tiny crystal around which a larger stone can form.

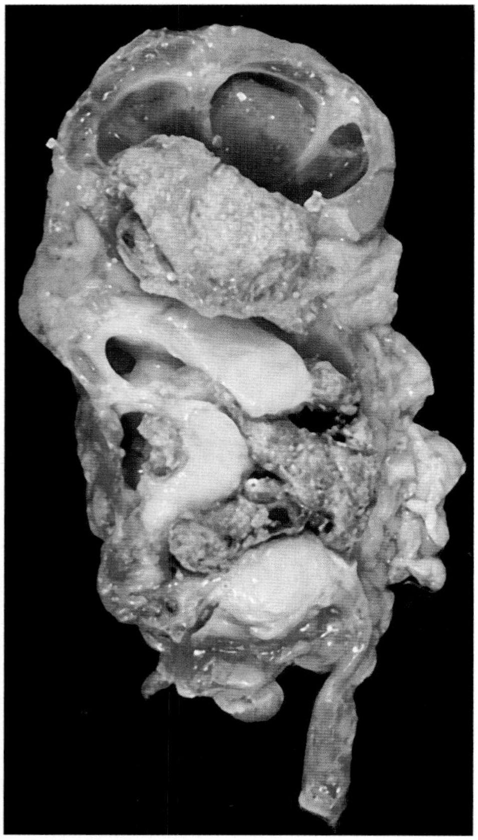

FIGURE 10.3 Staghorn calculus

Kidney stones are rarely a once-in-a-lifetime event. Most people who pass one stone pass at least one more, possibly many years later. Research suggests that the risk for eventual renal failure increases with each stone an individual passes, so people with a history of this condition need to be watchful about all aspects of kidney health.

Several inherited anomalies raise the risk of kidney stones. Other risk factors include the use of certain medications, a history of surgery or inflammation in the gastrointestinal tract, and urinary tract infections **(UTIs)** or blockages. **Diabetes** and a history of bariatric surgery or other GI tract procedures are other possible risk factors. These are an issue for people who are already genetically inclined toward forming stones, but they do not seem to be a big issue for people who are not.

Kidney stones can be composed of any of several substances, each one indicative of a different type of metabolic problem.

Types of Kidney Stones

- *Calcium stones*: These account for most kidney stones. They are composed of calcium oxalate or calcium phosphate and associated with problems with calcium metabolism or too much incoming calcium, usually in the form of calcium supplements or calcium-based antacids (Figure 10.4).

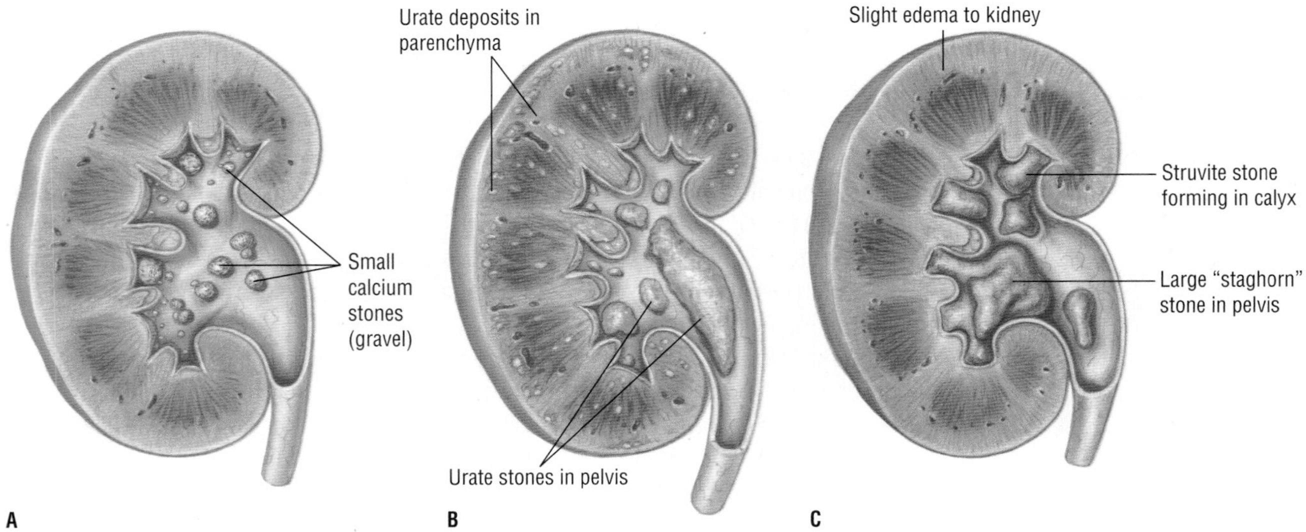

FIGURE 10.4 **A:** Calcium stones, **B:** Uric acid stones, and **C:** Struvite stone

- *Struvite stones*: These are composed of magnesium and ammonia and are associated with chronic UTIs.
- *Uric acid stones*: These form in the kidneys of people whose blood is abnormally acidic. They are associated with a diet high in meat and purine. People who have uric acid kidney stones are also at high risk for **gout**.
- *Cystine stones*: These are relatively rare. They are directly related to a genetic dysfunction with the metabolism of cystine, an amino acid.
- *Other stones*: These account for a tiny percentage of kidney stones. Genetic problems with metabolism and the use of protease inhibitors to treat **HIV/AIDS** are the primary causes of these stones.

Signs and Symptoms

Most kidney stones are completely silent; and they pass through the ureters without pain. If they get stuck or if they are large enough to scrape the delicate lining of the urinary tract, however, they cause hematuria. In addition, the kidney may swell as it continues to produce urine that cannot drain freely; this is extremely painful. The ureters contract in irritation, causing **renal colic**. The pain has a sudden onset, comes and goes in waves, and can be so severe that it causes nausea and vomiting as a sympathetic reaction. The pain often refers to the groin. Occasionally, the stone may be caused by or may lead to an infection in the kidneys; in these instances, fever and chills accompany the severe pain.

Renal colic: Severe pain caused by the impaction or passage of a kidney stone.

Percutaneous nephrolithotomy: A medical procedure in which an incision is made through the skin of the back directly to the kidney in order to remove a stone.

Extracorporeal shockwave lithotripsy: A medical procedure in which intense sound waves are used to break up stones in the body such as kidney stones and gallstones.

Treatment

The pain of kidney stones is so intense that long ago, people operated on them without anesthesia: "cutting for stone" was considered worth the pain just to get rid of them. Nowadays, several other options are available, and only a small percentage of kidney stone patients have to go through major surgery. If a person is unable to pass a stone without help, three main interventions are available.

- **Percutaneous nephrolithotomy** is a surgery conducted through a tiny tunnel in the back leading to the stone, which is either extracted or subjected to sonic waves that break it up.
- Ureteroscopic stone removal uses a flexible tube that is inserted into the urethra and snakes up to where the stone is lodged to remove it from the ureters.
- **Extracorporeal shockwave lithotripsy** is the use of sound waves to break up stones into a size that can be passed through the ureters with minimal risk of getting stuck. This procedure can leave the patient feeling bruised and battered from the extremity of the shock waves that are required to break up stones, but it can treat larger deposits than either of the other two options.

People who have passed a stone before will recognize the signs of another attack (Case History 10.1). They may be counseled to pass the stone at home, using over-the-counter painkillers and urinating into a strainer so the stone can be captured and analyzed later.

Prevention for persons susceptible to kidney stones depends on what the stones are made of. Possible interventions include removal of the parathyroid glands; medication to regulate metabolism; dietary adjustments; and most impor-

CASE HISTORY 10.1 Kidney Stones

I've had kidney stone attacks all my life. In 1944, I had an attack at night in bed. Once you've had a kidney stone attack, you never forget what it feels like. I knew immediately what was happening, and they rushed me via command car to a military hospital, 20 miles away from the Battle of the Bulge. The renal surgeon authorized an attempt to remove the stone with a tube. Back in those days, the tube was metal, not flexible—hence, the discomfort, which I've never forgotten. The procedure was unsuccessful because somehow I had already passed the stone.

WALTER B., AGED 77: "Once you've had a kidney stone, you never forget it."

Then, in the blizzard of 1978, I had my last attack. Boston was digging out from a huge snowstorm. No one was allowed to drive; the streets had to be clear for ambulances and fire trucks. The pain was God awful, just unbearable. They always say it's like having a baby—you just wouldn't believe it. I couldn't get to the hospital right away, so the doctor told me to drink some whiskey to dull the pain. Finally, I was given special permission to take a taxicab to the hospital.

When the stone was basketed at the hospital, it was sent to the kidney stone lab, where it was identified as a calcium stone. The medication consisted of allopurinol tablets and hydrochlorothiazide pills taken daily. There's been no sign of an attack since then.

tantly, adequate hydration. Kidney stone patients need to drink up to 1 gallon of water every day to keep stones moving through the system before they become big enough to cause problems. Patients are also frequently advised to limit caffeine, alcohol, and oxalate-rich foods (dark leafy vegetables, nuts, and chocolate) to reduce the risk of future stones.

Medications

- For calcium or uric acid stones, alkalinizing agents, including allopurinol, to change the pH of fluid in the kidneys
- For struvite stones, possibly long-term low-dose prophylactic antibiotics
- For cystine stones, medication to bind cystine
- Analgesics, including ibuprofen or narcotics as necessary

Massage Therapy Implications

RISKS	A person in the throes of passing a kidney stone attack is not a good candidate for massage; this is a medical situation that needs appropriate attention.
BENEFITS	A client who has fully recovered from kidney stones can enjoy the same benefits from massage as the rest of the population.

Polycystic Kidney Disease

Definition: What Is It?

Polycystic kidney disease (PKD) is a common inherited disorder that involves a genetic mutation to the cells that form tubules or collecting ducts in the kidneys, along with some other tissues.

Demographics

PKD affects about 600,000 people in the United States. Males and females are equally affected, as are all racial groups. It causes between 5% and 10% of all cases of **renal failure**.

Etiology: What Happens?

PKD can be autosomal recessive (a person must inherit the gene from both parents for the disease to manifest) or autosomal dominant (a person develops the disease if they inherit the gene from only one parent).

Autosomal recessive PKD (ARPKD) is present at birth. It is often seen with extensive liver damage called **congenital hepatic fibrosis**. It is usually more severe than autosomal dominant PKD (ADPKD), and it is associated with a high risk of infant mortality.

ADPKD is the most common version of the disease. It usually doesn't cause problems until adulthood. Usually, **hypertension** is the first indicator, followed by other symptoms that typically develop in a person's 30s or 40s.

In either form of PKD, a genetic anomaly causes certain cells in the kidneys to proliferate. They form hollow pockets on top of the nephrons that then fill with fluid (Figures 10.5 and 10.6). The cysts can be tiny or large, and both the kidneys

Congenital hepatic fibrosis: Liver damage present as a result of a recessive genetic trait.

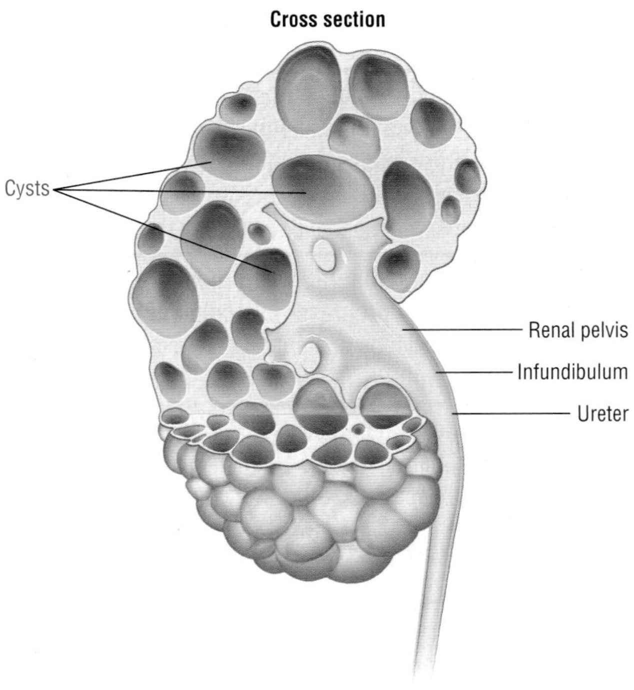

FIGURE 10.5 Polycystic kidney disease

are affected. As the cysts increase in size and number (affected kidneys can grow to huge dimensions), the rest of kidney function is seriously impaired. The remaining tubules or collecting ducts can be physically obstructed or heavily invested with scar tissue. Ultimately, a person with PKD will probably develop renal failure, and about half of all PKD patients eventually become candidates for a kidney transplant.

Complications

PKD opens the door to several serious complications. The genetic anomaly that causes cysts to develop in the kidneys can also affect the liver, leading to hepatomegaly and loss of liver function. Cysts in the kidneys and the liver may become infected, which can be difficult to diagnose correctly. The constant high blood pressure seen with PKD contributes to **atherosclerosis** and other cardiovascular complications. In addition, blood vessels may be unusually weak; thoracic and cerebral **aneurysms** and hemorrhagic **strokes** are more common for PKD patients than for the general population. Heart valves are often abnormal, which raises the risk for arterial and pulmonary **emboli**. Even the colon appears to be affected by this disease: **diverticular disease** is common among PKD patients.

The progressive kidney damage seen with PKD also has direct impact on the health of the whole urinary system. **Kidney stones**, infections in the cysts themselves, and **urinary tract infections** are all frequent complications.

The progressive loss of function with PKD means that many patients eventually develop end-stage renal failure (ESRF). At this point, **hemodialysis** becomes necessary, and a kidney transplant may be a lifesaving intervention. About one-half of all PKD patients will eventually seek a donor kidney. Fortunately, transplanted tissues do not develop cysts.

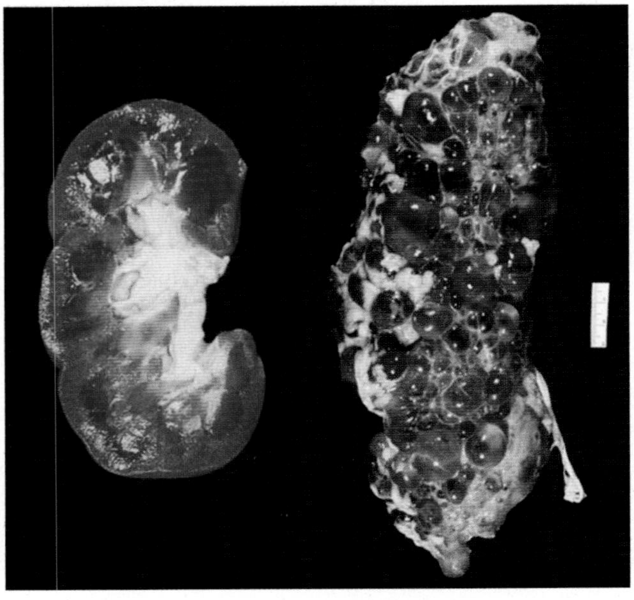

FIGURE 10.6 Normal kidney **(left)**; polycystic kidney **(right)**

Signs and Symptoms

Hypertension that is unusually high for young adults is often the first indicator for ADPKD; this may develop even while kidney function is normal. A reduction in urine concentration is predictable, along with chronic, intractable pain that is related to delicate kidney tissue that is stretched, compressed, and irritated. **Headaches** are a frequent complaint for PKD patients, along with extreme back and flank pain from kidney stones, UTIs, and infected cysts.

Treatment

As a genetic disorder, PKD has no treatment to correct the core problem. Treatment focuses instead on controlling complications and symptoms to preserve function for as long as possible. Managing pain and high blood pressure are high priorities, of course. Needle aspiration of large cysts using ultrasound imaging as a guide can relieve symptoms for months at a time, but cysts inevitably recur. Surgery may be considered for liver cysts.

Tracking the progress of PKD is important so that dialysis and kidney transplantation can be considered at the appropriate time.

Medications

- Antihypertensives, especially ACE inhibitors, but not calcium channel blockers
- Analgesics to manage headache and kidney-related pain; NSAIDs must be avoided
- Antibiotics for infection

Hemodialysis: A medical procedure in which blood is purified outside of the body, used when the kidneys cannot perform this function normally.

Massage Therapy Implications

RISKS	A person with PKD may have impaired ability to manage fluid, dangerously high blood pressure, and an increased risk for both liver damage and cerebral aneurysm, among other problems. All these factors may make rigorous circulatory massage a stimulus that is too challenging for their ability to adapt. Further, PKD patients may use particularly strong painkillers; this influences massage choices too, because pain sensation may be impaired.
BENEFITS	Massage therapy may help to drop blood pressure at least temporarily and reduce some of the anxiety and fear that may accompany a serious chronic and progressive condition like PKD. As long as a bodywork session is designed not to overly challenge a client's homeostatic capacity, massage can be a safe and helpful choice for a person with PKD.
RESEARCH	One case report documents an incident in which an elderly man received a "vigorous chair massage" and had a ruptured kidney cyst with internal hemorrhage.[1] This is an excellent reason to get a thorough client profile, even for chair massage or other nonclinical work. 1. Mufarrij AJ, Hitti E. Acute cystic rupture and hemorrhagic shock after a vigorous massage chair session in a patient with polycystic kidney disease. *American Journal of the Medical Sciences* 2011;342(1):76–78. http://www.ncbi.nlm.nih.gov/pubmed/21642815

Pyelonephritis

Definition: What Is It?

As the name implies, pyelonephritis is an infection of the nephrons in the kidney, although the renal pelvis may also be involved. These problems are usually a complication of a **urinary tract infection** but can be related to other problems.

Demographics

Chronic kidney infections are more common in infants and young children than they are in adults, often because of a structural problem in the urinary tract that is resolved later. It is estimated that up to 40% of children with UTIs have this structural anomaly, which allows bacteria to access the upper urinary tract.

Acute pyelonephritis is diagnosed about 250,000 times each year. Women with this condition outnumber men by about 5:1.

Etiology: What Happens?

The simplest form of kidney infection is one in which bacteria have moved from the lower urinary tract (urethra and bladder) into the upper urinary tract (ureters and kidneys). In this situation, the pathogen is nearly always *Escherichia coli*. More complex infections involve structural anomalies, urethral blockage, **pregnancy**, **diabetes**, or a neurogenic bladder (a bladder that has no motor control and so empties passively into a bag). Contaminated surgical or medical instruments such as **cystoscopes** and **catheters** can also introduce pathogens into the urinary tract. The causative agent for these complicated situations may be *Pseudomonas*, *Klebsiella*, or many other pathogens.

In some cases, bacteria access the kidneys via the bloodstream, rather than through the urinary tract.

> **Cystoscope:** A thin, lighted tube used to see inside the body with minimal damage.
>
> **Catheter:** A tube inserted into the body in order to drain fluid.
>
> **Sepsis:** An inflammation of the whole body in response to an infection. Can be fatal.
>
> **Vesicoureteral valve:** A valve in the ureters that prevents urine from passing from the bladder back up into the ureters.
>
> **Vesicoureteral reflux:** The flow of urine from the bladder backward into the kidneys.

Types of Pyelonephritis

- *Acute pyelonephritis*: This involves severe symptoms as the kidney is actively and aggressively attacked by bacteria. In some cases, bacteria can invade the capillaries of the kidney to lead to potentially life-threatening **sepsis**.
- *Chronic pyelonephritis*: This is usually the result of an incompletely treated infection. The bacteria continue to grow and destroy kidney tissue, but they do it slowly and silently, with little or no pain. The net result is a risk of permanent damage and lost function due to long-term inflammation and fibrosis.
- When chronic pyelonephritis occurs in children, it is typically related to a structural anomaly at the **vesicoureteral valve**. This condition, called **vesicoureteral reflux**, allows urine to back up into the kidney, which creates a high risk of long-term, silent, cumulative damage.
- *Emphysematous pyelonephritis*: This is a severe, life-threatening form of kidney infection involving necrosis and gas-filled pockets within the working tissues of the kidney. It is most often seen in patients with uncontrolled **diabetes**.

Signs and Symptoms

Acute pyelonephritis usually involves a rapid onset that begins with a UTI and ascends the urinary tract. Symptoms include fever, burning and frequent urination, cloudy and blood-tinged urine, extreme back pain, fatigue, nausea, and vomiting. In elderly patients, cognitive decline and disorientation are sometimes the leading signs of an infection. Symptoms typically develop over a day or two.

Chronic pyelonephritis symptoms in adults are often subtle. Therefore, many chronic kidney infections cause no symptoms, but damage in the kidney accumulates.

Treatment

It is important to treat UTIs to prevent them from complicating to a kidney infection, which can result in permanent scarring, hypertension, and an increased risk for renal failure.

Most kidney infections clear up with antibiotic therapy, but it is important to ensure that the infection has been fully eradicated before ending treatment. If the infection is extreme, the patient may need to be hospitalized. People with pyelonephritis along with diabetes, **spinal cord injury** survivors, and kidney transplant recipients need to be monitored especially closely.

Medications

- Antibiotics for bacterial infection

Massage Therapy Implications

RISKS	Acute kidney infections contraindicate most types of bodywork, mainly because they are so painful that adding another adaptive challenge could be unpleasant. Chronic renal infections carry less risk, but still require that massage therapists be sensitive to the fact that this client has a compromised ability to process fluid.
BENEFITS	Soothing, gentle massage during a low-grade, silent infection may be supportive but won't have much impact on the infection itself. Clients who have fully recovered from acute or chronic kidney infections can enjoy the same benefits from bodywork as the rest of the population.

Renal Cancer

Definition: What Is It?

Renal cancer is an umbrella term for any type of cancer that begins in kidney tissues. The vast majority of renal cancer cases are renal cell carcinoma (RCC). Synonyms for RCC include renal adenocarcinoma and **hypernephroma**.

Demographics

Renal cancer is diagnosed about 64,000 times a year in this country; men outnumber women with this disease by almost two to one. The average age at diagnosis is about 64 years, but it can certainly appear at a younger age, especially if it is related to an inherited genetic predisposition.

Some 14,000 people die each year from renal cancer, but about 200,000 survivors currently live in the United States.

Etiology: What Happens?

The kidneys are made primarily of epithelial cells, which grow fast, but are also more vulnerable to the genetic mutations that lead to cancer than other types of cells in the body. A layer of protective fat shields the kidneys from trauma. In addition, the kidneys and their adrenal glands are wrapped together by a dense layer of connective tissue called **Gerota fascia**. The fatty layer and Gerota fascia help to support and protect our delicate epithelial filters.

In RCC, cellular mutations in the renal tubules lead to the formation of highly vascularized, aggressive tumors (Figure 10.7). They begin in the renal cortex, but may extend into the renal fat, adrenal glands, the renal vein, and sometimes even the wall of the inferior vena cava. Renal cancer is much more serious when it gets through the Gerota fascia.

Specific causes for RCC have not been identified, but a genetic condition called **von Hippel-Lindau syndrome** is associated with a high risk for the disease. Other risk factors include cigarette smoking (which essentially doubles the chances of developing this disease), obesity, chronic **hypertension**, long-term dialysis, and excessive exposure to cadmium, coke ovens, and asbestos.

Whether a person inherits this condition or experiences a spontaneous genetic mutation, the net result is that their kidneys are prone to excessive cell growth, angiogenesis to support that growth, excellent tumor cell survival, and the tendency for those cells to proliferate and then travel to other parts of the body. RCC metastasizes readily to the lungs, bones, and liver. Staging protocols for renal cancer are covered in Sidebar 10.1.

Hypernephroma: The most common form of cancer of the kidneys.

Gerota fascia: The layer of connective tissue surrounding the kidneys and adrenal glands.

Von Hippel-Lindau syndrome: A genetic condition that increases the risk of several different kinds of cancer.

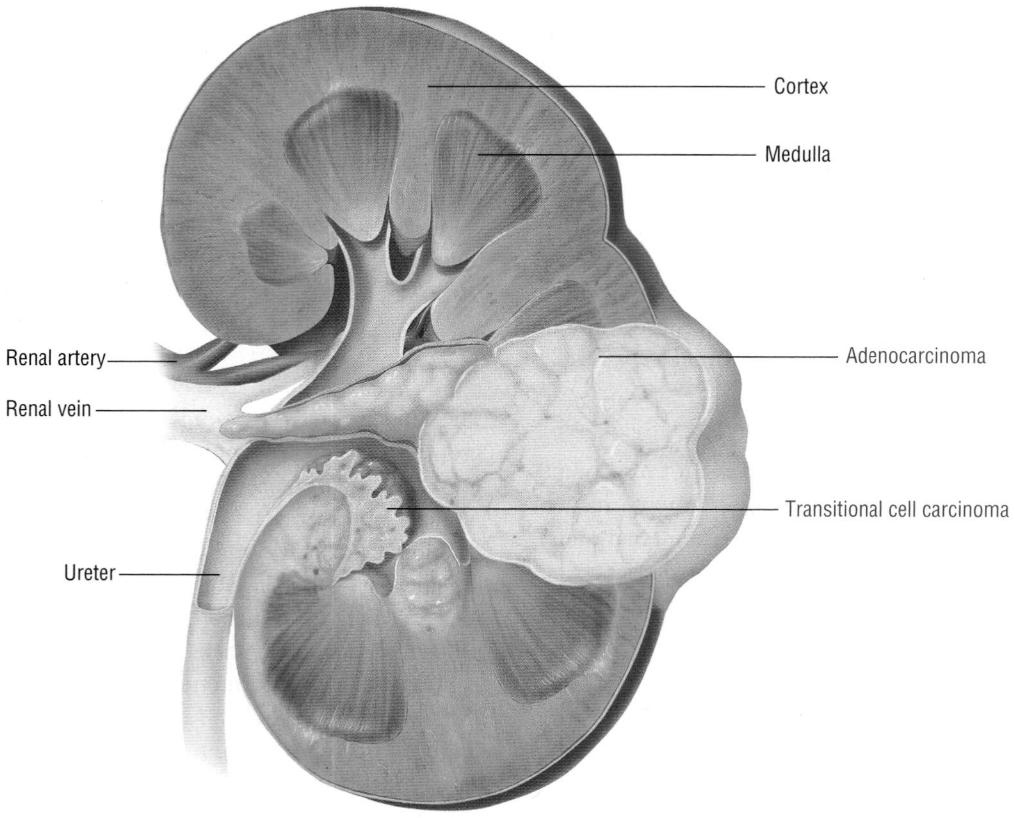

FIGURE 10.7 Renal cell carcinoma

SIDEBAR 10.1 Staging Renal Cancer

The seriousness of renal cancer is identified by whether growths have penetrated through the tough Gerota fascia that encloses the kidneys, renal fat, and adrenal glands. As with many cancers, renal cancer is staged using the TNM classifications and then translating those into stages 0 to IV. These stage identifications are used to identify the best treatment options for patients.

Tumor (T)	Node (N)	Metastasis (M)
Tx: Tumor cannot be assessed	Nx: Node involvement cannot be assessed	Mx: Metastasis cannot be assessed
T0: No evidence of primary tumor in situ	N0: No node involvement	M0: No distant metastasis is found
T1: Tumor is <7 cm, within the kidney.	N1: 1 regional node is involved.	M1: Distant metastasis is found.
T2: Tumor is >7 cm, within the kidney.	N2: More than 1 regional node is involved.	
T3: Tumor invades the renal vein, kidney fat, and/or adrenal glands		

The TNM classifications are translated into stages 0 to IV in this way:

Stage 0	T0, N0, M0
Stage I	T1, N0, M0
Stage II	T2, N0, M0
Stage III	T1–T2, N1, M0 *or* T3, N0–N1, M0
Stage IV	T any, N2, M0, *or* T any, N any, M1

Kidney tumors are also graded 1 through 4 on how much the cancer cells resemble healthy cells. The more the cancer cells look like normal cells, the lower the grade and the better the prognosis.

Types of Renal Cancer

- *Renal cell carcinoma*: This is the main focus of this discussion. It is the most common form of renal cancer, accounting for about 90% of all diagnoses, and it can be due to genetic or environmental influences. Several subtypes of RCC have been identified, each with a particular prognosis and treatment strategy.
- *Transitional cell carcinoma*: This is cancer that arises in the renal pelvis. It is essentially identical to **bladder cancer**, with the same histology, risk factors, and treatment challenges.
- *Wilms tumor*: This is a rare subtype of renal cancer that affects young children, mostly between 2 and 6 years old. It is also called **nephroblastoma**. It is usually found before it metastasizes and responds well to treatment, so the prognosis for this condition is usually very positive.

Signs and Symptoms

One of the distinguishing features of RCC is that it tends not to create any significant symptoms until it is advanced. Symptoms include blood in the urine, a palpable mass in the abdomen, flank pain, unintended weight loss, fever, fatigue, and malaise. In short, most of the signs of RCC mimic those of **polycystic kidney disease** or upper **urinary tract infections**.

Treatment

RCC is treated aggressively to achieve the best results. Surgery is often performed to remove the affected part of a kidney, the whole kidney, or the kidney plus adrenal gland and nearby lymph nodes. **Arterial embolization** may be used to shrink tumors before surgery. If the entire tumor is removed before metastasis, the prognosis for renal cancer is generally very good.

Unfortunately, RCC is resistant to most types of chemotherapy and biologic therapy, so these are not first-line interventions. Instead, drugs that interfere with angiogenesis at the tumor site are used, but they are also associated with a number of side effects that impact the health of the skin and other tissues.

Medications

- Traditional chemotherapy (many cases of renal cancer are resistant)
- Biologic therapies to alter immune system activity (has low success rate)
- Angiogenesis inhibitors to limit tumor growth

> **Nephroblastoma:** A type of kidney cancer that occurs primarily in children. Also called Wilms' tumor.
>
> **Arterial embolization:** A surgical procedure in which an artery is deliberately blocked in order to reduce blood flow to a tumor or other affected area.

Massage Therapy Implications

RISKS	Renal cancer is treated aggressively with drugs and surgery that can be extremely challenging to receive. Some drugs are associated with skin problems, including dry skin, hair loss, hair and skin discoloration, and problems with finger and toenails. Hand-foot syndrome reactions involving redness and peeling on the palms and soles may also happen. Any massage or bodywork choices must respect these challenges.
BENEFITS	Massage has many benefits to offer cancer patients, including reductions in anxiety and pain, better sleep and appetite, improved immune system function, and general improvement in quality of life. For more information on massage in the context of cancer, see Chapter 12.

Renal Failure

Definition: What Is It?

Renal failure means that for various reasons the kidneys are not functioning adequately. If the kidneys slow down suddenly (e.g., in response to shock or systemic infection), it is acute renal failure. If they sustain cumulative damage over the course of many months or years, it is chronic renal failure. In either case, although the name implies that they have ceased functioning altogether, the truth is that the kidneys are still working but they are unable to keep up with the body's demands.

Demographics

Some researchers suggest that as many as 10% of adult Americans (about 26 million people) are in some stage of kidney disease, although it is silent in early stages, so it usually goes undiagnosed. This number is expected to keep rising as the number of senior adults goes up, and our ability to extend the life expectancy of people with kidney disease continues to improve.

The distribution of renal failure is not even. Men develop end stage renal failure (ESRF) more often than women, and African Americans are diagnosed at about four times the rate of Whites. It appears that the per capita number of new cases of ESRF diagnosed each year is beginning to level off for most groups, and among Native Americans, unlike any other ethnic group, it has fallen significantly since about 2000.

Many people are living longer with ESRF, so it is increasingly common especially among people aged 60 and older. Currently, about 900,000 people in the United States are being treated for ESRF. Over 570,000 people are on dialysis, and some 100,000 people are on the transplant waiting list.

Etiology: What Happens?

The kidneys have several important functions: they produce EPO, the hormone that stimulates blood cell production; they manage electrolyte levels in the blood; they concentrate urine; and they control overall fluid levels. Any of these functions may be lost during renal failure. This can lead to **anemia**, peripheral and pulmonary **edema**, **pericarditis** with fluid in the pericardial sac (**cardiac tamponade**), and dangerous changes in circulating levels of calcium, phosphorus, and potassium. This has important effects on bone density, digestive capabilities, the inflammatory process, and heart rhythms. When the kidneys begin to fail, the repercussions can affect any or all of these functions.

Although the kidneys are able to heal from most short-term injury, any chronic or severe recurrent problems may eventually cause permanent damage to the delicate tissues, thereby interfering with kidney function. The two most common contributors to renal failure are long-term **hypertension** and untreated or undertreated **diabetes**. Both of these conditions damage the kidneys by exerting excessive mechanical pressure through the renal arteries, which then focus that pressure into the delicate Bowman capsule. Fortunately, the human body is equipped with 2 million nephrons, about twice as many as we absolutely need, so people can tolerate a lot of damage before problems develop.

To hear more of the author's thoughts on renal failure, visit http://thePoint.lww.com. thePoint®.

NOTABLE CASES Kidney disease has contributed to the deaths of many notable people, including actors Greta Garbo and Laurence Olivier, director and producer Alfred Hitchcock, cookbook author Julia Child, political leaders Ferdinand Marcos and Chiang Kai-shek, writers C.S. Lewis and Norman Mailer, and musicians Art Tatum and Barry White. Currently living celebrities with kidney disease include actors Tracy Morgan, Grizzwald Chapman, and George Lopez and musician Natalie Cole.

The major risk factors for renal failure include age, the presence of diabetes or hypertension, cardiovascular disease, obesity, high cholesterol, lupus, and any family history of kidney disease.

Types of Renal Failure

- *Acute renal failure*: Acute renal failure is also called acute kidney injury. It is identified when kidney function suddenly drops to 50% or less of normal levels; this may take place over several hours or days. It is often a short-term problem that can be corrected, but it can be life threatening. Causes of acute renal failure usually fall into one of three categories (Figure 10.8):
  - Prerenal problems: In this situation, blood flow into the kidneys drops and the nephrons essentially collapse from lack of fluid volume. Causative factors include a blockage in the renal artery, low blood volume (i.e., bleeding out), and blood poisoning followed by shock.
  - Intrinsic problems: These are problems that arise within the kidneys. They include a local infection with *E. coli* (also called **hemolytic uremic syndrome**), drug allergies, an embolism inside the kidney, or others.
  - Postrenal problems: When fluid is prevented from leaving the kidneys, damage to the nephrons can accumulate to dangerous levels. **Kidney stones**, **benign prostatic hypertrophy**, or tumors can create this kind of problem.
- *Chronic renal failure*: Chronic renal failure is also called chronic kidney disease. This describes impairment in kidney function that may persist for months or years before it causes any symptoms. Kidney function is measured in terms of glomerular filtration rate (GFR), that is, how efficiently fluid moves from the glomeruli into the nephrons. Normal GFR is 120 mL/min. Renal failure is a progression along a continuum of lost function and is discussed in these stages:
  - Stage I: Kidney damage is minor, and GFR is above 90 mL/min.

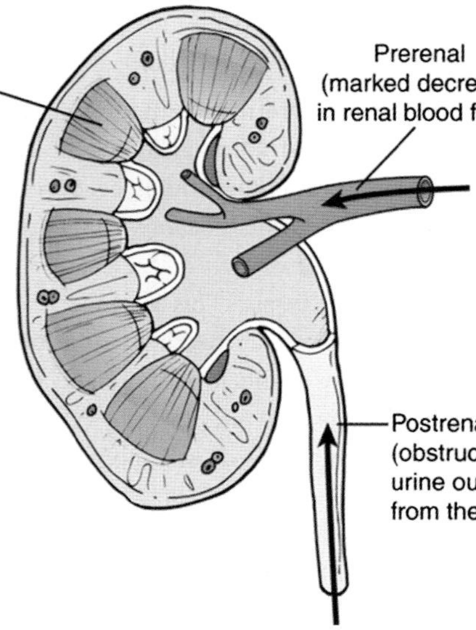

FIGURE 10.8 Acute renal failure: prerenal, intrinsic, or postrenal

Cardiac tamponade: Pathological compression of the heart, related to increased volume of the pericardium.

Hemolytic uremic syndrome: An infection in which red blood cells are destroyed, which in turn damages the kidneys.

- Stage II: Mild reduction in function; GFR is 60 to 89 mL/min.
- Stage III: Moderate reduction in function; GFR is 30 to 59 mL/min; chronic kidney disease is recognized at this stage.
- Stage IV: Severe reduction; GFR is 15 to 29 mL/min; dialysis may be recommended at this stage.
- Stage V: End-stage renal failure; GFR is less than 15 mL/min.

Chronic renal disease may also be diagnosed if the GFR is not abnormal, but if other signs of structural or functional problems are present. These would include abnormal urinalysis, imaging studies, or histological findings, along with symptoms that persist for 3 months or more.

Signs and Symptoms

Because the kidneys have so many functions, symptoms of renal failure affect virtually every major organ system of the body. Symptoms include decreased urine output, systemic and pulmonary edema from salt and water retention, arrhythmia from potassium retention, anemia from the lack of EPO, and osteomalacia from the lack of vitamin D, which is necessary for calcium metabolism. Rashes and skin discoloration arise from retention of toxic pigments in the blood. Other symptoms include lethargy, fatigue, **headaches**, loss of sensation in the hands and feet, **tremors**, **seizures**, easy bruising and bleeding, muscle **cramps**, and changes in mental and emotional states as the accumulation of wastes in the blood affects the brain (Figure 10.9).

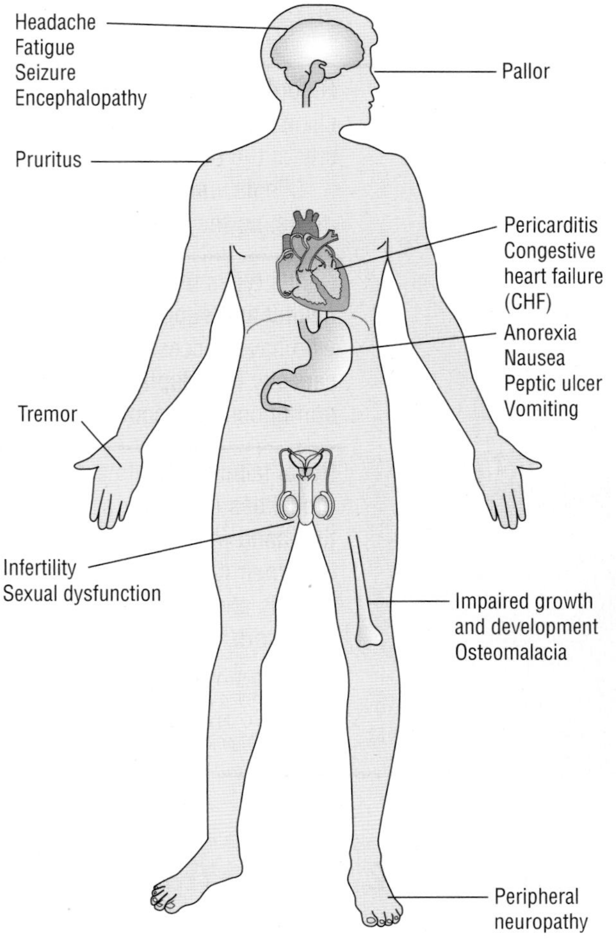

FIGURE 10.9 Effects of renal failure

Treatment

The treatment goal for acute renal failure is to restore renal blood flow as quickly as possible so that a minimum of permanent damage accrues. Treatment goals for chronic renal failure are to control the symptoms, prevent further complications, and slow the progress of the disease. This often means aggressively controlling blood pressure and blood sugar levels (if diabetes is part of the picture). Medication to control potassium and phosphorus levels is important to avoid heart problems. Fluid, protein, and salt intake may be restricted until kidney function can keep up with the body's demands. Diuretics are sometimes prescribed to help the kidneys process fluids.

It is important the people with chronic renal failure avoid taking most NSAIDs, because they can further damage the kidneys. Low-dose aspirin for its antiplatelet action in the context of heart disease is an exception. In addition to putting a greater load on the kidneys, these medications can interfere in the action of other drugs used to treat renal failure.

If a patient's kidneys are simply incompetent regardless of these interventions, dialysis may become necessary. This routes the blood through a machine or through the peritoneum to extract wastes. Dialysis can be a long-term intervention, but for many people, it is a stopgap measure to buy time while hoping for a suitable kidney to become available. For more information on kidney transplants, see Sidebar 10.2.

Medications

- Antihypertensive medication
- Antidiabetes medication, including glucose-lowering drugs and injected insulin
- Diuretics to shed excess fluid if necessary
- Phosphate- and potassium-lowering agents to manage arrhythmia
- EPO-stimulating drugs or analogues for anemia
- Iron salts for anemia

Massage Therapy Implications

RISKS	Rigorous massage is not a good choice for clients with significant renal function loss, and clients undergoing dialysis are at increased risk for infection, especially where the equipment enters the body, so a massage therapist must accommodate this special situation. Clients who have treated renal failure with a kidney transplant also take immunosuppressant drugs, so they are vulnerable to any pathogens carried by a massage therapist.
BENEFITS	Gentle types of massage or bodywork that do not demand a great adaptive change may be helpful and supportive for a person who is going through a very difficult process. Clients who have successfully undergone a transplant may receive any bodywork that is within their capacity for adaptation and that respects the fact that they are committed to a lifetime of immunosuppressant drugs.
RESEARCH	Renal failure patients are not good candidates for rigorous full body massage, but some modalities may offer some helpful benefits. Patients with serious pruritus during dialysis found that hand massage with some specific aromatherapy ingredients in the oil helped significantly with their itching.[1] An earlier study looked at acupressure with massage for ESRF patients on dialysis and found that their fatigue and depression scores were significantly improved with the bodywork.[2] 1. Shahgholian N, Dehghan M, Mortazavi M, et al. Effect of aromatherapy on pruritus relief in hemodialysis patients. *Iranian Journal of Nursing and Midwifery Research* 2010;15(4):240–244. http://www.ncbi.nlm.nih.gov/pmc/articles/PMC3203284/ 2. Cho YC, Tsay SL. The effect of acupressure with massage on fatigue and depression in patients with end-stage renal disease. *Journal of Nursing Research* 2004;12(1):51–59. http://www.ncbi.nlm.nih.gov/pubmed/15136963

SIDEBAR 10.2 Kidney Transplants: Many are Hopeful; Few are Chosen

The urinary system has about twice the capacity for urine production that any person actually needs. This is good news indeed, because it means that if it is necessary, we can get along with just one healthy kidney.

Kidney transplants replace a damaged organ with a healthy kidney from an appropriate donor. Transplants from living donors tend to have higher success rates than those from deceased donors, and the process of being a donor is safer and less intrusive than it used to be.

The new kidney is surgically implanted low in the abdomen, and the nonworking kidneys are usually left in place. Most kidney transplants use organs donated from people who have died, but if a good match is found, a kidney can be donated by a close relative or loved one.

Unfortunately, the shortage of suitable donated organs means that among the 100,000 people waiting for kidney transplants this year, only about 14,000 operations will be performed: 9,300 from deceased donors and 4,700 from living donors. Patients often wait several years for a match, and their ability to cope with surgery is impaired as they age. Almost 5,000 people on the waiting list die each year.

Bladder and Urinary Tract Disorders

Bladder Cancer

Definition: What Is It?

Bladder cancer is the growth of malignant cells in the urinary bladder. Transitional cells are most often affected. For this reason, the term **urothelial carcinoma** can refer to cancer that begins in the urinary bladder or in the transitional cells of the renal pelvis, ureters, or urethra. Urothelial carcinoma is by far the most common form of bladder cancer seen in the United States and is the main focus of this discussion.

Demographics

Bladder cancer is the sixth most common cancer in the United States, diagnosed in about 75,000 people each year, and causing about 15,000 deaths. Whites and smokers are

Urothelial carcinoma: A cancer of the kidneys, ureters, bladder, and urethra.

affected more often than other groups. It is usually a disease of mature people; the median age at diagnosis is 68 years. Men develop bladder cancer more often than women, at a ratio of about 3:1.

Etiology: What Happens?

Like most types of cancer, bladder cancer usually involves epithelial cells, in this case, the transitional epithelium that lines the urinary bladder. Because the kidneys filter environmental irritants out of the blood and into the urine, this delicate tissue is often bathed in toxic chemicals. Constant repetitive damage causes the mature cells to die. This stimulates rapid replication in the basal layer, and colonies of immature cells then migrate to the surface. These new cells are easily disrupted by genetic mutations and may become malignant growths that cause bleeding into the bladder.

Causes of bladder cancer vary according to medical history and geographic region. Persons who have undergone pelvic radiation for other problems are at an increased risk for developing bladder cancer, as are people who have had chronic infections, **bladder stones**, or catheter use. One type of chemotherapy used for **lymphoma** has been identified as a possible cause. In some developing countries, bladder cancer is associated with a parasitic infestation, **Schistosoma haematobium**.

Several genetic mutations that limit the body's ability to inhibit tumor growth or invasion have been linked to bladder cancer. These mutations are frequently triggered by exposure to carcinogenic substances or previous exposure to radiation in the pelvic area. In the United States and Europe, approximately half of bladder cancer cases are believed to be related to cigarette smoking. Other triggers include exposure to arsenic and workplace chemicals.

Most bladder cancer diagnoses are made when the cells affect only superficial layers of tissue. This is excellent news, because the survival rate for cancers caught early is much better than for cancers caught in stage III or later. Nevertheless, bladder cancer has an unusual habit of growing in several places and at different speeds all at the same time, so although it may be possible to catch one or two tumors, the invisible third, fourth, and fifth tumors may not become symptomatic for another several months (Figure 10.10). This means that the recurrence rate for bladder cancer is high: up to 80% of patients have at least one recurrence.

Two main types of bladder cancer tumors occur. Papillary bladder cell tumors are wart-like and attached to a stalk. Nonpapillary tumors are embedded in the bladder wall. These are less common, but more likely to become invasive.

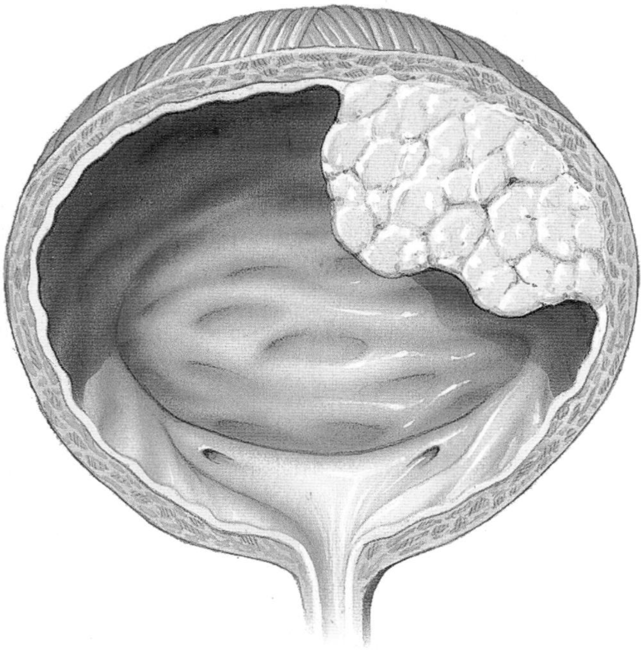

FIGURE 10.10 Bladder cancer.

Schistosoma haematobium: A parasitic flatworm that can infect the urinary system of humans.

Types of Bladder Cancer

- *Transitional cell carcinoma*: This accounts for about 90% of all bladder cancer diagnoses in the United States.
- *Squamous cell carcinoma*: This accounts for about 8% of diagnoses in the United States, but in developing countries, it is the most common type of bladder cancer. It can be caused by infection with Schistosoma.
- *Other types of bladder cancer*: Small cell carcinoma and adenocarcinoma of the bladder account for 1% to 2% of bladder cancer cases in the United States.

Signs and Symptoms

The earliest and most dependable sign of bladder cancer is hematuria. The urine of a bladder cancer patient is often visibly reddened or rust colored, although the patient has no particular pain in the early stages of the disease. If the tumors continue to grow and invade deeper layers of the bladder, secondary symptoms may develop. These are the result of mechanical pressure, including bladder irritability

NOTABLE CASES Bladder cancer has claimed many well-known personalities. Actors Jack Lemmon and Telly Savalas had this disease, as did Oz's scarecrow Ray Bolger, jazz pianist Mary Lou Williams, and singer Andy Williams.

10 Urinary System Conditions

SIDEBAR 10.3 Staging Bladder Cancer

Bladder cancer is staged with the traditional TNM classifications. Here is a simplified version:

Tumor (T)	Node (N)	Metastasis (M)
Ta: Noninvasive papillary tumor	Nx: Nodes cannot be assessed.	Mx: Metastasis cannot be assessed.
Tis (cancer in situ): Noninvasive flat, nonpapillary cells	N0: No nodes involved.	M0: No metastasis found.
T1: Cancer cells invaded urothelium but not muscle tissue	N1: One pelvic node involved; cells <2 cm	M1: Distant metastasis to organs or bones
T2: Cancer cells invaded muscle tissue	N2: 2 or more pelvic nodes are involved.	
T3: Cancer cells invade through muscular wall into connective tissue and exterior fat	N3: Nodes along the iliac artery are involved.	
T4: Cancer cells invade other tissues, including the prostate, uterus, pelvic wall, or abdominal wall.		

These delineations are translated to stages 0 to IV in this way:

Stage 0a	Ta, N0, M0
Stage 0 IS	T IS, N0, M0
Stage I	T1, N0, M0
Stage II	T2, N0, M0
Stage III	T3 or T4, N0, M0
Stage IV	T4, N0, M0; or any T, N3, M0; or any T, any N, M1

Bladder cancer cells are also graded according to their resemblance to normal cells. A lower grade (with cells that look like healthy cells) usually predicts a more positive outcome than a higher grade of cancer cell.

(painful urination, increased urinary frequency, reduced urine output) and compression on the rectum, pelvic lymph nodes, and any other structures that happen to be in the way.

Treatment

Bladder cancer treatment depends on the stage at diagnosis. See Sidebar 10.3 for bladder cancer staging protocols.

Surgeons can use a cystoscope and a variety of tools to remove abnormal tissue. More invasive surgeries may remove part or all of the bladder, and if signs of pelvic metastasis are present, other tissues as well. Men may lose the prostate gland; women may lose the uterus, ovaries, and parts of the vaginal wall. Pelvic lymph nodes are also removed, leading to the risk of lymphedema in the legs. Urine flow may be routed out of the body through a stoma, or a variety of surgeries have been developed to form artificial bladders from parts of the large or small intestines.

In addition to surgery, radiation therapy and chemotherapy may be used to treat bladder cancer. Chemotherapy may be administered intravenously, orally with pills, or through a site-specific bladder wash to distribute the medication directly to the target tissues.

Biologic therapies involve introducing substances into the bladder that stimulate immune system responses. The bacille Calmette-Guérin vaccine (sometimes used for **tuberculosis**) is successful in many cases. In other situations, interferon or other substances may be used.

Administering medication by bladder wash is most effective in combination with surgery to remove cancerous cells. After bladder cancer treatment is completed, it is especially important to be diligent about follow-up care because this cancer recurs in most patients.

Medications

- Chemotherapeutic agents intravenously, orally, or by bladder wash
- Biologic therapy by bladder wash to trigger immune system activity against cancer cells

Massage Therapy Implications

RISKS	Because bladder cancer has a high rate of recurrence, patients often undergo surgery in early stages. This may leave them with stomas, catheters, or other medical devices that must be accommodated for.
BENEFITS	The benefits of massage for bladder cancer patients are the same as those for any kind of cancer patients. While bodywork can promote pain reduction, anxiety reduction, and general support, massage therapists must work as part of a team, sharing information and concerns with the rest of the client's health care staff. A client who has successfully treated his bladder cancer can enjoy the benefits of any type of bodywork that is within his capacity for adaptation. More information on massage in the context of cancer can be found in Chapter 12.

Interstitial Cystitis

Definition: What Is It?

Interstitial cystitis (IC) is a condition in which the urinary bladder becomes irritated and inelastic. IC is often discussed as a part of a group of bladder issues referred to as painful bladder syndrome or bladder pain syndrome. These may also be connected to chronic pelvic pain syndrome, which is described as a subtype of **prostatitis**. One of these labels is usually used when a person has pelvic pain, but other causes of bladder discomfort like **bladder stones** or infection have been ruled out.

Demographics

This condition primarily affects women around age 40, but it has been seen in men and children as well. It is difficult to estimate how common it is because a universally agreed-upon definition of IC as it relates to chronic pelvic pain syndrome and painful bladder syndrome has yet to be found.

Some estimates suggest that about 1.2 million women and 82,000 men could be living with these conditions in this country.

Etiology: What Happens?

The bladder, as a hollow organ, shrinks when it is empty and expands when it is full. A healthy bladder can hold 8 to 12 oz. of urine. Normal urine is composed of water, excess salts and hormones extracted from the blood, nitrogenous wastes such as urea and uric acid, and other debris. It should not contain significant numbers of microorganisms. Protective mucous membranes shield the internal bladder wall from the acidity of urine.

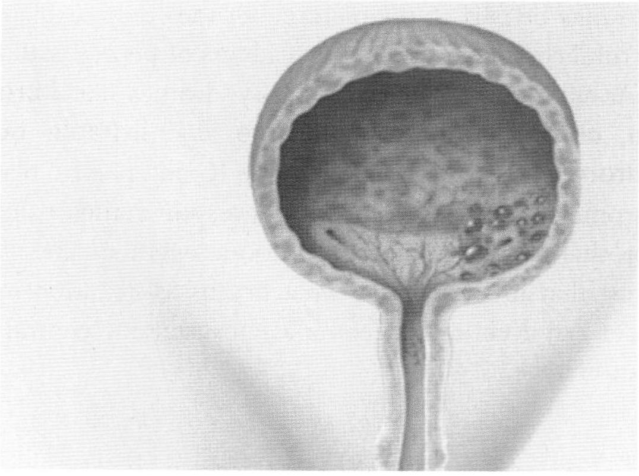

FIGURE 10.11 Interstitial cystitis: The bladder walls thicken and small hemorrhages develop in the lining.

IC occurs when the inner lining of the bladder no longer protects the organ from acidity. Many IC patients develop tiny bleeding areas called pinpoint hemorrhages or **glomerulations** in the bladder wall. About 10% of patients develop a deeper lesion called a **Hunner ulcer** inside the bladder. As the problem progresses, the muscular walls of the bladder become fibrotic and inelastic; this is especially true for people with Hunner ulcers. Patients find that they have little capacity for storing urine, even if their bladder is a normal size (Figure 10.11), and the bladder neck spasms, making urination difficult. It is common for IC patients to have to use the bathroom many times each day and all through the night.

The cause of IC is a mystery. One hypothesis is that this may be an autoimmune disease or allergy that weakens the protective mucous membrane in the bladder's epithelium. In this way, irritating chemicals from urine can infiltrate and damage the bladder wall. The presence of abnormal numbers of mast cells in some IC patients supports this idea. A pathologic thinning of the mucous membrane on the bladder wall is another factor to consider. IC does not respond to antibiotic therapy, so it is clear that no known strain of bacteria causes this problem. Other hypotheses suggest a neurological hypersensitivity to bladder fullness or trigger points in the perineum muscle that may refer pain into the pelvis.

Glomerulation: A tiny hemorrhage of the bladder.

Hunner ulcer: A star-shaped lesion in the wall of the bladder.

These may be part of the picture, but they don't explain the structural changes found in the bladders of people with IC.

As with some other chronic syndromes like **fibromyalgia**, **chronic fatigue syndrome**, and **irritable bowel syndrome**, it seems clear that some IC and painful bladder syndrome patients experience a progression in their pain sensation that can alter pain perception altogether. This would suggest that in these cases what begins as irritation in the bladder can eventually become a self-sustaining central sensitization issue.

Signs and Symptoms

Symptoms of IC include chronic pelvic pain, pain and burning on urination, increased urinary frequency and urgency, and painful intercourse. Symptoms are worst when the bladder is full, and they abate somewhat when the bladder is empty. Menstruation can exacerbate symptoms. Some patients find that symptoms occur in periods of flare and remission; others find that their daily experiences are all about the same.

Treatment

Because IC is a disease without a known cause, it is also without a known cure. IC treatment is generally aimed at symptomatic relief and the development of coping skills. Often, the diagnostic tool of bladder distension can give temporary relief, as can an **instillation**, or bladder wash. This is sometimes done with dimethylsulfoxide (DMSO), which can pass into the bladder wall to act as an anti-inflammatory and to block pain sensation. Lesions on the bladder wall may be removed with lasers or electrical wires. An oral medication to help repair the mucous lining has been approved, but it may take several months to be effective, and some patients don't respond to this intervention. Aspirin and other painkillers may be recommended, as are exercise, smoking cessation, and dietary changes to avoid highly acidic foods and drinks. Antidepressants can be effective pain modulators. Various nerve-stimulating devices may provide symptomatic relief. No single intervention is successful for all patients, and nothing has yet provided a permanent solution. IC may recur after months or even years of remission.

Some patients have such severe problems that surgery becomes an option. They may have a new bladder constructed from a segment of the colon, or they may have the bladder removed altogether and replaced with a stoma and external bag.

Medications

- Pentosan polysulfate sodium to help rebuild the bladder lining
- Bladder instillation with DMSO or other medications
- Analgesics, antidepressants, or antiseizure drugs for pain management

> **Instillation (bladder wash):** A medical procedure in which medication is administered directly into the bladder with a catheter.

Massage Therapy Implications

RISKS	The primary challenge for IC or irritable bladder patients who want to receive a massage is that they may need to interrupt the session to use the bathroom. If accommodations can be made for this, massage holds little risk for this clientele.
BENEFITS	Massage may be a useful intervention for the goal of relieving stress and anxiety, although it will probably have little direct effect on bladder irritation. Specific and educated touch to the lower abdomen with the intention of promoting freedom of movement between the organs may be helpful for bladder irritation, if the client can welcome the work. A person in remission from IC can enjoy all the benefits of massage as the rest of the population.
OPTIONS	A client with an external bag to act as a urine reservoir requires special positioning and care not to disrupt the stoma or the device. Consult with the client for best options.
RESEARCH	Myofascial work and other manual therapies for IC and pelvic pain have some evidence for a positive effect on pain, urgency, and frequency in IC patients.[1–4] Some of these studies are in the context of physical therapy and trigger point work on the perineum, which is not in the scope of massage therapy, but they yield useful information for interested massage therapists. 1. Gerald MP, Payne CK, Lukacz ES, et al. Randomized multicenter clinical trial of myofascial physical therapy in women with interstitial cystitis/painful bladder syndrome and pelvic floor tenderness. *Journal of Urology* 2012;187(6):2113–2118. http://www.ncbi.nlm.nih.gov/pmc/articles/PMC3351550/ 2. Oyama IA, Rejba A, Lukban JC, et al. Modified Thiele massage as therapeutic intervention for female patients with interstitial cystitis and high-tone pelvic floor dysfunction. *Urology* 2004;64(5):862–865. http://www.ncbi.nlm.nih.gov/pubmed/15533464. 3. Weiss JM. Pelvic floor myofascial trigger points: manual therapy for interstitial cystitis and the urgency-frequency syndrome. *Journal of Urology* 2001;166(6):2226–2231. http://www.ncbi.nlm.nih.gov/pubmed/11696740 4. Webster DC, Brennan T. Self-care strategies used for acute attack of interstitial cystitis. *Urologic Nursing* 1995;15(3):86–93. http://www.ncbi.nlm.nih.gov/pubmed/7481892

Urinary Tract Infection

Definition: What Is It?

A UTI is an infection that may occur anywhere in the lower urinary system. This discussion focuses on infections of the lower urinary tract, that is, the urethra (urethritis) and the bladder (cystitis).

Demographics

About one-half of all women have a UTI at least once. These are among the most common infections, leading to 6 to 8 million doctor visits each year in this country. They are most common among women, especially ages 20 to 40.

When men have a UTI, it is often a warning sign of a prostate problem or a sexually transmitted infection.

Etiology: What Happens?

Under normal circumstances, the environment in the bladder is essentially sterile. The urine contains waste products to be expelled from the body, but few or no living microorganisms should be present. Furthermore, the bladder is lined with a protective mucus-producing layer of cells that works to prevent infectious or noxious agents from harming the bladder walls.

Sometimes, foreign microorganisms are introduced into the urethra. *E. coli* are the causative agent behind close to 90% of UTIs. These strains of bacteria live normally and harmlessly in the digestive tract, but they can damage the urinary tract. Other pathogens can invade as well, but they are not typical. It is important to identify the correct causative agent, because not all of them respond to the same antibiotics.

UTIs are almost always a women's disorder, because the female urethra is short and close to the anus. People who must drain their bladder with a catheter are also at increased risk for UTI.

Chronic irritation can also contribute to the development of UTIs. "Honeymoon cystitis" is inflammation and subsequent infection brought about by repeated irritation of the urethra from sexual activity.

Some women are more susceptible to UTIs than others, although the reasons for this are not completely clear; they may have to do with immune system differences and shortages of certain types of antibodies. Some factors, however, are reliable predictors of who is at risk for developing a UTI:

- Spermicide use: Spermicide foams and jellies used with a diaphragm or alone have been shown to raise the risk of UTIs in some women.
- Diaphragm use: Women who use a diaphragm show statistically higher rates of UTIs than women who do not.
- Pregnancy: Pregnant women do not necessarily get more UTIs than women who are not pregnant, but the risk of having a simple infection complicate into a more dangerous one is higher for these patients.
- Diabetes: Elevated sugar levels in the urine make a hospitable environment for bacteria to grow in the bladder.
- Neurogenic bladder: A **neurogenic bladder** has lost motor function and does not empty as completely as a normal one. This raises the potential for infection, as does the presence of catheter tubes, which are used for people with limited bladder function.

If the bacteria that invade the urethra and bladder are able to travel up the ureters, they may complicate into a **kidney infection**. Chronic UTIs with progressive damage to the kidneys may contribute to chronic **renal failure**. Untreated kidney infections can also lead to the release of infectious bacteria in the blood and life-threatening septicemia.

Unfortunately, not all UTIs show symptoms, so they may be neglected, especially in children. It is possible for some people to have complications of this type of infection that can easily lead to permanent kidney damage or even to death.

Some basic precautions can help prevent UTIs, especially for women who are especially vulnerable to them. These include drinking lots of water and acidic juices, urinating whenever necessary rather than holding it for a more convenient time, wiping from front to back after a bowel movement to prevent the introduction of digestive bacteria into the urethra, taking showers rather than baths, emptying the bladder after sex, and avoiding feminine hygiene sprays and douches, which can aggravate the urethra.

Signs and Symptoms

The symptoms of UTIs are painful, burning urination; a frequent need to urinate; reduced bladder capacity; urinary urgency; and blood-tinged or cloudy urine. Pelvic, abdominal, or low back pain may also occur. Men with UTIs may have pain in the penis or scrotum. If severe flank or back pain and high fever develop, a kidney infection should be suspected.

Treatment

Many women find that blueberries and cranberries help to prevent UTIs; these berries contain chemicals that limit the ability of bacteria to cling to bladder walls. It is important, however, to avoid sweetened juice; the amount of sugar it takes to make cranberry juice sweet may actually make the bladder a more hospitable environment for infection. It is also important to realize that this is a preventive measure for UTI, but not an effective treatment option.

The first step in self-treatment of a UTI is to drown it: radically increasing fluid intake gives the body the much needed opportunity to fully and frequently empty the bladder—not

Neurogenic bladder: A condition in which there is a lack of motor control over the process of urination.

only of urine, but of bacteria as well. In subacute infection, hydrotherapy in the form of hot and cold **sitz baths** may be recommended.

UTIs usually respond well to antibiotics. With bladder infections, as with all types of bacterial infections, it is important to take the full prescription. Stopping too soon may result in recurrent infections with resistant bacteria, or it may allow the bacteria to invade the urinary tract further to lead to a much more potentially dangerous kidney infection. Antibiotics are often given along with a urinary painkiller.

People who have low-grade, chronic UTIs that do not clear up with normal treatments are sometimes successfully treated with long-term low doses of antibiotics. Structural problems with the way urine drains from the bladder may contribute to chronic infections; surgery may be recommended to correct these problems.

Sitz bath: A bath in which only the hips and buttocks are immersed, leaving the legs outside the tub.

Medications

- Antibiotics for bacterial infection
- Analgesics for pain management

Massage Therapy Implications

RISKS	UTIs are uncomfortable and, when acute, may involve fever and malaise. Clients may not be comfortable on a table for a full session in this state. Further, any but the most gentle bodywork is probably not welcome at this time.
BENEFITS	Noninvasive bodywork may be soothing during an infection, and any client who has fully recovered from a UTI can enjoy the same benefits from massage as the rest of the population.

Explore and Apply

LEVEL 1: Receive and Respond

1. What connects the kidneys to the bladder?
   a. Urethra
   b. Ureters
   c. Loop of Henle
   d. Bowman capsule

2. What happens inside the Bowman capsule?
   a. Plasma is pushed from the circulatory capillaries into the nephrons
   b. Urine is pushed from the renal pelvis into the bladder
   c. Plasma is reabsorbed by the loop of Henle
   d. Urine is filtered of hormonal wastes

3. What is the component found in the most common type of kidney stone?
   a. Phosphorus
   b. Cystine
   c. Oxalate
   d. Calcium

4. What is the best description of polycystic kidney disease?
   a. The result of long-term chronic renal infection
   b. The presence of multiple infected abscesses on the kidneys
   c. A genetic anomaly that causes hollow pockets in the kidneys
   d. A subtype of renal cancer that causes the formation of hollow tumors

5. Renal cancer has the best prognosis when it...
   a. Penetrates the Gerota fascia
   b. Is limited to the renal cortex
   c. Metastasizes to the lungs instead of the liver
   d. Encounters the layer of protective renal fat

6. What is another name for a bladder infection?
   a. Interstitial cystitis
   b. UTI
   c. Ureteritis
   d. Pyelonephritis

LEVEL 2: Application of Concepts

1. Your client has been diagnosed with end-stage renal failure. You work with him very gently during his appointments at the dialysis center. One day, you notice that he seems especially pale, and he complains of greater-than-normal fatigue. What may be happening?
   a. His liver is overloaded with toxins
   b. He is anemic due to lack of EPO
   c. He has encephalopathy from too many circulating toxins
   d. His spleen is at risk for rupture

2. Your new client is a young man who complains of sudden "grabbing pain" on one side in his midback. It comes in waves, but never goes away. It started 2 days ago, and it is beginning to refer into his groin. He's never had this before, and he assumes he strained his back playing Frisbee. As you interview him, he has a wave of pain that leaves him pale and sweating. It is clearly excruciating. What is your best strategy?
   a. Treat him normally and monitor his results
   b. Give only light massage to avoid exacerbating a problem
   c. Refer him to a chiropractor for a lumbar adjustment
   d. Delay his treatment until he has seen a doctor

3. Your client reports that he uses diuretics. What does this suggest?
   a. He has a problem shedding excess fluid; he is prone to edema
   b. He has a problem retaining fluid; he is prone to dehydration
   c. He has a problem filtering fluid; he is prone to toxicity
   d. He has a problem with digestion; he is prone to constipation

4. Your 62-year-old client reports midsession that her urine is rust colored, but that she has no pain on urination. She wants your advice on what to do. What is the best choice?
   a. Terminate the session and call her a cab to get to the hospital
   b. Finish the session as usual and encourage her to visit her doctor soon
   c. Finish the session as usual and suggest that she take cranberry pills for her urinary tract infection
   d. Inform her that she may have bladder cancer and needs to consult an oncologist as soon as possible

Explore and Apply (continued)

5. Your client has interstitial cystitis. What accommodation is most likely to be needed?
   a. She will probably need to use the restroom during the session
   b. She will not be able to tolerate massage to her abdomen
   c. She will probably have limited capacity for circulatory massage
   d. She will have a neurogenic bladder and a high risk of infection

Note to educators: Due to space considerations, these review questions only address the most important material from Chapter 11. The Test Bank provides a much more comprehensive selection of questions, all of which are keyed to the relevant chapter objectives.

What Would *You* Do?

A Kidney Donor

Your new client Antonia is a recent kidney donor; her surgery was 5 weeks ago. She is 42 and generally healthy, but she is having a lot of pain and fatigue and is hoping that a massage might help her regain her presurgery energy and activity level.

Make a list of questions that you need to ask to establish whether the massage that you practice is safe for this client. Use credible resources to gather other information about kidney donors and their recovery process that might inform your choices. Share your conclusions with a classmate.

A Client Facing a Bladder Cancer Diagnosis

Your long-time client Dennis is a 76-year-old retired factory worker, who is nervous and upset. He is being tested for bladder cancer tomorrow, largely because you encouraged him to tell his doctor about his symptoms. Now, he is hoping for an appointment that might help him relax before his ordeal.

What concerns do you have about working with Dennis today? Can you design a session that is safe for him and you? What would that look like?

At the Dialysis Center

You have volunteered to work at an outpatient dialysis facility where patients with ESRF are treated. The staff introduces you to Rick, a 56-year-old man on disability because he has lost one leg below the knee and ½ of the other foot due to diabetes. Rick is about 80 pounds overweight and a heavy smoker; the smell is very obvious. His hands are grimy, and he has a heavy, phlegmy cough.

You have agreed to offer a 30-minute gentle massage while he is receiving his dialysis treatment. Because of his foot situation, you will be working with his arms and hands and possibly his head and neck.

Make a list of any questions you want to ask. Whom will you ask—the staff or Rick?

Also, pay attention to whatever reactions and personal responses you have about working with Rick. Do you have any concerns? How can they be answered? When you discuss this prospective client with other students, are their reactions similar to yours?

Suggested Activities

1. For each condition covered in your curriculum, write down the following on a card:
   - A brief definition
   - Most common cause or contributing factor(s)
   - Major signs and symptoms
   - Risks and benefits of massage therapy
     - Variables that contribute to risks and benefits
     - Appropriate adaptations

   Use these as flash cards as you study.
2. For each condition covered in your curriculum, write one multiple-choice question. Share your questions with your classmates as you study together.
3. Quiz yourself using either the "labels off" feature in your enhanced e-book or the labeling exercise on thePoint® for Figures 10.1 and 10.2, be sure you can label each of the following: For Figure 10.1 Kidneys, Ureters, and Urinary bladder. For Figure 10.2 Bowman capsule, Glomerulus, and Collecting tubule.
4. In the student resources on thePoint®, find the labeling exercise, "Diseases of the Urinary Tract." Using the "labels off" function, identify the following problems:
   - Staghorn calculus
   - Small kidney stones
   - Acute renal failure
   - Renal artery stenosis
   - Adenocarcinoma
   - Transitional cell carcinoma (pelvis)
   - Transitional cell carcinoma (ureter)
   - Transitional cell carcinoma (bladder)
5. Use the student resources on thePoint® to find practice quiz questions and games.

11

Reproductive System Conditions

CHAPTER 11 / Abbreviated Chapter Objectives

Having completed assignments and classroom time related to Chapter 11, the learner is expected to be able to…

- Identify definitions of the key terms in the introduction and those connected to the conditions covered in your curriculum.
- Label the parts of the female and male reproductive systems.
- Name two sources of the hormones that govern the female reproductive cycle.
- Describe the pathway of an ovum from beginning to end (in the absence of a pregnancy).
- Identify the location where most ova are fertilized.
- Explain why the testes are located outside the pelvic cavity.
- Describe the pathway of a sperm cell from generation to ejaculation.
- Name the male organ that is most often involved in reproductive system disorders.
- Provide the following information for each condition covered in your curriculum:
  - Identify the definition of the condition.
  - List the most common causes or contributing factors to the condition.
  - List major signs and symptoms of the condition.
  - Identify possible risks and benefits of massage therapy, with:
    - Variables that contribute to risks and benefits
    - Appropriate adaptations for massage therapy

For detailed chapter objectives for each condition in this chapter, consult the student resource page at http://thePoint.lww.com/Werner6e. thePoint®

Introduction

Massage therapists are often short changed in their education about the reproductive system. This may be because of time constraints in the classroom, or the lingering stigma that confuses massage therapy with the sex industry, or a sense that much of this is not relevant to massage therapy practice. While massage is not a treatment of choice for most reproductive system diseases, many clients live with them, and the conditions themselves or their treatment options may have repercussions for bodywork choices.

Another stumbling block within the topic of reproductive system conditions is the perception that two perfectly normal, nonpathological states are often addressed as diseases: pregnancy and menopause. It is important for massage therapists (and other people too!) to understand that these are not diseases, but simply conditions that change the way the body functions. For that reason, massage therapists should be familiar enough with them to know when or if massage is appropriate.

Terminology for structures in the reproductive system can sometimes be confusing. Many resources now label structures by their location or function rather than by their traditional names, which commonly refer to the physicians or anatomists who first recorded them. Thus, fallopian tubes, named after the 16th century anatomist Gabriele Falloppio, may now be called oviducts or uterine tubes, which is more descriptive. Traditional names are still in common use, however. In this chapter, structures will be referred to by both traditional and functional or locational names, so that practitioners educated in either terminology may feel at home.

To hear the author's thoughts on reproductive disorders and massage, go to http://thePoint.lww.com/Werner6e. thePoint®

Function and Structure of the Female Reproductive System

Most of the female reproductive structures are low in the pelvis. In a healthy, nonpregnant woman with no scar tissue or other anomalies, the ovaries are typically behind the upper corners of where the pubic hair starts to grow. They are attached via the ovarian ligament to the uterus (Figure 11.1). The ovaries produce hormones, which are released into the bloodstream, and they release eggs, usually one each month during ovulation, which are released into the peritoneal space.

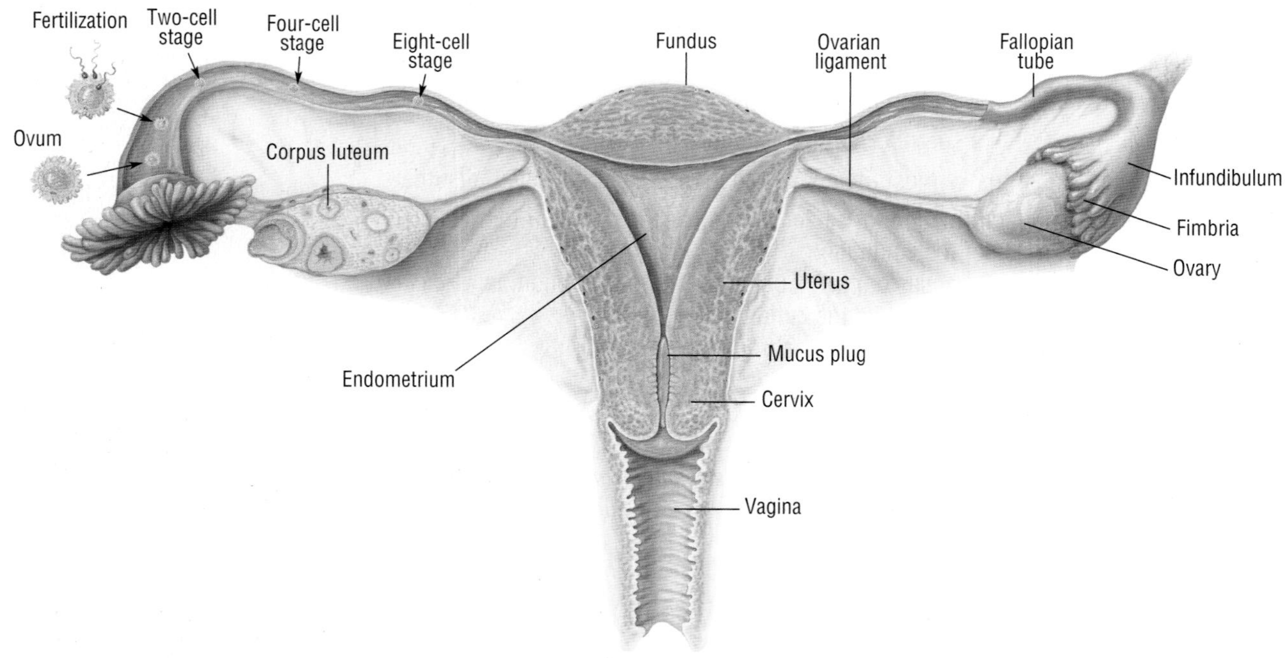

FIGURE 11.1 Female reproductive organs

Mittelschmerz is a German term for "middle pain." It refers to the sensation some women have when the dominant follicle on an ovary ruptures and the egg is released into the pelvic cavity. It is called "middle" because it occurs precisely in the middle (about day 14) of the menstrual cycle.

The **fimbriae** of the fallopian (uterine) tubes gently caress the ovaries, coaxing the released egg toward them. Once inside the tubes, the eggs make the 5-day journey to the uterus itself. If an egg is fertilized, it generally happens inside the uterine tube.

The uterine tubes lead to the uterus: a hollow organ that is built of crisscrossed layers of smooth muscle. The inside surface of the uterus, the **endometrium**, is made of delicate epithelial tissue that holds vast billowy supplies of specialized capillaries to provide a nest for that fertilized egg. If the egg is not fertilized, the uterus sheds the tissue and egg with it in the **menses**. Then, it begins to build a new nest for next month's candidate.

The timing of the ripening and release of eggs from the ovaries, and the building and shedding of the endometrial nest, are under the control of the endocrine system. Hormones secreted from the ovaries themselves and from the pituitary gland determine when and how these various events happen. Birth control pills and other hormonal applications work by introducing artificial hormones into the blood. These trick the pituitary into believing that the woman is always pregnant, so she doesn't ovulate. *To learn more, view the animation "Ovulation" at* http://thePoint.lww.com/Werner6e. thePoint®

Mittelschmerz: Pain upon ovulating.

Fimbriae: The fringe-like projections at the ends of the fallopian tubes (singular: fimbria).

Endometrium: The inner layers of the uterine wall.

Menses: The periodic discharge of blood and tissue from the uterus, usually as a result of ovulation not followed by pregnancy.

Estradiol: An estrogen produced in the ovaries.

Estriol: An estrogen produced in the ovaries, primarily during pregnancy.

Estrone: An estrogen produced in the ovaries that is less potent than estradiol.

Metabolite: Any product of metabolism.

Endogenous: Originating in the body.

Exogenous: Originating outside the body.

The relation between the reproductive system and the endocrine system is extremely tight; the female reproductive cycle is under the control of hormone secretions. Several of the conditions discussed in this chapter could be considered endocrine system disorders, but the tissue changes occur in reproductive system organs, so they are discussed here (Sidebar 11.1).

Female reproductive conditions that have significance for massage therapists generally have to do with growths or local tenderness deep in the abdomen. Although intrusive

SIDEBAR 11.1 What Is This Thing Called Estrogen?

Estrogen is not a single hormone but a group of closely related chemicals that includes **estradiol**, **estriol**, and **estrone**. These chemicals are synthesized from cholesterol primarily in the ovaries during a woman's fertile years. After menopause, they continue to be manufactured in peripheral tissues in much smaller amounts, using root chemicals secreted by the adrenal cortex.

Estrogens act on tissues all over the body. They are associated with sex organ function, but they also influence the growth, health, and activity of many organs, including the bones and heart. They influence cell production and differentiation. Estrogens are also associated with mood swings and emotional responsiveness.

The liver makes estrogens chemically able to stimulate biological activity in their target cells. This metabolism can occur in a variety of ways, with great implications for long-term health. Some "bad" estrogen **metabolites** are associated with tissue proliferation (i.e., cancer) of the breast, uterus, cervix, ovaries, and thyroid. "Good" estrogen metabolites are associated with healthy bone maintenance and cardiovascular protection.

What determines which estrogen metabolites are present in a woman's body? Two main factors are at work here: diet and estrogen exposure.

Diet

High-fat, low-fiber diets provide excessive cholesterol, thereby allowing the body to manufacture more estrogens than it otherwise could. With minimum fiber, fatty diets also prevent the binding of excessive estrogens to the molecules that would inactivate them. And by disrupting the healthy balance of bacteria in the intestines, poor diets allow some estrogens to reenter the circulation.

Estrogen Exposure

People are exposed to estrogen from internal production (**endogenous** estrogens) and external sources (**exogenous** estrogens). Endogenous estrogens have already

(sidebar continues on page 466)

11 Reproductive System Conditions

SIDEBAR 11.1 What Is This Thing Called Estrogen? (Continued)

been discussed as a function of diet and estrogen metabolism. Endogenous estrogen exposure is also increased by obesity, as hyperactive fat cells can contribute to estrogen production. Exogenous estrogen exposure is a topic that has only recently begun to be discussed. Oral birth control pills, hormone replacement therapy (HRT), and hormones in meat and dairy products, along with environmental chemicals such as pesticides, herbicides, plastics, and industrial solvents, all contribute to cumulative endogenous estrogen exposure.

Excessive estrogen exposure and the metabolism of "bad" estrogens have been identified as contributing factors in several cancers of hormone-dependent tissues. In addition, **estrogen dominance** may be a factor in other reproductive system disorders, including **premenstrual syndrome, endometriosis, uterine fibroids,** excessive **menopause** symptoms for women, and **benign prostatic hyperplasia** and **prostate cancer** for men. The good news is that estrogen exposure and metabolism can be influenced by diet and nutrition. Estrogen receptor sites in target tissues can bind with several estrogen-like substances (phytoestrogens, including soy, legumes, and other sources), and some nutritional supplements can help disable free estrogen metabolites before they influence cell proliferation or differentiation. Ultimately, these reproductive system disorders may be treated or even prevented when people take greater control over how much estrogen they are exposed to and how their bodies put that estrogen to use.

Estrogen dominance: A condition in which the ratio of estrogen to progesterone in the body is abnormally high.

Testis, testes: The male reproductive organ that produces sperm cells.

Epididymis: The winding duct that connects the testes to the vas deferens.

Flagellum, flagella: The whip-like "tail" that enables a sperm cell to swim.

Seminiferous tubules: The location in the testes where sperm cells develop.

Vas deferens: The secretory duct of the testicle, along which sperm travel from the testes.

Inguinal ring: The entrance to the inguinal canal, through which the vas deferens passes into the abdomen.

work in the vicinity of the uterus or ovaries is not generally done, sometimes these conditions can displace internal organs, making them vulnerable in places they wouldn't ordinarily be found. Obviously, this calls for special sensitivity on the part of massage therapists who do focused work with the abdomen.

Function and Structure of the Male Reproductive System

The male reproductive system consists of the **testes**, the **epididymis**, the spermatic cord, other glands that contribute to the production of semen, and the urethra, which expels semen through the penis (Figure 11.2). *To review the anatomy, see the animation "Male Reproductive Anatomy" at* http://thePoint.lww.com/Werner6e. thePoint®

Sperm cells are among the smallest of human cells and the only ones equipped with **flagella** for locomotion. They are manufactured in specialized tubes in the testes, the **seminiferous tubules**. Sperm cells grow and mature in the testes. The testes are suspended from the body in the scrotal sac, because sperm cells flourish best when the temperature is slightly lower than internal body temperature. Mature sperm cells are stored in the epididymis, a long tube that is coiled up behind the testes in the scrotum. Sperm cells leave the epididymis through the left and right **vas deferens**, which carries them through the **inguinal ring** into the abdomen. Along the way, other glands, including the seminal vesicles and prostate, contribute to the fluid that suspends and nourishes the sperm on their long journey toward the ovum. The left and right vas deferens join together at the urethra, and sperm leaves the penis via the urethra during ejaculation.

The most common disorders of the male reproductive system have to do with the prostate gland, which is in a position to obstruct the urethra during ejaculation or urination. While prostate massage is a protocol typically conducted by a urologist through the wall of the rectum during an examination (and is therefore outside the scope of practice of massage therapists), prostate problems can seriously diminish a person's quality of life. Consequently, some clients seek bodywork as a coping mechanism while managing their disorders. Massage conducted to maximize the benefits of parasympathetic effect and improve immune system function can be safe and appropriate choice.

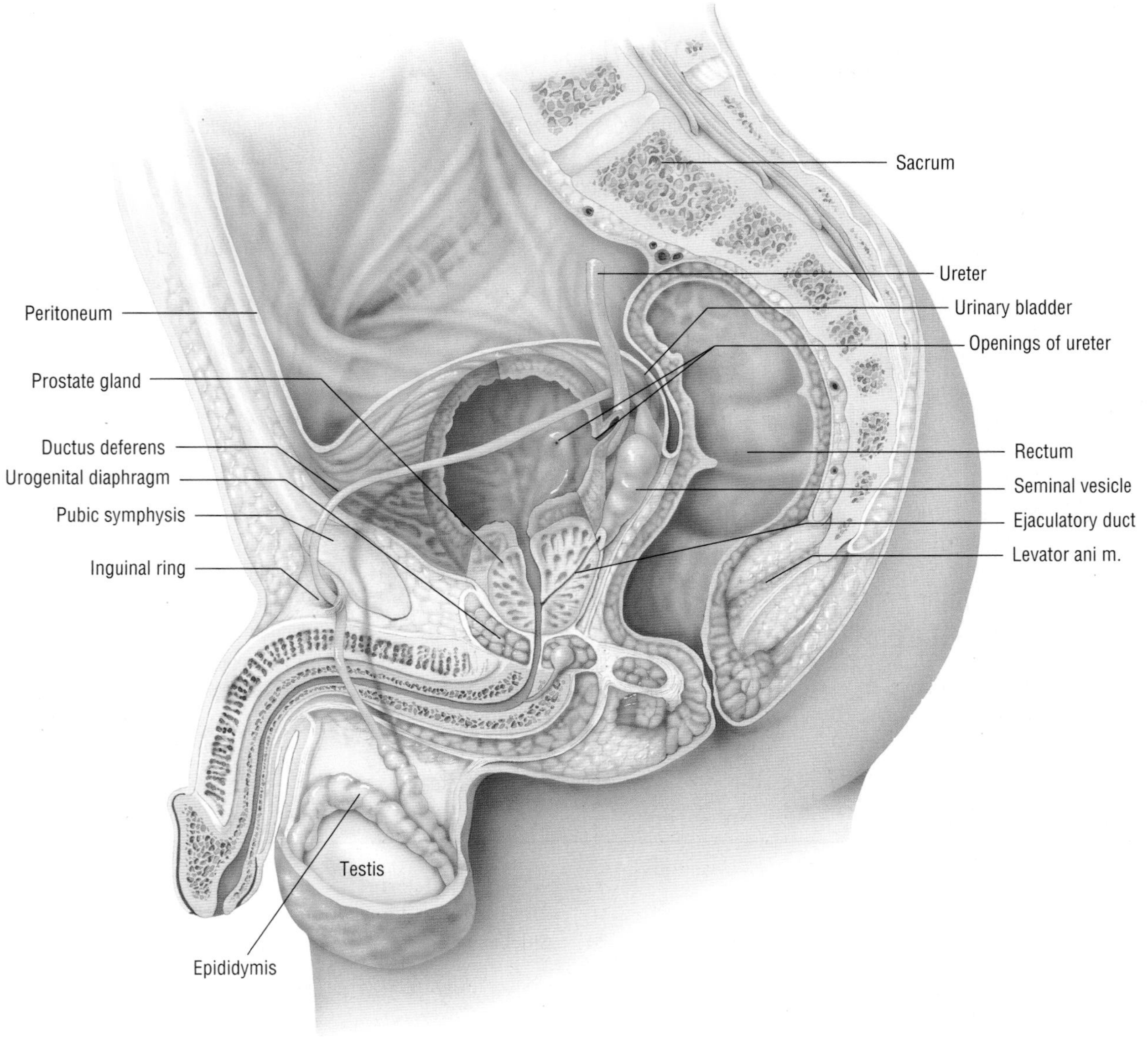

FIGURE 11.2 Male reproductive organs

Massage for Transgender Persons

In this chapter, the conditions are separated into groups according to whether women or men are likely to develop them. This is predicated on the concept that a clear division between what is male and female is obvious. In fact, this division is not always clear. Our sex organs dictate our biological state, but our gender is the product of psychological reality, and many people's gender identities don't completely conform to the bodies with which they were born.

In the context of pathology, this is not a huge issue. If a client has a problem, that problem is the central issue, regardless of whether that client identifies as male, female, or other. Our job in this situation, as in all situations, is to honor the needs of our clients and to create an experience of welcome, safety, and well-being. The unconditional positive regard that comes with being in a helping profession is an attitude that applies to every person, regardless of gender identity.

Reproductive System Conditions

Disorders of the Uterus

- Cervical cancer
  - Squamous cell carcinoma of the cervix
  - Adenocarcinoma of the cervix
  - Other types of cervical cancer
- Dysmenorrhea
  - Primary dysmenorrhea
  - Secondary dysmenorrhea
- Endometriosis
- Fibroid tumors
- Uterine cancer
  - Endometrial cancer
  - Uterine sarcoma

Disorders of Other Female Reproductive Structures

- Breast cancer
  - Ductal carcinoma
  - Lobular carcinoma
  - Inflammatory breast disease
  - Other types of breast cancer
- Ovarian cancer
  - Adenocarcinoma of the ovary
  - Germ cell ovarian cancer
  - Stromal cell ovarian cancer
- Ovarian cysts
  - Follicular cysts
  - Corpus luteum cysts
  - Polycystic ovaries
  - Endometriomas
  - Dermoid cysts
  - Cystadenomas

Disorders of the Male Reproductive System

- Benign prostatic hyperplasia
- Prostate cancer
- Prostatitis
  - Acute bacterial prostatitis
  - Chronic bacterial prostatitis
  - Chronic nonbacterial prostatitis/chronic pelvic pain syndrome
  - Asymptomatic inflammatory prostatitis
- Testicular cancer
  - Germ cell tumors
  - Stromal cell tumors

Other Reproductive System Conditions

- Menopause
- Pregnancy
- Premenstrual syndrome
- Sexually transmitted infections
  - Bacterial vaginosis
  - Chlamydia
  - Gonorrhea
  - Syphilis
  - Nongonococcal urethritis
  - Trichomoniasis
  - Molluscum contagiosum
  - Genital warts

Disorders of the Uterus

Cervical Cancer

Definition: What Is It?

Cervical cancer is the growth of malignant cells in the lining of the cervix, or "neck" of the uterus. While some types of abnormal cells grow slowly and don't present a serious threat, other types are aggressive and invasive.

Demographics

Although rates of cervical cancer diagnosis and death have been falling, it is still responsible for about 12,000 diagnoses and 4,000 deaths each year in the United States. Most women are diagnosed when they are over 30 years old.

On a global scale, more than 500,000 women are diagnosed with cervical cancer, and over 200,000 women die each year, mostly in low- to medium-income countries with limited access to preventive health care options.

Dysplasia: Abnormal tissue development.

For more information the history of cervical cancer, see Sidebar 11.2.

Etiology: What Happens?

Most cervical cancer is brought about directly by a viral infection, in this case with some of the 100+ varieties of the human papillomavirus (HPV) family. Being infected with HPV is not a dependable indicator of cervical cancer however: most of the viruses in this family are not associated with aggressive or invasive cancers.

When a woman is infected with HPV, the virus may trigger cellular changes in the lining of her cervix. Precancerous changes called **dysplasia** can be stimulated by both low-risk and high-risk types of HPV (Figure 11.3).

If a woman is infected with a low-risk type of virus, her abnormal cells may spontaneously resolve, and she may never know anything had happened. But if she is infected with an aggressive form of HPV, cancerous cells may grow in the lining of the cervix and then may spread throughout the uterus, the vagina, and into the pelvic cavity, affecting the bladder, colon, and inguinal lymph nodes. Ultimately, the cancer may travel to distant parts of the body.

HPVs that cause cervical cancer are sexually transmitted pathogens, transferred by direct skin-to-skin touching. While condoms have been seen to reduce the risk of developing

SIDEBAR 11.2 Cervical Cancer: History of a Disease

In the early part of the 20th century, cervical cancer was one of the leading causes of death by cancer for women in this country. This disease is virtually silent, causing no signs or symptoms until it has spread throughout the pelvic cavity and into the lymph system—by which time survival rates are very low.

Then from 1955 to 1992, a remarkable phenomenon occurred: rates of death by cervical cancer dropped by 74%.

What made the difference? A simple examination: the **Papanicolaou test**, which makes it possible to detect precancerous cells in the cervix before they spread. Because of the Pap test, women could have abnormal cells detected and removed before they had a chance to become malignant, and women could find and remove malignancies before they had a chance to spread throughout the pelvic cavity.

Higher mortality rates among women of low socioeconomic status in the United States and around the world point out the fact that many at-risk women still do not have access to this inexpensive and highly useful test.

Today in the United States, the recommended protocol for cervical cancer detection is to receive a traditional Pap test once a year. If a woman is over 30 years old, her doctor may recommend that she can have Pap tests less frequently. If a test is positive for abnormal cells, tests for HPV DNA may be conducted. These tests are most accurate for women over 30, but they can give very specific information about what type of virus may be present, which then dictates the best treatment options.

---

cervical cancer, they do not prevent the spread of all HPV, because skin still comes in contact during sexual activity.

Exposure to HPV is the central risk factor for developing cervical cancer. However, other factors may contribute to the likelihood of those abnormal cells becoming malignant. Sexual activity at an early age may increase the transmission rate of HPV, especially if a woman has multiple partners. Alternatively, if a woman has only one sexual partner but that person has a history of multiple partners, her risk of cervical cancer is increased. Smoking raises the risk of cervical cancer by roughly 100%. Increased risk is also seen with women who have had three or more children, who are overweight, or in those whose diet is low in fruits and vegetables.

Being the daughter of a woman who took **diethylstilbestrol**, a drug prescribed to prevent miscarriage from 1940 to 1971, increases the possibility of cervical cancer, as does immune system suppression through **HIV** infection or immunosuppressant drugs. Coinfection with **chlamydia** also raises the risk. Finally, socioeconomic standing is a major factor, as this often determines whether a woman has adequate access to early detection and care.

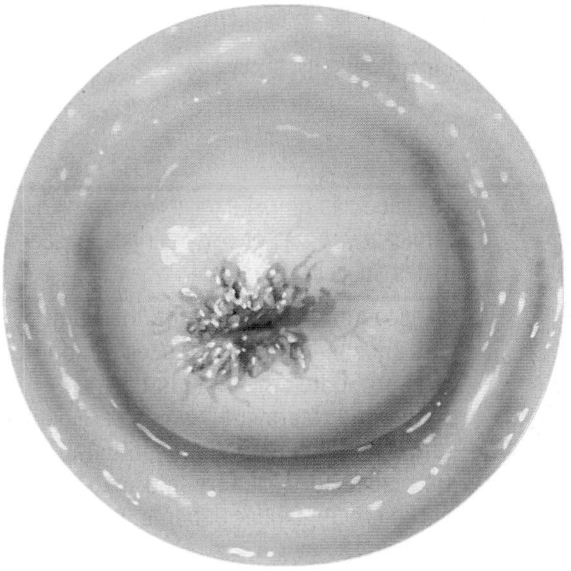

FIGURE 11.3 Lesions caused by HPV may lead to cervical cancer

A vaccine for certain types of HPV provides some protection from the transmission of HPV types 6 and 11 (the cause of some 90% of genital warts) and of HPV types 16 and 18 (the cause of about two-thirds of all cervical cancers). This vaccine does not prevent cervical cancer in a woman who has already been exposed to the virus. Furthermore, while it prevents most cervical cancers, it does not protect against all aggressive forms of HPV. For this reason, a woman who has had the vaccine series still must undergo routine cervical cancer screening.

Types of Cervical Cancer

- *Squamous cell carcinoma of the cervix*: This accounts for 80% to 90% of all diagnoses, and it tends to affect cells on the inferior part of the cervix.
- *Adenocarcinoma of the cervix*: This is more rare and typically begins in the mucus-producing cells at the superior aspect of the cervix. It is not associated with sexual activity.

NOTABLE CASES Argentinean political leader Eva Peron died of complications due to cervical cancer at age 33. Rumors suggest that it was purposely misdiagnosed as appendicitis when it could have been stopped earlier. The prolific award-winning comedian, writer, and actress Julia Sweeney is a cervical cancer survivor.

Papanicolaou test: A screening procedure for cervical cancer in which a few cells are removed from the cervix for examination under a microscope. Commonly called a Pap test.

Diethylstilbestrol: A synthetic estrogen. Formerly given to pregnant women in the mistaken belief that it would help prevent miscarriage.

SIDEBAR 11.3 Staging Cervical Cancer

The staging protocols for cervical cancer can be confusing, and as they are constantly under review, they change frequently. At this writing, the recommendations for cervical cancer divide this disease into precancerous and cancerous stages.

Precancer Staging
When abnormal cells are found in cervical cancer screening, they are classified into the following four subgroups:

- *Atypical squamous cells.* Cells look abnormal, but infection or irritation may be the cause.
  - *Atypical squamous cells of unknown significance.* The patient may be told to repeat the test in several weeks or months.
  - *High-grade atypical squamous cells.* They look suspicious and should be removed for further study.
- *Squamous intraepithelial lesions.* These lesions may be classified as low grade or high grade, but they all need further study.
- *Squamous cell carcinoma.* These cancerous cells must be removed.
- *Atypical glandular cells.* Mucus-producing cells are affected.

Cancer Staging
The staging protocol for invasive cervical cancer was developed by the Fédération Internationale de Gynécologie et d' Obstétrique, so it is sometimes called the FIGO system. Here is a simplified version:

- Stage 0. Cancer cells are found only in the superficial layer of the cervix.
- Stage I. Cancer cells are found only in the cervix. Lesions can range from microscopic to 5 cm in depth and 7 cm in width.
- Stage II. Cancer cells have moved from the cervix into the surrounding area, involving the upper vagina or tissue surrounding the uterus.
- Stage III. Cancer cells are found in the lower vagina and/or the pelvic wall. A growth may be big enough to block the flow of urine through the ureters. Pelvic lymph nodes may also be involved.
- Stage IV. Cancer cells are found in the bladder, rectum, or distant organs.

- *Other types of cervical cancer*: In very rare cases, melanoma, lymphoma, or sarcoma can develop at the cervix.

Signs and Symptoms

Early stages of cervical cancer have no symptoms to speak of. The cancer must be significantly advanced before any signs appear. These usually include bleeding or spotting between menstrual periods or after menopause, vaginal discharge, and pelvic or abdominal pain.

Treatment

Treatment for cervical cancer depends on the stage at which it is diagnosed (see Sidebar 11.3 for staging protocols). Most cases are found in stage 0 or I, which means treatment can be limited to removing the abnormal cells and watching carefully for further changes. Surgical interventions to remove dysplastic tissue include **cryotherapy**, **loop electrosurgical excision procedure**, laser surgery, **punch biopsy**, **cone biopsy**, and **endocervical curettage**.

Surgical procedures for cancer caught in later stages may range from full or partial hysterectomy (including a procedure that may preserve most of the uterus for the possibility of future childbearing) to full pelvic **exenteration**, in which virtually all of the pelvic organs are removed.

Radiation therapy and chemotherapy may also be employed with advanced or recurrent cases of cervical cancer.

Cryotherapy: a medical procedure that uses extremely cold temperatures to kill or slow the growth of cancerous tissue.

Loop electrosurgical excision procedure (LEEP): A medical procedure in which a wire loop heated by electricity is used to remove abnormal cells from the cervix or vagina.

Punch biopsy: The surgical removal of a cylindrical portion of tissue for examination.

Cone biopsy: The removal of a cone-shaped section of tissue from the cervix in order to examine it for cancer.

Endocervical curettage: A medical procedure in which the lining on the inside of the cervix is scraped with an instrument in order to obtain a tissue sample.

Exenteration: A radical surgery in which all the organ from the pelvic cavity are removed.

Medications

- Chemotherapeutic agents, if necessary

Massage Therapy Implications

RISKS	Massage has no risks for a woman with cervical dysplasia or early cervical cancer that is successfully treated.
BENEFITS	Massage has many benefits for women with advanced cervical cancer, as long as appropriate adjustments for the cancer and treatments, which can include surgery, radiation, and chemotherapy, are respected. For more information on working with cancer patients, see Chapter 12.

Dysmenorrhea

Definition: What Is It?

Dysmenorrhea is a technical term for painful menstrual periods. Generally, a woman is said to have dysmenorrhea if she has to limit her regular activities or requires medication to function for 1 day or more every cycle.

Demographics

Dysmenorrhea is a leading cause of lost time from school or work for women of childbearing age. It affects up to 50% of all menstruating women at one time or another. It was once thought that painful menstruation always decreases after childbirth. Research suggests that this is not always true, although the frequency and severity of symptoms does tend to decline with age.

Etiology: What Happens?

The female reproductive cycle is a complicated phenomenon, involving dozens of tightly interlocked processes that include proinflammatory chemicals, involuntary muscle contractions, and hormonal fluctuations that influence far more than the uterus alone. That said, it is a natural and healthy process that is not inherently painful.

Painful menstrual cramps can be a free-standing issue (primary dysmenorrhea) or a symptom of an underlying disorder (secondary dysmenorrhea). Ultimately, the result is the same: menstrual pain that is severe enough to limit activity every month.

In addition to pain being generated at the uterus, many women find that emotional stress—including the stress of anticipating menstrual pain—can exacerbate that pain. Add to this the problem of ligament laxity and subsequent muscle tightening that many women experience during their cycle, and pain associated with menstruation becomes a very complicated problem.

Types of Dysmenorrhea

- *Primary dysmenorrhea*: This usually starts within 3 months of **menarche**. Several factors can contribute, including excessive prostaglandin and vasopressin release (prostaglandins and vasopressin promote pain, inflammation, and smooth muscle contraction), the pain-spasm cycle created when the uterus contracts to expel its contents, and irritation as the round and broad ligaments that anchor the uterus are tugged.
- *Secondary dysmenorrhea*: This is a complication of some other pelvic disorder. Some of the most common problems that cause menstrual pain include **pelvic inflammatory disease** (PID), **fibroid tumors**, problems associated with intrauterine devices (IUDs), **sexually transmitted infections**, and **endometriosis**. **Torsion** or **ovarian cysts** can cause extreme menstrual pain, and pelvic adhesions, deposits of scar tissue from previous surgeries, or trauma may also contribute.

Menarche: The first occurrence of menstruation.

Torsion: Twisting. In the case of ovarian torsion, the ovary is rotated in such a way that the artery to the ovary becomes blocked.

Signs and Symptoms

Signs and symptoms of dysmenorrhea vary. They can include dull aches in the abdomen and low back or sharp pains and cramping in the pelvis and abdomen. These usually happen early in menstruation, but some women have symptoms during their whole period. **Headaches**, nausea, vomiting, diarrhea, and constipation are all possibilities, along with a frequent need to urinate.

Secondary dysmenorrhea typically begins after some years of relatively pain-free menstruation. Symptoms may not be limited to the menstrual period, menstrual flow may be irregular or abnormally heavy, pain medication is often not effective, and this condition is often accompanied by infertility.

Treatment

For most cases of dysmenorrhea, painkillers such as ibuprofen or naproxen provide some relief by inhibiting the secretion of prostaglandins. These are recommended along with warm or hot packs to the abdomen and increased exercise and stretching of the low back.

If painkillers, heat, and stretching are inadequate, more aggressive interventions may be considered. Narcotic painkillers may be prescribed. High-frequency TENS units have shown some success to manage symptoms. Low-dose birth control pills suppress ovulation, which in turn prohibits the secretion of prostaglandins in the uterus. If a structural condition, such as fibroid tumors, is at the root of the problem, surgery may be an option. And laparoscopic surgery for endometriosis may alleviate symptoms if that is the source of the problem.

Dysmenorrhea is often responsive to many alternative treatment options. A thorough nutritional analysis may reveal strategies for dealing with menstrual pain. Vitamin B1, vitamin E, fish oil, magnesium, and thiamine have all led to symptomatic improvement in small-scale trials. Dietary changes to reduce fats and animal proteins while increasing fiber and calcium are often recommended. Exercise and stretches can also relieve the pain in the left and right round ligaments that secure the uterus to the sacrum.

Medications

- Anti-inflammatories to manage inflammation and pain
- Narcotic analgesics if necessary (especially for secondary dysmenorrhea)
- Low-dose birth control pills to suppress ovulation

Massage Therapy Implications

RISKS	Intrusive abdominal work for an undiagnosed problem that causes menstrual pain or during a menstrual period should be avoided.
BENEFITS	Massage can be very helpful for primary dysmenorrhea by relieving stress, indirectly addressing the uterine pain-spasm cycle, and helping any muscle tightness brought about by ligament laxity that accompanies the menstrual cycle.
OPTIONS	Unlike most referred pain patterns, the tendency for the uterus to refer pain to the sacral area of the low back appears for many women to be reversible. In other words, gentle work around the skin of the sacrum can cause a reflexive relief of pain in the pelvic cavity. Massage to the abdomen when the client is not menstruating may improve tissue quality and help to maximize the mobility of abdominal adhesions that contribute to pain.
RESEARCH	Substantial research on using manual therapies to relieve primary menstrual pain has been conducted. This is a situation where using aromatherapy as part of the treatment plan appears to make a marked difference in outcomes for both pain levels and pain duration.[1–3] The use of acupressure without aromatherapy or essential oils was also found to reduce low back pain and distress among patients,[4] and the reduction in pain persisted for several months after the intervention was over. One systematic review of physiotherapy for menstrual pain suggests that much of the positive impact may be due to a placebo effect,[5] but this still points to the value of the therapeutic relationship in working with clients who have chronic pain problems. 1. Marzouk TM, El-Nemer AM, Baraka HN. The effect of aromatherapy abdominal massage on alleviating menstrual pain in nursing students: a prospective randomized cross-over study. *Evidence-Based Complementary and Alternative Medicine* 2013;2013:742421. http://www.hindawi.com/journals/ecam/2013/742421/ 2. Ou MC, Hsu TF, Lai AC, et al. Pain relief assessment by aromatic essential oil massage on outpatients with primary dysmenorrhea: a randomized, double-blind clinical trial. *Journal of Obstetrics and Gynaecology Research* 2012;38(5): 817–822. http://www.ncbi.nlm.nih.gov/pubmed/22435409 3. Apay SE, Arslan S, Akpinar RB, et al. Effect of aromatherapy massage on dysmenorrhea in Turkish students. *Pain Management Nursing* 2012;13(4):236–240. http://www.ncbi.nlm.nih.gov/pubmed/23158705 4. Chen HM, Wang HH, Chiu MH, et al. Effects of acupressure on menstrual distress and low back pain in dysmenorrheic young adult women: an experimental study. *Pain Management Nursing.* August 27, 2014 (E-pub ahead of print). 5. Kannan P, Claydon LS. Some physiotherapy treatments may relieve menstrual pain in women with primary dysmenorrhea: a systematic review. *Journal of Physiotherapy* 2014;60(1):13–21. http://www.journalofphysiotherapy.com/article/S1836-9553(14)00004-6/abstract

Endometriosis

Definition: What Is It?

Endometriosis is a condition in which cells from the endometrium implant elsewhere in the body. Growths usually begin in the pelvic cavity but may spread further into the abdomen and in rare cases above the diaphragm.

Demographics

It is estimated that anywhere from 8% to 10% of women of childbearing age have this disorder, although not all have symptoms. It appears to be a particular risk for women who had severe **acne** during adolescence, so this population is encouraged to seek help if they develop symptoms.

Etiology: What Happens?

Endometriosis involves the implantation and growth of endometrial cells anywhere outside the uterus. It was first described in 1921 by American gynecologist James Sampson, who noticed these growths in the peritoneal cavities of women undergoing abdominal surgery, but references to painful disorders of menstruation go back much further. Sampson hypothesized that the endometrial cells got out of the uterus via retrograde backflow through the uterine tubes.

Retrograde backflow is still a leading theory about the pathophysiology of this disorder, but since it has been found that most women have some endometrial cells in the pelvis during menstruation, clearly other factors are involved. These include **coelomic metaplasia** (the metamorphosis of some cells into endometrial cells, possibly triggered by inflammation), endometrial cells that are spread via surgical procedures (deposits located in the scar tissue from C-sections

> **Coelomic metaplasia:** A theory about the cause of endometriosis based on the fact that celomic epithelium is the common ancestor of endometrial and peritoneal cells and may undergo a change in formation later in life.

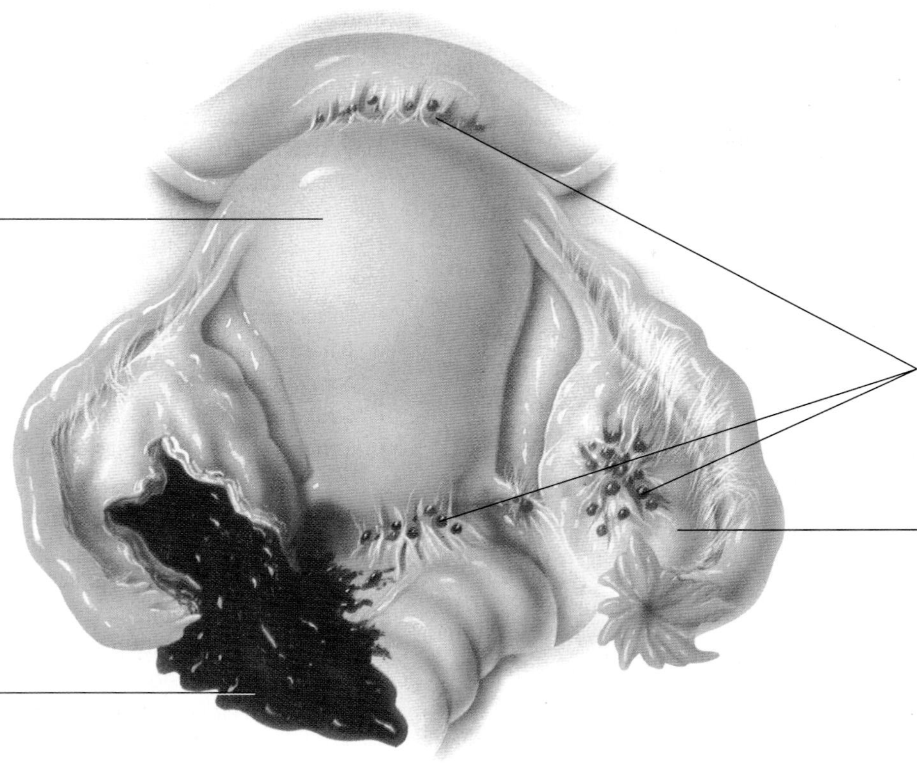

FIGURE 11.4 Sites of endometriosis

and laparoscopic procedures supports this theory), metastasis via blood or lymph (endometrial deposits are rarely found outside the abdominopelvic cavity, but this would be the mechanism), or immune system anomalies that promote inflammation but suppress activity against cells that are notably out of place. Exposure to exogenous estrogens may also promote rapid growth of these cells.

Wherever the endometrial cells land, if they are able to colonize the tissue, they do two things to start the disease process: they stimulate the growth of supplying blood vessels, and they proliferate in accordance with the hormonal commands in the body. But these growths cannot be shed with normal menstruation. Instead, they decay and accumulate in local areas, stimulating an inflammatory response. The body attempts to isolate them by surrounding the deposits with fibrous connective tissue. Eventually, multitudes of fibrous "blood blisters" called **endometriomas** accumulate (Figure 11.4).

Endometrial growths that are found early look like clear vesicles on the structures they have colonized. Later, these vesicles become bright red. Over a course of 10 or more years, they become thick, black, and scarred. Growths on ovaries that have darkened over time are sometimes called "chocolate cysts."

Growths appear in three main locations: on the ovaries, on the surface of the peritoneum, and in the area behind the uterus that links the rectum and vagina. While endometriosis can grow in these and other locations simultaneously, some scientists suggest that the lesions are different and can be classified by location. This may eventually lead to new treatment or prevention options.

Complications

Endometriosis can disrupt many functions in the pelvis, including a pain-free menstrual cycle; **dysmenorrhea** is a common complication. Accumulations of deposits and fibrous connective tissue can create adhesions in or on the uterine tubes and ovaries, which raise the risk of infertility or **ectopic pregnancy**. The collecting of blood in these deposits can deprive the rest of the body, resulting in **anemia**. **Uterine hyperplasia** is a condition that occasionally accompanies endometriosis; the normal endometrial lining becomes pathologically thickened, leading to excessive bleeding and further difficulties with fertility. Finally, the cysts and scarring associated with endometriosis can hide some of the early signs of ovarian or endometrial cancer, and these conditions are sometimes seen together, so it is important to be vigilant to this possibility.

Endometrioma: A type of cyst that forms when endometrial tissue grows on the ovaries.

Uterine hyperplasia: The excessive growth of cells of the lining of the uterus.

Signs and Symptoms

Very often, infertility is the complaint that brings a woman with endometriosis to a doctor for a first diagnosis. Other signs and symptoms of endometriosis are often nonexistent, at least in the early stages, but premenstrual spotting, a sensation of urinary urgency with painful urination, and diarrhea and rectal bleeding during menstruation may occur. Some cases include severe abdominal pain before, during, and after periods. Painful sexual activity is also common. Interestingly, the amount of pain a person has does not correlate with the size of her endometrial growths, so other factors are at play here as well. Leg pain, which can be unilateral or bilateral, is another common report from endometriosis patients.

Symptoms of endometriosis are cyclical, reaching a peak during menstruation. This feature has probably prevented a lot of women from seeking medical help, since traditionally it has been assumed that painful menstruation is a normal and expected. As women have become more proactive about health care, they have discovered that painful menstruation is not a given and have become more willing to explore the causes and possible solutions to their pain.

Treatment

Treatment for endometriosis depends on what outcome the woman desires. No permanent solution for this disorder exists until a woman is postmenopausal; even a complete hysterectomy won't protect a patient from endometriosis if any remaining microscopic deposits are stimulated with hormone replacement therapy.

Because many women wish to treat endometriosis to become pregnant, treatment options are often geared toward limiting symptoms and progression long enough to allow conception to take place. Symptoms disappear during pregnancy, but they usually recur after a baby is born.

Four main goals are at the center of medical intervention for endometriosis. These are to relieve pain, to stop the progression of established growths, to prevent the establishment of any new growths, and to maintain or restore fertility if that is the patient's wish. Nonsteroidal anti-inflammatory drugs (NSAIDs) or other analgesics may be adequate for pain relief. Hormone therapy that disrupts the secretion of estrogen may be employed to limit growths. These may be used alone or as a preparation for surgery. Surgical intervention may include the use of lasers or **electrocauterization** to **ablate** or cut out visible growths and to reduce adhesions between pelvic organs.

Medications

- Nonsteroidal anti-inflammatory drugs for pain and inflammation
- Narcotic analgesics if necessary for pain management
- Oral contraception to suppress estrogen and ovulation
- Other hormonal analogs to suppress ovulation

Massage Therapy Implications

RISKS	Endometriosis can cause scarring and adhesions in the pelvic cavity. This possibility requires special caution and care when doing anything more than superficial work on the abdomen.
BENEFITS	Many women with endometriosis live in a state of anxiety and frustration with their own body that may exacerbate their most painful symptoms. Massage therapy is frequently recommended along with other relaxation techniques for women who must learn to cope with the long-term consequences of a disorder that has no permanent cure.
OPTIONS	Special training in abdominal and pelvic bodywork may help to relieve pain and some other symptoms for women with endometriosis.
RESEARCH	Little research has addressed massage therapy for endometriosis, but one study found positive results for pain control specifically for this population.[1] 1. Valiani M, Ghasemi N, Bahadoran P, et al. The effects of massage therapy on dysmenorrhea caused by endometriosis. *Iranian Journal of Nursing and Midwifery Research* 2010;15(4):167–171. http://www.ncbi.nlm.nih.gov/pmc/articles/PMC3093183/

Electrocauterization: A medical procedure in which electricity is used to remove unwanted tissue or seal a blood vessel.

Ablation: A medical procedure in which tissue is removed.

Leiomyoma: A benign tumor that grows in smooth muscle tissue, such as in the uterus. Also called a fibroid tumor.

Fibroid Tumors

Definition: What Are They?

Fibroid tumors, or **leiomyomas**, are benign tumors that grow in or around the uterus. They can grow within the smooth muscle walls, or, more rarely, they can be suspended from a stalk into the pelvic cavity or uterus. Some even hang down into the vagina (Figure 11.5). Fibroids can

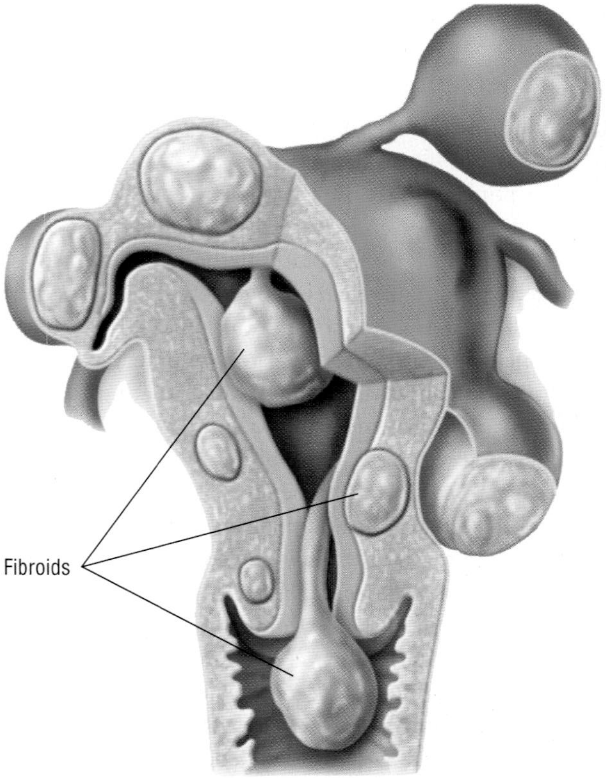

FIGURE 11.5 Fibroids

grow singly or in clusters, and they vary in size from being microscopic to weighing several pounds and completely filling the uterus.

Demographics

Uterine fibroids are extremely common. They occur in up to 50% of all women and contribute to about 200,000 hysterectomies each year.

Etiology: What Happens?

The pathophysiology of uterine fibroids is not well understood. While they sometimes run in families, they are not strictly genetically linked. They seem to be stimulated by estrogen; after menopause, many shrink and ultimately disappear. Many experts believe that fibroid tumors arise as a combination of genetic, environmental, and hormonal factors.

Histological studies show that the extracellular matrix of fibroid tumors lacks a key protein, and the collagen filaments are disorganized and not discretely formed. This is especially interesting because the same growth pattern has been observed in **keloid scars**. Both fibroids and keloids are about three times more common in African Americans than in the rest of the population.

Some evidence suggests that while fibroid tumors may be initially triggered by other factors, they may create a mechanical distortion in the uterine tissues that triggers other changes in the local extracellular matrix. These then signal chemical cascades that trigger the production of ever more extracellular matrix and disorganized collagen. This contributes to the textural stiffness of the tumors, which further distorts the local tissues, possibly leading to the rapid growth that is sometimes seen in this context.

Fibroids are typically classified by their location. Submucosal fibroids grow under the mucous lining of the uterus; they are the deepest type. Intramural fibroids grow within layers of the muscular wall of the uterus. Subserosal fibroids grow on the superficial aspect of the uterus, but deep to the peritoneum.

Complications

Fibroids are very seldom serious, but they can lead to some troubling consequences. The heavy periods they cause sometimes lead to **anemia**. They can cause infertility by obstructing uterine tubes or interfering with the implantation of a fertilized ovum. They can also interfere in late-stage pregnancies: if a fibroid is large enough, it can crowd the growing fetus or block the cervix. These problems can lead to premature births and a necessity for cesarean sections.

Pedunculate fibroids, the type that dangle into the uterus or vagina, can twist on their stalk. This causes extreme pain and requires surgery for removal. It is also possible for very large fibroids to outgrow their blood supply. This leads to necrosis, because tissue that is deprived of oxygen dies. The body slowly reabsorbs the necrotic mass, but it can be a long and painful process; more often, surgery is performed to remove the fibroid and associated dead tissue.

Signs and Symptoms

Usually, fibroids produce no symptoms at all. In extreme cases, the tumor may grow large enough to press on the sensory nerves inside the uterus. If they press on the bladder, they can cause urinary frequency; if on the rectum, they can cause difficulties with defecation. If they press on the fallopian (uterine) tubes, they may interfere with pregnancy. They can also cause heavy menstrual bleeding and occasionally bleeding between menstrual periods.

Fibroids typically grow slowly, but occasionally they grow fast, doubling their size within a few months. In this situation, a biopsy is recommended to rule out **uterine cancer**.

Pedunculate: Having a peduncle; suspended from a stalk.

Treatment

Fibroids seldom require treatment unless they cause pain and excessive bleeding or if they interfere with pregnancy.

Hormone therapy can shrink them, but they grow back when medication is stopped. Other options include minimally invasive procedures that remove parts of the tumors or blocking off the supplying arteries (**uterine artery embolization**), which may then be followed by a minimally invasive procedure to remove the fibroid. Surgical possibilities include laser ablation, myomectomy (the removal of the tumor while preserving the rest of the uterus), or full hysterectomy.

Medications

- Gonadotropin-releasing hormone inhibitors to help shrink the tumors before surgery
- Progesterone or progestin to counter the effects of estrogen

Massage Therapy Implications

RISKS	If a client knows she has large fibroid tumors, it is best not to disrupt them with intrusive massage low in the abdomen. Bodywork holds no other specific risks for a person with this condition.
BENEFITS	Massage has no direct impact on the presence of fibroid tumors. Most clients with this condition can enjoy all the benefits of bodywork as the rest of the population.

Uterine Cancer

Definition: What Is It?

Uterine cancer is the development of cancerous cells in the uterus. It is classified as endometrial cancer or uterine sarcoma.

Demographics

Uterine cancer is diagnosed in about 40,000 American women each year and leads to about 7,500 deaths. It is the fourth most common metastatic cancer in women (following lung, breast, and colorectal cancers), but it has a generally good prognosis because it is often found in early stages.

Uterine artery embolization: A medical procedure in which blood supply is cut off to a uterine body such as a fibroid tumor.

Etiology: What Happens?

Uterine cancer begins with a mutation in the DNA of the affected cells. Most often, these are cells in the endometrium, but uterine cancer can also develop in the connective tissue or muscle tissue of the uterus.

The primary trigger for many cases of uterine cancer appears to be exposure to excessive estrogen. That source can be endogenous (for instance, if the ovaries or fat cells produce more estrogen than can be tolerated) or exogenous (with hormone replacement therapy or other sources). Other factors, including race, age, and history of other cancers, also influence a woman's chance of developing uterine cancer.

When a new growth develops in the uterus, it tends to be fragile and easily disrupted. This leads to vaginal bleeding or spotting, especially in postmenopausal women; this is the most dependable early symptom of the disease.

Uterine cancer is often slow growing and not aggressive. When it does metastasize, however, it can use any of four mechanisms to spread. Direct contact can allow cells on the exterior of the uterus to become established on nearby organs, like the bladder or the colon. Cells from the uterus can also float through peritoneal fluid to land elsewhere in the region and set up new growth sites. Finally, both the lymphatic and circulatory systems can be recruited to carry cancerous cells outside the pelvis to the lungs, bones, or other areas.

Risk factors for uterine cancer have been extensively studied, and the most potent triggers all have to do with estrogen exposure. Uterine hyperplasia is a condition that develops in some perimenopausal women, especially when they supplement estrogen. This enlargement of the uterus can sometimes develop into cancer. Estrogen replacement therapy that is unopposed with progestin; obesity (abdominal fat cells can produce estrogen); a high-fat, low-fiber diet; never having had children; early menarche combined with late menopause; **polycystic ovarian disease**; and taking certain medication to reduce the risk of breast cancer recurrence can all increase the risk of uterine cancer.

Other risk factors for uterine cancer include age (it is mostly found in women over 50), race (it is most common among white women, but has a higher mortality rate among black women), and the genetic anomalies associated with a high risk of **colorectal cancer** and **breast cancer**. Type 2 **diabetes** is associated with uterine cancer; this is probably due to a tendency toward obesity, but the metabolic problems of diabetes itself may also have something to do with an increased risk of this disease. And a sedentary lifestyle with too much time sitting turns out to be risk factor for endometrial cancers as well.

Types of Uterine Cancer

- *Endometrial cancer*: This accounts for the vast majority of uterine cancer diagnoses. Its subtypes include the following:
    - *Adenocarcinoma*: This is the most common form of endometrial cancer. It involves cells that resemble normal endometrial cells. It tends not to be aggressive.

- *Adenosquamous carcinoma*: This involves squamous epithelial cells along with typical endothelial cells.
- *Papillary serous adenocarcinoma*: This is rare and potentially aggressive.
- *Clear cell adenocarcinoma*: This is the rarest form of endometrial cancer, and it has a high risk of being aggressive.

- *Uterine sarcoma*: This cancer originates from nonglandular tissues. While it progresses with essentially the same pattern as endometrial cancer, uterine sarcoma tends to be much more aggressive and has a poorer survival rate. Subtypes include the following:
  - *Stromal cell cancer*: This affects the connective tissue of the uterus.
  - *Leiomyosarcoma*: This starts in the smooth muscle cells of the uterus.
  - *Mixed müllerian sarcoma*: This combines features of adenocarcinomas and sarcomas.

Signs and Symptoms

Most women with uterine cancer are postmenopausal, so the most common early sign of this disease, vaginal spotting or bleeding, is easy to identify. While most women who have postmenopausal bleeding do not have uterine cancer, this early sign contributes to the excellent early detection rates for this disease: it is often found in stage I or II.

For women who still have a menstrual cycle, uterine cancer can be harder to identify early, but spotting between periods should be investigated.

Other signs and symptoms include vaginal discharge, pelvic pain, a pelvic mass, pain with sex, a change in bladder or bowel habits, and unintended weight loss.

Staging protocols for uterine cancer can be found in Sidebar 11.4.

NOTABLE CASES Actress ("Mrs. Robinson") Anne Bancroft succumbed to uterine cancer at age 73 in 2005. Actress and author (*Cancer Schmancer*) Fran Drescher is a uterine cancer survivor and outspoken advocate for uterine cancer patients.

Treatment

The mainstay of uterine cancer treatment is a hysterectomy, which is usually accompanied by the removal of the ovaries and uterine tubes as well. This may be followed by radiation and/or hormone therapy, depending on findings.

SIDEBAR 11.4 Staging Uterine Cancer

As with cervical cancer, the staging protocol for uterine cancer was developed by the Fédération Internationale de Gynécologie et d' Obstétrique, so it is sometimes called the FIGO system.

A simplified version of the tumor, node, metastasis (TNM) classifications for staging uterine cancer looks like this:

TUMOR	NODE	METASTASIS
T0: No signs of a tumor in the uterus	N0: No spread to nearby nodes	M0: No spread to distant nodes or tissues
Tis: Preinvasive cancer (in situ); cells are limited to the endometrium.	N1: Lymph nodes in the pelvis are involved.	M1: Spread to distant organs and lymph nodes
T1: Tumor is growing in the body of the uterus but not beyond.	N2: Lymph nodes along the aorta are involved.	
T2: The tumor has spread into supporting connective tissue of the cervix.		
T3: The cancer has spread from the uterus into nearby tissues, including superficial layers of the rectum and bladder.		
T4: The cancer has fully invaded other nearby organs or spread to distant organs.		

These are then translated into stages in this way:

Stage I	T1, N0, M0
Stage II	T2, N0, M0
Stage III	T3, N0, M0
Stage IV	T4, any N, M0, *or* any T, any N, M1

Lymph nodes near the aorta and in the groin are often dissected for signs of metastasis. Chemotherapy is used most often for uterine sarcomas or for women who are not good candidates for open surgery because of age or other health problems.

If a young woman is diagnosed with uterine cancer and wants to preserve her uterus for the possibility of childbearing, she may choose to have a **dilatation and curettage** procedure with progestin supplements instead of surgery. This option carries a high risk of recurrence, however, so it must be followed by careful surveillance.

Medications

- Chemotherapeutic agents
- Hormone therapy, including progesterone and progestin; **tamoxifen**; aromatase inhibitors (to reduce estrogen production at fat cells); and gonadotropin-releasing hormone inhibitors

Massage Therapy Implications

RISKS	Uterine cancer may be treated with any combination of surgery, chemotherapy, hormone therapy, or radiation. Any bodywork delivered in this setting must accommodate for the challenges of the disease as well as the challenges of its treatments.
BENEFITS	Bodywork has many demonstrated benefits for cancer patients, as long as appropriate adjustments are made. For more information on massage in the context of cancer, see Chapter 12.
RESEARCH	Women undergoing treatment for uterine cancer are susceptible to lymphedema in the legs because of disruption of the pelvic lymph nodes. Massage therapy has been used in this context to help control symptoms.[1] More on massage and lymphedema can be found in Chapter 12. 1. Salani R, Preston MM, Hade EM, et al. Swelling among women who need education about leg lymphedema: a descriptive study of lymphedema in women undergoing surgery for endometrial cancer. *International Journal of Gynecological Cancer* 2014;24(8):1507–1512. http://www.ncbi.nlm.nih.gov/pubmed/25078342

Disorders of Other Female Reproductive Structures

Breast Cancer

Definition: What Is It?

Breast cancer is the development of tumors in the epithelial or connective tissue of the breast. These growths may start out as nonmalignant, but may become invasive if neglected for a long period.

> **Dilatation and curettage:** Enlargement of the cervix and scraping of the endometrium to remove growths or other abnormal tissues.
>
> **Tamoxifen:** An antiestrogen drug used to treat breast cancer.
>
> **In situ:** In its own place. Carcinomas found *in situ* have not grown beyond where those cells would normally be found and are sometimes categorized as precancerous.
>
> **Stroma:** The connective tissue, fat, and blood cells that support an epithelial organ.

Demographics

About 230,000 new cases of invasive breast cancer are diagnosed in women, and about 2,300 cases in men each year in the United States. This does not include the 62,000 diagnoses found **in situ**. About 41,000 women and about 500 men die of this disease each year in this country. It is estimated that 2.5 million breast cancer survivors are alive in the United States today.

Etiology: What Happens?

Breasts are constructed of 15 to 20 lobes where milk is produced in lactating women, ducts that deliver milk to the nipple, and the **stroma** that provides support and the bulk of breast tissue. The lobes and ducts are made of epithelial cells; the stroma is connective tissue and lipid cells. Although cancer may grow in any of these tissues, malignant cells are most likely to grow in the epithelial lobes and ducts.

Many types of breast cancer begin as in situ growths that eventually develop malignant characteristics. It can take a long time for a tumor to become large enough to notice; it is estimated that it takes several years for a growth to reach a diameter of 1 cm.

As tumors grow, cells may invade the circulatory or lymphatic system. The proximity of the axillary lymph nodes makes these a common site for the spread of malignant cells (Figure 11.6).

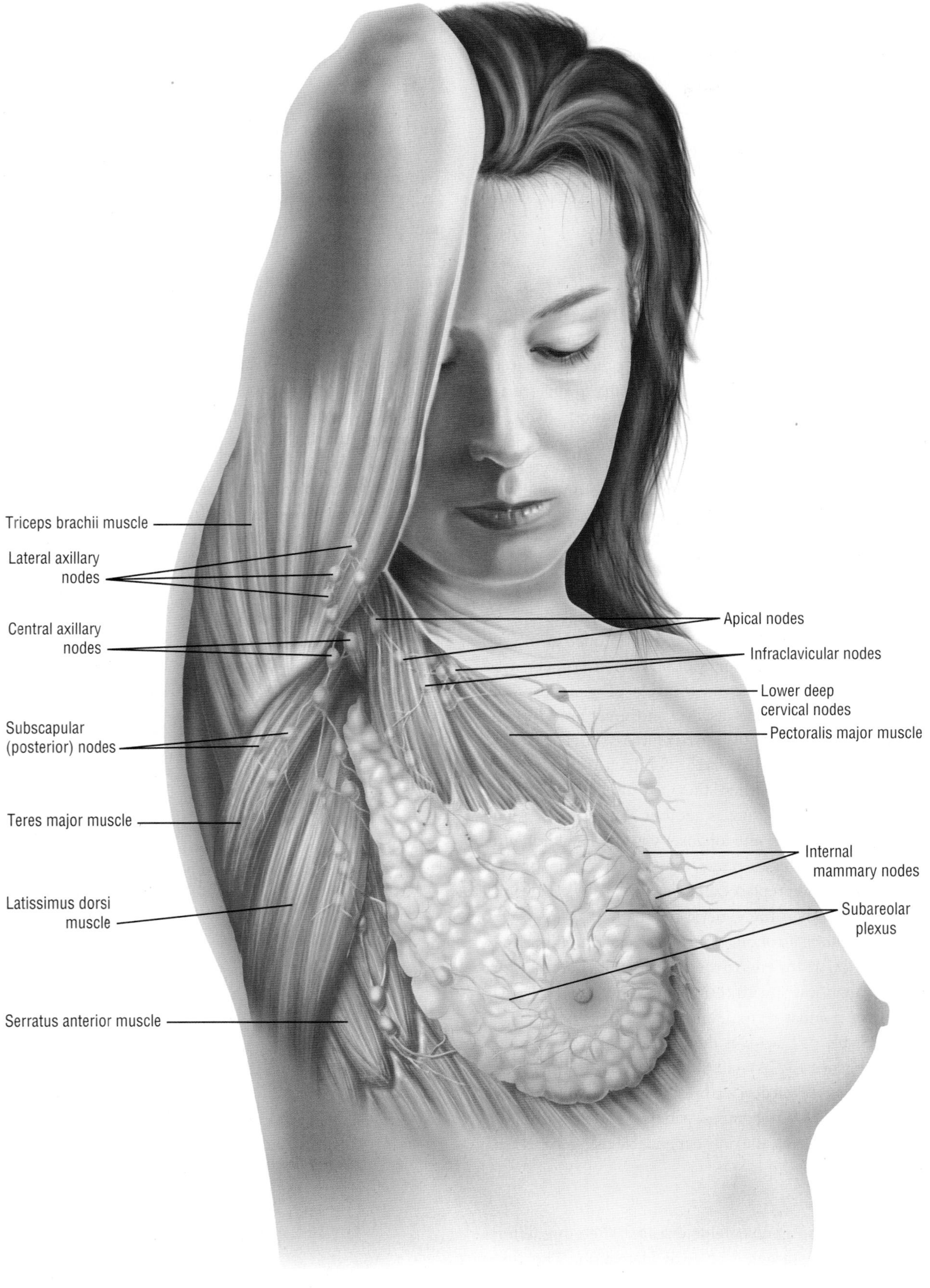

FIGURE 11.6 Breast cancer: proximity of lymph nodes

Breast cancer usually metastasizes to nearby lymph nodes in the axilla and thoracic cavity first; invasion of chest muscles, bones, and skin follows. Finally, distant metastatic sites include the liver, lung, and brain. If the cancer is not successfully treated, complications may include spinal cord pressure, bone **fractures**, pleural effusion, and bronchial obstruction.

NOTABLE CASES The list of well-known people with breast cancer is long and varied. It includes activist Gloria Steinem, singer Olivia Newton-John, journalist Linda Ellerbee, and—as a demonstration that breast cancer is not just a woman's disease—"Shaft" actor Richard Roundtree. Perhaps, the most eloquent breast cancer patient in recent years was columnist Molly Ivins, who declared, "Having breast cancer is massive amounts of no fun. First they mutilate you; then they poison you; then they burn you. I have been on blind dates better than that." Molly Ivins died from inflammatory breast disease in 2007.

Risk Factors

One of the most challenging things about breast cancer is that no dependable profile of the women most likely to get it has ever been developed. Some cancers, such as **lung, colon,** and **skin cancer,** can be directly linked to diet or environmental factors; breast cancer cannot. Although some risk factors have been identified as increasing the chance that a woman may develop breast cancer, most women with these risk factors (outside of genetic predisposition) never develop the disease, and most breast cancer patients don't carry most of these risk factors (outside of age).

Age is the leading risk factor for breast cancer: most patients are diagnosed when they are over 50 years old. Prolonged estrogen exposure is another factor: women with early menarche and late menopause; who had children after age 30 or not at all; who are obese, especially after menopause; or who use hormone replacement therapy are at greater risk for breast cancer than the general population. Women who have more than one alcoholic drink every day, who have a history of radiation treatments to the chest, or who have a history of lobular carcinoma in situ (LCIS) are also more likely than the rest of the population to develop breast cancer.

One reliable risk factor is the presence of two abnormal breast cancer genes, BRCA1 and BRCA2. About 80% of women carrying these genes will develop breast cancer, but they account for only 5% to 10% of diagnosed patients. For the other 90% of breast cancer patients, the only dependable risk factor is age.

Prevention

Breast cancer is not a preventable disease. Therefore, efforts for prevention are targeted at early detection. The three main courses for early detection are self-examination, breast examination by a professional, and mammograms, which use radiation to look for unusually dense masses in the breast tissue. MRI or ultrasound imaging is typically saved for high-risk women who are under 40 years old.

Women who have a personal or family history of breast cancer, who are positive for the breast cancer genes, or who are otherwise considered at high risk for this disease may be counseled to test earlier and more often than the general public.

It is important to emphasize that a mammogram is not a definitive test for breast cancer. Mammogram interpretations vary widely, and mammograms may miss the subtle changes in breast tissue that only women who perform monthly self-examinations may notice. Therefore, an "all clear" from a mammogram does not rule out breast cancer.

Types of Breast Cancer

- *Ductal carcinoma*: This is the most common type of breast cancer, accounting for 70% to 80% of diagnoses. It can occur in situ, in which case cells affect only the epithelial lining of the ducts, or it can become invasive (Figure 11.7). Ductal carcinoma in situ (DCIS) is associated with the development of small, calcified deposits in the breasts and a slightly increased risk for invasive breast cancer.
- *Lobular carcinoma*: This is less common than ductal carcinoma, accounting for 5% to 10% of tumors. It can be limited to the epithelial lining of the lobes (LCIS), but this condition carries a significant risk of becoming invasive

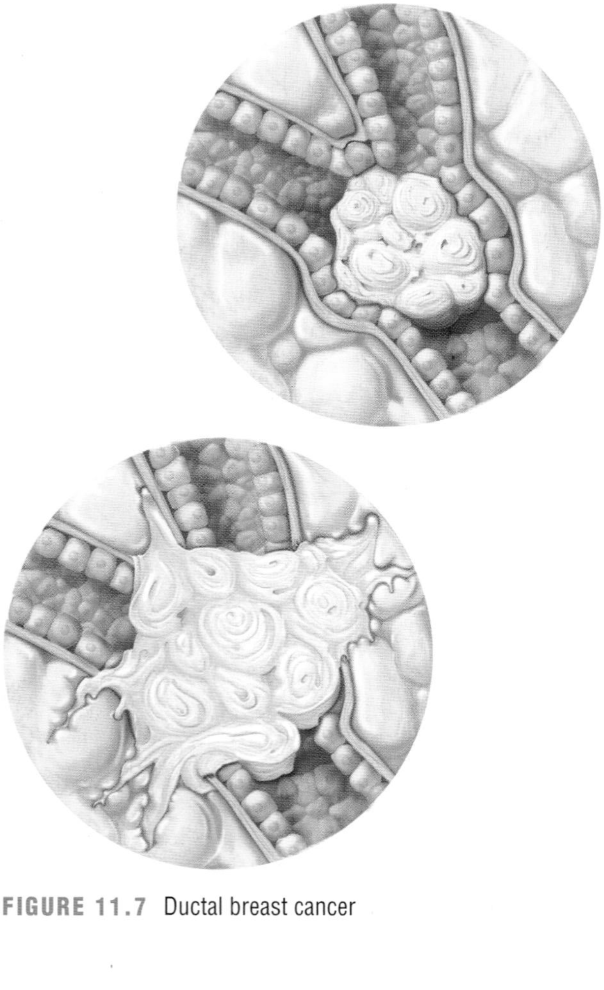

FIGURE 11.7 Ductal breast cancer

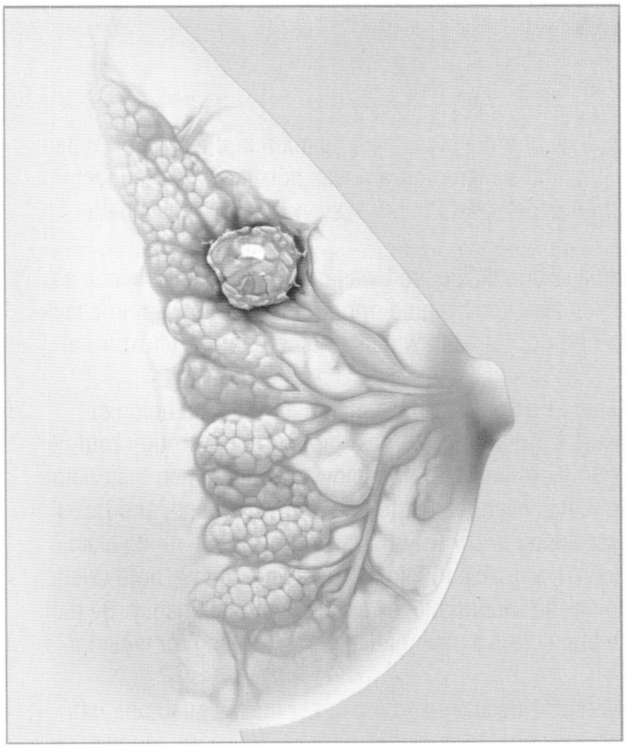

FIGURE 11.8 Lobular breast cancer

(Figure 11.8). Lobular carcinoma also has a higher incidence of appearing in both breasts than ductal carcinoma.

- *Inflammatory breast disease*: This is a form of breast cancer that is relatively rare in the West. It resembles a local infection or insect bite, with warm, red, itching skin.
- *Other types of breast cancer*: Collectively, these account for only 10% to 15% of diagnoses. Paget disease of the breast affects specifically the nipple and presents with eczema-like changes in the skin. Medullary carcinoma is a rare malignancy of the connective tissues in the breast. Tubular carcinoma refers to the shape of the mutated cells. And mucinous carcinoma is a rare type with a good prognosis.

Signs and Symptoms

Early symptoms of breast cancer are subtle. Breast tissue is soft and loose, especially in women over 50, so tumors have

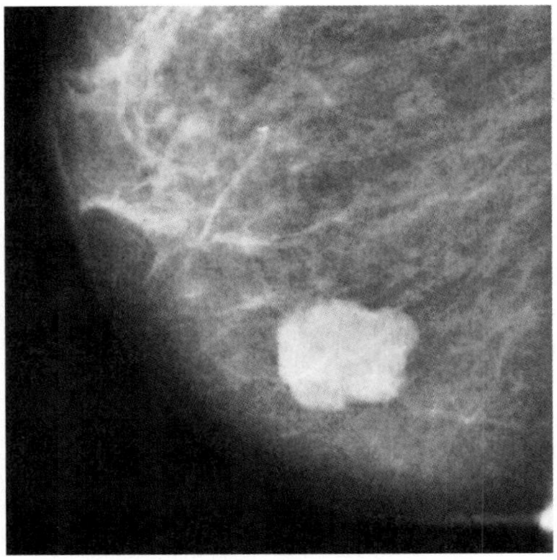

FIGURE 11.9 Mammogram showing a breast cancer tumor: note the irregular shape and borders of growth

ample room to grow without causing pain. Sometimes, self-examination can find changing textures or lumps before a mammogram can show them, and sometimes, a mammogram reveals thickenings or minute calcifications that are too subtle to feel (Figure 11.9). Self-exams may also find nonmalignant breast changes that can easily be mistaken for breast cancer (see Sidebar 11.5).

Advanced cases of breast cancer show asymmetrical breast growth, inverted nipples that may have discharge, and sometimes a characteristic "orange peel" texture of the skin on the breast. Advanced cases may also cause symptoms in other parts of the body that are damaged by the growth of invasive tumors: bone pain, weight loss, spinal cord compression, and swelling in the arms may be the result of tumors far from the original site of the cancer (Case History 11.1).

Mastitis: Inflammation of the mammary gland of the breast.

Ductal ectasia: A condition in which the milk ducts of the breast becomes clogged.

Fat necrosis: The death of fat cells, often in the breast.

SIDEBAR 11.5 Nonmalignant Breast Changes

Not all breast growths are malignant. Most growths in breast tissue are cysts or benign tumors; many fall into the classification of fibrocystic breast changes. Some of these growths carry a risk of eventually becoming malignant, but for the most part, they are not serious conditions and can easily be distinguished from malignancies with testing procedures that include mammograms, fine-needle aspiration, ultrasound, or biopsy.

Breasts can also be affected by infection (called **mastitis** if a woman is lactating or **ductal ectasia** if she is not). Injury from trauma, surgery, or radiation may cause **fat necrosis**. Breast infections and fat necrosis can be serious, requiring medical intervention for the best outcomes.

CASE HISTORY 11.1 Breast Cancer

Right before my 57th birthday, I found a lump in my left breast while doing a breast examination in the shower. When I went in for my mammogram, the doctor said he couldn't feel it, and the mammogram was normal. A subsequent ultrasound did not reveal anything, and the technician also could not feel what I felt. So, even though I knew better, this gave me a sense of security that all was well.

Until January, I could still feel the lump, and by now, my husband could also, so I was not imagining it. I made an appointment with a surgeon. He not only felt what I had felt (which was a thickening, more than a lump), but in checking my previous mammogram, he found pinpoints of calcium in the right breast, which are sometimes indicators of cancer. Three days later, I had bilateral biopsies.

During the biopsies, a frozen section was done on the thickening on the left side, which meant the pathologist could tell right away whether the tissue was malignant. (The tissue from the right breast biopsy went through routine pathology, and I had to wait for several days for those results.) So there I was, in the recovery room, when the doctor came in and told me that the left breast biopsy revealed a malignancy. Then, he left to talk to my husband, and I was by myself. The greatest feeling I had was just incredible sadness. I don't know why I wasn't angry or anything else; I was just so sad. After a few minutes, I was able to join my husband and we both cried.

CAROL E., 60 YEARS OLD:
"When you have had breast cancer, the thought of possible recurrence is always with you. It makes you look at what is really important in life."

After 3 days, the call came saying the second biopsy showed no malignancy. By that time, I was thankful that only one breast had a malignancy. Strange thing for which to be thankful.

My diagnosis was a stage I infiltrated ductal carcinoma, upper medial quadrant, left breast. After I got a second opinion, surgery was scheduled for the following Monday. Before that, I had to have chest x-rays, a bone scan, and a radiation oncology consult, as I had opted to have conservative surgery (a lumpectomy followed by 6 weeks of radiation).

The surgeon performed a lumpectomy and also did an axillary dissection—removal of some lymph nodes in the armpit. It is during this surgery that a nerve in my armpit was either severed or damaged. This produces numbness in the underarm and inner upper arm that can be permanent. The lymph nodes removed (16 in my case) were tested for malignancy, and later I learned that they showed no cancer. Chances were that the cancer had been confined to the breast tissue. Good news indeed!

But then, the surgeon called and said that the margins of the tissue removed were not clean—meaning that there were still some cancer cells in the breast. So back to surgery for another resection of the breast. My surgeon did not usually do this, but he felt that there was very little cancer left, and a mastectomy could still be avoided. Unfortunately, the margins on that sample weren't clean either. The following week again found me in surgery having a total mastectomy. Three major surgeries in 3 weeks with general anesthetic each time are a lot to cope with, but you do what you have to do.

Because I had a mastectomy, and because my lymph nodes were negative for cancer cells, I did not have to have any radiation. I also did not have to have chemotherapy. A big relief!

I do take tamoxifen and amitriptyline, a mild antidepressant, to help break the cycle of chronic nerve pain that I have had in my left arm—an unusual and difficult complication. About 8 months ago, I also started on Neurontin, an antiseizure drug that can also work on nerve pain, and in my case, it has really helped. So, after almost 2 years, the pain in my arm is under control. I have no lymphedema. However, this could happen at any time.

I do not feel that the doctors emphasize enough how vulnerable the affected arm is. Infections can develop very easily, and I have to be really careful, especially working in the garden. It seems that little burns and scratches take forever to heal. I should not lift more than 10 pounds with the affected arm and should not have any needle sticks or even have my blood pressure taken on that arm. Once I awoke after minor surgery to find a blood pressure cuff on my left arm, and was I upset! I thought that I had taken enough precautions that this should not have happened. The prescription for medication post surgery had been clipped over the warning note! The next time I had an anesthetic, I wrote on my left arm with a surgical pen, and that did not come off!

When you have had breast cancer, the thought of recurrence is always with you. Breast cancer does not follow any rules; it can come back at any time. It is a lifelong commitment always to be on the watch and take really good care of yourself. This makes you look at what is really important in life. You try not to put off things that you want to say or do. Life is precious, and I am glad to still have it!

SIDEBAR 11.6 Staging Breast Cancer

Although the progression of cancer from stage to stage has been categorized for the sake of convenience, it is impossible to predict exactly how this disease will progress in each patient. Every person who develops breast cancer will undergo a unique disease process, unlike anybody else's.

Here is a simplified version of TNM classifications for breast cancer:

TUMOR	NODE	METASTASIS
T0: No tumors found	N0: No nodes involved	M0: No metastasis
Tis: Cancer in situ; first layer of tissue involved; could be DCIS or LCIS	N1: One to three lymph nodes involved on affected side; not attached to each other or to other tissues	M1: Distant metastasis
T1: ≥1 tumors, <2 cm in diameter	N2: Four to nine nodes on same side as tumor involved; nodes attached to each other or to surrounding tissues	
T2: ≥1 tumors, 2–5 cm in diameter	N3: ≥10 axillary nodes involved or nodes from other groups (e.g., infraclavicular, supraclavicular, internal mammary nodes)	
T3: ≥1 tumors >5 cm in diameter		
T4: Tumors invaded chest wall or skin		

These are translated into stages I–IV in this way:

Stage 0	T IS, N0, M0
Stage I	T 1, N0, M0
Stage IIA	T0–T2, N0–N1, M0
Stage IIB	T2–T3, N0–N1, M0
Stage IIIA	T0–T3, N1–N2, M0
Stage IIIB	T4, N0–N2, M0
Stage IIIC	Any T, N3, M0
Stage IV	Any T, any N, M1

Treatment

Treatment for breast cancer depends on the stage of the disease when it is found; staging protocols are discussed in Sidebar 11.6. An early step in treatment then is to determine the stage of the disease. This usually begins with a **sentinel node biopsy**.

Several options for treatment are often used in combination for best results:

Sentinel node biopsy: A biopsy of the first lymph node to receive lymph drainage from a malignant tumor; used to determine whether the cancer has spread.

Postmastectomy pain syndrome: A condition characterized by chronic pain in the axilla, shoulder, arm, or chest wall following breast surgery.

- *Surgery*: Lumpectomies, partial mastectomies, total mastectomies, and modified mastectomies are surgical options for removing tumors and nearby lymph nodes. Lymph nodes are examined for signs of further metastasis. Lymphedema and **postmastectomy pain syndrome** from damaged nerves are possible adverse effects of surgery.
- *Radiation therapy*: Radiation is aimed at tumors to slow or stop growth or to shrink tumors to make them easier to remove surgically. Radiation may be applied externally or internally, with radioactive pellets that are surgically placed around the tumors and removed later.
- *Chemotherapy*: Chemotherapy may be used before surgery to reduce the size of a growth for a better chance of full removal, after surgery as a protective measure, or instead of surgery when tumors are determined to be inoperable.

- *Hormone therapy*: Some breast cancer tumors have been found to be sensitive to estrogen levels; they need access to this hormone to grow. Medications called **selective estrogen receptor modulators** can block estrogen receptor sites or inhibit estrogen production to limit these growths.
- *Biologic therapy*: Monoclonal antibodies may be used to attack potential cancer cells and reduce the risk of recurrence.

All of these treatment options have serious potential side effects that may influence choices about massage and bodywork. These are discussed in detail in Chapter 12.

Medications

- Chemotherapeutic drugs
- Hormone therapy to block receptor sites on cells and to disable growth-promoting proteins
- Biologic therapy: monoclonal antibodies to reduce the risk of recurrence
- Bisphosphonates to promote bone density
- Antiemetics to limit chemotherapy-induced vomiting

Selective estrogen receptor modulators: A group of medications developed to reduce the risk of estrogen-dependent cancers and conditions.

Massage Therapy Implications

RISKS

The risks of massage and bodywork in the context of breast cancer are the same as those for all other cancers: accessible tumors, unstable bones, compromised organs, challenges of treatment, and surgical equipment must all be accommodated. For more information about working with clients who have cancer, see Chapter 12.

BENEFITS

Breast cancer was one of the first types of cancer studied for possible benefits offered by massage therapy. Among these patients, it was found that massage can improve sleep, soothe anxiety, reduce depression, and help to manage pain. As long as appropriate precautions are taken, it is clear that massage and bodywork have much to offer this population.

RESEARCH

The research on massage therapy in the context of breast cancer is far reaching and generally positive. While it isn't shown to "treat" the cancer itself, carefully administered massage therapy has been seen to successfully address anxiety, depression, pain, nausea, constipation, negative self-image, fatigue, immune system function, and quality of life in patients with this disease.[1–4] Studies range from case reports and small-scale pilot studies to larger randomized controlled trials and systematic reviews. Lee et al.[5] concluded that the quality of current research is still too sporadic to proclaim that massage is an effective treatment for the symptoms of breast cancer and treatment, but that it shows promise in this context. Another review[6] looked at research on reflexology, as compared to no treatment or simple rest. Pain, nausea, and vomiting were decreased in the treatment groups, but the risk of bias was high; they conclude that more methodologically rigorous research is needed.

1. Fernandez-Lao C, Cantarero-Villanueva I, Diaz-Rodriguez L, et al. Attitudes towards massage modify effects of manual therapy in breast cancer survivors: a randomised clinical trial with crossover design. *European Journal of Cancer Care* 2012;21(2):233–241. http://www.ncbi.nlm.nih.gov/pubmed/22060159
2. Fernandez-Lao C, Cantarero-Villanueva I, Diaz-Rodriguez L, et al. The influence of patient attitude toward massage on pressure pain sensitivity and immune system after application of myofascial release in breast cancer survivors: a randomized, controlled crossover study. *Journal of Manipulative and Physiological Therapeutics* 2012;35(2):94–100. http://www.ncbi.nlm.nih.gov/pubmed/22018755
3. Mustian KM, Roscoe JA, Palesh OG, et al. Polarity therapy for cancer-related fatigue in patients with breast cancer receiving radiation therapy: a randomized controlled pilot study. *Integrative Cancer Therapies* 2011;10(1):27–37. http://www.ncbi.nlm.nih.gov/pmc/articles/PMC3085180/
4. Krohn M, Listing M, Tjahjono G, et al. Depression, mood, stress, and Th1/Th2 immune balance in primary breast cancer patients undergoing classical massage therapy. *Supportive Care in Cancer* 2011;19(9):1303–1311. http://www.ncbi.nlm.nih.gov/pubmed/20644965
5. Lee MS, Lee EN, Ernst E. Massage therapy for breast cancer patients: a systematic review. *Annals of Oncology* 2011;22(6):1459–1461. http://annonc.oxfordjournals.org/content/22/6/1459.long
6. Kim JI, Lee MS, Kang JW, et al. Reflexology for the symptomatic treatment of breast cancer: a systematic review. *Integrative Cancer Therapies* 2010;9(4):326–330. http://www.ncbi.nlm.nih.gov/pubmed/21106613

Ovarian Cancer

Definition: What Is It?

Ovarian cancer is the growth of malignant tumors on the ovaries. Several varieties of ovarian cancer have been identified, but most of them begin in the epithelial cells of these organs. The tumors may take a long time to become established, but once they do, some types may grow quickly and metastasize readily through the peritoneal cavity to the pelvic wall and other organs.

Demographics

Ovarian cancer is diagnosed in about 24,000 women in this country each year. Although the number of women with this disease is low compared to those of other cancers, its mortality rate is high: ovarian cancer kills about 14,000 women every year.

Etiology: What Happens?

The ovaries, by definition, are made primarily of cells that are primed for reproduction; this makes it vulnerable to the DNA mutations that can lead to malignancy and metastasis. Furthermore, ovaries are located in close contact with several other organs, so the seeding of malignant cells via direct contact, through the peritoneal cavity, or through the circulatory or lymph systems happens easily. This all develops without major symptoms, which is why most diagnoses of ovarian cancer are made at stage III or IV (Figure 11.10).

Although the specific triggers for the growth of tumors on the ovaries are unknown, some of the most important risk factors for developing the disease have been identified:

- *Familial history*: A significant risk factor for ovarian cancer is having it in the family. Women who have a first-degree relative (mother, sister, or daughter) with ovarian cancer have a roughly one in three chance of developing the cancer themselves. Having a second-degree relative (grandmother, aunt, half-sister) with ovarian cancer also increases the chance of developing the disease. Families with a history of breast or colorectal cancer have statistically higher rates of ovarian cancer than the general population. This is true even more consistently if identified breast or colorectal cancer genes are present.
- *Reproductive history*: Women who never have a break in their menstrual cycle (i.e., never been pregnant or taken birth control pills) are at significantly increased risk for this disease. This supports a theory that ovarian cancer may be related to ovulation trauma: the ovaries must heal every time an egg is released, and this wear and tear may trigger genetic mutations in ovary cells. In addition, women who have taken fertility drugs without conceiving and bearing a child may also be at increased risk, although the statistics for these women have been inconsistent.

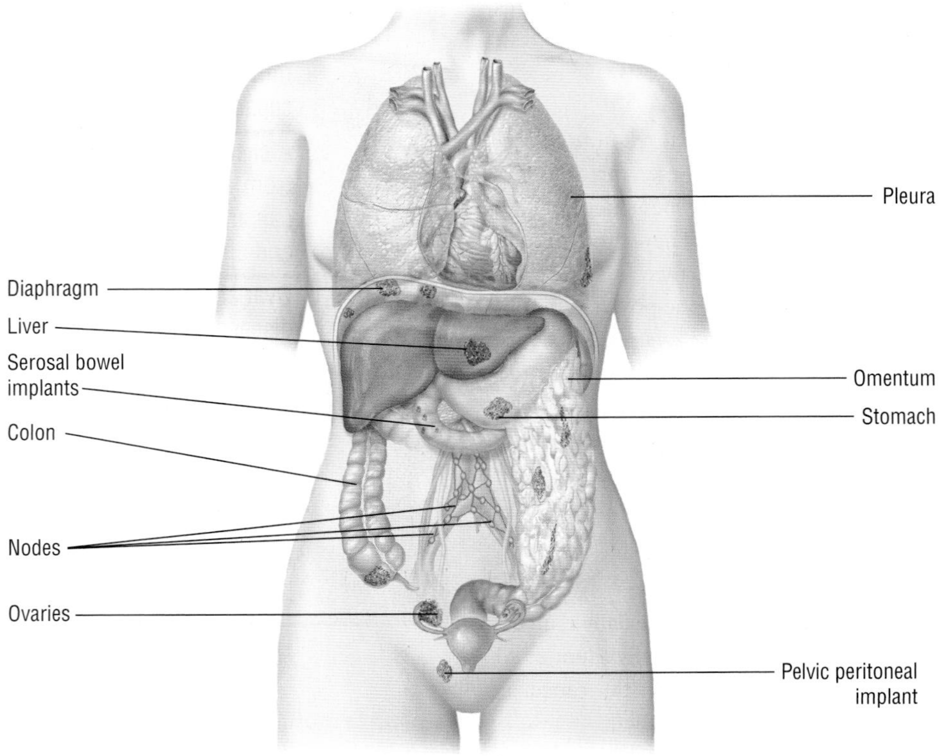

FIGURE 11.10 Metastasis of ovarian cancer

- *Hormone replacement therapy*: Women who have employed HRT have a higher chance of developing ovarian cancer than others. This is most likely when a woman who had a hysterectomy used estrogen alone for more than 10 years.
- *Other*: Other risks include exposure to radiation or asbestos, the use of talcum powder on the genitals, a high-fat diet, a history of **endometriosis,** and age; the chance of developing ovarian cancer goes up considerably between ages 40 and 60.

NOTABLE CASES Mary Tudor, also known as "Bloody Mary" for her relentless persecution of Protestants during her time as Queen of England, is believed to have died of uterine or ovarian cancer at age 42. More recently, civil rights activist Coretta Scott King and actors Madeline Kahn and Gilda Radner succumbed to ovarian cancer. Oscar-winning actor Kathy Bates and US Congresswoman Rosa DeLauro are both long-term ovarian cancer survivors.

Ovarian cancer survivor, triathlete, and licensed massage therapist Jenn Sommerman's response to her experience is this: "I am doing 50 triathlons in all 50 states by the time I am 50 years old to raise $100,000 for ovarian cancer research. As a survivor, I am passionate about finding a method of early detection for this deadly 'silent killer.'"

Jenn met her goal in 2013 and continues to bring attention to this important cause. Her comment: "Completing all 50 states and raising over $100,000 for the Ovarian Cancer Research Fund was more fulfilling than I could have imagined. I know the campaign had an impact on many women and that lives were saved as a result. I raced for women in treatment, those who lost the fight, and for those yet to be diagnosed."

Types of Ovarian cancer

- *Adenocarcinoma of the ovary*: These epithelial cell tumors comprise about 90% of all ovarian cancer diagnoses. Several subcategories have been identified with varying growth patterns. Some are entirely benign; some are not threatening, but others aggressively invade other pelvic and abdominal organs, often without major early symptoms.
- *Germ cell ovarian cancer*: These rare tumors occur most often in women under 30 years old. Several subtypes have been identified, but the prognosis is generally positive.
- *Stromal cell ovarian cancer*: These rare tumors can be benign or malignant. They grow in the connective tissue and hormone-producing cells of the ovaries, so symptoms often have to do with excessive estrogen or testosterone. The prognosis for stromal cell ovarian cancer is usually good.

Signs and Symptoms

The feature that makes ovarian cancer an especially dangerous disease is that early symptoms are practically silent or so subtle that they are easily passed over. When the cancer is finally identified, it has often already metastasized.

Symptoms of ovarian cancer include a feeling of heaviness in the pelvis; vague abdominal discomfort, including bloating, nausea, diarrhea, and constipation; urinary frequency or urgency; vaginal bleeding; a change in menstrual cycles; and weight gain or loss. Because the most common age for women to be affected by ovarian cancer is also the time when symptoms of perimenopause develop, these signals are easily ignored. Later symptoms can include a palpable abdominal mass, increased girth around the abdomen, and ascites—the accumulation of fluid in the peritoneum.

Treatment

Ovarian cancer is generally treated according to stage (see Sidebar 11.7 for staging protocols). Surgery and chemotherapy are the usual first-line strategies. Surgery removes the ovaries (**oophorectomy**) and often the uterine tubes and uterus as well. Surgical "debulking" removes of as much cancerous tissue as possible. This may involve taking out parts of the large or small intestines or other structures. Chemotherapy can be administered orally at home, intravenously, or directly into the peritoneum, where it can have immediate access to malignant tumors. Radiation is seldom used for ovarian cancer itself, but may sometime be employed as **adjunctive therapy**.

Medications

- Chemotherapeutic agents by mouth, IV, or directly into the peritoneum
- Biologic therapies are sometimes used but have not been approved for ovarian cancer treatment

Massage Therapy Implications

RISKS	Ovarian cancer patients typically undergo treatments that are rife with possible adverse effects. Any bodywork offered in this setting must be carefully gauged to these patients' capacity for adaptation and general fragility.
BENEFITS	A client who is in treatment or recovery from ovarian cancer may find that massage can ameliorate the challenges of surgery and chemotherapy.
RESEARCH	Ovarian cancer is a serious, life-threatening disease. Having a positive, hopeful attitude may add to both the quality of life and the life expectancy of patients. Massage therapy has been seen to significantly impact hopelessness scores for the better in ovarian cancer patients.[1] 1. Gross AH, Cromwell J, Fonteyn M, et al. Hopelessness and complementary therapy use in patients with ovarian cancer. *Cancer Nursing* 2013;36(4):256–264. http://www.ncbi.nlm.nih.gov/pubmed/23086133

Oophorectomy: Surgical removal of the ovaries.

Adjunctive therapy: A secondary treatment used to support the primary treatment method for a condition.

SIDEBAR 11.7 Staging Ovarian Cancer

The Fédération Internationale de Gynécologie et d' Obstétrique (FIGO) has developed the most commonly used staging system for ovarian cancer. The tumors are described as being superficial or deep, and the capsule around the tumor is either intact or ruptured. Here is a simplified version of the FIGO system for ovarian cancer staging:

STAGE	SUBDIVISIONS OF STAGES
I: Growth limited to ovaries	IA: One ovary affected; tumor deep; capsule intact; no ascites IB: Two ovaries affected; tumors deep; capsules intact IC: Tumor(s) superficial; capsule(s) ruptured; cancer cells in peritoneal fluid
II: One or both ovaries involved; extensions into pelvis	IIA: Metastases to uterus and/or uterine tubes IIB: Metastases to other pelvic organs IIC: Metastases to uterus, tubes, other pelvic organs
III: One or both ovaries involved; cells in peritoneal fluid; possible metastases in abdomen	IIIA: Metastases limited to pelvis; no lymph nodes involved IIIB: Tumors <2 cm outside pelvis; no lymph nodes involved IIIC: Tumors >2 cm outside pelvis; lymph nodes may be involved
IV: Distant metastases	Metastases in liver or lungs

Ovarian Cysts

Definition: What Are They?

A variety of cysts may grow on the ovaries. They may be related to endometriosis, or they may be types of precancerous growths that eventually develop into ovarian cancer. Most cysts however arise from normal ovaries, either just before or just after ovulation. For this reason, they are often called functional cysts.

Demographics

Most women have an ovarian cyst at some point. Most of them are functional cysts and completely benign and resolve without intervention. Some cysts are associated with other health problems, however. Some 5% to 7% of women in their childbearing years have polycystic ovarian syndrome (PCOS), which is connected to several other disease processes, and **ovarian cancer** can begin as cystadenomas, so it is important to pursue an accurate diagnosis for persistent symptoms.

Etiology: What Happens?

Each month, a fertile woman develops several follicles (pockets where eggs are held) on one of her ovaries. As her cycle progresses, a single follicle becomes dominant and the others recede. At the appropriate hormonal signal, the follicle ruptures, releasing a mature ovum into the pelvic cavity. From there, the egg is drawn into the uterine tubes for the journey toward the uterus.

Every follicle that develops could become a cyst, either before ovulation or after. Sometimes, the hormonal signal (a surge in luteinizing hormone) doesn't occur, and the follicle doesn't rupture completely. Consequently, a blister forms on the ovary, locking the egg inside. Sometimes, the ruptured follicle (now called the **corpus luteum**) seals up behind the discharged ovum, trapping the hormones that should flow freely from it. This kind of blister may eventually break and bleed into the pelvic cavity.

The reasons some women develop cysts and others do not are complex and multifactorial. Estrogen dominance may play a role, as well as hypersensitivity to gonadotropin-stimulating hormone. Infertility treatments (which drastically alter hormone levels) can also cause ovarian cysts to develop.

Size is the major factor that determines whether or not ovarian cysts cause any trouble. They can grow big enough to interfere with blood flow; they may also rest on the bladder. In rare cases, they grow to huge dimensions. An ovarian cyst that hangs from a stalk sometimes gets twisted; this is called torsion. Large cysts can also cause the whole ovary to twist. If torsion develops, acute abdominal pain, nausea, and fever develop; medical intervention is necessary, as the tissue may become necrotic. The risk of **peritonitis** is high in this situation.

Perhaps, the most serious complicating factor of ovarian cysts is that their early symptoms, subtle as they may be, mimic an advanced case of ovarian cancer. This is a threatening cancer

Corpus luteum: A temporary hormone-secreting structure in an ovary that exists where a follicle containing an egg used to be.

that has few early symptoms. By the time a person can feel a firm, painless swelling in her pelvis, the disease is dangerously advanced. Therefore, if a client displays any of these symptoms but has not been examined, it is important for her to get more information as soon as possible.

Types of Ovarian Cysts

- *Follicular cysts*: When a follicle that holds a mature egg doesn't rupture completely, a blister forms at the site; this occurs before ovulation (Figure 11.11). Follicular cysts rarely get bigger than 2 to 3 inches across, and they usually spontaneously recede within two menstrual cycles. Follicular cysts are the most common ovarian cysts.
- *Corpus luteum cysts*: Blisters can form over the corpus luteum, which blocks the hormones that should be secreted from the ovaries. This happens after ovulation. Corpus luteum cysts delay subsequent ovulations and produce symptoms mimicking pregnancy (nausea, vomiting, breast tenderness) until they spontaneously resolve, usually within a month or two. Corpus luteum cysts are less common than follicular cysts, but they can be more serious, as they may rupture and bleed.
- *Polycystic ovaries*: This condition is characterized by enlarged ovaries with multiple small cysts that are immature follicles that don't ovulate (Figure 11.12). The changes in hormone secretion that this condition produces may lead to loss of menstrual cycle, **acne,** and hirsutism. Polycystic ovarian syndrome (PCOS) is also closely linked to poor insulin sensitivity, high triglycerides, low high-density lipoproteins, and other signs associated with **metabolic syndrome, diabetes,** and heart disease. A genetic anomaly leading to the overproduction of androgens has been identified as a contributing factor to PCOS.
- *Endometriomas*: These are pockets of endometrial cells on the ovaries as a part of **endometriosis.** They are sometimes called chocolate cysts.
- *Dermoid cysts*: In dermoid cysts, also called teratomas, some primitive cells have been isolated from the rest of the body, and these develop into various types of tissues. Dermoid cysts may contain teeth, hairs, bone fragments, and other types of tissue. They are usually harmless in women, although they can limit ovarian function. Men can develop them too, but for males, teratomas are a much more serious condition that may be connected to testicular cancer.
- *Cystadenomas*: These are usually benign fluid-filled cysts on the surface of the ovary, but they bear watching, because they can develop malignant characteristics.

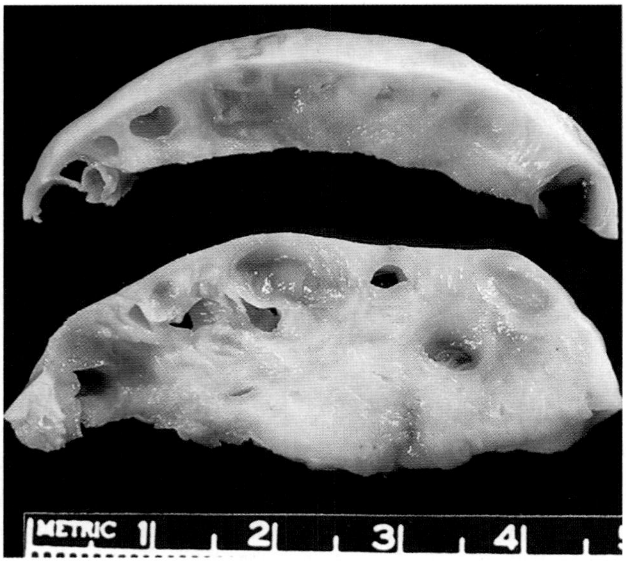

FIGURE 11.12 Polycystic ovary

Follicular cyst

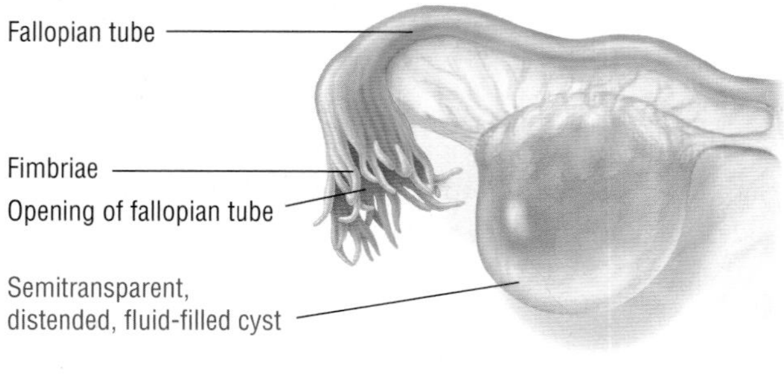

FIGURE 11.11 Follicular cysts form at the site of egg release, blocking ovulation

Signs and Symptoms

Most ovarian cysts have no symptoms until the cyst is injured in some way. Some women, however, have a dull ache in the lower abdomen on the affected side. A firm, painless swelling may develop in the pelvis, and occasionally, an ovarian cyst causes pain with intercourse. Large cysts may cause low back pain or, through pressure on the lumbar plexus, pain in the legs.

In the absence of these signs, a person might never know a cyst is present unless it grows big enough to interfere with other functions or if it twists or ruptures.

Treatment

Follicular and corpus luteum cysts are often treated with watchful waiting to make sure they resolve. Oral contraceptives may be used to alter hormonal secretions and prevent new cysts from forming.

Hirsutism: Abnormally strong presence of bodily and facial hair in a male pattern, especially in women.

Teratoma: A tumor that contains tissues not normally found in the tissue in which it arises. Usually found in the ovaries and testes.

Surgery may be recommended if hormone treatment is not successful. This can be in the form a closed **laparoscopy** or an open **laparotomy**, depending on the type of cyst and the risks involved. In some cases, complete removal of the ovaries and uterus is recommended because some types of cysts tend to recur and can develop into cancer.

Medications

- Oral birth control pills
- Luteinizing hormone analogs for PCOS
- Antiandrogenizing hormones if birth control pills are unsuccessful

Massage Therapy Implications

RISKS	Ovarian cysts locally contraindicate intrusive abdominal massage. Cysts can be quite large, and they can cause the pelvic contents to shift so that structures are vulnerable outside of their usual locations. Pressure may cause them to rupture and bleed, which can be a medical emergency. Clients with PCOS are at increased risk for diabetes and metabolic syndrome, each of which has its own set of cautions for bodywork.
BENEFITS	While massage is unlikely to change the course of ovarian cysts for the better, simple precautions can allow clients with this condition to receive many benefits from bodywork. A history of ovarian cysts with no current symptoms carries no cautions for massage.

Disorders of the Male Reproductive System

Benign Prostatic Hyperplasia

Definition: What Is It?

Benign prostatic hyperplasia (BPH) is a condition in which the prostate gland of mature men grows new cells and becomes enlarged. This growth late in life is not related to **prostate cancer,** hence the name "benign." For more information on BPH vocabulary, see Sidebar 11.8.

Demographics

Nearly 50% of men over 60 years old have some level of BPH, 70% of men over 70 have it, 80% of men over 80 have it, and so on. Approximately 14 million men in the United States have been diagnosed with this condition, although many of them do not experience significant symptoms.

Etiology: What Happens?

The prostate gland of a preadolescent male is very small. As a boy enters puberty, this pea-sized gland that wraps around the urethra just below the bladder grows approximately to the size of a walnut. It stays that size until a man is 25 to 40 years old, and then some prostates begin to grow again.

It is unclear why some prostate glands grow and others do not. Theories about triggers for late prostate growth involve the hormonal changes that come with maturity. One possible factor may be the formation of **dihydrotestosterone**

> **Laparoscopy:** Examination of the abdominal contents with a scope passed through the abdominal wall.
>
> **Laparotomy:** An incision into the abdominal wall.
>
> **Dihydrotestosterone:** A form of testosterone.

SIDEBAR 11.8 Vocabulary Check: Hypertrophy versus Hyperplasia—A Small But Important Difference

In discussions of prostate enlargement, the terms *hypertrophy* and *hyperplasia* are sometimes used interchangeably. This is understandable, because both of them suggest an increase in size. But they mean two different things, and it is important to be accurate.

Hypertrophy means each cell in the tissue under discussion gets larger, but the structure does not grow new cells. For instance, when we exercise and our muscles get bigger, it is because each muscle cell is expanding—we are not adding to our total number of muscle cells.

Hyperplasia means the cells stay the same size, but we grow more of them. This is the case with tumors, for instance. BPH then describes a prostate that grows new cells—not cancerous ones—but because its symptoms are so similar to those of prostate cancer, it is wise to track this process carefully.

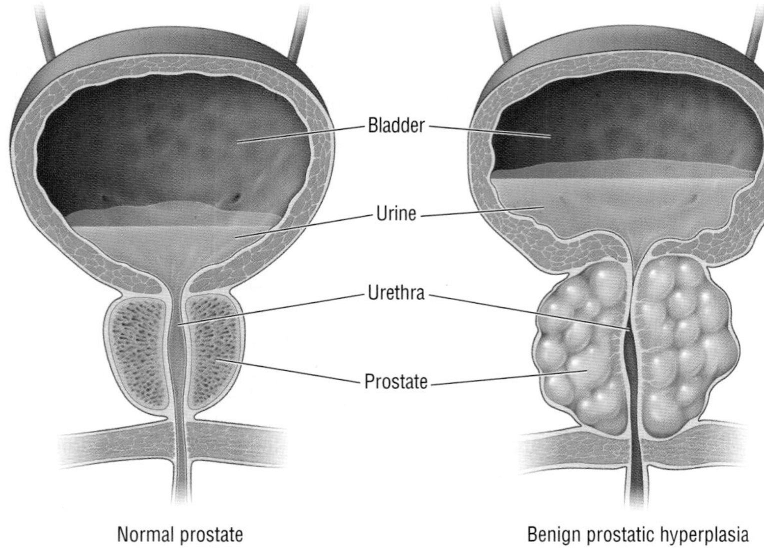

FIGURE 11.13 Benign prostatic hyperplasia

(DHT). This hormone is a form of testosterone that has been seen to increase prostate size. Another theory is that as men age, they produce less testosterone to balance out their normal levels of estrogen plus estrogen from outside sources; this may lead to **hyperplasia**, as estrogen is also associated with prostate growth.

Regardless of the cause of prostate growth, BPH may lead to mechanical pressure on the urethra (Figure 11.13). This occurs for two reasons: the prostate is surrounded by a tough fascial capsule that does not allow it to expand outward, and the tissue usually affected by BPH is in the **periurethral** and **transitional** sections of the gland. This helps to distinguish BPH from prostate cancer, which typically begins on the outer borders of the prostate.

The extent of prostate growth does not always correspond with the sense of pressure on the urethra; some men have advanced BPH with no urinary symptoms at all, while others have minimal amounts of prostate growth and severe urethral constriction.

Complications

Mechanical pressure on the urethra makes it difficult to expel urine from the body. Long-term consequences can include pathological changes in the bladder, which can become stiff, inelastic, and irritable. The risk of **urinary tract infections, pyelonephritis,** and **bladder stones** is much higher in men who cannot urinate easily; these are common complications of BPH.

> **Hyperplasia:** An increase in the number of cells in a tissue or organ, outside of tumor formation.
>
> **Periurethral:** Related to the tissues that surround the urethra.
>
> **Transitional:** The transitional portion of the prostate surrounds part of the urethra. It continues to grow throughout life and is responsible for BPH.

Signs and Symptoms

Signs and symptoms of BPH, when any develop at all, involve difficulties with urination. Weak flow, interrupted flow, frequency, and a feeling that the bladder is never completely emptied are often reported. Leaking or dribbling urine between visits to the bathroom is common. Some men find it difficult to initiate urination, and they must strain or push to start their flow. Other men find that they need to urinate more frequently, especially at night. BPH does not typically cause pelvic pain, which distinguishes it from **prostatitis**.

One rare but serious sign of BPH is an abrupt obstruction of the urethra, called acute urinary retention. In this situation, the urethra is suddenly completely obstructed and urine has no way to get out of the body. This situation is often associated with the use of over-the-counter cold or allergy medications. It is a medical emergency and must be treated in a hospital.

Treatment

BPH is treated according to severity. If it does not seriously affect a man's ability to urinate, it may be left untreated but closely monitored for signs of further growth.

A number of options have been developed to limit prostate growth, including medications and a variety of minimally invasive surgeries.

Medications for BPH include drugs designed to lower levels of DHT and alpha-blockers. These medications were originally developed to treat high blood pressure, and they help the prostate and bladder neck to relax. The side effects of these medications can be significant however, including inability to achieve erection, lowered sex drive, lowered sperm counts, dizziness, fatigue, and others.

Surgical options for BPH include a variety of techniques that cut away, vaporize, burn, microwave, or otherwise remove small sections of the prostate gland to relieve pressure on the urethra. These are done by way of the urethra as minimally invasive procedures.

Medications

- Hormones to alter prostate cell behavior
- Alpha-blockers to relax smooth muscle tissue and improve urinary symptoms

Massage Therapy Implications

RISKS	If a client with BPH reports any symptoms of a urinary tract or kidney infection, it is important that he get appropriate care as soon as possible. Otherwise, massage carries no specific risks for a client with BPH.
BENEFITS	Most bodywork is safe and appropriate for clients who have BPH, as long as they are comfortable receiving it, but massage is unlikely to have a direct effect on prostate size.
OPTIONS	Practitioners trained in visceral manipulation report that clients with BPH may experience some symptomatic relief with careful abdominopelvic bodywork. It is important to work knowledgeably in this area and to rule out the risk of prostate cancer.

Prostate Cancer

Definition: What Is It?

Prostate cancer is the growth of malignant tumor cells in the prostate gland. This cancer often grows slowly, but some versions of it can be aggressive. Prostate cancer can metastasize to other parts of the body, most often the bladder, rectum, and bones of the pelvis.

Demographics

Prostate is the second leading cause of death by cancer for men: each year, about 233,000 cases of prostate cancer are diagnosed in this country, and about 29,000 men die of the disease. That said, the 5-year survival rate for prostate cancer is 98.9%, and 2.5 million men in the United States have successfully treated or are living with this condition.

Most prostate cancer patients are men over 65; it is rare in men under 40. It is both more common and more serious in African American men than in other races.

Etiology: What Happens?

The prostate is a doughnut-shaped gland that lies inferior to the bladder and encircles the male urethra. It produces the fluid that allows for the motility and viability of sperm. The prostate also controls the release of urine from the bladder. Some enlargement of the prostate in later years is a guarantee for most men. Simple enlargement with no malignant cells is **benign prostatic hyperplasia** (BPH). But sometimes the growth and thickening of the prostate gland is not benign; it indicates prostate cancer.

When cancerous cells begin to form a tumor in the prostate, they can exert direct or indirect pressure on the urethra. This can lead to a number of different problems, from difficulty in urinating to urgency, frequency, **nocturia**, painful ejaculation, and **urinary tract infections**. Because the symptoms of prostate cancer are similar to those of BPH, these signs may be ignored until the urethra is seriously restricted. (Compare & Contrast 11.1.) Prostate cancer often grows slowly, and it can stay silent long enough for cells to metastasize before it is detected.

Three main red flags for prostate cancer risk have been identified from findings in biopsied tissues; these are sometimes called precancerous conditions. **Prostatic intraepithelial neoplasia** can be rated as low grade or high grade; and **proliferative inflammatory atrophy** has also been associated with an increased risk. Men whose biopsies return these findings don't have prostate cancer per se, but they need to be more diligent than others about tracking their prostate health.

The triggers for prostate cancer are unknown. However, for tumors to grow, they must have access to testosterone

NOTABLE CASES Prostate cancer is often so treatable that many of the first people who were willing to publicize their disease are still living. Politicians Bob Dole, Rudolf Giuliani, and John Kerry are all prostate cancer survivors. This puts them in company with former President of South Africa Nelson Mandela, former Secretary of State Colin Powell, and musician, artist, and activist Harry Belafonte.

Sadly, the diagnosis of prostate cancer came too late for actor Telly Savalas, musician Frank Zappa, and two-time Nobel Prize winner Linus Pauling, PhD.

Nocturia: The need to wake and urinate during the night.

Prostatic intraepithelial neoplasia (PIN): The presence of abnormal cells in the epithelium of the prostate.

Proliferative inflammatory atrophy: A condition of the prostate and other tissues involving chronic inflammation, which leads to cellular proliferation and an increased risk of cancer.

COMPARE & CONTRAST 11.1 Prostate Dysfunction

When the prostate gland becomes enlarged or irritated, symptoms are predictable: restriction of urinary flow, bladder irritation, and a risk of urinary tract infection that can complicate to pyelonephritis. The causes of prostate enlargement, however, are not so consistent. BPH can be hard to distinguish from prostate cancer, and prostatitis adds to the general confusion. Here are some general guidelines about similarities and differences with these conditions:

CHARACTERISTICS	PROSTATE CANCER	BENIGN PROSTATIC HYPERPLASIA	PROSTATITIS
Who gets it?	Usually affects men older than 50 but can occur in younger men with certain risk factors.	Very common in mature men; incidence increases with age.	Can occur in males of any age; leading cause of visits to urologist for young men.
Signs and symptoms	Restricted urinary flow; pain with pressure on other structures or bone damage; blood in urine possible.	Restricted urinary flow, bladder irritation.	Symptoms vary with causes, but usually significant pelvic pain.
Diagnosis	DRE, PSA tests, ultrasound to evaluate risk of prostate cancer; findings confirmed with biopsy.	DRE, PSA tests, and tests to measure urinary flow usually confirm BPH.	DRE, examinations of urine, semen, prostate secretions to evaluate type of prostatitis.
Treatment	Determined by age of patient, stage of cancer. Options include surgery, chemotherapy, radiation, watchful waiting.	Medications to limit prostate growth may be prescribed; surgery to enlarge passageway for urethra may be performed.	Antibiotics for infections; otherwise treated symptomatically.
Implications for massage	Therapists must adapt to chosen treatment options (see Chapter 12).	Massage has no direct effect on BPH and is safe as long as no infection is present and client is comfortable on table.	After any infection is treated, massage is safe. Some pelvic pain may be referred from trigger points.

DRE, digital rectal exam; PSA, prostate-specific antigen.

from fully functional testes. This disease is not seen in men who have been physically or chemically castrated, and removal of the testes shrinks cancerous tumors.

Men with prostate cancer in their immediate family are more likely than others to develop this disease. Likewise, men from families whose women have breast cancer have a higher-than-average risk. Heredity is estimated to account for about 5% to 10% of prostate cancer cases.

Signs and Symptoms

Signs of prostate cancer are similar to those for BPH: an enlarged prostate, obstruction of the urethra with resulting difficulty in urination, and susceptibility to urinary tract and **kidney infections**. In addition, men with prostate cancer may also have pain while urinating or ejaculating, blood in the urine, and an inability to maintain an erection. Low back pain and pain that refers into the upper thighs may follow as the growths become large enough to put mechanical pressure on pelvic nerves or erode into bone tissue.

One possible sign of prostate cancer is a positive PSA (prostate-specific antigen) blood test. Its usefulness is somewhat debatable, since many variables may cause PSA levels to rise or fall, but when levels are higher than normal, this blood test can serve as a warning sign to consider the possibility of prostate cancer. For more information on PSA tests, see Sidebar 11.9.

SIDEBAR 11.9 What Does a PSA Test Tell?

One of the diagnostic procedures for prostate cancer is a blood test to measure levels of a substance called prostate-specific antigen (PSA). PSA is a protein secreted by the prostate gland. Under certain circumstances, levels of this protein can rise; one of those circumstances is the growth of malignant tumors in the prostate gland.

PSA tests can be used to predict the possibility of prostate cancer, to monitor the effectiveness of prostate cancer treatment, and to detect the recurrence of prostate cancer. However, lots of things can elevate PSA levels, including infection or inflammation, ejaculation within the past 24 hours, riding a bicycle, and some herbs and medications. Any of these can falsely elevate PSA levels in a blood test.

A "normal" PSA test shows fewer than four nanograms of this protein per milliliter of blood (ng/mL). Even at this level, up to 15% of men tested still have prostate cancer, so this rating system may be recalibrated. PSA readings show the following for the risk of prostate cancer:

PSA LEVELS	% DIAGNOSED WITH PROSTATE CANCER
<4 ng/mL	15%
4–10 ng/mL	25%
>10 ng/mL	>50%

A PSA test is just the beginning of gathering information about the risk of prostate cancer. Other variables include whether the PSA is free or attached to other blood proteins: higher ratios of free PSA indicate a higher chance for a nonmalignant situation, while higher ratios of attached PSA are associated with an increased risk of prostate cancer. PSA velocity (how the levels change over time), PSA density (the relationship between PSA and the size of the prostate), and other factors can yield more information about the risk of prostate cancer.

Overall, a basic PSA reading can be influenced by so many noncancer factors, and the treatments for early prostate cancer are so fraught with possible risks and complications that doing PSA testing is considered by some to be more harmful than not.

Treatment

Treatment options for prostate cancer depend on the stage at which it is diagnosed. For information on staging prostate cancer, see Sidebar 11.10. Treatments include watchful waiting; radiation from surgically implanted pellets (**brachytherapy**), external beams, or precisely aimed protons; surgery to remove part or all of the prostate, seminal vesicles, or testes; and hormone therapy to counteract elevated levels of testosterone. Chemotherapy is generally reserved for very advanced cases. The "training" of white blood cells or specially developed stem cells to attack cancer cells is another strategy that is new but showing promising results. One pilot study of men with low-risk prostate cancer showed that when they underwent an intense change in diet and lifestyle (moving to a plant-based diet and adding exercise), gene expression in the prostate was modulated, leading to less malignant characteristics.

> **Brachytherapy:** a medical procedure in which radioactive materials are implanted directly into tissue.

Most treatment options for prostate cancer have daunting side effects, including temporary or permanent incontinence, erectile dysfunction, sterility, and the development of feminine characteristics. For these reasons, elderly men or men with other health problem who have slow-growing tumors may opt not to treat their disease because their quality of life would be so seriously affected.

Medications

- Hormone therapy to interfere with cancer cell receptors or suppress testosterone production
- Analgesics for pain management
- Bisphosphonates to maintain or recover bone density
- Chemotherapeutic agents for advanced disease
- Biologic therapy to sensitize white blood cells to attack cancer cells

Massage Therapy Implications

RISKS	Any massage therapists who number elderly men among their clientele will have some clients living with the threat of prostate cancer. This condition can be slow growing and relatively nonthreatening; but it can also be aggressive. Any bodywork must accommodate not only prostate cancer but also whatever treatment options the client has chosen to pursue. Clients who have chosen brachytherapy are best delaying massage until the radioactive pellets have been removed.
BENEFITS	Massage therapy is a wonderful option to deal with the often underaddressed issues related to cancer: depression, anxiety, insomnia, and general pain. For more information on massage in the context of cancer, see Chapter 12.

SIDEBAR 11.10 Staging Prostate Cancer

Most specialists in the United States use the TNM staging system for prostate cancer, in combination with a cancer cell rating system called the Gleason scale. This rates cells according to their appearance and aggressiveness; a low score suggests a less threatening problem, and a higher score means a more threatening problem. The Gleason ratings range from 2 to 10, but may be doubled if multiple neoplasms are found in the prostate.

Prostate cancer, like some other cancers, sometimes cannot be fully staged until surgery is conducted and tissue is examined. The following is a combination of clinical staging (based on best estimates without surgery) and pathological staging (based on findings during or after surgery).

TUMOR	TUMOR SUBSTAGE	NODE	METASTASIS
T1: Tumor cannot be palpated or found with transrectal ultrasound	T1A: Tumor found with treatment for BPH; affects <5% of tissue	N0: No nodes involved	M0: No metastasis
	T1B: Tumor found with treatment for BPH; affects >5% of tissue	N1: ≥1 regional nodes involved	M1: Distant metastasis
	T1C: Tumor found with needle biopsy, elevated PSA levels		
T2: Tumor palpable with DRE; confined to the prostate	T2A: <50% of one side is affected.		
	T2B: >50% of one side is affected.		
	T2C: Both sides affected		
T3: Tumors outside prostate and/or on seminal vesicles	T3A: Tumors outside prostate but not on seminal vesicles		
	T3B: Tumors on seminal vesicles		
T4: Tumors on other tissues, including bladder and wall of pelvis			

The TNM ratings are then combined with Gleason scores to stage prostate cancer from stage I to IV in this way:

STAGE	TUMOR	NODE	METASTASIS	PSA	GLEASON SCORE
I	T1A or 2A	N0	M0	<10	<6
II	T1–T2	N0–N1	M0	10–20	2–10
III	T3	N1	M0	Any	Any
IV	Any	N1	M0	Any	Any
IV	Any	Any	M1	Any	Any

BPH, benign prostatic hyperplasia; DRE, digital rectal exam

Prostatitis

Definition: What Is It?

Prostatitis is a condition in which the prostate becomes painful and possibly inflamed. Unlike **benign prostatic hyperplasia**, prostatitis usually involves significant pain throughout the pelvis and groin. While occasionally connected to a specific infection, it is often difficult to identify and treat the causes of prostatitis.

Demographics

Prostatitis in its several forms accounts for 2 million visits to urologists each year. It is estimated that 50% of all American men will experience symptoms at some point. Prostatitis is the most common prostate problem in men under 50.

Etiology: What Happens?

The prostate of an adult man is a walnut-sized gland that surrounds the urethra just distal to the urinary bladder of males. It is composed of ducts and channels into which epithelial cells secrete seminal fluid, a constituent of semen. The seminal fluid is expressed into the urethra during ejaculation.

The draining channels in the prostate are arranged in a basically horizontal plane around the periphery of the organ.

This allows material to become stagnant within the gland if it is not frequently expelled. Furthermore, bladder reflux, which allows urine to collect in the prostate, can cause irritation or even direct bacterial exposure to these delicate epithelial tissues, leading to a risk of prostate stones that can block channels and acute or chronic infection that may be difficult to treat.

Prostatitis is an umbrella term for four basic types of problems. These classes of prostatitis were outlined by the National Institutes of Health in 1995 to create a framework for more efficient study of this often mysterious and difficult problem.

Types of Prostatitis

- *Type 1, Acute bacterial prostatitis*: This is an acute infection of the prostate. This may be accompanied by abscesses, which may require surgical removal.
- *Type 2, Chronic bacterial prostatitis*: This is a recurrent, low-grade infection of the prostate. The most common infectious agent for types 1 and 2 is *Escherichia coli*.
- *Type 3, Chronic nonbacterial prostatitis/chronic pelvic pain syndrome (CPPS)*: This is prostate irritation with no demonstrable infection. Another term for this condition is **prostatodynia**. Subgroups of this class include the following, although these distinctions are becoming less important and may be discarded because the treatment strategies are the same.
  - *Type 3a, Inflammatory chronic pelvic pain syndrome*: White blood cells are found in the semen, expressed prostatic secretions, or urine.
  - *Type 3b, Noninflammatory chronic pelvic pain syndrome*: White blood cells are not found in semen, expressed prostatic secretions, or urine. This is by far the most commonly reported version of prostatitis. It is not well understood, because no specific causative factors have been identified. Some experts suggest that CPPS may be due to bacteria that are difficult to culture and treat; others think that chronic hypertonicity or trigger points are referring pain from the perineal muscle; this suggests that some cases may be related to myofascial pain.
- Type 4, *Asymptomatic inflammatory prostatitis*: This has no subjective symptoms, but white blood cells are found in prostate secretions or in prostate tissue during an evaluation for other disorders.

> **Prostatodynia:** Chronic pelvic pain in men that is not the result of an infection or other obvious cause. Also called chronic pelvic pain syndrome (CPPS).

Signs and Symptoms

Acute bacterial prostatitis has all of the signs and symptoms of a **urinary tract infection**: pain and burning with urination along with urinary frequency and urgency. In addition, pain in the pelvis, perineum, testicles, and penis may be present, along with penile discharge, painful ejaculation, possible erectile dysfunction, low back pain, and fever. The prostate, palpated by a doctor through the wall of the rectum, is painful and palpably hot.

Chronic bacterial prostatitis, which indicates recurrent low-grade infection, produces the same symptoms, but with less severity.

CPPS has the same profile without the element of fever, and although pelvic pain is present, palpation of the prostate shows no inflammation.

Treatment

Acute bacterial prostatitis responds well to antibiotics, but chronic bacterial prostatitis does not. Antibiotics cannot easily access the interior of the prostate; treatment may take 6 weeks or more of antibiotic therapy, and infection frequently recurs.

If prostate stones are discovered, they are surgically removed, typically with laser surgery through the urethra.

Chronic pelvic pain is often treated with a short or long course of antibiotics just in case some bacteria were missed and then dealt with symptomatically. Alpha-blockers relax the smooth muscle tissue in the bladder for easier urination; anti-inflammatories, frequent ejaculations, and sitz baths (a bath just for the pelvic area) to help relax the perineal muscle are also recommended. Antianxiety medications are sometimes prescribed. Biofeedback techniques to increase awareness of tightness in the perineal muscle have some success. Some urologists suggest teaching patients to use a tool for self-massage of perineal trigger points. Devices that modulate perineal nerves may work for some patients as well. For many men, however, CPPS is a stubborn disorder with no simple answers; it can have a long-term and severe impact on their quality of life.

Medications

- Antibiotics for bacterial infection
- Anti-inflammatories and analgesics for chronic pain
- Alpha-blockers to improve urine flow
- Antianxiety medication for chronic pain

Massage Therapy Implications

RISKS	When acute infection with fever and inflammation is present, invasive or rigorous massage is inappropriate.
BENEFITS	Massage is unlikely to have a direct impact on prostate irritation, but anything that can improve the quality of life for a patient with a chronic, nonacute problem can be helpful.
OPTIONS	It is possible that some pelvic pain is related to trigger points in the perineal muscle that refer to the pelvic cavity. That makes this a musculoskeletal condition. In most massage laws, however, work on the perineal muscle is not within the scope of practice for massage therapists.
RESEARCH	One group[1] conducted a feasibility study, comparing myofascial physical therapy (which addresses trigger points on the perineum) to global therapeutic massage for patients with CPPS. Both groups had relief, but the myofascial physical therapy group had greater relief that lasted for longer. 1. Fitzgerald MP, Anderson RU, Potts J, et al. Randomized multicenter feasibility trial of myofascial physical therapy for the treatment of urological chronic pelvic pain syndromes. *Journal of Urology* 2013;189(1 Suppl):S75–S85. http://www.ncbi.nlm.nih.gov/pubmed/23234638

Testicular Cancer

Definition: What Is It?

Testicular cancer is growth of malignant cells in the testicles. These cells usually grow slowly, but they may metastasize through the lymph or blood systems to the bones, liver, lungs, and brain.

Demographics

Testicular cancer is diagnosed about 8,800 times per year and causes about 400 deaths per year in this country. It is most often found in white men between 20 and 55 years old, but it has been found in males of any age and race.

Although it is a relatively rare disease, diagnostic rates of testicular cancer have been rising for several decades in the United States and other developed countries. Researchers suggest that this may be connected to environmental endocrine disruptors.

Cryptorchidism: The failure of one or both of the testes to descend.

Seminoma: The most common type of testicular cancer.

Nonseminoma: A type of testicular cancer.

Embryonic carcinoma: A rare cancer of the ovaries and testes.

Yolk sac tumor: A rare form of cancer, usually found in the ovaries or testes of children under the age of 2.

Choriocarcinoma: A very invasive cancer, usually of the placenta, but which also occurs sometimes in the ovaries and testes.

This is a highly treatable cancer with an excellent cure rate. Five years after diagnosis, over 95% of all patients are alive, and about 230,000 testicular cancer survivors live in the United States at this time.

Etiology: What Happens?

As with many other cancers, testicular cancer begins with a mutation to fast-growing cells that causes them to pile up into tumors that can invade healthy tissue. The causes or contributing factors of testicular cancer are not well understood. The only consistent risk factor is that males who were born with **cryptorchidism** have a slightly higher risk of developing this disease. Other risk factors include other congenital abnormalities, age, race, personal or family history of testicular cancer, and **HIV** status: men who are HIV positive have a slightly higher risk of testicular cancer than others.

Types of Testicular Cancer

- *Germ cell tumors*: These are tumors that arise within the sperm and hormone-producing cells of the testicle. Germ cell tumors are further classified into **seminomas** and **nonseminomas**.
  - *Seminomas*: These are the most common variety of testicular cancer, accounting for 40% to 45% of diagnoses. They tend to grow slowly and are highly sensitive to radiation.
  - *Nonseminomas*: These are several different types of testicular tumors, some of which are more aggressive than others. **Embryonic carcinomas**, **yolk sac tumors**, and **teratomas** are growths that resemble the growth pattern of embryos. **Choriocarcinoma** is the most aggressive form of testicular cancer and has the poorest prognosis.

- *Stromal cell tumors*: These are growths within the supportive tissue for the testicle. They are quite rare and account for only 5% or less of testicular cancers.

Signs and Symptoms

Testicular cancer usually begins with a painless lump on the testicle (Figure 11.14). It may be accompanied by a feeling of fullness or heaviness or fluid in the scrotum. A dull ache in the low abdomen or groin may develop, along with enlargement and tenderness at the breasts. If any of these symptoms persist for more than 2 weeks, the person should consult his physician as soon as possible.

Later signs of testicular cancer indicate metastasis: coughing and shortness of breath if tumors have invaded the lungs, painless lumps in the neck if the cervical lymph nodes are affected, and so on.

Treatment

The treatment options for testicular cancer depend on the stage at diagnosis (see Sidebar 11.11), but they usually begin with surgery to remove the affected testicle and any secondary tumors that are found. If the cancer is identified as a seminoma, radiation therapy follows surgery; these cancer cells are extremely sensitive to radiation, and this protocol is usually completely successful. If the cancer was a mixed tumor or a nonseminoma, chemotherapy may be used following surgery.

Depending on the findings in the removed tissue, a second surgery may be conducted to take lymph nodes from the pelvis or abdomen. This is a more invasive procedure that has a higher risk of complications, including damage to the nerves that control ejaculation, which can be permanent.

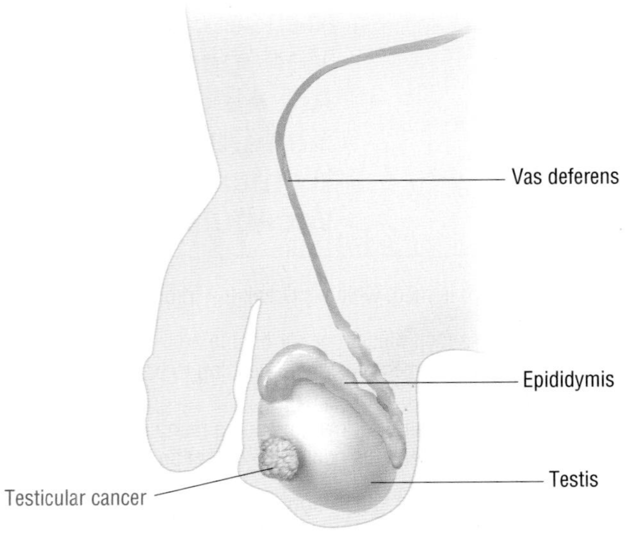

FIGURE 11.14 Testicular cancer: the earliest sign is usually a painless lump on the testicle

SIDEBAR 11.11 Staging Testicular Cancer

Testicular cancer is staged differently from most other cancers; instead of progressing from stage 0 to stage IV, it is usually discussed as stages 0 to III. Specialists use highly defined and detailed staging protocols to make appropriate treatment plans and prognoses. These often include measurements of cancer markers and hormones in the blood along with tumor, node, and metastatic progress. The following is a simplified version of testicular cancer staging:

- Stage 0. This is cancer in situ: preinvasive germ cell cancer.
- Stage I. The testicle and spermatic cord are affected; no spread to lymph nodes; blood tests are normal.
- Stage II. Nearby lymph nodes are invaded.
- Stage IIA. The nodes show signs of microscopic invasion. This is sometimes called "nonbulky stage II."
- Stage IIB. The nodes are larger than 5 cm; this can be called "bulky stage II."
- Stage III. Distant lymph nodes and other tissues are invaded.
- Stage IIIA. Only lymph nodes are invaded, but growths are smaller than 2 cm (nonbulky stage III).
- Stage IIIB. Other tissues are invaded, usually the central nervous system and/or lungs. Lymph node metastases are larger than 2 cm (bulky stage III).

Follow-up care after testicular cancer treatment is critical to make sure no metastases were missed. Furthermore, testicular cancer survivors have a small but significant risk of developing cancer in the other testicle.

The survival rate for testicular cancer is so high, and the treatments available are so effective that no invasive early screening protocols for this disease have been demonstrated to improve life expectancy. Nonetheless, many men are taught to conduct testicular self-examinations, just as women are taught to do breast self-examinations. In this way, any changes in the tissue may be identified and investigated as quickly as possible.

NOTABLE CASES Perhaps, the most famous public figure with testicular cancer is bicyclist Lance Armstrong, who was diagnosed with a combination of nonseminoma growths that had metastasized to his lungs and brain. Other familiar names include Olympic figure skater Scott Hamilton, the subject of the movie "Brian's Song" football player Brian Piccolo, and actor and comedian Richard Belzer, who, coincidentally, produced a CD titled "Another Lone Nut."

Medications

- Chemotherapeutic agents

11 Reproductive System Conditions

Massage Therapy Implications

RISKS	Most testicular cancer patients undergo cycles of radiation or chemotherapy. Any bodywork must be adjusted for these challenges.
BENEFITS	Many testicular cancer patients are encouraged to exercise; this is a good sign that massage is also appropriate. Any bodywork that supports, rather than challenges, a client's capacity for adaptation is safe and appropriate in this setting, as it can help with pain, anxiety, depression, and other common cancer complications. For more information on massage in the context of cancer, see Chapter 12.

Other Reproductive System Conditions

Menopause

Definition: What Is It?

Menopause is a specific event: it describes the moment the ovaries permanently stop secreting enough hormones to initiate a menstrual cycle. The time leading up to this event and for a year after the last menstrual period is called perimenopause, and many of the symptoms associated with declining hormone secretion occur during this period. Menopause itself is not conclusively identified until a full year after the last menstrual period.

It is important to point out that menopause is not a disease: it is a normal part of aging that every woman, if she lives long enough, will experience. Nevertheless, it can cause significant symptoms that impact function and quality of life. For more information on women's "men-" vocabulary, see Sidebar 11.12.

Demographics

The average age for the onset of perimenopausal symptoms is 47.5 years; the average age at which the transition is final is 51.4 years. It is estimated that about 46 million women in the United States are postmenopausal, and with the increasing number of mature Americans, about 50 million women will be postmenopausal by 2020.

Etiology: What Happens?

In addition to ripening several eggs each month and releasing at least one for the possibility of fertilization, the ovaries secrete a variety of chemicals (mostly estrogen and progesterone) into the bloodstream. They do this under the control of hypothalamus and pituitary secretions of follicle-stimulating hormone (FHS) and luteinizing hormone (LH).

As ovaries age, they become less sensitive to these hormones. Consequently, FHS levels go up, but estrogen and progesterone levels go down. It is misleading to refer to estrogen and progesterone as only two hormones, as both of these substances are produced in various chemical forms, each of which is metabolized and used in different ways.

Estrogens and progesterones influence sex organs either to support a pregnancy or to shed the endometrial lining of the uterus. When the ovaries lose function, either as a normal part of aging or because their function has been interrupted by surgery, radiation, or drugs (this is called "induced menopause"), these processes come to a stop. When a woman no longer ovulates, she no longer grows an endometrial lining in her uterus, and she no longer sheds that lining during menstruation. But ovarian hormones also work on many other tissues in the body in ways that are still being explored.

- *Bone density*: The role of estrogens and progesterones in maintaining bone density is complex. Estrogen inhibits osteoclast activity, that is, it helps to prevent the thinning of bone tissue. But some forms of progesterone are involved in maintaining bone density as well, stimulating

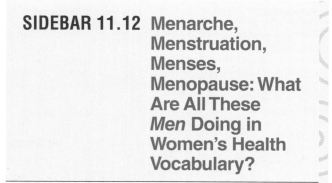

SIDEBAR 11.12 Menarche, Menstruation, Menses, Menopause: What Are All These *Men* Doing in Women's Health Vocabulary?

The root word is mēn, which is Greek for "month."

- Menarche is mēn plus arche, or beginning.
- Menstruation is mēn plus atus, meaning to be menstruant.
- Menses is the plural for mēn, meaning many months.
- Menopause is mēn plus pausis, or cessation.

Another anatomic application of the moon analogy is "meniscus": this describes crescent moon–shaped cartilaginous structures found in the knee and the jaw.

osteoblast activity. In other words, estrogen prevents bone from being dissolved, while progesterone helps it to build up. When both of these are in short supply, women can lose up to 20% of their bone mass during the 1st years of hormonal fluctuation.

- *Cardiovascular health*: As women age, the types of cholesterol in their blood change. Premenopausal women have a higher proportion of HDLs (the "good" cholesterols), and postmenopausal women have higher levels of low-density lipoproteins and triglycerides (the "bad" types of cholesterol). In other words, the blood lipids of postmenopausal women resemble that of men, which helps to explain why heart disease is the number one killer of both men and women. Further, estrogens appear to have a role in healthy endothelial growth, which influences the inner layer of blood vessels.
- *Protection from some types of cancer*: This is an extremely complex issue that reflects just how little is understood about the effects of different types of estrogens and progesterones on different types of tissues. High levels of some types of estrogen have a statistical link with lower rates of **colorectal cancer** but with higher rates of some other types of cancer, including **breast** and **ovarian cancers**. Ultimately, it may be found that whether hormone levels are dangerous or protective depends on the chemical variation of the hormone, where it comes from, how it is metabolized, where it is used, and other variables that haven't even been considered yet.
- *Central nervous system functions*: Estrogen seems linked to mood, **depression**, and basic cognitive function. Supplementing low doses of estrogen has been seen to be effective for dealing with the mild depression, **insomnia**, and short-term memory loss that may accompany perimenopause, but it is not effective for more severe depressive disorders.

When the ovaries decrease hormonal production, a woman becomes dependent on other tissues to secrete enough hormones to provide for her daily function. Some fat cells and other tissues continue to produce estrogen after the ovaries atrophy, but at a fraction of previous levels. Further, while some estrogen production continues after menopause, most progesterone production does not. Combine this with exposure to excessive exogenous estrogens, and it is clear to see how the premenopausal ratio between estrogens and progesterones is lost.

Signs and Symptoms

The symptoms of perimenopause are related to changes in hormone secretion. Symptoms generally subside when hormone levels stabilize, but this may not happen until years after a final menstrual period.

The signs and symptoms of menopause vary with each individual, but some of the most common ones are hot flashes (some of us call them power surges), night sweats, insomnia, mood swings, urinary urgency, loss of urinary continence, decreased sex drive, vaginal dryness or itchiness, confusion, short-term memory loss, and poor concentration. Some of these symptoms may be interrelated: for instance, insomnia may have to do with night sweats and hot flashes; depression and decreased sex drive may have to do with a change in self-perception as a woman becomes no longer fertile. But for some women, the symptoms of perimenopause are directly linked to hormonal disruption, and taking steps to smooth out the hormonal shifts can alleviate a lot of discomfort. "Genitourinary syndrome of menopause" or GSM is a term that encompasses changes in sex drive, vaginal dryness, and urinary discomfort. It has been coined so that women and their doctors may be able to discuss some of these issues more comfortably.

The long-term consequences of menopause include pathological thinning of bones and decreased resistance to heart disease, although these phenomena are controllable.

Treatment

Treatment options for the symptoms of perimenopause and the long-term consequences of reduced estrogen and progesterone secretion are many and varied. Estrogen replacement therapy provides supplements of various types of estrogens. This seems to be adequate for some women, but it doesn't address the lost balance between estrogens and progesterones that are implicated in many health issues. Further, it is appropriate only for women who have had a hysterectomy, because unopposed estrogen stimulates potentially dangerous endometrial growth.

While hormone replacement therapy can address some symptoms of perimenopause and it can reduce the risk of osteoporosis and colorectal cancer, it is also associated with some increased risk of other problems. This is especially true for women who have supplemented hormones for prolonged periods. (See Sidebar 11.13 for more information on HRT risks and benefits.)

If a woman decides not to supplement hormones to treat her menopausal symptoms, she may consider other options. Medications to support bone density and decrease the risk of heart disease are possibilities, as are a variety of herbal preparations. It is important to note that using herbs to treat symptoms of perimenopause is not risk free. Options include black cohosh (which should be avoided when other estrogen supplements are used), red clover, dong quai (which should not be used along with blood thinners), ginseng, wild yam, and kava (which have been associated with a risk of liver problems).

Medications

- Hormone replacement therapy (estrogen only for women with no uterus; estrogen and progesterone for women with a uterus)
- Herbal preparations (these may cause problematic interactions with other medications)
- Statins and other cardiovascular disease treatments if necessary
- Bisphosphonates for osteoporosis if necessary

Massage Therapy Implications

RISKS	Massage and bodywork have no risks for women who are fundamentally healthy while they go through perimenopause.
BENEFITS	While massage is unlikely to have a direct impact on perimenopausal processes, it may help to mitigate some of its symptoms, including mood disruptions, insomnia, and fatigue.
OPTIONS	Menopause can be both tremendously challenging as a basic part of a woman's self-definition changes and wonderfully fulfilling, as her commitments to children and parents are often tapering off, and she may be able to devote more of her time, energy, creative drive, and focus to her own purposes. Massage can be a way to reinforce a sense of physical joy and wholeness during a time of great transition.
RESEARCH	Massage therapy, with and without aromatherapy, has good support in the evidence for helping to deal with many of the symptoms of perimenopause. Taavoni et al.[1] found improved psychological scores for all participants in their study. Similar findings using a different scale for menopausal symptoms were found by Darsareh et al.[2] in 2011. Another study found that massage therapy improved insomnia and quality of life scores, as compared to passive movement or control.[3] These findings are not surprising, but another study is: Saetung et al.[4] found that traditional Thai massage led to an increase in biomarkers for bone formation—in other words, this type of massage may assist with improving bone density. 1. Taavoni S, Darsareh F, Joolaee S, et al. The effect of aromatherapy massage on the psychological symptoms of postmenopausal Iranian women. *Complementary Therapies in Medicine* 2013;21(3):158–163. http://www.ncbi.nlm.nih.gov/pubmed/23642946 2. Darsareh F, Taavoni S, Joolaee S, et al. Effect of aromatherapy massage on menopausal symptoms: a randomized placebo-controlled clinical trial. *Menopause* 2012;19(9):995–999. http://www.ncbi.nlm.nih.gov/pubmed/22549173 3. Oliveira DS, Hachul H, Goto V, et al. Effect of therapeutic massage on insomnia and climacteric symptoms in postmenopausal women. *Climacteric* 2012;15(1):21–29. http://www.ncbi.nlm.nih.gov/pubmed/22017318 4. Saetung S, Chailurkit LO, Ongphiphadhanakul B. Thai traditional massage increases biochemical markers of bone formation in postmenopausal women: a randomized crossover trial. *BMC Complementary and Alternative Medicine* 2013;13:69. http://www.ncbi.nlm.nih.gov/pmc/articles/PMC3770450/

SIDEBAR 11.13 Hormone Replacement Therapy

The Women's Health Initiative was a study of 161,809 postmenopausal American women between 50 and 79 years of age. The goal was to track these participants over 8 years to gather information about health trends for older women. One question they pursued concerned the benefits and risks of the most common version of HRT: concentrated equine estrogens (Premarin) plus medroxyprogesterone acetate (progestin) for women who had not had a hysterectomy. This hormone supplement regimen has traditionally been prescribed to reduce perimenopausal symptoms like hot flashes and vaginal dryness and to reduce the risk of heart disease and osteoporosis.

After 5 years of following the study participants, researchers found some surprising results. While the relative risk of osteoporosis and colorectal cancer went down as expected, all other health concerns being tracked actually increased, as follows:

Heart attack	Increased	29%
Breast cancer	Increased	26%
Stroke	Increased	41%
Blood clot in leg or lung	Increased	111%
Dementia	Increased	105%
Hip fractures (as measure of osteoporosis)	Decreased	33%
Colorectal cancer	Decreased	37%

The cardiovascular risks rose within 2 years of beginning HRT, and the increase in breast cancer risk was found after 4 years. Protection against osteoporosis was lost within 2 years of stopping therapy. These findings were so significant that it was considered unethical to keep women on HRT without informed consent, and this branch of the study was concluded in 2002.

When the results of the WHI became public, thousands of women stopped using HRT. Interestingly, within a year, the per capita diagnosis rate of breast cancer began to decline. That trend continued over several years, and statistical analysis suggests that the two phenomena are related.

Researchers have continued to look at this issue, and current findings suggest that HRT for women at the onset of perimenopause does help to manage symptoms and to reduce the risk of colorectal cancer and osteoporosis. However, the general recommendation is to encourage women to use the lowest possible dosage of hormones for the shortest period possible.

Pregnancy

Definition: What Is It?

Pregnancy, obviously, is the condition in which a woman carries a fetus.

Demographics

In the United States, about 60 million women are in their childbearing years (age 15 to 44). Each year, almost 6 million women know that they become pregnant, and about 4 million babies are born. Just under 2 million pregnancies do not lead to live births; they are interrupted by miscarriage, elective termination, stillbirth, or other complications.

Etiology: What Happens?

The physiologic changes that occur when a woman is pregnant are wide ranging and complex, and this text will not pursue all of them fully. Instead, the most common or dangerous complications of pregnancy will be discussed, and several symptoms that many pregnant women experience that are especially pertinent to massage and bodywork will be examined.

Types of Pregnancy Complications

- *Asthma*: Many pregnant women have **asthma**, and incomplete control of this condition has serious repercussions for both mother and baby. It has been linked to low birth weight and prematurity, an increased risk of **cerebral palsy** and mental disability, and preeclampsia. Well-controlled asthma, by contrast, is not associated with significant risks.
- *Thromboembolism*: This is a combination of **deep vein thrombosis** and **pulmonary embolism**. Pregnant and newly postpartum women have approximately ten times more risk of blood clots than the nonpregnant population. The risk increases as the pregnancy develops and is highest in the first few days after the baby is delivered.
- *Gestational diabetes*: Pregnancy-related diabetes is diagnosed with a glucose tolerance test, in which the woman drinks a sweet beverage, and then her urine is examined for elevated levels of glucose. Gestational diabetes is usually identified in the 5th or 6th month of pregnancy (between 24 and 26 weeks of gestation). It is estimated to affect up to 9.2% of all pregnancies each year.

  If diabetes develops during pregnancy, risks to the baby and mother are significant. The rerouting of nutrients in the blood can cause babies to grow abnormally large in a condition called **macrosomia**, which may require a **cesarean section**. Babies born to women with gestational diabetes also have a high risk of respiratory distress syndrome, early hypoglycemia, and later obesity and type 2 **diabetes**.

  A woman who develops gestational diabetes has a high risk of doing so again with subsequent pregnancies and of developing type 2 diabetes later in life.
- *Pregnancy-induced hypertension*: This is a condition that generally starts mildly but can quickly become life-threatening both for the baby and the mother. It occurs in three categories: **hypertension** alone; **preeclampsia**, which is hypertension along with elevated proteins in the urine and possible systemic edema; and **eclampsia**, which is the same condition along with convulsions or coma. Preeclampsia affects 6% to 8% of all pregnancies each year.

  Most cases of pregnancy-induced hypertension occur during a first pregnancy, in teens, or in women over 40. Other women at risk include those who are obese prior to pregnancy, those who have a personal or family history of chronic high blood pressure, women carrying multiple babies, and women who have an underlying disease that can affect the circulatory system, including diabetes, **lupus**, and **scleroderma**. Treatment includes medication to bring down the blood pressure, strict bed rest, and, where appropriate, early delivery of the baby.

  A complication of pregnancy-induced hypertension is **HELLP syndrome**: **hemolysis** with elevated liver enzymes and low platelet count. This disorder of impaired blood cells and poor liver function can result in bleeding and severe liver damage. Other complications of pregnancy-induced hypertension for mothers include **renal failure**, **hemorrhagic stroke**, liver damage, and retinal detachment leading to blindness. Risks to the baby include reduced growth from circulatory impairment and **placenta abruptio**.
- *Ectopic pregnancy*: An ectopic pregnancy occurs when a fertilized egg implants and grows outside of the uterus. Most ectopic pregnancies develop in the uterine tubes; some implant in the peritoneum, on the ovaries, or on the cervix.

Macrosomia: A condition in which a fetus grows abnormally large as a result of gestational diabetes.

Cesarean section: A surgical procedure in which a mother's abdomen is cut open in order to remove the infant directly.

Preeclampsia: A condition occurring in pregnant women characterized by hypertension along with elevated proteins in the urine and sometimes systemic swelling.

Eclampsia: Convulsions caused by pregnancy-induced hypertension.

HELLP syndrome: A mnemonic for hemolysis, elevated liver enzymes, and low platelet count. Associated with pregnancy-induced hypertension.

Hemolysis: The destruction of red blood cells.

Placenta abruptio: A condition in which the placenta prematurely separates from the uterus.

Risk factors for ectopic pregnancy include IUD use; a history of **pelvic inflammatory disease**, **endometriosis**, or **sexually transmitted infection**; and adhesions from previous abdominal surgeries. Ectopic pregnancies cannot come to term; the uterine tube inevitably ruptures, killing the fetus and endangering the life of the mother. Ectopic pregnancies that are recognized early (usually by ultrasound and testing for hormone levels) may be terminated by medication or laparoscopic surgery, preserving the ovary and uterine tube for the chance of a future successful pregnancy.

Signs and Symptoms

Pregnancy creates a wide array of signs and symptoms, and some of them have specific implications for massage. Here are some of the complaints of pregnant women that bodywork practitioners can influence:

- *Loose ligaments*: Pregnant women often experience ligament laxity, even early in fetal growth. This can lead to joint instability, including subluxations of the vertebrae and the sacroiliac joints. Muscles then work hard to stabilize the joints, causing spasm and pain.
- *Fatigue*: Pregnant women carry a lot of extra weight. The baby itself is only a fraction of the whole load, which includes the placenta, amniotic fluid, 40% more blood, and any extra fat she may accumulate during her pregnancy. In addition to carrying extra weight, a pregnant woman tends to have low blood pressure and low blood sugar, and she secretes hormones that signal her to get a lot of rest. This is a command that many pregnant women don't have the luxury of obeying, at least if they're trying to hold a job until the baby is born.
- *Shifting proprioception*: Pregnant women change their size every day. This is true especially in the last trimester, when the baby grows at an astounding rate. The result is that a pregnant woman never knows exactly how much room she takes up. Her sense of where in space her body ends and the rest of the world begins is very shaky. This, along with newly loose ligaments and a shifted center of gravity, may make a pregnant woman clumsy and prone to injury. Massage provides an extraordinary sense of where bodies are in space. It can improve proprioceptive senses by giving continuous and accurate feedback about boundaries.
- *Depression*: Many women experience **anxiety** and **depression** in a new pattern when they are pregnant. This condition can significantly alter her quality of life and interfere with her ability to bond with and enjoy her child.

Treatment

No medical treatment for an uncomplicated pregnancy is necessary.

Treatment for pregnancy complications obviously depends on the situation. They may include anticoagulants, antihypertensive drugs, steroids and other anti-inflammatories for asthma, antidepressants, and others.

Massage Therapy Implications

RISKS

First trimester: from the time a woman knows she is pregnant until she delivers, intrusive work in the abdomen must be avoided.

Second trimester: this is the most stable, least risky phase of pregnancy. At some point during this time, it will no longer be comfortable for a client to lay prone without special accommodations in the way of support cushions, extensive bolstering, or a specially designed pregnancy table.

Third trimester: during this time, a woman may not be able to lay prone or supine, as reclining allows the fetus to compress major blood vessels, which can lead to dizziness and/or muscle cramps (Figure 11.15). In addition, the risk of blood clots causing deep vein thrombosis and the possibility of pulmonary embolism is high at this time and through the first few weeks postpartum. Any fever, edema, dizziness, headache, or nausea during this time requires immediate medical attention.

BENEFITS

As long as a pregnancy is not complicated by diabetes, hypertension, or other disorders, massage is a wonderful gift for a person whose body doesn't quite belong to herself for a while. Particularly for issues of anxiety, fatigue shifting proprioception, and musculoskeletal pain, massage can be a powerful intervention.

OPTIONS

Specific guidelines for positioning pregnant clients are discussed in the *risks* section. Some experts suggest having the mother lay only on her left side in the late stage of pregnancy. Special training for working with pregnant and postpartum women is widely available and highly recommended. This is a precious group of clients who require some particular skills for the safest and most effective bodywork.

RESEARCH

Much of the research on record about pregnancy and massage has to do with massage during childbirth or immediate postpartum massage of the uterus to promote contractions and limit bleeding; this is usually performed by a labor nurse or birth attendant. One review of the literature supports massage therapy to reduce prematurity and low birth weight and as an effective method to help with mild signs of postpartum depression.[1] Another review found promising evidence of massage as an intervention for pregnancy-related insomnia, but not enough research has been conducted to make a solid judgment.[2]

1. Deligiannidis KM, Freeman MP. Complementary and alternative medicine therapies for perinatal depression. *Best Practice & Research. Clinical Obstetrics & Gynaecology* 2014;28(1):85–95. http://www.ncbi.nlm.nih.gov/pmc/articles/PMC3992885/
2. Hollenbach D, Broker R, Herlehy S, et al. Non-pharmacological interventions for sleep quality and insomnia during pregnancy: a systematic review. *Journal of the Canadian Chiropractic Association* 2013;57(3):260–270. http://www.ncbi.nlm.nih.gov/pmc/articles/PMC3743652/

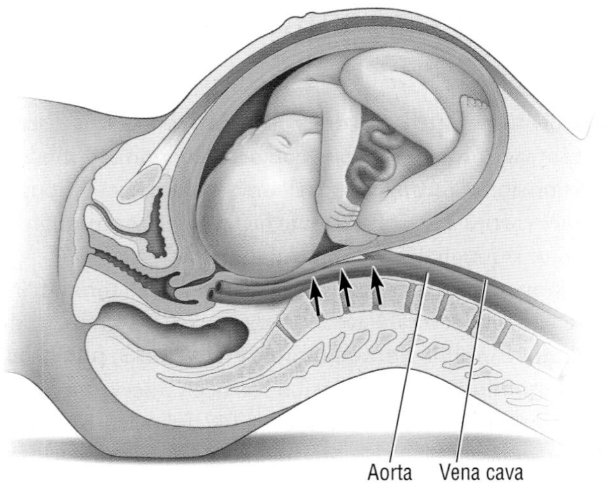

FIGURE 11.15 Pregnancy: a late-term fetus can obstruct blood flow through the iliac arteries or vena cava

Premenstrual Syndrome

Definition: What Is It?

Premenstrual syndrome (PMS) is a collection of signs and symptoms that combine to interfere with a woman's ability to function normally during the luteal phase of the menstrual cycle: the time between ovulation and menstruation.

Demographics

Up to 75% of American women between the onset of menarche and **menopause** report some symptoms of PMS, and 3% to 8% report symptoms of **premenstrual dysphoric disorder (PMDD)**. Women who are obese are three times more likely than others to have PMS, and those who smoke are two times more likely to have this condition.

Etiology: What Happens?

PMS is one of the most common and least well-understood conditions that women experience. It has been described since ancient times; it was recognized as a specific pattern in 1931 and finally named in 1953. Nonetheless, the etiology of this condition remains mysterious. Several factors seem to contribute to it, and each woman's experience is unique. This makes it difficult to predict or treat, as no single approach is universally successful.

Some of the hypotheses for the causes or triggers of PMS include the following:

- *Hormonal hypersensitivity*: The precipitous drop in hormones just before a period occurs in every menstruating woman, but some appear to be especially sensitive to the change. In addition, exposure to environmental estrogens in animal fats and other sources may cause the endometrial lining to become overactive, leading to an even more extreme fluctuation in hormonal levels.
- *Nutritional deficiencies*: Some women with PMS are deficient in specific nutrients, notably calcium, magnesium, folic acid, vitamin B_6, and some essential fatty acids.
- *Neurotransmitter imbalance*: Plunging estrogen and progesterone levels have been seen to suppress the secretion of serotonin, a neurotransmitter that is strongly related to mood swings and depression. **Opioid peptides** are other brain chemicals that appear to be adversely affected by hormone disruption.
- *Other factors*: Some factors that may contribute to PMS are more vague but definitely a part of the picture for many women. Genetic predisposition may be a factor, but it is unclear whether the problem is passed on through heredity or the likelihood to seek help for it is passed on through environmental influence. Cultural expectations, general stress, and a number of unrelated disorders may also contribute to PMS.

Signs and Symptoms

PMS is identified when symptoms are present in the 10 days leading up to a period and disappear within the first days after a period begins. This distinguishes it from **dysmenorrhea**, which occurs only after the menstrual period begins.

More than 150 signs and symptoms have been documented among PMS patients. These have been loosely categorized into physical and emotional indicators of this disorder.

- *Physical manifestations*: The most common physical signs and symptoms associated with PMS include bloating, breast tenderness, **acne**, salt, and sugar cravings (along with **binge eating**), **headaches** (including migraines), backaches, **insomnia**, and digestive upset, that is, diarrhea and/or constipation. Less common physical manifestations include sinus problems, heart palpitations, and dizziness. **Asthma**, hay fever, migraines, and **seizures** all tend to get worse during the luteal phase for women who live with these challenges.
- *Emotional manifestations*: These include confusion, poor concentration, **depression, anxiety, panic attacks**, mood swings, and general irritability.

It is important to point out that PMS or PMDD symptoms are restricted to the luteal phase of the menstrual cycle. If they occur outside of this pattern, other causes must be pursued.

Premenstrual dysphoric disorder (PMDD): A condition characterized by debilitating depression and anxiety during the period before menstruation more severe than PMS.

Opioid peptides: Chemicals that bind to opioid receptors in the brain.

Treatment

PMS is typically treated symptomatically. Conventional physicians often prescribe low-dose birth control in the form of pills or other delivery systems to control estrogen and progesterone levels, diuretics to control water retention, or antidepressants to address serotonin levels. Most women are also strongly advised to make sure that they get the best sleep they can muster during their difficult time and to exercise regularly.

Health professionals who focus on nutritional aspects of PMS often recommend that patients follow a low-fat vegetarian diet to avoid excessive estrogen exposure and that they avoid salt, sugar, caffeine, and alcohol. Many herbal remedies have been reputed to help PMS; some of the more common herbal recommendations include borage or evening primrose (for essential fatty acids), *Crocus sativus* (saffron), black cohosh, and chasteberry.

Ultimately, PMS usually can be successfully managed so that a woman doesn't have to lose function for 10 days every month, but it is unlikely to spontaneously disappear until the onset of menopause.

Medications

- Hormone supplements that suppress ovulation
- Diuretics to manage water retention
- Herbal remedies

Massage Therapy Implications

RISKS	Because PMS is not related to underlying infection, structural problems, neoplasm, or other dysfunctions, massage and bodywork carry no specific risks for clients with this condition.
BENEFITS	Massage and other types of bodywork may help to reduce depression and anxiety and to address some other physical symptoms that make PMS so uncomfortable.
RESEARCH	Massage therapy is a nonpharmacological intervention that many women with PMS are willing to pursue,[1] but while massage might improve mood and a sense of well-being, it has not yet been demonstrated to be an effective intervention for this specific population. 1. Tolossa FW, Bekele ML. Prevalence, impacts and medical managements of premenstrual syndrome among female students: cross-sectional study in College of Health Sciences, Mekelle University, Mekelle, northern Ethiopia. *BMC Womens Health* 2014;14:52. http://www.ncbi.nlm.nih.gov/pmc/articles/PMC3994244/

Sexually Transmitted Infections

Definition: What Are They?

Sexually transmitted infections (STIs) are contagious diseases that spread through intimate contact. The primary mode of transmission is through vaginal, oral, or anal sex, although a mother carries a risk of infecting her baby either through the blood or through direct contact during birth.

More than 20 infectious diseases are spread through intimate contact. Several have been discussed elsewhere in this book; they include **herpes simplex**, **HIV/AIDS**, **pubic lice**, and **hepatitis B**. This discussion has been reserved for some common bacterial STIs (Figure 11.16), followed by a brief look at some viral and protozoan infections.

Demographics

Some STIs are so common that it's hard to estimate the true number of infected people. Others became much rarer with aggressive public information campaigns and the increased accessibility of barrier methods of birth control. They remain a significant public health issue however, and some have become more common and more antibiotic resistant in the last decade. Table 11.1 gives a brief overview of the statistics on some of the most closely tracked STIs in the United States.

Etiology: What Happens?

The pathophysiology of each STI discussed here is covered in the discussion of the infectious agents. Most are spread through sexual activity with an infected partner, but some may also be shared from mother to fetus.

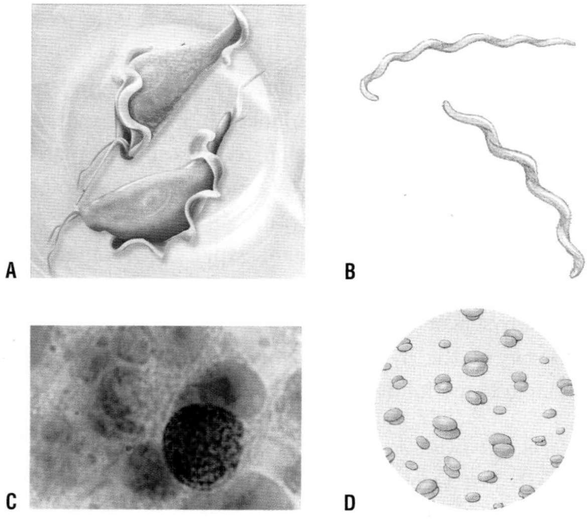

FIGURE 11.16 Pathogens behind common STIs: **(A)** trichomoniasis, **(B)** syphilis, **(C)** chlamydia, and **(D)** gonorrhea

TABLE 11.1 Common STIs

Infection	Incidence	Who is Most Affected
Chlamydia	Almost three million new infections per year	Most new infections are seen in newly sexually active young women and in men who have sex with men (MSM).
Gonorrhea	820,000 new diagnoses per year	Almost two-thirds of new infections are among people 15 to 24 years old.
Syphilis	55,000 infections per year, more than doubled since 2000	Biggest increase is among MSM.
Trichomoniasis	Almost four million probably have it, although only 30% may develop symptoms.	This is seen in older patients more often than in younger ones.
Genital warts	About 79 million have HPV, with 14 million new infections per year. Of those, 360,000 develop highly contagious genital warts.	HPV is an equal opportunity infection.
Bacterial vaginosis	New infection numbers are unknown.	Most common vaginal infection among women 15–44

The transmission of STIs can be prevented, but the only completely successful method is to practice abstinence or to have sex with one partner who is known to be uninfected. Barrier methods of birth control (male or female condoms) provide protection from some but not all STIs: molluscum contagiosum, genital warts, and syphilis may spread to areas not covered by condoms. And of course, other methods of birth control (spermicidal cream, birth control pills, IUDs, and other hormonal applications) provide no protection from STIs.

Types of Sexually Transmitted Infections

- *Bacterial vaginosis*: This condition is exclusive to women. It involves an imbalance in the normal bacterial environment of the vagina with the result of foul-smelling discharge, irritation, and an increased risk of catching and transmitting other STIs, **pelvic inflammatory disease** (PID), and complicated **pregnancy**. It is caused by bacteria, which distinguishes this condition from **candida**-related vaginitis. The triggers for bacterial vaginosis are not well understood, but having multiple partners and frequent douching are seen to increase the incidence of this condition. It is treated with antibiotics.
- *Chlamydia*: This is a bacterial infection with *Chlamydia trachomatis*. These bacteria have an affinity for columnar mucus-producing cells. These infections can develop at any site of sexual contact: the reproductive tract, the mouth and throat, and the anus.

While chlamydia quietly attacks columnar mucus cells in the reproductive tract, it also invades the uterus and uterine tubes, where a chronic low-grade infection and inflammatory response may lead to permanent scarring and infertility. This is one variety of PID.

NOTABLE CASES Of the conditions discussed here, only syphilis (sometimes called "Cupid's disease") is potentially life-threatening. Before penicillin was available, it was treated with near-lethal doses of mercury or arsenic. One theory behind the death of Napoleon Bonaparte is that he died of poisoning in an attempt to cure syphilis. Other notable figures whose lives were shortened by this infection include Franz Schubert, Christopher Columbus, Scott Joplin, and Al Capone.

Chlamydia is often silent; three-quarters of infected women and about half of infected men report no symptoms. When symptoms are present, they include vaginal or penile discharge, pain and burning during urination, and painful intercourse. Because this often resembles a bladder infection, chlamydia is often missed as a diagnosis.

The primary complication of a chlamydia infection for a woman is PID and the risk of ectopic pregnancy or

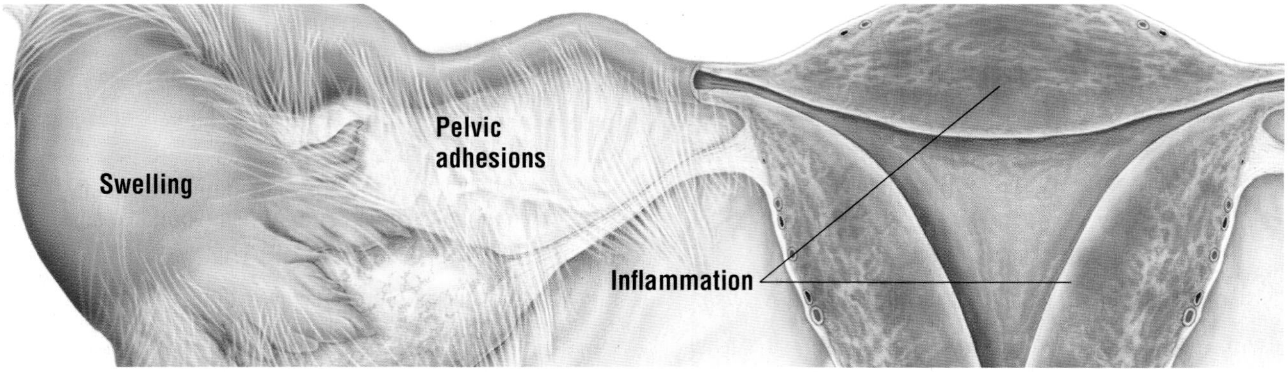

FIGURE 11.17 Pelvic inflammatory disease is a frequent complication of STIs. It can lead to chronic pelvic pain, infertility, and potentially dangerous infection

lifelong infertility (Figure 11.17). An infection in a man may cause **epididymitis**, swelling of the testicles, and a risk of infertility for him too. A baby born to a woman with undiagnosed chlamydia has a risk of exposure in the birth canal that may lead to conjunctivitis or life-threatening pneumonia. A chlamydia infection also increases the risk of HIV transmission.

Chlamydia is treatable with appropriate antibiotics, as long as sexual partners are treated too. It often appears with gonorrhea, which requires a different antibiotic treatment, so it is important to get a thorough diagnosis. Exposure and treatment for chlamydia does not impart immunity, so any future exposure to this pathogen can lead to a new infection that requires treatment.

- *Gonorrhea*: This is an infection with *Neisseria gonorrhoeae*, a diplococcal bacterium. It is spread through intimate contact, affecting mucous membranes of the throat, vagina, and rectum. It is rarely transmitted by any contact other than sex; it is unusual for a pregnant mother with gonorrhea to pass it to her child. Once inside the body, gonorrhea may infect tissues other than mucous membranes; **gonococcal arthritis** is an infection of joints that can lead to permanent damage.

  Gonorrhea is often silent, especially in women. If symptoms do appear in a woman, they typically include vaginal discharge, urinary discomfort, and painful intercourse. An infection from oral sex may lead to lesions in the mouth and a sore throat.

  Male symptoms of gonorrhea include burning on urination, a yellow-white discharge from the penis, and **orchitis**.

  This infection is responsive to antibiotics, although it has developed resistance to a number of them, and in geographic areas where more antibiotic resistance has been noted, it appears to be spreading faster than in other areas. It is frequently comorbid with chlamydia, which requires concurrent treatment with a different antibiotic.

- *Syphilis*: This infection with the bacterial spirochete *Treponema pallidum* spreads easily through sexual contact and from mother to unborn child. It travels through the blood and may affect joints, bones, blood vessels, and the central nervous system if it is untreated. This bacterium is very fragile outside a host and does not survive when exposed to air or sunlight.

  Syphilis moves through the system in predictable stages. It is communicable only in the first two stages of infection. In the late stage, although it may cause very serious problems in the infected person, it is no longer contagious.

  - Primary syphilis is detectable 10 days to 3 months after exposure, when a characteristic **chancre** appears. A chancre is usually not acutely painful, and if it appears inside the vaginal canal, a woman may not be aware of it. The tissue in chancres is very contagious. A typical lesion heals in 3 to 6 weeks.
  - Secondary syphilis takes the form of a rash of open brownish sores that appear several weeks after the chancre heals. This rash is often on the soles of the feet or palms of the hands, but it may be anywhere. These lesions are also highly infectious. The rash associated with secondary syphilis may come and go for 1 to 2 years before the infection becomes latent.
  - In some people, syphilis becomes a silent infection after the secondary stage and may produce no further symptoms. No skin lesions appear, and the infection is no longer contagious. However, about one-third of people with secondary syphilis develop tertiary syphilis, a condition in which the bacteria invade other body systems. At this point, the infection may attack the bones and joints, causing rheumatic pain, or the blood vessels, causing a risk of aneurysm. Most significantly, syphilis may attack the central nervous

Epididymitis: Inflammation of the epididymis.
Gonococcal arthritis: A joint infection caused by gonorrhea.
Orchitis: Inflammation of the testes.
Chancre: The primary lesion of syphilis.

system, leading to a range of problems including blindness, loss of hearing, stroke, meningitis, or psychosis.

Like other bacterial STIs, syphilis significantly increases the transmission rate of HIV. A pregnant woman with syphilis, if she doesn't miscarry, has a nearly 100% chance of spreading the disease to her newborn through the bloodstream. Babies born with syphilis may not have symptoms immediately, but may develop vision or central nervous system problems along with syphilitic rhinitis; their mucus secretions are highly contagious.

Syphilis is sensitive to penicillin, and a single dose is typically adequate. Treatment must be administered before organ damage takes place, however. Syphilitic damage to the central nervous system, blood vessels, and other structures is irreversible.

- *Nongonococcal urethritis*: This is a bacterial infection of the urinary tract by an agent other than gonorrhea. It is often related to chlamydia, *Ureaplasma urealyticum*, or *Mycoplasma genitalium*. It is usually an STI but can also be related to prostatitis, urinary tract infection, or catheter use. If it is identified as a bacterial infection, it can be successfully treated with antibiotics.
- *Trichomoniasis*: This infectious agent is a protozoan parasite called *Trichomonas vaginalis*. It causes vaginal discharge, pain, itching, and an increased risk of HIV transmission. Pregnant women with "trich" are more likely to have preterm babies. Trichomoniasis is highly treatable with antibiotics, but reinfection is common.
- *Molluscum contagiosum virus* (MCV): This is a generally benign condition that is commonly seen among children, in whom it is not an STI. When MCV appears as an STI, it appears on the thighs, buttocks, groin, external genitalia, and anus. It is treated by removing the growths with topical chemicals or cryotherapy.

Condylomata acuminata: Genital warts.

- *Genital warts*: These are also called **condylomata acuminate**. They can grow on the vulva, the walls of the vagina, the perineum, or the cervix of a woman or on the penis, scrotum, or anus of a man. Oral infections may grow in the mouth or throat. Genital warts have a high transmission rate; exposure leads to infection about two-thirds of the time. They are typically small, but they can grow in clusters large enough to interfere with a pregnancy. Many types of HPV can cause genital warts, and some of them are associated with cervical, penile, or vulvar cancer. Genital warts can be removed, but over-the-counter medications that treat common warts are inappropriate for these lesions, which grow on sensitive, delicate tissues. The HPV vaccine that is discussed in cervical cancer is available for boys and girls and prevents most forms of genital warts.

Medications

- Antibiotics for bacterial and protozoan infections
- Antiviral medications for viral infections
- Topical applications for genital warts and molluscum contagiosum

Massage Therapy Implications

RISKS	Most STIs are only spread through sexual contact, which makes communicability for massage therapists a nonissue. Exceptions to this rule include herpes simplex, molluscum contagiosum, genital warts, and open syphilis lesions. These can travel by skin-to-skin contact, and lesions may not be confined to genitalia.
BENEFITS	Clients who are under treatment for STIs, or who have fully recovered from an infection, can enjoy all the benefits from bodywork as the rest of the population.

Explore and Apply

LEVEL 1: Receive and Respond

1. The hormones that govern the female reproductive cycle are secreted by the…
   a. Pituitary and hypothalamus
   b. Uterus and ovaries
   c. Ovaries and pituitary
   d. Uterus and hypothalamus

2. If an ovum is fertilized, this is most likely to happen in the…
   a. Peritoneum
   b. Uterine tube
   c. Uterus
   d. Ovary

3. Where do sperm cells mature?
   a. In the testes
   b. In the vas deferens
   c. In the penis
   d. In the epididymis

4. Primary dysmenorrhea is another term for…
   a. Lack of menstruation due to scarring and pelvic fibrosis
   b. Painful menstruation not due to an underlying disorder
   c. Excessive menstrual flow and resulting anemia
   d. Painful menstruation due to endometriosis

5. What is the situation that most often prompts women to be diagnosed for endometriosis?
   a. Infertility
   b. Yeasty pelvic discharge
   c. Premature perimenopausal symptoms
   d. Pregnancy

6. This condition is usually silent unless it puts pressure on other tissues or obstructs a successful pregnancy. It often spontaneously resolves after menopause. What is it?
   a. Fibroid tumor
   b. Uterine cancer
   c. Cervical warts
   d. Ovarian cyst

7. This condition is strongly linked to genetics and family history. It is rarely caught early, and its early signs and symptoms are extremely subtle. What is it?
   a. Breast cancer
   b. Endometriosis
   c. Syphilis
   d. Ovarian cancer

8. What is true of the most common type of prostatitis?
   a. It is a chronic pain syndrome but not an infection
   b. It is an acute bacterial infection
   c. It is a precancerous condition leading to prostate cancer
   d. It is a chronic bacterial infection

9. What is true about the most common type of testicular cancer?
   a. It is highly resistant to treatment
   b. It is easily treatable if caught early
   c. It is usually found among men over 50
   d. It is related to a history of sexually transmitted infection

10. Which condition carries the most concern for a woman who is pregnant?
    a. Eczema
    b. Hay fever
    c. Asthma
    d. Hives

11. Which of these cannot be treated successfully with antibiotics?
    a. Genital warts
    b. Syphilis
    c. Gonorrhea
    d. Chlamydia

LEVEL 2: Application of Concepts

1. Your client tells you she had cervical cancer cells removed 2 years ago, with no need for further treatment. What is your best strategy?
   a. Work normally but avoid low abdominal work to avoid disrupting any suspicious cells
   b. Refuse to work with her without a doctor's note
   c. Work normally because massage poses no specific risks for her situation
   d. Refuse to work with her until the requisite three years of being cancer free have passed

2. Your client has painful menstrual cramps on the day of her appointment. What is the most likely accommodation you will make for her?
   a. Work deeply in the abdomen to interrupt the pain-spasm cycle in her uterus
   b. Reschedule the massage for after her period
   c. Work only lightly on her extremities to avoid disrupting inflamed tissues
   d. Work normally with special focus on gentle work to the low abdomen and low back

3. Your 45-year-old client asks you for advice for preventing breast cancer. She is reluctant to see the doctor, and she has never had a mammogram. She is nervous because she knows breast cancer runs in her family. What is your best strategy?
   a. Suggest that she visit the American Cancer Society website for information on how to prevent breast cancer
   b. Recommend that she visits a psychotherapist to share her concerns and work through her fears
   c. Inform her that breast cancer isn't a preventable disease, but it is successfully treated if found early so she should seek a doctor or clinic where she feels comfortable to do this
   d. Educate her in how to do her own breast exam so she can screen herself for any suspicious changes

4. Your client is a 76-year-old man who complains that he has to get up to urinate frequently at night, and he often feels that he cannot fully empty his bladder. What two conditions might he be dealing with?
   a. Prostate cancer and BPH
   b. Prostatitis and BPH
   c. Bladder cancer and BPH
   d. Interstitial cystitis and prostate cancer

5. Myofascial trigger points in the pelvic floor are a contributing factor to symptoms of chronic pelvic pain syndrome (CPPS). How does this impact massage therapists?
   a. Massage therapists can legitimately claim to treat CPPS
   b. Deep, specific abdominal work is the best way to access these trigger points
   c. Perineal trigger points are outside the massage therapy scope of practice
   d. Digital massage of levator ani trigger points is within the scope of practice for every massage therapist

6. Your 52-year-old client suddenly becomes warm in the middle of a session. Her skin becomes visibly reddened, and she breaks into an all-over sweat. What is probably happening, and what should you do about it?
   a. She is inappropriately sexually aroused; terminate the session
   b. She is having a hot flash; ask how to make her comfortable
   c. She is developing a fever; tell her to go home and take aspirin
   d. She is having an allergic reaction to the lubricant; terminate the session and send her home to shower as quickly as possible

7. Your client, a 25-year-old woman, reports that she has felt bloated, with a headache, indigestion, and low back pain, for several days. She says it is not a new pattern; this happens to her regularly. What condition is she probably dealing with?
   a. Premenstrual syndrome
   b. Polycystic ovarian syndrome
   c. Chronic pelvic pain syndrome
   d. Genitourinary syndrome

Note to educators: Due to space considerations, these review questions only address the most important material from Chapter 11. The Test Bank provides a much more comprehensive selection of questions, all of which are keyed to the relevant chapter objectives.

Explore and Apply (continued)

What Would *You* Do?

A Client with Menstrual Cramps

Sage is a new client who is transgender. He has visible feminine characteristics, but he identifies as a male. While Sage has not undergone any surgical procedures, he has recently begun supplementing male hormones in an effort to adjust his outward appearance to his gender identity. Sage also has extreme menstrual cramps that make it hard to function several days each month.

Work with a partner to role-play being both a client and a therapist in this situation. What are some of the issues you can expect to make this session different from a typical one?

A client who wants to get pregnant

Julia is looking for a massage therapist to help her with a special problem. She has endometriosis that has contributed to great difficulty in conceiving a child. She read on some website that massage helps to reestablish fertility for women like her, and she wants you to help her.

Work with a partner to role-play being both client and therapist in this situation. Pay special attention to the language you use to discuss her goals.

A client with an upset tummy

Your client Tamara has been looking forward to her session. She is 24 years old and physically fit, although perhaps a bit underweight. She complains that for several days she has been feeling bloated and uncomfortable in her abdomen, and she hopes you can help resolve her discomfort.

After warming up her abdomen with rocking, gentle clockwise strokes and petrissage—all of which she received with pleasure—you begin to work more deeply. As you begin to trace the pathway of her colon in the lower right quadrant, she gasps and doubles up in pain.

Tamara ends up in the emergency department, where it is established that an ovarian cyst has ruptured on the right side.

Could this be related to the massage? Could it have been anticipated? What might you do differently the next time?

A client with urinary symptoms

Jon has been coming for massage for several years. Now in his 60s, he is beginning to slow down a bit. He has shared several health concerns with you, and today he brings another: he can't sleep well anymore because he has to get up to go to the bathroom at least twice every night—but even then, he still doesn't feel like he has fully emptied his bladder.

Jon hates to go to the doctor, and he trusts you implicitly. He knows you can recommend some supplements or vitamins that will ease his symptoms.

Work with a partner to practice having an appropriate conversation with this client. Where are you likely to stray out of your scope of practice? How can you avoid this kind of problem, while still being a warm, empathetic health care provider?

Suggested Activities

1. For each condition covered in your curriculum, write down the following on a card:
   - A brief definition
   - Most common cause or contributing factor(s)
   - Major signs and symptoms
   - Risks and benefits of massage therapy
     - Variables that contribute to risks and benefits
     - Appropriate adaptations

   Use these as flash cards as you study.
2. For each condition covered in your curriculum, write one multiple-choice question. Share your questions with your classmates as you study together.
3. Quiz yourself using either the "labels off" feature in your enhanced e-book or the labeling exercise on thePoint® for Figures 11.1 and 11.2. For Figure 11.1, be sure you can label each of the following: Ovary, Fimbriae, Uterine (fallopian) tube, Endometrium, and Broad ligament. For Figure 11.2, be sure you can label each of the following: Testis, Epididymis, Vas deferens, Prostate gland, and Urethra.

Use the student resources on thePoint® to find practice quiz questions and games.

12

Principles of Cancer

CHAPTER 12 / Abbreviated Chapter Objectives

Having completed assignments and classroom time related to Chapter 12, the learner is expected to be able to...

- Identify the definitions of all of the highlighted vocabulary words.
- Name which type of cancer is diagnosed most often and which type of cancer is the leading cause of death in the United States.
- List the steps in metastasis in correct order.
- Define external versus internal factors in the development of cancer.
- List at least three internal factors in the development of cancer.
- Define "carcinogen" and list at least four known carcinogens.
- Identify at least five viruses associated with cancer development.
- Identify at least one bacterium associated with cancer development.
- Recognize 10 common signs that indicate the possibility of cancer.
- In the "TNM" protocol, identify what each letter stands for and describe the staging system.
- In the "0 to IV" protocol, define what stage 0 and stage IV mean and describe the staging system.
- Define what "grading" means for cancer prognosis.
- List and describe at least eight treatment options for cancer.
- List 10 strategies for cancer prevention.
- Compare lymphedema to typical edema and describe how it must be treated differently.
- Identify four risks for massage therapy in the context of cancer.
- Identify four risks for massage therapy in the context of cancer treatment.
- Describe appropriate massage therapy modifications for the following circumstances:
  - Bone fragility
  - Undiagnosed lump
  - Subclavicular port
  - Chemotherapy-induced neuropathy
  - Radiation burns
  - Implanted radioactive pellets
  - A sore that comes and goes in the same place
- Identify at least five well-supported benefits for massage therapy in the context of cancer.

Principles of Cancer

Cancer is not a single disorder. It comprises more than 100 diseases that have one thing in common: normal body cells mutate slightly and begin to replicate uncontrollably. When the malignant cells begin in epithelial tissue, the cancer is called **carcinoma**. When the original cells are muscle or connective tissue, the cancer is a type of **sarcoma**. Carcinomas and sarcomas typically involve solid tumors. Cancers of the blood and lymph (leukemia, myeloma, lymphoma) usually do not; these are called **hematologic** cancers.

The principles laid out here are designed to provide background information for the discussions that appear throughout this book, which include **skin cancer**; **osteosarcoma**, **leukemia**, and **myeloma**; **lymphoma**; **laryngeal** and **lung cancer**; **esophageal**, **stomach**, **colorectal**, **liver**, and **pancreatic cancer**; **thyroid cancer**; **kidney** and **bladder cancer**; and **cervical**, **uterine**, **breast**, **ovarian**, **prostate**, and **testicular cancer**.

Massage therapy education has had a history of overstating the risks of receiving bodywork if a client has cancer, leading to therapists turning clients away for fear of making their clients' situations worse. While it is appropriate to be conservative and to "do no harm," it is also appropriate to use massage to provide many benefits to people who are going through a difficult time. To quote Tracy Walton's Massage Contraindication and Cancer Principle, "Skilled massage therapy is safe for people with cancer and will not spread the disease. Specific massage adjustments are based on *clinical presentations* of cancer, not the presence of a cancer diagnosis." In other words, the guidelines for massage and bodywork for clients with cancer are determined by the circumstances presented in each case—not by the fact that cancer is present.

For more of the author's views on massage therapy in the context of cancer, visit http://thePoint.lww.com/Werner6e. thePoint®

> **Carcinoma:** Any kind of malignant tumor that arises in epithelial tissue.
>
> **Sarcoma:** Any kind of malignant tumor that arises in muscle or connective tissue.
>
> **Hematologic:** Having to do with blood.
>
> **Oncogene:** Any of a family of genes that normally code for proteins related to cell growth, but which can encourage the development of cancer if mutated or abnormally activated.
>
> **Tumor suppressor gene:** A gene that suppresses or protects against cancer. Also called an antioncogene.

Cancer Statistics

Cancer is the second leading cause of death in the United States, coming in behind cardiovascular disease. A man's lifetime chance of developing cancer is just under 1:2; a woman's lifetime chance is just over 1:3. This is usually a disease of mature people: 77% of all cases are diagnosed in people over 55.

An estimated 1.7 million cases are diagnosed each year, but this does not include cancers found in situ, or nonmelanoma skin cancers. About 585,000 people die from cancer each year in this country, that's about 1,600 each day. The good news is that in 1977, the overall average 5-year survival rate for cancer was 49%, and now it is 68%. This is a remarkable change, due largely to better early screening procedures and improved treatment options. The result is that 13.7 million living Americans have a history of at least one type of cancer, and many will enjoy a full life expectancy.

Nonmelanoma skin cancer is the most common variety diagnosed (and these statistics do not reflect the countless moles that are removed as a safeguard against melanoma development), but lung cancer is the leading cause of death by cancer for both men and women. Other leading causes of death in the United States include breast and ovarian cancer for women, prostate cancer for men, and cancer of the colon, rectum, and pancreas for both genders. In other countries, most cancer deaths are due to lung cancer as a result of smoking, and liver and cervical cancers as a result of infection with hepatitis B or C, and human papilloma virus, respectively.

Steps in Metastasis

It is still unclear exactly why or how a healthy cell changes into a malignant cell. One thing that all cancers have in common is that the DNA of a cell mutates so that the cell acquires certain growth properties.

The following is a simplified version of the process of cancer development, as it is currently understood:

- *Oncogene activation*: An **oncogene** is a gene that initiates malignant characteristics within a cell. Oncogene activation is the beginning of the changes that cause certain cells to become malignant. The trigger for activation may be toxic environmental exposures, diet, genetic predisposition, or some combination of factors, but it is often not clear. Oncogenes are typically inhibited by the activity of **tumor suppressor genes**. Eventually, it may be found that a lack of tumor suppressor genes (instead of or in addition to a surfeit of oncogenes) may be a significant factor in cancer risk.
- *Local invasion*: Mutated cells invade healthy tissue. They often do this without creating an inflammatory response because they secrete chemicals that suppress immune system reactions against them.

- *Proliferation:* The mutated cells proliferate, often piling up into distinct and disorganized masses called tumors. As masses of cells accumulate, they begin to lose the characteristics that define their tissue type. This lack of differentiation is associated with aggressiveness of the tumor.
- *Angiogenesis:* This is the growth of blood vessels to supply a tumor. Any growth of more than 1 or 2 cm^3 requires a dedicated blood supply. Some cancer cells seem especially well supplied with the chemical messengers that command the body to build new capillaries. The more highly invested a tumor is with blood vessels, the more likely it is to have metastasized.
- *Migration:* Cancer cells break off the primary tumor and travel to new areas. The circulatory or lymphatic system may be used as a transfer medium, but cancer cells can also spread through direct contact with other organs or in peritoneal fluid.
- *Colonization:* When cancer cells land in a new target tissue, they must begin the process over again, starting with proliferation. This requires that the cells be able to adhere to the new tissue and that they secrete the correct enzymes to suppress an immune system attack, create new blood vessels, and erode the new extracellular matrix. The first tumor that grows in the disease process is called the primary tumor; other tumors that grow from metastasis of the primary tumor are called secondary tumors. In other words, cancer that began in the ovary and spread to the bladder is called ovarian cancer with metastasis to the bladder—or "mets to the bladder."

Causes of Cancer

Triggers for oncogene activation vary by tissue type and individual case. Causes of cancer are slowly being narrowed to some identifiable factors. These are generally discussed as *internal* or *external* factors.

Internal Factors

Every cell in the body has a built-in capacity for self-destruction. This is a natural and healthy process called apoptosis, or programmed cell death. A specific gene in some cancer cells has been found to inhibit apoptosis. Therefore, some cancers may be as much related to cells that refuse to die as it is to new cells coming to life.

Some cancers are brought about by or connected to inherited characteristics. This means an inherited gene is likely to cause cellular mutations sometime in the future. Such genes have been identified for a small percentage of breast and colorectal cancers. It may also mean that a person has a genetic susceptibility to environmental factors that might not be a threat to someone else.

Other internal factors may include hormonal activity (some hormones appear to stimulate malignant cell division; others may suppress it) and immune system problems in recognizing and fighting off cancer cells.

External Factors

Carcinogens are chemical or environmental agents that have been identified as cancer causers. The National Toxicology Program is a consortium of several government entities including the National Institutes of Health, the Centers for Disease Control and Prevention, and the Food and Drug Administration. This organization lists 240 substances as known or highly probable carcinogens. This list includes the hydrocarbons in cigarette smoke; compounds created when meats are grilled over high heat; and several substances found in dyes, inks, and paint. Radiation from the sun, radon gas, gamma rays, or x-rays and CT scans can cause cancer, as can exposure to asbestos, benzene, nickel, cadmium, uranium, and vinyl chloride.

In addition to environmental irritants and pollutants, some pathogens have been determined to cause certain types of cancer. Others simply have a strong statistical link with the development of various cancers, but the cause-and-effect relationship has not been defined. Cancer-related pathogens include viruses, bacteria, and animal parasites.

Viruses

- *HTLV-1* (human T-cell lymphotropic virus) resembles HIV; it is a retrovirus that is spread through intimate fluids. It can cause lymphocytic leukemia and non-Hodgkin lymphoma.
- *HPV* (human papillomavirus) is a large group of viruses associated with various types of warts. A few viruses in this group can cause cancer of the cervix, penis, anus, vagina, vulva, mouth, and throat. At this point, it is not possible to tell from early cellular changes whether the HPV involved is dangerous, so all dysplastic cells are removed if they are found. Vaccines against some forms of HPV are available.
- *HHV-8* (human herpesvirus 8) can cause Kaposi sarcoma, a type of skin cancer. HHV-8 is active only when the immune system is suppressed. Consequently, Kaposi sarcoma is an indicator disease for HIV infection or other immune-suppressing conditions.
- *HIV* (human immunodeficiency virus) is indirectly associated with cancer via suppressed immune system function that would otherwise protect against both HPV and HHV-8.
- *EBV* (Epstein-Barr virus) is another herpesvirus. It resides in B cells and usually causes **mononucleosis** in its first infection. EBV is associated with an increased risk of nasopharyngeal cancer, Burkitt lymphoma, Hodgkin lymphoma, and stomach cancer.
- *HBV* and *HCV* (**hepatitis B** and **C** viruses) open the door to liver cancer through chronic long-term inflammation that interrupts function in epithelial cells.

Bacteria

- *Helicobacter pylori*, which is also associated with peptic ulcers, has been seen to convert nitrites in foods to potential carcinogens. It is implicated in stomach cancer and lymphoma.
- *Others* include *Borrelia burgdorferi* (the spirochete that causes **Lyme disease**) and *Campylobacter jejuni*, which have both been associated with digestive tract lymphomas.

Animal Parasites

- *Liver flukes* are associated with cancer in bile ducts. These flatworms are spread through the consumption of raw or undercooked fish.
- *Schistosoma haematobium* can cause cancer of the urinary bladder. These tiny worms are spread through contaminated water. They are not found in the United States but may be carried by those who travel to areas where the parasites are common.

It is often a combination of external and internal factors that tips the scales in favor of developing cancer. Exposure to carcinogens in certain combinations can also be dangerous. For example, heavy smoking combined with excessive alcohol consumption is an especially potent combination for developing cancers of the mouth or upper gastrointestinal tract. Very often, many years or even decades may pass between the initial exposure to a carcinogen and the development of distinguishable tumors. This makes it difficult to pin down precise causes of cancer that are consistent from person to person.

Signs and Symptoms

Signs and symptoms of cancer vary widely, depending on the site. One of the most insidious features of this disease is that it is often painless until it is far advanced. Tumors begin to cause pain when they press on nerve endings or when they cause a blockage in a tube or duct that in turn presses on nerve endings. A list of common signs that are red flags for the possibility of cancer includes the following:

- A change in bowel or bladder habits; blood in the stool or urine
- A sore that does not heal or that comes and goes in the same place; a change in a wart or a mole
- Other skin changes in color, itching, or hair growth
- White patches inside the mouth or on the tongue
- Uterine bleeding between periods or postmenopause
- Thickening or lump in the breast or elsewhere
- A prostate exam that shows enlargement
- Indigestion or swallowing difficulty
- Persistent cough or hoarseness; coughing up blood
- Unexplained weight loss
- Fatigue; anemia
- Unexplained fever
- Unexplained, unremitting pain

Cancer screening recommendations vary for types of cancer, risk factors, genetic history, and other issues. The most successful screening protocols aim to do two things: to find cancerous cells while treatment is most likely to be completely successful and to lead to an increased survival rate. Not all screening protocols accomplish these goals equally well, and some procedures carry risks themselves, including exposure to radiation, perforation of hollow organs, false-negative results, false-positive results, and overdiagnosis that may lead to anxiety and unnecessary interventions, even surgery, for the patient. For more details on cancer screening recommendations, see Sidebar 12.1.

If suspicious changes are noted during screening, tissue samples are taken and analyzed for the presence of malignant cells; this is called a **biopsy**. If these tests are positive, further examinations of the patient follow to determine how far the cancer has developed.

Staging

Most types of cancer develop in predictable enough patterns that they can be staged, or given a label that indicates how far the cancer has advanced. Staging is based on collected knowledge about how cancer grows and how readily various types of cancer may metastasize. Some variables include the location of the primary tumor, the size and number of tumors, lymph node involvement, the characteristics of cells in the examined tissue, and the presence or absence of distant growths. Some cancers can be staged with typical screening mechanisms; others cannot be accurately staged until surgery is performed. Staging may be further qualified by the use of A and B designations to allow for differences in patterns of progression. Accurate cancer staging allows care providers to choose treatment strategies with the best chances for success.

Several staging protocols have been developed, but most cancers are rated by the TNM system, which may be

Biopsy: The process of removing tissue from a patient for examination.

False positive: A test result that mistakenly reports the presence of a condition when it is actually absent.

False negative: A test result that mistakenly reports the absence of a condition when it is actually present.

SIDEBAR 12.1 Cancer Screening: Who, What, Where, When, Why?

The science of early cancer detection is far from fully developed or universally accepted. A survey of several medical agencies yields significantly different guidelines for individuals to follow in the attempt to be vigilant against early signs of cancer. One of the concerns with making screening recommendations is the risk of **false positives** or the identification of nonthreatening growths as cancerous. These findings may lead to unnecessary interventions and even dangerous surgeries. At the other end of the spectrum is the risk of **false negatives**, where a screening test misses an important finding, and the patient misses the opportunity for early treatment. Screening recommendations are further complicated by differences for low-risk and high-risk populations.

The following is a brief synopsis of the leading recommendations for early cancer detection.

Cancer Type	Low-Risk Population Recommendations	High-Risk Population Recommendations
Breast cancer	*Self-exam.* Monthly after age 20 onward *Clinical exam.* Every 3 y from ages 20–39; annually from 40 onward *Mammogram.* Opinions vary; most suggest exams every 1–3 y starting at age 40 or 50.	This includes women with the identified breast cancer genes, women who have first-degree relatives with breast cancer, or women who have had breast or other types of cancer before. Screening schedules are matched to individual cases.
Cervical cancer	When a woman reaches age 21, she should have a pelvic exam and Pap test. This should be repeated every 3–5 y, or by her doctor's recommendation, for as long as she has a cervix. Testing can be suspended after age 65 if she has never had a positive test. Pap tests look for dysplastic cells; HPV tests look for the DNA of the human papilloma virus. Both tests can be conducted at the same appointment, and an "all clear" on both is a sign that cancer risk is very low.	This includes women who have shown signs of cervical dysplasia in pelvic exams or Pap tests. Screening should continue on a yearly basis until patients have three normal tests in a row. Screening can be discontinued if a patient has had a hysterectomy, ***unless*** the surgery was related to cervical cancer.
Skin cancer	Several agencies recommend a regular self-exam for changes in skin, with a clinical visual exam every 3 y from age 20–40 and annually from age 40 onward.	This includes fair-skinned people and anyone previously diagnosed with any type of skin cancer or precancerous condition; clinical exams should be scheduled on an as-needed basis.
Prostate cancer	Traditionally, a PSA test and DRE have been recommended yearly for men over 50 y old with high PSA readings and every 2 y for men with low PSA tests. However, prostate cancer screening is somewhat controversial because many cancers are slow growing and not threatening, so men may go through risky, painful, expensive procedures to treat a problem that isn't truly a problem. For this reason, the U. S. Preventive Services Task Force now recommends against PSA testing: the potential benefit does not outweigh the harms.	This includes African American men and men with a father, brother, or son who have prostate cancer, testing should begin at age 40–45.
Colorectal cancer	From age 50–75, patients should choose one: • FOBT every year • Sigmoidoscopy every 5 y plus FOBT every 3 y • Colonoscopy every 10 y. After age 75, screening is based on the patient's history. With no history of colorectal cancer, screening may be suspended.	This includes people with a history of colon polyps, IBD, or a family history of hereditary colorectal cancer; screening should begin before age 50.
Lung, ovarian, and endometrial cancer	No effective noninvasive screening measures have been developed to detect these cancers in early stages. Postmenopausal women with any vaginal bleeding or spotting should consult with their doctor.	Some screening techniques may find these cancers, but they tend to be invasive procedures that are reserved for patients with a high risk for developing them.

DRE, digital rectal examination; FOBT, fecal occult blood test; IBD, inflammatory bowel disease; PSA, prostate-specific antigen.

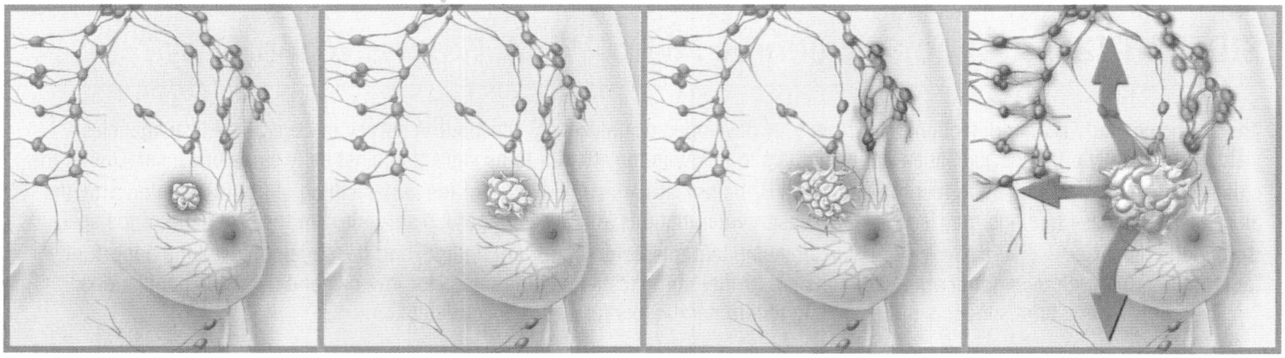

Stage I	Stage II	Stage III	Stage IV
T (< 2 cm)	**T** (> 2 cm)	**T** (> 5 cm)	**T** (any size)
N (no axillary metastasis)	**N** (axillary metastasis nonfixed)	**N** (axillary metastasis fixed)	**N** (supra- or infraclavicular nodes)
M (no metastasis)	**M** (no metastasis)	**M** (no metastasis)	**M** (distant metastasis)

FIGURE 12.1 Cancer staging, using breast cancer as an example

translated into the stage 0 to IV system (Figure 12.1). In addition, cancer cells may be rated by grade, which describes their appearance and potential aggressiveness.

- *TNM system:* The TNM system rates cancer progression by evaluations of tumors, nodes, and metastasis. These are further explained in Tables 12.1 to 12.3.
- *Stage 0 to IV system:* TNM ratings are often translated to the more familiar stages 0 to IV. Cancers have varying growth patterns though, so the exact translation from TNM to stages 0 to IV varies by type. Stage 0 typically means that malignant cells are restricted to the first layer of affected tissue; stage IV means that distant metastasis has occurred. The 0 to IV staging system is explained in more detail in Table 12.4.
- *Grade:* Another predictor for how cancer grows is the grade of tumor cells. This refers to two issues: how well differentiated the cells are (the higher the differentiation, the better the prognosis) and the propensity for proliferation, or aggressiveness. Cancer grading is explained further in Table 12.5.

Not all cancers lend themselves to the TNM or 0 to IV staging systems. Leukemia and lymphoma do not involve primary tumors, so their staging systems refer to blood counts, symptoms, and grade of cancer cells. Some cancers may be discussed in other terms, such as whether the lesion is operable or whether it has reached nearby organs.

Treatment

Decisions on how to treat cancer depend on the stage, the age, general health, and wishes of the patient, and what kind of cancer is present. Within each tumor, different kinds of cells may require different modes of attack. This makes

TABLE 12.1 T: Tumor

Tumor	Definition
Tx	Tumor cannot be evaluated.
T0	No evidence of primary tumor
Tis	In situ: tumor has not spread to nearby tissue.
T1, T2, T3, T4	These refer to the size and extent of primary tumor(s).

TABLE 12.2 N: Node

Node	Definition
Nx	Node involvement cannot be evaluated.
N0	No cancer is found in nearby nodes.
N1, N2, N3	These refer to the number and extent of regional lymph nodes invaded by cancer cells.

TABLE 12.3 M: Metastasis

Metastasis	Definition
Mx	Metastasis cannot be evaluated.
M0	No distant metastasis can be found.
M1	Distant metastasis is found.

successful treatment of cancer a matter of finding the correct combination of therapies.

Neoadjuvant therapy is the use of an intervention before main treatment begins, to increase the chances for success. Radiation to shrink tumors before surgery is an example of neoadjuvant therapy. **Adjuvant** therapy is the use of an intervention after the main treatment is completed to increase the chance for complete success, or to reduce the risk of future recurrence. Using **tamoxifen** after breast cancer is an example of adjuvant therapy. **Palliative** therapy is given to treat the symptoms of cancer rather than the cancer itself. For example, surgery to reduce tumor size and take pressure off of tissues might be conducted, not to cure the cancer, but to relieve pain and improve quality of life.

- *Surgery:* Cancer surgeries are performed to remove malignant tumors with a layer of healthy tissue around them when possible: this is called a "clean margin." A sample of nearby lymph nodes is often taken as well to examine them for signs of metastasis. If a **sentinel lymph node** can be identified (this is a node through which most or all of the lymph from an area passes before going on to other nodes), it can be taken alone for examination.
- *Radiofrequency thermal ablation:* This is a procedure in which instruments are inserted through the skin to the depth of a targeted tumor, and an electrical current essentially "microwaves" cancerous material. It is used for tumors that are not easily accessible for traditional surgery, especially in liver cancer. It may find applications in treatment for kidney and prostate cancer as well.
- *Chemotherapy:* A variety of **cytotoxic** drugs have been developed for use in cancer treatment. These drugs specifically target any fast-growing cells in the body. Therefore, in addition to killing cancer cells, they may cause several side effects.
- *Stem cell implantation:* Cells from healthy bone marrow may be harvested to implant as a treatment for leukemia, or after a very extreme course of cytotoxic drugs is administered. These cellular blanks have the potential to grow into whatever kinds of cells the body needs to replace.
- *Radiation therapy:* Radiation therapy involves high-energy rays that are focused on tumors to kill them or slow their growth. The radiation may be applied from an external machine, which requires daily outpatient visits for several weeks, or it may come from small radioactive pellets implanted close to the tumor. **Stereotactic radiotherapy** involves doses of rays from several directions at once.
- *Hormone therapy:* Some tumors depend on certain hormones to grow. Therapies to limit the secretion of these hormones or to change the way they affect the body are used in the treatment of these cancers.

TABLE 12.4 Numerical Staging

Stage	Definition
0	Cancer in situ: cells have not penetrated tissue beyond original layers of affected tissue.
I, II, III	These refer to the size and extent of tumors, nodal involvement, and invasion of adjacent tissues.
IV	Cancer has spread to another organ. By convention, stage IV often means metastasis to other side of diaphragm or into the central nervous system.

TABLE 12.5 Grading Cancer

Grade	Definition
Gx	Grade cannot be assessed.
G1	Cells are well differentiated (low grade).
G2	Cells are moderately well differentiated (intermediate grade).
G3	Cells are poorly differentiated (high grade).
G4	Cells are undifferentiated (high grade).

Neoadjuvant: A treatment administered prior to the primary therapy.

Adjuvant: A substance added to a medication that affects the action of the drug in a predictable way.

Tamoxifen: An anti-estrogen agent used in the treatment of breast cancer.

Palliative: Describing any treatment aimed at relieving symptoms rather than treating the underlying condition.

Sentinel lymph node: The first lymph node to receive lymph drainage from a malignant tumor.

Cytotoxic: Describing a substance that is toxic to cells.

Stereotactic radiotherapy: A targeted form of radiotherapy in which beams of radiation from various positions are all aimed at one place.

- *Hypothermia:* In some cases, specifically with precancerous cells on the skin or cervix, potentially malignant cells may be killed by freezing them off the affected structure.
- *Hyperthermia:* Raising the body's temperature has been seen to make some cancer cells more vulnerable to the effects of chemotherapy. Drugs are sometimes administered through warmed intravenous fluids or when the core temperature has been raised.
- *Biologic (targeted) therapy:* These strategies work to support the immune system in various ways to identify and fight cancer more aggressively. The main categories of biologic therapies are monoclonal antibodies, cytokines, therapeutic vaccines, a bacterium called bacillus Calmette-Guérin, cancer-killing viruses, gene therapy, and adoptive T-cell transfer.
- *Photodynamic therapy*: This approach uses a drug along with a specific type of light, often a laser, to kill cancer cells. It requires that patients avoid sunlight and bright indoor lights for at least 6 weeks.

Prevention

Several organizations publish lists of preventive measures individuals can take to reduce their cancer risk. A simplified compilation of these recommendations follows:

- Stop smoking and other tobacco use.
- Achieve and maintain healthy weight.
- Adopt a physically active lifestyle.
- Consume a healthy diet, with an emphasis on plant foods.
- Limit alcohol consumption.
- Avoid known carcinogens like radon and hazardous materials.
- Use sunscreen or clothing to protect the skin from ultraviolet radiation.
- Practice safe sex. (This is as a precaution against contracting HPV, which is associated with cervical cancer. However, barrier methods such as condoms do *not* reliably protect against the spread of this virus. Therefore, "safe sex" in this context means to have relations only with an uninfected partner.)
- Vaccinate against cancer-causing pathogens when possible.
- Know your family history if possible, and use early cancer screening methods.

Massage?

Although it has traditionally been believed that circulatory types of massage carry the risk of aiding metastasis by boosting blood and lymph flow, research shows that cancerous growths can take years to become established before they are detectable by palpation. It seems far-fetched to suppose that a 60-minute massage could contribute to that process any more significantly than a brisk walk around the block or a long hot shower. Nonetheless, it is obviously inappropriate to manipulate a diagnosed tumor or any undiagnosed swelling or thickening of tissue.

Massage for persons undergoing cancer treatment, however, has a vital and useful role. Five symptoms of cancer and cancer treatment that are common in most patients include pain, anxiety, nausea, fatigue, and depression: all of these can be addressed with massage. In addition, constipation, altered body image, and poor sleep are problems that massage and bodywork can help with. Massage in various forms is being researched in all of these contexts. Perhaps most of all, massage provides for a basic human need: nurturing, caring, informed touch at a time when many cancer patients feel isolated, anxious, and dehumanized. The benefits massage has to offer are well accepted and frequently requested by patients.

It is important to bear in mind that the complications associated with cancer and various cancer treatments can have serious implications for the choice of bodywork modalities, especially when multiple treatments are employed. One way to clarify choices about massage for cancer patients is to determine whether certain risks are brought about by the cancer itself or by cancer treatment.

Massage Risks for Cancer

- *Tumor sites:* Massage should not disrupt any site where tumors or undiagnosed lesions are located close to the surface of the body. Further, a person with any kind of pelvic or abdominal cancer is not a good candidate for intrusive abdominal work.
- *Bone involvement:* When cancer metastasizes to bones, they can become brittle and unstable. This can make a person extremely vulnerable to fractures. Bones are an extremely common site of metastasis, especially the axial skeleton: the cranium, vertebrae, ribs, and pelvis. The risk of bony involvement is difficult to overstate: this must be rigorously screened.
- *Vital organ involvement:* A client who has cancer or metastasis in a vital organ (this includes the lungs, liver, brain, kidneys, and heart) may have compromised function of any of those organs. This risk must be evaluated to predict if or how well the patient may be able to adapt to bodywork. Accommodations might include changing positions to allow easier breathing, taking care with pressure if blood clotting is an issue, and adding help to get on and off the table if any risk of falling is present.
- *Deep vein thrombosis:* A potential complication of both cancer and cancer treatment, the risk of **deep vein thrombosis**, is a red flag for massage. This risk may persist for up to 6 months after treatment is concluded.

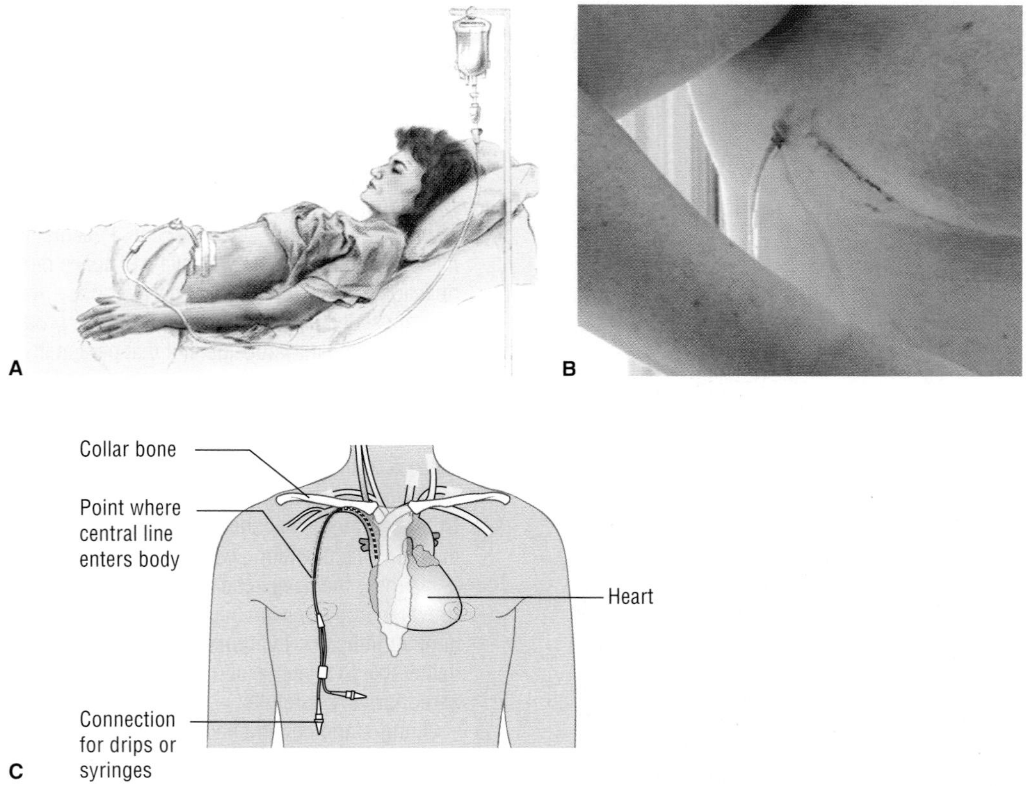

FIGURE 12.2 **A:** Abdominal chemotherapy port allows the delivery of drugs directly into the peritoneal cavity. **B:** Postsurgical drain. **C:** PICC line.

Massage Risks for Cancer Treatment

Cancer treatment is often aggressive and leaves side effects that may seem more extreme or even hazardous than the cancer itself. It is crucial for massage therapists working with this population to be well informed about making appropriate adaptations. Among the most common side effects that can develop with a variety of cancer treatments are low white blood cell count (which reduces resistance to infection), low platelet count (leading to easy bruising and bleeding), and factors that contribute to the risk of venous thromboembolism.

- *Surgery:* Several complications of cancer surgery can have implications for massage. Postsurgical infection obviously contraindicates massage until the client is out of danger. Constipation is a frequent postsurgical complaint, but intrusive abdominal massage may be inappropriate, depending on the cancer site. Any constipation related to an intestinal obstruction or abdominal tumor contraindicates massage. Experts suggest waiting at least six weeks after radiation to the abdomen to do any work here. In the absence of these cautions, gentle work to the abdomen can give significant relief to patients who are constipated.

  Medical devices may be present after surgery, including ports, peripherally inserted central catheters (PICC lines), drains, or ostomies. Inguinal catheters in particular increase clotting risk. Devices should be locally avoided, and the client must be positioned in ways that minimize the risk of their disruption (Figure 12.2).
- *Lymphedema*: The removal and examination of local lymph nodes for signs of metastasis is an important part of cancer staging. When regional lymph nodes are surgically removed for staging purposes, **lymphedema** may develop (Figures 12.3 and 12.4). Both the surgery to

Lymphedema: Swelling caused by the buildup of proteins in the body's interstitial spaces.

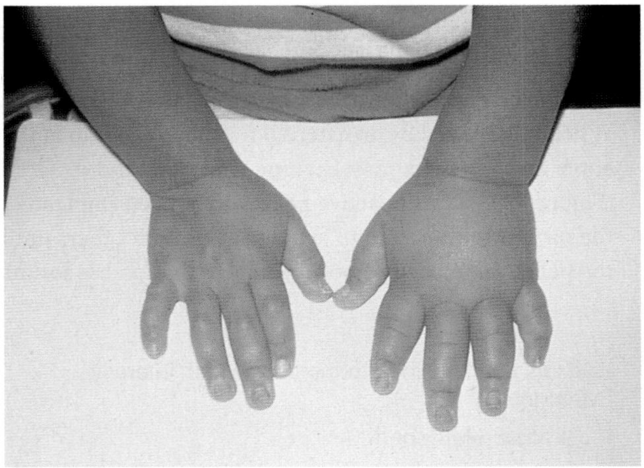

FIGURE 12.3 Lymphedema

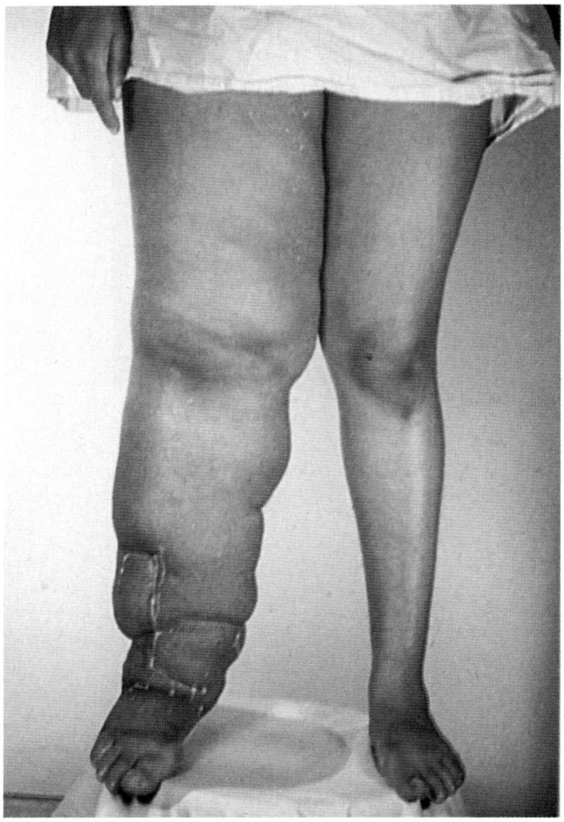

FIGURE 12.4 Extreme lymphedema

remove sample nodes and the treatment to kill cancer that might be growing in remaining nodes can lead to this serious complication. Massage therapists with special training can help to treat lymphedema, but uneducated touch here can make a bad situation much worse.

Lymphedema describes the accumulation of protein-rich fluid in interstitial spaces as a result of lymph system dysfunction. (This distinguishes it from simple edema, which is typically related to venous insufficiency or local trauma.) The chemistry of interstitial fluid is such that when it doesn't flow freely into nearby lymph vessels, it attracts water. That is, a small amount of fluid retention can become a significant problem in a short period. For more on lymphedema, see Sidebar 12.2.

- *Radiation therapy:* Radiation can create several problems. When it is applied by an external machine, the skin at the entry and exit sites may become thin, red, and irritated (Figure 12.5). If radioactive pellets have been implanted, the patient is often told to avoid contact with others until the pellets have been removed or the radiation has lost its

Hydrophilic: Inclined to mix with water. Literally, "water loving"
Indurated: Hardened

SIDEBAR 12.2 Lymphedema

Lymphedema is the accumulation of protein-rich, **hydrophilic** interstitial fluid in the extremities. It can develop in the days or weeks after cancer surgery or radiation therapy, or it can suddenly appear decades later; all that is required is an insufficiency in lymph node function. Patients most at risk for this problem are those who have had nodes removed, had radiation therapy following surgery, who are overweight, and who are sedentary. Once the shift in tissue proteins occurs, the symptoms may subside, but that person is considered always to have lymphedema; from that point forward, it is either well controlled or not.

The most subtle sign of lymphedema is a feeling of fullness in the affected limb. Having trouble removing rings from one's hand may be an early indicator of an episode. Other symptoms can include redness, heat, and pain; these indicate infection along with fluid retention. Often, however, it is simply the deep ache and loss of function of a limb that grows to large or even huge proportions. Pitting edema is another indicator. Lymphedematous limbs are particularly vulnerable to bacterial and fungal infections and must be cared for very carefully.

Long-standing lymphedema can lead to fibrosclerotic changes in the interstitial spaces of the superficial fascia. As a result, the tissue and skin on the affected limb become **indurated**, or hardened. Once this stage is reached, it is very difficult to reverse.

Standard treatment options for lymphedema are limited. Compression machines, bandages, and supportive clothing are often unsatisfactory. Lymphedema is of particular relevance for massage therapists, because it would seem tempting to use Swedish massage, reputed to influence fluid flow, to help resolve it. However, because of the chemical imbalance in the interstitial spaces, any kind of work that compresses blood vessels or causes redness only makes lymphedema worse. For a client with a history of lymphedema, only the lightest touch or holding, for anywhere within the affected quadrant of the body, is appropriate unless a practitioner has specialized skills. Various kinds of bodywork techniques have been developed to address lymphedema, but they employ extensive knowledge of the anatomy and physiology of the lymph system to maximize benefits while minimizing risks. Practitioners who learn these techniques, however, are likely to find an eager group of clients hoping to benefit from their work and acceptance in the medical community.

Clients with a history of lymphatic impairment carry a lifelong risk of lymphedema. It is crucial that massage therapists bear this in mind. Even in client with no lymphedema history, a short massage with medium pressure, if given against lymphatic flow, can lead to an acute episode and a potentially devastating chronic condition. While gentle massage to the rest of the body may be safe, massage of the affected limb and quadrant of the trunk must be conducted extremely conservatively. Precise modifications in pressure, stroke direction, and other details are necessary, and these take special training.

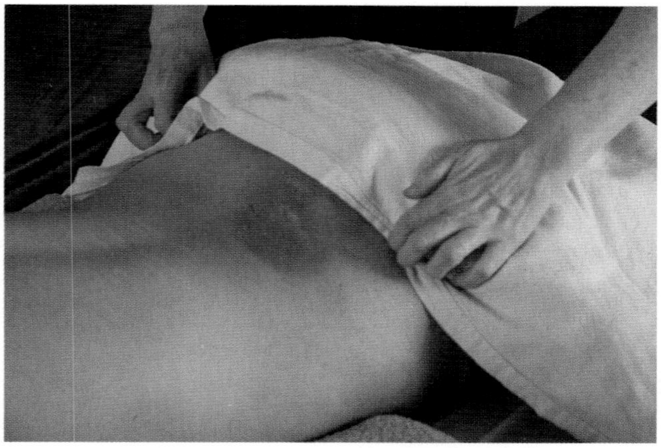

FIGURE 12.5 Skin damage from radiation

potency. The gastrointestinal tract may be irritated, leading to nausea, vomiting, and diarrhea: this calls for our best soothing massage. Bone marrow suppression can lead to anemia, fatigue, poor clotting, and susceptibility to infection. Irradiated lymph nodes can be damaged, leading to a risk of lymphedema. Finally, externally or internally applied radiation can cause fatigue that is extreme enough to interfere with fulfilling a treatment series.

- *Chemotherapy:* Chemotherapeutic drugs may be administered orally or through intravenous drips. They often suppress bone marrow activity, leading to anemia, an elevated risk of infection, and clotting problems. Anemia causes fatigue and coldness; massage therapy needs to accommodate for these symptoms. Low platelet counts calls for care in order to avoid inadvertent capillary injury and bruising.

  Gastrointestinal tract irritation, mouth sores, **hand-foot syndrome,** and hair loss are other side effects of drugs that kill fast-growing cells. Other complications of chemotherapy include **neuropathy**, constipation, skin rashes, and mood changes. Some of these are so serious it impacts patients' ability to finish treatment and therefore their chances of survival. Massage therapy may be able to address fatigue and neuropathy to improve treatment tolerance and make chemotherapy less taxing.

  Some varieties of chemotherapy are eliminated through the skin. It may not be appropriate for a patient to be extensively touched skin to skin during this process, but gloves can be used. In many hospital settings, the risk of infection among immune-compromised patients is considered to be so high that using gloves is a standard protocol regardless of chemotherapy type.

Hand-foot syndrome: A complication of chemotherapy in which the palms and soles become red, swollen, numb, and flaky. Also called palmar-plantar erythrodysesthesia.

- *Other therapies:* Other cancer treatments may also hold cautions for massage. Hormone treatments may increase the risk of blood clots, biologic therapies may cause fatigue and flulike symptoms, cryotherapy can leave irritated areas on the skin, and so on.

No matter what kind of cancer or cancer treatments a person is going through, it is vital for his or her massage therapist to communicate with the rest of the health care team to provide the best benefits that bodywork has to offer with minimal risks. For more information on the role of massage and bodywork for cancer patients, please consult the works cited at the end of this chapter, and consider pursuing formal certification as a specialist for this population. This training will provide specific guidance on interviewing for relevant information and anticipating appropriate bodywork modifications.

Massage Benefits for Cancer Patients

Cancer has been a focal point of massage therapy research since the early 1990s when some brave people challenged the concept that massage had no safe role for cancer patients. While the results of the research have some variations, the general themes are these: expertly performed massage for cancer patients can...

- Improve sleep
- Increase appetite
- Relieve constipation
- Improve mood
- Reduce anxiety
- Decrease depression
- Alleviate pain

These benefits can be applied to both cancer and cancer treatments, as long as appropriate adjustments for the risks listed above are employed. Further, massage must of course be gauged to fit within a client's typical activity levels and capacity for adaptation, which may vary greatly from one person to another. Even though massage alone is unlikely to reverse the course of cancer, by interfering with some of the most common and debilitating side effects of the disease and its treatments, bodywork can without doubt improve the quality of life for people who face this challenge.

Research on Massage Therapy and Cancer

Research about massage therapy in the context of cancer is being produced at such a rate that a synopsis of findings is likely to be outdated before it is even written down. Recent studies look at the effects of massage therapy on cancer-related pain, fatigue, anxiety, depression, well-being of patients and their caregivers, and where massage therapy fits with other complementary and conventional interventions. Some of these are references in the "research" section of each cancer-related item in this text.

Many reviews of massage and cancer studies come to the conclusion that massage therapy shows promise, or appears to be effective for certain goals, but that study sizes are small, the risk of bias is high, or other limitations are obstacles to making stronger statements. It would be great to have bigger, more rigorous studies with lots of participants, but in the meantime, even the smaller studies are useful to help educate ourselves, our clients, and their health care teams about what massage therapy can do. Appendix B, "Evidence-Informed Practice," has some guidelines about finding and using research studies to help our practice and our clients achieve the best possible outcomes.

Bibliography

1. MacDonald G. *Medicine hands, massage therapy for people with cancer.* © Gayle MacDonald 1999, 2007, 2014. Scotland: Findhorn Press; 2007.
2. Society for Oncology Massage: S4OM.org
3. Walton T. *Medical conditions and massage therapy, a decision tree approach*. Philadelphia: Lippincott Williams & Wilkins, a Wolters Kluwer Business 2011.

Explore and Apply

LEVEL 1: Receive and Respond

1. A carcinoma is cancer of what kind of tissue?
   a. Epithelial
   b. Connective
   c. Nerve
   d. Muscle

2. Cancer cells can travel through blood, lymph, and peritoneal fluid or by direct contact with healthy tissue. This process is called…
   a. Local invasion
   b. Oncogene activation
   c. Migration
   d. Colonization

3. Which is the list of potential carcinogens?
   a. Radiation, asbestos, and benzene
   b. Radon, hormones, and genes
   c. Hormones, genes, and immune system cells
   d. Radon, herpes zoster, and uranium

4. Match the following cancer treatments to their descriptions:
   a. Surgery — Using tools to remove the cancerous material
   b. Chemotherapy — Using immune system activity to attack specific classes of cells
   c. Radiation — Using drugs that kill fast-growing cells
   d. Biologic therapy — Using high-energy rays to kill cells or to slow their growth

5. Of the following, which is the most likely to be protective against cancer risk?
   a. Maintain a healthy weight
   b. Get enough vitamin A
   c. Meditate daily
   d. Avoid saturated fats

LEVEL 2: Application of Concepts

1. Your client is between chemotherapy cycles for breast cancer. Her prognosis is good; they caught the cancer early, but she is exhausted from her treatment. She would like to receive massage therapy to help with her fatigue. What is the best response?
   a. Welcome her to a session that is more conservative than for a healthier client, but that puts emphasis on the relaxation benefits that massage can offer
   b. Require that she gets permission from her doctor to receive massage while she goes through this challenging treatment; delay her session until she is cleared
   c. Carefully inform her that massage therapy is contraindicated for a person with cancer because of the risk for unintended metastasis, and let her know that when she is cancer free, she can visit you for an excellent treatment
   d. Provide a session that puts emphasis on circulatory flow in her limbs so that the toxins from her chemotherapy can be processed and expelled

2. Your client had a sentinel node biopsy and it came back clear. What does this mean?
   a. The rest of her lymph nodes will have to be removed
   b. The risk of metastasis is low
   c. Distant metastasis has been confirmed
   d. She has been diagnosed with lymphedema

3. Your client is in the final weeks of his life, after a long battle with colorectal cancer. What limitations for massage does he have?
   a. None; he should be able to receive any kind of bodywork that he wants
   b. Only his family should work with him at this time; a massage therapist is not qualified to work in this situation
   c. He has the same limitations as other clients do for his safety and well-being
   d. People who are at the end of life should receive massage only on their hands and feet to avoid overstimulating their organ systems

4. Your client has radioactive pellets embedded in his prostate gland to help treat prostate cancer. What accommodations are needed for massage?
   a. This client needs to receive massage only in the prone position
   b. This client needs to receive massage only in the supine position
   c. This client needs to receive massage specifically to the abdomen and pelvis so that his treatment has the best chance of being successful
   d. This client needs to delay massage until after the pellets have been removed

5. Your client has a lesion on his scalp that looks like a basal cell carcinoma. What is your best choice?
   a. Calmly inform him that he has a BCC on his scalp, and he should have it removed as soon as possible
   b. Let him know you see a sore on his scalp and suggest that he get it looked at before his next appointment
   c. Ignore it; this is not a significant problem
   d. Terminate the session and let him know you cannot work with him until this situation is dealt with

Note to educators: Due to space considerations, these review questions only address the most important material from Chapter 12. The Test Bank provides a much more comprehensive selection of questions, all of which are keyed to the relevant chapter objectives.

What Would *You* Do?

Massage Therapists Are Role Models

Review the list of behaviors and activities that reduce the risk of cancer. Being brutally honest, analyze how many of these you follow, and where you have room for growth. What habits are on display for your clients to see? Discuss these with a partner, and strategize how you plan to be a role model for good health and cancer prevention for your clients.

What is a Legitimate Claim?

A man calls asking about massage therapy for his wife, who is recovering from surgery for colorectal cancer two weeks ago. Make a list of the information you need to gather to form a session strategy. What are some realistic benefits that you can offer while assuaging any worry that you might inadvertently harm his wife? Role-play this conversation with a partner.

Suggested Activities

1. Quiz yourself using the "labels off" feature in your enhanced e-book, or the labeling exercise on thePoint® for Figure 12.1. Be sure you can identify the changes that occur in the "T, N, M" headings for the progressive stages of cancer.
2. Use the student resources on thePoint® to find practice quiz questions and games.

APPENDIX A
Medications

It is the rare massage therapist who has *no* clients who use any medications. Massage therapists are always encouraged to ask about what medications, prescription or otherwise their clients might be taking. Traditionally, this has been to help discover what conditions a client might have that could influence the way massage needs to be conducted. But the possible interactions between bodywork and medications themselves are a related but separate topic.

When we work with clients who use medication, we must balance the intended effects of the drugs, medical interactions, all possible side effects, and the potential for bodywork to tip the scales for better or worse. In many cases, a conversation with the primary care provider is in order—not to ask permission to do massage, but to investigate whether the general changes massage brings about carry any concern or risk in the presence of prescription drugs.

Some excellent resources about bodywork in the context of pharmaceuticals include these excellent books:

Wible J. *Pharmacology for massage therapy*. Philadelphia, PA: Lippincott Williams & Wilkins; 2005.

Wible J. *Drug handbook for massage therapy*. Philadelphia, PA: Lippincott Williams & Wilkins; 2009.

Persad R. *Massage therapy and medications*. Toronto, ON: Curties-Overzet Publications; 2001.

The list of medication classes under discussion here includes the following:

- Antianxiety drugs
- Antidepressant drugs
- Anti-inflammatory/analgesic drugs
- Autonomic nervous system (ANS) drugs
- Cardiovascular drugs
- Cancer drugs
- Clotting management drugs
- Diabetic drugs
- Muscle relaxant drugs
- Thyroid supplemental drugs
- Others

Within each description, the following information is provided:

- Basic mechanism of the drugs
- Bodywork cautions associated with the medication or the condition they treat
- Common name brands

The discussion of specific medications in this appendix has been largely informed by the findings of the IMS Institute for Healthcare Informatics review of the use of medicines in the United States in 2013.[1] A listing of the top 25 most-prescribed medications in the United States is provided in Table A.1, just to give a sense of what kinds of prescription drugs massage clients are likely to report using. This list is ordered by how often the drug is prescribed. The main ingredient of the drug is named, along with the common brand, and its location in this appendix.

---

[1]Medicine use and shifting costs of healthcare. ©IMS Health Incorporated and its affiliates. URL: http://www.imshealth.com/deployedfiles/imshealth/Global/Content/Corporate/IMS%20Health%20Institute/Reports/Secure/IIHI_US_Use_of_Meds_for_2013.pdf. Accessed Winter 2015.

TABLE A.1 The Top 25 Medicines by Prescriptions Dispensed in 2013

	Main Ingredient	Common Name Brands	Location in Appendix A
1	Acetaminophen/hydrocodone	Vicodin, Lortab	Anti-inflammatory and analgesic drugs —Narcotics and mixed narcotics
2	Levothyroxine	Synthroid	Thyroid supplement drugs —Levothyroxine sodium
3	Lisinopril	Zestril, Prinivil	Cardiovascular drugs —ACE inhibitors
4	Metoprolol	Lopressor	Cardiovascular drugs —Beta blockers
5	Simvastatin	Zocor	Cardiovascular drugs —Antilipemic drugs
6	Amlodipine	Norvasc	Cardiovascular drugs —Calcium channel blockers
7	Metformin	Glucophage	Diabetes management drugs —Oral glucose management drugs
8	Omeprazole	Prilosec	Other common drugs —Omeprazole
9	Atorvastatin	Lipitor	Cardiovascular drugs —Antilipemic drugs
10	Albuterol	Proventil	Autonomic nervous system drugs —Adrenergic drugs
11	Amoxicillin	Amoxil	Other common drugs —Antibiotics
12	Hydrochlorothiazide	Microzide	Cardiovascular drugs —Diuretics
13	Alprazolam	Xanax	Antianxiety drugs —Benzodiazepines
14	Azithromycin	Zithromax	Other common drugs —Antibiotics
15	Fluticasone	Flonase, Flovent HFA	Anti-inflammatory and analgesic drugs —Steroidal anti-inflammatories
16	Furosemide	Lasix	Cardiovascular drugs —Diuretics
17	Gabapentin	Neurontin	Other common drugs —Gabapentin
18	Sertraline	Zoloft	Antianxiety drugs —SSRIs
19	Zolpidem	Ambien	Muscle relaxant drugs —Centrally acting skeletal muscle relaxants
20	Tramadol	Ultram	Anti-inflammatory and analgesic drugs —Narcotics and mixed narcotics
21	Citalopram	Celexa	Antianxiety drugs —SSRIs
22	Prednisone	Deltasone	Anti-inflammatory and analgesic drugs —Steroidal anti-inflammatories
23	Acetaminophen/oxycodone	Percocet	Anti-inflammatory and analgesic drugs —Narcotics and mixed narcotics
24	Ibuprofen	Advil, Motrin, Nuprin	Anti-inflammatory and analgesic drugs —NSAIDs
25	Pravastatin	Pravachol	Cardiovascular drugs —Antilipemic drugs

Source: IMS Health, National Prescription Audit, December 2013.

Antianxiety Drugs

These medications are used to alter the sympathetic *flight-or-fight* response that is so prevalent for many people with anxiety disorders. They act on the central nervous system, but their effects may be far reaching. Common side effects of antianxiety medications include CNS depression, poor reflexes, dry mouth, and feeling unusually exhausted. All of these side effects impact decisions about bodywork. While most of the time side effects are mild and easily tolerated, they can become a medical emergency. Clients should be encouraged to report any troubling symptoms to their primary physician.

Classes of Antianxiety Drugs

Benzodiazepines
Buspirone HCl

Benzodiazepines

Common examples	Valium, Ativan, Xanax, Halcion, Dalmane, Restoril, Librium, Tranxene, Serax
Basic mechanism	It is believed that these medications mimic the inhibitory action of the neurotransmitter GABA, making neurons harder to activate, and by suppressing the emotional component of anxiety in the limbic system. Benzodiazepines are used for short-term anxiety, seizures, insomnia, and convulsions. They are potentially addictive.
Implications for massage	When a person's sympathetic response is suppressed, she is more prone to slide into a deep parasympathetic state. This is fine, until she tries to sit up and falls off the table because of orthostatic hypotension. Massage in the presence of these drugs must be conducted conservatively to respect the client's reduced ability to adapt to external changes. Using more stimulation throughout the massage will help the client to avoid dizziness and fatigue at the end of the massage.

Buspirone HCl

Common example	BuSpar
Basic mechanism	The mechanism of this medication is not well understood. It appears to bind up serotonin and dopamine receptors in the brain, leading to calmer affect without the CNS side effects seen with benzodiazepines. It is less addictive as well. BuSpar is used for short-term anxiety and for chronic problems like general anxiety disorder (GAD).
Implications for massage	The systemic side effects with BuSpar are less than those with other antianxiety medications, but the rules are the same: clients need to move carefully after a session because of sympathetic suppression, and more stimulating massage throughout the session will aid in avoiding dizziness and fatigue.

Antidepressant Drugs

The exact causes of depression remain under dispute, and so do the exact working mechanisms of antidepressant medications. The main classes of antidepressants include tricyclics, MAOIs, SSRIs, and some atypical antidepressants. As a whole, these drugs prolong the availability of various types of neurotransmitters in synapses in the brain, although why exactly this makes a difference is still an issue of some contention. It takes time for the body to adapt to these changes, however; 4 weeks or more are often needed for the drugs to take effect.

Antidepressants all have some side effects, although these are usually temporary and mild. Agitation at the beginning of treatment is common, along with increased anxiety, headaches, and insomnia; these often fade quickly. Other side effects include dry mouth, constipation, reduced sexual function, bladder problems, increased heart rate, and dizziness. If these symptoms don't subside, or if they become a significant issue, patients should consult with their prescribing doctors as soon as possible.

Two types of antidepressants are associated with significant health risks: MAOIs have dangerous interactions with decongestants and some food groups that lead to dangerously high blood pressure and a risk of stroke; and Serzone has been associated with liver toxicity.

Dizziness, drowsiness, and light-headedness are common side effects to many antidepressants. Massage may exacerbate these symptoms, so the therapist should take care not to overtreat, especially when a client is just starting new course of drugs.

Classes of Medications

Tricyclics
Monoamine oxidase inhibitors (MAOIs)
Selective serotonin reuptake inhibitors (SSRIs)
Atypical antidepressants

Tricyclics

Common examples	Imipramine/Tofranil, amitriptyline/Elavil, nortriptyline/Pamelor, desipramine/Norpramin, clomipramine/Anafranil, doxepin/Sinequan, protriptyline/Vivactil
Basic mechanism	Tricyclics block the reuptake of norepinephrine and serotonin at synapses; this leads to *downregulation* and more normal function of the postsynaptic receptors, but it may take 4 weeks or more before improvement is noticed.
Implications for massage	Like other antidepressants, tricyclics may have dizziness as a side effect. Clients may need some gently stimulating strokes at the end of the session to come back to full alertness. Of all the antidepressants, tricyclics tend to have the most extreme side effects.

Monoamine Oxidase Inhibitors

Common examples	Nardil, Parnate, Marplan
Basic mechanism	MAOIs work by inhibiting monoamine oxidase, an enzyme that breaks down the neurotransmitters, but are used less often than other antidepressants because of the risk of dangerous interactions with some substances, notably decongestants, and aged cheeses, red wine, pickles, and other foods with tyramine.
Implications for massage	MAOIs and other antidepressants have the tendency to cause excessive drowsiness and dizziness; massage must be performed and concluded appropriately.

Selective Serotonin Reuptake Inhibitors

Common examples	Prozac, Zoloft, Luvox, Paxil, Celexa, Lexapro
Basic mechanism	These drugs all work to keep serotonin present in CNS synapses for a longer period of time. The theory is that this will lead to a more normalized uptake of serotonin from presynaptic neurons and a decrease in symptoms. SSRIs are used to treat various types of anxiety disorders and eating disorders as well as depression.
Implications for massage	SSRIs often have fewer side effects than other antidepressants, but therapists should be alert for signs of excessive dizziness or drowsiness and compensate appropriately.

Atypical Antidepressants

Common examples	Effexor, Cymbalta, Serzone, Wellbutrin, Remeron, Ludiomil, Desyrel, Symbyax
Basic mechanism	These drugs are similar to other antidepressants, although they focus on serotonin, norepinephrine, or dopamine uptake.
Implications for massage	In addition to the general guidelines about massage and antidepressants, Serzone, in particular, is associated with a risk of liver toxicity. Clients with signs of jaundice, chronic nausea, or other abdominal discomfort should immediately consult their primary care provider.

Anti-inflammatory and Analgesic Drugs

Inflammation is frequently a source of nerve irritation at acute or chronic sites of tissue damage. Consequently, many analgesics work to reduce pain sensation by reducing or inhibiting the inflammatory process. Other analgesics alter pain perception in the central nervous system and do not affect inflammation.

Regardless of the site of drug activity, analgesics and anti-inflammatories change tissue response. It is important to work extremely conservatively with clients who take these medications, because information therapists gather about temperature, muscle guarding, local blood flow, and other signs will be altered, and overtreatment is a significant risk. Although it is inappropriate to suggest that clients skip or change their medication for massage, it is important to be aware when these drugs are at their peak of activity so that therapists may be prepared for the changes in tissue and the effects on clients.

Classes of Drugs

Salicylates
Acetaminophen
NSAIDs
Steroidal anti-inflammatories
Narcotics and mixed narcotics

Salicylates

Common examples	Aspirin, Bayer, Empirin, Doans Pills, Trilisate, Dolobid
Basic mechanism	Salicylates inhibit prostaglandin synthesis, which then reduces pain sensitivity and inflammatory response. They also reduce fever by acting on the hypothalamus and promoting peripheral vasodilation. (They do not reduce a normal temperature.) In addition, aspirin works to inhibit platelet aggregation (see *anticoagulants*).
Implications for massage	Reduced pain perception and inhibited inflammation means that compromised tissue may not send a strong signal about pain; bodywork needs to be conducted conservatively to avoid overtreatment and deep tissue massage used with caution. Also the tendency for peripheral vasodilation raises the risk for hypotension (dizziness and lethargy) and chilling during and after a massage.

Acetaminophen

Common examples	Tylenol, Anacin
Basic mechanism	The mechanism for acetaminophen is not thoroughly understood. It is clear that these medications act on the heat-regulating center of the hypothalamus to reduce fever. These drugs reduce pain sensation, possibly in both the CNS and in the peripheral tissues, but do *not* influence inflammation.
Implications for massage	As with other pain medications, caution must be used to avoid overtreatment.

NSAIDs

Common examples	Celebrex, Lodine, ibuprofen/Advil, Relafen, indomethacin/Indocin, Aleve, Ansaid, Ketoprofen, Mobic, Clinoril
Basic mechanism	All of these medications work to inhibit prostaglandin synthesis at sites of tissue damage to reduce inflammation and the pain associated with it.
Implications for massage	NSAIDs are effective for pain and inflammation, but they are also associated with stomach and kidney damage; clients need to consult their doctor if they have any discomfort (bear in mind that kidney pain may present as low back pain). Regular use of Vioxx and Celebrex has been shown in some studies to increase the risk of cardiovascular disease, including heart attack and stroke. Massage therapists carry the responsibility to avoid overtreatment, even if the client doesn't report feeling pain.

Steroidal Anti-inflammatories

Common examples	Cortisone, Beconase, hydrocortisone, Depo-Medrol, Prednisol, prednisone, Decadron, fluticasone
Basic mechanism	These synthetic analogs to glucocorticoids produced in the adrenal cortex all work to undo the main symptoms of inflammation: they reduce pain, heat, redness, and edema in the short run. The mechanism by which they do this is not well understood, although some researchers suggest that they change local cellular activity leading to suppressed production of prostaglandins, histamine, and other inflammatory substances.
Implications for massage	Steroidal anti-inflammatories are powerful but have several serious side effects. In addition to altering tissue response (which requires extra caution with massage), they suppress immune system activity. Long-term use is associated with weakened connective tissues, fat deposition, muscle wasting, reduced bone density, fluid retention, hypertension, and easy bruising. Topical applications of steroid creams can lead to thinning skin. All of these features influence bodywork choices. Deep tissue massage should not be used when these drugs are used long term, and myofascial techniques should be used with great caution. Steroidal anti-inflammatories may also be prescribed in inhalant form for the treatment of asthma. While these medications specifically target the lung, long-term use may have negative impact on other tissues.

Narcotics and Mixed Narcotics

Common examples	Codeine, Demerol, Oxycontin, Darvon, Percocet, Lortab, vicodin fentanyl/Duragesic, Dilaudid, MS Contin, morphine, Ultram
Basic mechanism	Narcotics bind to opiate receptors in the brain to mimic the action of pain-killing endorphins. This leads to a reduced sensation of pain without loss of consciousness, along with suppression of the cough reflex, and GI tract sluggishness. Narcotics are potentially addictive; mixed narcotics were developed to minimize the risk of dependence, but have proven to be addictive also.
Implications for massage	A client taking these medications has a problem that is too extreme to be managed with less intrusive analgesics. Interference with pain perception is more complete, and appropriate caution is called for. Furthermore, clients taking narcotic analgesics may be prone to mood swings and difficulties with accurate communication. Deep tissue massage should not be used, and stimulation during or at the end of the session is needed to prevent side effects of dizziness and fatigue. Avoid massaging around the area of transdermal patches.

Autonomic Nervous System Drugs

ANS drugs work to stimulate or block the action of the sympathetic or parasympathetic nervous systems. They are used for a wide variety of diseases including gastrointestinal, urinary, cardiac, and respiratory conditions. They can work directly on the receptors to stimulate or block them, or they can work to increase or decrease the associated neurotransmitters.

Classes of Drugs

Cholinergic (increase parasympathetic nervous system actions)

Anticholinergic (block the actions of the parasympathetic nervous system)

Adrenergic (increase sympathetic nervous system actions)

Adrenergic blockers (block sympathetic nervous system actions)

Cholinergics

Common examples	Urecholine, Carbastat, pilocarpine, Aricept
Basic mechanism	These drugs mimic the action of the parasympathetic system.
Massage implications	Since these drugs do the exact thing that massage is usually meant to do (activate the parasympathetic nervous system), care should be taken not to overtreat. Stimulating forms of massage should be used throughout the session so the client is alert at the end, rather than dizzy and in a deep parasympathetic lethargy.

Anticholinergic Drugs

Common examples	Atropine, Transderm Scop, scopolamine, Anaspaz, Librax, Cogentin, Bentyl, Ditropan, Detrol, Artane
Basic mechanisms	The actions of these drugs can vary. They are often organ specific and may suppress or stimulate parasympathetic nervous system receptors.
Implications for massage	These drugs affect the parasympathetic response of the client and therefore the effects of massage. Looking up the drug, target organ, and side effects as well as talking with the client about how the drug affects them will help determine if the parasympathetic response is stimulated or blocked. Massage can then be given with these individual effects in mind.

Adrenergic Drugs

Common examples	Dopamine, epinephrine, Isuprel, albuterol, terbutaline, Serevent, Neo-Synephrine
Basic mechanism	These drugs stimulate the sympathetic nervous system.
Implications for massage	The goal of massage to induce a parasympathetic response is more difficult to achieve with the actions of these drugs. Longer, slower massages may be needed. Be cautious with strokes that stimulate, such as tapotement and friction.

Adrenergic Blockers

Common examples	Cardura, Minipress, Flomax, Migranal, Coreg, Normodyne, Betagan, Corgard, Inderal, Betapace
Basic mechanism	These drugs block the action of the sympathetic nervous system at various receptor sites and include alpha- and beta blockers. They can be very specific to the target organ but may have side effects that are systemic.
Implication for massage	Blocking the sympathetic nervous system means the client may be susceptible to going into a deep parasympathetic state with massage. Caution should be used to be certain the client is awake and not experiencing dizziness or other effects.

Cardiovascular Drugs

Most of the drugs used to treat cardiovascular disease work in some way to minimize a sympathetic response or to dilate peripheral blood vessels. The overriding rule when a client uses these substances is that their slide into a parasympathetic state may be intensified by massage, leaving the client dizzy, fatigued, and lethargic. Ending a session with strokes that are more stimulating may help to ameliorate these effects, as long as they fit into a protocol that is suitable for a person with compromised cardiovascular health. Clients should be instructed to sit up and move slowly after their massage, in order to minimize dizziness or discomfort.

Hydrotherapeutic techniques can present a greater challenge to maintain homeostasis than many other modalities. Many clients with cardiovascular diseases should avoid total immersions in favor of smaller, localized hydrotherapy applications.

Classes of Drugs

Beta blockers
Calcium channel blockers
Angiotensin-converting enzyme (ACE) inhibitors
Digitalis
Antiangina drugs
Antilipemic drugs
Diuretics

Beta Blockers

Common examples	Inderal, Normodyne, Levatol, Corgard, Tenormin, metoprolol/Lopressor/Toprol, sotalol, Coreg, Betagan
Basic mechanism	These affect beta receptors at the heart, bronchi, blood vessels, and the uterus. They lower blood pressure and cardiac output. They are used to treat angina, hypertension, anxiety, and some other disorders. Beta blockers may be selective for action on the heart only or nonselective for a more general effect.
Implications for massage	Beta blockers can lead to excessively low blood pressure, especially when the client is in a relaxed state. Hydrotherapy is generally safer with local applications than systemic immersions in hot tubs, saunas, or other facilities.

ACE Inhibitors

Common examples	Lotensin, captopril, Vasotec, Monopril, Accupril, Altace, Zestril
Basic mechanism	ACE inhibitors work by limiting the action of an enzyme that is employed in the renin-angiotensin system: the loop between blood pressure and kidney function. They promote the excretion of sodium and water, reducing load on the heart. They are used to control hypertension and heart failure.
Implications for massage	As with other drugs for cardiovascular disease, excessive hypotension is a possible side effect. Clients may experience fatigue, dizziness, and lethargy if gentle invigorating strokes are not administered toward the end of the session.

Calcium Channel Blockers

Common examples	Norvasc, Cardene, Isoptin, Procardia, Plendil, verapamil
Basic mechanism	These drugs block the movement of calcium ions in smooth and cardiac muscle tissue. The result is vasodilation and more efficient myocardial function. They are used for hypertension and long-term (not acute) angina.
Implications for massage	Side effects of these drugs include flushing, dizziness, and hypotension. Massage should be conducted to minimize the risk of exacerbating these: less emphasis on big, draining strokes and more emphasis on smaller, less circulatory strokes is appropriate.

Digitalis

Common examples	Digitek, digoxin/Lanoxin, Lanoxicaps
Basic mechanism	Digitalis increases the force of the heartbeat by boosting calcium in cardiac muscle cells; it also slows the heartbeat through action in the CNS. It is used to treat arrhythmia and heart failure.
Implications for massage	Clients who take any form of digitalis to control heart failure are not good candidates for rigorous circulatory massage. Invigorating strokes to conclude a session must be chosen to support alertness rather than circulatory flow.

Antilipemic Drugs

Common examples	LoCholest, Prevalite, Questran, Lopid, Lipitor, Lescol, Zocor, Crestor, Mevacor, Pravachol, Zetia, Tricor, Niaspan, Vytorin
Basic mechanism	Cholesterol-lowering drugs work by sequestering bile or by inhibiting cholesterol synthesis. Bile-sequestering drugs promote the excretion of bile in stool, requiring the liver to use more cholesterol in bile manufacturing; this lowers blood cholesterol. Cholesterol synthesis inhibitors interfere with enzyme activity in the liver that leads to cholesterol synthesis. Both approaches lead to lower LDL (low density lipoprotein) levels.
Implications for massage	A common side effect for all these drugs is constipation as they influence the GI tract. Massage may help to relieve this symptom, but if a client has abdominal pain and has had no bowel movement for several days, an acute bowel impaction is possible; this is a medical emergency. Other side effects (which are not always listed) may include muscle soreness, cramping, and weakness. If a client taking an antilipemic drug has these problems, the prescribing doctor should be consulted before the massage therapist works to resolve them. On rare occasions, these drugs can cause a life-threatening muscle wasting disease called rhabdomyolysis. Symptoms include worsening muscle pain and weakness. If your client has these symptoms, refer them to the physician immediately.

Diuretics

Common examples	chlorthalidone/Thalitone, Lasix, Bumex, Lozol, spironolactone/Aldactone, Demadex, Zaroxolyn, Dyazide, Maxzide, hydrochlorothiazide
Basic mechanism	Some diuretics prevent sodium from being reabsorbed in the kidney. As it is processed into urine, sodium then pulls water along with it. Other medications target specific parts of the nephron to prevent water and salt reabsorption, but can control the loss of other electrolytes more carefully.
Implications for massage	Rigorously applied massage may put an extra load on the kidneys. Resting hypotension may also be a problem for people taking these medications. General diuretics may cause a loss of potassium that can contribute to muscle cramps. This needs to be addressed by a doctor rather than by a massage therapist.

Antiangina Medication

Common examples	Apo-ISDN, IMDUR, Monoket, Nitrodisc, Nitrostat, Transderm-Nitro, nitroglycerin
Basic mechanism	Antiangina drugs reduce myocardial oxygen demand, or they increase the supply of oxygen to the heart, or both. Chronic angina is treated with beta blockers or calcium channel blockers, which is discussed elsewhere. Acute angina is typically treated with various nitrates. These cause vasodilation, especially of veins, leading to decreased load on the heart. They are typically dissolved under the tongue for fast action or applied with a skin patch or ointment for longer-lasting effect.
Implications for massage	If a client has a transdermal patch for antiangina medication, that area and the adjacent tissue must be avoided so that dosage is not influenced. Clients taking these medications have the same risk of hypotension, flushing, and dizziness seen with other cardiovascular drugs.

Cancer Drugs

Cancer drugs or chemotherapy drugs are a large group that acts in a wide variety of ways on the body. While the goal is to attack the cancer cells, cancer drugs are generally toxic to the whole body. Newer drugs can target cancer cells more carefully, but still tax the body as a whole. Massage should be applied very conservatively and circulatory massage minimized. Timing of the session should be related to excretion rates of the drug and discussed with the client's physician in detail.

Classes of Drugs

Alkylating drugs
Antimetabolite drugs
Antibiotic antineoplastics
Hormonal antineoplastics
Natural antineoplastics
Other antineoplastic drugs

Cancer Drugs

Common examples	This is a limited list of the most commonly seen drugs: Cytoxan, dacarbazine/DTIC-Dome, CeeNU, thiotepa/Thioplex, cisplatin, methotrexate, fluorouracil, dactinomycin, tamoxifen, Teslac, vinblastine, vincristine, aldesleukin, alpha interferons.
Basic mechanism	Targets the cancer cells and kills them, or blocks the growth of the cells, or blocks the vascular feeding of the cells
Implications for massage	Always consult with the physician. Massage application should be very conservative. Be aware of methods of excretions (some excrete through the skin) and take appropriate precautions. If radioactive elements are implanted in the body, check with the physician on any limits to the time that should be spent in close proximity to the client.

Clotting Management Drugs

Medications to manage blood clots come in three basic forms: anticoagulants to prevent the formation of new clots by acting on clotting factors, antiplatelet medications to prevent the clumping of platelets to form new clots, and thrombolytics, which are used to dissolve preexisting clots. Thrombolytics are used only in emergency situations (i.e., in early treatment for heart attack or ischemic stroke), and so won't be discussed here. Other clot management drugs are used for chronic problems or to lower the risk of future clots.

Classes of Drugs

Anticoagulants
Antiplatelet drugs

Anticoagulants

Common examples	Heparin, Lovenox, Coumadin
Basic mechanism	Heparin and Lovenox are injected anticoagulants; Coumadin is an oral medication. All of them alter the formation of clotting factors in the liver to prevent the formation of new clots, although they do not help to dissolve preexisting clots. These medications are used for people with atrial fibrillation, a high risk of deep vein thrombosis (DVT), or for people using hemodialysis. Heparin may also be used in orthopedic surgery to reduce the risk of postsurgical DVT.
Implications for massage	All blood-clotting medications carry a risk for bruising, even with relatively light massage. Furthermore, the need for these medications indicates a tendency to form blood clots that may contraindicate all but the lightest forms of bodywork.

Antiplatelet Drugs

Common examples	Aspirin, Empirin, Pletal, Plavix
Basic mechanism	These drugs prevent platelets from clumping at the site where a clot might otherwise form.
Implications for massage	Although these are typically less powerful than anticoagulants, the risk of bruising must still be respected for clients who take antiplatelet drugs.

Diabetes Management Drugs

Because type 2 diabetes is so prevalent in the United States, the chances that a massage therapist might have diabetic clients are excellent. When type 2 diabetes cannot be managed by diet and exercise alone, other interventions are used. They often start with diabetes management drugs and may eventually culminate with the supplementation of insulin in various forms. Type 1 diabetes is also fairly common and is managed with the use of insulin in various forms.

The implications for diabetes and massage therapists are many and complicated. While many diabetics manage their disease well and minimize their risk for secondary complications, others are prone to several problems that pose serious cautions for massage: systemic atherosclerosis, an increased risk of stroke, diabetic ulcers, and peripheral neuritis to name a few.

Furthermore, massage appears to lower blood glucose. While this is an advantage to diabetic clients, this challenge to homeostasis may sometimes be overwhelming enough to trigger a hypoglycemic episode. Massage therapists with diabetic clients should be aware of signs of hypo- and hyperglycemia and should consult with those clients about how best to address their needs in an emergency.

Classes of Drugs

Insulin
Oral glucose management drugs

Insulin

Common examples	Humulin, Humalog, Lantus, Novolog, Novolin
Basic mechanism	Insulin is a protein-based hormone that would be destroyed by digestive juices if taken orally. Consequently, it is administered by injection, either through multiple daily injections or through an insulin pump. It decreases blood glucose by helping to deliver glucose to cells that need this clean-burning fuel to do their jobs.
Implications for massage	Clients who supplement insulin vary their injection sites; these areas need to be locally avoided in order not to interfere with normal uptake of the drug. Length of time for peak effect of the drug varies with the type of insulin; it is best to avoid the injection area for at least that amount of time. If uncertain, avoid it for 24 hours. Because blood glucose stability is an issue for diabetic clients, it is best for them to receive massage in the middle of their insulin cycle, rather than at the end or at the beginning. It might also be useful for a new client to check blood glucose before and after the session, so that if he or she needs to take in sugar in an easily accessible form, the therapist can plan ahead and have some juice, milk, or candy available.

Oral Glucose Management Drugs

Common examples	Diabinese, Glucotrol, glyburide, Glucophage, Precose
Basic mechanism	These drugs work in a variety of ways to inhibit the production of sugar in the liver, to improve the output of insulin in the pancreas, and to increase the sensitivity of insulin receptors on target cells.
Implications for massage	Of these drugs, Glucophage may have the least risk for setting up a hypoglycemic episode. Nonetheless, any clients who manage their diabetes with any combination of drugs and insulin must be monitored carefully for blood glucose stability. As with insulin, it is safest to work with these clients *after* the peak of drug activity.

Muscle Relaxant Drugs

Muscle relaxants are prescribed to deal with acute spasms related to trauma or anxiety or to help with chronic spasticity from central nervous system damage as seen with multiple sclerosis, stroke, spinal cord injury, or cerebral palsy. They can act on the brain, on the spinal cord, or in the muscle tissue itself.

A client who takes muscle relaxants is *not* inherently relaxed, although his or her tissues may seem that way. These drugs interfere with muscle protection reflexes, and so the risk of overtreatment with deep tissue work, range of motion exercises, or stretching is significant.

Classes of Drugs

Centrally acting skeletal muscle relaxants
Peripherally acting skeletal muscle relaxants

Centrally Acting Skeletal Muscle Relaxants

Common examples	Soma, chlorzoxazone/Lorzone, Flexeril, Skelaxin, Norflex, baclofen, Valium, Robaxin, Zanaflex, Ambien
Basic mechanism	These medications are central nervous system depressants. They suppress reflexes that would tighten muscles in response to stretching or damage. They are used to control painful acute spasms related to trauma or anxiety or to promote sleep.
Implications for massage	These drugs enforce a parasympathetic state, which may then be intensified by massage. Therapists should take care that clients are not overly exhausted at the end of a session. In addition, the protective stretch reflex is inhibited under these medications; therapists should not try to create an increased range of motion while the client is in this altered state.

Peripherally Acting Skeletal Muscle Relaxants

Common examples	Dantrium
Basic mechanism	This drug interferes with calcium release at the sarcoplasmic reticulum of muscle cells, leading to weaker contractions. It is used to treat chronic spasticity associated with central nervous system damage, but the overall weakness that ensues makes it a questionable choice for patients whose strength is borderline.
Implications for massage	A client taking Dantrium will have a compromised stretch reflex and falsely hypotonic muscles; massage must be conducted conservatively.

Thyroid Supplement Drugs

Hypothyroidism is typically treated with supplements to replace thyroid secretions T3 and T4. Levothyroxine sodium is chemically identical to the thyroid secretion T4 and is meant to be converted to bioactive T3. While many hypothyroidism patients successfully treat their disease with levothyroxine sodium, some supplement T3 instead of or in addition to T4. This substance has traditionally been available in the form of dessicated animal glands, but a synthetic form of T3 has recently become available.

Classes of Drugs

Levothyroxine sodium
Dessicated extract
Liothyronine sodium

Levothyroxine Sodium

Common examples	Synthroid, Eltroxin, Levo-T, Levothroid, Levoxyl
Basic mechanism	Synthetic thyroid hormones mimic the action of naturally occurring thyroid hormones to boost protein synthesis in cells, promote the use of glycogen stores, increase heart rate and cardiac output, and increase urine output.
Implications for massage	New users of synthetic thyroid supplements may go through a period of nervousness, agitation, and insomnia, which massage may help to improve. If these symptoms persist, the dosage may not be correct, and the person should consult with the prescribing physician. Someone who has been taking synthetic thyroid supplements for a long time probably has no significant side effects and no implications for massage therapy.

Dessicated Extract

Common examples	Armour Thyroid, Nature-Throid, thyroid USP, Westhroid
Basic mechanism	These forms of thyroid hormone have the same action as synthetic supplements: they mimic the action of naturally occurring thyroid hormones to boost protein synthesis in cells, promote the use of glycogen stores, increase heart rate and cardiac output, and increase urine output. The difference is that the potency of these dosages is more difficult to predict, so users may experience significant fluctuation of symptoms.
Implications for massage	As with synthetic hormones, a new user may experience increased anxiety, insomnia, or agitation, all of which indicate massage. If symptoms persist, the person needs to consult with the physician. Otherwise, massage is perfectly appropriate for clients who supplement thyroid hormones.

Liothyronine Sodium

Common examples	Cytomel, Triostat
Basic mechanism	These synthetic forms of T3 are prescribed for patients who don't have success with levothyroxine sodium. They are meant to mimic the action of naturally occurring thyroid hormones to boost protein synthesis in cells, promote the use of glycogen stores, increase heart rate and cardiac output, and increase urine output.
Implications for massage	As with other hormone supplements, anxiety, insomnia, or agitation may occur until dosage is correctly gauged. If symptoms persist, the person needs to consult with the physician. Otherwise, massage is perfectly appropriate for clients who supplement thyroid hormones.

Other Common Drugs

These are commonly prescribed medications that are not included in the classes listed above.

Antibiotics

Common examples	Amoxicillin, azithromycin
Basic mechanism	Antibiotics hinder or kill susceptible bacteria.
Implications for massage	Massage is contraindicated in acute, active infection. If the patient is recovering, massage may be given with caution depending on the individual's condition. Nausea is a possible side effect of antibiotics, and the therapist should limit rocking or strokes that may exacerbate that symptom.

Omeprazole

Common examples	Prilosec, Losec
Basic mechanism	Inhibits activity of acid (proton) pump block formation of gastric acid
Implications for massage	Clients who use these medications are dealing with GERD or ulcers. It is important to make sure that massage therapy doesn't exacerbate symptoms. Dizziness is a possible side effect; be alert for signs of it, and make sure the client feels safe and not at risk for a fall. If the client has constipation and gas, abdominal massage may help. Avoid any rashes, and recommend that the client report them to his or her physician.

Gabapentin

Common examples	Neurontin, Gralise, Horizant
Basic mechanism	Prevents and treats partial seizures and treats neuropathy and postherpetic neuralgia
Implications for massage	The main caution for clients on gabapentin has to do with the painful conditions that may call for its use. Neuropathy and postherpetic neuralgia may be exacerbated by massage. Side effects of gabapentin include dizziness, sleepiness, and vasodilation. These may require care in getting on and off the table. The sedating effect of gabapentin on the central nervous system may increase the relaxing effects of massage.

APPENDIX B
Evidence-Informed Practice

As discussed in Chapter 1, evidence-informed practice is the habit of making clinical decisions that balance three things: practitioner expertise, client goals and values, and the best research evidence that is available. How much each of those three things influence treatment choices may change with each client on each day, but to offer the best that massage therapy has to give, it is essential that each of them be included in the decision-making process.

The main part of *A Massage Therapist's Guide to Pathology* is dedicated to broadening your knowledge: the "practitioner expertise" circle. In this appendix, we focus on the "best research evidence" circle and introduce some key concepts about research literacy: the ability to find, read, critique, and apply research findings. But before we get to that, we need a little background (Figure B.1).

The Scientific Method

Humans share a basic need to understand their world. We do this by making observations and then seeing if they're correct. Research is simply the use of the scientific method to test our observations.

The scientific method is a widely applicable set of steps that can be adjusted for any scientific study, from physics to biology. For the context of massage, it can be described as five basic steps. A published research article, *Massage Therapy for Lyme Disease Symptoms: A Prospective Case Study,*[1] provides clear examples of these steps. (One note: this article is a bit unusual because it is a case study, which usually does not include an experimental element. But it is a clear and useful example for this discussion.)

1. **Form a question about the natural world, based on observation and looking at what other experts have said on the topic.**
   Lyme disease is a common illness resulting in joint pain, headache, and other symptoms. Evidence suggests that massage therapy is an effective treatment for several of those symptoms. Would massage also have a positive impact for someone with Lyme disease?
2. **Develop a testable hypothesis about how massage or bodywork might influence that observation.**
   It is possible that massage therapy could be an effective treatment for someone who has Lyme disease (LD) symptoms.
3. **Carry out an experiment that tests your hypothesis. Try to control the circumstances around your test so that you can accurately connect the experiment to the outcomes.**
   This was a five-phase study of a 21-year-old college student.
   - i. *Intake and interview after 9 days with no treatment for LD.*
   - ii. *Six massage therapy sessions were given over a 3-week period.*
   - iii. *A 1-week period with no massage.*
   - iv. *Six massage therapy sessions were given over a 3-week period, as in phase II.*
   - v. *A 9-day period with no massage, followed by a qualitative interview.*
4. **Analyze your results, and draw appropriate conclusions.**
   Scores for all three symptoms decreased during the two treatment periods and increased during the nontreatment periods. This study presents evidence that massage therapy can be an effective treatment for the symptoms of Lyme disease, at least for this client. We also observed that the more massage the client received, the lower her symptom scores were. This suggests that ongoing massage therapy could be even more effective.

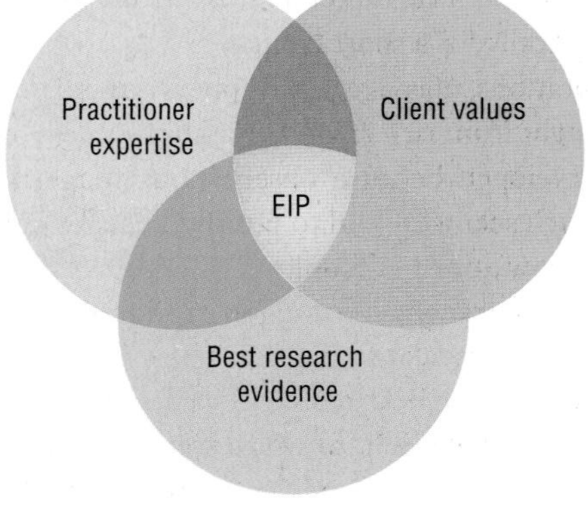

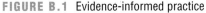

FIGURE B.1 Evidence-informed practice

[1]Thomason MJ, Moyer CA. Massage therapy for Lyme disease symptoms: a prospective case study. *International Journal of Therapeutic Massage and Bodywork* 2012;5(4):9–14. http://www.ncbi.nlm.nih.gov/pmc/articles/PMC3528190/

5. **Communicate your results.**
This case study was published in ***The International Journal of Therapeutic Massage and Bodywork*** *in 2012.*

STUDENT ACTIVITY

Write down a brief five-step scientific method process involving any experiment about massage that you would like to do.

It is important to point out that the scientific method can be much broader and complex than what is presented here, but this model provides a good starting point for this discussion.

The Language Barrier

Many people who are new to research become frustrated with trying to read scientific articles because the language seems so dense, obscure, and impersonal. A couple of issues contribute to this. One is that good scientists are not always gifted writers; that is not their primary focus. But also, the language of research is extremely precise so that every reader is likely to understand it in the same way. For this reason, similar words like "efficacy" and "effectiveness" have different meanings, "bias" does not mean fabric cut on a 45-degree angle, and "double blinded" does not mean that someone wore a two-layered blindfold.

Table B.1 provides some basic vocabulary words that will help readers begin to make sense of research articles. It is not comprehensive, but it provides a strong start.

Is Massage an Art or a Science?

The practice of massage is as old as the human instinct to rub tired muscles or to stroke a fussy child. But massage therapy as an organized health care intervention has only been investigated scientifically for a short time.

For generations, massage practitioners around the world have been taught from rich cultural traditions. Most of these modalities developed because observations suggested that welcomed touch seems to lead to positive changes in health. Variations in how touch is employed have yielded tremendous diversity that ranges from qigong to lomilomi to proprioceptive neuromuscular facilitation.

More recently, our field has developed some capacity to rigorously question the extent to which some of these revered historical modalities really work or whether some are better than others to achieve specific goals. We have even begun to examine whether some of the proposed mechanisms for those techniques are accurate, and the answers are sometimes surprising.

The application of the scientific process to the art of massage sometimes creates tension in the field. Many people feel that if massage therapy is to hold a credible place in the health care system, then it needs to meet the same standards for scientific credibility that we expect from conventional health care interventions. Others are concerned that the art of massage may be lost if we become restrained to only using what shows up well in research, especially since some types of research are not well designed to highlight the benefits that we know from experience that massage therapy has to offer. It may be comforting to know that massage therapy is not the only health care field that struggles with this level of self-analysis. Much of the medical field continues to wrestle with this task.

Changing one's point of view is always challenging, but it is a process that is necessary for a profession to grow. There was a time when people were taught to interpret personality traits by palpating the bumps on the head, and that bleeding a patient with high fever would release her evil spirits. We no longer apply spiderwebs to toothache. We don't rub dead mice on our warts, and it's been a long time since anyone recommended trepanation (drilling a hole through the skull) to treat migraines.

All of these interventions were well-accepted traditions in their time, but each was eventually abandoned. Why? Because rigorous inquiry discovered it was ineffective or because something better (that stood up to examination) came along. If the field of massage therapy is likewise to grow in credibility, we too must be willing to test our traditions and change them when they are shown to be misguided.

It can feel threatening to have one's beloved customs challenged, but the profession becomes stronger when we are brave enough to question which interventions work and which do not. Discovering *how* they work is another question altogether, and it will not be surprising if we find out that much of what we think we are doing (like rehydrating fascia, or breaking down scar tissue, or triggering a parasympathetic response) turns out to be incorrect. This doesn't mean that a modality has no effect; it means its mechanism is something other than what we thought. Understanding the true mechanisms of massage will allow us to deliver even more effective treatments, so that our clients can expect the best possible outcomes. In addition, it will allow us to describe our work in terms that our health care colleagues can find credible.

Of course, a further confounding challenge is tied up in the value of the therapeutic encounter. Research in massage and other fields shows that when patients or clients believe that their caregiver is skilled and invested in their well-being, then outcomes are usually more positive than otherwise.[2,3] This can sometimes muddy the water in research findings, but it is excellent news for massage therapists: we certainly

[2]Bishop MD, et al. Patient expectations of benefit from interventions for neck pain and resulting influence on outcomes. *The Journal of Orthopaedic and Sports Physical Therapy* 2013;43(7):457–465.

[3]Boulanger K, et al. The development and validation of the client expectations of massage scale. *International Journal of Therapeutic Massage and Bodywork* 2012;5(3):3–15.

TABLE B.1 Research Literacy Vocabulary

Research Term	Definition	In context...
Anecdotes, anecdotal evidence	Informal stories, not rigorously analyzed	Any sentence that begins "I have a client who..." is an anecdote.
Bias	Influence or prejudice in a particular direction; any threat to objectivity	If a client is asked to provide a pain level on a VAS to a therapist who just gave her a treatment, the scores may be inaccurate because the client wants to please the therapist.
Confound	Something that interferes or confuses the connection between the treatment and the outcome	If a client starts a new medication or exercise routine while undergoing a massage therapy trial, it could confound the results.
Control group	A group of subjects who do not receive the treatment being studied	If both a control group and an intervention group have lower pain scores over time, then it is not clear how well the intervention worked.
Double blinding	Neither the participants nor the scientists collecting the data know who is in the intervention arm and who is in the control arm of a study	Double-blinding works best in drug trials where subjects don't know whether they're getting the medication or a placebo, and scientists don't know which group is the source of the data.
Empirical evidence	Evidence based on practical experimentation and observation, rather than on theory or logic	It used to be thought that even careful massage was too dangerous for cancer patients. Empirical evidence has shown otherwise.
IRB (institutional review board)	Also called independent ethics committee or ethical review board: a formal committee that oversees the ethical considerations of human experimentation	While massage therapy research seems to be benign, it is always important to have oversight to make sure that the rights and welfare of human subjects are respected.
Likert scale	A scale in which a patient or subject in a study indicates a level of agreement with statements that are arranged in order from more to less strong or vice versa	See Figure B.2.
Randomization	Using chance to determine which group (treatment or control) the subjects of a study are assigned to. The purpose of randomization is to reduce the risk of bias.	Randomization is often challenging in massage studies, because people who are not assigned to the massage group tend to drop out. This potentially confounds the findings.
Sham	Something that appears to be an active treatment, but doesn't include the components that are meant to make it work	It is difficult to conduct a "sham massage," but comparing massage to an ultrasound treatment (in which the participant and ultrasound technician are unaware that the ultrasound machine has been disabled) is an example of using a sham in a massage therapy study.
Validity	A judgment of how well aspects of a study actually do what they are intended to do	Clients with low back pain (LBP) often have a history of injury, surgery, medication use, and other factors. These complicated clients may be excluded from LBP studies. This means that the external validity of these may be challenged.
Visual analog scale	A scale in which a patient or a subject reports a subjective experience along a continuum, provided by a 10-cm line	See Figure B.3.

How interested are you in the topic of research literacy? (Circle one)

Not at all interested	Not very interested	Neutral	Somewhat interested	Very interested

Research literacy is...

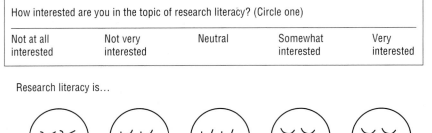

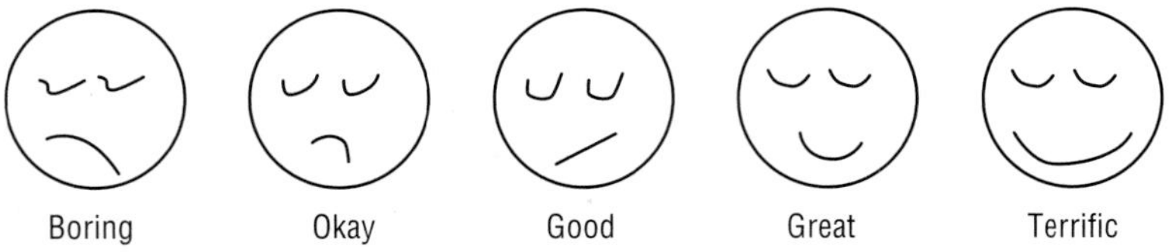

FIGURE B.2 **Top:** Likert scale. **Bottom:** Likert scale alternative.

need to bring our best to the table, but the simple act of being present and compassionate sets the stage for success.

The takeaway message is this: art and science are not mutually exclusive. The beauty of evidence-informed practice is that the influence of research findings is balanced with practitioner expertise and client goals. The profession of massage therapy has some work to do before it calls itself evidence informed. That work begins with creating a constituency of massage therapists who are research literate: able to find, read, critique, and apply research findings.

Finding Research

When a scientist or a scientific team writes an article, they are reporting on the results of their scientific process. They use a particular format to organize their material, and then, they submit their article to a journal that has a readership that might be interested. Before any academic article goes to print however, it goes through editorial and peer review. That means a group of people with appropriate expertise examine every aspect of the paper, looking for weaknesses that need to be defended. By the time an article gets to press, it has usually been thoroughly vetted and revised. Even so, mistakes sometimes get through peer review, so it is not realistic to suppose that every published article is free of flaws.

Until recently, most rigorous research articles were published in small journals that were locked behind paywalls

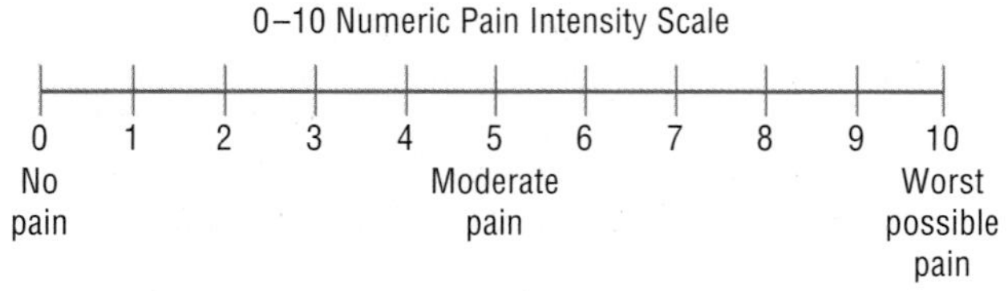

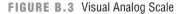

FIGURE B.3 Visual Analog Scale

and mostly inaccessible to people without an association with an academic institution, unable to pay for subscriptions, or lacking access to a medical school library. A movement toward open-sourced publishing and a commitment from the National Institutes of Health to make all taxpayer-funded research freely available has changed that picture, and now we can access many articles that at one time might have been out of reach.

Beginners in the world of research literacy will find two resources that are especially useful. Google Scholar (scholar.google.com) is a search engine that filters out most commercial material. It brings up academic articles, books, magazines, dissertations, and other materials that might be pertinent on any topic, but not all of it is "primary resources," that is, research written by the scientific teams who conduct it.

PubMed (pubmed.gov) is a search engine that links almost entirely to primary resource material. It provides links to articles and abstracts on life sciences and biomedical topics. PubMed is maintained by the U.S. Library of Medicine.

PubMed searches in particular can be overwhelming, so it is extremely useful to take advantage of the Quick Start Guide and tutorials that are available on the opening page (Figure B.4). In this way, users can learn to use filters to see only articles published in English, or only those that offer free full access, or those released within a specific time period.

PubMed and Google Scholar both have features that allow users to request automatic alerts when articles on specific topics are published. In this way, you can have links to pertinent articles delivered to your inbox on a regular basis.

While many articles are now available without a fee, this is not true for all of them. Some important research is sometimes difficult to access unless users are willing to pay for access. When this is the case, it is worthwhile to check at your local public library or, if you have a nearby medical school, to see if they can

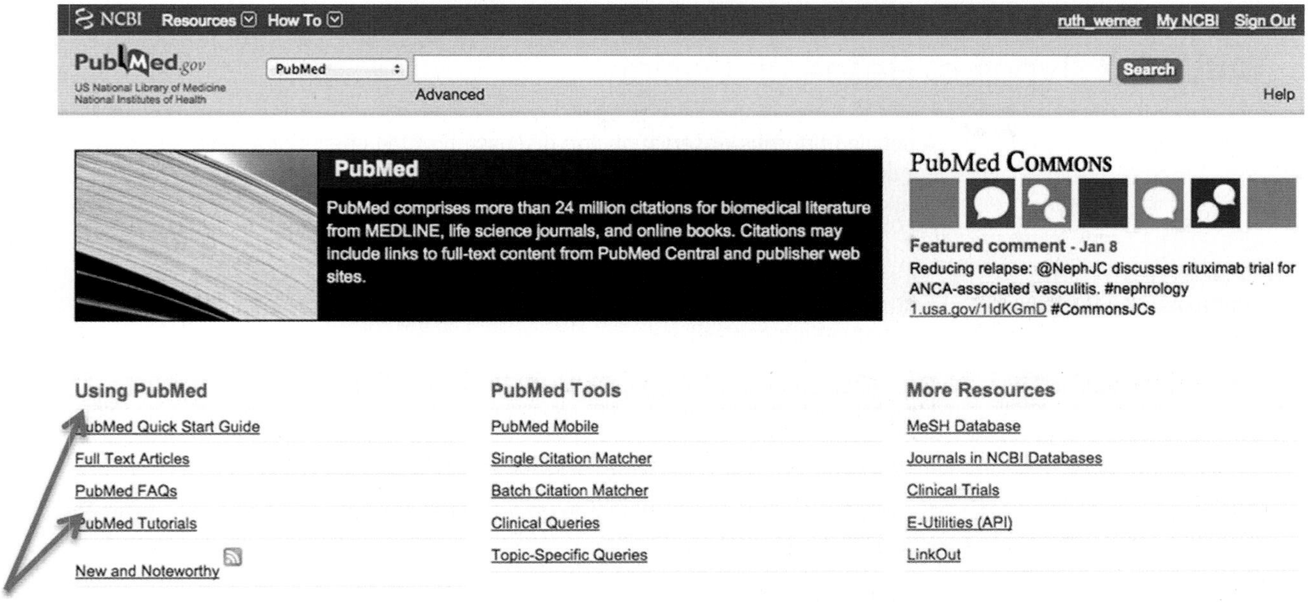

FIGURE B.4 PubMed tutorials and Quick Start Guide

provide you with the article in question. Once you have it in your hands, making sense of it is the next challenge.

> **STUDENT ACTIVITY**
>
> *Conduct a search on PubMed for "massage and arthritis." Use filters for publication dates and for free full access.*

Reading Research

Structure of a Journal Article: IMRaD

Most research articles follow a standard format, which describes a project in an organized way. The format is sometimes called IMRaD, an acronym that stands for *introduction, methods, results, and discussion.*

I = Introduction

"I" stands for "introduction," which is the first part of the body of an article. The author uses the introduction to explain the importance of a certain problem, to share an observation, and to offer a testable hypothesis and prediction for what is expected to happen in the study.

M = Methods

"M" stands for the "methods" section of the article. This segment describes exactly how the experiment is conducted. This is where the study design is described, along with the timeline, the population of participants, a description of the intervention, measurement or survey tools, and a plan for how the data will be analyzed.

R = Results

"R" stands for the "results" section of the article. This is where the researcher reports what happens, without interpretation. This may be done as a verbal description and/or with charts or graphs to display data.

aD = and Discussion

"a" stands for "and"; "D" stands for "discussion." In this section, the researcher examines the meaning of the results; whether the hypothesis was confirmed or not and why; and what this means for future research. Any weaknesses or limitations in a study are shown here. It is important for the discussion to relate the study to other evidence, and to demonstrate why the findings are important. Many of the best studies provide some ideas for clinical application,

The IMRaD format is typically bracketed by an abstract at the beginning, which is a snapshot of the project that gives enough information for potential readers to decide if they want to read the whole paper, and by references at the end, which shows what other articles were cited in the paper.

Research Design

Part of research literacy is the ability to recognize different research designs. This helps us understand how best to use the information that each study yields. Table B.2 is a short list of study types that are frequently represented

TABLE B.2 Types of Research Design

Case report	A detailed rigorous observation and discussion of the effects of a treatment or a condition in one patient
Case series	A collection of similar case reports (usually four or more) with a unifying component such as a treatment approach or condition
Comparative effectiveness study	A study that compares one intervention to others (as opposed to a strict no-intervention control)
Crossover study	A research study in which each subject is examined under at least two conditions, for instance, while receiving a series of massage sessions and receiving no massage
Descriptive study	A study whose results are reported without statistical testing
Effectiveness study	A study that examines whether an intervention is effective in an environment that is similar to or is a real-life setting
Efficacy study	A study that examines whether an intervention is effective in a controlled environment: one that is free of bias and designed to yield the clearest possible outcomes. (This is not always applicable in usual care settings.)
Feasibility study	A study that examines some component of a research design for the practicality of including it in research design
Mechanistic study	A study that examines the exact route by which an intervention produces an effect
Meta-analysis	A method of statistical analysis that combines results from multiple similar trials. Meta-analyses are considered to provide the most rigorous possible conclusions about an intervention.
Mixed methods study	A study that collects and combines quantitative and qualitative data
Pilot study	An initial look at a hypothesis; pilot studies are typically small in scale and designed to determine whether a larger more robust study is justified.
Qualitative research	Studies in which data reflect qualities, or descriptive observation properties, rather than objectively defined measures. Qualitative research often includes semistructured interviews and open-ended questions.
Quantitative research	Studies in which specific, objective, precise measures are collected and reported such as temperature, angles, units of time
Randomized control trial (RCT)	Studies in which most, if not all, aspects of the design are controlled for bias, using randomization and control groups. RCTs are often considered the "gold standard" in research, but this design tends to be problematic for research about massage therapy and other patient-centered disciplines like nursing.
Systematic review	A careful literature review focused on a research question with strict search and inclusion criteria

in massage therapy research. These are not always mutually exclusive; studies often have aspects of more than one design type.

In addition to study design, research is also discussed as a hierarchy of credibility. This mainly has to do with both power (the number of subjects involved) and validity (the rigor of the scientific method). Figure B.5 is a representation of one version of the "research pyramid" that shows how anecdotes and case reports form the base of our knowledge base, and systematic review and meta-analyses provide our most credible, widely applicable information.

STUDENT ACTIVITY

Find an article on PubMed and identify where on the research pyramid it fits.

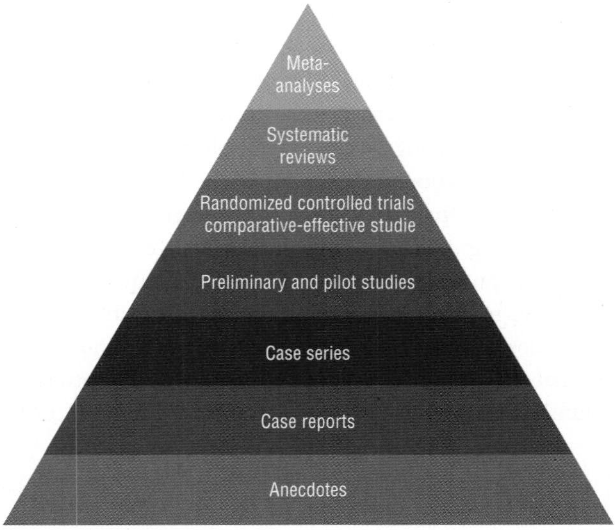

FIGURE B.5 The hierarchy of evidence

Critiquing Research

Being able to identify weaknesses in published works may be the most challenging aspect of research literacy. It is an important one, because not all research is created equal, and some projects with obvious bias, unaddressed confounds, or other challenges sometimes make it through peer review and get published in reputable journals. However, being truly adept at research evaluation takes a level of knowledge that is beyond the scope of this appendix. For more information about critiquing published research, please consult the resources listed at the end.

In the meantime, simply reading a lot of articles about topics that are meaningful to you will help you begin to recognize what distinguishes top-tier research from projects with inherent problems. As with any new skill, practice makes better, which eventually approaches perfect.

STUDENT ACTIVITY

Read a paper and identify a weakness in it.

Applying Findings

The final step in research literacy is applying findings to practice. The research boxes that have been included in the text have highlighted some examples for how that might happen.

The application of findings can go beyond making specific treatment plans, however; findings can support creating relationships with other caregivers, or they can create new working opportunities when findings suggest that massage can be safe and effective in various settings.

Good research opens many doors for massage therapists. In the early 1980s, for instance, it was considered unsafe to work with clients who had a history of cancer; now, massage therapists can build entire careers by offering research-demonstrated benefits to this population. As this field continues to mature, high-quality research that identifies its strengths and demonstrates its value will help continue to define the place of massage therapy in health care.

STUDENT ACTIVITY

How would you apply this finding?
"Conclusions: The study demonstrated that participants who have osteoarthritis (OA) of the knee benefit from the self-massage intervention therapy. Further studies are needed to clarify the long-term effects of self-massage on the progression and symptoms of knee OA."[4]

Where to Go From Here?

Becoming research literate allows massage therapists to claim evidence-informed practice: the highest standard of best practices. Research literacy is a skill that is within the reach of every massage therapist, and it needs to become an entry-level expectation for the whole profession. This appendix dips just a toe in the ocean of what is possible to know in the world of massage therapy research.

A number of other excellent and readily accessible resources exist for massage therapists who are ready to expand their research literacy skills. Two especially important books are these:

Menard M. *Making sense of research*. 2nd ed. Toronto, ON: Curties-Overzet Publications; 2010.

Dryden T, Moyer C, eds. *Massage therapy: Integrating research and practice*. Champaign, IL: Human Kinetics; 2012.

In addition, several organizations have the promotion of research literacy within their vision or mission, and they offer many free resources:

- **The Massage Therapy Foundation** (www.massagetherapyfoundation.org) is an organization dedicated to advancing the massage therapy profession through supporting scientific research, education, and community service, with a vision that the practice of massage therapy is evidence informed and accessible to everyone. The Capitalize Foundation has

4 Atkins DV, Eichler DA. The effects of self-massage on osteoarthritis of the knee: a randomized, controlled trial. *International Journal of Therapeutic Massage and Bodywork* 2013;6(1):4–14. http://www.ncbi.nlm.nih.gov/pmc/articles/PMC3577640/

developed many valuable resources for massage therapists, including an annual case report contest for students and practitioners, information on how to write good case reports, podcasts on research, research literacy continuing education classes, and much more.

- *The International Journal of Therapeutic Massage and Bodywork* (published by the Massage Therapy Foundation) is the only open-sourced academic journal that is specifically about massage therapy research. It is available at www.ijtmb.org. Registration and all use is free.
- **Project to Enhance Research Literacy** is a program of the Center for Optimal Integration, under the auspices of the Academic Consortium for Complementary and Alternative Health Care. At the PERL site, free learning materials have been contributed from academic programs that won grants from the National Institutes of Health to enhance research literacy and to increase the use of research in clinical decision making. Access is available here: http://www.optimalintegration.org/project-perl/perl.php.
- **Project for Open Education in Massage** (http://poem-massage.org). POEM's mission is to change lives through making professional massage and high-quality, valid knowledge about massage universally accessible. POEM provides a supportive learning environment and educational opportunities that are free of charge. This project is administered by Ravensara S. Travillian, PhD, NA-C, LMP.

APPENDIX C
Extra Conditions—At a Glance

Abortion, Spontaneous and Elective

Definition: What Is It?

An elective abortion is the intentional termination of a pregnancy; a spontaneous abortion is an unintentional termination. In either case, the fetus and placenta are detached from the uterine wall and cannot continue to develop.

Etiology: What Happens?

A pregnancy can be electively terminated in different ways, depending on the stage. If it happens within the first 12 weeks, an elective abortion is usually conducted with medication or vacuum suction. In the 13th to 15th weeks, a D&C (dilation and curettage) may be performed. Later terminations are brought about by inducing premature labor. They can be very difficult and require hospitalization.

Spontaneous abortion is called miscarriage if it happens in the first 14 weeks of pregnancy and stillbirth if it happens late in gestation. Several factors may contribute to the spontaneous disruption of a pregnancy. Some of these are controllable, but many of them are not.

Controllable factors that may raise the risk of miscarriage include smoking; untreated infections of the reproductive tract; untreated diabetes or thyroid disorders; exposure to toxic chemicals, especially solvents; and progesterone deficiency in the early weeks of pregnancy. An immune system response that causes blood in fetal vessels to clot can be controlled with low doses of aspirin or other blood thinners.

Uncontrollable factors include structural problems in the uterus (fibroid tumors or a weak cervix), the fertilization of multiple eggs, age, autoimmune disease, an immune system rejection of fetal tissue, failure of the fetus to implant into the endometrium, or what is perhaps the most common cause of miscarriage: the fetus is simply missing key genetic information that would allow it to continue to develop. When the moment comes that the needed genes are missing, the fetus dies.

Signs and Symptoms

When the endometrial lining of the uterus is disrupted in any way but a normal menses, the endometrium is traumatized. This is true for elective and spontaneous abortions and also for childbirth. Symptoms of this trauma can include pain (local and referred), bleeding, and cramping. These are generally self-limiting, that is, the symptoms resolve themselves with time, unless complications develop.

Complications

Complications of elective abortions or miscarriages can include infection from incomplete shedding of the uterine lining; damage to the uterus, bladder, or colon from surgical instruments; and possible hemorrhaging. Depression or anxiety disorders are other frequent complications. The later the gestational age of the fetus, the higher the risk of complications from elective or spontaneous abortion.

Treatment

Spontaneous abortions that are complete require no treatment. Elective abortions, or spontaneous abortions that are incomplete or complicated, may require procedures ranging from medication to stimulate uterine contraction, to dilation and curettage, to open surgery. Other treatments are determined by the needs of the woman and may include antibiotics for infection, analgesics, counseling, or other interventions.

Medications

- For medical abortion: drugs that mimic hormonal activity, administered orally, by injection, or via the vagina
- Analgesics, including NSAIDs or codeine
- Ergot alkaloids to promote uterine contraction
- Prostaglandins, oxytocin, or other medication to control bleeding

Massage Therapy Implications

RISKS	Intrusive abdominal work is not indicated for a woman recovering from a recent pregnancy loss until the bleeding has stopped and she is free from any signs of complications.
BENEFITS	Gentle bodywork can be supportive and helpful during an extremely stressful time.

Acromegaly

Definition: What Is It?

Acromegaly ("acro-" means extremities, "megaly" means enlargement) is a disorder involving the production of too much growth hormone in adults. It is usually related to the development of a slow-growing benign tumor on the pituitary gland, although it can occasionally be connected to tumors elsewhere.

Etiology: What Happens?

The pituitary gland secretes growth hormone (GH), under the command of the hypothalamus. The secretion of GH stimulates in turn the release of a chemical from the liver: insulin-like growth factor I (IGF-I). GH and IGF-I stimulate the metabolism of fuel into new cells for growth (in young people) and for repair (in older people).

A tumor on the pituitary gland leads to the release of excessive amounts of GH and IGF-I. This stimulates the production of new tissues, resulting in bone enlargement, which can cause joint distortion and pain, and enlargement and weakening of the heart. In addition, the tumor itself can exert mechanical pressure on the pituitary and other brain structures, causing a variety of problems. The type of tumor associated with acromegaly is not cancerous, but it is dangerous for the symptoms it causes.

Signs and Symptoms

Often, the earliest symptoms of acromegaly are **headaches** and vision problems brought about by pressure inside the cranium. The hands and feet may grow, and facial changes include enlarged mandibles and spaces between teeth. Joint pain, fatigue, hyperhidrosis (excessive sweatiness) with body odor, and **obstructive sleep apnea** (probably related to an enlarged tongue) are frequent problems. Skin tags are common, along with a deeper voice. If a tumor grows to a significant size, other central nervous system symptoms may occur, including cranial nerve damage.

Complications

Many acromegaly patients develop painful **osteoarthritis**. If the tumor interferes other pituitary functions, other endocrine-related dysfunctions might include oily skin, heavy menstrual periods, growth of body hair, and breast discharge. Because the sudden growth of new tissues can stress the heart, some of the most serious complications of acromegaly are connected to cardiovascular challenge. **High blood pressure** is common, along with a pathologic enlargement of the heart: cardiomegaly. Eventually, untreated acromegaly patients may experience **heart failure**.

Some acromegaly patients develop insulin resistance or **diabetes mellitus**. A higher-than-average risk of **colorectal cancer** has also been observed among this population. Women are more prone to **uterine fibroid tumors** as well.

Treatment

Surgery for acromegaly is most successful when the pituitary tumor is small. This transsphenoidal surgery is conducted through the nose or upper lip. Postsurgical radiation may be recommended. Other therapies focus on attempts to balance the GH/IGF-I balance that is lost when the pituitary gland becomes hyperactive.

Medications

- Somatostatin analogs to suppress GH production and shrink the tumor
- GH receptor antagonists to interfere with GH activity and normalize IGF-I secretion
- Dopamine agonists to lower GH and IGF-I secretion

Massage Therapy Implications

RISKS	Serious or extreme cases of acromegaly carry a risk of heart failure; this requires adaptation of bodywork choices. Acromegaly patients also have higher-than-average rates of colorectal cancer and diabetes: these must be investigated for safety.
BENEFITS	Massage is unlikely to change the course of acromegaly, but within safety limits, it can certainly improve a patient's quality of life. Clients who have successfully treated their pituitary tumor with no long-term damage can enjoy the same benefits from massage as the rest of the population.

Addison Disease

Definition: What Is It?

Addison disease involves the destruction of the adrenal cortex, limiting the secretion of any combination of cortisol, aldosterone, or androgenic hormones. It can be related to an infection, but it is usually an autoimmune condition.

Etiology: What Happens?

The adrenal glands are composed of two main regions: the medulla and the cortex. The adrenal cortex produces hormones in three main classes: glucocorticoids, mineralocorticoids, and androgens. Glucocorticoids, of which cortisol is the most well-known, do many things. They create and prolong stress responses; influence the metabolism of proteins, fats, and sugars; suppress immune system activity; and do several other important jobs. Mineralocorticoids help to maintain blood pressure by affecting water and salt retention at the kidneys. Aldosterone is the primary mineralocorticoid. Androgens are male sex hormones; women secrete much of their androgens from the adrenal cortex, while men secrete most of theirs from the testes.

Addison disease develops when autoimmune disease or infection destroys much of the adrenal cortex and interferes with the secretion of adrenal cortex hormones. Pituitary disruption can also suppress adrenal cortex secretion.

Signs and Symptoms

Signs and symptoms of adrenal cortex insufficiency include muscle weakness and fatigue, low blood pressure, hypoglycemia, irritability, and **depression**. When aldosterone levels are low, salt craving and dehydration develop. Low androgen levels in women result in the loss of pubic and axillary hair; men, who secrete most of their androgens from the testes, are not affected in this way.

A link between corticotropin-releasing hormone (which increases when the adrenals are low functioning) and melanocyte-stimulating hormone means that Addison disease often involves patches of darkened skin and mucous membranes where melanocytes become overactive.

Types of Addison Disease

- *Primary Addison disease*: This is usually an autoimmune attack on the adrenal glands, called idiopathic adrenal insufficiency. If other glands are affected, it is called polyendocrine deficiency syndrome. About 20% of primary Addison disease in the United States is related to **tuberculosis**, but in countries where TB is more common, this percentage is much higher. Adrenal damage can also occur because of cancer metastasis, chronic fungal infections, local hemorrhage, and other more obscure reasons.
- *Secondary Addison disease*: This occurs when pituitary secretions of adrenocorticotropic hormone (ACTH) from the pituitary are abnormally low. If ACTH levels drop, then cortisol secretion also drops. This can happen when a person who supplements steroidal hormones suddenly stops taking his or her medication or when the pituitary is affected by a tumor or surgery.

Complications

An addisonian crisis involves a sudden onset of sharp abdominal pain, severe nausea, vomiting, and diarrhea. Low back pain and pain in the arms and legs may occur, along with dangerously low blood pressure, high potassium levels, and loss of consciousness. An addisonian crisis is a medical emergency.

Treatment

Addison disease is highly treatable with oral or injected doses of steroids to replace the missing hormones. Salt supplementation is recommended for patients low on aldosterone, especially during hot weather or with excessive physical work that involves sweating.

Medications
- Oral or injected corticosteroids to replace depleted cortisol
- Synthetic mineralocorticoid (fludrocortisone acetate) to replace depleted aldosterone
- Androgen replacement therapy for women with Addison disease

Massage Therapy Implications

RISKS	Addison disease often involves weakness and low blood pressure, and the treatment involves taking steroids that carry potentially serious side effects. Massage therapists must make adjustments accordingly.
BENEFITS	While massage is unlikely to change the prognosis of Addison disease, within the limits of client adaptation, it can certainly add to a client's quality of life.

Amputation

Definition: What Is It?

Amputation is the removal of part of an extremity, usually due to vascular disease, trauma, or cancer.

Etiology: What Happens?

The leading reason for amputation in this country is the vascular compromise that accompanies **diabetes**. In this situation, poor circulation not only leads to dead and dying tissue but also impedes the ability to fight off infection. At this point, amputation becomes a lifesaving intervention.

Signs and Symptoms

The signs and symptoms of amputation are obvious: part or all of an extremity is surgically removed.

Complications

The postsurgical complications of amputation can be serious. Phantom limb pain, pain at the wound site, neuropathy, and central sensitization can all develop after a person loses a limb. Any of these may interfere with the ability to use a prosthesis and cause great difficulties with activities of daily living.

The postural, gait, and center of gravity adjustments that follow such an event may also lead to other musculoskeletal injuries.

Treatment

Physical and occupational therapy frequently help people with amputations to learn how best to cope with a new limitation, how to care for the surgical wound, and how to use a prosthetic for the best results. Pain management may include narcotic analgesics, NSAIDs, and massage.

Medications
- Narcotic analgesics
- NSAIDs

Massage Therapy Implications

RISKS	The primary risk for massage for a person who has had an amputation is inadvertently making stump or phantom pain worse. Careful handling of the wound site and good communication with the client can keep this risk to a minimum.
BENEFITS	Massage therapy that focuses on scar tissue mobility may be extremely helpful to clients with stump pain or problems with their prostheses. Sometimes, massage therapists can conduct skin checks more easily than clients, and with careful palpation, we may be able to isolate the nerve endings that may alleviate some phantom pain. In addition, massage therapy may help with some of the depressive symptoms that often accompany this situation.
OPTIONS	Some clients find relief when their massage therapist builds a "pretend limb" out of pillows and makes massaging motions over it as the client watches.

Avascular Necrosis

Definition: What Is It?

Avascular necrosis (AVN) is a condition in which blood supply to a bone is impeded by some combination of factors. Bone tissue and blood vessels disintegrate and are never fully replaced. The resulting weakness leads to a high risk of **fractures**, **osteoarthritis**, and **dislocation** or joint collapse.

Etiology: What Happens?

Several factors may work together to interrupt blood flow to a bone, including trauma or tiny emboli made of blood clots, fat cells, or nitrogen bubbles: this can be a complication of decompression sickness or "the bends."

Other conditions that can lead to AVN include excessive alcohol consumption, steroids for autoimmune disease or organ transplant patients, **hemophilia**, **sickle cell disease**, **HIV**, and **pancreatitis**.

Because it relies on only one major blood source, the head of the femur is particularly vulnerable to interruptions in blood flow. The end result of AVN often involves serious damage to this important structure. Damage is usually unilateral.

Signs and Symptoms

AVN often has a slow onset. It may begin with loss of range of motion, limping, and joint pain just during movement, but the pain worsens and becomes prevalent even during rest. Pain may refer to the lateral thigh or knee. In later stages, AVN shows all the signs of osteoarthritis. Eventually, it may lead to total collapse of the joint.

Types of Avascular Necrosis

- Legg-Calvé-Perthes *disease (LCPD)*: This is a type of AVN that is almost exclusive to young children. This rare condition affects boys about four times more often than girls and is typically diagnosed between ages 3 and 10. Most cases of LCPD have an excellent prognosis, but children may temporarily need braces, crutches, and surgery to reshape the head of the femur.
- *Osteonecrosis of the jaw*: This is a rare form of AVN that affects the mandible. It is related to the use of bisphosphonate drugs used to treat **osteoporosis** or the bone loss that sometimes develops with cancer or cancer treatments.

Treatment

Treatment options for AVN are determined by several variables, including age, cause, and severity. Nonsurgical treatments include the use of physical therapy, braces, or crutches to temporarily relieve weight-bearing stress. Electrical stimulation of the bone may be recommended to stimulate healthy new growth.

Many AVN patients eventually undergo some kind of surgery to decompress the medullary canal, to remove dead tissue, to reshape the bone for better strength, or to replace a ruined joint (**joint replacement surgery**).

Medications

- Anti-inflammatories to control inflammation and pain (this does not include aspirin for young children)
- Anticholesterol drugs to limit the risk of fat emboli

Massage Therapy Implications

RISKS	Avascular necrosis involves severely damaged bone with loss of range of motion and the risk of fracture. Any massage needs to be adjusted for this vulnerability at and around the affected area. AVN is often a complication of an underlying disorder: this must be pursued in case other cautions for massage exist.
BENEFITS	As long as the rest of circulation is healthy, massage anywhere away from the affected area may help to manage some of the compensatory postural and movement patterns that develop when walking is painful.

Bladder Stones

Definition: What Are They?

Bladder stones are hard accretions of minerals that form in the urinary bladder, which can in turn cause bladder irritation.

Etiology: What Happens?

The most common type of bladder stones are formed from uric acid when urine in the bladder becomes concentrated and stagnant. Urine stagnation can be a result of anything that interferes with bladder emptying, such as **benign prostatic enlargement** and neurogenic bladder. Diverticula in the bladder can also create pockets of stagnant urine where bladder stones may form.

Most bladder stones form in the bladder itself. Kidney stones that are small enough to pass through the ureter into the bladder also tend to be small enough to exit the bladder through the urethra. Occasionally though, a stone formed in the kidney may pass into the bladder, where additional layers of minerals are deposited, causing the stone to grow. Young children with diets low in phosphorus can also develop bladder stones, although this occurs less and less as maternal and infant nutrition improve globally.

Signs and Symptoms

Bladder stones are often silent. Symptoms occur when they irritate the lining of the bladder or block the normal flow of urine. Painful, frequent, or difficult urination; dark, cloudy, or bloody urine; and abdominal pain are common symptoms when this happens.

Complications

Untreated bladder stones can lead to infection and permanent damage to the bladder.

Treatment

Many bladder stones pass from the body without intervention. In the case of smaller bladder stones that do not block the flow of urine, a physician may recommend increased water intake to help the stone to pass. If the stone is larger, it is usually broken up in a procedure called cystolitholapaxy.

During cystolitholapaxy, the stone is viewed with a cystoscope inserted into the bladder via the urethra. It is then broken up using a laser, ultrasound, or mechanical vibration. The small pieces then pass from the body during urination. Very rarely, a stone must be surgically removed.

Treatment for bladder stones also includes treatment for the underlying cause, if necessary.

Massage Therapy Implications

RISKS	Care should be taken when massaging the abdomen of a client with bladder stones, as the area can be tender. While massage has no particular impact on bladder stones specifically, the underlying cause of the stones should be taken into account. Clients who experience the need to urinate frequently may feel more comfortable with a massage of shorter duration.
BENEFITS	Clients with silent bladder stones, or with a history of this condition, can enjoy the same benefits of massage as the general population.

Bronchiectasis

Definition: What Is It?

Bronchiectasis is a condition in which the bronchi and bronchioles of the lungs become permanently dilated, thickened, and unable to clear mucus. It is related to a wide variety of underlying disorders.

Etiology: What Happens?

In this condition, chronic or repeated irritation to the proximal and medium-sized bronchi causes the smooth muscle and elastin in these tubes to degenerate. The structures become rigidly open and thickened, and the ability to clear mucus is seriously impaired. This allows the lungs to become a growth medium for bacteria or other pathogens, leading to more mucus production, and a vicious circle of lung dysfunction.

Bronchiectasis is considered part of the chronic obstructive pulmonary disease (COPD) group, along with chronic bronchitis and emphysema, but instead of being related closely to cigarette smoking, it is most often connected to repeated infections (especially **pneumonia** or pertussis), congenital disorders (especially **cystic fibrosis**), autoimmune disease, **gastroesophageal reflux disease**, or other conditions.

Signs and Symptoms

Signs and symptoms of bronchiectasis typically begin with a productive cough. Shortness of breath and chest pain are frequently present. During an infection, mucus may be thick, opaque, and foul smelling. Lung sounds called crackles may be audible with a stethoscope.

Complications

Bronchiectasis has several serious possible complications. Increased vulnerability to infection raises the risk of lung abscesses or life-threatening **pneumonia**. Rarely, extreme coughing can damage an artery in the lung leading to excessive bleeding into the sputum; this is called hemoptysis. Progressive respiratory failure can develop as the lungs lose function. And resistance in the pulmonary circuit can put an excessive load on the right side of the heart, leading to cor pulmonale or right-sided **heart failure**.

Treatment

Treatment for bronchiectasis is directed at improving lung clearance, controlling infection, addressing underlying conditions, and improving the strength of breathing muscles. Patients are counseled to avoid smoking and secondhand smoke and to keep current on immunizations for flu and pneumonia. Physical therapy often includes aggressive manual clapping over the thorax; this may also be accomplished with devices that range from an inflatable percussive vest to a handheld inhaling instrument that sends vibrations into the chest. If the bronchiectasis is limited to a focal area of the lung and other interventions are not successful, resection surgery may be recommended. Patients at risk for cor pulmonale may supplement oxygen.

Medications

Medications may vary according to other conditions that contribute to lung damage.

- Antibiotics to treat and prevent bacterial and mycoplasma infections
- Expectorants to assist lung clearing
- Inhaled medications
  - Bronchodilators
  - Corticosteroids
  - Beta agonists for smooth muscle relaxation
- Immunosuppressant drugs to treat autoimmune diseases
- Medications to treat gastroesophageal reflux disease

Massage Therapy Implications

RISKS	A person with bronchiectasis may be at significantly increased risk for developing respiratory infections; massage should be rescheduled if either the client or the therapist shows any signs of respiratory infection. Patients may also have a variety of underlying disorders, any of which may require adaptation for massage.
BENEFITS	Pulmonary physical therapy is a mainstay of bronchiectasis treatment, and massage may be adapted to fit into this context as well. Any bodywork that improves resilience, immune system activity, and fatigue will be welcomed, as long as it respects other challenges that the patient faces.

Carditis

Definition: What Is It?

Technically, carditis is inflammation of the heart. In reality, this term refers to any of three sites of inflammation: the pericardium, the myocardium, or the endocardium, especially where it covers the heart valves.

Etiology: What Happens?

Carditis is often related to an infection. Many viruses, bacteria, and fungi can colonize the layers of the heart, and each pathogen has its own pattern of symptoms, damage, and response to treatment. Other causes of inflammation in and around the heart include autoimmune activity (especially with **systemic lupus erythematosus**, **scleroderma**, and **sarcoidosis**), trauma, or reactions to medications.

Signs and Symptoms

Signs and symptoms of carditis vary according to the causative factors and the part of the heart that is affected. Some forms of myocarditis are practically silent in early stages, but most acute viral and bacterial infections cause a predictable set of symptoms including fever, malaise, dyspnea, and stabbing chest pain. Pain often refers to the left arm, shoulder, and scapula. Many patients find that inhalation becomes painful, but sitting with the trunk in flexion relieves pain: this is a characteristic sign of carditis. Heart rhythms may become abnormal, and sounds from the friction of scarred layers of pericardium rubbing together may be audible through a stethoscope.

Types of Carditis

- *Pericarditis*: This is inflammation of the pericardial sac, but it may penetrate to the myocardial cells as well. It is usually due to a viral or bacterial infection. Damage to healthy cells comes about both through pathogenic activities and through immune system responses. While most cases of pericarditis are short-lived, two serious complications can develop: cardiac tamponade, where the pericardial sac fills with fluid that puts mechanical pressure on the heart and can lead to circulatory failure, and constrictive pericarditis, where enough scar tissue builds between the visceral and parietal layers of the pericardium that a normal heartbeat is inhibited.
- *Myocarditis*: This is inflammation of the myocardium. It is often related to a viral attack, but autoimmune diseases can cause it as well. The net result is that myofibers are destroyed and replaced with noncontractile connective tissue. The prognosis of myocarditis is unpredictable: it can go to full recovery with no long-term ill effects, or it can lead to **heart failure**.
- *Endocarditis*: This is inflammation of the endocardium, especially where it covers the valves of the heart. People with a history of heart or valve problems are at heightened risk for developing an infection here, so they are often counseled to use prophylactic antibiotics before undergoing any dental procedures or other types of surgery.

Pathogens tend to colonize the heart valves downstream from blood flow, where they trigger the growth of structures called vegetations. These are formed of platelets, fibrin, pathogens, and immune system cells. Vegetations can be large enough to occlude a valve opening, but they tend to be delicate and easily breakable. Fragments that enter the bloodstream become **arterial emboli** and can have serious repercussions.

Treatment

Most forms of carditis are treated with bed rest, good nutrition, and drugs to address infection, autoimmune activity, or the risk of heart failure. Pericardiocentesis is a procedure using a long thin needle to extract excess fluid from the pericardial sac: this is used to treat cardiac tamponade. Surgery to replace damaged valves or to repair or remove a seriously scarred pericardium is sometimes recommended.

Medications

- NSAIDs to manage pain and inflammation
- Antibiotics for bacterial infection (note: these may be given intravenously for several weeks)
- Narcotic analgesics if necessary
- Steroidal anti-inflammatories to manage autoimmune disease (note: these must be avoided in the presence of infection)
- Beta-blockers, ACE inhibitors, diuretics, and other hypertension management drugs in the presence of heart failure

Massage Therapy Implications

RISKS	Whichever type of carditis is present, it is an indication that the homeostatic processes of the body are impaired. Any kind of bodywork that requires significant adaptation should be postponed until the inflammation has subsided and the patient is restored to health.
BENEFITS	Bodywork that does not present a challenge to homeostasis may be soothing and welcome during a time of significant fear and stress. Clients who have fully recovered from carditis and are cleared for physical activity can enjoy the same benefits from massage as the rest of the population.

Charcot-Marie-Tooth Syndrome

Definition: What Is It?

Charcot-Marie-Tooth syndrome (CMT) is a collection of genetic neurologic conditions that affect the myelin or long axons of the peripheral nervous system. It affects about 125,000 people in the United States.

Etiology: What Happens?

The inherited genetic mutations that cause CMT can be dominant, recessive, X-linked, or spontaneous. Each type of CMT involves a different mutation, but the ultimate results on the body are the same. Most versions lead to problems with the production of the myelin sheath by Schwann cells in the peripheral nervous system. Areas of unstable myelin develop, the myelin breaks down, and then Schwann cells proliferate, make extra myelin that may be defective, and the cycle begins again. Ultimately, poorly myelinated axons have slowed conduction, and sensation is impaired. In a slightly different form of CMT, the damage occurs not to the myelin but to the nerve fibers themselves. All forms of CMT lead to poor conduction of motor impulses and some sensory messages.

Interestingly, the sensory deficit brought about by the most common type of CMT is restricted to texture and pressure sensation. Pain and temperature-sensitive neurons are not myelinated and so are usually unaffected by this disease.

Signs and Symptoms

CMT symptoms usually develop by adolescence or early adulthood. Weakness and muscle wasting in the feet and lower legs are common early signs. Clumsiness, frequent tripping, and falls may be the first things parents notice. As the muscles of the foot atrophy, the flexor tendons may distort the foot into an extremely high arch (**pes cavus**) with **hammertoe**, along with a risk of sores and infections at the foot. Foot drop and an exaggerated gait to accommodate for this weakness may develop.

Many CMT patients don't report numbness or loss of sensation, but this may be because pain and temperature sensation are usually intact, and the other sensations (texture, pressure) had never fully developed. Some patients experience pain with nerve degeneration and severe muscle cramps.

CMT is often slowly progressive and may eventually affect the muscles of the hand and arm. In rare cases, it impairs the action of the phrenic nerve, leading to problems with breathing.

Treatment

As a genetic disorder, CMT has no specific treatment. Instead, symptoms and complications are addressed with orthotics; crutches, canes or braces; medication to manage pain; and therapy to enhance strength and stability.

Medications
- NSAIDs for pain and inflammation
- Tricyclic antidepressants for neuropathic pain and depression
- Anticonvulsant medications for pain and sedation
- Botox to reduce muscle spasm

Massage Therapy Implications

RISKS	CMT patients have some reduced sensation in the affected limbs. Fortunately, pain and temperature sensation tend to remain intact, but care must be taken to respect the fact that pressure and texture sensation may be impaired. The pain related to CMT is mainly related to nerve damage and muscle spasm. Carelessly applied massage may make either of these situations worse.
BENEFITS	CMT patients are often engaged in extensive physical and occupational therapy to counteract progressive muscle weakness, contracture of tendons, and postural instability. Massage, with respect for cramping, nerve pain, and loss of sensation, could have a useful place here as well.

Conjunctivitis

Definition: What Is It?

Conjunctivitis, also known as pink eye, is the inflammation of the conjunctiva (covering membrane) of the eye. It is common around the world and among people of all ages. It has a wide variety of causes, the most common of which are viral, bacterial, or allergic.

Etiology: What Happens?

Viral and bacterial conjunctivitis are both highly contagious. They are most commonly spread when a person comes into contact with the infected tears, eye secretions, or respiratory discharge of an infected person and then touches his or her own eye. In this way, a person with one infected eye can also infect the other.

Allergic conjunctivitis is noninfectious and often accompanies other allergic reactions. Other causes of conjunctivitis include air pollution, swimming pool chlorine, and mechanical problems such as blocked tear ducts.

Signs and Symptoms

Conjunctivitis is called "pink eye" due to the characteristic pink or reddish appearance of the sclera of the eye and the inside of the eyelid. Other symptoms include itchy or painful eyes; sticky, viscous, or watery discharge that may crust over; increased tears; and sensitivity to light. These symptoms may appear in one or both eyes.

Types of Conjunctivitis

- *Viral conjunctivitis*: This is the most common type of conjunctivitis; it is infectious, but usually does not require treatment.
- *Bacterial conjunctivitis*: This type is more common in children under the age of five; it is infectious and can be treated with antibiotics.
- *Allergic conjunctivitis*: This is a noninfectious form of conjunctivitis generally found in people who show other signs of allergic conditions, such as **allergic sinusitis** (hay fever) **or eczema**.

Treatment

Bacterial conjunctivitis is typically treated with oral or topical antibiotics. When removal of an allergen is not possible, antihistamines may be used to treat mild cases allergy-related conjunctivitis, and corticosteroids may be prescribed for acute cases. The majority of viral conjunctivitis cases clear up without treatment. Artificial tears and cool compresses can reduce discomfort due to dry and inflamed eyes.

Medications

- Oral or topical antibiotics
- Antihistamines for allergic conjunctivitis
- Artificial tears if necessary

Massage Therapy Implications

RISKS	Unless a person has been formally diagnosed with a noninfectious form of conjunctivitis, all cases must be treated as highly contagious, making massage a contraindication. Note that a physician's permission to return to work or school is *not* equivalent to clearance to receive massage. (For confirmed cases of allergic conjunctivitis, also see the section on **allergic reactions**.)
BENEFITS	After the condition has resolved, clients can experience the same benefits from massage as the rest of the population.

Cushing Syndrome

Definition: What Is It?

Cushing syndrome is a condition in which cortisol levels in the blood are excessively high for a prolonged period, leading to tissue changes and possible death. It is also called hypercortisolism.

Etiology: What Happens?

Cortisol, the principal glucocorticoid hormone, is secreted by the adrenal cortex. It has many functions, including working with the stress response, immune system activity, fluid retention, metabolism of food into energy, and balancing insulin activity. Cortisol production is controlled by a chain that begins in the hypothalamus, which signals the pituitary gland to release adrenocorticotropic hormone, or ACTH. ACTH stimulates the adrenal glands to release cortisol. When cortisol levels are dangerously high for a prolonged period, many tissues throughout the body are affected.

The most common forms of Cushing syndrome occur when ACTH levels are abnormally high (endogenous hypercortisolism) or as a reaction to cortisol-based medication (exogenous hypercortisolism).

Signs and Symptoms

Perhaps the most well-recognized sign of Cushing syndrome is the development of fatty deposits around the neck and face (giving rise to a "moon face" presentation) and around the abdomen and upper back. Arms and legs typically become thin and weak.

High levels of cortisol can damage supportive collagen. This is reflected in bone thinning and in the development of very thin, delicate skin, often with purple stretch marks.

Other effects of hypercortisolism include **high blood pressure**; high blood glucose with an increased risk of developing **diabetes**; mood changes that involve irritability, **anxiety**, and **depression**; severe **acne**; slowed healing with suppressed immune system activity; the development of excessive body hair (hirsutism) and disrupted menstrual cycles for women; and decreased fertility, decreased sex drive, and erectile dysfunction for men.

Types of Cushing Syndrome

- *Endogenous hypercortisolism*: This develops when too much ACTH is secreted by the pituitary gland or other tissues, or when the adrenal glands themselves secrete too much cortisol. It can come about because of a benign tumor on the pituitary gland (this is called Cushing disease), or because tumor cells in other tissues produce abnormal levels of ACTH. Rarely, Cushing syndrome is related to tumors on the adrenal glands themselves.
- *Exogenous hypercortisolism*: Patients who have autoimmune diseases or who are organ transplant recipients may take cortisol-based steroid medications to control their disease or to prevent tissue rejection. These medications have serious side effects, including bone thinning, diabetes, mood swings, and high blood pressure: this is exogenous hypercortisolism, and it is the most common form of Cushing syndrome.

Treatment

Cushing syndrome is treated according to its cause. Exogenous Cushing syndrome is treated by reevaluating the correct dose of corticosteroid drugs to achieve the best benefits with the least risk. Pituitary adenomas are usually surgically removed; radiation therapy may be part of this treatment course. Cushing syndrome brought about by tumor cells secreting ACTH is treated by dealing with the tumors, but drugs that inhibit cortisol may also be used.

Medications

- Adrenal steroid inhibitors to limit cortisol production
- Supplements of hydrocortisone (postsurgery for pituitary tumor)
- Chemotherapeutic agents for adrenal carcinoma

Massage Therapy Implications

RISKS	Hypercortisolism affects the body in many ways that influence decisions about bodywork: hypertension, brittle bones, a risk of diabetes, and immune system suppression are just a few issues. The cause and treatment options for a client with Cushing syndrome may require significant adaptations to design a safe bodywork session.
BENEFITS	As long as massage stays within the average physical challenges of a person with Cushing syndrome, it can be a useful treatment option. Clients who have successfully treated their Cushing syndrome can enjoy the same benefits from massage as the rest of the population.

Diabetes Insipidus

What Is It?

Diabetes insipidus is a condition in which a person cannot adequately concentrate urine. The result is extreme thirst and increased output of extremely diluted urine.

What Does It Look Like?

Thirst and increased urine output are the main signs of diabetes insipidus. Other indicators may include chronic dehydration, nocturia, bed wetting, and enlarged bladder.

Massage Therapy Implications

RISKS	Massage has no particular risks for a person with treated diabetes insipidus, as long as he or she is comfortable on a table or chair.
BENEFITS	A client under treatment for diabetes insipidus can enjoy the same benefits from massage as the rest of the population.

Diabetes Insipidus

Definition: What Is It?

Diabetes insipidus (DI) is a problem in the brain or in the kidneys leading to a failure to concentrate urine appropriately. It is a relatively rare condition that is often linked to underlying trauma or disorders. It is unrelated to diabetes mellitus.

Etiology: What Happens?

Fluid levels in the body are controlled through a feedback loop that employs the thirst mechanism; a hormone made in the hypothalamus and stored in the pituitary gland called antidiuretic hormone, or ADH; and the kidneys. When a person takes in more fluid than he or she needs, the kidneys extract it from the blood and excrete it as urine. ADH limits urine production and increases concentration. Without adequate ADH, or without sensitivity to ADH in the kidneys, the urine is not adequately concentrated.

Whether DI begins in the kidneys or in the brain, the result is the same: urine is too diluted. This means that the patient expels anywhere from 2.5 to 15 L of urine everyday and must replace that fluid by drinking.

Signs and Symptoms

Polyuria (frequent urination) and polydipsia (frequent thirst) are the two leading indicators for this disease. Nocturia (needing to urinate in the nighttime) is frequent, and even adults may experience bed wetting. Many patients develop an enlarged bladder to accommodate excessive urine flow. Signs of dehydration may also develop, including sunken eyes, muscle weakness, hypotension, rapid heartbeat, and headache.

Types of Diabetes Insipidus

- *Central diabetes insipidus*: This is the most common form of DI, and it is the result of a reduction of ADH production in the hypothalamus or a reduction of ADH release from the pituitary. It can be the result of brain tumors, **traumatic brain injury**, or a postsurgical complication of brain surgery.
- *Nephrogenic diabetes insipidus*: This is a problem with ADH sensitivity at the collecting tubules in the kidney. It can be idiopathic, but it may be related to lithium toxicity, too much calcium in the blood (hypercalcemia), too much potassium in the blood (hyperkalemia), or rare diseases of the kidneys.
- *Gestational diabetes insipidus*: This condition develops during pregnancy, when placental enzymes destroy ADH in the mother. It resolves after the birth of the infant.
- *Dipsogenic diabetes insipidus*: This is the result of too much fluid intake, which can alter the activity of ADH. It may be related to a psychiatric disorder that causes a person to drink too much water or other liquids.

Treatment

DI is treated according to its type and cause. If it is related to a tumor, surgery may be recommended. Central DI is treated with a synthetic form of ADH. Nephrogenic DI is treated with drugs that change the way the kidneys respond to ADH. Dipsogenic DI may be treated with counseling or other psychiatric interventions.

Medications

- Desmopressin (synthetic ADH) to activate urinary concentration in kidneys
- Hydrochlorothiazide to decrease urinary volume
- Ibuprofen, indomethacin, to reduce the delivery of urinary solute to the tubules of the kidney

Massage Therapy Implications

RISKS	Massage has no particular risks for a person with treated diabetes insipidus, as long as he or she is comfortable on a table or chair.
BENEFITS	A client under treatment for diabetes insipidus can enjoy the same benefits from massage as the rest of the population.

Ehlers-Danlos Syndrome

Definition: What Is It?

Ehlers-Danlos syndrome (EDS) is a group of genetic disorders that lead to problems in the production of various types of connective tissue proteins. It affects about 50,000 people in the United States, but it is very mild and not easily recognized in many cases.

Etiology: What Happens?

EDS is the result of genetic mutations that affect the production of collagen, elastin, and some other parts of the extracellular matrix that forms the bulk of connective tissues. Most people with this disorder experience hypermobility of the joints, along with chronic joint pain, delicate skin, and poor wound healing.

EDS is an inherited disorder, but that inheritance may be through autosomal dominant, recessive, or X-linked chromosomes. The most common versions are autosomal dominant, which means a child needs to inherit only one chromosome from a parent to develop this disorder.

Signs and Symptoms

The signs and symptoms of EDS are determined the type of genetic mutation that is present. Most symptoms are related to extremely delicate skin, hypermobile joints, and chronic joint pain. Common signs include easy bruising, poor wound healing, frequent joint **dislocations**, and eye problems, including myopia, detached retina, and damage to the connective tissue that maintains the globular shape of the eyeball. The risk of mitral valve prolapse is higher for EDS patients than for the rest of the population. Rarer signs of EDS include extreme **postural deviations** and slack, baggy skin.

Types of Ehlers-Danlos Syndrome

- *Classic EDS* involves delicate skin that is fragile and prone to bruising, slow wound healing, and joints that are loose and vulnerable to injury.
- *Hypermobility EDS* names its most prominent feature. Patients are prone to multiple dislocations, joint pain, and early-onset osteoarthritis

- *Arthrochalasia EDS* is a different genetic anomaly than hypermobility EDS, but the result is the same: easy joint disruptions, including hip dysplasia and frequent subluxations.
- *Dermatosparaxis EDS* involves very loose and baggy skin that sags and wrinkles, even in childhood.
- *Kyphoscoliosis EDS* leads to a severe, progressive curvature of the spine.
- *Vascular EDS* affects the connective tissues in blood vessels and other tubes with serious repercussions: midsized blood vessels and the gastrointestinal tract are vulnerable to damage or even rupture. This is a life-shortening version of the disease.

Treatment

EDS is treated according to symptoms or related problems. People with hypermobile joints are taught how to preserve joint function and are discouraged from stretching joints beyond a healthy range of motion. Skin wounds are typically treated with bandages or wound glue rather than sutures, because the skin is so delicate. Any surgery or dental work is conducted with extreme care because of poor wound healing and because people with a risk of mitral valve prolapse are also at risk for endocardial bacterial infections (**endocarditis**).

Medications

- Over-the-counter and prescription analgesics asneeded
- Medications to manage blood pressure in weak vessels

Massage Therapy Implications

RISKS	Most EDS patients have hypermobile joints; bodywork that challenges range of motion must be done with respect for this problem. Skin and cardiovascular health may inform modality choices.
BENEFITS	Because joints tend to be loose, EDS patients may experience muscle tightness, pain, and inefficient movement. Massage that can reduce pain and increase ease of movement—without compromising joint integrity or other tissue weaknesses—is helpful and appropriate.

Fractures

Definition: What Are They?

Fractures are any variety of broken bone, from a hairline crack to a complete break with protrusion through the skin.

The three basic classes are simple fracture (the bone is completely broken but little or no damage has occurred to the surrounding soft tissues), incomplete fractures (the bone is cracked but not completely broken), and compound fractures (the bone is completely broken and a great deal of soft tissue damage has occurred). Beyond that, fractures are named for the type or shape of the lesion.

Etiology: What Happens?

When a bone undergoes more mechanical stress than it can accommodate, it cracks or breaks altogether. This typically occurs as a trauma, a result of **osteoporosis**, or because of overuse. If a bone is appropriately stabilized during the healing process, osteocytes can lay down a thickened area of new growth over the break site, leading to a structure that is actually denser than before it was broken. Fractures become problematic when they affect the growth plate in children, or when the healing process is slowed due to age, nutrition, unrelenting stress, or other factors.

Signs and Symptoms

Big bone breaks are usually obvious: they are painful, they usually follow a specific traumatic event, and they severely limit the function of the adjacent joints. But some fractures can be difficult to identify, particularly if they are accompanied by a lot of soft tissue trauma. Sprained ankles and shin splints are two conditions that frequently hide minor bone fractures.

Types of Fractures

- *Avulsion fractures*: These occur when a bone fragment of bone is pulled away. This is an occasional complication of **Osgood-Schlatter** disease, for example.
- *Comminuted fractures*: These involve a bone that shatters into multiple pieces.
- *Compression fractures*: These involve collapsed vertebral bodies. They are often associated with low bone density, as seen with osteoporosis and **osteogenesis imperfecta**.
- *Greenstick fractures*: These involve bending and partial breakage of the bone.
- *Malunion fractures*: These occur when the bone fragments heal in a nonanatomic position.
- *Stress fractures*: These are common minor cracks that occur with chronic overuse. They can be difficult to identify without x-rays or other imaging tests.

Treatment

Most fractures heal well if the bones are immobilized with a cast or other device. More complicated situations may call for pins, plates, screws, or reparative surgery. Grafts of bone tissue or bone paste along with electrical stimulation to the site may help to speed healing when recovery is impaired.

Medications

- NSAIDs for pain and inflammation

Massage Therapy Implications

RISKS	Acute fractures locally contraindicate massage, until the bones are stabilized and other soft tissue damage is addressed.
BENEFITS	Swelling is a frequent complication of casting. Any lymphatic work to decrease fluid retention may help with both comfort and efficiency of circulatory turnover in the compromised area. Massage elsewhere to the body while a fracture is healing can help address the challenge of having impaired movement, as well as any limping or other compensations that may occur. A person who has fully recovered from a fracture can enjoy the same benefits from massage as the rest of the population.

Guillain-Barré Syndrome

Definition: What Is It?

Guillain-Barré syndrome (GBS) is a condition involving acute inflammation and destruction of the myelin layer of peripheral nerves. It usually starts in the extremities and moves toward the trunk, but some variants of this syndrome affect only cranial nerves or have other patterns. It is the most frequently seen form of acute neuromuscular paralysis in the Western Hemisphere.

Etiology: What Happens?

GBS is not fully understood, but it is believed that for many patients, a triggering infection stimulates an immune system attack mistakenly directed against the myelin sheaths of peripheral nerves. This disorder has also been seen in conjunction with pregnancy, surgery, and administration of certain vaccines, specifically the swine flu vaccine that was distributed in 1976.

Regardless of what initiates the disease process, the result is that the myelin sheaths on peripheral nerves are attacked and destroyed by macrophages and lymphocytes. It can primarily affect motor or sensory neurons, or both. The damage progresses proximally and may also involve cranial nerves. This can be life threatening if the nerves that control breathing are damaged; many GBS patients spend time on a ventilator before they recover.

Signs and Symptoms

When GBS first appears, it often involves symmetrical weakness or tingling in the affected limbs. Reflexes become dull or disappear altogether. Loss of sensation progresses proximally, although pain frequently develops in the hips and pelvis. If the GBS affects cranial nerves of the face, facial weakness, pain, and difficulty with speech and swallowing may develop. If GBS attacks cranial nerves, then autonomic symptoms may develop. These can include variable heart rate and blood pressure, flushing, excessive sweating, or lack of sweating. As the disease progresses, the nerves that supply respiratory muscles are affected, and dangerous problems with breathing develop.

GBS symptoms usually peak 2 or 3 weeks after onset, and they may persist for several weeks before they begin to subside. Full recovery can take 18 months or more. Some patients experience permanent weakness after GBS, and a small number of patients don't survive.

Types of Guillain-Barré Syndrome

- *Acute inflammatory demyelinating polyradiculoneuropathy*: This is the most common form, accounting for 90% of GBS diagnoses.
- *Acute motor axonal neuropathy*: This affects motor neurons only. It is most common in children and has a good prognosis.
- *Acute motor-sensory axonal neuropathy*: This affects motor and sensory function. It is most common in adults and has a poorer recovery rate than other forms of GBS.
- *Miller-Fisher syndrome*: This is a rare variant of GBS that involves only the cranial nerves. It leads to poor control of the eyes and other facial muscles.

Treatment

Two treatment options have been successfully used to shorten recovery time for GBS patients: plasmapheresis and injections of high concentrations of immunoglobulin (donated antibodies).

Other interventions for GBS patients are dictated by patients' individual needs. About one-third of patients require the use of a ventilator until the respiratory nerves regain full function. Pain management is problematic because powerful pain medications can depress the nervous system; massage and other nondrug options are often recommended for this purpose. Once the acute inflammation has passed, occupational and physical therapy is used to help the patient regain as much muscle function as possible.

Medications

- Immunomodulators to inhibit antibody production
- Anticoagulants to reduce risk of deep vein thrombosis and pulmonary embolism
- NSAIDs for pain management
- Narcotics for pain management if NSAIDs are insufficient

Massage Therapy Implications

RISKS	A GBS patient may have weakness, pain, and numbness that progressively move from the extremities toward the trunk. Any massage must respect the many challenges that this person is undergoing, including the disease process and any medical efforts to control it. This includes medications, assisted ventilation, and other interventions.
BENEFITS	When a person has begun to recover from a GBS attack, physical and occupational therapy are often employed to speed recovery and prevent muscle atrophy. Massage at this stage may be useful to limit pain, improve circulation, and reduce fatigue and anxiety. Clients who have recovered from GBS can enjoy the same benefits from massage as the rest of the population.

Glomerulonephritis

Definition: What Is It?

Glomerulonephritis is a relatively rare but serious situation involving inflammation and scarring of the glomeruli in the kidneys. This can occur as a result of toxic exposure, as a complication of a bacterial infection, or related to autoimmune disease. Some cases are idiopathic.

Etiology: What Happens?

"Glomerulus" is the diminutive form of the Latin word *glomus*, for "ball of yarn," which is an excellent description of the tufts of capillary loops that allow for diffusion and filtration in the kidneys. These points of interface between circulatory capillaries and nephrons act as filters to keep vital blood components in the bloodstream while allowing water and wastes to exit into the urinary system.

When the body launches an immune system attack against an invader, one consequence can be the formation of "immune complexes": sticky clumps of antigens and antibodies. Ordinarily, these would be consumed by macrophages, but occasionally, they can develop in or get caught by the glomeruli, leading to a localized inflammatory reaction: glomerulonephritis. Triggers for this process can include bacterial infections (especially with *Streptococcus*), toxic exposures, or autoimmune disorders.

Acute or chronic inflammation in the glomeruli can compromise their effectiveness and allow important substances to leave the body through the urine, while allowing metabolic wastes to accumulate in the bloodstream. Inflammation in the kidneys leads to an accumulation of scar tissue where only soft, pliable epithelium should be; consequently, the kidneys become progressively less able to manage fluids in the body, which may lead to chronic **renal failure**.

Signs and Symptoms

Early symptoms of glomerulonephritis include abnormalities in the urine such as high protein levels or red blood cells. Hematuria, or blood in the urine, can be observed as dark- or rust-colored urine. Protein in the urine makes it look foamy. Occasionally, no observable signs develop, and glomerulonephritis is found only when a routine analysis reveals higher-than-normal levels of protein or blood in the urine.

Hypertension that does not respond to normal interventions is both a symptom and a complication of glomerulonephritis. Later symptoms are indicators of renal failure, including general malaise, skin discoloration, itching, fatigue, **anemia**, low urine output, systemic **edema**, and, in very severe cases, lethargy, confusion, and coma.

Treatment

The treatment for glomerulonephritis depends on the cause and is generally geared toward symptom abatement and improved kidney function. Controlling high blood pressure is the first priority; this may be done with antihypertensive drugs, as well as by restricting salt and protein intake. If glomerulonephritis is a complication of a general infection, antibiotics may lead to a complete recovery. If it is an autoimmune or other inflammatory problem, steroids or other immunosuppressant drugs may be used to limit damage to the nephrons. In some cases, plasmapheresis is recommended to remove inflammatory immune complexes.

Medications

- Diuretics to promote urine production
- ACE inhibitors or angiotensin II receptor antagonists to control hypertension
- Antibiotics in the presence of bacterial infection
- Steroidal anti-inflammatories or immunosuppressants for autoimmune diseases

Massage Therapy Implications

RISKS	Glomerulonephritis is an inflammatory condition that impairs the body's ability to manage circulatory turnover in the kidneys. Any bodywork that emphasizes fluid flow may exceed a client's ability to adapt.
BENEFITS	Noncirculatory types of massage or bodywork may be appropriate for glomerulonephritis patients to receive, as long as the contributing factors and medications are identified and accommodated.

Hemochromatosis

Definition: What Is It?

Hemochromatosis is a group of inherited conditions in which the body absorbs too much iron from the diet or elsewhere. Excessive iron can cause damage to many tissues, but the liver is particularly at risk. This disease affects white northern Europeans far more than any other ethnic group.

Etiology: What Happens?

All cells require iron to function. This vital mineral is absorbed from food; the small intestine controls how much iron is taken in from a typical daily diet. For most people, this is around 10% of the amount that is consumed each day.

The body has no mechanism to unload excessive iron outside of bleeding. Women who menstruate can shed excess iron, but other individuals cannot. If more iron is absorbed than can be stored normally, the excess iron in the blood and other organs promotes free-radical formation. This can lead to cellular injury and tissue damage.

In various forms of hemochromatosis, the body absorbs too much iron. Iron then accumulates in various tissues, but it is especially hazardous in the liver, pancreas, heart, joints, and pituitary gland. It can take many years of pathologic iron deposition to develop the symptoms of this disease.

Untreated hemochromatosis can lead to many serious complications, including irregular heartbeat, **diabetes**, **osteoarthritis**, **osteoporosis**, **cirrhosis**, **gallstones**, and some types of cancer.

Types of Hemochromatosis

- *Primary hemochromatosis*: This is the most common form of the condition. It is the result of an inherited genetic defect that allows the absorption of too much iron from the diet.
- *Secondary hemochromatosis*: This can occur when a person receives blood transfusions too frequently, usually as a treatment for some type of **anemia**. Secondary hemochromatosis can also develop as a complication of liver disease.
- *Neonatal hemochromatosis*: This is a rare birth defect related to liver failure in late-term fetuses and newborn infants. It may be related to a maternal immune system attack on the fetal liver.

Signs and Symptoms

Early signs and symptoms of hemochromatosis are often vague, often leading to a long delay between the onset of symptoms and a successful treatment regimen. Symptoms include joint pain, especially in the hand, fatigue, abdominal pain, loss of sex drive, irregular heartbeat, and memory problems. The skin may also take on an abnormal bronze or gray tone.

Treatment

The highest priority in hemochromatosis treatment is to get circulating levels of iron down to normal numbers. Phlebotomy (bloodletting) is the most common way to go about this. Fortunately, it is possible for hemochromatosis patients to do this in the context of blood donation, as often as every 8 weeks if the condition is severe enough.

Patients who recognize and treat their condition early enough to avoid organ damage can expect normal life expectancy. Others are at increased risk for several disorders including diabetes and erectile dysfunction, but cirrhosis and liver cancer are the most common long-term complications.

Medications

- Chelating agents may be used to remove iron from the blood, but this is rare, as phlebotomy is a simpler, less expensive, and very effective way to treat this disease.

Massage Therapy Implications

RISKS	The safety of massage therapy for clients with hemochromatosis depends on the success of treatment options to control the progression of the disease. If extensive liver or joint damage has accrued, then massage must be adapted to the needs of the client.
BENEFITS	A client who successfully manages this disease requires no special adaptations for massage therapy and can enjoy the same benefits as the rest of the population.

Hematoma

Definition: What Is It?

The term hematoma (literally, "blood tumor") refers to extensive bleeding and pooling of blood in a confined area. The bleeding is all internal; this term does not apply to skin injuries that allow blood to escape.

Etiology: What Happens?

When a blood vessel is internally damaged, blood leaks out into whatever interstitial space is available. In the best of circumstances, clotting factors thicken the blood quickly and plug the leaky vessel. Then, the immune system reabsorbs the leaked blood, and the injury is fully healed.

The leakage of blood from damaged superficial capillaries is called a bruise, or ecchymosis. The familiar injury that happens when a person hammers his or her thumb or catches his or her finger in the door is called a subungual hematoma. Inside the cranium, hematoma can be a result of **traumatic brain injury** or a ruptured **aneurysm**. Blood can also accumulate between muscle sheaths as a result of trauma or a complication of **hemophilia**.

One possible complication of a hematoma is **heterotopic ossification**: the development of a chip of calcified material where blood has pooled.

Signs and Symptoms

Symptoms depend on size and location but generally include pain and inflammation. The texture of the affected area may change: it is indurated in a new injury and gradually becomes softer as the blood is reabsorbed. A superficial bruise is obvious with purple-blue discoloration that fades to green and yellow as it resolves.

Treatment

A hematoma in the cranium is a medical emergency, but other sites of damage may be treated more simply with the RICE protocol. People who take blood thinners are at increased risk for hematomas, so this should be watched carefully.

Medications

- NSAIDs, if necessary

Massage Therapy Implications

RISKS	Pain and the risk of blood clots make deep hematomas at least a local contraindication for massage. Bruises carry less risk.
BENEFITS	Massage elsewhere to the body when a hematoma is mild is safe. After the acute phase has past, gentle massage around the edges of the injury, along with hydrotherapy, may help to speed healing.

Heterotopic Ossification

Definition: What Is It?

Heterotopic ossification describes a condition in which calcifications form in soft tissue. The most common form is seen most often in adolescents and young adults and usually affects the quadriceps and brachialis muscles.

Etiology: What Happens?

The most common variety of heterotopic ossification follows an injury with bleeding into the muscle belly or between fascial sheets a **hematoma**. Eventually, a formation develops at the site of the contusion that looks and feels like a bone embedded in soft tissue. Bone-like growths can be suspended within muscle or other soft tissue, but in many cases, they are attached continuously or by a stalk to nearby periosteum.

Other forms of heterotopic ossification are associated with disorders that either limit mobility or promote excessive growth of bone tissue. **Spinal cord injury**, **traumatic brain injury**, **ankylosing spondylitis**, **Paget disease**, and some autoimmune disorders carry an increased risk for developing this condition. **Hip replacement surgery** also carries a significant risk of developing bony deposits in surrounding soft tissues.

Signs and Symptoms

In the acute stage of trauma-based heterotopic ossification, the area feels bruised; within a few days, it may feel hard and locally very tender. The range of motion in the nearby joint is limited: if it occurs in the brachialis, the elbow doesn't fully extend, and when it occurs in the quadriceps, the knee can't fully flex. Eventually, little or no local pain may be present, but a dense, unyielding mass develops where nothing hard should be.

Treatment

Treatment for heterotopic ossification tends to be conservative. Patients are recommended to rest and isolate the injured area in the acute stage to limit further bleeding. Later in the process, passive stretching is employed for range of motion, followed by exercises to restore normal muscle strength.

If a fully mature and calcified mass interferes with muscle or tendon function, it can be surgically removed. This kind of surgery is avoided if possible, however, because many patients have a postsurgical recurrence of the growth.

Medications

- NSAIDs against pain and blood clotting to prevent heterotopic ossification from developing or recurring

Massage Therapy Implications

RISKS	Heterotopic ossification locally contraindicates rigorous massage because of the risk of increased internal bleeding: this is true for both a new and mature injury.
BENEFITS	Gentle massage around the edges of a calcium deposit may stimulate bony reabsorption. Massage elsewhere is safe and appropriate.

Hyperparathyroidism

Definition: What Is It?

Hyperparathyroidism is a condition in which the parathyroid glands produce too much hormone. It affects about 100,000 people in this country each year. Women are affected about twice as often as men, and it is most common in people over 60 years old.

Etiology: What Happens?

The parathyroid glands are tiny glands located behind or close to the thyroid gland. They secrete parathyroid hormone (PTH). Unlike many endocrine glands that operate under control of the hypothalamus and pituitary, the parathyroids are essentially self-regulating: they release PTH when plasma calcium is low and stop when plasma calcium is high.

PTH has several functions in blood calcium maintenance. It causes the demineralization of cortical bone to increase plasma calcium and phosphate; it increases the absorption of calcium in the intestines, and the reabsorption of calcium in the kidneys; and it promotes the conversion of vitamin D into a usable form.

The etiology of hyperparathyroidism depends on the type; these are described below. Regardless of the version, this disorder causes the secretion of excessive amounts of PTH, leading to elevated blood calcium. This can be a minor abnormality that produces no symptoms and requires no treatment, or it can be severe and potentially life threatening.

Signs and Symptoms

Signs and symptoms of hyperparathyroidism are related to elevated plasma calcium levels. They include muscle weakness and fatigue at the mild end of the scale and nausea, vomiting, diarrhea, depression, and confusion at the more severe end.

Types of Hyperparathyroidism

- *Primary hyperparathyroidism*: This is the most common form and is usually related to the growth of one or more adenomas (benign epithelial tumors) on the parathyroid glands. Very rarely, it may be related to parathyroid cancer.
- *Secondary hyperparathyroidism*: This form of the disease is usually related to kidney dysfunction. It is almost always seen with end-stage renal failure but may also develop because of an extreme deficiency in calcium or vitamin D.
- *Tertiary hyperparathyroidism*: This is a situation where long-term dysfunction becomes self-sustaining, and the parathyroids continue to produce too much hormone after other contributing factors have been resolved.

Complications

The complications of hyperparathyroidism may be among the first indicators of the disease. They include **hypertension**, bradycardia, osteopenia that affects cortical bone (this distinguishes it from **osteoporosis**, which affects mainly trabecular bone), **kidney stones**, and pseudogout.

Treatment

Surgery to remove the affected parathyroid gland or glands is the most common treatment option for hyperparathyroidism that requires treatment. Patients may need to supplement calcium and vitamin D after surgery, especially as the bones quickly pull calcium from the blood to add density in a condition called "hungry bone syndrome." In addition, patients are advised to hydrate well, to exercise within tolerance, and to avoid any diuretics if possible.

Medications

- Hormone replacement therapy if surgery is not an option
- Bisphosphonates to improve bone density
- Calcimimetic drugs for secondary hyperparathyroidism

Massage Therapy Implications

RISKS	A person with hyperparathyroidism may have kidney problems too: these must be addressed for best safety. Patients may also have significant bone thinning in cortical bone, which requires adjustments in depth of bodywork.
BENEFITS	Massage won't change the course of hyperparathyroidism, but it can improve the quality of life for people with this condition. A client who has a mild case that is under observation, or who has fully recovered from surgery, can enjoy the same benefits from massage as the rest of the population.

Hypoparathyroidism

Definition: What Is It?

Hypoparathyroidism is a rare condition in which the parathyroid glands don't produce an adequate amount of parathyroid hormone.

Etiology: What Happens?

Calcium in plasma and extracellular fluid is extremely important for many body functions, including regulating muscle contraction, blood clotting, nerve transmission, and kidney function. Normal levels of circulating calcium are usually extremely stable. Special cells in the parathyroid glands (as well as a few other areas) are sensitive to calcium, and when these levels drop, parathyroid hormone (PTH) is released.

Parathyroid hormone has several jobs: it activates osteoclasts to pull calcium off bone and add it to plasma; it influences kidney function to retain calcium and eliminate phosphorus; and it stimulates the kidneys to metabolize vitamin D for calcium absorption. When PTH is in short supply, these functions are lost. Consequently, the kidneys pull excessive calcium out of the blood, leading to high urinary calcium and a risk of **kidney stones**. Circulating calcium levels drop, along with the ability to absorb this important mineral from the diet, while phosphorus levels go up. Lack of plasma calcium prevents bones from increasing their density, changes muscle contractions, and ultimately affects the central nervous system.

Hypoparathyroidism can be the result of a congenital birth defect or a complication of an autoimmune attack against several endocrine glands. The most common form, however, is related to a history of neck surgery or radiation that damages the parathyroid glands. This condition is permanent; while it is treatable, it never resolves.

Signs and Symptoms

Signs and symptoms of hypoparathyroidism often begin with tingling and paresthesia in the lips, fingers, and toes. Skin and hair become dry, and severe and long-lasting muscle cramps called tetany may occur. Severe muscle cramping at the larynx and bronchi is rare but may be life threatening. Excessive calcium processing in the kidneys raises the risk for kidney stones. **Headache**, fatigue, mood swings, and irritability are common. Children born with this condition may have abnormal calcification of teeth and bones and delayed growth patterns.

Treatment

Hypoparathyroidism is typically treated with calcium and vitamin D supplements. Surgical implant of parathyroid tissue has been used, but the results are inconsistent compared with the simpler strategy of supplementation.

Medications
- Supplements of calcium and vitamin D
- Synthetic parathyroid hormone is under investigation

Massage Therapy Implications

RISKS	Hypoparathyroidism is easily treatable and not usually life threatening; it carries no specific risks for massage as long as the bodywork does not trigger painful muscle cramps.
BENEFITS	Massage is unlikely to improve the course of this condition, but it may improve the quality of life of the person who lives with hypoparathyroidism.

Ichthyosis

Definition: What Is It?

Ichthyosis vulgaris or common ichthyosis (from the Greek for "fish condition") is a group of problems that lead to the formation of dried, scaly skin. It is usually an inherited genetic anomaly, but it can develop as a symptom or complication of another underlying disorder.

Etiology: What Happens?

Ichthyosis develops when a normal waterproofing protein is impaired, usually because of a genetic anomaly. The normal balance between new skin cell production and old skin cell exfoliation is upset, and the result is the development of small scales of dead cells. The old scales are firmly attached to new cells underneath, so the risk of skin cracking and bleeding is high.

People with ichthyosis may also be vulnerable to **eczema**, **allergic sinusitis**, and **asthma**.

This is usually a genetic disorder, but acquired ichthyosis can develop as a symptom or a complication of other diseases, including cancer (especially **lymphoma**), Hansen disease (also called leprosy), **lupus**, **sarcoidosis**, thyroid dysregulation, and some other conditions.

Signs and Symptoms

The hallmark of ichthyosis is dry skin with irregular polyhedral scales. It is most common on the extensor side of the extremities and the abdomen, but it can develop elsewhere. Ichthyosis symptoms tend to be worst during cold, dry weather.

Types of Ichthyosis

Ichthyosis vulgaris accounts for the vast majority of ichthyosis diagnoses. Rarer types include the following:

- *Lamellar ichthyosis*: This is a severe, potentially disfiguring variety with deep painful cracks, especially on the palms or soles.
- *X-linked ichthyosis*: This is mild and seen in males.
- *Epidermolytic hyperkeratosis*: This rare version affects babies with massive blistering and peeling of superficial skin.

Treatment

Soothing lotions and moisturizers along with mild applications of salicylic acid to remove loosened scales are often recommended.

Medications
- Hypoallergenic moisturizers to manage ichthyosis vulgaris
- Tretinoins to slow the production of new skin cells
- Steroidal anti-inflammatories to manage itchiness

Massage Therapy Implications

RISKS	Skin that is bleeding or oozing locally contraindicates massage.
BENEFITS	If the skin is intact, clients with ichthyosis can enjoy the extra moisturizing that massage may offer, along with the wonderful experience of having their skin be carefully tended. Be sure to use a hypoallergenic lubricant.

Impetigo

Definition: What Is It?

Impetigo is usually a streptococcal infection of the skin, although staph can sometimes also be involved. It occurs mostly among infants and young children, but adults can get it too.

Etiology: What Happens?

Most cases of impetigo in the United States are caused by *Staphylococcus aureus*. In a typical infection, the bacteria gains access through a minor skin injury. Lesions are usually restricted to the epidermis and don't cause permanent scarring, but one type of impetigo can penetrate to deeper layers of the skin. Scratching the itchy infected blisters allows the bacteria to spread over large areas.

Impetigo can lead to serious complications including **renal failure**, **meningitis**, **cellulitis**, and blood poisoning. For this reason, it is usually treated quickly and aggressively.

Signs and Symptoms

Impetigo lesions usually occur around the nose and mouth, but it can infect the skin anywhere on the body. The characteristic presentation is a cluster of small red sores that blister, then rupture, and form yellow or honey-colored crusts. Left untreated, these sores heal in 2 to 3 weeks, leaving no scars.

Types of Impetigo

- *Impetigo contagiosa*: This is the most common version; sores are itchy but not painful.
- *Bullous impetigo*: This involves large, painless, delicate blisters on the trunk, arms, and legs; it may be accompanied by fever, diarrhea, and general weakness.
- *Ecthyma*: This version penetrates to deep layers of the skin and can cause permanent scarring.

Treatment

For prevention, chapped skin should be treated with lubricant to prevent damage, and all other wounds should be cleaned thoroughly, treated with antibacterial ointment, and covered.

Patients are counseled to keep lesions clean and dry and to remove crusts as soon as possible. The patient's bedding and towels must be strictly isolated during the infection. Children should avoid contact with others for at least 24 hours after they begin treatment.

Antibiotics are the mainstay of medical treatment for impetigo, but the increasing incidence of **methicillin-resistant *Staphylococcus aureus*** (MRSA) in these infections has made antibiotic choice more challenging.

Medications

- Topical over-the-counter or prescription antibiotic ointment
- Oral or parenteral antibiotics for severe cases

Massage Therapy Implications

RISKS	Because of the risk of communicability, impetigo systemically contraindicates massage until the lesions have healed completely. If a client reports that someone in his or her house has impetigo, it is best to reschedule the appointment after the infection is over.
BENEFITS	A client who has fully recovered from impetigo can enjoy the same benefits of bodywork as the rest of the population.

Jaundice

Definition: What Is It?

Jaundice, from the French *jaune* (yellow), is also called ***icterus***. It is a condition involving a yellowish tinge to skin, mucous membranes, and the sclera of the eyes, brought about by liver dysfunction.

Etiology: What Happens?

Bilirubin is dark pigmented material that is a product of dead erythrocytes. The spleen sends bilirubin to the liver via the portal vein. One of the many functions of the liver is to use bilirubin to make bile. Bile drips from the liver to the gallbladder, which squirts it into the duodenum when fatty food is present. Bile helps hold particles of fat in suspension, so that fat-dissolving enzymes from the pancreas can break them down effectively. In this way, bilirubin gets into the digestive tract, where it is also a coloring agent for feces.

If dark reddish-brown bilirubin can't leave the liver, it accumulates in the bloodstream and the tissues. Eventually, it can visibly stain the skin, mucous membranes, and the sclera of the eyes.

Signs and Symptoms

Yellow-tinted skin, mucous membranes, and sclera of the eye are the main signs of jaundice. Urine often becomes dark, as the kidneys pull bilirubin out of the bloodstream and deposit it in urine. In contrast, stools tend to become light or clay-colored because the bilirubin doesn't enter the GI tract.

Other signs and symptoms are related to underlying liver disease, which may involve **hepatitis**, **cirrhosis**, or other problems.

Types of Jaundice

- *Neonatal jaundice*: Also called kernicterus, this occurs in newborn babies if their livers are not mature enough to keep up with the turnover of fetal red blood cells. It takes a few days to catch up with this extra workload. Treatment is usually exposure to sunlight or full-spectrum "bili-lights," which stimulate liver activity.
- *Hemolytic jaundice*: In this situation, red blood cells break down too fast, overwhelming the spleen and liver with too much material: this is seen with **sickle cell disease**, mismatched blood transfusions, and some infections.
- *Hepatic jaundice*: This describes internal liver dysfunction due to **cirrhosis**, **liver cancer**, infection, or a congenital malfunction of enzyme systems.
- *Extrahepatic jaundice*: This is related to a mechanical obstruction outside the liver. **Gallstones**, **pancreatic cancer**, or tumors in the GI tract are usually responsible.

Complications

Jaundice is a sign of liver dysfunction, which is often slowly progressive. Left untreated, it can lead to liver failure and the need for a liver transplant. Untreated neonatal jaundice can lead to brain damage as metabolic wastes accumulate in the bloodstream.

Treatment

Jaundice is treated according to the cause. Antiviral medications can reduce the impact of viral hepatitis; gallbladder surgery can correct an obstructed bile duct; other interventions are also tied to underlying causes.

Massage Therapy Implications

RISKS	A person with jaundice predictably has some liver dysfunction. Problems may be mild or severe, but they must be addressed before any rigorous or challenging bodywork can be done. If the condition is due to infection, hygienic precautions must be especially scrupulously observed.
BENEFITS	Gentle or energetic bodywork may be well received by a person dealing with a liver problem. A person who has fully recovered from jaundice can enjoy the same benefits from massage as the rest of the population.

Lichen Planus in Brief

What Is It?

Lichen planus is an idiopathic, noncontagious inflammatory condition of the skin and mucous membranes. It usually affects the wrists, ankles, shins, and mouth, although it can be found elsewhere.

What Does It Look Like?

The distinguishing feature of lichen planus is a raised shiny, purplish, angular bumps that may be intensely itchy. Lesions may be arranged in rows or clusters, and they may be marked with thin, lacy white lines. In the mouth, lesions may develop on the tongue, gums, or cheeks, and they appear as tiny white dots or lines. Larger lesions may be ulcerated and painful.

Massage Therapy Implications

RISKS	The only risk for a client with lichen planus is that massage may exacerbate itching.
BENEFITS	Massage probably won't improve the prognosis for lichen planus, but clients can enjoy the same general benefits from bodywork as the rest of the population.

Lichen Planus

Definition: What Is It?

Lichen planus is a noncontagious inflammatory condition involving small, flat, hard lesions on the skin. It may also affect some mucous membranes.

Etiology: What Happens?

Lichen planus is an idiopathic disease that most often affects middle-aged people. It often appears with autoimmune conditions or in conjunction with allergic reactions to medications, leading experts to theorize that it is somehow connected to immune system dysfunction.

Signs and Symptoms

Lichen planus lesions are small, purplish, flat-topped, angular bumps that usually appear on the wrists, ankles, shins, and in the mouth, but they are also found on the low back, neck, and genitals. The bumps may be intensely itchy. They may form where the skin has been damaged, so people prone to this condition are advised to be careful about skin injuries. Skin lesions may be covered with fine lacey white lines; this is called Wickham's striae. This form of the disease usually disappears in 6 to 18 months.

When lichen planus occurs in the mouth, it looks like patches of white dots or lines on the tongue, gums, or cheeks. Larger lesions may become painful ulcerations. Oral lichen planus is associated with an increased risk of **squamous cell carcinoma**, so it is useful to be aware of this condition. Mouth lesions tend to last longer than the skin form: it persists here for up to 5 years.

Treatment

Lichen planus is typically treated with steroids or antihistamines to address itching. Severe cases may call for systemic steroids or medication in combination with UV radiation.

Medications

- Topical or oral corticosteroids for itching on the skin and in the mouth
- Antihistamines for itching
- PUVA: psoralen with UV radiation

Massage Therapy Implications

RISKS	The only risk for a client with lichen planus is that massage may exacerbate itching.
BENEFITS	Massage probably won't improve the prognosis for lichen planus, but clients can enjoy the same general benefits from bodywork as the rest of the population.

Malaria

Definition: What Is It?

Malaria is a vector-borne infection of blood cells. The causative agents are a group of single-celled parasites from the genus of protozoa called Plasmodium, and the vector is the bite of an infected female mosquito from the Anopheles species. Globally, malaria infects about 500 million people each year and causes about a million deaths. In North America, it is relatively rare but not unheard of.

Etiology: What Happens?

When a mosquito infected with malaria-causing protozoa bites a human, an immature form of the parasites is introduced into the bloodstream. They travel to the liver, where they grow for 6 to 9 days. At that time, they reenter into the bloodstream, where they begin to invade healthy red blood cells.

The protozoa feed on hemoglobin and replicate inside the RBCs. The infected cells rupture, releasing toxic wastes and more protozoa. These go back to the liver to grow, and then, newly released protozoa invade more erythrocytes. Each cycle damages more liver cells and destroys more erythrocytes. When an uninfected mosquito bites this person, immature parasites enter the insect to begin the cycle again.

Signs and Symptoms

The signs and symptoms of malaria include extreme fluctuations between fever and chills (these reflect whether red blood cells are being invaded or rupturing), in cycles that may recur over several days.

When enough red blood cells have been invaded, anemia develops. Malaria is a type of hemolytic **anemia**: a situation in which red blood cells are destroyed faster than they can be replaced. **Jaundice** is another complication: this is related to the rapid destruction of erythrocytes that allows bilirubin to accumulate in the skin and mucous membranes. In some forms of the infection, the central nervous system, lungs, and kidneys may also be damaged.

A typical infection with the less virulent protozoa lasts about 2 weeks and then subsides, but some parasites may remain in the liver to launch a new episode months or years later.

Treatment

The treatment options for malaria are limited, and the most common and aggressive parasites are developing resistance to chloroquine, the most frequently used and cost-effective treatment option. Most malaria patients can be treated successfully if they have full access to all the drugs necessary and if they take the drugs according to prescription.

Medications

- Topical applications of DEET to prevent mosquito bites
- Antimalarial medications, including:
  - Chloroquine, hydroxychloroquine, and doxycycline to prevent or treat some types of malaria
  - Quinine to treat but not prevent new infection

Massage Therapy Implications

RISKS	Malaria carries a risk of brain, liver, and kidney damage. For this reason, any client who may be dealing with this disease must be fully treated before receiving any kind of rigorous bodywork.
BENEFITS	People who have had malaria may have long-term organ damage. Any bodywork that is conducted within these parameters may be safe and supportive. People who successfully treated malaria with no long-term repercussions may enjoy the same benefits from massage as the rest of the population.

Marfan Syndrome

Definition: What Is It?

Marfan syndrome is the result of a genetic mutation that leads to the production of dysfunctional fibrillin, a key connective tissue fiber.

Etiology: What Happens?

Marfan syndrome is a result of the production of faulty protein fibers with the consequence that certain connective tissues throughout the body may be weak or otherwise dysfunctional. The musculoskeletal system, the meninges, the heart and aorta, and the eyes are most at risk for problems related to Marfan syndrome.

Signs and Symptoms

Marfan syndrome affects several body systems. In the musculoskeletal system, it can lead to abnormally long extremities and digits. One sign of this disorder is the wrist test: persons with Marfan syndrome can overlap the thumb and fifth digit (little finger) of one hand while encircling the opposite wrist. Ligament laxity, joint hypermobility, and anomalies in the shape of the thorax are also common. A protruding sternum is called pectus carinatum; a sunken sternum is called pectus excavatum. **Scoliosis** and **hyperkyphosis** are also possible indicators of Marfan syndrome. These bony anomalies can be severe enough to interfere with breathing and raise the risk of **pneumonia**.

In the cardiovascular system, Marfan syndrome can weaken the aortic and mitral valves of the heart. Prolapsed valves lead to the regurgitation of blood and an irregular heartbeat. An enlarged aorta with a risk of a dissecting **aneurysm** is a potential cause of death for Marfan syndrome patients.

In the nervous system, patients may experience dural ectasia: a situation in which the dura mater stretches and weakens with age.

Other symptoms include stretch marks on the skin, hernias, and eye problems that range from myopia to dislocated lens, detached retina, and possible blindness.

Treatment

Marfan syndrome is treated according to the symptoms. Surgery may be needed for heart valves, to correct an aortic aneurysm, to deal with postural deviation, or to repair a deformed thorax.

Medications
- Beta-blockers to reduce cardiac load
- Prophylactic antibiotics to prevent infection of the valves of the heart

Massage Therapy Implications

RISKS	Marfan syndrome patients have fragile connective tissues. Hypermobility in the joints and a risk of blood vessel weakness require accommodations in bodywork.
BENEFITS	As long as the challenges of massage are kept within the client's ability to adapt, a person with Marfan syndrome can enjoy the same benefits from massage as the rest of the population.

Myasthenia Gravis

Definition: What Is It?

First described by Wilhelm Erb in 1890, MG is an autoimmune disease that involves the destruction of receptor sites at neuromuscular junctions. It is a progressive disease, but it is usually manageable with medical and surgical intervention. It diagnosed most often in women under 40 and men over 60, and it affects about 36,000 people in the United States.

Etiology: What Happens?

Acetylcholine (ACh), a neurotransmitter associated with increased excitability, is a key player in the cascade of events that translates electrical stimulation from the brain into chemical reactions in the muscles. In myasthenia gravis, antibodies attack the ACh receptor sites. Then, the receptor sites don't function correctly, and the muscle loses the ability to respond and ultimately to contract. Symptoms develop when about 70% of receptors have been lost.

It is not clear why antibodies attack the neuromuscular junction, but many experts believe the thymus may be involved in some way because the vast majority of MG patients show signs of thymus disruption.

Signs and Symptoms

Most people with MG report weakness and fatigability in affected muscles. The process begins most often around the eyes, face, and throat. Early signs include a flattened smile, droopy eyelids (ptosis), blurred vision, and difficulty with eating, swallowing, and speech.

Symptoms tend to fluctuate during the day and are worst early in the morning and late at night. Repetitive activity, emotional stress, overexertion, exposure to heat, and some medications can make symptoms much worse.

One very serious consequence of MG is called a myasthenic crisis. In this situation, an event like a respiratory infection or a reaction to medication triggers a sudden and rapid loss of strength in the muscles that control respiration. Patients need assisted ventilation until the crisis passes.

Treatment

Treatment of MG is intended to boost nerve transmission and to suppress immune system activity at neuromuscular junctions. Surgery is occasionally recommended to remove an abnormal thymus gland. In extreme situations, plasmapheresis may be conducted to remove faulty antibodies from the blood, but this is a temporary solution.

Medications
- Cholinesterase inhibitors to increase the availability of ACh at neuromuscular junctions
- Corticosteroids to suppress immune system activity

Massage Therapy Implications

RISKS	Excessive heat may aggravate MG symptoms, so this must be avoided. People with MG may treat it with immunosuppressant drugs, so they are at higher risk than the general population for picking up infections.
BENEFITS	Because MG involves motor paralysis but not sensory deficit, carefully applied massage can be safe and supportive.

Multiple System Atrophy

Definition: What Is It?

Multiple system atrophy (MSA) is a fairly rare progressive disease that involves degeneration of neurons in the brain that control several autonomic functions. It usually affects adults in their 50s and typically progresses from onset of symptoms to death over the course of about 10 years.

Etiology: What Happens?

MSA occurs when oligodendrocytes (insulating cells in the central nervous system) accumulate an abnormal amount of a protein called alpha-synuclein. This interferes with several functions, including the production of dopamine, which is why MSA can sometimes be difficult to distinguish from **Parkinson disease**. The cause of the buildup of alpha-synuclein is not clear. Neither heredity nor toxic exposure appears to be a factor. MSA can progress in different parts of the brain, which can influence how symptoms develop.

Signs and Symptoms

Signs and symptoms of MSA vary according to the location of the damage. And because this disease is progressive, symptoms can evolve and encompass more and more of autonomic function. This can cause difficulty with maintaining appropriate blood pressure: it tends to be too high when a person is laying down, and too low when a person is standing—leading to syncope, or fainting spells. Heart rate may be extremely variable. The digestive system may be impaired, from swallowing to peristalsis to continence. Bladder control is likewise vulnerable. Loss of muscle control of the limbs, along with rigidity, tremor, and flexion of the trunk, raise the risk of falls.

Types of Multiple System Atrophy

Specialists sometimes discuss MSA as two types. It is possible to begin with one version and progress to have symptoms of another version.

- MSA-P is a version that resembles Parkinson disease in many ways. Its primary symptoms are rigidity, bradykinesia, and tremor.
- MSA-C is named for its focus on cerebellar damage. Leading symptoms of this type of MSA include loss of motor control for gait and limb movement, slurred speech, and difficulties swallowing.

Treatment

MSA has no cure and does not enter remission. Treatment is aimed solely at managing symptoms. Patients who have difficulty with regulating their heart rate may have a pacemaker surgically implanted. A speech pathologist may be employed to help with speech and swallowing skills.

Medications

- Blood pressure medication to either raise or lower blood pressure
- Parkinsonism drugs to improve dopamine uptake and muscle control
- Dietary fiber or laxatives for constipation
- Drugs to manage bladder control

Massage Therapy Implications

RISKS	A client with MSA may have any number of problems that massage might exacerbate, including low blood pressure, high blood pressure, incontinence, balance and coordination problems, and others.
BENEFITS	Using a massage chair rather than a table, and aiming for short sessions to track the client's tolerance, is probably a good strategy for working with people who have MSA. The relaxation provided by massage may help to mitigate some stress-related symptoms, as long as the work is within the client's ability to adapt.

Osteogenesis Imperfecta

Definition: What Is It?

Osteogenesis imperfecta (OI) is a group of genetic disorders that change the quality or the quantity of certain collagen fibers, leading to bones that are pathologically thin and possibly brittle. About 50,000 people in the United States have OI; men and women are affected equally.

Etiology: What Happens?

Type I collagen provides the scaffolding for bones and invests connective tissues of organ capsules, fascia, the cornea and sclera, tendons, meninges, and skin. Osteogenesis imperfecta is the result of a genetic mutation that alters the quality or quantity of type I collagen fibers. Consequently, the creation of healthy bone tissue is impaired.

This mutation is autosomal dominant (a person can inherit the trait from just one parent), but about a third of all cases seem to be the result of spontaneous mutations.

Signs and Symptoms

The primary feature of OI is having bones that fracture extremely easily, especially in infancy and early childhood. Children with OI are sometimes mistaken for victims of child abuse because their radiographs show a history of multiple broken bones. Other possible signs include brittle teeth, ligament laxity, easy bruising, short stature, bowed long bones, extreme **postural deviations** (especially hyperkyphosis with scoliosis), hearing loss, and low muscle mass.

Having poorly formed or inadequate type 1 collagen can lead several problems outside of the musculoskeletal system, including heart valve weakness, dilation of the aorta, distortions of the sclera with vision loss, and muscle weakness. An especially serious complication occurs when ligament laxity allows the odontoid process of C_2 to narrow the foramen magnum or put pressure on the brainstem; this is called basilar invagination.

Treatment

The main goals of OI treatment are to maintain health and independence, to preserve bone density, and to minimize cardiovascular problems. Children and adults are encouraged to be physically active within safety parameters. A healthy diet is strongly promoted to control weight and assist with bone density.

Surgery to straighten and support bowed long bones may be conducted, and other assistive devices, from crutches to braces to wheelchairs, may be used to improve mobility. TENS units or nerve blocks may be used for pain if other drugs are not sufficient.

Medications

- NSAIDs for pain management
- Bisphosphonates to promote bone density

Massage Therapy Implications

RISKS	OI involves bones that are abnormally brittle. Very severe versions of the disease can lead to fractures with little or no trauma. It is imperative that any massage therapist working with an OI patient be fully informed about this risk.
BENEFITS	People with OI are directed to manage stress and to exercise to maintain muscle mass and control weight. Carefully conducted massage that stays within the client's ability to adapt may have a role here, as long as the fragility of the bones and other tissues is respected.

Osteomalacia

Definition: What Is It?

Osteomalacia, which technically means "bone softening," is a condition in which bone tissue breaks down faster than it can rebuild. It is distinguished from osteoporosis by the fact that it involves problems with the bone-building process, rather than the dismantling of previously healthy bones. When osteomalacia is seen in children, it is often called by its traditional name, rickets.

Etiology: What Happens?

Healthy bone tissue is formed within units called osteoids. Type I collagen forms the scaffolding of the osteoids, and minerals collect around the fibers. In osteomalacia, some osteoids don't mineralize completely or correctly, leading to gaps within healthy bone tissue, bone weakness, a high risk of fractures, and bowing in the weight-bearing long bones of the leg.

Osteomalacia has several contributing factors, but they all lead to problems with building bone density. The nutrients that are deficient in some cases of osteomalacia include calcium, vitamin D, and phosphate. Some people with **celiac disease** or a history of stomach or small intestine surgeries are incapable of absorbing these important nutrients from their diet. Certain thyroid, kidney, and liver diseases can interfere with bone development. Long-term exposure to toxins, use of some antiseizure drugs, and overuse of over-the-counter antacids have also been seen to trigger osteomalacia.

Signs and Symptoms

The leading symptom of osteomalacia in adults is progressive deep, achy bone pain, especially in the legs, pelvis, and low back. Muscle weakness and general fatigue are often present as well. A waddling gait may develop as the leg bones begin to bow.

X-rays of people with osteomalacia may show characteristic zones where the bone tissue forms abnormally. These seams of low-density bone often resemble stress fractures. In children, this is especially visible at the growth plates, which stay wide and irregular. Eventually, the long bones of the leg weaken and bow outward.

Treatment

Osteomalacia is treated according to its cause. Vitamin and mineral supplements and treating other underlying conditions that contribute to the problem are the highest priorities.

Medications

- Vitamin or mineral supplements

Massage Therapy Implications

RISKS	In adults, osteomalacia is frequently associated with underlying disorders that must be addressed to work safely. This condition involves weak bones with a high risk of fracture, so any bodywork or massage must be adapted for that vulnerability.
BENEFITS	As long as the pressure is appropriate for the client and other underlying problems have been addressed, massage may be a useful strategy to deal with the deep pain and muscle weakness that frequently accompany this condition.

Osteomyelitis

Definition: What Is It?

Osteomyelitis is an acute or chronic bone infection.

Etiology: What Happens?

The infectious agents that cause osteomyelitis are usually varieties of bacteria including **MRSA** (methicillin-resistant *Staphylococcus aureus*), *Streptococcus*, *Enterobacter*, and some others. The pathogens access the bones through a variety of routes. Compound **fractures** allow environmental agents to directly access bones. Osteomyelitis is an occasional surgical complication as well. Sometimes, a relatively minor skin wound becomes a portal of entry for pathogens to gain deep access. And in some cases, a condition like **pneumonia** or a **urinary tract infection** can allow pathogens to travel elsewhere in the body, leading to bone infections.

Some populations are particularly vulnerable to osteomyelitis. Long-term users of any surgical tubing like central lines or dialysis are at risk, as are people who are **HIV** positive or otherwise immunosuppressed, **sickle cell anemia** patients, people with advanced **diabetes**, those with **peripheral artery disease**, intravenous drug users, and those who have undergone **joint replacement surgeries**.

Signs and Symptoms

Osteomyelitis can be acute or chronic. A chronic situation generally involves a long-lasting infection that persistently recurs despite aggressive treatment.

Acute bone infections typically show a slow onset. When they occur in children, the long bones of the extremities are usually affected. In adults, the vertebrae or pelvic bones are the most common infection sites. In either case, fever, lethargy, irritability, edema, and limited movement of the affected area are seen in conjunction with redness and swelling at the affected bone.

Treatment

Intravenous antibiotics are the first recourse to treat osteomyelitis, but surgery to remove necrotic tissue may follow.

If this condition becomes a chronic situation that is resistant to treatment, chronic skin ulcers or sinuses may develop where the internal infection seeps to the surface. Inadequately treated osteomyelitis may lead to extensive loss of bone and soft tissue, raising the risk for fractures, loosening of implanted joint prostheses, spinal cord compression, **deep vein thrombosis**, and other serious complications.

Medications

- Antibiotics for bacterial infection; these are typically administered intravenously for several weeks.

Massage Therapy Implications

RISKS	A person with osteomyelitis has an active and potentially dangerous infection. Most massage is inappropriate until this situation has been resolved. A person who has recently had surgery to treat osteomyelitis may need special considerations during recovery.
BENEFITS	Bodywork that focuses on soothing, parasympathetic support during recovery from infection may be safe and appropriate, as long as local skin problems are avoided. Clients who have fully recovered from osteomyelitis can enjoy the same benefits from massage as the rest of the population.

Paget Disease

Definition: What Is It?

Paget disease, also called osteitis deformans, is a condition in which bone is reabsorbed much faster than normal. It is replaced with disorganized fibrous connective tissue, which never completely matures, leaving the affected bones weakened and distorted. Paget disease is most common in people over age 50 of northern European descent.

Etiology: What Happens?

Normal bone activity involves osteoclasts and osteoblasts that keep each other in balance. In Paget disease, the osteoclasts become huge and hyperactive. Osteoblasts also increase activity, but they don't change in size or form. The result is that bony tissue is broken down and replaced at an accelerated pace, but the new tissue is extremely brittle and disorganized. The cause or trigger for this change in cellular behavior is not fully understood. A genetic component seems clear because it runs in families, but the precise mutation has not been found.

Paget disease can occur in one bone or several. The vertebrae, pelvis, leg, and skull bones are affected most often. Once established, the lesions may grow, but they do not appear to spread to other bones.

Signs and Symptoms

Paget disease usually has no symptoms until it is advanced enough to cause visible changes to the affected bones. Later signs and symptoms include deep bone pain, palpable heat where the bone is affected, and problems related to a change in bone shape in the affected area. These can include a loss of hearing and chronic **headaches** if the skull is affected, pinched nerves and vertebral **fractures** if the disease is in the spine, and a visible change in the shape of long bones, which may become bowed and distorted.

Complications

The most common complications of Paget disease are **arthritis** and fractures in the affected bones. If the cranial bones press on parts of the central nervous system, deafness, headaches, or vision problems could develop. Teeth can loosen if the disease distorts the mandible. **Heart failure** may occur because the heart must pump blood through whole massive networks of vessels in the new, useless fibrous tissue. A small number of Paget disease patients may develop a rare but aggressive form of bone cancer.

Treatment

Treatment for Paget disease includes recommendations for exercise and physical therapy to maintain function and healthy bone mass. Medications can address symptoms of the disease, but may not interrupt the progress. Surgery may become necessary to repair fractures or replace joint surfaces when the bones become badly distorted.

Medications

- NSAIDs for pain and inflammation
- Bisphosphonates to inhibit osteoclast activity
- Calcitonin, if bisphosphonates aren't successful

Massage Therapy Implications

RISKS	People with Paget disease have bones that are severely compromised. This fragility must be accommodated with modality and positioning choices.
BENEFITS	Early stage Paget disease may be treated with physical therapy to maintain flexibility and bone density. Massage in this context, and in coordination with the rest of the health care team, may be safe and appropriate.

Peritonitis

Definition: What Is It?

Peritonitis refers to inflammation of the peritoneum. It is usually an infection that has become established in the peritoneal space, where pathogens can grow easily. Other irritants may also cause inflammation of the peritoneum, including gastric juice from a perforated peptic ulcer or bile from the gallbladder or injured liver.

Etiology: What Happens?

Peritonitis that is related to infection can begin when pathogenic agents gain access to the peritoneal space. This can happen in a variety of ways: mechanical perforation (as in a knife wound or a complication of surgery), with the rupture of an abdominal or pelvic abscess (**pelvic inflammatory disease**), or with organ damage related to underlying disease (perforating **ulcers**, acute appendicitis, **Crohn disease**, **ulcerative colitis**, or **diverticulitis**). Peritonitis can also happen spontaneously; this is an occasional complication of ascites: massive abdominal fluid retention that is seen with **cirrhosis** and some other disorders. Experts theorize that in this case, bacteria seep into the abdominal fluid through the gut wall or mesenteric lymph nodes.

One form of peritonitis is related to peritoneal dialysis. This is a procedure that uses the peritoneum as a filter for blood dialysis, but it carries a significant risk of contamination and infection.

Once bacteria establish residence in the peritoneal space, they promote the production of scar tissue. This can lead to severe adhesions and cysts that serve to protect bacteria from immune system response.

Signs and Symptoms

Dull, diffuse abdominal pain is the most common sign of peritonitis. It can have a fast or insidious onset, depending on underlying causes. Anorexia and nausea are often present, along with fever and rapid heart rate.

Treatment

If the abdominal inflammation or infection can be treated without surgery, this is obviously the preferred course. Open or laparoscopic surgery may be required, however, to repair perforations or ruptures.

Medications

- Oral or intravenous antibiotics for bacterial infection

Massage Therapy Implications

RISKS	Acute peritonitis is a medical emergency and contraindicates massage until the crisis is over.
BENEFITS	A client who has fully recovered from peritonitis can enjoy the same benefits from massage as the rest of the population.

Pelvic Inflammatory Disease

Definition: What Is It?

Pelvic inflammatory disease (PID) can involve infection of the uterus (endometritis), infection of the uterine tubes (salpingitis), or abscesses on the ovaries (oophoritis).

Etiology: What Happens?

PID is usually the result of a bacterial infection that begins in the vagina. The infectious agent is often a **sexually transmitted infection**:

Chlamydia or gonorrhea or both. Other possible causes include irritation from an IUD or incomplete elective or spontaneous **abortion**.

Common complications of PID include infertility, **ectopic pregnancy**, and chronic pelvic pain. PID becomes dangerous when the infection backs up from the vagina to the uterus and into the fallopian tubes, where it can start growing in the open pelvic cavity. Occasionally, PID causes the growth of tuboovarian abscesses. If an abscess ruptures, it releases infectious material into the pelvis. In either case, life-threatening **peritonitis** is the result.

Types of Pelvic Inflammatory Disease

- *Acute PID*: This is a high-grade infection with symptoms that include fever, low back pain, nausea, vomiting, lethargy, painful intercourse, and heavy vaginal discharge.
- *Chronic PID*: This condition involves long-term low-grade inflammation that can cause subtle symptoms but can also lead to extensive scarring of the uterine tubes and a high risk of infertility or ectopic pregnancy.

Signs and Symptoms

The signs and symptoms of PID depend on whether the infection is acute or chronic. They are described above.

Treatment

PID is usually a fairly simple bacterial infection. Caught early, it responds well to antibiotics and bed rest, although some women need hospitalization and intravenous antibiotics. Sexual activity must be curtailed for several weeks, and the woman's sexual partner or partners should also be treated for gonorrhea or Chlamydia if either of those is causing the infection.

Medications

- Antibiotics for bacterial infection

Massage Therapy Implications

RISKS	Acute PID contraindicates any but the most gentle, noninvasive bodywork until the infection has been resolved. Chronic PID (if it is identified at all) calls for special caution for abdominal work, and of course, any other massage must fit within the client's capacity for adaption.
BENEFITS	Massage is unlikely to have a direct positive impact on PID, but it may be a helpful and soothing coping mechanism for a woman going through a difficult time. Clients who have fully recovered from PID can enjoy all the same benefits from massage as the rest of the population.

Pityriasis Rosea

Definition: What Is It?

Pityriasis rosea is an idiopathic, self-limiting rash that usually affects teenagers and young adults. Its name derives from the Greek for "pink bran" because the lesions are round, pinkish, and slightly itchy.

Etiology: What Happens?

The etiology of pityriasis rosea is unclear, but it seems to have a strong link with a viral trigger: many cases erupt after a recent upper respiratory tract infection. It does not appear to be contagious, however, so the rash may be a side effect of viral exposure rather than the result of direct damage to the tissues. It is rare for a person to have pityriasis rosea more than once.

Signs and Symptoms

Pityriasis rosea typically begins with a single round pinkish lesion on the trunk; this is called the "herald patch." This is followed within the next 2 weeks with many similar lesions, often in a symmetrical "Christmas tree" pattern on the body. The lesions, which are not intensely itchy, are usually confined to the back, chest, or abdomen. It is most common among people between 10 and 35 years old. The rash lasts 2 to 8 weeks and then spontaneously disappears, leaving little or no discoloration.

It is useful to get a professional diagnosis for pityriasis rosea because this noncontagious rash resembles both ringworm and secondary syphilis: both potentially communicable conditions that require treatment to eradicate.

Treatment

Often, no treatment is prescribed for this benign, self-limiting condition. Home care may include avoiding harsh or drying soaps and using soothing lotion. Exposure to ultraviolet light may be recommended, as this appears to speed healing. When medication is prescribed, it is to deal with symptoms only.

Medications

- Corticosteroid cream for itching
- Antihistamines for itching

Massage Therapy Implications

RISKS	It is important to work with this condition only when a definitive diagnosis has been obtained, because pityriasis resembles other skin conditions that are potentially communicable. Massage may exacerbate itching, so this rash may be a local contraindication while it is present.
BENEFITS	Massage won't speed healing or otherwise directly improve pityriasis rosea, but if it can be conducted without making the itching worse, a client with this condition can enjoy the same benefits of bodywork as the rest of the population.

Pleurisy

Definition: What Is It?

Pleurisy refers to inflammation of the pleurae: the epithelial membranes that line the thoracic cavity. Pleuritis is a synonym.

Etiology: What Happens?

The outer surface of each lung is covered by an epithelial membrane called the visceral pleura; the inner surface of the thoracic cavity is lined with a similar membrane called the parietal pleura. In normal conditions, the visceral and parietal layers of the pleurae secrete a small amount of lubricating fluid that allows the two surfaces to slip and slide easily over each other with every breath. Pleurisy develops when the visceral and parietal layers develop inflammation. This causes the layers to stick together, making breathing painful. Further, prolonged inflammation can allow the pleural space to fill with fluid. This compresses the lungs and creates a risk of empyema: infection in the pleural space.

Causes of pleurisy include **pneumonia**, chest trauma, the congestion that occurs with heart failure, inhaled chemicals or toxins, autoimmune diseases (specifically **rheumatoid arthritis** and **lupus**), **lung cancer**, **pulmonary embolism**, and abdominal problems that can put pressure on the thoracic cavity, including **pancreatitis**, **gallstones**, and **cirrhosis**.

Signs and Symptoms

Pleurisy typically involves stabbing chest pain with inhalation. The pain is usually unilateral and has a sudden onset in conjunction with a predisposing factor: a respiratory infection, a flare of autoimmune disease, a chest trauma, or something else. It is important to get a confirmed diagnosis of pleurisy: chest muscle strains or costochondritis look similar but require different treatment options.

Treatment

Pleurisy is treated according to underlying causes. Drugs can treat bacterial infections, autoimmune diseases, and emboli. Other causes may have to be treated with a combination of medication and surgical procedures.

Nonpharmacological interventions for pleurisy start with external splinting of the chest wall but may include thoracentesis (needle aspiration of the pleural space); decortication, a procedure to remove infectious material and scar tissue; or pleurodesis, which introduces an irritant to the pleural space that essentially "glues" the layers together in order to prevent future episodes of pleural effusion.

Medications

- Aspirin, ibuprofen, and NSAIDs to control pain and inflammation
- Antibiotics for bacterial infections
- Anticoagulants for pulmonary embolism
- Immunosuppressants for autoimmune disease

Massage Therapy Implications

RISKS	Pleurisy is sometimes a sequence of serious underlying diseases that have implications for massage: these must be explored before safety is assured.
BENEFITS	A client whose pleurisy is identified and being treated may be a good candidate for any bodywork that he or she can tolerate, as long as infections are no longer communicable. Massage that focuses on breathing muscles and awareness may be welcomed. A client who has fully recovered from pleurisy can enjoy the same benefits of massage as the rest of the population.

Polymyalgia Rheumatica

Definition: What Is It?

The name polymyalgia rheumatica (PMR) describes "multiple muscle and joint pain," and this is an apt label for a condition that involves aching, stiff sore muscles and joints that persist for months or years and then spontaneously goes away. This idiopathic condition mostly affects women of northern European ancestry between 50 and 80 years old.

Etiology: What Happens?

The etiology of PMR is poorly understood, but most experts agree that it involves a combination of genetic predisposition, exposure to an environmental trigger, and abnormal monocyte activation along with the presence of several proinflammatory cytokines. Signs of recent infection with a variety of common viruses are common with PMR, so some researchers theorize that these are the trigger.

An episode of PMR typically affects the neck, shoulders, hip, and proximal limbs. Joint muscles are painful, possibly because the fasciae, bursae, and synovial capsules are mildly inflamed. Fortunately, joint inflammation is nonerosive, that is, no permanent damage occurs.

Signs and Symptoms

Deep, aching pain of the neck, shoulders, and hips is the hallmark of PMR. The pain usually has a short onset, developing over a matter of a few days. It is worst after periods of inactivity, and morning stiffness persists for an hour or more every day. PMR may begin on one side, but it becomes bilateral. Proximal joints are the first site of pain, but the muscles of the upper arms and thighs are usually also stiff and painful. Range of motion becomes limited as well.

Some people experience low-grade fever, malaise, fatigue, and weight loss when PMR begins. Distal edema happens to some, with accompanying carpal tunnel syndrome if edema affects the wrists.

Types of Polymyalgia Rheumatica

- *Giant cell arteritis (GCA)*: While GCA isn't exactly a subtype of PMR, these problems are frequently seen together, and most experts agree that they are somehow linked. About 20% of people with PMR develop GCA, and about 60% of people with GCA had PMR first.

GCA is also called temporal arteritis or cranial arteritis. In this situation, the medium-sized blood vessels in the head and face become inflamed. The risk of permanent vision loss or stroke is significant. Symptoms of GCA include jaw and scalp pain, headache pain, and visual impairment. These are signals that a person must seek immediate medical help to decrease inflammation.

Treatment

PMR usually goes away by itself 2 to 3 years after it begins, but the quality of life for patients is severely impacted during the process. It responds to long-term, low-dose steroids, so this is the treatment of choice. Vitamin D and calcium supplements may be suggested to deal with the bone thinning that accompanies long-term steroid use. PMR patients are counseled to stay as active as possible: this condition puts no limitations on physical activity, as long as pain isn't exacerbated.

Medications

- Corticosteroids to control inflammation (low dose, for up to 3 years)
- High-dose steroids for giant cell arteritis

Massage Therapy Implications

RISKS	Massage that is too vigorous may exacerbate pain for a client with PMR rather than relieve it. People with PMR are also likely to be taking long-term corticosteroids, which have some cautions for massage. Clients with symptoms of giant cell arteritis (which can include headache) must see a health care provider right away.
BENEFITS	Gentle massage that is soothing and nonchallenging may help decrease pain and stiffness in clients with PMR.

Pulmonary fibrosis

Definition: What Is It?

Pulmonary fibrosis (PF) is a condition in which scar tissue progressively invades the lungs, interfering with function and potentially shortening life span. While it is sometimes a sequela of some other disorder, PF is usually idiopathic.

Etiology: What Happens?

It is not clear why scar tissue develops in the lungs of most people with pulmonary fibrosis. It does not appear to be associated with severe inflammation. Some experts suggest that epithelial injury in the lung can trigger a cascade of fibroblastic hyperactivity, which leads to the development of excessive scar tissue. One theory builds on the observation that the majority of people with PF also have **gastroesophageal reflux disorder**, so it is perhaps possible that the inhalation of minute amounts of stomach acid may stimulate the fibroblastic activity seen with this condition.

As scar tissue accumulates, a distinctive honeycomb pattern can be identified in imaging tests: this shows the distribution of scar tissue within functioning lung tissue.

The prognosis for PF is grave: the mean survival rate is 2 to 5 years after diagnosis. Most patients die of respiratory collapse.

Signs and Symptoms

This condition is marked by a gradual onset of a chronic, nonproductive cough, along with difficulty with breathing. Most patients have abnormal breath sounds. Fatigue and unintended weight loss are common. Many patients develop clubbed fingertips, which is a sign of long-term oxygen deprivation.

Treatment

Many patients with pulmonary fibrosis have several other conditions that may contribute to symptoms, including **GERD**, **obstructive sleep apnea**, **emphysema**, **chronic bronchitis**, and **coronary artery disease**. It is a high priority to manage these comorbidities.

Oxygen supplementation is used for patients who show low O_2 saturation at rest or with exercise.

Patients who are under 60 years old and whose condition does not respond to other treatments may be considered for lung transplant.

Medications

Some medication protocols have been found to reduce symptoms, but not to expand life expectancy. The medications that pulmonary fibrosis patients use include

- Biological response modifiers to suppress fibroblastic activity
- Anticoagulants
- Steroidal anti-inflammatories
- Immunosuppressants

Massage Therapy Implications

RISKS	Massage therapy is unlikely to make pulmonary fibrosis worse, but patients may be uncomfortable on the table without support for coughing or easy breathing. Be aware that these clients may have several other conditions that require adjustments and that their medications should be documented.
BENEFITS	Massage therapy is unlikely to make pulmonary fibrosis better, but gentle work with the muscles involved in inspiration may help to alleviate unnecessary inefficiencies and increase a sense of easier breathing. In addition, massage therapy may also help to manage symptoms of anxiety that are almost inevitable with a progressive, often terminal condition of this kind.

Rheumatic Heart Disease

Definition: What Is It?

Rheumatic heart disease is a complication of a bacterial infection, usually with *Streptococcus pyogenes*. The vast majority of people with rheumatic heart disease experienced this infection in early childhood as strep throat. For reasons that are not clear, about 0.3% to 3.0 % of people who have strep throat develop a condition called rheumatic fever several weeks later. Rheumatic fever is a systemic condition that causes joint pain and inflammation, rash, and sometimes uncontrollable twitching called Sydenham's chorea. Of the people who develop rheumatic fever, anywhere from 39% to 60% are at risk to develop rheumatic heart disease.

Thanks to effective antibiotics against strep throat and improved health care delivery systems, rheumatic heart disease is now rare in developed countries. However, this condition can cause extensive damage to the heart, and it is still the leading reason behind mitral valve replacement surgeries in the United States.

Etiology: What Happens?

Rheumatic heart disease does not mark a resurgence of a streptococcal infection. Rather, most experts believe that an immune system mistake causes B cells and T cells to misidentify normal tissues as outposts of bacteria. This makes rheumatic heart disease, for all intents and purposes, an autoimmune disorder.

These immune system attacks against healthy tissues are typically initiated by repeated exposure to *S. pyogenes*. That is, each repeated episode of strep throat raises the risk that the immune system will 1 day cause rheumatic fever and then rheumatic heart disease. The whole heart may be affected, but the worst outcomes occur when the endocardium that covers the mitral valve is attacked. This can lead to mitral valve stenosis, atrial fibrillation, a high risk of **thromboembolism**, **stroke**, **heart failure**, and even death.

Signs and Symptoms

Signs and symptoms of rheumatic heart disease are similar to those for more typical versions of heart failure: shortness of breath, chest discomfort, edema, and cough. In addition, palpitations may develop, and abnormal heart sounds, including murmurs in a new pattern, may be heard through a stethoscope.

Treatment

The mainstay of treatment for rheumatic heart disease is bed rest and management of issues relating to congestive heart failure. Surgery to correct damaged valves may be recommended.

Medications

- Prophylactic antibiotics against recurring infection with *S. pyogenes*
- Salicylates for pain and inflammation
- In acute cases, steroidal anti-inflammatories
- Diuretics for heart failure management

Massage Therapy Implications

RISKS	Rheumatic heart disease can lead to mitral valve stenosis, congestive heart failure, and death. These extremes are rare but not unheard of in the United States. Any massage that presents significant challenges to homeostasis may be too intense for a person with a compromised system to withstand.
BENEFITS	Massage for a person with a heart weakened by rheumatic heart disease can be restorative and beneficial as long as the client's limited ability to adapt is respected. Massage that presents challenges no greater than the client's typical daily activities is likely to be safe and appropriate.

Sarcoidosis

Definition: What Is It?

Sarcoidosis is an idiopathic disease in which abnormal immune system activity leads to the formation of tiny clumps of white blood cells and other matter called granulomas. These trigger an inflammatory response that can cause extensive tissue damage and scarring. Sarcoidosis can affect any organ system, but it is most often associated with lung and skin problems.

Etiology: What Happens?

The exact triggers that begin the process of sarcoidosis are not fully understood. Most experts suggest that a combination of genetic predisposition and environmental exposures to pathogens or irritating substances creates a reaction that leads to granulomas, inflammation, scarring, and damage in a variety of tissues.

The majority of people diagnosed with sarcoidosis have it in their lungs, supporting the theory that the trigger may be an inhaled pathogen or irritant. The granulomas can develop in virtually any tissues, however, including the skin, lymph nodes, kidneys, liver, bones, heart, and brain.

Unlike many autoimmune diseases, sarcoidosis does not appear to run in cycles of flare and remission. Rather, the majority of people diagnosed with this disease have it in a relatively mild or harmless form that runs through its course over several years and then spontaneously resolves with no permanent damage. Some people develop serious organ damage, however. Sarcoidosis is very rarely fatal.

Signs and Symptoms

Signs and symptoms of sarcoidosis vary according to severity and which tissues are affected. Many people have no specific symptoms; their diagnosis is the evidence of the disease found on a chest x-ray taken for some other reason. Some patients begin with fever, fatigue, weight loss, and malaise. Lung damage may cause dyspnea and chest pain. If lymph nodes are affected, they become enlarged; this is most consistent in the thorax. Eyes may become painful with excessive tearing and light sensitivity. The risk of permanent damage to the eye is significant, and symptoms here should be reported as quickly as possible. Skin lesions vary from discoloration to a rash on the lower leg to large nodules or ulcers that may appear on the face or hands.

Types of Sarcoidosis

- *Lofgren syndrome*: This form of sarcoidosis involves enlarged lymph nodes, especially in the thorax. Erythema nodosum is a rash of red or purplish bumps that appear over the ankles and shins. Joint pain, especially at the ankles, is common with this type. Lofgren syndrome is typically acute and short-lived and is associated with a positive prognosis for the disease.
- *Lupus pernio*: This involves dramatic and potentially disfiguring plaques and nodules on the face, inside the nasal passages, and on the digits.
- *Subcutaneous nodular sarcoidosis*: Also called Darier-Roussy sarcoidosis, this involves small flesh-colored or purplish nodules on the extremities or trunk. The lesions are not painful. This form of sarcoidosis usually signals a mild course of the disease.

Complications

Complications of sarcoidosis happen in fewer than half of the people diagnosed with this disease, but they can be serious. **Pulmonary fibrosis** can permanently limit lung function and raise the risk of **pneumonia**. If this disease affects the eyes, then color sensitivity can be lost, while glaucoma, cataracts, light sensitivity, and even blindness can develop. Changes with how calcium is managed in the body can lead to kidney damage. It is rare, but sarcoidosis can affect the nervous system, affecting the pituitary and hypothalamus or causing damage to cranial nerve VII (this is a type of **Bell palsy**). In the heart, it interferes with the electrical conduction system.

Treatment

Many cases of sarcoidosis are subtle enough that they don't require intrusive treatment before they simply dissipate. Treatments are aimed at controlling symptoms and complications, preventing progression, and limiting lung damage.

Medications

- NSAIDs for Lofgren syndrome
- Bronchodilators for lung dysfunction
- Steroidal anti-inflammatories to suppress inflammation and immune system activity
- TNF-alpha inhibitors (infliximab) to suppress immune system activity
- Antirejection drugs to suppress immune system activity
- Antimalarial drugs to manage calcium processing and skin lesions

Massage Therapy Implications

RISKS	Sarcoidosis sometimes involves skin lesions that may be portals of entry for infection. Patients with lung damage may be uncomfortable lying flat for prolonged periods. Some patients may use immunosuppressant drugs to manage this disease, so they may be vulnerable to infection.
BENEFITS	Activity limitations for sarcoidosis patients are related mainly to lung involvement: it is safe for them to exercise within tolerance. This means that forms of bodywork that stay within those parameters are also likely to be safe. While massage is unlikely to alter the course of this condition, it may improve a patient's quality of life. People who have a history of sarcoidosis that has resolved can enjoy the same benefits from massage as the rest of the population.

Definition: What Is It?

Sjögren syndrome is a common systemic disorder involving chronic inflammation that affects exocrine glands, especially tear ducts and salivary glands. The term "sicca" refers to dry eyes and mouth, so Sjögren syndrome is sometimes called sicca syndrome.

Etiology: What Happens?

While the etiology of Sjögren syndrome is not completely understood, it is clear that this condition is related to autoimmune activity against some specific tissues. This condition affects tear ducts and parotid salivary glands most often, but the lungs, kidneys, skin, and nervous system may all be involved.

Several possible viral infections have been implicated in triggering the development of Sjögren syndrome, including Epstein-Barr virus, cytomegalovirus, **hepatitis C**, and **HIV**. An inappropriate immune system reaction following exposure to one of these pathogens can lead to the destruction of working cells in targeted tissues. In the worst cases, the chronic inflammation and immune system hyperactivity appear to increase the risk of a type of **lymphoma**.

Since 90% of Sjögren syndrome patients are women, it is believed that sex hormones may play a part in how the condition develops.

Signs and Symptoms

The primary symptom of Sjögren syndrome is sicca: dry eyes and dry mouth. These symptoms are common without a diagnosis of this autoimmune disorder, however, so they are not conclusive in a diagnosis.

Repercussions of chronic dry mouth can include a sore or cracked tongue, dry lips, changes in olfaction and taste, and difficulty in talking, chewing, and swallowing.

Other symptoms can include dry sinuses, itchy, dry skin, dryness of the esophagus, and an increased risk of **kidney stones**. Many patients report fatigue and joint pain as well.

Unlike other autoimmune diseases, Sjögren syndrome does not tend to show cycles of flare and remission. Instead, it is steadily progressive for most patients.

Other signs of advanced disease, although these tend to be rare.

Types of Sjögren Syndrome

- *Primary Sjögren syndrome*: This occurs as a freestanding disorder.
- *Secondary Sjögren syndrome*: This describes Sjögren syndrome that appears as a part of some other disorder. The most common conditions that it accompanies are **rheumatoid arthritis**, **scleroderma**, and **lupus**.

Treatment

Treatment for Sjögren syndrome is largely guided by symptoms. Surgery to improve the function of salivary glands is a possibility. Artificial tears and skin moisturizers are often suggested. Other treatments focus on whatever conditions might accompany Sjögren syndrome.

Medications

- Over-the-counter and prescription eye drops
- Immunosuppressant drugs to quell autoimmune activity

Massage Therapy Implications

RISKS	Sjögren syndrome patients may be uncomfortable if a face cradle puts pressure on their eyes, which may feel gritty and dry. Similarly, being prone for a prolonged period may cause their mouth to become uncomfortably dry; it is a good idea to keep water nearby for the client's comfort. The medications used to control other autoimmune diseases that include sicca symptoms may require some adaptation of massage.
BENEFITS	Massage has no specific benefits to offer Sjögren syndrome patients. As long as the client is comfortable, people with this condition can enjoy the same benefits of massage as the rest of the population.

Thromboangiitis Obliterans

Definition: What Is It?

Also called Buerger disease, thromboangiitis obliterans (TAO) is a condition of small arteries and veins in the feet, hands, toes, and fingers. It is seen most often in people between 20 and 50 years old. It leads to painful ulcers on the fingers and toes, with a high risk of gangrene and amputation. Unlike other conditions that affect circulation, TAO is not related to atherosclerotic plaques, hypercoagulability, or diabetes.

Etiology: What Happens?

Thromboangiitis obliterans is a condition in which small arteries and veins in the extremities (almost exclusively the hands, feet, fingers, and toes) become inflamed and blocked by tiny blood clots. The result is nonhealing ulcers on the digits, a high risk for gangrene infection, and a need for **amputation**.

While the exact etiology of TAO is unknown, one unifying factor in all patients is tobacco use. Cigarettes are the most common form of use, but this disease has been seen in tobacco chewers and cigar smokers as well. Even the use of nicotine patches has been seen to stimulate progression of the disease. Experts theorize that some people have a genetic predisposition toward vascular inflammation and the development of tiny blood clots, and this tendency is triggered by nicotine exposure.

Signs and Symptoms

Signs and symptoms of TAO include intermittent claudication, resting pain, **Raynaud phenomenon**, paresthesia in the affected limbs, painful ulcers on the digits, and possible gangrene, which means amputation will probably be necessary. Most TAO patients have these signs in more than one extremity.

Treatment

Treatment for TAO begins and ends with the cessation of tobacco use. People with TAO are also counseled to be extremely careful about footwear, to treat infections on the feet or hands very aggressively, and to avoid vasoconstrictive drugs and extreme cold environments.

Surgical intervention to replace damaged blood vessels is sometimes attempted, but the success rate is relatively low. Sympathectomy to alter vasoconstriction and pain sensation may be recommended. This procedure has some short-term benefits, but long-term benefits have not been established.

Medications

Medical treatment for TAO has not had a great deal of success. Some options include the following:

- NSAIDs for inflammation and pain management
- Vasodilators
- Anticoagulants

Massage Therapy Implications

RISKS	TAO involves pain, poor circulation, and damaged skin at the hands and feet. Any massage or bodywork must be adapted to accommodate these complications.
BENEFITS	People with TAO have no limitations on exercise outside of their own tolerance. Their proximal limbs and trunk are likely to be healthy, and careful massage in these areas is probably safe and appropriate. In addition, TAO patients are probably dealing with smoking cessation. Any stress relief that massage provides during this difficult time can be welcome.

Uterine Prolapse

Definition: What Is It?

Uterine prolapse describes a situation in which the uterus protrudes into the vaginal canal. It can range from very mild to complete descent of the organ. It is almost exclusively seen in postmenopausal women who have vaginally delivered children, especially if any of those children were over 9 pounds at birth.

Etiology: What Happens?

The uterus is held in suspension in the pelvic cavity by fasciae, supporting ligaments, and the tone and tightness of the muscles in the pelvic floor, which is determined by healthy nerve transmission to the muscles involved. If the fasciae, ligaments, muscles, and nerves are damaged, then the integrity of the pelvic floor can be compromised. A history of childbirth can weaken this important group of structures, but multiple other factors are often involved. Among these are neuropathy, pelvic tumors, general connective tissue weakness, and any condition that adds to intra-abdominal pressure, like obesity, chronic obstructive pulmonary disease, or long-term constipation.

When the pelvic floor is seriously compromised and the ligaments that should stabilize the uterus become loose, the uterus can protrude into the vaginal space. This can occur on a continuum of severity, so minor cases cause no symptoms or problems, but major cases can cause the whole uterus to descend out of the pelvic cavity.

Signs and Symptoms

Mild cases of uterine prolapse cause no symptoms. More severe cases can involve a feeling of fullness and discomfort in the vagina, low back pain, problems with voiding the bladder or the rectum, and painful sexual intercourse. Vaginal spotting may be present if the cervix develops ulcerations.

Complications

Complications from uterine prolapse are mostly related to long-term severe cases that are not adequately treated. They can include a risk of **urinary tract infection**, permanent incontinence, ulcerations on the cervix, and prolapse of other pelvic organs, including the bladder (cystocele) and rectum (rectocele).

Treatment

If the extent of uterine prolapse is mild and no symptoms or complications have arisen, no treatment is recommended. A more serious situation calls for treatment, which often begins with the use of a pessary: this is a device that is inserted into the vagina to give mechanical support to the cervix and the rest of the uterus. It is removed for sexual activity and for frequent cleaning. Pessaries can be a temporary or permanent solution to uterine prolapse. If they are unsuccessful, surgery may be recommended.

Surgery for uterine prolapse ranges from to reattaching loosened ligaments, to inserting a sling to support the uterus, to full hysterectomy. It can be conducted via the vagina, as open abdominal surgery, or laparoscopically.

Medications

- Estrogen replacement therapy (ERT) to improve muscle tone in the pelvic floor—if risks for ERT don't outweigh benefits
- Topical estrogen applied via pessary
- Postsurgical analgesics

Massage Therapy Implications

RISKS	Massage has few risks for a client with uterine prolapse, unless she has an extreme situation that has not been treated by a physician.
BENEFITS	While massage may not influence the process or prognosis of uterine prolapse, it may improve the quality of life of a person undergoing this type of physical challenge. A person who has undergone surgery to repair a prolapsed uterus and has fully recovered can enjoy the same benefits from massage as the rest of the population.

Bibliography

Chapter 1

1. Healthcare Wide Hazards: (Lack of) Universal Precautions. Occupational Safety & Health Administration. https://www.osha.gov/SLTC/etools/hospital/hazards/univprec/univ.html. Accessed Summer 2014.
2. Dermal Absorption as an Exposure Route. Children's Environmental Health Project; 2000. http://www.cape.ca/children/derm2.html
3. Guideline for hand hygiene in health-care settings. *Morbidity and Mortality Weekly Report* 2002;51(RR-16). http://www.cdc.gov/mmwr/pdf/rr/rr5116.pdf
4. WHO Guidelines on Hand Hygiene in Health Care. World Health Organization; 2009. http://whqlibdoc.who.int/publications/2009/9789241597906_eng.pdf
5. Laundry: Washing Infected Material. Healthcare-Associated Infections. Centers for Disease Control and Prevention; 2011. http://www.cdc.gov/HAI/prevent/laundry.html
6. Viruses. Microbe World. American Society for Microbiology; 2014. http://www.microbeworld.org/index.php?option=com_content&view=category&layout=blog&id=77&Itemid=72
7. Aiello AE, Larson EL, Levy SB. Consumer antibacterial soaps: effective or just risky? *Clinical Infectious Diseases* 2007;45(Suppl 2):S137–S147. http://cid.oxfordjournals.org/content/45/Supplement_2/S137.long
8. Best TM, Gharaibeh B, Huard J. Stem cells, angiogenesis and muscle healing: a potential role in massage therapies? *Postgraduate Medical Journal* 2013;89(1057):666–670. http://www.ncbi.nlm.nih.gov/pubmed/24129034
9. Crane JD, Ogborn DI, Cupido C, et al. Massage therapy attenuates inflammatory signaling after exercise-induced muscle damage. *Science Translational Medicine* 2012;4(119):119ra113. http://www.ncbi.nlm.nih.gov/pubmed/24129034
10. Davidson L, Knight R. Neuropathogenesis of Prion disease. *Future Neurology* 2014;9(2):135–147. http://www.medscape.com/viewarticle/822701
11. Donoyama N, Wakuda T, Tanitsu T, et al. Washing hands before and after performing massages? Changes in bacterial survival count on skin of a massage therapist and a client during massage therapy. *Journal of Alternative and Complementary Medicine* 2004;10(4):684–686. http://www.ncbi.nlm.nih.gov/pubmed/15353027
12. Jabbar U, Leischner J, Kasper D, et al. Effectiveness of alcohol-based hand rubs for removal of Clostridium difficile spores from hands. *Infection Control and Hospital Epidemiology* 2010;31(6):565–570. http://www.ncbi.nlm.nih.gov/pubmed/20429659
13. Khan S. Inflammatory Response. Khan Academy. https://www.khanacademy.org/science/biology/immunology/v/inflammatory-response. Accessed Summer 2014.
14. King DG. Inflammation. Southern Illinois University School of Medicine; 2013. http://www.siumed.edu/~dking2/intro/inflam.htm
15. King MW. Extracellular Matrix. The Medical Biochemistry Page; 2013. http://themedicalbiochemistrypage.org/extracellularmatrix.html
16. Ramachandran TS. Prion-Related Diseases. Medscape; 2012. http://emedicine.medscape.com/article/1168941-overview
17. Rutala WA, Weber DJ, HICPAC. Guideline for Disinfection and Sterilization in Healthcare Facilities, 2008. Centers for Disease Control and Prevention; 2008. http://www.cdc.gov/hicpac/pdf/guidelines/Disinfection_Nov_2008.pdf
18. Siegel JD, Rhinehart E, Jackson M, et al.; HICPAC. Management of Multidrug-Resistant Organisms in Healthcare Settings, 2006. Centers for Disease Control and Prevention; 2006. http://www.cdc.gov/hicpac/pdf/guidelines/MDROGuideline2006.pdf
19. Siegel JD, Rhinehart E, Jackson M, et al.; HICPAC. 2007 Guideline for Isolation Precautions: Preventing Transmission of Infectious Agents in Healthcare Settings. Centers for Disease Control and Prevention; 2007. http://www.cdc.gov/hicpac/pdf/isolation/Isolation2007.pdf
20. Waites KB. Mycoplasma Infections. Medscape; 2013. http://emedicine.medscape.com/article/223609-overview
21. Waters-Banker C, Dupont-Versteegden EE, Kitzman PH, Butterfield TA. Investigating the mechanisms of massage efficacy: the role of mechanical immunomodulation. *Journal of Athletic Training* 2014;49(2):266–273. http://www.ncbi.nlm.nih.gov/pubmed/24641083

Chapter 2

Acne Vulgaris

1. Acne Lesions and Classification. Dermnet. http://www.dermnet.com/videos/acniform-eruptions/acne/acne-lesions-and-classification/. Accessed Summer 2014.
2. What Causes Acne? AcneNet. American Academy of Dermatology; 2011. http://www.skincarephysicians.com/acnenet/acne.html
3. Acne. American Skin Association; 2012. http://www.americanskin.org/resource/acne.php
4. Fulton J. Acne Vulgaris. Medscape; 2013. http://emedicine.medscape.com/article/1069804-overview
5. Keri JE, Nijhawan RI. Diet and Acne. Medscape; 2008. http://www.medscape.com/viewarticle/579326
6. Thielitz A, Gollnick H. Overview of New Therapeutic Developments for Acne. Medscape; 2009. http://www.medscape.com/viewarticle/587306

Animal Parasites

1. Parasites—Scabies. Centers for Disease Control and Prevention; 2010. http://www.cdc.gov/parasites/scabies/

2. Parasites—Lice. Centers for Disease Control and Prevention; 2013. http://www.cdc.gov/parasites/lice/
3. Pubic Lice (Crabs). MedicineNet; 2014. http://www.medicinenet.com/pubic_lice_crabs/article.htm
4. Barr M. Scabies. Medscape; 2013. http://emedicine.medscape.com/article/1109204-overview
5. Flinders DC, Schweinitz Pd. Pediculosis and scabies. *American Family Physician* 2004;69(2):341–348. http://www.aafp.org/afp/2004/0115/p341.html
6. Guenther L. Pediculosis (Lice). Medscape; 2014. http://emedicine.medscape.com/article/225013-overview
7. Mersch J. Lice. eMedicineHealth: WebMD; 2014. http://www.emedicinehealth.com/lice/article_em.htm
8. Perlstein D. Head Lice Infestation (Pediculosis). MedicineNet; 2012. http://www.medicinenet.com/head_lice/article.htm
9. Stöppler MC. Scabies. MedicineNet; 2012. http://www.medicinenet.com/scabies/article.htm

Burns

1. Mass Casualties: Burns. Emergency Preparedness and Response. Centers for Disease Control and Prevention; 2013. http://www.bt.cdc.gov/masscasualties/burns.asp
2. Cho YS, Jeon JH, Hong A, et al. The effect of burn rehabilitation massage therapy on hypertrophic scar after burn: a randomized controlled trial. *Burns* 2014;40(8):1513–1520. http://www.ncbi.nlm.nih.gov/pubmed/24630820
3. Cox RD. Chemical Burns. Medscape; 2013. http://emedicine.medscape.com/article/769336-overview
4. Jenkins JA. Emergent Management of Thermal Burns. Medscape; 2014. http://emedicine.medscape.com/article/769193-overview
5. Morien A, Garrison D, Smith NK. Range of motion improves after massage in children with burns: a pilot study. *Journal of Bodywork and Movement Therapies* 2008;12(1):67–71. http://www.ncbi.nlm.nih.gov/pubmed/19083657
6. Roh YS, Cho H, Oh JO, et al. Effects of skin rehabilitation massage therapy on pruritus, skin status, and depression in burn survivors. *Journal of Korean Academy of Nursing* 2007;37(2):221–226. http://kan.or.kr/kor/shop_sun/files/memoir_img/200702/221.pdf

Decubitus Ulcers

1. NPUAP Pressure Ulcer Stages/Categories. National Pressure Ulcer Advisory Panel; 2007. http://www.npuap.org/resources/educational-and-clinical-resources/npuap-pressure-ulcer-stagescategories/
2. What Are Bed Sores (Pressure Ulcers)? What Causes Bed Sores? Medical News Today; 2009. http://www.medicalnewstoday.com/artiUlcerStages/Categoriescles/173972.php
3. Pressure Ulcer. MedlinePlus: National Library of Medicine; 2012. http://www.nlm.nih.gov/medlineplus/ency/article/007071.htm
4. Bedsores (pressure sores). Diseases and Conditions. Mayo Clinic; 2014. http://www.mayoclinic.org/diseases-conditions/bedsores/basics/definition/con-20030848
5. Duimel-Peeters IG, Halfens RJ, Berger MP, et al. The effects of massage as a method to prevent pressure ulcers. A review of the literature. *Ostomy Wound Management* 2005;51(4):70–80. http://www.o-wm.com/content/the-effects-massage-a-method-prevent-pressure-ulcers-a-review-literature?page=0,0
6. Duimel-Peeters IG, Halfens R JG, Ambergen AW, et al. The effectiveness of massage with and without dimethyl sulfoxide in preventing pressure ulcers: a randomized, double-blind cross-over trial in patients prone to pressure ulcers. *International Journal of Nursing Studies* 2007;44(8):1285–1295. http://www.ncbi.nlm.nih.gov/pubmed/17553503
7. Kirman CN. Nonsurgical Treatment of Pressure Ulcers. Medscape; 2012. http://emedicine.medscape.com/article/1293614-overview
8. Revis DR. Pressure Ulcers and Wound Care. Medscape; 2014. http://emedicine.medscape.com/article/190115-overview
9. Stevens J. Pressure Sores (Decubitus Ulcers). Continuum of Care. University of New Mexico School of Medicine. http://coc.unm.edu/common/manual/Pressure_Sores.pdf. Accessed Summer 2014.
10. Werdin F, Tennenhaus M, Schaller HE, et al. Evidence-based management strategies for treatment of chronic wounds. *Eplasty* 2009;9:e19. http://www.medscape.com/viewarticle/709000

Dermatitis, Eczema

1. Nummular Dermatitis. American Academy of Dermatology. http://www.aad.org/dermatology-a-to-z/diseases-and-treatments/m---p/nummular-dermatitis. Accessed Summer 2014.
2. Sebhorrheic Dermatitis. EczemaNet. American Academy of Dermatologists; 2006. http://www.skincarephysicians.com/eczemanet/seborrheic_dermatitis.html
3. AAD Clinical Guidelines. American Academy of Dermatology; 2014. http://www.aad.org/education/clinical-guidelines
4. Adisen E, Onder M. Allergic contact dermatitis from Laurus nobilis oil induced by massage. *Contact Dermatitis* 2007;56(6):360–361. http://www.ncbi.nlm.nih.gov/pubmed/17577382
5. Berke R, Singh A, Guralnick M. Atopic dermatitis: an overview. *American Family Physician* 2012;86(1):35–42. http://www.aafp.org/afp/2012/0701/p35.html
6. Danby SG, AlEnezi T, Sultan A, et al. Effect of olive and sunflower seed oil on the adult skin barrier: implications for neonatal skin care. *Pediatric Dermatology* 2013;30(1):42–50. http://www.ncbi.nlm.nih.gov/pubmed/22995032
7. Grimm L. The Many Manifestations of Eczema. Medscape; 2013. http://reference.medscape.com/features/slideshow/eczema
8. Hoffjan S, Stemmler S. On the role of the epidermal differentiation complex in ichthyosis vulgaris, atopic dermatitis and psoriasis. *British Journal of Dermatology* 2007;157(3):441–449. http://www.medscape.com/viewarticle/564078_4
9. Kedrowski DA, Warshaw EM. Hand dermatitis: a review of clinical features, diagnosis, and management. *Dermatology Nursing* 2008;20(1):17–25; quiz 26. http://www.medscape.com/viewarticle/572227
10. Lakshmi C. Allergic contact dermatitis (type IV hypersensitivity) and type I hypersensitivity following aromatherapy with ayurvedic oils (Dhanwantharam thailam, Eladi coconut oil) presenting as generalized erythema and pruritus with flexural eczema. *Indian Journal of Dermatology* 2014;59(3):283–286. http://www.e-ijd.org/article.asp?issn=0019-5154;year=2014;volume=59;issue=3;spage=283;epage=286;aulast=Lakshmi
11. Larson D, Jacob SE. Tea tree oil. *Dermatitis* 2012;23(1):48–49. http://www.ncbi.nlm.nih.gov/pubmed/22653070
12. Perry AD, Trafeli JP. Hand dermatitis: review of etiology, diagnosis, and treatment. *Journal of the American Board of Family Medicine* 2009;22(3):325–330. http://www.medscape.com/viewarticle/710375

13. Treadwell PA. Eczema and infection. *Pediatric Infectious Disease Journal* 2008;27(6):551–552. http://www.medscape.com/viewarticle/578781

Fungal Infections

1. Andrews S. Tinea in Emergency Medicine. Medscape; 2013. http://emedicine.medscape.com/article/787217-overview
2. Berman K. Tinea Capitis. MedlinePlus. National Library of Medicine; 2012. http://www.nlm.nih.gov/medlineplus/ency/article/000878.htm
3. Berman K. Tinea Versicolor. MedlinePlus. National Library of Medicine; 2012. http://www.nlm.nih.gov/medlineplus/ency/article/001465.htm
4. Berman K. Jock Itch. MedlinePlus. National Library of Medicine; 2013. http://www.nlm.nih.gov/medlineplus/ency/article/000876.htm
5. Burkhart CG. Tinea Versicolor. Medscape; 2013. http://emedicine.medscape.com/article/1091575-overview
6. Kao GF. Tinea Capitis. Medscape; 2013. http://emedicine.medscape.com/article/1091351-overview
7. Lesher JL. Tinea Corporis. Medscape: 2013. http://emedicine.medscape.com/article/1091473-overview
8. Robbins CM. Tinea Pedis. Medscape; 2013. http://emedicine.medscape.com/article/1091684-overview
9. Tosti A. Onychomycosis. Medscape; 2014. http://emedicine.medscape.com/article/1105828-overview
10. Wiederkeh M. Tinea Cruris. Medscape; 2013. http://emedicine.medscape.com/article/1091806-overview

Herpes Simplex

1. Genital Herpes—CDC Fact Sheet. Centers for Disease Control and Prevention; 2014. http://emedicine.medscape.com/article/1091806-overview
2. Eastern JS. Dermatalogic Manifestations of Herpes Simplex. Medscape; 2013. http://emedicine.medscape.com/article/1132351-overview
3. Kramer A, Schwebke I, Kampf G. How long do nosocomial pathogens persist on inanimate surfaces? A systematic review *BMC Infectious Diseases* 2006;6:130. http://www.biomedcentral.com/1471-2334/6/130
4. Omori MS. Herpetic Whitlow. Medscape; 2014. http://emedicine.medscape.com/article/788056-overview
5. Salvaggio MR. Herpes Simplex. Medscape; 2012. http://emedicine.medscape.com/article/218580-overview

Rosacea

1. Frequently Asked Questions. National Rosacea Society. http://www.rosacea.org/patients/faq.php. Accessed Summer 2014.
2. Rosacea. American Osteopathic College of Dermatology. http://www.aocd.org/?page=Rosacea. Accessed Summer 2014.
3. All About Rosacea. National Rosacea Society. http://www.rosacea.org/patients/allaboutrosacea.php. Accessed Summer 2014.
4. Banasikowska AK. Rosacea. Medscape; 2013. http://emedicine.medscape.com/article/1071429-overview
5. Cole GW. Rosacea. MedicineNet; 2010. http://www.medicinenet.com/rosacea/article.htm
6. Jarmuda S, O'Reilly N, Zaba R, et al. Potential role of Demodex mites and bacteria in the induction of rosacea. *Journal of Medical Microbiology* 2012;61(Pt 11):1504–1510. http://jmm.sgmjournals.org/content/early/2012/08/28/jmm.0.048090-0.full.pdf
7. Oakley A, Ngan V. Rosacea. DermNet New Zealand Trust; 2014. http://dermnetnz.org/acne/rosacea.html
8. Wilkin J, Dahl M, Detmar M, et al. Standard grading system for rosacea: report of the National Rosacea Society Expert Committee on the classification and staging of rosacea. *Journal of the American Academy of Dermatology* 2004;50(6):907–912. http://www.rosacea.org/grading/gradingsystem.php

Scar Tissue

1. Acne Scars. AcneNet. American Academy of Dermatologists; 2011. http://www.skincarephysicians.com/acnenet/scarring.html. Accessed Summer 2014.
2. Cole GW. Scars. MedicineNet; 2013. http://www.medicinenet.com/scars/article.htm
3. Fearmonti R, Bond J, Erdmann D, et al. A review of scar scales and scar measuring devices. *Eplasty* 2010;10:e43. http://www.medscape.com/viewarticle/726034_4
4. Shin TM, Bordeaux JS. The role of massage in scar management: a literature review. *Dermatologic Surgery* 2012;38(3):414–423. http://www.ncbi.nlm.nih.gov/pubmed/22093081
5. Wilk I, Kurpas D, Mroczek B, et al. Application of tensegrity massage to relive complications after mastectomy—case report. *Rehabilitation Nursing* 2014 (electronic publication ahead of print). http://www.ncbi.nlm.nih.gov/pubmed/24668661
6. Wong T, McGrath JA, Navsaria H. The role of fibroblasts in tissue engineering and regeneration. *British Journal of Dermatology* 2007;156(6):1149–1155. http://www.medscape.com/viewarticle/558003

Seborrheic Keratosis

1. Seborrheic Keratoses. American Academy of Dermatology. http://www.aad.org/dermatology-a-to-z/diseases-and-treatments/q---t/seborrheic-keratoses. Accessed Summer 2014.
2. Basal Cell Carcinoma. Diseases and Conditions. Mayo Clinic; 2013. http://www.mayoclinic.org/diseases-conditions/basal-cell-carcinoma/basics/definition/con-20028996
3. Seborrheic Keratosis. Diseases and Conditions. Mayo Clinic; 2014. http://www.mayoclinic.org/diseases-conditions/seborrheic-keratosis/basics/definition/con-20028396
4. Balin AK. Seborrheic Keratosis. Medscape; 2014. http://emedicine.medscape.com/article/1059477-overview
5. Nordqvist C. What is seborrheic keratosis? Medical News Today; 2013. http://www.medicalnewstoday.com/articles/266748.php

Skin Cancer

1. Bowen's Disease. American Osteopathic College of Dermatology. http://www.aocd.org/?page=BowensDisease. Accessed Summer 2014.
2. What You Need To Know About Melanoma and Other Skin Cancers. National Cancer Institute. http://www.cancer.gov/cancertopics/wyntk/skin. Accessed Summer 2014.
3. Types of Melanoma. Skin Cancer Foundation. http://www.skincancer.org/skin-cancer-information/melanoma/types-of-melanoma, Accessed Summer 2014.
4. Four Types of Melanoma. SkinCancerNet. American Academy of Dermatology; 2010. http://www.skincarephysicians.com/skincancernet/four_types.html

5. Basal Cell Carcinoma. Diseases and Conditions. Mayo Clinic; 2013. http://www.mayoclinic.org/diseases-conditions/basal-cell-carcinoma/basics/definition/con-20028996
6. How is melanoma skin cancer staged? American Cancer Society; 2013. http://www.cancer.org/cancer/skincancer-melanoma/detailedguide/melanoma-skin-cancer-staging
7. Leukoplakia. Diseases and Conditions. Mayo Clinic; 2013. http://www.mayoclinic.org/diseases-conditions/leukoplakia/basics/definition/con-20023802
8. Skin Cancer Statistics. Centers for Disease Control and Prevention; 2013. http://www.cdc.gov/cancer/skin/statistics/index.htm
9. Skin Cancer: Basal and Squamous Cell. American Cancer Society; 2013. http://documents.cancer.org/acs/groups/cid/documents/webcontent/003139-pdf.pdf
10. What are the survival rates for melanoma skin cancer by stage? American Cancer Society; 2013. http://www.cancer.org/cancer/skincancer-melanoma/detailedguide/melanoma-skin-cancer-survival-rates
11. Intraocular (Uveal) Melanoma Treatment. National Cancer Institute; 2014. http://www.cancer.gov/cancertopics/pdq/treatment/intraocularmelanoma/healthprofessional/allpages
12. Campbell SM, Louie-Gao Q, Hession ML, et al. Skin cancer education among massage therapists: a survey at the 2010 meeting of the American Massage Therapy Association. *Journal of Cancer Education* 2013;28(1):158–164. http://www.ncbi.nlm.nih.gov/pubmed/22915212
13. Gandey A. Malignant Melanomas Often Look Noticeably Different From Other Moles. Medscape; 2008. http://www.medscape.com/viewarticle/569114
14. Lober BA, Lober CW. Actinic keratosis is squamous cell carcinoma. *Southern Medical Journal* 2000;93(7):650–655. http://www.medscape.com/viewarticle/410575
15. McIntyre WJ, Downs MR, Bedwell SA. Treatment options for actinic keratoses. *American Family Physician* 2007;76(5):667–671. http://www.aafp.org/afp/2007/0901/p667.html
16. Spencer JM. Actinic Keratosis. Medscape; 2014. http://emedicine.medscape.com/article/1099775-overview
17. Trotter SC, Louie-Gao Q, Hession MT, et al. Skin cancer education for massage therapists: a novel approach to the early detection of suspicious lesions. *Journal of Cancer Education* 2014;29(2):266–269. http://www.ncbi.nlm.nih.gov/pubmed/24407881

Staph Infections of the Skin

1. Boils and Carbuncles. Diseases and Conditions. Mayo Clinic; 2013. http://www.mayoclinic.org/diseases-conditions/boils-and-carbuncles/basics/definition/con-20024235
2. MRSA and the Workplace. Workplace Safety & Health Topics. Centers for Disease Control and Prevention; 2013. http://www.cdc.gov/niosh/topics/mrsa/
3. General Information About MRSA in Healthcare Settings. Methicillin-resistant Staphylococcus aureus (MRSA) Infections. Centers for Disease Control and Prevention; 2013. http://www.cdc.gov/mrsa/healthcare/index.html
4. MRSA Tracking. Methicillin-resistant *Staphylococcus aureus* (MRSA) Infections. Centers for Disease Control and Prevention; 2013. http://www.cdc.gov/mrsa/tracking/index.html
5. Understanding Styes—the Basics. WebMD; 2014. http://www.webmd.com/eye-health/understanding-stye-basics
6. Baorto EP. *Staphylococcus aureus* Infection. Medscape; 2014. http://emedicine.medscape.com/article/971358-overview
7. Green BN, Johnson CD, Egan JT, et al. Methicillin-resistant *Staphylococcus aureus*: an overview for manual therapists. *Journal of Chiropractic Medicine* 2012;11(1):64–76. http://www.ncbi.nlm.nih.gov/pmc/articles/PMC3315869/
8. Jovanovic M. Hidradenitis Suppurativa. Medscape; 2014. http://emedicine.medscape.com/article/1073117-overview
9. Lanigan MD. Pilonidal Cyst and Sinus. Medscape; 2012. http://emedicine.medscape.com/article/788127-overview
10. Martinez JM. MRSA Skin Infection in Athletes. Medscape; 2013. http://emedicine.medscape.com/article/108972-overview
11. Ray GT, Suaya JA, Baxter R. Incidence, microbiology, and patient characteristics of skin and soft-tissue infections in a U.S. Population: a retrospective population-based study. *BMC Infectious Diseases* 2013;13(1):252. http://www.biomedcentral.com/1471-2334/13/252
12. Satter EK. Folliculitis. Medscape; 2013. http://emedicine.medscape.com/article/1070456-overview

Strep Infections of the Skin

1. Group A Streptococcal Infections. National Institute of Allergy and Infectious Diseases; 2012. http://www.niaid.nih.gov/topics/streptococcal/Pages/Default.aspx
2. GAS Frequently Asked Questions. Group A Streptococcal (GAS) Disease. Centers for Disease Control and Prevention; 2014. http://www.cdc.gov/groupAstrep/about/faqs.html
3. Davis L. Erysipelas. Medscape; 2014. http://emedicine.medscape.com/article/1052445-overview
4. Herchline TE. Cellulitis. Medscape; 2014. http://emedicine.medscape.com/article/214222-overview
5. Schwartz RA. Dermatologic Manifestations of Necrotizing Fasciitis. Medscape; 2014. http://emedicine.medscape.com/article/1054438-overview

Warts

1. Human Papilloma Virus. Stanford University. http://virus.stanford.edu/papova/HPV.html. Accessed Summer 2014.
2. Warts. American Academy of Dermatology. http://www.aad.org/dermatology-a-to-z/diseases-and-treatments/u---w/warts. Accessed Summer 2014.
3. Seed Warts: Minute and Irritating. Warts Information Center. http://www.warts.org/seed-warts.html. Accessed Summer 2014.
4. Common Warts. Diseases and Conditions. Mayo Clinic; 2012. http://www.mayoclinic.org/diseases-conditions/common-warts/basics/definition/con-20021715
5. Bhatia AC. Molluscum Contagiosum. Medscape; 2012. http://emedicine.medscape.com/article/910570-overview
6. Lipke MM. An armamentarium of wart treatments. *Clinical Medicine and Research* 2006;4(4):273–293. http://www.clinmedres.org/content/4/4/273.full
7. Miller KE. Duct tape more effective than cryotherapy for warts. *American Family Physician* 2003;67(3):614–615. http://www.aafp.org/afp/2003/0201/p614.html
8. Gearhart PA. Human Papillomavirus. Medscape; 2014. http://emedicine.medscape.com/article/219110-overview
9. Shenefelt PD. Nongenital Warts. Medscape; 2012. http://emedicine.medscape.com/article/1133317-overview

Chapter 3

Adhesive Capsulitis

1. A Patient's Guide to Adhesive Capsulitis. eOrthopod. http://www.eorthopod.com/content/adhesive-capsulitis. Accessed Summer 2014.
2. Ewald A. Adhesive capsulitis: a review. *American Family Physician* 2011;83(4):417–422. http://www.aafp.org/afp/2011/0215/p417.html
3. Guler-Uysal F, Kozanoglu E. Comparison of the early response to two methods of rehabilitation in adhesive capsulitis. *Swiss Medical Weekly* 2004;134(23–24):353–358. http://www.smw.ch/docs/pdf200x/2004/23/smw-10630.pdf
4. Ho CY, Sole G, Munn J. The effectiveness of manual therapy in the management of musculoskeletal disorders of the shoulder: a systematic review. *Manual Therapy* 2009;14(5):463–474. http://www.ncbi.nlm.nih.gov/pubmedhealth/PMH0028749/
5. Jewell DV, Riddle DL, Thacker LR. Interventions associated with an increased or decreased likelihood of pain reduction and improved function in patients with adhesive capsulitis: a retrospective cohort study. *Physical Therapy* 2009;89(5):419–429. http://ptjournal.apta.org/content/89/5/419.long
6. Page P, Labbe A. Adhesive capsulitis: use the evidence to integrate your interventions. *North American Journal of Sports Physical Therapy* 2010;5(4):266–273. http://www.ncbi.nlm.nih.gov/pmc/articles/PMC3096148/
7. Roy A. Adhesive Capsulitis in Physical Medicine and Rehabilitation. Medscape; 2012. http://emedicine.medscape.com/article/326828-overview
8. Shiel WC. Frozen Shoulder (Adhesive Capsulitis). MedicineNet; 2014. http://www.onhealth.com/frozen_shoulder/article.htm
9. Sokk J, Gapeyeva H, Ereline J, et al. Shoulder muscle strength and fatigability in patients with frozen shoulder syndrome: the effect of 4-week individualized rehabilitation. *Electromyography and Clinical Neurophysiology* 2007;47(4–5):205–213. http://www.ncbi.nlm.nih.gov/pubmed/17711038

Baker Cyst

1. A Patient's Guide to Popliteal Cysts. eOrthopod. http://www.eorthopod.com/content/popliteal-cysts. Accessed Summer 2014.
2. Baker's Cyst—Topic Overview. WebMD; 2012. http://www.webmd.com/pain-management/tc/bakers-cyst-topic-overview
3. Bui-Mansfield LT. Baker Cyst Imaging. Medscape; 2013. http://emedicine.medscape.com/article/387399-overview
4. Nordqvist C. What is a Baker's Cyst (Popliteal Cyst)? What Causes a Baker's Cyst? Medical News Today; 2010. http://www.medicalnewstoday.com/articles/184714.php
5. Wheeless CR. Baker's Cyst/Popliteal Cyst. Wheeless' Textbook of Orthopaedics. Duke Orthopaedics; 2012. http://www.wheelessonline.com/ortho/bakers_cyst_popliteal_cysts

Bunion

1. Bunions. OrthoInfo. American Academy of Orthopaedic Surgeons; 2012. http://orthoinfo.aaos.org/topic.cfm?topic=a00155
2. What to do about bunions. Harvard Women's Health Watch; 2012. http://www.health.harvard.edu/newsletters/Harvard_Womens_Health_Watch/2011/June/what-to-do-about-bunions
3. Bunions. Diseases and Conditions. Mayo Clinic; 2014. http://www.mayoclinic.org/diseases-conditions/bunions/basics/definition/con-20014535
4. Laughlin RT. Bunion. Medscape; 2014. http://emedicine.medscape.com/article/1235796-overview
5. Radovic PA. Bunions (Hallux Valgus). MedicineNet.com; 2014. http://www.medicinenet.com/bunions/article.htm
6. Torkki M, Malmivaara A, Seitsalo S, et al. Surgery vs orthosis vs watchful waiting for hallux valgus: a randomized controlled trial. *JAMA* 2001;285(19):2474–2480. http://www.ncbi.nlm.nih.gov/pubmed/11368700

Bursitis

1. Bursitis, Tendinitis, and Other Soft Tissue Rheumatic Syndromes. Department of Orthopaedics and Sports Medicine, University of Washington. http://www.orthop.washington.edu/?q=patient-care/articles/arthritis/bursitis-tendinitis-and-other-soft-tissue-rheumatic-syndromes.html. Accessed Summer 2014.
2. Bursitis. Diseases and Conditions. Mayo Clinic; 2011. http://www.mayoclinic.org/diseases-conditions/bursitis/basics/definition/con-20015102
3. Hip Bursitis. OrthoInfo. American Academy of Orthopaedic Surgeons; 2014. http://orthoinfo.aaos.org/topic.cfm?topic=a00409
4. Lohr KM. Bursitis. Medscape; 2014. http://emedicine.medscape.com/article/2145588-overview
5. Shiel WC. Bursitis. MedicineNet; 2013. http://www.onhealth.com/bursitis/article.htm

Carpal Tunnel Syndrome

1. Carpal Tunnel Syndrome Fact Sheet. Disorders A-Z. National Institute of Neurological Disorders and Stroke; 2014. http://www.ninds.nih.gov/disorders/carpal_tunnel/detail_carpal_tunnel.htm
2. Ashworth NL. Carpal tunnel syndrome. *Clinical Evidence (Online)* 2010;2010. http://www.ncbi.nlm.nih.gov/pubmed/21718565
3. Elliott R, Burkett B. Massage therapy as an effective treatment for carpal tunnel syndrome. *Journal of Bodywork and Movement Therapies* 2013;17(3):332–338. http://www.ncbi.nlm.nih.gov/pubmed/23768278
4. Fuller DA. Orthopedic Surgery for Carpal Tunnel Syndrome. Medscape; 2012. http://emedicine.medscape.com/article/1243192-overview
5. Lowe W. Suggested variations on standard carpal tunnel syndrome assessment tests. *Journal of Bodywork and Movement Therapies* 2008;12(2):151–157. http://www.ncbi.nlm.nih.gov/pubmed/19083667
6. Madenci E, Altindag O, Koca I, et al. Reliability and efficacy of the new massage technique on the treatment in the patients with carpal tunnel syndrome. *Rheumatology International* 2012;32(10):3171–3179. http://www.ncbi.nlm.nih.gov/pmc/articles/PMC3456919/

Compartment Syndrome

1. Burning Thigh Pain (Meralgia Paresthetica). OrthoInfo. American Academy of Orthopaedic Surgeons; 2007. http://orthoinfo.aaos.org/topic.cfm?topic=A00340
2. Compartment Syndrome. OrthoInfo. American Academy of Orthopaedic Surgeons; 2009. http://orthoinfo.aaos.org/topic.cfm?topic=A00204

3. Chronic exertional compartment syndrome. Diseases and Conditions. Mayo Clinic; 2013. http://www.mayoclinic.org/diseases-conditions/chronic-exertional-compartment-syndrome/basics/definition/con-20026471
4. Blackman PG, Simmons LR, Crossley KM. Treatment of chronic exertional anterior compartment syndrome with massage: a pilot study. *Clinical Journal of Sport Medicine* 1998;8(1):14–17. http://www.ncbi.nlm.nih.gov/pubmed/9448951
5. Bong MR, Polatsch DB, Jazrawi LM, et al. Chronic exertional compartment syndrome: diagnosis and management. *Bulletin (Hospital for Joint Diseases (New York, N.Y.))* 2005;62(3–4):77–84. http://www.ncbi.nlm.nih.gov/pubmed/16022217
6. Bouché R. Chronic Compartment Syndrome. American Academy of Podiatric Sports Medicine. http://www.aapsm.org/chroniccompartment.html. Accessed Summer 2014.
7. Rasul AT. Acute Compartment Syndrome. Medscape; 2013. http://emedicine.medscape.com/article/307668-overview
8. Wedro B. Compartment Syndrome. MedicineNet; 2014. http://www.medicinenet.com/compartment_syndrome/article.htm

Disc Disease

1. Award-winning paper questions assumptions about how herniated discs happen. Medical News Today; 2013. http://www.medicalnewstoday.com/releases/264840.php
2. Herniated disk. Diseases and Conditions. Mayo Clinic; 2014. http://www.mayoclinic.org/diseases-conditions/herniated-disk/basics/definition/con-20029957
3. Avery RM. Massage therapy for cervical degenerative disc disease: alleviating a pain in the neck? *International Journal of Therapeutic Massage and Bodywork* 2012;5(3):41–46. http://ijtmb.org/index.php/ijtmb/article/view/146/232
4. Baldwin NG. Lumbar disc disease: the natural history. *Neurosurgical Focus* 2002;13(2):E2. http://www.medscape.com/viewarticle/442526
5. Jordan J, Konstantinou K, O'Dowd J. Herniated lumbar disc. *Clinical Evidence (Online)* 2011;2011. http://www.ncbi.nlm.nih.gov/pmc/articles/PMC3275148/
6. Keller G. The effects of massage therapy after decompression and fusion surgery of the lumbar spine: a case study. *International Journal of Therapeutic Massage and Bodywork* 2012;5(4):3–8. http://www.ncbi.nlm.nih.gov/pubmed/23429839
7. Sahrakar K. Lumbar Disc Disease. Medscape; 2013. http://emedicine.medscape.com/article/249113-overview
8. Ullrich PF. What's a Herniated Disc, Pinched Nerve, Bulging Disc...? Spine-Health; 2009. http://www.spine-health.com/conditions/herniated-disc/whats-a-herniated-disc-pinched-nerve-bulging-disc
9. Wang HQ, Samartzis D. Clarifying the nomenclature of intervertebral disc degeneration and displacement: from bench to bedside. *International Journal of Clinical and Experimental Pathology* 2014;7(4):1293–1298. http://www.ncbi.nlm.nih.gov/pmc/articles/PMC4014210/
10. Windsor RE. Cervical Discogenic Pain Syndrome. Medscape; 2014. http://emedicine.medscape.com/article/93761-overview

Dupuytren Contracture

1. Dupuytren's Contracture. OrthoInfo. American Academy of Orthopaedic Surgeons; 2011. http://orthoinfo.aaos.org/topic.cfm?topic=A00008
2. Dupuytren's contracture. Diseases and Conditions. Mayo Clinic; 2012. http://www.mayoclinic.org/diseases-conditions/dupuytrens-contracture/basics/definition/con-20024378
3. Dupuytren's disease (Morbus Dupuytren or Dupuytren's contracture). International Dupuytren Society; 2014. http://www.mayoclinic.org/diseases-conditions/dupuytrens-contracture/basics/definition/con-20024378
4. Barnes CJ. Knuckle Pads. Medscape; 2014. http://emedicine.medscape.com/article/1074379-overview
5. Christie WS, Puhl AA, Lucaciu OC. Cross-frictional therapy and stretching for the treatment of palmar adhesions due to Dupuytren's contracture: a prospective case study. *Manual Therapy* 2012;17(5):479–482. http://www.ncbi.nlm.nih.gov/pubmed/22123331
6. Hart MG, Hooper G. Clinical associations of Dupuytren's disease. *Postgraduate Medical Journal* 2005;81(957):425–428. http://www.ncbi.nlm.nih.gov/pmc/articles/PMC1743313/pdf/v081p00425.pdf
7. Mathew SD. Dupuytren Contracture. Medscape; 2013. http://emedicine.medscape.com/article/329414-overview
8. Murphy K. Straightening Bent Fingers, No Surgery Required. The New York Times; 2007. http://www.nytimes.com/2007/07/24/health/24hand.html?_r=4&

Ganglion Cyst

1. Ganglion Cysts. American Society for Surgery of the Hand; 2012. http://handcare.assh.org/Hand-Anatomy/Details-Page/ArticleID/27970/Ganglion-Cysts.aspx
2. Ganglion Cyst of the Wrist and Hand. OrthoInfo. American Academy of Orthopaedic Surgeons; 2013. http://orthoinfo.aaos.org/topic.cfm?topic=A00006
3. Ganglion cyst. Diseases and Conditions. Mayo Clinic; 2013. http://www.mayoclinic.org/diseases-conditions/ganglion-cyst/basics/definition/con-20023936
4. Genova R. Ganglion Cyst. Medscape; 2012. http://emedicine.medscape.com/article/1243454-overview

Gout

1. Questions and Answers about Gout. Health Information. National Institute of Arthritis and Musculoskeletal and Skin Diseases; 2012. http://www.niams.nih.gov/Health_Info/Gout/default.asp
2. Nordqvist C. What is gout? What causes gout? Medical News Today; 2014. http://www.medicalnewstoday.com/articles/144827.php
3. Rothschild BM. Gout and Pseudogout. Medscape; 2014. http://emedicine.medscape.com/article/329958-overview

Hammertoe

1. Hammertoe. Foot Health Facts. American College of Foot and Ankle Surgeons. http://www.foothealthfacts.org/footankleinfo/hammertoes.htm. Accessed Summer 2014.
2. Hammertoe. Health Education. Hartford HealthCare Medical Group. http://www.hartfordhealthcaremedicalgroup.org/ed_podiatry_hammertoe.php. Accessed Summer 2014.
3. Hammertoe and mallet toe. Diseases and Conditions. Mayo Clinic; 2013. http://www.mayoclinic.org/diseases-conditions/hammertoe-and-mallet-toe/basics/definition/con-20019378
4. Watson A. Hammertoe Deformity. Medscape; 2014. http://emedicine.medscape.com/article/1235341-overview

Hernia

1. Hernia. A.D.A.M. Medical Encyclopedia. U.S. National Library of Medicine; 2013. http://www.ncbi.nlm.nih.gov/pubmedhealth/PMH0001956/
2. Inguinal Hernia. National Digestive Diseases Information Clearinghouse. National Institute of Diabetes and Digestive and Kidney Diseases; 2014. http://digestive.niddk.nih.gov/ddiseases/pubs/inguinalhernia/index.aspx
3. Erickson KM. Abdominal Hernias. Medscape; 2014. http://emedicine.medscape.com/article/189563-overview
4. Humphries AD, Liang MK, Fordis M. Surgical Management of Inguinal Hernia. Effective Health Care Program. Agency for Healthcare Research and Quality; 2013. http://effectivehealthcare.ahrq.gov/index.cfm/search-for-guides-reviews-and-reports/?productid=1590&pageaction=displayproduct#toc
5. Kohn GP, Price RR, Demeester SR, et al. Guidelines for the Management of Hiatal Hernia. Society of American Gastrointestinal and Endoscopic Surgeons; 2013. http://www.sages.org/publications/guidelines/guidelines-for-the-management-of-hiatal-hernia/
6. Qureshi WA. Hiatial Hernia. Medscape; 2013. http://emedicine.medscape.com/article/178393-overview
7. Shah AR. Hernia Reduction. Medscape; 2013. http://emedicine.medscape.com/article/149608-overview

Joint Disruptions

1. Dislocation. MedlinePlus. U.S. National Library of Medicine; 2012. http://www.nlm.nih.gov/medlineplus/ency/article/000014.htm
2. Snapping Hip. OrthoInfo. American Academy of Orthopaedic Surgeons; 2013. http://orthoinfo.aaos.org/topic.cfm?topic=A00363
3. Banit D. Atlantoaxial Instability. Medscape; 2012. http://emedicine.medscape.com/article/1265682-overview
4. Buyukyilmaz F, Asti T. The effect of relaxation techniques and back massage on pain and anxiety in Turkish total hip or knee arthroplasty patients. *Pain Management Nursing* 2013;14(3):143–154. http://www.ncbi.nlm.nih.gov/pubmed/23972865
5. Ebert JR, Joss B, Jardine B, et al. Randomized trial investigating the efficacy of manual lymphatic drainage to improve early outcome after total knee arthroplasty. *Archives of Physical Medicine and Rehabilitation* 2013;94(11):2103–2111. http://www.ncbi.nlm.nih.gov/pubmed/23810354
6. Malanga GA. Patellar Injury and Dislocation. Medscape; 2012. http://reference.medscape.com/article/90068-overview
7. McMillan SR. Hip Dislocation in Emergency Medicine. Medscape; 2014. http://emedicine.medscape.com/article/823471-overview
8. Peter WF, Nelissen RG, Vliet Vlieland TP. Guideline recommendations for post-acute postoperative physiotherapy in total hip and knee arthroplasty: are they used in daily clinical practice? *Musculoskeletal Care* 2014;12(3):125–131. http://www.ncbi.nlm.nih.gov/pubmed/24497426
9. Polansky R. Finger Dislocation Joint Reduction. Medscape; 2013. http://emedicine.medscape.com/article/109206-overview
10. Tamai J. Developmental Dysplasia of the Hip. Medscape; 2014. http://emedicine.medscape.com/article/1248135-overview

Joint Replacement Surgery

1. Standard Shoulder Replacement vs. Reverse Shoulder Replacement. Cleveland Clinic. http://my.clevelandclinic.org/orthopaedics-rheumatology/treatments-procedures/hic-total-shoulder-joint-replacement.aspx. Accessed Summer 2014.
2. Shoulder Joint Replacement. OrthoInfo. American Academy of Orthopaedic Surgeons; 2011. http://orthoinfo.aaos.org/topic.cfm?topic=A00094
3. Joint Replacement Surgery: Information for Multicultural Communities. Health Information. National Institute of Arthritis and Musculoskeletal and Skin Diseases; 2012. http://www.niams.nih.gov/Health_Info/Joint_Replacement/default.asp
4. Preparing for Joint Replacement Surgery. OrthoInfo. American Academy of Orthopaedic Surgeons; 2014. http://orthoinfo.aaos.org/topic.cfm?topic=A00220
5. Total Joint Replacement. OrthoInfo. American Academy of Orthopaedic Surgeons; 2014. http://orthoinfo.aaos.org/topic.cfm?topic=A00233
6. Buyukyilmaz F, Asti T. The effect of relaxation techniques and back massage on pain and anxiety in Turkish total hip or knee arthroplasty patients. *Pain Management Nursing* 2013;14(3):143–154. http://www.ncbi.nlm.nih.gov/pubmed/23972865
7. Shiel WC. Total Hip Replacement. MedicineNet.com; 2012. http://www.medicinenet.com/total_hip_replacement/article.htm
8. Shiel WC. Total Knee Replacement. MedicineNet.com; 2014. http://www.medicinenet.com/total_knee_replacement/article.htm
9. Wojcik B, Jablonski M, Gebala E, et al. A comparison of effectiveness of fascial relaxation and classic model of patients rehabilitation after hip joint endoprosthetics. *Ortopedia, Traumatologia, Rehabilitacja* 2012;14(2):161–178. http://www.ncbi.nlm.nih.gov/pubmed/22619101

Lyme Disease

1. Lyme Disease. American Lyme Disease Foundation; 2010. http://www.aldf.com/lyme.shtml
2. Lyme Disease. Diseases and Conditions. Mayo Clinic; 2012. http://www.mayoclinic.org/diseases-conditions/lyme-disease/basics/definition/con-20019701
3. Other Tick-Borne Diseases. American Lyme Disease Foundation; 2013. http://www.aldf.com/majorTick.shtml
4. Lyme Disease. Centers for Disease Control and Prevention; 2014. http://www.cdc.gov/lyme/
5. Post-Treatment Lyme Disease Syndrome. Centers for Disease Control and Prevention; 2014. http://www.cdc.gov/lyme/postLDS/
6. Meyerhoff JO. Lyme Disease. Medscape; 2014. http://emedicine.medscape.com/article/330178-overview
7. Thomason MJ, Moyer CA. Massage therapy for lyme disease symptoms: a prospective case study. *International Journal of Therapeutic Massage and Bodywork* 2012;5(4):9–14. http://www.ncbi.nlm.nih.gov/pmc/articles/PMC3528190/

Morton Neuroma

1. Morton's neuroma. Diseases and Conditions. Mayo Clinic; 2013. http://www.mayoclinic.org/diseases-conditions/mortons-neuroma/basics/definition/con-20026482

2. Berry K. Physical Medicine and Rehabilitation for Morton Neuroma. Medscape; 2014. http://emedicine.medscape.com/article/308284-overview
3. Davis F. Therapeutic massage provides pain relief to a client with Morton's neuroma: a case report. *International Journal of Therapeutic Massage and Bodywork* 2012;5(2):12–19. http://www.ncbi.nlm.nih.gov/pmc/articles/PMC3390214/

Muscular Dystrophy

1. Developing gene therapy for Duchenne muscular dystrophy. About Muscular Dystrophy. Muscular Dystrophy Campaign; 2013. http://www.muscular-dystrophy.org/research/grants/current_grants/7005_developing_gene_therapy_for_duchenne_muscular_dystrophy
2. Muscular Dystrophy. University of Maryland Medical Center; 2013. http://umm.edu/health/medical/altmed/condition/muscular-dystrophy
3. Muscular Dystrophy: Hope Through Research. Disorders A-Z. National Institute of Neurological Disorders and Stroke; 2014. http://www.ninds.nih.gov/disorders/md/detail_md.htm
4. Bushby K, Finkel R, Birnkrant DJ, et al. Diagnosis and management of Duchenne muscular dystrophy, part 1: diagnosis, and pharmacological and psychosocial management. *Lancet Neurology* 2010;9(1):77–93. http://www.thelancet.com/journals/lancet/article/PIIS1474-4422(09)70271-6/abstract
5. Carter GT. Rehabilitation Management of Neuromuscular Disease. Medscape; 2014. http://emedicine.medscape.com/article/321397-overview
6. Do TT. Muscular Dystrophy. Medscape; 2014. http://emedicine.medscape.com/article/1259041-overview
7. Klingler W, Jurkat-Rott K, Lehmann-Horn F, et al. The role of fibrosis in Duchenne muscular dystrophy. *Acta Myologica* 2012;31(3):184–195. http://www.ncbi.nlm.nih.gov/pubmed/23620650
8. Turner C, Hilton-Jones D. The myotonic dystrophies: diagnosis and management. *Journal of Neurology, Neurosurgery, and Psychiatry* 2010;81(4):358–367. http://www.ncbi.nlm.nih.gov/pubmed/20176601
9. Zhu Y, Romitti PA, Conway KM, et al. Complementary and alternative medicine for Duchenne and Becker muscular dystrophies: characteristics of users and caregivers. *Pediatric Neurology* 2014;51(1):71–77. http://www.ncbi.nlm.nih.gov/pubmed/24785967

Myofascial Pain Syndrome

1. Myofascial Pain Syndrome. Diseases and Conditions. Mayo Clinic; 2012. http://www.mayoclinic.org/diseases-conditions/myofascial-pain-syndrome/basics/definition/con-20033195
2. Myofascial Pain Syndrome (Muscle Pain). WebMD; 2013. http://www.webmd.com/pain-management/guide/myofascial-pain-syndrome
3. Bodes-Pardo G, Pecos-Martin D, Gallego-Izquierdo T, et al. Manual treatment for cervicogenic headache and active trigger point in the sternocleidomastoid muscle: a pilot randomized clinical trial. *Journal of Manipulative and Physiological Therapeutics* 2013;36(7):403–411. http://www.ncbi.nlm.nih.gov/pubmed/2384520
4. Bronfort G, Haas M, Evans R, et al. Effectiveness of manual therapies: the UK evidence report. *Chiropractic and Osteopathy* 2010;18:3. http://www.ncbi.nlm.nih.gov/pmc/articles/PMC2841070/
5. Elliott R, Burkett B. Massage therapy as an effective treatment for carpal tunnel syndrome. *Journal of Bodywork and Movement Therapies* 2013;17(3):332–338. http://www.ncbi.nlm.nih.gov/pubmed/23768278
6. Finley JE. Physical Medicine and Rehabilitation for Myofascial Pain. Medscape; 2013. http://emedicine.medscape.com/article/313007-overview
7. Jaeger B. Myofascial trigger point pain. *Alpha Omegan* 2013;106(1–2):14–22. http://www.ncbi.nlm.nih.gov/pubmed/24864393
8. Moraska A, Chandler C. Changes in clinical parameters in patients with tension-type headache following massage therapy: a pilot study. *Journal of Manual and Manipulative Therapy* 2008;16(2):106–112. http://www.ncbi.nlm.nih.gov/pmc/articles/PMC2565109/
9. Phillips CD. Cervical Myofascial Pain. Medscape; 2012. http://emedicine.medscape.com/article/305937-overview

Osgood-Schlatter Disease

1. Patient Johns Hopkins Sports Medicine Guide to Osgood-Schlatter Disease. Johns Hopkins Medicine. http://www.hopkinsortho.org/osgood-schlatter_.html. Accessed Summer 2014.
2. Osgood-Schlatter Disease (Knee Pain). OrthoInfo. American Academy of Orthopaedic Surgeons; 2007. http://orthoinfo.aaos.org/topic.cfm?topic=a00411
3. Antich TJ, Brewster CE. Osgood-Schlatter disease: review of literature and physical therapy management. *Journal of Orthopaedic and Sports Physical Therapy* 1985;7(1):5–10. http://www.ncbi.nlm.nih.gov/pubmed/18802290
4. Strickland J, Coleman N, Brunswic M, et al. Osgood-Schlatter's Disease: An Active Approach Using Massage and Stretching. European Database of Sport Science; 2008. http://ecss.de/asp/edss/C13/13-3736.pdf
5. Sullivan JA. Osgood-Schlatter Disease. Medscape; 2014. http://emedicine.medscape.com/article/1993268-overview

Osteoarthritis

1. Osteoarthritis. Disease Center. Arthritis Foundation. http://www.arthritis.org/conditions-treatments/disease-center/osteoarthritis/. Accessed Summer 2014.
2. Osteoarthritis. Health Information. National Institute of Arthritis and Musculoskeletal and Skin Diseases; 2013. http://www.niams.nih.gov/Health_Info/Osteoarthritis/default.asp
3. Abramson SB, Attur M. Developments in the scientific understanding of osteoarthritis. *Arthritis Research and Therapy* 2009;11(3):227. http://www.ncbi.nlm.nih.gov/pubmed/19519925
4. Atkins DV, Eichler DA. The effects of self-massage on osteoarthritis of the knee: a randomized, controlled trial. *International Journal of Therapeutic Massage and Bodywork* 2013;6(1):4–14. http://www.ncbi.nlm.nih.gov/pmc/articles/PMC3577640/
5. Lozada CJ. Osteoarthritis. Medscape; 2014. http://emedicine.medscape.com/article/330487-overview
6. Perlman AI, Ali A, Njike VY, et al. Massage therapy for osteoarthritis of the knee: a randomized dose-finding trial. *PLoS One* 2012;7(2):e30248. http://www.ncbi.nlm.nih.gov/pmc/articles/PMC3275589/
7. Perlman AI, Sabina A, Williams AL, et al. Massage therapy for osteoarthritis of the knee: a randomized controlled trial. *Archives of Internal Medicine* 2006;166(22):2533–2538. http://archinte.jamanetwork.com/article.aspx?articleid=769544

8. Peungsuwan P, Sermcheep P, Harnmontree P, et al. The effectiveness of Thai exercise with traditional massage on the pain, walking ability and QOL of older people with knee osteoarthritis: a randomized controlled trial in the community. *Journal of Physical Therapy Science* 2014;26(1):139–144. http://www.ncbi.nlm.nih.gov/pmc/articles/PMC3927027/
9. Reginster JY, Bruyere O, Neuprez A. Current role of glucosamine in the treatment of osteoarthritis. *Rheumatology (Oxford)* 2007;46(5):731–735. http://www.medscape.com/viewarticle/557058

Osteoporosis

1. Live with Osteoporosis. National Osteoporosis Foundation. http://nof.org/live/treating. Accessed Summer 2014.
2. Secondary Osteoporosis. International Osteoporosis Foundation. http://www.iofbonehealth.org/secondary-osteoporosis. Accessed Summer 2014.
3. Osteoporosis Overview. NIH Osteoporosis and Related Bone Diseases National Resource Center. National Institute of Arthritis and Musculoskeletal and Skin Diseases; 2012. http://www.niams.nih.gov/Health_Info/Bone/Osteoporosis/overview.asp
4. Guo Z, Chen W, Su Y, et al. Isolated unilateral vertebral pedicle fracture caused by a back massage in an elderly patient: a case report and literature review. *European Journal of Orthopaedic Surgery and Traumatology: Orthopedie Traumatologie* 2013;23(Suppl 2):S149–S153. http://www.ncbi.nlm.nih.gov/pubmed/23412164
5. Jacobs-Kosmin D. Osteoporosis. Medscape; 2013. http://emedicine.medscape.com/article/330598-overview
6. Sefton JM, Yarar C, Berry JW. Six weeks of massage therapy produces changes in balance, neurological and cardiovascular measures in older persons. *International Journal of Therapeutic Massage and Bodywork* 2012;5(3):28–40. http://www.ncbi.nlm.nih.gov/pubmed/23087776
7. Werner R. Osteoporosis and Hyperkyphosis: What Does Calcium Have to Do With It? Massage and Bodywork. Associated Bodywork and Massage Professionals; 2006. http://www.massagetherapy.com/articles/index.php/article_id/1260/Osteoporosis-and-Hyperkyphosis:-What-Does-Calcium-Have-to-Do-With-It

Osteosarcoma

1. Bone Tumor. OrthoInfo. American Academy of Orthopaedic Surgeons; 2010. http://orthoinfo.aaos.org/topic.cfm?topic=A00074
2. Ewing's Sarcoma. OrthoInfo. American Academy of Orthopaedic Surgeons; 2011. http://orthoinfo.aaos.org/topic.cfm?topic=A00082
3. Bone Cancer. Diseases and Conditions. Mayo Clinic; 2013. http://www.mayoclinic.org/diseases-conditions/bone-cancer/basics/definition/con-20028192
4. What is Ewing's sarcoma? Bone Cancer Information. Bone Cancer Research Trust; 2013. http://bcrt.org.uk/bci_what_is_ewings_sarcoma.php
5. What are the survival rates for osteosarcoma? American Cancer Society; 2014. http://www.cancer.org/cancer/osteosarcoma/detailedguide/osteosarcoma-survival-rates
6. Chansky HA. Metastatic Bone Disease. Medscape; 2014. http://emedicine.medscape.com/article/1253331-overview
7. Choy E. Osteogenic Sarcoma Staging. Medscape; 2013. http://emedicine.medscape.com/article/2007306-overview
8. Mehlman CT. Osteosarcoma. Medscape; 2012. http://emedicine.medscape.com/article/1256857-overview

Patellofemoral Pain Syndrome

1. Juhn MS. Patellofemoral pain syndrome: a review and guidelines for treatment. *American Family Physician* 1999;60(7):2012–2022. http://www.aafp.org/afp/1999/1101/p2012.html
2. Potter PJ. Patellofemoral Syndrome. Medscape; 2014. http://emedicine.medscape.com/article/308471-overview
3. Servi JT. Patellofemoral Joint Syndromes. Medscape; 2013. http://emedicine.medscape.com/article/90286-overview
4. Witvrouw E, Callaghan MJ, Stefanik JJ, et al. Patellofemoral pain: consensus statement from the 3rd International Patellofemoral Pain Research Retreat held in Vancouver, September 2013. *British Journal of Sports Medicine* 2014;48(6):411–414. http://www.medscape.com/viewarticle/821085

Pes Planus, Pes Cavus

1. Flat Feet. Health Information. University of Maryland Medical Center; 2014. http://umm.edu/health/medical/ency/articles/flat-feet
2. Buchanan M. Pes Planus. Medscape; 2012. http://emedicine.medscape.com/article/1236652-overview
3. Turner NS. Pes Cavus. Medscape; 2012. http://emedicine.medscape.com/article/1236538-overview
4. Wheeless CR. Pes Cavus. Wheeless' Textbook of Orthopaedics. Duke Orthopaedics; 2012. http://www.wheelessonline.com/ortho/pes_cavus
5. Wheeless CR. Pes Planus/Flat Foot. Wheeless' Textbook of Orthopaedics. Duke Orthopaedics; 2013. http://www.wheelessonline.com/ortho/pes_planus_flat_foot

Plantar Fasciitis

1. Plantar Fasciitis and Bone Spurs. OrthoInfo. American Academy of Orthopaedic Surgeons; 2010. http://orthoinfo.aaos.org/topic.cfm?topic=a00149
2. Glatter RD. Plantar Fasciitis: Evidence-Based Management. Medscape. American Academy of Emergency Medicine; 2007. http://www.medscape.com/viewarticle/562437
3. Goff JD, Crawford R. Diagnosis and treatment of plantar fasciitis. *American Family Physician* 2011;84(6):676–682. http://www.aafp.org/afp/2011/0915/p676.html
4. Moghtaderi A, Khosrawi S, Dehghan F. Extracorporeal shock wave therapy of gastroc-soleus trigger points in patients with plantar fasciitis: a randomized, placebo-controlled trial. *Advanced Biomedical Research* 2014;3:99. http://www.ncbi.nlm.nih.gov/pmc/articles/PMC4007320/
5. Schwartz EN, Su J. Plantar fasciitis: a concise review. *Permanente Journal* 2014;18(1):e105–e107. http://www.ncbi.nlm.nih.gov/pmc/articles/PMC3951039/
6. Young CC. Plantar Fasciitis. Medscape; 2014. http://emedicine.medscape.com/article/86143-overview

Postural Deviations

1. Hyperkyphosis/Scheuermann's Disease. http://neckandback.com/conditions/hyperkyphosis-scheuermanns-disease. Accessed Summer 2014.
2. Scoliosis. Health Encyclopedia. University of Rochester Medical Center. http://www.urmc.rochester.edu/Encyclopedia/Content.aspx?ContentTypeID=85&ContentID=P07815. Accessed 2014.

3. Brauser D. Hyperkyphosis Associated With Increased Mortality in Older Women With Vertebral Fractures. Medscape; 2009. http://www.medscape.com/viewarticle/703647
4. Brooks WJ, Krupinski EA, Hawes MC. Reversal of childhood idiopathic scoliosis in an adult, without surgery: a case report and literature review. *Scoliosis* 2009;4:27. http://www.ncbi.nlm.nih.gov/pmc/articles/PMC2808297/
5. Dalton E. Straight Talk: Symptomatic Scoliosis. Massage and Bodywork. Associated Massage and Bodywork Professionals; 2003. http://www.massageandbodywork.com/Articles/AprilMay2006/scoliosis.html
6. Graham DI. The Treatment of Scoliosis by Massage. *Annals of Surgery* 1887;6(6):485–492. http://www.ncbi.nlm.nih.gov/pmc/articles/PMC1430433/
7. Hughes S. Replica Skeleton Shows King Richard III Had Scoliosis. Medscape; 2014. http://www.medscape.com/viewarticle/826117
8. LeBauer A, Brtalik R, Stowe K. The effect of myofascial release (MFR) on an adult with idiopathic scoliosis. *Journal of Bodywork and Movement Therapies* 2008;12(4):356–363. http://www.ncbi.nlm.nih.gov/pubmed/19083694
9. Mehlman CT. Idiopathic Scoliosis. Medscape; 2012. http://emedicine.medscape.com/article/1265794-overview

Shin Splints

1. Shin Splints. WebMD; 2012. http://www.webmd.com/fitness-exercise/shin-splints
2. Shin splints. Diseases and Conditions. Mayo Clinic; 2014. http://www.mayoclinic.org/diseases-conditions/shin-splints/basics/definition/con-20023428
3. Shin splints—self-care. MedlinePlus; 2014. http://www.nlm.nih.gov/medlineplus/ency/patientinstructions/000654.htm
4. Cutler N. Massage for Anterior Shin splints. Institute for Integrative Healthcare; 2006. http://www.integrativehealthcare.org/mt/archives/2006/02/massage_for_ant.html
5. Shiel WC. Shin Splints. MedicineNet; 2014. http://www.medicinenet.com/shin_splints/article.htm
6. Stickley CD, Hetzler RK, Kimura IF, et al. Crural fascia and muscle origins related to medial tibial stress syndrome symptom location. *Medicine and Science in Sports and Exercise* 2009;41(11):1991–1996. http://www.medscape.com/viewarticle/711305
7. Walker B. Shin Pain, Shin Splints and Shin Splints Exercises and Stretches. InjuryFix. http://injuryfix.com/archives/shin-splints.php. Accessed Summer 2014.
8. Winters M, Eskes M, Weir A, et al. Treatment of medial tibial stress syndrome: a systematic review. *Sports Medicine* 2013;43(12):1315–1333. http://www.ncbi.nlm.nih.gov/pubmed/23979968

Spasms, Cramps

1. Muscle Spasms, Cramps, and Charley Horse. WebMD; 2012. http://www.webmd.com/pain-management/muscle-spasms-cramps-charley-horse
2. Albertin A, Kerppers, II, Amorim CF, et al. The effect of manual therapy on masseter muscle pain and spasm. *Electromyography and Clinical Neurophysiology* 2010;50(2):107–112. http://www.ncbi.nlm.nih.gov/pubmed/20405786
3. Halpin S. Case report: the effects of massage therapy on lumbar spondylolisthesis. *Journal of Bodywork and Movement Therapies* 2012;16(1):115–123. http://www.ncbi.nlm.nih.gov/pubmed/22196437
4. Loyola DP, Camargos S, Maia D, et al. Sensory tricks in focal dystonia and hemifacial spasm. *European Journal of Neurology* 2013;20(4):704–707. http://www.ncbi.nlm.nih.gov/pubmed/23216586
5. Minasny B. Understanding the process of fascial unwinding. *International Journal of Therapeutic Massage and Bodywork* 2009;2(3):10–17. http://www.ncbi.nlm.nih.gov/pubmed/21589734
6. Minetto MA, Holobar A, Botter A, et al. Origin and development of muscle cramps. *Exercise and Sport Sciences Reviews* 2013;41(1):3–10. http://www.medscape.com/viewarticle/777550
7. Pierson MJ. Changes in temporomandibular joint dysfunction symptoms following massage therapy: a case report. *International Journal of Therapeutic Massage and Bodywork* 2011;4(4):37–47. http://www.ncbi.nlm.nih.gov/pubmed/22211156
8. Wedro B. Muscle Spasms. MedicineNet; 2014. http://www.medicinenet.com/muscle_spasms/article.htm

Spondylolisthesis

1. Dawson EG. What is Spondylolisthesis; 2013. http://www.spineuniverse.com/conditions/spondylolisthesis/spondylolisthesis
2. Froese BB. Lumbar Spondylolysis and Spondylolisthesis. Medscape; 2012. http://emedicine.medscape.com/article/310235-overview
3. Guo Z, Chen W, Su Y, et al. Isolated unilateral vertebral pedicle fracture caused by a back massage in an elderly patient: a case report and literature review. *European Journal of Orthopaedic Surgery and Traumatology: Orthopedie Traumatologie* 2013;23(Suppl 2):S149–S153. http://www.ncbi.nlm.nih.gov/pubmed/23412164
4. Halpin S. Case report: the effects of massage therapy on lumbar spondylolisthesis. *Journal of Bodywork and Movement Therapies* 2012;16(1):115–123. http://www.ncbi.nlm.nih.gov/pubmed/22196437
5. Irani Z. Spondylolisthesis Imaging. Medscape; 2013. http://emedicine.medscape.com/article/396016-overview
6. Litao A. Lumbosacral Spondylolysis. Medscape; 2013. http://emedicine.medscape.com/article/95691-overview
7. Meryerding HW. Spondylolisthesis. *Journal of Bone and Joint Surgery* 1931;13(1):39–48. http://jbjs.org/content/13/1/39
8. Pearson A, Blood E, Lurie J, et al. Degenerative spondylolisthesis versus spinal stenosis: does a slip matter? Comparison of baseline characteristics and outcomes (SPORT). *Spine (Phila Pa 1976)* 2010;35(3):298–305. http://www.ncbi.nlm.nih.gov/pmc/articles/PMC2887281/

Spondylosis

1. Cervical Spondylosis and Spondylotic Cervical Myelopathy. The Merck Manual; 2014. http://www.merckmanuals.com/professional/neurologic_disorders/spinal_cord_disorders/cervical_spondylosis_and_spondylotic_cervical_myelopathy.html
2. Al-Shatoury HAH. Cervical Spondylosis. Medscape; 2012. http://emedicine.medscape.com/article/306036-overview
3. Cheng YH, Huang GC. Efficacy of massage therapy on pain and dysfunction in patients with neck pain: a systematic review and meta-analysis. *Evidence-based Complementary and Alternative Medicine* 2014;2014:204360. http://www.ncbi.nlm.nih.gov/pmc/articles/PMC3950594/

4. Ding Q, Yan M, Zhou J, et al. Clinical effects of innovative tuina manipulations on treating cervical spondylosis of vertebral artery type and changes in cerebral blood flow. *Journal of Traditional Chinese Medicine* 2012;32(3):388–392. http://www.journaltcm.com/modules/Journal/contents/stories/123/15.pdf
5. Nordqvist C. What is Cervical Spondylosis (Cervical Osteoarthritis)? What Causes Cervical Spondylosis? Medical News Today; 2009. http://www.medicalnewstoday.com/articles/172015.php
6. Sherman KJ, Cook AJ, Wellman RD, et al. Five-week outcomes from a dosing trial of therapeutic massage for chronic neck pain. *Annals of Family Medicine* 2014;12(2):112–120. http://www.annfammed.org/content/12/2/112.long
7. Vokshoor A. Spondylolisthesis, Spondylolysis, and Spondylosis. Medscape; 2012. http://emedicine.medscape.com/article/1266860-overview
8. Walker KA. Drugs, Medications, and Injections for Spondylosis. SpineUniverse; 2012. http://www.spineuniverse.com/conditions/spondylosis/drugs-medications-injections-spondylosis

Sprains

1. Sprains, Strains, and Other Soft-Tissue Injuries. OrthoInfo. American Academy of Orthopaedic Surgeons; 2007. http://orthoinfo.aaos.org/topic.cfm?topic=A00304
2. Fong DT, Chan YY, Mok KM, et al. Understanding acute ankle ligamentous sprain injury in sports. *Sports Medicine, Arthroscopy, Rehabilitation, Therapy and Technology* 2009;1:14. http://www.ncbi.nlm.nih.gov/pmc/articles/PMC2724472
3. Guillodo Y, Le Goff A, Saraux A. Adherence and effectiveness of rehabilitation in acute ankle sprain. *Annals of Physical Rehabilitation Medicine* 2011;54(4):225–235. http://www.sciencedirect.com/science/article/pii/S1877065711000467
4. Harrison L. Should POLICE Replace RICE as the Ankle Therapy of Choice? Medscape; 2014. http://www.medscape.com/viewarticle/823217
5. Hupperets MD, Verhagen EA, van Mechelen W. Effect of unsupervised home based proprioceptive training on recurrences of ankle sprain: randomised controlled trial. *BMJ* 2009;339:b2684. http://www.ncbi.nlm.nih.gov/pmc/articles/PMC2714677/
6. Stecco A, Stecco C, Macchi V, et al. RMI study and clinical correlations of ankle retinacula damage and outcomes of ankle sprain. *Surgical and Radiologic Anatomy* 2011;33(10):881–890. http://www.ncbi.nlm.nih.gov/pubmed/21305286
7. Williams GN, Allen EJ. Rehabilitation of syndesmotic (high) ankle sprains. *Sports Health* 2010;2(6):460–470. http://www.ncbi.nlm.nih.gov/pmc/articles/PMC3438867/

Strains

1. Muscle Strains in the Thigh. OrthoInfo. American Academy of Orthopaedic Surgeons; 2014. http://orthoinfo.aaos.org/topic.cfm?topic=a00366
2. Best TM, Gharaibeh B, Huard J. Stem cells, angiogenesis and muscle healing: a potential role in massage therapies? *British Journal of Sports Medicine* 2013;47(9):556–560. http://bjsm.bmj.com/content/early/2012/11/28/bjsports-2012-091685.short
3. Crane JD, Ogborn DI, Cupido C, et al. Massage therapy attenuates inflammatory signaling after exercise-induced muscle damage. *Science Translational Medicine* 2012;4(119):119ra113. http://www.ncbi.nlm.nih.gov/pubmed/22301554
4. Haas C, Butterfield TA, Zhao Y, et al. Dose-dependency of massage-like compressive loading on recovery of active muscle properties following eccentric exercise: rabbit study with clinical relevance. *British Journal of Sports Medicine* 2013;47(2):83–88. http://bjsm.bmj.com/content/47/2/83.short
5. Shiel WC. Muscle Strain. eMedicineHealth; 2014. http://www.emedicinehealth.com/muscle_strain/article_em.htm
6. Tol JL, Hamilton B, Best TM. Palpating muscles, massaging the evidence? An editorial relating to 'Terminology and classification of muscle injuries in sport: the Munich consensus statement'. *British Journal of Sports Medicine* 2013;47(6):340–341. http://bjsm.bmj.com/content/47/6/340.full
7. Waters-Banker C, Dupont-Versteegden EE, Kitzman PH, et al. Investigating the mechanisms of massage efficacy: the role of mechanical immunomodulation. *Journal of Athletic Training* 2014;49(2):266–273. http://www.natajournals.org/doi/full/10.4085/1062-6050-49.2.25

Temporomandibular Joint Syndrome

1. Prolotherapy: An Expert Interview With Paul H. Goodley, MD. Medscape; 2009. http://www.medscape.com/viewarticle/707539
2. TMJ disorders. Diseases and Conditions. Mayo Clinic; 2012. http://www.mayoclinic.org/diseases-conditions/tmj/basics/definition/con-20043566
3. TMJ Disorders. National Institute of Dental and Craniofacial Research; 2013. http://www.nidcr.nih.gov/OralHealth/Topics/TMJ/TMJDisorders.htm
4. de Toledo EG Jr, Silva DP, de Toledo JA, et al. The interrelationship between dentistry and physiotherapy in the treatment of temporomandibular disorders. *Journal of Contemporary Dental Practice* 2012;13(5):579–583. http://www.ncbi.nlm.nih.gov/pubmed/23250156
5. Miernik M, Wieckiewicz M, Paradowska A, et al. Massage therapy in myofascial TMD pain management. *Advances in Clinical and Experimental Medicine* 2012;21(5):681–685. http://www.advances.am.wroc.pl/pdf/2012/21/5/681.pdf
6. Pierson MJ. Changes in temporomandibular joint dysfunction symptoms following massage therapy: a case report. *International Journal of Therapeutic Massage and Bodywork* 2011;4(4):37–47. http://ijtmb.org/index.php/ijtmb/article/view/110/201
7. Tsai V. Temporomandibular Joint Syndrome. Medscape; 2014. http://emedicine.medscape.com/article/809598-overview

Tendinopathies

1. Tendinopathy: a complete guide. The Sports Injury Doctor. http://www.sportsinjurybulletin.com/archive/. Accessed Summer 2014.
2. Tendonitis and Tenosynovitis. Patient.co.uk. http://www.patient.co.uk/health/tendonitis-and-tenosynovitis. Accessed Summer 2014.
3. What is Tendinosis? Tendinosis.org. http://www.tendinosis.org/index.shtml. Accessed Summer 2014.
4. Bass E. Tendinopathy: why the difference between tendinitis and tendinosis matters. *International Journal of Therapeutic Massage and Bodywork* 2012;5(1):14–17. http://ijtmb.org/index.php/ijtmb/article/view/153/212
5. Cook JL, Khan KM. What is the most appropriate treatment for patellar tendinopathy? *British Journal of Sports Medicine* 2001;35(5):291–294. http://www.ncbi.nlm.nih.gov/pmc/articles/PMC1724394/

6. DeBerardino TM. Supraspinatus Tendonitis. Medscape; 2013. http://emedicine.medscape.com/article/93095-overview
7. Foster MR. Tenosynovitis. Medscape; 2013. http://emedicine.medscape.com/article/2189339-overview
8. Gonzalez P. Biceps Tendinopathy. Medscape; 2013. http://emedicine.medscape.com/article/327227-overview
9. Hyman GS. Jumper's Knee. Medscape; 2013. http://emedicine.medscape.com/article/89569-overview
10. Joseph MF, Taft K, Moskwa M, Denegar CR. Deep friction massage to treat tendinopathy: a systematic review of a classic treatment in the face of a new paradigm of understanding. *Journal of Sport Rehabilitation* 2012;21(4):343–353. http://www.ncbi.nlm.nih.gov/pubmed/22234925
11. Meals RA. De Quervain Tenosynovitis. Medscape; 2013. http://emedicine.medscape.com/article/1243387-overview
12. Sagimbeni AJ. Achilles Tendon Injuries. Medscape; 2014. http://emedicine.medscape.com/article/309393-overview
13. Steele M. Tendonitis. Medscape; 2012. http://emedicine.medscape.com/article/809692-overview
14. Wasielewski NJ, Kotsko KM. Does eccentric exercise reduce pain and improve strength in physically active adults with symptomatic lower extremity tendinosis? A systematic review. *Journal of Athletic Training* 2007;42(3):409–421. http://www.ncbi.nlm.nih.gov/pmc/articles/PMC1978463/
15. Wilson JJ, Best TM. Common overuse tendon problems: a review and recommendations for treatment. *American Family Physician* 2005;72(5):811–818. http://www.aafp.org/afp/2005/0901/p811.html

Thoracic Outlet Syndrome

1. Thoracic Outlet Syndrome. Nicholas Institute of Sports Medicine and Athletic Trauma. http://www.nismat.org/patients/injury-evaluation-treatment/head-neck-back/thoracic-outlet-syndrome-more-than-just-a-pain-in-the-neck. Accessed Summer 2014.
2. Thoracic Outlet Syndrome. OrthoInfo. American Academy of Orthopaedic Surgeons; 2011. http://orthoinfo.aaos.org/topic.cfm?topic=a00336
3. NINDS Thoracic Outlet Syndrome Information Page. Disorders A-Z. National Institute of Neurological Disorders and Stroke; 2011. http://www.ninds.nih.gov/disorders/thoracic/thoracic.htm
4. Thoracic outlet syndrome. Diseases and Conditions. Mayo Clinic; 2013. http://www.mayoclinic.org/diseases-conditions/thoracic-outlet-syndrome/basics/definition/con-20040509
5. Lawande M, Patkar DP, Pungavkar S. Pictorial essay: role of magnetic resonance imaging in evaluation of brachial plexus pathologies. *Indian Journal of Radiology and Imaging* 2012;22(4):344–349. http://www.ncbi.nlm.nih.gov/pmc/articles/PMC3698898/
6. Matullo KS, Duncan IC, Richmond J, et al. Characterization of a first thoracic rib ligament: anatomy and possible clinical relevance. *Spine (Phila Pa 1976)* 2010;35(23):2030–2034. http://www.medscape.com/viewarticle/732226
7. Singh MK. Neurologic Thoracic Outlet Syndrome. Medscape; 2012. http://emedicine.medscape.com/article/1143532-overview
8. Streit RS. NTOS symptoms and mobility: a case study on neurogenic thoracic outlet syndrome involving massage therapy. *Journal of Bodywork and Movement Therapies* 2014;18(1):42–48. http://www.ncbi.nlm.nih.gov/pubmed/24411148
9. Thompson RW. Challenges in the treatment of thoracic outlet syndrome. *Texas Heart Institute Journal* 2012;39(6):842–843. http://www.ncbi.nlm.nih.gov/pmc/articles/PMC3528229/

Whiplash

1. Whiplash. Diseases and Conditions. Mayo Clinic; 2012. http://www.mayoclinic.org/diseases-conditions/whiplash/basics/definition/con-20033090
2. Angst F, Gantenbein AR, Lehmann S, et al. Multidimensional associative factors for improvement in pain, function, and working capacity after rehabilitation of whiplash associated disorder: a prognostic, prospective outcome study. *BMC Musculoskeletals Disorders* 2014;15:130. http://www.medscape.com/viewarticle/825023
3. Bismil Q, Bismil M. Myofascial-entheseal dysfunction in chronic whiplash injury: an observational study. *JRSM Short Reports* 2012;3(8):57. http://www.ncbi.nlm.nih.gov/pmc/articles/PMC3434435/
4. Cobo EP, Mesquida ME, Fanegas EP, et al. What factors have influence on persistence of neck pain after a whiplash? *Spine (Phila Pa 1976)* 2010;35(9):E338–E343. http://www.medscape.com/viewarticle/721609
5. Hunter OK. Cervical Sprain and Strain. Medscape; 2014. http://emedicine.medscape.com/article/306176-overview
6. Kumar S, Ferrari R, Narayan Y. Looking away from whiplash: effect of head rotation in rear impacts. *Spine (Phila Pa 1976)* 2005;30(7):760–768. http://www.medscape.com/viewarticle/502445

Chapter 4

Addiction

1. Drug Addiction. Diseases and Conditions. Mayo Clinic; 2011. http://www.mayoclinic.org/diseases-conditions/drug-addiction/basics/definition/con-20020970
2. Epidemic: Responding to America's Prescription Drug Abuse Crisis. Office of National Drug Control Policy; 2011. http://www.whitehouse.gov/sites/default/files/ondcp/policy-and-research/rx_abuse_plan.pdf
3. Understanding Drug Abuse and Addiction. DrugFacts. National Institute of Drug Abuse; 2012. http://www.drugabuse.gov/publications/drugfacts/understanding-drug-abuse-addiction
4. Principles of Drug Addiction Treatment: A Research-Based Guide (Third Edition). National Institute on Drug Abuse; 2012. http://www.drugabuse.gov/publications/principles-drug-addiction-treatment-research-based-guide-third-edition/principles-effective-treatment
5. Women and Alcohol. National Institute on Alcohol Abuse and Alcoholism; 2013. http://pubs.niaaa.nih.gov/publications/womensfact/womensfact.htm
6. Black S, Jacques K, Webber A, et al. Chair massage for treating anxiety in patients withdrawing from psychoactive drugs. *Journal of Alternative and Complementary Medicine* 2010;16(9):979–987. http://www.ncbi.nlm.nih.gov/pubmed/20799900
7. Marley D. Chemical Addiction, Drug Use, and Treatment. Medscape. http://www.medscape.org/viewarticle/418525. Accessed Summer 2014.
8. Prater CD, Zylstra RG, Miller KE. Successful pain management for the recovering addicted patient. *Primary Care Companion to the Journal of Clinical Psychiatry* 2002;4(4):125–131. http://www.ncbi.nlm.nih.gov/pmc/articles/PMC315480/

9. Reader M, Young R, Connor JP. Massage therapy improves the management of alcohol withdrawal syndrome. *Journal of Alternative and Complementary Medicine* 2005;11(2):311–313. http://www.ncbi.nlm.nih.gov/pubmed/15865498
10. Thompson W. Alcoholism. Medscape; 2014. http://emedicine.medscape.com/article/285913-overview

Alzheimer Disease

1. Alzheimer's Myths. Alzheimer's Association. http://www.alz.org/alzheimers_disease_myths_about_alzheimers.asp. Accessed Summer 2014.
2. About Alzheimer's Disease: Treatment. Alzheimer's Disease Education and Referral Center. National Institute on Aging. http://www.nia.nih.gov/alzheimers/topics/treatment. Accessed Summer 2014.
3. About Alzheimer's Disease: Symptoms. Alzheimer's Disease Education and Referral Center. National Institute on Aging. http://www.nia.nih.gov/alzheimers/topics/symptoms. Accessed Summer 2014.
4. 10 Early Signs and Symptoms of Alzheimer's. Alzheimer's Association. http://www.alz.org/alzheimers_disease_10_signs_of_alzheimers.asp. Accessed Summer 2014.
5. Alzheimer's Facts and Figures. Alzheimer's Association; 2014. http://www.alz.org/alzheimers_disease_facts_and_figures.asp
6. Alzheimer's disease. Diseases and Conditions. Mayo Clinic; 2014. http://www.mayoclinic.org/diseases-conditions/alzheimers-disease/basics/definition/con-20023871
7. Anderson HS. Alzheimer Disease. Medscape; 2014. http://emedicine.medscape.com/article/1134817-overview
8. Behrman S, Chouliaras L, Ebmeier KP. Considering the senses in the diagnosis and management of dementia. *Maturitas* 2014;77(4):305–310. http://www.ncbi.nlm.nih.gov/pubmed/24495787
9. Harris M, Richards KC. The physiological and psychological effects of slow-stroke back massage and hand massage on relaxation in older people. *Journal of Clinical Nursing* 2010;19(7–8):917–926. http://www.ncbi.nlm.nih.gov/pubmed/20492036
10. Rowe M, Alfred D. The effectiveness of slow-stroke massage in diffusing agitated behaviors in individuals with Alzheimer's disease. *Journal of Gerontological Nursing* 1999;25(6):22–34. http://www.ncbi.nlm.nih.gov/pubmed/10603811
11. Walter C, Edwards NE, Griggs R, et al. Differentiating Alzheimer disease, Lewy body, and Parkinson dementia using DSM-5. *Journal for Nurse Practitioners* 2014;10(4):262–270. http://www.medscape.com/viewarticle/823809

Amyotrophic Lateral Sclerosis

1. Amyotrophic Lateral Sclerosis (ALS). American Speech-Language-Hearing Association. http://www.asha.org/public/speech/disorders/ALS.htm. Accessed Summer 2014.
2. Amyotrophic lateral sclerosis. A.D.A.M. Medical Encyclopedia. U.S. National Library of Medicine; 2012. http://www.ncbi.nlm.nih.gov/pubmedhealth/PMH0001708/
3. Amyotrophic Lateral Sclerosis (ALS) Fact Sheet. Disorders A-Z. National Institute of Neurological Disorders and Stroke; 2014. http://www.ninds.nih.gov/disorders/amyotrophiclateralsclerosis/detail_ALS.htm
4. Armon C. Amyotrophic Lateral Sclerosis. Medscape; 2014. http://emedicine.medscape.com/article/1170097-overview
5. Blatzheim K. Interdisciplinary palliative care, including massage, in treatment of amyotrophic lateral sclerosis. *Journal of Bodywork and Movement Therapies* 2009;13(4):328–335. http://www.ncbi.nlm.nih.gov/pubmed/19761955
6. Brites D, Vaz AR. Microglia centered pathogenesis in ALS: insights in cell interconnectivity. *Frontiers in Cellular Neuroscience* 2014;8:117. http://www.ncbi.nlm.nih.gov/pmc/articles/PMC4033073/
7. Carter GT. Rehabilitation Management of Neuromuscular Disease; 2014. http://emedicine.medscape.com/article/321397-overview
8. Coggrave M, Norton C, Cody JD. Management of faecal incontinence and constipation in adults with central neurological diseases. *Cochrane Database of Systematic Reviews* 2014;(1):CD002115. http://www.ncbi.nlm.nih.gov/pubmed/24420006
9. McClurg D, Lowe-Strong A. Does abdominal massage relieve constipation? *Nursing Times* 2011;107(12):20–22. http://www.ncbi.nlm.nih.gov/pubmed/21520798
10. Negahban H, Rezaie S, Goharpey S. Massage therapy and exercise therapy in patients with multiple sclerosis: a randomized controlled pilot study. *Clinical Rehabilitation* 2013;27(12):1126–1136. http://www.ncbi.nlm.nih.gov/pubmed/23828184
11. Pan W, Chen X, Bao J, et al. The use of integrative therapies in patients with amyotrophic lateral sclerosis in Shanghai, China. *Evidence-Based Complementary and Alternative Medicine* 2013;2013:613596. http://www.ncbi.nlm.nih.gov/pmc/articles/PMC3865630/

Anxiety Disorders

1. Generalized Anxiety Disorder (GAD). Understanding the Facts: Anxiety and Depression Association of America. http://www.adaa.org/understanding-anxiety/generalized-anxiety-disorder-gad. Accessed Summer 2014.
2. DSM-5: Changes to the Diagnostic and Statistical Manual of Mental Disorders. Understanding the Facts: Anxiety and Depression Association of America. http://www.adaa.org/understanding-anxiety/DSM-5-changes
3. Social anxiety disorder (social phobia). Diseases and Conditions. Mayo Clinic; 2011. http://www.mayoclinic.org/diseases-conditions/social-anxiety-disorder/basics/definition/con-20032524
4. Obsessive-compulsive disorder (OCD). Diseases and Conditions. Mayo Clinic; 2013. http://www.mayoclinic.org/diseases-conditions/ocd/basics/definition/con-20027827
5. Bogels SM, Knappe S, Clark LA. Adult separation anxiety disorder in DSM-5. *Clinical Psychology Review* 2013;33(5):663–674. http://www.sciencedirect.com/science/article/pii/S0272735813000469
6. Brasic JR. Pediatric Obsessive-Compulsive Disorder. Medscape; 2012. http://emedicine.medscape.com/article/1826591-overview
7. Burstein M, Ameli-Grillon L, Merikangas KR. Shyness versus social phobia in US youth. *Pediatrics* 2011;128(5):917–925. http://pediatrics.aappublications.org/content/128/5/917.long
8. Cutshall SM, Wentworth LJ, Engen D, et al. Effect of massage therapy on pain, anxiety, and tension in cardiac surgical patients: a pilot study. *Complementary Therapies in Clinical Practice* 2010;16(2):92–95. http://www.ncbi.nlm.nih.gov/pubmed/20347840

9. Hatayama T, Kitamura S, Tamura C, et al. The facial massage reduced anxiety and negative mood status, and increased sympathetic nervous activity. *Biomedical Research* 2008;29(6):317–320. https://www.jstage.jst.go.jp/article/biomedres/29/6/29_6_317/_pdf
10. Morgan AJ, Jorm AF. Outcomes of self-help efforts in anxiety disorders. *Expert Review of Pharmacoeconomics and Outcomes Research* 2009;9(5):445–459. http://www.medscape.com/viewarticle/711635
11. Price C. Body-oriented therapy in recovery from child sexual abuse: an efficacy study. *Alternative Therapies in Health and Medicine* 2005;11(5):46–57. http://www.ncbi.nlm.nih.gov/pmc/articles/PMC1933482/
12. Sherman KJ, Ludman EJ, Cook AJ, et al. Effectiveness of therapeutic massage for generalized anxiety disorder: a randomized controlled trial. *Depression and Anxiety* 2010;27(5):441–450. http://www.ncbi.nlm.nih.gov/pmc/articles/PMC2922919/
13. Yates WR. Pediatric Specific Phobia. Medscape; 2013. http://emedicine.medscape.com/article/917056-overview
14. Yates WR. Anxiety Disorders. Medscape; 2014. http://emedicine.medscape.com/article/286227-overview

Attention Deficit Hyperactivity Disorder

1. Attention Deficit Hyperactivity Disorder. Health and Education. National Institute of Mental Health; 2012. http://www.nimh.nih.gov/health/publications/attention-deficit-hyperactivity-disorder/index.shtml
2. Brooks M. 'Meta-Cognitive' Therapy Effective for Adult ADHD. Medscape; 2010. http://www.medscape.com/viewarticle/718932
3. DeSimone EM. Adult ADHD: treatment of a grown-up disorder. *US Pharmacist* 2014;39(1):52–57. http://www.medscape.com/viewarticle/822549
4. Hamre HJ, Witt CM, Kienle GS, et al. Anthroposophic therapy for attention deficit hyperactivity: a two-year prospective study in outpatients. *International Journal of General Medicine* 2010;3:239–253. http://www.ncbi.nlm.nih.gov/pubmed/20830200
5. Maddigan B, Hodgson P, Heath S, et al. The effects of massage therapy & exercise therapy on children/adolescents with attention deficit hyperactivity disorder. *Canadian Child and Adolescent Psychiatry Review* 2003;12(2):40–43. http://www.ncbi.nlm.nih.gov/pmc/articles/PMC2538473/
6. Rabiner D. New Diagnostic Criteria for ADHD. Attention Deficit Disorder Association. http://www.add.org/?page=DiagnosticCriteria. Accessed Summer 2014.
7. Scudder L. The Changing Epidemiology of ADHD: an expert interview with Susanna Visser, MS. Medscape; 2011. http://www.medscape.com/viewarticle/735440
8. Soreff S. Attention Deficit Hyperactivity Disorder. Medscape; 2014. http://emedicine.medscape.com/article/289350-overview

Autism Spectrum Disorders

1. Autism Spectrum Disorder. American Psychiatric Association; 2013. http://www.dsm5.org/Documents/Autism%20Spectrum%20Disorder%20Fact%20Sheet.pdf
2. Autism Spectrum Disorder (ASD): Overview. Health & Research. Eunice Kennedy Shriver National Institute of Child Health and Human Development; 2014. http://www.nichd.nih.gov/health/topics/autism/Pages/default.aspx
3. Facts About ASD. Autism Spectrum Disorder (ASD); 2014. http://www.cdc.gov/ncbddd/autism/facts.html
4. Autism Spectrum Disorder (ASD): Condition Information. Health & Research. Eunice Kennedy Shriver National Institute of Child Health and Human Development; 2014. http://www.nichd.nih.gov/health/topics/autism/conditioninfo/Pages/default.aspx
5. Brasic JR. Autism. Medscape; 2014. http://emedicine.medscape.com/article/912781-overview
6. Carpenter L. DSM-5 Autism Spectrum Disorder Guidelines & Criteria Exemplars. University of Washington; 2013. https://depts.washington.edu/dbpeds/Screening%20Tools/DSM-5(ASD.Guidelines)Feb2013.pdf
7. Lee MS, Kim JI, Ernst E. Massage therapy for children with autism spectrum disorders: a systematic review. *Journal of Clinical Psychiatry* 2011;72(3):406–411. http://www.ncbi.nlm.nih.gov/pubmed/21208598
8. McLay LL, France K. Empirical research evaluating non-traditional approaches to managing sleep problems in children with autism. *Developmental Neurorehabilitation* 2014 (electronic publication ahead of print). http://www.ncbi.nlm.nih.gov/pubmed/24724691
9. Silva L, Schalock M. Treatment of tactile impairment in young children with autism: results with qigong massage. *International Journal of Therapeutic Massage and Bodywork* 2013;6(4):12–20. http://www.ncbi.nlm.nih.gov/pmc/articles/PMC3838308/

Bell Palsy

1. Bell's Palsy Fact Sheet. Disorders A-Z. National Institute of Neurological Disorders and Stroke; 2014. http://www.ninds.nih.gov/disorders/bells/detail_bells.htm
2. Gronseth GS, Paduga R. Evidence-based guideline update: steroids and antivirals for Bell palsy: report of the Guideline Development Subcommittee of the American Academy of Neurology. *Neurology* 2012;79(22):2209–2213. http://www.neurology.org/content/early/2012/11/07/WNL.0b013e318275978c.full.pdf+html
3. Lindsay RW, Robinson M, Hadlock TA. Comprehensive facial rehabilitation improves function in people with facial paralysis: a 5-year experience at the Massachusetts Eye and Ear Infirmary. *Physical Therapy* 2010;90(3):391–397. http://ptjournal.apta.org/content/90/3/391.long
4. Manikandan N. Effect of facial neuromuscular re-education on facial symmetry in patients with Bell's palsy: a randomized controlled trial. *Clinical Rehabilitation* 2007;21(4):338–343. http://www.ncbi.nlm.nih.gov/pubmed/17613574
5. Shafshak TS. The treatment of facial palsy from the point of view of physical and rehabilitation medicine. *Europa Medicophysica* 2006;42(1):41–47. http://www.ncbi.nlm.nih.gov/pubmed/16565685
6. Taylor DC. Bell Palsy. Medscape; 2013. http://emedicine.medscape.com/article/1146903-overview
7. Teixeira LJ, Valbuza JS, Prado GF. Physical therapy for Bell's palsy (idiopathic facial paralysis). *Cochrane Database of Systematic Reviews* 2011;(12):CD006283. http://www.ncbi.nlm.nih.gov/pubmed/22161401

Bipolar

1. Bipolar Disorder in Adults. Health and Education. National Institute of Mental Health; 2012. http://www.nimh.nih.gov/health/publications/bipolar-disorder-in-adults/index.shtml

2. Mixed Features Specifier. American Psychiatric Association; 2013. http://www.dsm5.org/Documents/Mixed%20Features%20Specifier%20Fact%20Sheet.pdf
3. Cheney T. The Bipolar Lens. Psychology Today; 2013. http://www.psychologytoday.com/blog/the-bipolar-lens/201301/insiders-tips-how-not-treat-bipolar-disorder
4. Tartakovsky M. Bipolar Disorder Fact Sheet. Psych Central; 2009. http://psychcentral.com/lib/bipolar-disorder-fact-sheet/0001561

Cerebral Palsy

1. Prevalance and Incidence of Cerebral Palsy. MyChild; http://cerebralpalsy.org/about-cerebral-palsy/prevalence-of-cerebral-palsy/. Accessed Summer 2014.
2. Cerebral Palsy. Diseases and Conditions. Mayo Clinic; 2013. http://www.mayoclinic.org/diseases-conditions/cerebral-palsy/basics/definition/con-20030502
3. Cerebral Palsy: Hope Through Research. Disorders A-Z. National Institute of Neurological Disorders and Stroke; 2014. http://www.ninds.nih.gov/disorders/cerebral_palsy/detail_cerebral_palsy.htm
4. Cerebral Palsy (CP). Centers for Disease Control and Prevention; 2014. http://www.cdc.gov/ncbddd/cp/index.html
5. Glew GM, Fan MY, Hagland S, et al. Survey of the use of massage for children with cerebral palsy. *International Journal of Therapeutic Massage and Bodywork* 2010;3(4):10–15. http://www.ncbi.nlm.nih.gov/pmc/articles/PMC3088521/
6. Macgregor R, Campbell R, Gladden MH, et al. Effects of massage on the mechanical behaviour of muscles in adolescents with spastic diplegia: a pilot study. *Developmental Medicine and Child Neurology* 2007;49(3):187–191. http://www.ncbi.nlm.nih.gov/pubmed/17355474
7. Powell L, Cheshire A, Swaby L. Children's experiences of their participation in a training and support programme involving massage. *Complementary Therapies in Clinical Practice* 2010;16(1):47–51. http://www.ncbi.nlm.nih.gov/pubmed/20129410
8. Thorogood C. Rehabilitation and Cerebral Palsy. Medscape; 2013. http://emedicine.medscape.com/article/310740-overview
9. Werner R. Adults with Cerebral Palsy: It's Not Just a Children's Condition. Massage and Bodywork; 2012(November/December). http://www.abmp.com/textonlymags/article.php?article=558

Complex Regional Pain Syndrome

1. Description—Four Stages of CRPS. American RSDHope. http://www.rsdhope.org/crps-stages.html. Accessed Summer 2014.
2. Reflex Sympathetic Dystrophy/Complex Regional Pain Syndromes (SRPS): State-of-the-Science. News from NINDS. National Institute of Neurological Disorders and Stroke; 2011. http://www.ninds.nih.gov/news_and_events/proceedings/reflex_sympathetic_dystrophy_2001.htm
3. Complex regional pain syndrome. Diseases and Conditions. Mayo Clinic; 2014. http://www.mayoclinic.org/diseases-conditions/complex-regional-pain-syndrome/basics/definition/con-20022844
4. Duman I, Ozdemir A, Tan AK, et al. The efficacy of manual lymphatic drainage therapy in the management of limb edema secondary to reflex sympathetic dystrophy. *Rheumatology International* 2009;29(7):759–763. http://www.ncbi.nlm.nih.gov/pubmed/19030864
5. Lee J, Nandi P. Early aggressive treatment improves prognosis in complex regional pain syndrome. *Practitioner* 2011;255(1736):23–26. http://www.ncbi.nlm.nih.gov/pubmed/21370711
6. Safaz I, Tok F, Taskaynatan MA, et al. Manual lymphatic drainage in management of edema in a case with CRPS: why the(y) wait? *Rheumatology International* 2011;31(3):387–390. http://www.ncbi.nlm.nih.gov/pubmed/19823831
7. Singh MK. Physical Medicine and Rehabilitation for Complex Regional Pain Syndromes. Medscape; 2013. http://emedicine.medscape.com/article/328054-overview
8. Weeler AH. Complex Regional Pain Syndromes. Medscape; 2012. http://emedicine.medscape.com/article/1145318-overview

Depression

1. Massage Therapy for Depression. Reproductive Psychiatry Resource and Information Center. MGH Center for Women's Mental Health; 2010. http://womensmentalhealth.org/posts/massage-therapy-for-depression/
2. Depression. Health and Education. National Institute of Mental Health; 2011. http://www.nimh.nih.gov/health/publications/depression/index.shtml
3. Major Depression. A.D.A.M Medical Encyclopedia. U.S. National Library of Medicine; 2014. http://www.ncbi.nlm.nih.gov/pubmedhealth/PMH0001941/
4. Babaee S, Shafiei Z, Sadeghi MM, et al. Effectiveness of massage therapy on the mood of patients after open-heart surgery. *Iranian Journal of Nursing and Midwifery Research* 2012;17(2 Suppl 1):S120–S124. http://www.ncbi.nlm.nih.gov/pmc/articles/PMC3696961/
5. Falkensteiner M, Mantovan F, Muller I, Them C. The use of massage therapy for reducing pain, anxiety, and depression in oncological palliative care patients: a narrative review of the literature. *ISRN Nursing* 2011;2011:929868. http://www.ncbi.nlm.nih.gov/pmc/articles/PMC3168862/
6. Halverson JL. Depression. Medscape; 2014. http://emedicine.medscape.com/article/286759-overview
7. Hou WH, Chiang PT, Hsu TY, et al. Treatment effects of massage therapy in depressed people: a meta-analysis. *Journal of Clinical Psychiatry* 2010;71(7):894–901. http://www.ncbi.nlm.nih.gov/pubmed/20361919
8. Joy S. Postpartum Depression. Medscape; 2014. http://reference.medscape.com/article/271662-overview
9. Li YH, Wang FY, Feng CQ, et al. Massage therapy for fibromyalgia: a systematic review and meta-analysis of randomized controlled trials. *PLoS One* 2014;9(2):e89304. http://www.ncbi.nlm.nih.gov/pmc/articles/PMC3930706/
10. Munk N, Kruger T, Zanjani F. Massage therapy usage and reported health in older adults experiencing persistent pain. *Journal of Alternative and Complementary Medicine* 2011;17(7):609–616. http://www.ncbi.nlm.nih.gov/pubmed/21668368
11. Oliveira DS, Hachul H, Goto V, et al. Effect of therapeutic massage on insomnia and climacteric symptoms in postmenopausal women. *Climacteric* 2012;15(1):21–29. http://www.ncbi.nlm.nih.gov/pubmed/22017318
12. Vale S. Depressive symptoms, risk of stroke and the stress response. *Stroke* 2007;38(6):e34. http://stroke.ahajournals.org/content/38/6/e34.full

13. Varghese FP, Brown ES. The hypothalamic-pituitary-adrenal axis in major depressive disorder: a brief primer for primary care physicians. *Primary Care Companion to the Journal of Clinical Psychiatry* 2001;3(4):151–155. http://www.ncbi.nlm.nih.gov/pmc/articles/PMC181180/

Dystonia

1. Dystonia. Diseases and Conditions. Mayo Clinic; 2012. http://www.mayoclinic.org/diseases-conditions/dystonia/basics/definition/con-20033527
2. Dystonias Fact Sheet. Disorders A-Z. National Institute of Neurological Disorders and Stroke; 2012. http://www.ninds.nih.gov/disorders/dystonias/detail_dystonias.htm
3. What is Dystonia? Dystonia Medical Research Foundation; 2012. http://50.115.120.214/~dystonia/images/uploads/DMRF_What_Is_Dystonia_brochure_FINAL.pdf
4. Garcia L. My battle with spasmodic torticollis: a healing experience. *Holistic Nursing Practice* 2006;20(6):275–281. http://www.ncbi.nlm.nih.gov/pubmed/17099415
5. Kang Y, Lu S, Li J, et al. Primary massage using one-finger twining manipulation for treatment of infantile muscular torticollis. *Journal of Alternative and Complementary Medicine* 2011;17(3):231–237. http://www.ncbi.nlm.nih.gov/pubmed/21381962
6. Kruer MC. Torticollis. Medscape; 2014. http://emedicine.medscape.com/article/1152543-overview
7. Loyola DP, Camargos S, Maia D, et al. Sensory tricks in focal dystonia and hemifacial spasm. *European Journal of Neurology* 2013;20(4):704–707. http://www.ncbi.nlm.nih.gov/pubmed/23216586
8. Moberg-Wolff EA. Dystonias. Medscape; 2014. http://emedicine.medscape.com/article/312648-overview
9. Nordqvist C. What is dystonia? What causes dystonia? Medical News Today; 2014. http://www.medicalnewstoday.com/articles/171354.php

Eating Disorders

1. Body image. WomensHealth.gov. Office on Women's Health, U.S. Department of Health and Human Services; 2009. http://www.womenshealth.gov/body-image/
2. Eating Disorders. Health & Education. National Institute of Mental Health; 2011. http://www.nimh.nih.gov/health/publications/eating-disorders/index.shtml
3. Anorexia nervosa fact sheet. WomensHealth.gov. Office on Women's Health, U.S. Department of Health and Human Services; 2012. http://www.womenshealth.gov/publications/our-publications/fact-sheet/anorexia-nervosa.html
4. Binge Eating Disorder Fact Sheet. WomensHealth.gov. Office on Women's Health, U.S. Department of Health and Human Services; 2012. http://www.womenshealth.gov/publications/our-publications/fact-sheet/binge-eating-disorder.html
5. Bulimia nervosa fact sheet. WomensHealth.gov. Office on Women's Health, U.S. Department of Health and Human Services; 2012. http://www.womenshealth.gov/publications/our-publications/fact-sheet/bulimia-nervosa.html
6. Feeding and Eating Disorders. DSM5.org. American Psychiatric Association; 2013. http://www.dsm5.org/Documents/Eating%20Disorders%20Fact%20Sheet.pdf
7. Eating Disorder Information. Academy for Eating Disorders; 2014. http://aedweb.org/web/index.php/education/eating-disorder-information/eating-disorder-information-2
8. Chu SM, Gustafson KE, Leiszler M. Female Athlete Triad: clinical evaluation and treatment. *American Journal of Lifestyle Medicine* 2013;7(6):387–394. http://www.medscape.com/viewarticle/814607
9. Fogarty S, Smith CA, Touyz S, et al. Patients with anorexia nervosa receiving acupuncture or acupressure; their view of the therapeutic encounter. *Complementary Therapies in Medicine* 2013;21(6):675–681. http://www.ncbi.nlm.nih.gov/pubmed/24280477
10. Smith C, Fogarty S, Touyz S, et al. Acupuncture and acupressure and massage health outcomes for patients with anorexia nervosa: findings from a pilot randomized controlled trial and patient interviews. *Journal of Alternative and Complementary Medicine* 2014;20(2):103–112. http://www.ncbi.nlm.nih.gov/pubmed/24102480
11. Varga M, Thege BK, Dukay-Szabo S, et al. When eating healthy is not healthy: orthorexia nervosa and its measurement with the ORTO-15 in Hungary. *BMC Psychiatry* 2014;14:59. http://www.ncbi.nlm.nih.gov/pmc/articles/PMC3943279/

Encephalitis

1. West Nile Virus. Diseases and Conditions. Mayo Clinic; 2012. http://www.mayoclinic.org/diseases-conditions/west-nile-virus/basics/definition/con-20023076
2. Encephalitis. Diseases and Conditions. Mayo Clinic; 2014. http://www.mayoclinic.org/diseases-conditions/encephalitis/basics/definition/con-20021917
3. Meningitis and Encephalitis Fact Sheet. Disorders A-Z. National Institute of Neurological Disorder and Stroke; 2014. http://www.ninds.nih.gov/disorders/encephalitis_meningitis/detail_encephalitis_meningitis.htm
4. Cunha BA. West Nile Encephalitis. Medscape; 2014. http://emedicine.medscape.com/article/234009-overview
5. Gondim FdAA. Viral Encephalitis. Medscape; 2013. http://reference.medscape.com/article/1166498-overview

Fibromyalgia

1. 2010 Fibromyalgia Diagnostic Criteria—Exceprt. American College of Rheumatology; 2010. http://www.rheumatology.org/ACR/practice/clinical/classification/fibromyalgia/fibro_2010.asp
2. Fibromyalgia and Complementary Health Approaches. National Center for Complementary and Alternative Medicine; 2013. http://nccam.nih.gov/health/pain/fibromyalgia.htm
3. Questions and Answers About Fibromyalgia. National Institute of Arthritis and Musculoskeletal and Skin Diseases; 2014. http://www.niams.nih.gov/Health_Info/Fibromyalgia/
4. Boomershine CS. Fibromyalgia. Medscape; 2014. http://emedicine.medscape.com/article/329838-overview
5. Castro-Sanchez AM, Mataran-Penarrocha GA, Granero-Molina J, et al. Benefits of massage-myofascial release therapy on pain, anxiety, quality of sleep, depression, and quality of life in patients with fibromyalgia. *Evidence-Based Complementary and Alternative Medicine* 2011;2011:561753. http://www.ninds.nih.gov/disorders/spina_bifida/detail_spina_bifida.htm
6. Grimm L. Fibromyalgia: Slideshow. Medscape; 2014. http://reference.medscape.com/features/slideshow/fibromyalgia?src=wnl_ref_clinfo&uac=78486SY#11
7. Kalichman L. Massage therapy for fibromyalgia symptoms. *Rheumatology International* 2010;30(9):1151–1157. http://www.ncbi.nlm.nih.gov/pubmedhealth/PMH0029074/

8. Li YH, Wang FY, Feng CQ, et al. Massage therapy for fibromyalgia: a systematic review and meta-analysis of randomized controlled trials. *PLoS One* 2014;9(2):e89304. http://www.ncbi.nlm.nih.gov/pmc/articles/PMC3930706/
9. Smith HS, Harris R, Clauw D. Fibromyalgia: an afferent processing disorder leading to a complex pain generalized syndrome. *Pain Physician* 2011;14(2):E217–E245. http://www.painphysicianjournal.com/linkout_vw.php?issn=1533-3159&vol=14&page=E217

Headache

1. IHS Classification ICHD-II. International Headache Society. http://ihs-classification.org/en/02_klassifikation/. Accessed Winter 2014.
2. Headaches and Complementary Health Approaches. Health Info. National Center for Complementary and Integrative Health; 2012. https://nccih.nih.gov/health/pain/headachefacts.htm
3. Cluster headache. Diseases and Conditions. Mayo Clinic; 2013. http://www.mayoclinic.org/diseases-conditions/cluster-headache/basics/definition/con-20031706
4. Headache: Hope Through Research. Disorders A-Z. National Institute of Neurological Disorders and Stroke; 2014. http://www.ninds.nih.gov/disorders/headache/detail_headache.htm
5. Blanda M. Cluster Headache. Medscape; 2014. http://emedicine.medscape.com/article/1142459-overview
6. Chatchawan U, Eungpinichpong W, Sooktho S, et al. Effects of Thai traditional massage on pressure pain threshold and headache intensity in patients with chronic tension-type and migraine headaches. *Journal of Alternative and Complementary Medicine* 2014;20(6):486–492. http://www.ncbi.nlm.nih.gov/pubmed/24738648
7. Chawla J. Migraine Headache. Medscape; 2014. http://emedicine.medscape.com/article/1142556-overview
8. Hopper D, Bajaj Y, Kei Choi C, et al. A pilot study to investigate the short-term effects of specific soft tissue massage on upper cervical movement impairment in patients with cervicogenic headache. *Journal of Manual and Manipulative Therapy* 2013;21(1):18–23. http://www.ncbi.nlm.nih.gov/pmc/articles/PMC3578191/
9. Lopez JI. Pediatric Headache. Medscape; 2014. http://emedicine.medscape.com/article/2110861-overview
10. Mitchell WG. Childhood Migraine Variants. Medscape; 2014. http://emedicine.medscape.com/article/1178141-overview
11. Moraska A, Chandler C. Changes in psychological parameters in patients with tension-type headache following massage therapy: a pilot study. *Journal of Manual and Manipulative Therapy* 2009;17(2):86–94. http://www.ncbi.nlm.nih.gov/pmc/articles/PMC2700492/
12. Noudeh YJ, Vatankhah N, Baradaran HR. Reduction of current migraine headache pain following neck massage and spinal manipulation. *International Journal of Therapeutic Massage and Bodywork* 2012;5(1):5–13. http://www.ncbi.nlm.nih.gov/pmc/articles/PMC3312646/
13. Singh MK. Muscle Contraction Tension Headache. Medscape; 2013. http://emedicine.medscape.com/article/1142908-overview
14. Youssef EF, Shanb AS. Mobilization versus massage therapy in the treatment of cervicogenic headache: a clinical study. *Journal of Back and Musculoskeletal Rehabilitation* 2013;26(1):17–24. http://www.ncbi.nlm.nih.gov/pubmed/23411644

Herpes Zoster

1. Shingles (Herpes Zoster). Centers for Disease Control and Prevention; 2014. http://www.cdc.gov/shingles/hcp/clinical-overview.html
2. Shingles. Diseases and Conditions. Mayo Clinic; 2014. http://www.mayoclinic.org/diseases-conditions/shingles/basics/definition/con-20019574
3. Varicella (Chickenpox). Vaccine Safety. Centers for Disease Control and Prevention; 2014. http://www.cdc.gov/vaccinesafety/vaccines/varicella/
4. Anderson WE. Varicella-Zoster Virus. Medscape; 2014. http://emedicine.medscape.com/article/231927-overview
5. Janniger CK. Herpes Zoster. Medscape; 2014. http://emedicine.medscape.com/article/1132465-overview
6. McElveen WA. Postherpetic Neuralgia. Medscape; 2014. http://emedicine.medscape.com/article/1143066-overview

Huntington Disease

1. What is Huntington's Disease (HD)? Huntington's Disease Society of America. http://www.hdsa.org/about/our-mission/what-is-hd.html. Accessed Winter 2015.
2. Huntington's Disease: Hope Through Research. Disorders A-Z. National Institute of Neurological Disorders and Stroke; 2015. http://www.ninds.nih.gov/disorders/huntington/detail_huntington.htm
3. Im W, Kim M. Cell therapy strategies vs. paracrine effect in Huntington's disease. *Journal of Movement Disorders* 2014;7(1):1–6. http://www.ncbi.nlm.nih.gov/pmc/articles/PMC4051721/
4. Nance M, Paulsen JS, Rosenblatt A, et al. A Physician's Guide to the Management of Huntington's Disease. Huntington's Disease Society of America; 2011. http://www.hdsa.org/images/content/1/6/16692/HDSAPhysDeskRef_11_web.pdf
5. Sharon I. Huntington Disease Dementia. Medscape; 2014. http://emedicine.medscape.com/article/289706-overview

Meniere Disease

1. Meniere's Disease in Brief. Meniere's Disease Information Center. http://www.menieresinfo.com/start.html. Accessed Winter 2015.
2. NIDCD Fact Sheet: Ménière's Disease. National Institute on Deafness and Other Communication Disorders; 2010. http://www.nidcd.nih.gov/staticresources/health/hearing/MeineresFS.pdf
3. Ménière's disease. A.D.A.M. Medical Encyclopedia. U.S. National Library of Medicine; 2013. http://www.ncbi.nlm.nih.gov/pubmedhealth/PMH0001721/
4. Li JC. Meniere Disease (Idiopathic Endolymphatic Hydrops). Medscape; 2014. http://emedicine.medscape.com/article/1159069-overview
5. Orji F. The influence of psychological factors in Meniere's disease. *Annals of Medical and Health Sciences Research* 2014;4(1):3–7. http://www.ncbi.nlm.nih.gov/pmc/articles/PMC3952292/

Meningitis

1. Encephalitis. Diseases and Conditions. Mayo Clinic; 2014. http://www.mayoclinic.org/diseases-conditions/encephalitis/basics/definition/con-20021917
2. Meningitis. Centers for Disease Control and Prevention; 2014. http://www.cdc.gov/meningitis/clinical-resources.html

3. Chihara S. Common Organisms by Patient Population in Bacterial Meningitis. Medscape; 2013. http://emedicine.medscape.com/article/1953111-overview
4. Hasbun R. Meningitis. Medscape; 2015. http://emedicine.medscape.com/article/232915-overview
5. Wan C. Viral Meningitis. Medscape; 2013. http://emedicine.medscape.com/article/1168529-overview

Obsessive-Compulsive Disorders

1. OCD And Related Disorders Community. HealthyPlace.com. http://www.healthyplace.com/ocd-related-disorders/. Accessed Summer 2014.
2. Disorders Related to OCD. International OCD Foundation; 2012. http://www.ocfoundation.org/relateddisorders.aspx
3. Obsessive-Compulsive Disorder. NIH Fact Sheets. National Institutes of Health; 2013. http://report.nih.gov/nihfactsheets/viewfactsheet.aspx?csid=54&key=o#o
4. Obsessive Compulsive and Related Disorders. American Psychiatric Association; 2013. http://www.dsm5.org/Documents/Obsessive%20Compulsive%20Disorders%20Fact%20Sheet.pdf
5. Elston DM. Trichotillomania. Medscape; 2014. http://emedicine.medscape.com/article/1071854-overview
6. Goodman WK. Obsessive-Compulsive Disorder. OCD Information & Treatment. Psych Central; 2013. http://psychcentral.com/disorders/ocd/
7. Murphy DL, Timpano KR, Wheaton MG, et al. Obsessive-compulsive disorder and its related disorders: a reappraisal of obsessive-compulsive spectrum concepts. *Dialogues in Clinical Neuroscience* 2010;12(2):131–148. http://www.ncbi.nlm.nih.gov/pmc/articles/PMC3181955/
8. Scheinfeld NS. Excoriation Disorder. Medscape; 2013. http://emedicine.medscape.com/article/1122042-overview

Parkinson Disease

1. Parkinson's Disease: Hope Through Research. Disorders A-Z. National Institute of Neurological Disorders and Stroke; 2014. http://www.ninds.nih.gov/disorders/parkinsons_disease/detail_parkinsons_disease.htm
2. Parkinson's Disease. Diseases and Conditions. Mayo Clinic; 2014. http://www.mayoclinic.org/diseases-conditions/parkinsons-disease/basics/definition/con-20028488
3. Coggrave M, Norton C, Cody JD. Management of faecal incontinence and constipation in adults with central neurological diseases. *Cochrane Database of Systematic Reviews* 2014;(1):CD002115. http://www.ncbi.nlm.nih.gov/pubmed/24420006
4. Craig LH, Svircev A, Haber M, et al. Controlled pilot study of the effects of neuromuscular therapy in patients with Parkinson's disease. *Movement Disorders* 2006;21(12):2127–2133. http://www.ncbi.nlm.nih.gov/pubmed/17044088
5. Donoyama N, Ohkoshi N. Effects of traditional Japanese massage therapy on various symptoms in patients with Parkinson's disease: a case-series study. *Journal of Alternative and Complementary Medicine* 2012;18(3):294–299. http://www.ncbi.nlm.nih.gov/pubmed/22385078
6. Duval C, Lafontaine D, Hebert J, et al. The effect of Trager therapy on the level of evoked stretch responses in patients with Parkinson's disease and rigidity. *Journal of Manipulative and Physiological Therapeutics* 2002;25(7):455–464. http://www.ncbi.nlm.nih.gov/pubmed/12214187
7. Hauser RA. Parkinson Disease. Medscape; 2014. http://emedicine.medscape.com/article/1831191-overview
8. Paterson C, Allen JA, Browning M, et al. A pilot study of therapeutic massage for people with Parkinson's disease: the added value of user involvement. *Complementary Therapies in Clinical Practice* 2005;11(3):161–171. http://www.ncbi.nlm.nih.gov/pubmed/16005833
9. Rao SS, Hofmann LA, Shakil A. Parkinson's disease: diagnosis and treatment. *American Family Physician* 2006;74(12):2046–2054. http://www.aafp.org/afp/2006/1215/p2046.html
10. Svircev A, Craig LH, Juncos JL. A pilot study examining the effects of neuromuscular therapy on patients with Parkinson's disease. *Journal of the American Osteopathic Association* 2005;105(1):26. http://www.jaoa.osteopathic.org/content/105/1/26.1.long

Peripheral Neuropathy

1. About Peripheral Neuropathy: Facts. The Neuropathy Association. http://www.neuropathy.org/site/PageServer?pagename=About_Facts. Accessed Winter 2015.
2. Alcoholic Neuropathy. A.D.A.M. Medical Encyclopedia. U.S. National Library of Medicine; 2013. http://www.nlm.nih.gov/medlineplus/ency/article/000714.htm
3. Peripheral Neuropathy Fact Sheet. Disorders A-Z. National Institute of Neurological Disorders and Stroke; 2014. http://www.ninds.nih.gov/disorders/peripheralneuropathy/detail_peripheralneuropathy.htm
4. Peripheral Neuropathy. Diseases and Conditions. Mayo Clinic; 2014. http://www.mayoclinic.org/diseases-conditions/peripheral-neuropathy/basics/definition/con-20019948
5. Aslam A, Singh J, Rajbhandari S. Pathogenesis of painful diabetic neuropathy. *Pain Research and Treatment* 2014;2014:412041. http://www.ncbi.nlm.nih.gov/pmc/articles/PMC4026988/
6. Cunningham JE, Kelechi T, Sterba K, et al. Case report of a patient with chemotherapy-induced peripheral neuropathy treated with manual therapy (massage). *Supportive Care in Cancer* 2011;19(9):1473–1476. http://www.ncbi.nlm.nih.gov/pubmed/21766161
7. Poncelet AN. An algorithm for the evaluation of peripheral neuropathy. *American Family Physician* 1998;57(4):755–764. http://www.aafp.org/afp/1998/0215/p755.html
8. Singh NN. HIV-Associated Distal Painful Sensorimotor Polyneuropathy. Medscape; 2013. http://emedicine.medscape.com/article/1167783-overview

Polio

1. Post-Polio Syndrome Fact Sheet. Disorders A-Z. National Institute of Neurological Disorders and Stroke; 2014. http://www.ninds.nih.gov/disorders/post_polio/detail_post_polio.htm
2. Poliomyelitis. World Health Organization; 2014. http://www.who.int/mediacentre/factsheets/fs114/en/
3. Atwal A, Spiliotopoulou G, Coleman C, et al. Polio survivors' perceptions of the meaning of quality of life and strategies used to promote participation in everyday activities. *Health Expectations* 2014 (electronic publication ahead of print). http://www.ncbi.nlm.nih.gov/pubmed/24438097
4. Kedlaya D. Postpolio Syndrome. Medscape; 2013. http://emedicine.medscape.com/article/306920-overview
5. Vidyadhara S. Poliomyelitis. Medscape; 2014. http://emedicine.medscape.com/article/1259213-overview

Seizure Disorders

1. Partial (Focal) Seizures. Epilepsy Center. Johns Hopkins Medicine. http://www.hopkinsmedicine.org/neurology_neurosurgery/centers_clinics/epilepsy/seizures/types/partial-focus-seizures.html. Accessed Winter 2014.
2. Generalized Seizures. Epilepsy Center. Johns Hopkins Medicine. http://www.hopkinsmedicine.org/neurology_neurosurgery/centers_clinics/epilepsy/seizures/types/generalized-seizures.html. Accessed Winter 2014.
3. Epilepsy Frequently Asked Questions. Centers for Disease Control and Prevention; 2013. http://www.cdc.gov/epilepsy/basics/faqs.htm
4. Seizures and Epilepsy: Hope Through Research. Disorders A-Z. National Institute of Neurological Disorders and Stroke; 2014. http://www.ninds.nih.gov/disorders/epilepsy/detail_epilepsy.htm
5. Get Seizure Smart. CDC Features. Centers for Disease Control and Prevention; 2014. http://www.cdc.gov/features/getseizuresmart/
6. Dalal K, Devarajan E, Pandey RM, et al. Role of reflexology and antiepileptic drugs in managing intractable epilepsy—a randomized controlled trial. *Forschende Komplementarmedizin (2006)* 2013;20(2):104–111. http://www.ncbi.nlm.nih.gov/pubmed/23636029
7. Ko DY. Epilepsy and Seizures. Medscape; 2014. http://emedicine.medscape.com/article/1184846-overview
8. Nouri S. Epilepsy and the Autonomic Nervous System. Medscape; 2013. http://emedicine.medscape.com/article/1186872-overview
9. Segan S. Absence Seizures. Medscape; 2013. http://reference.medscape.com/article/1183858-overview
10. Shafer PO. About Epilepsy: The Basics. Epilepsy Foundation; 2014. http://www.epilepsy.com/learn/about-epilepsy-basics
11. Tejani NR. Febrile Seizures. Medscape; 2014. http://emedicine.medscape.com/article/801500-overview

Sleep Disorders

1. Insomnia. Sleep Problems & Disorders. National Sleep Foundation. http://sleepfoundation.org/sleep-disorders-problems/insomnia. Accessed Winter 2014.
2. Narcolepsy and Sleep. Sleep Topics. National Sleep Foundation. http://sleepfoundation.org/sleep-topics/sleep-related-problems/narcolepsy-and-sleep. Accessed Winter 2014.
3. Periodic Limb Movements in Sleep. Sleep Problems & Disorders. National Sleep Foundation. http://sleepfoundation.org/sleep-disorders-problems/sleep-related-movement-disorders/periodic-limb-movement-disorder. Accessed Winter 2014.
4. Restless Legs Syndrome (RLS) and Sleep. Sleep Problems & Disorders. National Sleep Foundation. http://sleepfoundation.org/sleep-disorders-problems/restless-legs-syndrome. Accessed Winter 2014.
5. Sleep Aids and Insomnia. Sleep Problems & Disorders. National Sleep Foundation. http://sleepfoundation.org/sleep-disorders-problems/insomnia/sleep-aids-and-insomnia. Accessed Winter 2014.
6. Sleep Apnea. Diseases and Conditions. Mayo Clinic; 2012. http://www.mayoclinic.org/diseases-conditions/sleep-apnea/basics/definition/con-20020286
7. Key Sleep Disorders. Sleep and Sleep Disorders. Centers for Disease Control and Prevention; 2013. http://www.cdc.gov/sleep/about_sleep/key_disorders.htm
8. Sleep Disorders and Complementary Health Approaches: What You Need To Know. Health Info. National Center for Complementary and Alternative Medicine; 2014. http://nccam.nih.gov/health/sleep/ataglance.htm
9. Restless Legs Syndrome Fact Sheet. Disorders A-Z. National Institute of Neurological Disorders and Stroke; 2014. http://www.ninds.nih.gov/disorders/restless_legs/detail_restless_legs.htm
10. Narcolepsy Fact Sheet. Disorders A-Z. National Institute of Neurological Disorders and Stroke; 2014. http://www.ninds.nih.gov/disorders/narcolepsy/detail_narcolepsy.htm
11. Hill R, Baskwill A. Positive effects of massage therapy on a patient with narcolepsy. *International Journal of Therapeutic Massage and Bodywork* 2013;6(2):24–28. http://ijtmb.org/index.php/ijtmb/article/view/205/256
12. Lubit RH. Sleep Disorders. Medscape; 2014. http://emedicine.medscape.com/article/287104-overview
13. Oliveira D, Hachul H, Tufik S, et al. Effect of massage in postmenopausal women with insomnia: a pilot study. *Clinics (Sao Paulo)* 2011;66(2):343–346. http://www.ncbi.nlm.nih.gov/pmc/articles/PMC3059875/

Spina Bifida

1. Frequently Asked Questions About Spina Bifida. Spina Bifida Association. http://www.kintera.org/site/c.liKWL7PLLrF/b.2642327/k.5899/FAQ_About_Spina_Bifida.htm. Accessed Fall 2014.
2. Spina bifida. March of Dimes; 2014. http://www.marchofdimes.org/baby/spina-bifida.aspx#
3. Spina Bifida Fact Sheet. Disorders A-Z. National Institute of Neurological Disorders and Stroke; 2014. http://www.ninds.nih.gov/disorders/spina_bifida/detail_spina_bifida.htm
4. Spina Bifida. Centers for Disease Control and Prevention; 2014. http://www.cdc.gov/ncbddd/spinabifida/facts.html
5. Adzick NS, Thom EA, Spong CY, et al. A randomized trial of prenatal versus postnatal repair of myelomeningocele. *New England Journal of Medicine* 2011;364(11):993–1004. http://www.nejm.org/doi/full/10.1056/NEJMoa1014379?query=featured_home&&
6. Foster MR. Spina Bifida. Medscape; 2014. http://emedicine.medscape.com/article/311113-overview
7. Samdup DZ, Smith RG, Il Song S. The use of complementary and alternative medicine in children with chronic medical conditions. *American Journal of Physical Medicine and Rehabilitation* 2006;85(10):842–846. http://www.ncbi.nlm.nih.gov/pubmed/16998432

Spinal Cord Injury

1. Spinal Cord Injury Facts and Figures at a Glance. National Spinal Cord Injury Statistical Center; 2013. https://www.nscisc.uab.edu/PublicDocuments/fact_figures_docs/Facts%202013.pdf
2. Spinal Cord Injury: Hope Through Research. Disorders A-Z. National Institute of Neurological Disorders and Stroke; 2014. http://www.ninds.nih.gov/disorders/sci/detail_sci.htm
3. Benzel EC. Spinal Cord Injury (SCI): Damage Control and Treatment. SpineUniverse; 2012. http://www.spineuniverse.com/conditions/spinal-cord-injury/spinal-cord-injury-sci-damage-control-treatment
4. Benzel EC. Drugs and Medications for Spinal Cord Injury. Spine Universe; 2014. http://www.spineuniverse.com/conditions/spinal-cord-injury/drugs-medications-spinal-cord-injury

5. Cardenas DD, Felix ER. Pain after spinal cord injury: a review of classification, treatment approaches, and treatment assessment. *PM & R* 2009;1(12):1077–1090. http://www.ncbi.nlm.nih.gov/pubmed/19797006
6. Chase T, Jha A, Brooks CA, et al. A pilot feasibility study of massage to reduce pain in people with spinal cord injury during acute rehabilitation. *Spinal Cord* 2013;51(11):847–851. http://www.ncbi.nlm.nih.gov/pmc/articles/PMC3815956/
7. Coggrave M, Norton C. Management of faecal incontinence and constipation in adults with central neurological diseases. *Cochrane Database of Systematic Reviews* 2013;(12):CD002115. http://www.ncbi.nlm.nih.gov/pubmed/24347087
8. Coggrave M, Norton C, Cody JD. Management of faecal incontinence and constipation in adults with central neurological diseases. *Cochrane Database of Systematic Reviews* 2014;(1):CD002115. http://www.ncbi.nlm.nih.gov/pubmed/24420006
9. Heutink M, Post MW, Wollaars MM, et al. Chronic spinal cord injury pain: pharmacological and non-pharmacological treatments and treatment effectiveness. *Disability and Rehabilitation* 2011;33(5):433–440. http://www.ncbi.nlm.nih.gov/pubmed/20695788
10. Janssen TW, Prakken ES, Hendriks JM, et al. Electromechanical abdominal massage and colonic function in individuals with a spinal cord injury and chronic bowel problems. *Spinal Cord* 2014;52(9):693–696. http://www.ncbi.nlm.nih.gov/pubmed/24937700
11. Kedlaya D. Heterotopic Ossification in Spinal Cord Injury. Medscape; 2013. http://emedicine.medscape.com/article/322003-overview
12. Manella C, Backus D. Gait characteristics, range of motion, and spasticity changes in response to massage in a person with incomplete spinal cord injury: case report. *International Journal of Therapeutic Massage and Bodywork* 2011;4(1):28–39. http://www.ijtmb.org/index.php/ijtmb/article/view/108/157
13. Stephenson RO. Autonomic Dysreflexia in Spinal Cord Injury. Medscape; 2014. http://emedicine.medscape.com/article/322809-overview

Stroke

1. Spinal Cord Injury Facts and Figures at a Glance. National Spinal Cord Injury Statistical Center; 2013. https://www.nscisc.uab.edu/PublicDocuments/fact_figures_docs/Facts%202013.pdf
2. Spinal Cord Injury: Hope Through Research. Disorders A-Z. National Institute of Neurological Disorders and Stroke; 2014. http://www.ninds.nih.gov/disorders/sci/detail_sci.htm
3. Benzel EC. Spinal Cord Injury (SCI): Damage Control and Treatment. SpineUniverse; 2012. http://www.spineuniverse.com/conditions/spinal-cord-injury/spinal-cord-injury-sci-damage-control-treatment
4. Benzel EC. Drugs and Medications for Spinal Cord Injury. SpineUniverse; 2014. http://www.spineuniverse.com/conditions/spinal-cord-injury/drugs-medications-spinal-cord-injury
5. Cardenas DD, Felix ER. Pain after spinal cord injury: a review of classification, treatment approaches, and treatment assessment. *PM & R* 2009;1(12):1077–1090. http://www.ncbi.nlm.nih.gov/pubmed/19797006
6. Chase T, Jha A, Brooks CA, et al. A pilot feasibility study of massage to reduce pain in people with spinal cord injury during acute rehabilitation. *Spinal Cord* 2013;51(11):847–851. http://www.ncbi.nlm.nih.gov/pmc/articles/PMC3815956/
7. Coggrave M, Norton C. Management of faecal incontinence and constipation in adults with central neurological diseases. *Cochrane Database of Systematic Reviews* 2013;(12):CD002115. http://www.ncbi.nlm.nih.gov/pubmed/24347087
8. Coggrave M, Norton C, Cody JD. Management of faecal incontinence and constipation in adults with central neurological diseases. *Cochrane Database of Systematic Reviews* 2014;(1):CD002115. http://www.ncbi.nlm.nih.gov/pubmed/24420006
9. Heutink M, Post MW, Wollaars MM, et al. Chronic spinal cord injury pain: pharmacological and non-pharmacological treatments and treatment effectiveness. *Disability and Rehabilitation* 2011;33(5):433–440. http://www.ncbi.nlm.nih.gov/pubmed/20695788
10. Janssen TW, Prakken ES, Hendriks JM, et al. Electromechanical abdominal massage and colonic function in individuals with a spinal cord injury and chronic bowel problems. *Spinal Cord* 2014;52(9):693–696. http://www.ncbi.nlm.nih.gov/pubmed/24937700
11. Kedlaya D. Heterotopic Ossification in Spinal Cord Injury. Medscape; 2013. http://emedicine.medscape.com/article/322003-overview
12. Manella C, Backus D. Gait characteristics, range of motion, and spasticity changes in response to massage in a person with incomplete spinal cord injury: case report. *International Journal of Therapeutic Massage and Bodywork* 2011;4(1):28–39. http://www.ijtmb.org/index.php/ijtmb/article/view/108/157
13. Stephenson RO. Autonomic Dysreflexia in Spinal Cord Injury. Medscape; 2014. http://emedicine.medscape.com/article/322809-overview

Trauma- and Stressor-Related Disorders

1. Posttraumatic Stress Disorder. DSM5.org. American Psychiatric Association; 2013. http://www.dsm5.org/Documents/PTSD%20Fact%20Sheet.pdf
2. Posttraumatic Stress Disorder: PTSD Information and Treatment. Psych Central; 2014.
3. Collinge W, Kahn J, Soltysik R. Promoting reintegration of National Guard veterans and their partners using a self-directed program of integrative therapies: a pilot study. *Military Medicine* 2012;177(12):1477–1485. http://www.ncbi.nlm.nih.gov/pmc/articles/PMC3645256/
4. Friedman MJ. Trauma and Stress-Related Disorders in DSM-5. International Society for Traumatic Stress Studies. http://www.istss.org/AM/Template.cfm?Section=Expert_Training_ISTSS_Conferences&Template=/CM/ContentDisplay.cfm&ContentID=5910%20
5. Gore TA. Posttraumatic Stress Disorder. Medscape; 2014. http://emedicine.medscape.com/article/288154-overview
6. Longacre M, Silver-Highfield E, Lama P, et al. Complementary and alternative medicine in the treatment of refugees and survivors of torture: a review and proposal for action. *Torture* 2012;22(1):38–57. http://www.irct.org/Files/Filer/TortureJournal/22_1_2012/Complementary-alternative-1-2012.pdf

Traumatic Brain Injury

1. Mild TBI/Concussion Overview. CEMM Virtual Library. Center of Excellence for Medical Multimedia. http://

www.traumaticbraininjuryatoz.org/Mild-TBI/Mild-TBI-Concussion-Overview. Accessed Fall 2014.

2. Moderate to Severe TBI Overview. CEMM Virtual Library. Center of Excellence for Medical Multimedia. http://www.traumaticbraininjuryatoz.org/Moderate-to-Severe-TBI/Moderate-to-Severe-TBI-Overview. Accessed Fall 2014.
3. TBI Statistics. BrainTrauma.org. Brain Trauma Foundation. https://www.braintrauma.org/tbi-faqs/tbi-statistics/. Accessed Fall 2014.
4. Concussion and Mild TBI. CDC's Injury Center. Centers for Disease Control and Prevention; 2014. http://www.cdc.gov/concussion/index.html
5. Traumatic Brain Injury: Hope Through Research. Disorders A-Z. National Institute of Neurological Disorders and Stroke; 2014. http://www.ninds.nih.gov/disorders/tbi/detail_tbi.htm
6. Dawodu ST. Traumatic Brain Injury (TBI)—Definition, Epidemiology, Pathophysiology. Medscape; 2013. http://emedicine.medscape.com/article/326510-overview
7. Hartvigsen J, Boyle E, Cassidy JD, et al. Mild traumatic brain injury after motor vehicle collisions: what are the symptoms and who treats them? A population-based 1-year inception cohort study. *Archives of Physical Medicine and Rehabilitation* 2014;95(Suppl 3):S286–S294. http://www.ncbi.nlm.nih.gov/pubmed/24581914
8. Hoffman SW, Shesko K, Harrison CR. Enhanced neurorehabilitation techniques in the DVBIC Assisted Living Pilot Project. *NeuroRehabilitation* 2010;26(3):257–269. http://www.ncbi.nlm.nih.gov/pubmed/20448315
9. Kolias AG, Guilfoyle MR, Helmy A, et al. Traumatic brain injury in adults. *Practical Neurology* 2013;13(4):228–235. http://www.medscape.com/viewarticle/808434
10. Krafft RM. Trigeminal neuralgia. *American Family Physician* 2008;77(9):1291–1296. http://www.aafp.org/afp/2008/0501/p1291.html
11. Laureys S, Owen AM, Schiff ND. Brain function in coma, vegetative state, and related disorders. *Lancet, Neurology* 2004;3(9):537–546. http://www.coma.ulg.ac.be/papers/vs/PVS_MCS_LIS_LancetN04.pdf
12. Pangilinan PH. Classification and Complications of Traumatic Brain Injury. Medscape; 2014. http://emedicine.medscape.com/article/326643-overview

Tremor

1. ET vs. Parkinson's disease. How do they differ? International Essential Tremor Foundation; 2010. http://essentialtremor.org/wp-content/uploads/2013/07/ETvsPD092012.pdf
2. Tremor Fact Sheet. Disorders A-Z. National Institute of Neurological Disorders and Stroke; 2014. http://www.ninds.nih.gov/disorders/tremor/detail_tremor.htm
3. Ahmed A, Sweeney P. Tremors. Cleveland Clinic; 2014. http://www.clevelandclinicmeded.com/medicalpubs/diseasemanagement/neurology/tremors/Default.htm
4. Burke DA. Essential Tremor. Medscape; 2014. http://emedicine.medscape.com/article/1150290-overview
5. Chen JJ, Swope DM. Essential tremor: diagnosis and treatment. *Pharmacotherapy* 2003;23(9):1105–1122. http://www.medscape.com/viewarticle/461397
6. Puschmann A, Wszolek ZK. Diagnosis and treatment of common forms of tremor. *Seminars in Neurology* 2011;31(1):65–77. http://www.medscape.com/viewarticle/739106_4
7. Riou N. Massage therapy for essential tremor: quieting the mind. *Journal of Bodywork and Movement Therapies* 2013;17(4):488–494. http://www.ncbi.nlm.nih.gov/pubmed/24139008

Trigeminal Neuralgia

1. Treatment Options for Trigeminal Neuralgia. Facial Pain Association. http://fpa-support.org/treatment-options-trigeminal-neuralgia/. Accessed Winter 2015.
2. Trigeminal Neuralgia. Diseases and Conditions. Mayo Clinic; 2012. http://www.mayoclinic.org/diseases-conditions/trigeminal-neuralgia/basics/definition/con-20043802
3. Trigeminal Neuralgia Fact Sheet. Disorders A-Z. National Institute of Neurological Disorders and Stroke; 2014. http://www.ninds.nih.gov/disorders/trigeminal_neuralgia/detail_trigeminal_neuralgia.htm
4. Cheshire WP. Trigeminal neuralgia: for one nerve a multitude of treatments. *Expert Review of Neurotherapeutics* 2007;7(11):1565–1579. http://www.medscape.com/viewarticle/567262
5. Cole CD, Liu JK, Apfelbaum RI. Historical perspectives on the diagnosis and treatment of trigeminal neuralgia. *Neurosurgical Focus* 2005;18(5):E4. http://www.medscape.com/viewarticle/505379
6. Kaufman AM, Patel M. Your Complete Guide to Trigeminal Neuralgia. Center for Cranial Nerve Disorders, University of Manitoba; 2001. http://www.umanitoba.ca/cranial_nerves/trigeminal_neuralgia/manuscript/index.html
7. Singh MK. Trigeminal Neuralgia. Medscape; 2014. http://emedicine.medscape.com/article/1145144-overview

Vestibular Balance Disorders

1. Balance Procedures Manual. Centers for Disease Control and Prevention; 2003. http://www.cdc.gov/nchs/data/nhanes/nhanes_03_04/BA.pdf
2. Balance Disorders. Health Info. National Institute on Deafness and Other Communication Disorders; 2014. http://www.nidcd.nih.gov/health/balance/pages/balance_disorders.aspx
3. Boston ME. Labyrinthitis. Medscape; 2014. http://www.cdc.gov/nchs/data/nhanes/ba.pdf
4. Hubbard JE. Myofascial trigger points. What physicians should know about these neurological imitators. *Minnesota Medicine* 2010;93(5):42–45. http://www.minnesotamedicine.com/Past-Issues/Past-Issues-2010/May-2010/Clinical-Hubbard-May-2010
5. Li JC. Benign Paroxysmal Positional Vertigo. Medscape; 2014. http://emedicine.medscape.com/article/884261-overview
6. McDonnell MN, Hillier SL. Vestibular rehabilitation for unilateral peripheral vestibular dysfunction. *Cochrane Database of Systematic Reviews* 2015;(1):Cd005397. http://www.ncbi.nlm.nih.gov/pubmedhealth/PMH0013445/
7. Samy HM. Dizziness, Vertigo, and Imbalance. Medscape; 2014. http://emedicine.medscape.com/article/2149881-overview

Chapter 5

Anemia

1. Anemia. American Society of Hematology. http://www.hematology.org/Patients/Anemia/. Accessed Winter 2015.
2. Iron and Iron Deficiency. Nutrition for Everyone. Centers for Disease Control and Prevention; 2011. http://www.cdc.gov/nutrition/everyone/basics/vitamins/iron.html

3. What is Pernicious Anemia? Health Topics. National Heart, Lung, and Blood Institute; 2011. http://www.nhlbi.nih.gov/health/health-topics/topics/prnanmia/
4. What is Anemia? Health Topics. National Heart, Lung, and Blood Institute; 2012. http://www.nhlbi.nih.gov/health/health-topics/topics/anemia/
5. What is Aplastic Anemia? Health Topics. National Heart, Lung, and Blood Institute; 2012. http://www.nhlbi.nih.gov/health/health-topics/topics/aplastic/
6. Anemia. Diseases and Conditions. Mayo Clinic; 2014. http://www.mayoclinic.org/diseases-conditions/anemia/basics/definition/con-20026209
7. Artz AS. Anemia in Elderly Persons. Medscape; 2013. http://emedicine.medscape.com/article/1339998-overview
8. Braden CD. Chronic Anemia. Medscape; 2013. http://emedicine.medscape.com/article/780176-overview
9. Halfdanarson TR, Litzow MR, Murray JA. Hematologic manifestations of celiac disease. *Blood* 2007;109(2):412–421. http://www.bloodjournal.org/content/109/2/412?sso-checked=true
10. Maakaron JE. Anemia. Medscape; 2014. http://emedicine.medscape.com/article/198475-overview

Aneurysm

1. Abdominal Aneurysm. Vascular and Interventional Radiology. Johns Hopkins Medicine. http://www.hopkinsmedicine.org/vascular/conditions/Abdominal. Accessed Winter 2015.
2. What is an Aneurysm? Health Topics. National Heart, Lung, and Blood Institute; 2011. http://www.nhlbi.nih.gov/health/health-topics/topics/arm/
3. Aneurysm. A.D.A.M. Medical Encyclopedia. U.S. National Library of Medicine; 2012. http://www.ncbi.nlm.nih.gov/pubmedhealth/PMH0002109/
4. Cerebral Aneurysms Fact Sheet. Disorders A-Z. National Institute of Neurological Disorders and Stroke; 2014. http://www.ninds.nih.gov/disorders/cerebral_aneurysm/detail_cerebral_aneurysms.htm
5. Aortic Aneurysm Fact Sheet. Division for Heart Disease and Stroke Prevention. Centers for Disease Control and Prevention; 2014. http://www.cdc.gov/dhdsp/data_statistics/fact_sheets/fs_aortic_aneurysm.htm
6. What You Should Know About Cerebral Aneurysms. About Stroke. American Stroke Association; 2014. http://www.strokeassociation.org/STROKEORG/AboutStroke/TypesofStroke/HemorrhagicBleeds/What-You-Should-Know-About-Cerebral-Aneurysms_UCM_310103_Article.jsp
7. Nelson BP. Thoracic Aneurysm. Medscape; 2013. http://emedicine.medscape.com/article/761627-overview
8. O'Connor RE. Abdominal Aortic Aneurysm Rupture. Medscape; 2013. http://emedicine.medscape.com/article/756735-overview

Atherosclerosis

1. Heart Disease: Scope and Impact. Heart Disease Statistics. The Heart Foundation. http://www.theheartfoundation.org/heart-disease-facts/heart-disease-statistics/. Accessed Winter 2015.
2. High Cholesterol and Complementary Health Practices: What the Science Says. NCCIH Clinical Digest for Health Professionals. National Center for Complementary and Integrative Health; 2013. https://nccih.nih.gov/health/providers/digest/cholesterol-science
3. Coronary Artery Disease. Heart Information Center. Texas Heart Institute; 2014. http://www.texasheart.org/HIC/Topics/Cond/CoronaryArteryDisease.cfm
4. Peripheral Vascular Disease. Heart Information Center. Texas Heart Institute; 2014. http://www.texasheart.org/HIC/Topics/Cond/pvd.cfm
5. What is Atherosclerosis? Health Topics. National Heart, Lung, and Blood Institute; 2014. http://www.nhlbi.nih.gov/health/health-topics/topics/atherosclerosis/
6. Boudi FB. Noncoronary Atherosclarosis Overview of Atherosclerosis. Medscape; 2014. http://emedicine.medscape.com/article/1950759-overview
7. Boudi FB. Risk Factors for Coronary Artery Disease. Medscape; 2014. http://emedicine.medscape.com/article/164163-overview
8. Desai R. Atherosclerosis—Part 1. Khan Academy; 2012. https://www.khanacademy.org/science/health-and-medicine/circulatory-system-diseases/blood-vessel-diseases/v/atherosclerosis-part-1
9. Mohamad TN. Primary and Secondary Prevention of Coronary Artery Disease. Medscape; 2014. http://emedicine.medscape.com/article/164214-overview
10. Murphy SL, Xu J, Kochanek KD. Deaths: final data for 2010. *National Vital Statistics Reports* 2013;61(4). http://www.cdc.gov/nchs/data/nvsr/nvsr61/nvsr61_04.pdf
11. Rimmerman CM. Coronary Artery Disease. Center for Continuing Education. Cleveland Clinic; 2013. http://www.clevelandclinicmeded.com/medicalpubs/diseasemanagement/cardiology/coronary-artery-disease/Default.htm

Heart Attack

1. Heart Attack. Heart Disease. Centers for Disease Control and Prevention; 2013. http://www.cdc.gov/heartdisease/heart_attack.htm
2. What is a Heart Attack. Health Topics. National Heart, Lung, and Blood Institute; 2013. http://www.nhlbi.nih.gov/health/health-topics/topics/heartattack/
3. Burke AP. Pathology of Acute Myocardial Infarction. Medscape; 2013. http://emedicine.medscape.com/article/1960472-overview
4. Kondur AK. Complications of Myocardial Infarction. Medscape; 2014. http://emedicine.medscape.com/article/164924-overview
5. Zafari M. Myocardial Infarction. Medscape; 2014. http://emedicine.medscape.com/article/155919-overview

Heart Failure

1. Heart Failure Statistics. Learn About Heart Failure. Emory Heart and Vascular Center. http://www.emoryhealthcare.org/heart-failure/learn-about-heart-failure/statistics.html. Accessed Winter 2015.
2. Heart Failure Medications. American Heart Association; 2012. http://www.heart.org/HEARTORG/Conditions/HeartFailure/PreventionTreatmentofHeartFailure/Heart-Failure-Medications_UCM_306342_Article.jsp
3. Heart Failure. HeartFailure.org; 2013. http://www.heartfailure.org/heart-failure/
4. Heart Failure Overview. A.D.A.M. Medical Encyclopedia. U.S. Library of Medicine; 2013. http://www.ncbi.nlm.nih.gov/pubmedhealth/PMH0001211/
5. What is Heart Failure. Health Topics. National Heart, Lung, and Blood Institute; 2014. http://www.nhlbi.nih.gov/health/health-topics/topics/hf/

6. Heart Failure Fact Sheet. Division for Heart Disease and Stroke Prevention. Centers for Disease Control and Prevention; 2014. http://www.cdc.gov/dhdsp/data_statistics/fact_sheets/fs_heart_failure.htm
7. Chen WL, Liu GJ, Yeh SH, et al. Effect of back massage intervention on anxiety, comfort, and physiologic responses in patients with congestive heart failure. *Journal of Alternative and Complementary Medicines* 2013;19(5):464–470. http://www.ncbi.nlm.nih.gov/pmc/articles/PMC3651680/
8. Jones J, Thomson P, Lauder W, et al. Reflexology has no immediate haemodynamic effect in patients with chronic heart failure: a double blind randomised controlled trial. *Complementary Therapies in Clinical Practice* 2013;19(3):133–138. http://www.ncbi.nlm.nih.gov/pubmed/23890459
9. Leduc O, Crasset V, Leleu C, et al. Impact of manual lymphatic drainage on hemodynamic parameters in patients with heart failure and lower limb edema. *Lymphology* 2011;44(1):13–20. http://www.ncbi.nlm.nih.gov/pubmed/21667818
10. Torpy JM, Lynm C, Glass RM. JAMA patient page. Heart failure. *JAMA* 2007;297(22):2548. http://jama.jamanetwork.com/article.aspx?articleid=207470

Hemophilia

1. Hemophilia A. Bleeding Disorders. National Hemophilia Foundation. http://www.hemophilia.org/Bleeding-Disorders/Types-of-Bleeding-Disorders/Hemophilia-A. Accessed Winter 2015.
2. Hemophilia B. Bleeding Disorders. National Hemophilia Foundation. https://www.hemophilia.org/Bleeding-Disorders/Types-of-Bleeding-Disorders/Hemophilia-B. Accessed Winter 2014.
3. Von Willebrand Disease. Bleeding Disorders. National Hemophilia Foundation. http://www.hemophilia.org/Bleeding-Disorders/Types-of-Bleeding-Disorders/Von-Willebrand-Disease. Accessed Winter 2015.
4. Hemophilia in Pictures. World Federation of Hemophilia; 2005. http://www1.wfh.org/en/pdf/english.pdf
5. What is Von Willebrand Disease? Health Topics. National Heart, Lung, and Blood Institute; 2011. http://www.nhlbi.nih.gov/health/health-topics/topics/vwd/
6. What is Hemophilia. Health Topics. National Heart, Lung, and Blood Institute; 2013. http://www.nhlbi.nih.gov/health/health-topics/topics/hemophilia/
7. Beyer R, Ingerslev J, Sorensen B. Muscle bleeds in professional athletes—diagnosis, classification, treatment and potential impact in patients with haemophilia. *Haemophilia* 2010;16(6):858–865. http://www.ncbi.nlm.nih.gov/pubmed/20491962
8. Brookes L, Josephson NC. Hemophilia: Current Management, Unmet Needs. Medscape Oncology; 2014. http://www.medscape.com/viewarticle/818239
9. Grethlein SJ. Acquired Hemophilia. Medscape; 2014. http://emedicine.medscape.com/article/211186-overview
10. Zaiden RA. Hemophilia A. Medscape; 2014. http://emedicine.medscape.com/article/779322-overview

Hypertension

1. The Seventh Report of the Joint National Committee on Prevention, Detection, Evaluation, and Treatment of High Blood Pressure. National Heart, Lung, and Blood Institute; 2003. http://www.nhlbi.nih.gov/files/docs/guidelines/express.pdf
2. High Blood Pressure (Hypertension). Texas Heart Institute; 2014. http://www.texasheart.org/HIC/Topics/Cond/hbp.cfm
3. High Blood Pressure Fact Sheet. Division for Heart Disease and Stroke Prevention. High Blood Pressure Fact Sheet; 2014. http://www.cdc.gov/dhdsp/data_statistics/fact_sheets/fs_bloodpressure.htm
4. Cambron JA, Dexheimer J, Coe P. Changes in blood pressure after various forms of therapeutic massage: a preliminary study. *Journal of Alternative and Complementary Medicine* 2006;12(1):65–70. http://www.ncbi.nlm.nih.gov/pubmed/16494570
5. Desai R. What is Hypertension? Khan Academy. Khan Academy; 2012. https://www.khanacademy.org/science/health-and-medicine/circulatory-system-diseases/hypertension/v/what-is-hypertension
6. Elliott WJ. New Targets in Global Cardiovascular Risk Reduction: Considering the Whole Patient. Medscape Cardiology; 2008. http://www.medscape.org/viewarticle/576630
7. Givi M. Durability of effect of massage therapy on blood pressure. *International Journal of Preventive Medicine* 2013;4(5):511–516. http://www.ncbi.nlm.nih.gov/pmc/articles/PMC3733180/
8. Madhur MS. Hypertension. Medscape; 2014. http://emedicine.medscape.com/article/241381-overview
9. Olney CM. The effect of therapeutic back massage in hypertensive persons: a preliminary study. *Biological Research for Nursing* 2005;7(2):98–105. http://brn.sagepub.com/content/7/2/98
10. Supa'at I, Zakaria Z, Maskon O, et al. Effects of Swedish massage therapy on blood pressure, heart rate, and inflammatory markers in hypertensive women. *Evidence-Based Complementary and Alternative Medicine* 2013;2013:171852. http://www.ncbi.nlm.nih.gov/pubmed/24023571
11. Wood S. HEAT-PPCI in Print: 'It's Pretty Bloody Detailed'. Medscape; 2014. http://www.medscape.com/viewarticle/827877
12. Xiong XJ, Li SJ, Zhang YQ. Massage therapy for essential hypertension: a systematic review. *Journal of Human Hypertension* 2015;29(3):143–151. http://www.ncbi.nlm.nih.gov/pubmed/24990417
13. Yang X, Zhao H, Wang J. Chinese massage (Tuina) for the treatment of essential hypertension: a systematic review and meta-analysis. *Complementary Therapies in Medicine* 2014;22(3):541–548. http://www.ncbi.nlm.nih.gov/pubmed/24906593

Leukemia

1. Acute Lymphoblastic Leukemia. Disease Information & Support. Leukemia & Lymphoma Society. http://www.lls.org/#/diseaseinformation/leukemia/acutelymphoblasticleukemia. Accessed Winter 2015.
2. Acute Myeloid Leukemia. Disease Information & Support. Leukemia & Lymphoma Society. http://www.lls.org/#/diseaseinformation/leukemia/acutemyeloidleukemia. Accessed Winter 2015.
3. Chronic Lymphocytic Leukemia. Disease Information & Support. Leukemia & Lymphoma Society. http://www.lls.org/#/diseaseinformation/leukemia/chroniclymphocyticleukemia/. Accessed Winter 2015.
4. Chronic Myeloid Leukemia. Disease Information & Support. Leukemia & Lymphoma Society. http://www.lls.org/#/diseaseinformation/leukemia/chronicmyeloidleukemia. Accessed Winter 2015.

5. Leukemia: What is Leukemia. Health Topics A-Z. NIH Senior Health. http://nihseniorhealth.gov/leukemia/whatisleukemia/01.html. Accessed Winter 2015.
6. Definition of Philadelphia Chromosome (Ph). MedicineNet; 2012. http://www.medicinenet.com/script/main/art.asp?articlekey=4870
7. What You Need to Know About Leukemia. National Cancer Institute; 2013. http://www.cancer.gov/publications/patient-education/wyntk-leukemia/AllPages
8. Stringer J, Swindell R, Dennis M. Massage in patients undergoing intensive chemotherapy reduces serum cortisol and prolactin. *Psycho-oncology* 2008;17(10):1024–1031. http://www.ncbi.nlm.nih.gov/pubmed/18300336
9. Wesa KM, Cassileth BR. Is there a role for complementary therapy in the management of leukemia? *Expert Review of Anticancer Therapy* 2009;9(9):1241–1249. http://www.ncbi.nlm.nih.gov/pmc/articles/PMC2792198/

Myeloma

1. Multiple Myeloma: A Study of K-25 Workers. Centers for Disease Control and Prevention; 2009. http://www.cdc.gov/niosh/pgms/worknotify/pdfs/k25_7-06-09.pdf
2. 10 Steps to Better Care. About Myeloma. International Myeloma Foundation; 2011. http://myeloma.org/ArticlePage.action?tabId=1&menuId=352&articleId=3525&aTab=-1
3. A Snapshot of Myeloma. Research & Funding. National Cancer Institute; 2014. http://www.cancer.gov/researchandfunding/snapshots/myeloma
4. Hu W. Myeloma. eMedicineHealth; 2013. http://www.emedicinehealth.com/myeloma/article_em.htm
5. Kuehl WM, Bergsagel PL. Molecular pathogenesis of multiple myeloma and its premalignant precursor. *Journal of Clinical Investigation* 2012;122(10):3456–3463. http://www.jci.org/articles/view/61188
6. Shah D. Multiple Myeloma. Medscape; 2014. http://emedicine.medscape.com/article/204369-overview

Raynaud Syndrome

1. Raynaud's. Raynaud's & Scleroderma Association. http://www.raynauds.org.uk/raynauds/raynauds. Accessed Winter 2015.
2. Questions and Answers about Raynaud's Phenomenon. Health Info. National Institute of Arthritis and Musculoskeletal and Skin Diseases; 2012. http://www.niams.nih.gov/Health_Info/Raynauds_Phenomenon/default.asp
3. What is Raynaud's? Health Topics. National Heart, Lung, and Blood Institute; 2014. http://www.nhlbi.nih.gov/health/health-topics/topics/raynaud/
4. The Cold Facts on Raynaud's and Strategies for a Warmer Life. Raynaud's Association; 2014. http://www.raynauds.org/wp-content/uploads/2014/06/Raynauds-Guide-PDF.pdf
5. Hansen-Dispenza H. Raynaud Phenomenon. Medscape; 2014. http://emedicine.medscape.com/article/331197-overview
6. Herrick AL. Pathogenesis of Raynaud's phenomenon. *Rheumatology (Oxford)* 2005;44(5):587–596. http://rheumatology.oxfordjournals.org/content/44/5/587.full

Sickle Cell Disease

1. A Century of Progress: Milestones in Sickle Cell Disease Research and Care. National Heart, Lung, and Blood Institute; 2010. http://www.nhlbi.nih.gov/files/docs/public/blood/Tagged2NHLBISickleCellTimeline.pdf
2. Questions and Answers About Sickle Cell Trait. Spotlight on Research. National Heart, Lung, and Blood Institute; 2010. http://www.nhlbi.nih.gov/news/spotlight/fact-sheet/questions-and-answers-about-sickle-cell-trait
3. What is Sickle Cell Anemia? Health Topics. National Heart, Lung, and Blood Institute; 2012. http://www.nhlbi.nih.gov/health/health-topics/topics/sca/
4. Sickle Cell Disease. Yesterday, Today, & Tomorrow: NIH Research Timelines. National Institutes of Health; 2013. http://report.nih.gov/nihfactsheets/ViewFactSheet.aspx?csid=116&key=S
5. Sickle Cell Disease (SCD). Centers for Disease Control and Prevention; 2014. http://www.cdc.gov/NCBDDD/sicklecell/index.html
6. Stem Cell Transplant for Sickle Cell Disease. WebMD; 2014. http://www.webmd.com/cancer/bone-marrow-transplant-for-sickle-cell-disease
7. Lemanek KL, Ranalli M, Lukens C. A randomized controlled trial of massage therapy in children with sickle cell disease. *Journal of Pediatric Psychology* 2009;34(10):1091–1096. http://jpepsy.oxfordjournals.org/content/34/10/1091.long
8. Maakaron JE. Sickle Cell Anemia. Medscape; 2014. http://emedicine.medscape.com/article/205926-overview
9. Majumdar S, Thompson W, Ahmad N, et al. The use and effectiveness of complementary and alternative medicine for pain in sickle cell anemia. *Complementary Therapies in Clinical Practice* 2013;19(4):184–187. http://www.ncbi.nlm.nih.gov/pubmed/24199970
10. Neville KA, Panepinto JA. Pharmacotherapy of Sickle Cell Disease. World Health Organization; 2011. http://www.who.int/selection_medicines/committees/expert/18/applications/Sicklecell.pdf
11. Sanders KA, Labott SM, Molokie R, et al. Pain, coping and health care utilization in younger and older adults with sickle cell disease. *Journal of Health Psychology* 2010;15(1):131–137. http://www.ncbi.nlm.nih.gov/pubmed/20064892

Thrombophlebitis

1. Deep Vein Thrombosis. OrthoInfo. American Academy of Orthopaedic Surgeons; 2009. http://orthoinfo.aaos.org/topic.cfm?topic=A00219
2. What is Deep Vein Thrombosis? Health Topics. National Heart, Lung, and Blood Institute; 2011. http://www.nhlbi.nih.gov/health/health-topics/topics/dvt/
3. Thrombophlebitis. Medline Plus. U.S. National Library of Medicine; 2014. http://www.nlm.nih.gov/medlineplus/ency/article/001108.htm
4. Thrombophlebitis. Diseases and Conditions. Mayo Clinic; 2014. http://www.mayoclinic.org/diseases-conditions/thrombophlebitis/basics/definition/con-20021437
5. Data and Statistics. Deep Vein Thrombosis (DVT)/Pulmonary Embolism (PE)—Blood Clot Forming in a Vein. Centers for Disease Control and Prevention; 2014. http://www.cdc.gov/ncbddd/dvt/data.html
6. Beckman MG, Hooper WC, Critchley SE, et al. Venous thromboembolism: a public health concern. *American Journal of Preventive Medicine* 2010;38(4 Suppl):S495–S501. http://www.ajpmonline.org/article/S0749-3797(09)00946-5/fulltext
7. Bieri D, Heath J, Samios R. The effects of faradism under pressure on venous pressure. *Australian Journal of Physiotherapy* 1970;16(4):159–160. http://www.ncbi.nlm.nih.gov/pubmed/25028255

8. Geersing GJ, Zuithoff NP, Kearon C, et al. Exclusion of deep vein thrombosis using the Wells rule in clinically important subgroups: individual patient data meta-analysis. *BMJ* 2014;348:g1340. http://www.ncbi.nlm.nih.gov/pmc/articles/PMC3948465/
9. Jerjes-Sanchez C. Venous and arterial thrombosis: a continuous spectrum of the same disease? *European Heart Journal* 2005;26(1):3–4. http://eurheartj.oxfordjournals.org/content/26/1/3.full
10. Ouellette DR. Pulmonary Embolism. Medscape; 2014. http://emedicine.medscape.com/article/300901-overview
11. Palm MD. Thrombophlebitis. Medscape; 2014. http://emedicine.medscape.com/article/1086399-overview
12. Reyes N, Grosse S, Grant A. Deep Vein Thrombosis & Pulmonary Embolism. Travelers' Health. Centers for Disease Control and Prevention; 2013. http://wwwnc.cdc.gov/travel/yellowbook/2014/chapter-2-the-pre-travel-consultation/deep-vein-thrombosis-and-pulmonary-embolism

Thrombus/Embolism

1. Thrombus or Embolus. StrokeSTOP. University of Massachusetts Medical School. http://www.umassmed.edu/strokestop/module_one/thrombus_embolus.html. Accessed Winter 2015.
2. What is Thrombosis? North American Thrombosis Forum; 2012. http://natfonline.org/patients/what-is-thrombosis/
3. Blood Clots. A.D.A.M. Medical Encyclopedia. U.S. National Library of Medicine; 2014. http://www.nlm.nih.gov/medlineplus/ency/article/001124.htm
4. Crump C, Paluska SA. Venous thromboembolism following vigorous deep tissue massage. *Physician and Sportsmedicine* 2010;38(4):136–139. http://www.ncbi.nlm.nih.gov/pubmed/21150153
5. Kirkland L. Cholesterol Embolism. Medscape; 2013. http://www.healthline.com/health/arterial-embolism#Overview1
6. Lim DC, Jayanthi HK, Money-Kyrle A, et al. Massaging the outcome: an unusual presentation of pulmonary embolism. *BMJ Case Reports* 2009;2009. http://www.ncbi.nlm.nih.gov/pmc/articles/PMC3029203/
7. Macon BL, Boskey E. Arterial Embolism. Healthline; 2014. http://www.healthline.com/health/arterial-embolism#Overview1
8. Oulette DR. Pulmonary Embolism. Medscape; 2014. http://emedicine.medscape.com/article/300901-overview
9. Park H, Kim HJ, Cha MJ, et al. A case of cerebellar infarction caused by acute subclavian thrombus following minor trauma. *Yonsei Medical Journal* 2013;54(6):1538–1541. http://synapse.koreamed.org/DOIx.php?id=10.3349/ymj.2013.54.6.1538
10. Previtali E, Bucciarelli P, Passamonti SM, et al. Risk factors for venous and arterial thrombosis. *Blood Transfusion* 2011;9(2):120–138. http://www.ncbi.nlm.nih.gov/pmc/articles/PMC3096855/

Varicose Veins

1. Hemorrhoids—Topic Overview. WebMD; 2012. http://www.webmd.com/digestive-disorders/tc/hemorrhoids-topic-overview
2. Esophageal Cancer. Diseases and Conditions. Mayo Clinic; 2013. http://www.mayoclinic.org/diseases-conditions/esophageal-varices/basics/definition/con-20027505
3. What are Varicose Veins? Health Topics. National Heart, Lung, and Blood Institute; 2014. http://www.nhlbi.nih.gov/health/health-topics/topics/vv/
4. Alaiti S. Sclerotherapy. Medscape; 2013. http://emedicine.medscape.com/article/300901-overview
5. Cole GW, Nabili SN. Varicose Veins and Spider Veins. MedicineNet; 2014. http://www.medicinenet.com/varicose_veins/article.htm
6. Pereira de Godoy JM, Braile DM, de Fatima Guerreiro Godoy M. Lymph drainage in patients with joint immobility due to chronic ulcerated lesions. *Phlebology* 2008;23(1):32–34. http://www.ncbi.nlm.nih.gov/pubmed/18361267
7. Thornton SC. Hemorrhoids. Medscape; 2014. http://emedicine.medscape.com/article/775407-overview
8. Vandy F, Wakefield TW. Treatments, with emphasis on powered phlebectomy for branch varicosities. *Interventional Cardiology* 2012;4(5):527–536. http://www.medscape.com/viewarticle/778728
9. Weiss R. Varicose Veins and Spider Veins. Medscape; 2014. http://emedicine.medscape.com/article/1085530-overview
10. White WM. Varicocele. Medscape; 2014. http://emedicine.medscape.com/article/438591-overview
11. Wright N, Fitridge R. Varicose veins—natural history, assessment and management. *Australian Family Physician* 2013;42(6):380–384. http://www.racgp.org.au/afp/2013/june/varicose-veins/

Chapter 6

Allergies

1. Allergic Reactions: Tips to Remember. Conditions and Treatments. American Academy of Allergy Asthma & Immunology. http://www.aaaai.org/conditions-and-treatments/library/at-a-glance/allergic-reactions.aspx. Accessed Winter 2014.
2. Begin P. Unproven and Non-Standardized Tests for Food Allergy. Food Allergy Research and Education. http://www.foodallergy.org/document.doc?id=238. Accessed Winter 2014.
3. Crawford GH, Katz KA, Ellis E, et al. Use of aromatherapy products and increased risk of hand dermatitis in massage therapists. *Archives of Dermatology* 2004;140(8):991–996. http://www.ncbi.nlm.nih.gov/pubmed/15313817
4. Green TE. Acute Angiodema Overview of Angiodema Treatment. Medscape; 2012. http://emedicine.medscape.com/article/756261-overview
5. Johnson RF, Peebles RS. Anaphylactic shock: pathophysiology, recognition, and treatment. *Seminars in Respiratory and Critical Care Medicine* 2004;25(6):695–703. http://www.medscape.com/viewarticle/497498
6. Lakshmi C. Allergic contact dermatitis (type IV hypersensitivity) and type I hypersensitivity following aromatherapy with ayurvedic oils (Dhanwantharam thailam, Eladi coconut oil) presenting as generalized erythema and pruritus with flexural eczema. *Indian Journal of Dermatology* 2014;59(3):283–286. http://www.ncbi.nlm.nih.gov/pmc/articles/PMC4037951/
7. Sicherer SH. Food Allergies. Medscape; 2014. http://emedicine.medscape.com/article/135959-overview
8. Trattner A, David M, Lazarov A. Occupational contact dermatitis due to essential oils. *Contact Dermatitis* 2008;58(5):282–284. http://www.ncbi.nlm.nih.gov/pubmed/18416758

Ankylosing Spondylitis

1. Ankylosing Spondylitis (AS). Arthritis Facts. Arthritis Foundation. http://www.arthritis.org/arthritis-facts/disease-center/ankylosing-spondylitis.php. Accessed Winter 2014.

2. Questions and Answers About Ankylosing Spondylitis. Health Info. National Institute of Arthritis and Musculoskeletal and Skin Diseases; 2013. http://www.niams.nih.gov/health_info/Ankylosing_Spondylitis/default.asp
3. Ankylosing Spondylitis. Diseases and Conditions. Mayo Clinic; 2014. http://www.mayoclinic.org/diseases-conditions/ankylosing-spondylitis/basics/definition/con-20019766
4. Brent LH. Ankylosing Spondylitis and Undifferentiated Spondyloarthropathy. Medscape; 2014. http://emedicine.medscape.com/article/332945-overview
5. Chunco R. The effects of massage on pain, stiffness, and fatigue levels associated with ankylosing spondylitis: a case study. *International Journal of Therapeutic Massage and Bodywork* 2011;4(1):12–17. http://www.ncbi.nlm.nih.gov/pmc/articles/PMC3088527/
6. Dean LE, Jones GT, MacDonald AG, et al. Global prevalence of ankylosing spondylitis. *Rheumatology (Oxford)* 2014;53(4):650–657. http://www.medscape.com/viewarticle/823006
7. MacGill M. What is ankylosing spondylitis? How can AS be managed? Medical News Today; 2014. http://www.medicalnewstoday.com/articles/248217.php
8. Peh WC. Imaging in Ankylosing Spondylitis. Medscape; 2014. http://emedicine.medscape.com/article/386639-overview
9. Reveille JD. Spondylarthritis (Spondylarthropathy). American College of Rheumatology; 2012. https://www.rheumatology.org/Practice/Clinical/Patients/Diseases_And_Conditions/Spondylarthritis_(Spondylarthropathy)/

Chronic Fatigue Syndrome

1. Chronic Fatigue Syndrome. New York Medical College Center for Hypotension. https://www.nymc.edu/FHP/Centers/Syncope/cfs.htm. Accessed Winter 2014.
2. Chronic Fatigue Syndrome (CFS). Centers for Disease Control and Prevention; 2012. http://www.cdc.gov/cfs/general/index.html
3. Alraek T, Lee MS, Choi TY, et al. Complementary and alternative medicine for patients with chronic fatigue syndrome: a systematic review. *BMC Complementary and Alternative Medicine* 2011;11:87. http://www.ncbi.nlm.nih.gov/pmc/articles/PMC3201900/
4. Bayliss K, Goodall M, Chisholm A, et al. Overcoming the barriers to the diagnosis and management of chronic fatigue syndrome/ME in primary care: a meta synthesis of qualitative studies. *BMC Family Practice* 2014;15:44. http://www.ncbi.nlm.nih.gov/pmc/articles/PMC3973969/
5. Cunha BA. Chronic Fatigue Syndrome. Medscape; 2014. http://emedicine.medscape.com/article/235980-overview
6. Hitt E. Chronic Fatigue Syndrome Not Linked to XMRV. Medscape; 2011. http://www.medscape.com/viewarticle/741121
7. Jones JF, Maloney EM, Boneva RS, et al. Complementary and alternative medical therapy utilization by people with chronic fatiguing illnesses in the United States. *BMC Complementary and Alternative Medicine* 2007;7:12. http://www.ncbi.nlm.nih.gov/pmc/articles/PMC1878505/
8. McCleary KK, Vernon SD. Chronic fatigue syndrome. *Pain Practitioner* 2010;20(1):14–19. http://www.um.es/lafem/Actividades/CursoBiologia/Consultas/Actual-chronicfatigue.pdf
9. Simon H. Chronic Fatigue Syndrome. Health Information. University of Maryland Medical Center; 2013. http://umm.edu/health/medical/reports/articles/chronic-fatigue-syndrome
10. White PD, Goldsmith K, Johnson AL, et al. Recovery from chronic fatigue syndrome after treatments given in the PACE trial. *Psychological Medicine* 2013;43(10):2227–2235. http://www.ncbi.nlm.nih.gov/pmc/articles/PMC3776285/

Crohn Disease

1. What is Crohn's Disease? Crohn's & Colitis Foundation of America. http://www.ccfa.org/what-are-crohns-and-colitis/what-is-crohns-disease/. Accessed Winter 2014.
2. Crohn's Disease. Health Info. National Institute of Diabetes and Digestive and Kidney Diseases; 2014. http://www.niddk.nih.gov/health-information/health-topics/digestive-diseases/crohns-disease/Pages/facts.aspx
3. Inflammatory Bowel Disease (IBD). eMedicineHealth; 2014. http://www.emedicinehealth.com/inflammatory_bowel_disease_ibd/article_em.htm
4. Inflammatory bowel disease (IBD). Centers for Disease Control and Prevention; 2014. http://www.cdc.gov/ibd/
5. Bhandari BM, Kroser JA, Bloomfeld RS, et al. Inflammatory Bowel Disease. Patient Education and Resource Center. American College of Gastroenterology. http://patients.gi.org/topics/inflammatory-bowel-disease/. Accessed Winter 2014.
6. Ghazi LJ. Crohn Disease. Medscape; 2014. http://emedicine.medscape.com/article/172940-overview
7. Rendi M. Crohn Disease Pathology. Medscape; 2013. http://emedicine.medscape.com/article/1986158-overview
8. Rowe WA. Inflammatory Bowel Disease. Medscape; 2014. http://emedicine.medscape.com/article/179037-overview

Edema

1. Edema Overview. Heart Failure Health Center. WebMD; 2012. http://www.webmd.com/heart-disease/heart-failure/edema-overview
2. Edema. Diseases & Conditions. Cleveland Clinic; 2012. http://my.clevelandclinic.org/health/diseases_conditions/hic_Edema
3. Edema. Diseases and Conditions. Mayo Clinic; 2014. http://www.mayoclinic.org/diseases-conditions/edema/basics/definition/con-20033037
4. Brodovicz KG, McNaughton K, Uemura N, et al. Reliability and feasibility of methods to quantitatively assess peripheral edema. *Clinical Medicine and Research* 2009;7(1–2):21–31. http://www.ncbi.nlm.nih.gov/pmc/articles/PMC2705274/
5. Ebert JR, Joss B, Jardine B, et al. Randomized trial investigating the efficacy of manual lymphatic drainage to improve early outcome after total knee arthroplasty. *Archives of Physical Medicine and Rehabilitation* 2013;94(11):2103–2111. http://www.ncbi.nlm.nih.gov/pubmed/23810354
6. Hwang O, Ha K, Choi S. The effects of PNF techniques on lymphoma in the upper limbs. *Journal of Physical Therapy Science* 2013;25(7):839–841. http://www.ncbi.nlm.nih.gov/pmc/articles/PMC3820393/
7. O'Brien JG, Chennubhotla SA, Chennubhotla RV. Treatment of edema. *American Family Physician* 2005;71(11):2111–2117. http://www.aafp.org/afp/2005/0601/p2111.html
8. Priollet P. Venous edema of the lower limbs. Phlebolymphology; 2010. http://www.phlebolymphology.org/venous-edema-of-the-lower-limbs/

9. Warren AG, Janz BA, Borud LJ, et al. Evaluation and management of the fat leg syndrome. *Plastic and Reconstructive Surgery* 2007;119(1):9e–15e. http://www.ncbi.nlm.nih.gov/pubmed/17255648

Fever

1. Affronti M, Mansueto P, Soresi M, et al. Low-grade fever: how to distinguish organic from non-organic forms. *International Journal of Clinical Practice* 2010;64(3):316–321. http://www.medscape.com/viewarticle/716202
2. Dalal S, Zhukovsky DS. Pathophysiology and management of fever. *Journal of Supportive Oncology* 2006;4(1):9–16. http://d.yimg.com/kq/groups/15854266/652670728/name/feb+neu+2.pdf
3. Davis CP. Fever in Adults. eMedicineHealth; 2014. http://www.emedicinehealth.com/fever_in_adults/article_em.htm
4. Kaneshiro NK. Fever. A.D.A.M. U.S. National Library of Medicine; 2014. http://www.nlm.nih.gov/medlineplus/ency/article/003090.htm

HIV/AIDS

1. HIV-1 Drug Resistance in ARV-naive Populations. HIV Drug Resistance Database. Stanford University. http://hivdb.stanford.edu/surveillance/map/. Accessed Winter 2015.
2. Alternative HIV Treatment. Treatment and Care. AVERT. http://www.avert.org/alternative-hiv-treatment.htm. Accessed Winter 2015.
3. Antiretroviral Drugs Side Effects. Treatment and Care. AVERT. http://www.avert.org/antiretroviral-drugs-side-effects.htm. Accessed Winter 2015.
4. USA HIV & AIDS Statistics. Global Epidemic. AVERT. http://www.avert.org/usa-hiv-aids-statistics.htm. Accessed Winter 2015.
5. Stress Management Interventions May Enhance Immune Function in People With HIV. Research. National Center for Complementary and Integrative Health; 2008. https://nccih.nih.gov/research/results/spotlight/060208.htm
6. Preventing HIV and AIDS. The Patient Education Institute; 2013. http://www.nlm.nih.gov/medlineplus/tutorials/aids/hp249104.pdf
7. Tuberculosis and HIV. HIV/AIDS. World Health Organization; 2014. http://www.who.int/hiv/topics/tb/en/
8. Pre-exposure Prophylaxis (PrEP) for HIV Prevention. Centers for Disease Control and Prevention; 2014. http://www.cdc.gov/hiv/pdf/PrEP_fact_sheet_final.pdf
9. Global Summary of the AIDS Epidemic | 2013. World Health Organization; 2014. http://www.who.int/hiv/data/epi_core_dec2014.png?ua=1
10. Hillier SL, Louw Q, Morris L, et al. Massage therapy for people with HIV/AIDS. *Cochrane Database of Systematic Reviews* 2010;(1):CD007502. http://www.ncbi.nlm.nih.gov/pubmed/20091636
11. Kennedy R. HIV AIDS (HIVP-AIDS) (HIV Potentiated AIDS). The Doctors' Medical Library. http://www.medical-library.net/hiv_aids.html. Accessed Winter 2015.
12. Kumar P. Long term non-progressor (LTNP) HIV infection. *Indian Journal of Medical Research* 2013;138(3):291–293. http://www.ncbi.nlm.nih.gov/pmc/articles/PMC3818590/
13. Mohammed I, Nasidi A. The pathophysiology and clinical manifestations of HIV/AIDS. In: AIDS in Nigeria: a nation on the threshold. Harvard University; 2004. http://www.apin.harvard.edu/AIDS_in_Nigeria.html
14. Poland RE, Gertsik L, Favreau JT, et al. Open-label, randomized, parallel-group controlled clinical trial of massage for treatment of depression in HIV-infected subjects. *Journal of Alternative and Complementary Medicine* 2013;19(4):334–340. http://www.ncbi.nlm.nih.gov/pmc/articles/PMC3627430/

Lupus

1. Understanding Lupus. Get Answers. Lupus Foundation of America. http://www.lupus.org/answers/topic/understanding-lupus. Accessed Winter 2015.
2. Handout on Health: Systemic Lupus Erythematosus. Health Information. National institute of Arthritis and Musculoskeletal and Skin Diseases; 2013. http://www.niams.nih.gov/Health_Info/Lupus/default.asp
3. Systemic Lupus Erythematosus. A.D.A.M. Medical Encyclopedia. U.S. National Library of Medicine; 2014. http://www.ncbi.nlm.nih.gov/pubmedhealth/PMH0001471/
4. Bartels CM. Systemic Lupus Erythematosus (SLE). Medscape; 2014. http://emedicine.medscape.com/article/332244-overview
5. Greidinger EL. Mixed Connective-Tissue Disease. Medscape; 2013. http://emedicine.medscape.com/article/335815-overview
6. Schwartz RA. Dermatologic Manifestations of Mixed Connective Tissue Disease. Medscape; 2014. http://emedicine.medscape.com/article/1066445-overview
7. Somers EC, Marder W, Cagnoli P, et al. Population-based incidence and prevalence of systemic lupus erythematosus: the Michigan Lupus Epidemiology and Surveillance program. *Arthritis and Rheumatology* 2014;66(2):369–378. http://onlinelibrary.wiley.com/doi/10.1002/art.38238/full
8. van Vollenhoven RF, Mosca M, Bertsias G, et al. Treat-to-target in systemic lupus erythematosus: recommendations from an international task force. *Annals of the Rheumatic Diseases* 2014;73(6):958–967. http://ard.bmj.com/content/73/6/958.full

Lymphangitis

1. Lymphangitis. A.D.A.M. Medical Encyclopedia. U.S. National Library of Medicine; 2013. http://www.ncbi.nlm.nih.gov/pubmedhealth/PMH0004551/
2. Feied C, Smith M, Handler J, et al. Erysipelas Cellulitis Lymphangitis. National Center for Emergency Medicine Informatics. http://www.ncemi.org/cse/cse1111.htm. Accessed Winter 2015.
3. Pitetti RD. Lymphangitis. Medscape; 2014. http://emedicine.medscape.com/article/966003-overview

Lymphoma

1. Hodgkin Lymphoma (HL). Lymphoma Research Foundation. http://www.lymphoma.org/site/pp.asp?c=bkLTKaOQLmK8E&b=6300137. Accessed Winter 2015.
2. What You Need to Know About Non-Hodgkin Lymphoma. Patient Education Publications. National Cancer Institute; 2007. http://www.cancer.gov/publications/patient-education/wyntk-non-hodgkin-lymphoma/AllPages
3. What You Need to Know About Hodgkin Lymphoma. Patient Education Publications. National Cancer Institute; 2013. http://www.cancer.gov/publications/patient-education/wyntk-hodgkin/AllPages
4. Adult Hodgkin Lymphoma Treatment (PDQ). Cancer Topics. National Cancer Institute; 2014. http://www.cancer.

gov/cancertopics/pdq/treatment/adulthodgkins/Patient/AllPages

5. Burkitt Lymphoma. MedlinePlus. U.S. National Library of Medicine; 2014. http://www.nlm.nih.gov/medlineplus/ency/article/001308.htm
6. Hodgkin Disease. American Cancer Society; 2015. http://www.cancer.org/acs/groups/cid/documents/webcontent/003105-pdf.pdf
7. Non-Hodgkin Lymphoma. American Cancer Society; 2015. http://www.cancer.org/acs/groups/cid/documents/webcontent/003126-pdf.pdf
8. Breitbart W, Poppito S, Rosenfeld B, et al. Pilot randomized controlled trial of individual meaning-centered psychotherapy for patients with advanced cancer. *Journal of Clinical Oncology* 2012;30(12):1304–1309. http://www.ncbi.nlm.nih.gov/pmc/articles/PMC3646315/
9. Gajra A. B-Cell Lymphoma. Medscape; 2014. http://emedicine.medscape.com/article/202677-overview
10. Habermann TM, Thompson CA, LaPlant BR, et al. Complementary and alternative medicine use among long-term lymphoma survivors: a pilot study. *American Journal of Hematology* 2009;84(12):795–798. http://www.ncbi.nlm.nih.gov/pmc/articles/PMC3154703/
11. Lash BW. Hodgkin Lymphoma. Medscape; 2014. http://emedicine.medscape.com/article/201886-overview
12. Vinjamaram S. Non-Hodgkin Lymphoma. Medscape; 2014. http://emedicine.medscape.com/article/203399-overview

Mononucleosis

1. Mononucleosis. Health Information. Cleveland Clinic. http://my.clevelandclinic.org/health/diseases_conditions/hic-mononucleosis. Accessed Winter 2015.
2. Mononucleosis. Diseases and Conditions. Mayo Clinic; 2012. http://www.mayoclinic.org/diseases-conditions/mononucleosis/basics/definition/con-20021164
3. Epstein-Barr Virus and Infectious Mononucleosis. Centers for Disease Control and Prevention; 2014. http://www.cdc.gov/epstein-barr/index.html
4. Bennett NJ. Pediatric Mononucleosis and Epstein-Barr Virus. Medscape; 2014. http://emedicine.medscape.com/article/963894-overview
5. Cunha BA. Infectious Mononucleosis. Medscape; 2014. http://emedicine.medscape.com/article/222040-overview
6. Doerr S. Mononucleosis (Mono). eMedicineHealth; 2014. http://www.emedicinehealth.com/mononucleosis/article_em.htm

Multiple Sclerosis

1. About MS. National Multiple Sclerosis Society. http://www.nationalmssociety.org/For-Professionals/Clinical-Care/About-MS. Accessed Winter 2014.
2. What is MS? National Multiple Sclerosis Society. http://www.nationalmssociety.org/What-is-MS. Accessed Winter 2014.
3. Multiple Sclerosis. A.D.A.M Medical Encyclopedia. U.S. National Library of Medicine; 2014. http://www.ncbi.nlm.nih.gov/pubmedhealth/PMH0001747/
4. Multiple Sclerosis: Hope Through Research. Disorders A-Z. National Institute of Neurological Disorders and Stroke; 2014. http://www.ninds.nih.gov/disorders/multiple_sclerosis/detail_multiple_sclerosis.htm
5. Coggrave M, Norton C, Cody JD. Management of faecal incontinence and constipation in adults with central neurological diseases. *Cochrane Database of Systematic Reviews* 2014;(1):CD002115. http://www.ncbi.nlm.nih.gov/pubmed/24420006
6. Finch P, Bessonnette S. A pragmatic investigation into the effects of massage therapy on the self efficacy of multiple sclerosis clients. *Journal of Bodywork and Movement Therapies* 2014;18(1):11–16. http://www.ncbi.nlm.nih.gov/pubmed/24411144
7. Goldenberg MM. Multiple sclerosis review. *P & T* 2012; 37(3):175–184. http://www.ncbi.nlm.nih.gov/pmc/articles/PMC3351877/
8. Loma I, Heyman R. Multiple sclerosis: pathogenesis and treatment. *Current Neuropharmacology* 2011;9(3):409–416. http://www.ncbi.nlm.nih.gov/pmc/articles/PMC3151595/
9. Luzzio C. Multiple Sclerosis. Medscape; 2014. http://emedicine.medscape.com/article/1146199-overview
10. Marquez-Rebollo C, Vergara-Carrasco L, Diaz-Navarro R, et al. Benefit of endermology on indurations and panniculitis/lipoatrophy during relapsing-remitting multiple sclerosis long-term treatment with glatiramer acetate. *Advances in Therapy* 2014;31(8):904–914. http://www.ncbi.nlm.nih.gov/pubmed/25047757
11. McClurg D, Hagen S, Hawkins S, et al. Abdominal massage for the alleviation of constipation symptoms in people with multiple sclerosis: a randomized controlled feasibility study. *Multiple Sclerosis* 2011;17(2):223–233. http://www.ncbi.nlm.nih.gov/pubmed/20940182
12. Schreiner TL. Pediatric Multiple Sclerosis. Medscape; 2013. http://emedicine.medscape.com/article/2091406-overview
13. Schroeder B, Doig J, Premkumar K. The effects of massage therapy on multiple sclerosis patients' quality of life and leg function. *Evidence-Based Complementary and Alternative Medicine* 2014;2014:640916. http://www.hindawi.com/journals/ecam/2014/640916/

Polymyalgia Rheumatica

1. Polymyalgia Rheumatica and Giant Cell Arteritis. Health Info. National Institute of Arthritis and Musculoskeletal and Skin Diseases; 2012. http://www.niams.nih.gov/Health_Info/Polymyalgia/default.asp
2. Polymyalgia Rheumatica. Diseases and Conditions. Mayo Clinic; 2012. http://www.mayoclinic.org/diseases-conditions/polymyalgia-rheumatica/basics/definition/con-20023162
3. Ameer F, McNeil J. Polymyalgia rheumatica: clinical update. *Australian Family Physician* 2014;43(6):373–376. http://www.racgp.org.au/afp/2014/june/polymyalgia-rheumatica/
4. Kermani TA, Warrington KJ. Advances and challenges in the diagnosis and treatment of polymyalgia rheumatica. *Therapeutic Advances in Musculoskeletal Disease* 2014;6(1):8–19. http://www.ncbi.nlm.nih.gov/pmc/articles/PMC3897167/
5. Saad ER. Polymyalgia Rheumatica. Medscape; 2014. http://emedicine.medscape.com/article/330815-overview

Psoriasis

1. Types of Psoriaisis. National Psoriasis Foundation. http://www.psoriasis.org/learn_types. Accessed Winter 2015.
2. Psoriasis Triggers. PsoriasisNet; 2005. http://www.skincarephysicians.com/psoriasisnet/triggers.html
3. Psoriasis Pictures, Symptoms, Causes and Treatments. MedicineNet; 2013. http://www.medicinenet.com/psoriasis_symptoms_treatment_pictures_slideshow/article.htm

4. Azfar RS, Gelfand JM. Psoriasis and metabolic disease: epidemiology and pathophysiology. *Current Opinion in Rheumatology* 2008;20(4):416–422. http://www.medscape.com/viewarticle/576496
5. Lui H. Plaque Psoriasis. Medscape; 2015. http://emedicine.medscape.com/article/1108072-overview
6. Parisi R, Symmons DP, Griffiths CE, et al. Global epidemiology of psoriasis: a systematic review of incidence and prevalence. *Journal of Investigative Dermatology* 2013;133(2):377–385. http://www.nature.com/jid/journal/v133/n2/full/jid2012339a.html

Rheumatoid Arthritis

1. What People With Rheumatoid Arthritis Need to Know About Osteoarthritis. NIH Osteoporosis and Related Bone Diseases National Resource Center. National Institute of Arthritis and Musculoskeletal and Skin Diseases; 2012. http://www.niams.nih.gov/Health_Info/Bone/Osteoporosis/Conditions_Behaviors/osteoporosis_ra.asp
2. Rheumatoid Arthritis and Complementary Health Approaches. Health Info. National Center for Complementary and Alternative Medicine; 2013. http://nccam.nih.gov/health/RA/getthefacts.htm
3. Rheumatoid Arthritis. A.D.A.M Medical Encyclopedia. U.S. National Library of Medicine; 2014. http://www.ncbi.nlm.nih.gov/pubmedhealth/PMH0001467/
4. Handout on Health: Rheumatoid Arthritis. Health Info. National Institute of Arthritis and Musculoskeletal and Skin Diseases; 2014. http://www.niams.nih.gov/Health_Info/Rheumatic_Disease/default.asp
5. Cubick EE, Quezada VY, Schumer AD, et al. Sustained release myofascial release as treatment for a patient with complications of rheumatoid arthritis and collagenous colitis: a case report. *International Journal of Therapeutic Massage and Bodywork* 2011;4(3):1–9. http://www.ncbi.nlm.nih.gov/pmc/articles/PMC3184472/
6. Field T, Diego M, Delgado J, et al. Rheumatoid arthritis in upper limbs benefits from moderate pressure massage therapy. *Complementary Therapies in Clinical Practice* 2013;19(2):101–103. http://www.ncbi.nlm.nih.gov/pubmed/23561068
7. Shiel WC. Juvenile Ideiopathic Arthritis (Juvenile Rheumatoid Arthritis). eMedicineHealth; 2014. http://www.emedicinehealth.com/juvenile_rheumatoid_arthritis/article_em.htm
8. Shiel WC. Rheumatoid Arthritis. eMedicineHealth; 2014. http://www.emedicinehealth.com/rheumatoid_arthritis/article_em.htm
9. Vivar N, Van Vollenhoven RF. Advances in the treatment of rheumatoid arthritis. *F1000Prime Reports* 2014;6:31. http://www.ncbi.nlm.nih.gov/pmc/articles/PMC4017904/

Scleroderma

1. What is Scleroderma? Scleroderma Foundation. http://www.scleroderma.org/site/PageServer?pagename=patients_whatis#.VMVrX2TF8pw. Accessed Winter 2015.
2. Scleroderma. Health Info. National Institute of Arthritis and Musculoskeletal and Skin Diseases; 2012. http://www.niams.nih.gov/Health_Info/Scleroderma/default.asp
3. Scleroderma. A.D.A.M. Medical Encyclopedia. U.S. National Library of Medicine; 2014. http://www.ncbi.nlm.nih.gov/pubmedhealth/PMH0001465/
4. Bongi SM, Del Rosso A, Passalacqua M, et al. Manual lymph drainage improving upper extremity edema and hand function in patients with systemic sclerosis in edematous phase. *Arthritis Care and Research (Hoboken)* 2011;63(8):1134–1141. http://www.ncbi.nlm.nih.gov/pubmed/21523925
5. Jimenez SA. Scleroderma. Medscape; 2014. http://emedicine.medscape.com/article/331864-overview
6. Poole JL. Musculoskeletal rehabilitation in the person with scleroderma. *Current Opinion in Rheumatology* 2010;22(2):205–212. http://www.ncbi.nlm.nih.gov/pubmed/21523925

Ulcerative Colitis

1. What is Ulcerative Colitis. Crohn's & Colitis Foundation of America. http://www.ccfa.org/what-are-crohns-and-colitis/what-is-ulcerative-colitis/. Accessed Winter 2015.
2. Inflammatory Bowel Disease. Patient Education & Resource Center. American College of Gastroenterology. http://patients.gi.org/topics/inflammatory-bowel-disease/. Accessed Winter 2015.
3. Ulcerative Colitis. American Society of Colon & Rectal Surgeons; 2012. http://www.fascrs.org/patients/conditions/ulcerative_colitis/
4. Ulcerative Colitis. Health Topics. National Institute of Diabetes and Digestive and Kidney Diseases; 2014. http://www.niddk.nih.gov/health-information/health-topics/digestive-diseases/ulcerative-colitis/Pages/facts.aspx
5. Basson MD. Ulcerative Colitis. Medscape; 2014. http://emedicine.medscape.com/article/183084-overview
6. Diamanti A, Knafelz D, Panetta F, et al. Thalidomide as rescue therapy for acute severe ulcerative colitis. *European Review for Medical and Pharmacological Sciences* 2014;18(12):1690–1693. http://www.europeanreview.org/article/7500
7. Kerr M. The Difference Between Crohn's, UC, and IBD. Healthline; 2012. http://www.healthline.com/health/crohns-disease/crohns-ibd-uc-difference
8. Rawsthorne P, Clara I, Graff LA, et al. The Manitoba Inflammatory Bowel Disease Cohort Study: a prospective longitudinal evaluation of the use of complementary and alternative medicine services and products. *Gut* 2012;61(4):521–527. http://www.ncbi.nlm.nih.gov/pubmed/21836028
9. Rowe WA. Inflammatory Bowel Disease. Medscape; 2015. http://emedicine.medscape.com/article/179037-overview

Chapter 7

Acute Bronchitis

1. Acute Bronchitis. MedlinePlus. U.S. National Library of Medicine. http://www.nlm.nih.gov/medlineplus/acutebronchitis.html. Accessed Winter 2015.
2. What is Bronchitis? Health Topics. National Heart, Lung, and Blood Institute; 2011. http://www.nhlbi.nih.gov/health/health-topics/topics/brnchi/
3. Bronchitis (Chest Cold). Get Smart: Know When Antibiotics Work. Centers for Disease Control and Prevention; 2013. http://www.cdc.gov/getsmart/antibiotic-use/URI/bronchitis.html
4. Bronchitis—acute. A.D.A.M. Medical Encyclopedia. U.S. National Library of Medicine; 2014. http://www.ncbi.nlm.nih.gov/pubmedhealth/PMH0002078/
5. Fayyaz J. Bronchitis. Medscape; 2014. http://emedicine.medscape.com/article/297108-overview
6. Llor C, Moragas A, Bayona C, et al. Efficacy of anti-inflammatory or antibiotic treatment in patients with non-complicated

acute bronchitis and discoloured sputum: randomised placebo controlled trial. *BMJ* 2013;347:f5762. http://www.ncbi.nlm.nih.gov/pmc/articles/PMC3790568/

Asthma

1. Asthma. The Ohio State University Wexner Medical Center. http://wexnermedical.osu.edu/patient-care/healthcare-services/lung-pulmonary/asthma. Accessed Winter 2015.
2. Asthma. Conditions & Treatments. American Academy of Allergy Asthma & Immunology. http://www.aaaai.org/conditions-and-treatments/asthma.aspx. Accessed Winter 2015.
3. Asthma and Exercise: Tips to Remember. Conditions & Treatments. American Academy of Allergy Asthma & Immunology. http://www.aaaai.org/conditions-and-treatments/library/asthma-library/asthma-and-exercise.aspx. Accessed Winter 2015.
4. Asthma in Adults Fact Sheet. American Lung Association; 2012. http://www.lung.org/lung-disease/asthma/resources/facts-and-figures/asthma-in-adults.html
5. Asthma and Complementary Health Approaches. Health Info. National Center for Complementary and Integrative Health; 2013. https://nccih.nih.gov/health/asthma/facts
6. What is Asthma? Health Topics. National Heart, Lung, and Blood Institute; 2014. http://www.nhlbi.nih.gov/health/health-topics/topics/asthma/
7. Institute of Medicine Committee on the Assessment of Asthma and Indoor Air. *Clearing the air: asthma and indoor air exposures*. Washington, DC: National Academies Press; 2000. Copyright 2000 by the National Academy of Sciences. All rights reserved.; Book NBK224477 [bookaccession]. http://www.ncbi.nlm.nih.gov/books/NBK224477/
8. Morris MJ. Asthma. Medscape; 2014. http://emedicine.medscape.com/article/296301-overview

Chronic Bronchitis

1. Understanding Chronic Bronchitis. Lung Disease. American Lung Association. http://www.lung.org/lung-disease/bronchitis-chronic/understanding-chronic-bronchitis.html. Accessed Winter 2015.
2. What is Bronchitis? Health Topics. National Heart, Lung, and Blood Institute; 2011. http://www.nhlbi.nih.gov/health/health-topics/topics/brnchi/
3. Global Strategy for the Diagnosis, Management, and Prevention of Chronic Obstructive Pulmonary Disease. Global Initiative for Chronic Obstructive Lung Disease; 2011. http://www.goldcopd.org/uploads/users/files/GOLD_Report_2011_Feb21.pdf
4. What Are Lung Function Tests? Health Topics. National Heart, Lung, and Blood Institute; 2012. http://www.nhlbi.nih.gov/health/health-topics/topics/lft/
5. Chronic Obstructive Pulmonary Disease Among Adults—United States, 2011. *Morbidity and Mortality Weekly Report* 2012;61(46):938–943. http://www.cdc.gov/mmwr/preview/mmwrhtml/mm6146a2.htm?s_cid=mm6146a2_w
6. What is COPD? Health Topics A-Z. National Institutes of Health Senior Health; 2013. http://nihseniorhealth.gov/copd/whatiscopd/01.html
7. Faner R, Tal-Singer R, Riley JH, et al. Lessons from ECLIPSE: a review of COPD biomarkers. *Thorax* 2014;69(7):666–672. http://www.medscape.com/viewarticle/826747
8. Mosenifar Z. Chronic Obstructive Pulmonary Disease. Medscape; 2014. http://emedicine.medscape.com/article/297664-overview
9. Qaseem A, Wilt TJ, Weinberger SE, et al. Diagnosis and management of stable chronic obstructive pulmonary disease: a clinical practice guideline update from the American College of Physicians, American College of Chest Physicians, American Thoracic Society, and European Respiratory Society. *Annals of Internal Medicine* 2011;155(3):179–191. http://annals.org/article.aspx?articleid=479627

Common Cold

1. What Causes Cold Symptoms. Understanding Colds. http://www.commoncold.org/undrstn4.htm. Accessed Winter 2015.
2. Anatomy of the Nose. Understanding Colds. http://www.commoncold.org/undrstnd.htm. Accessed Winter 2015.
3. Common Colds: Protect Yourself and Others. Health & Research Topics. National Institute of Allergy and Infectious Diseases; 2011. http://www.niaid.nih.gov/topics/commonCold/Pages/default.aspx
4. Catching a Cold When It's Warm. News in Health. National Institutes of Health; 2012. http://newsinhealth.nih.gov/issue/jun2012/feature2
5. Common Cold and Runny Nose. Get Smart: Know When Antibiotics Work. Centers for Disease Control and Prevention; 2013. http://www.cdc.gov/getsmart/antibiotic-use/URI/colds.html
6. Common Cold. Diseases and Conditions. Mayo Clinic; 2013. http://www.mayoclinic.org/diseases-conditions/common-cold/basics/definition/con-20019062
7. How Long Do Viruses Live on Surfaces? 2014. http://hubpages.com/hub/How-Long-Do-Viruses-Live
8. Sexton DJ. Up To Date: Wolters Kluwer Health. Patient Information: The Common Cold in Adults (Beyond the Basics); 2014. http://www.uptodate.com/contents/the-common-cold-in-adults-beyond-the-basics

Cystic Fibrosis

1. Cystic Fibrosis. Lung Disease. American Lung Association. http://www.lung.org/lung-disease/cystic-fibrosis/. Accessed Winter 2015.
2. Information for Adults With Cystic Fibrosis. Cystic Fibrosis Foundation. http://www.cff.org/Adults/. Accessed Winter 2015.
3. Facts About Cystic Fibrosis. Science Ambassador Program. Centers for Disease Control and Prevention; 1995. http://www.cdc.gov/excite/ScienceAmbassador/ambassador_pgm/lessonplans/high_school/Am%20I%20a%20Carrier%20for%20Cystic%20Fibrosis/Cystic_Fibrosis_Fact_Sheet.pdf
4. What is Cystic Fibrosis? Health Topics. National Heart, Lung, and Blood Institute; 2013. http://www.nhlbi.nih.gov/health/health-topics/topics/cf/
5. Frequently Asked Questions. About Cystic Fibrosis. Cystic Fibrosis Foundation; 2014. http://www.cff.org/AboutCF/Faqs/
6. Cystic Fibrosis. Genetics Home Reference. U.S. National Library of Medicine; 2015. http://ghr.nlm.nih.gov/condition/cystic-fibrosis
7. Huth MM, Zink KA, Van Horn NR. The effects of massage therapy in improving outcomes for youth with cystic fibrosis: an evidence review. *Pediatric Nursing* 2005;31(4):328–332. http://www.ncbi.nlm.nih.gov/pubmed/16229132
8. Lee A, Holdsworth M, Holland A, et al. The immediate effect of musculoskeletal physiotherapy techniques and massage

on pain and ease of breathing in adults with cystic fibrosis. *Journal of Cystic Fibrosis* 2009;8(1):79–81. http://www.cysticfibrosisjournal.com/article/S1569-1993(08)00111-2/pdf

9. Sharma GD. Cystic Fibrosis. Medscape; 2014. http://emedicine.medscape.com/article/1001602-overview
10. Smyth AR, Bell SC, Bojcin S, et al. European cystic fibrosis society standards of care: best practice guidelines. *Journal of Cystic Fibrosis* 2014;13(Suppl 1):S23–S42. http://www.cysticfibrosisjournal.com/article/S1569-1993(14)00085-X/fulltext#s0005
11. Tsui LC, Dorfman R. The cystic fibrosis gene: a molecular genetic perspective. *Cold Spring Harbor Perspectives in Medicine* 2013;3(2):a009472. http://perspectivesinmedicine.org/content/3/2/a009472.full

Emphysema

1. Lung Sections. National Institute for Occupational Safety and Health. http://www.cdc.gov/niosh/topics/surveillance/ords/pdfs/LungSections.pdf. Accessed Winter 2015.
2. What is COPD? Health Topics. National Heart, Lung, and Blood Institute; 2013. http://www.nhlbi.nih.gov/health/health-topics/topics/copd/
3. Chronic Obstructive Pulmonary Disease (COPD). NIH Fact Sheets Home. National Institutes of Health; 2013. http://report.nih.gov/nihfactsheets/ViewFactSheet.aspx?csid=77
4. Chronic Obstructive Pulmonary Disease. A.D.A.M. Medical Encyclopedia. U.S. National Library of Medicine; 2014. http://www.ncbi.nlm.nih.gov/pubmedhealth/PMH0001153/
5. Chronic Obstructive Pulmonary Disease (COPD) Fact Sheet. American Lung Association; 2014. http://www.lung.org/lung-disease/copd/resources/facts-figures/COPD-Fact-Sheet.html
6. Boka K. Emphysema. Medscape; 2014. http://emedicine.medscape.com/article/298283-overview
7. Dias OM, Baldi BG, Costa AN, et al. Combined pulmonary fibrosis and emphysema: an increasingly recognized condition. *Jornal Brasileiro de Pneumologia* 2014;40(3):304–312. http://www.ncbi.nlm.nih.gov/pmc/articles/PMC4109203/
8. Khan AN. Emphysema Imaging. Medscape; 2014. http://emedicine.medscape.com/article/355688-overview

Influenza

1. Who's at Risk. U.S. Department of Health & Human Services. http://www.flu.gov/at-risk/index.html. Accessed Winter 2015.
2. 2009 H1N1 Flu ("Swine Flu") and You. Centers for Disease Control and Prevention; 2010. http://www.cdc.gov/h1n1flu/qa.htm
3. The Flu, the Common Cold, and Complementary Health Approaches. Health Info. National Center for Complementary and Integrative Health; 2013. https://nccih.nih.gov/health/flu/ataglance.htm
4. Key Facts About Influenza (Flu) & Flu Vaccine. Influenza (Flu). Centers for Disease Control and Prevention; 2014. http://www.cdc.gov/flu/keyfacts.htm
5. Flu Symptoms & Severity. Influenza (Flu). Centers for Disease Control & Prevention; 2014. http://www.cdc.gov/flu/about/disease/symptoms.htm
6. Vaccination: Who Should Do It, Who Should Not and Who Should Take Precautions. Influenza (Flu). Centers for Disease Control and Prevention; 2014. http://www.cdc.gov/flu/protect/whoshouldvax.htm
7. Derlet RW. Influenza. Medscape; 2015. http://emedicine.medscape.com/article/219557-overview
8. Sandrock CE. Influenza Antiviral Therapy. Medscape; 2015. http://emedicine.medscape.com/article/1966844-overview

Laryngeal Cancer

1. Voice Box (Laryngeal) Cancer. Patient Health. American Academy of Otolaryngology—Head and Neck Surgery; 2012. http://www.entnet.org/content/voice-box-laryngeal-cancer
2. Throat Cancer. Diseases and Conditions. Mayo Clinic; 2012. http://www.mayoclinic.org/diseases-conditions/oral-and-throat-cancer/basics/definition/con-20042850
3. Laryngeal and Hypopharyngeal Cancers. American Cancer Society; 2015. http://www.cancer.org/acs/groups/cid/documents/webcontent/003108-pdf.pdf
4. Johnson JT. Malignant Tumors of the Larynx. Medscape; 2014. http://emedicine.medscape.com/article/848592-overview
5. Stevenson MM. Oral Cavity and Laryngeal Cancer Staging. Medscape; 2013. http://emedicine.medscape.com/article/2048034-overview

Lung Cancer

1. Lung Cancer Fact Sheet. Lung Disease. American Lung Association; 2014. http://www.lung.org/lung-disease/lung-cancer/resources/facts-figures/lung-cancer-fact-sheet.html
2. What You Need To Know About Lung Cancer. Patient Education Publications. National Cancer Institute; 2014. http://www.cancer.gov/publications/patient-education/wyntk-lung-cancer
3. Lung Cancer (Non-Small Cell). American Cancer Society; 2015. http://www.cancer.org/acs/groups/cid/documents/webcontent/003115-pdf.pdf
4. Deng GE, Rausch SM, Jones LW, et al. Complementary therapies and integrative medicine in lung cancer: Diagnosis and management of lung cancer, 3rd ed: American College of Chest Physicians evidence-based clinical practice guidelines. *Chest* 2013;143(5 Suppl):e420S–e436S. http://www.ncbi.nlm.nih.gov/pubmed/23649450
5. Pozo CL, Morgan MA, Gray JE. Survivorship issues for patients with lung cancer. *Cancer Control* 2014;21(1):40–50. http://www.ncbi.nlm.nih.gov/pubmed/24357740
6. Ramlogan-Steel CA, Steel JC, Morris JC. Lung cancer vaccines: current status and future prospects. *Translational Lung Cancer Research* 2014;3(1):46–52. http://www.medscape.com/viewarticle/826300
7. Stevenson MM. Small Cell Lung Cancer Staging. Medscape; 2013. http://emedicine.medscape.com/article/2006716-overview
8. Stöppler MC. Lung Cancer. eMedicineHealth; 2013. http://www.emedicinehealth.com/lung_cancer/article_em.htm

Pneumonia

1. Pneumonia. Lung Disease. American Lung Association. http://www.lung.org/lung-disease/pneumonia/. Accessed Winter 2015.
2. What is Pneumonia? Health Topics. National Heart, Lung, and Blood Institute; 2011. http://www.nhlbi.nih.gov/health/health-topics/topics/pnu/
3. Pneumonia. Diseases & Conditions. Cleveland Clinic; 2012. http://my.clevelandclinic.org/health/diseases_conditions/hic_Pneumonia

4. Pneumonia Can Be Prevented—Vaccines Can Help. Diseases & Conditions. Centers for Disease Control and Prevention; 2014. http://www.cdc.gov/Features/Pneumonia/
5. Pneumonia: an infection of the lungs. Centers for Disease Control and Prevention; 2014. http://www.cdc.gov/pneumonia/index.html
6. Pneumonia. FastStats. Centers for Disease Control and Prevention; 2014. http://www.cdc.gov/nchs/fastats/pneumonia.htm
7. Kamangar N. Bacterial Pneumonia. Medscape; 2014. http://emedicine.medscape.com/article/300157-overview
8. Mosenifar Z. Viral Pneumonia. Medscape; 2015. http://emedicine.medscape.com/article/300455-overview

Sinusitis

1. Sinusitis: Tips to Remember. Conditions & Treatments. American Academy of Allergy Asthma & Immunology. http://www.aaaai.org/conditions-and-treatments/library/At-a-glance/sinusitis.aspx. Accessed Winter 2015.
2. 20 Questions About Your Sinuses. Patient Health Information. American Academy of Otolaryngology—Head and Neck Surgery. http://www.entnet.org/?q=node/1374. Accessed Winter 2015.
3. Sinusitis. National Institute of Allergy and Infectious Diseases; 2012. http://www.niaid.nih.gov/topics/sinusitis/Documents/sinusitis.pdf
4. Nasal Wash Treatment. Health Information. National Jewish Health; 2012. http://www.nationaljewish.org/healthinfo/medications/lung-diseases/alternative/nasal-wash-treatment.aspx
5. Seasonal Allergies and Complementary Health Practices: What the Science Says. NCCIH Clinical Digest. National Center for Complementary and Integrative Health; 2013. https://nccih.nih.gov/health/providers/digest/allergies-science
6. An Overview of Sinusitis. WebMD; 2014. http://www.webmd.com/allergies/sinusitis-and-sinus-infection
7. Sinusitis. A.D.A.M Medical Encyclopedia. U.S. National Library of Medicine; 2014. http://www.ncbi.nlm.nih.gov/pubmedhealth/PMH0001670/
8. Help for Sinus Pain and Pressure: Nasal Saline Irrigation and Neti Pots. WebMD; 2014. http://www.webmd.com/allergies/sinus-pain-pressure-11/neti-pots
9. Becker DG. Allergic and Non-Allergic Sinusitis for the Primary Care Physician. Pathophysiology, Evaluation and Treatment; 2010. http://www.beckerentcenter.com/documents/book10.pdf
10. Pfaar O, Raap U, Holz M, et al. Pathophysiology of itching and sneezing in allergic rhinitis. *Swiss Medical Weekly* 2009;139(3–4):35–40. http://www.smw.ch/docs/PdfContent/smw-12468.pdf
11. Radojicic C. Sinusitis. Center for Continuing Education. Cleveland Clinic. http://www.clevelandclinicmeded.com/medicalpubs/diseasemanagement/allergy/rhino-sinusitis/. Accessed Winter 2015.

Tuberculosis

1. Detailed Explanation of TB. Health & Research Topics. National Institute of Allergy and Infectious Diseases; 2009. http://www.niaid.nih.gov/topics/tuberculosis/Understanding/WhatIsTB/pages/detailed.aspx
2. Tuberculosis (TB). Health & Research Topics. National Institute of Allergy and Infectious Diseases; 2010. http://www.niaid.nih.gov/topics/tuberculosis/Understanding/Pages/overview.aspx
3. Tuberculosis: General Information. Centers for Disease Control and Prevention; 2011. http://www.cdc.gov/tb/publications/factsheets/general/tb.htm
4. BCG Vaccine. Centers for Disease Control and Prevention; 2011. http://www.cdc.gov/tb/publications/factsheets/prevention/bcg.htm
5. TB Elimination: Extensively Drug-Resistant Tuberculosis (XDR TB). Centers for Disease Control and Prevention; 2013. http://www.cdc.gov/tb/publications/factsheets/drtb/xdrtb.pdf
6. Questions and Answers About Tuberculosis. Centers for Disease Control and Prevention; 2014. http://www.cdc.gov/tb/publications/faqs/pdfs/qa.pdf
7. Tuberculosis. World Health Organization; 2014. http://www.who.int/mediacentre/factsheets/fs104/en/
8. Trends in Tuberculosis, 2013. Centers for Disease Control and Prevention; 2014. http://www.cdc.gov/tb/publications/factsheets/statistics/TBTrends.htm
9. Batra V. Pediatric Tuberculosis. Medscape; 2014. http://emedicine.medscape.com/article/969401-overview
10. Todar K. Mycobacterium tuberculosis and Tuberculosis. Todar's Online Textbook of Bacteriology; 2012. http://textbookofbacteriology.net/tuberculosis.html

Chapter 8

Candidiasis

1. Candidiasis. Fungal Diseases. Centers for Disease Control and Prevention; 2014. http://www.cdc.gov/fungal/diseases/candidiasis/index.html
2. Hidalgo JA. Candidiasis. Medscape; 2014. http://emedicine.medscape.com/article/213853-overview
3. Kalyoussef S. Pediatric Candidiasis. Medscape; 2014. http://emedicine.medscape.com/article/962300-overview
4. Khan MS, Malik A, Ahmad I. Anti-candidal activity of essential oils alone and in combination with amphotericin B or fluconazole against multi-drug resistant isolates of Candida albicans. *Medical Mycology* 2012;50(1):33–42. http://www.ncbi.nlm.nih.gov/pubmed/21756200
5. Pankhurst CL. Candidiasis (oropharyngeal). *Clinical Evidence (Online)* 2013;2013:1304. http://www.ncbi.nlm.nih.gov/pmc/articles/PMC2907793/

Celiac Disease

1. What is Celiac Disease. Celiac Disease Foundation. http://celiac.org/celiac-disease/what-is-celiac-disease/. Accessed Winter 2015.
2. Celiac Disease. Health Topics. National Institute of Diabetes and Digestive and Kidney Diseases; 2012. http://www.niddk.nih.gov/health-information/health-topics/digestive-diseases/celiac-disease/Pages/facts.aspx
3. Celiac Disease—Sprue. A.D.A.M. Medical Encyclopedia. U.S. National Library of Medicine; 2014. http://www.ncbi.nlm.nih.gov/pubmedhealth/PMH0001280/
4. Brooks M. Celiac Disease Diagnosis Up 4-Fold Worldwide. Medscape Medical News; 2010. http://www.medscape.com/viewarticle/726127
5. Gasbarrini G, Mangiola F. Wheat-related disorders: a broad spectrum of 'evolving' diseases. *United European*

Gastroenterology Journal 2014;2(4):254–262. http://www.ncbi.nlm.nih.gov/pmc/articles/PMC4114114/

6. Halfdanarson TR, Litzow MR, Murray JA. Hematologic manifestations of celiac disease. *Blood* 2007;109(2):412–421. http://www.bloodjournal.org/content/109/2/412?sso-checked=true
7. Picco MF. I have celiac disease. Do I need to be concerned about sunscreens, shampoos and cosmetics that contain gluten? Diseases and Conditions. Mayo Clinic. http://www.mayoclinic.org/diseases-conditions/celiac-disease/expert-answers/celiac-disease/faq-20057879. Accessed Winter 2015.
8. Rubio-Tapia A, Ludvigsson JF, Brantner TL, et al. The prevalence of celiac disease in the United States. *American Journal of Gastroenterology* 2012;107(10):1538–1544; quiz 1537, 1545. http://www.nature.com/ajg/journal/v107/n10/full/ajg2012219a.html

Cirrhosis

1. Cirrhosis. University of California San Francisco Medical Center. http://www.ucsfhealth.org/conditions/cirrhosis/. Accessed Winter 2015.
2. Cirrhosis: A Patient's Guide. VA Hepatitis C Resource Centers; 2007. http://www.hepatitis.va.gov/pdf/cirrhosis_handbook.pdf
3. North American Indian Childhood Cirrhosis. Genetics Home Reference. U.S. National Library of Medicine; 2011. http://ghr.nlm.nih.gov/condition/north-american-indian-childhood-cirrhosis
4. Cirrhosis. Health Topics. National Institute of Diabetes and Digestive and Kidney Diseases; 2014. http://www.niddk.nih.gov/health-information/health-topics/liver-disease/cirrhosis/Pages/facts.aspx
5. Cirrhosis. Liver Disease Information. American Liver Foundation; 2015. http://www.liverfoundation.org/abouttheliver/info/cirrhosis
6. Non-Alcoholic Fatty Liver Disease. Liver Disease Information. American Liver Foundation; 2015. http://www.liverfoundation.org/abouttheliver/info/nafld/
7. LaBrecque DR, Abbas Z, Anania F, et al. World Gastroenterology Organisation global guidelines: nonalcoholic fatty liver disease and nonalcoholic steatohepatitis. *Journal of Clinical Gastroenterology* 2014;48(6):467–473. http://journals.lww.com/jcge/Fulltext/2014/07000/World_Gastroenterology_Organisation_Global.4.aspx
8. Mauss S, Berg T, Rockstroh J, et al. *Hepatology 2014: a clinical textbook*. Flying Publisher. http://emedicine.medscape.com/article/185856-overview
9. Wolf DC. Cirrhosis. Medscape; 2014. http://emedicine.medscape.com/article/185856-overview

Colorectal Cancer

1. Colon Polyps. Health Topics. National Institute of Diabetes and Digestive and Kidney Diseases. http://www.niddk.nih.gov/health-information/health-topics/digestive-diseases/colon-polyps/Pages/overview.aspx. Accessed Winter 2015.
2. Colon and Rectal Cancer. Cancer Topics. National Cancer Institute. http://www.cancer.gov/cancertopics/types/colon-and-rectal. Accessed Winter 2015.
3. SEER Stat Fact Sheets: Colon and Rectum Cancer. Surveillance, Epidemiology, and End Results Program. National Cancer Institute. http://seer.cancer.gov/statfacts/html/colorect.html. Access Winter 2015
4. Colon and Rectum Cancer Staging. American Joint Committee on Cancer; 2009. https://cancerstaging.org/references-tools/quickreferences/Documents/ColonLarge.pdf
5. Colorectal Cancer Overview. American Cancer Society; 2014. http://www.cancer.org/acs/groups/cid/documents/webcontent/003047-pdf.pdf
6. Colorectal Cancer and Continence. International Foundation for Functional Gastrointestinal Disorders; 2014. http://www.aboutincontinence.org/site/what-is-incontinence/causes-of-incontinence/cancer
7. Colon Cancer Treatment. National Cancer Institute; 2015. http://www.cancer.gov/cancertopics/pdq/treatment/colon/HealthProfessional
8. Andrea C, Fausto P, Francesca BK, et al. Which strategy after first-line therapy in advanced colorectal cancer? *World Journal of Gastroenterology* 2014;20(27):8921–8927. http://www.ncbi.nlm.nih.gov/pmc/articles/PMC4112862/
9. Cagir B. Rectal Cancer. Medscape; 2014. http://emedicine.medscape.com/article/281237-overview
10. Connolly A. Cancerous Colon Tissue. Khan Academy; 2011. https://www.khanacademy.org/science/health-and-medicine/healthcare-misc/v/cancerous-colon-tissue
11. Guerin A, Mody R, Fok B, et al. Risk of developing colorectal cancer and benign colorectal neoplasm in patients with chronic constipation. *Alimentary Pharmacology and Therapeutics* 2014; 40(1):83–92. http://www.medscape.com/viewarticle/827211
12. Khiewkhern S, Promthet S, Sukprasert A, et al. Effectiveness of aromatherapy with light Thai massage for cellular immunity improvement in colorectal cancer patients receiving chemotherapy. *Asian Pacific Journal of Cancer Prevention* 2013;14(6): 3903–3907. http://www.ncbi.nlm.nih.gov/pubmed/23886205

Diverticular Disease

1. What I need to know about Diverticular Disease. Health Topics. National Institute of Diabetes and Digestive and Kidney Diseases; 2012. http://www.niddk.nih.gov/health-information/health-topics/digestive-diseases/diverticular-disease/Pages/ez.aspx
2. Diverticular Disease. WebMD; 2014. http://www.webmd.com/digestive-disorders/diverticular-disease
3. Diverticula, Diverticulosis, Diverticulitis: What's the Difference? International Foundation for Functional Gastrointestinal Disorders; 2014. http://www.iffgd.org/site/gi-disorders/other/diverticulosis/difference
4. Hobson KG, Roberts PL. Etiology and pathophysiology of diverticular disease. *Clinics in Colon and Rectal Surgery* 2004;17(3):147–153. http://www.ncbi.nlm.nih.gov/pmc/articles/PMC2780060/
5. Humes DJ, Spiller RC. Review article: the pathogenesis and management of acute colonic diverticulitis. *Alimentary Pharmacology and Therapeutics* 2014;39(4):359–370. http://www.medscape.com/viewarticle/820353
6. Joffe S. Imaging in Diverticulitis of the Colon. Medscape; 2013. http://emedicine.medscape.com/article/367320-overview
7. Shahedi K. Diverticulitis. Medscape; 2015. http://emedicine.medscape.com/article/173388-overview

Esophageal Cancer

1. What You Need To Know About Cancer of the Esophagus. National Cancer Institute; 2014. http://www.cancer.gov/publications/patient-education/wyntk-esophagus-cancer

2. Baldwin KM. Esophageal Cancer. Medscape; 2014. http://emedicine.medscape.com/article/277930-overview
3. Fischbach LA, Graham DY, Kramer JR, et al. Association between *Helicobacter pylori* and Barrett's esophagus: a case-control study. *American Journal of Gastroenterology* 2014;109(3):357–368. http://www.ncbi.nlm.nih.gov/pmc/articles/PMC4046944/
4. Rhodes TD. Esophageal Cancer Staging. Medscape; 2013. http://emedicine.medscape.com/article/2003224-overview

Gallstones

1. Understanding Gallstones. Patient Center. American Gastroenterological Association. http://www.gastro.org/patient-center/digestive-conditions/gallstones. Accessed Winter 2015.
2. Dieting and Gallstones. Weight-control Information Network. National Institute of Diabetes and Digestive and Kidney Diseases; 2008. http://win.niddk.nih.gov/publications/gall stones.htm
3. Gallstones. A.D.A.M. Medical Encyclopedia. U.S. National Library of Medicine; 2013. http://www.ncbi.nlm.nih.gov/pubmedhealth/PMH0001318/
4. Bonheur JL. Biliary Obstruction. Medscape; 2014. http://emedicine.medscape.com/article/187001-overview
5. Heuman DM. Gallstones (Cholelithiasis). Medscape; 2015. http://emedicine.medscape.com/article/175667-overview
6. Kennedy M. Pediatric Gallstones (Cholelithiasis). Medscape; 2013. http://emedicine.medscape.com/article/927522-overview

Gastroenteritis

1. Viral Gastroenteritis. Health Information. National Institute of Diabetes and Digestive and Kidney Diseases; 2012. http://www.niddk.nih.gov/health-information/health-topics/digestive-diseases/viral-gastroenteritis/Pages/facts.aspx
2. Norovirus. Centers for Disease Control and Prevention; 2014. http://www.cdc.gov/norovirus/
3. Rotavirus. Centers for Disease Control and Prevention; 2014. http://www.cdc.gov/rotavirus/index.html
4. Bonheur JL. Bacterial Gastroenteritis. Medscape; 2014. http://emedicine.medscape.com/article/176400-overview
5. Diskin A. Emergent Treatment of Gastroenteritis. Medscape; 2015. http://emedicine.medscape.com/article/775277-overview
6. Tablang MVF. Viral Gastroenteritis. Medscape; 2014. http://emedicine.medscape.com/article/176515-overview
7. Wedro B. Gastroenteritis (Stomach Flu). eMedicineHealth; 2014. http://www.emedicinehealth.com/gastroenteritis/article_em.htm

Gastroesophageal Reflux Disease

1. Gastroesophageal Reflux (GER) and Gastroesophageal Reflux Disease (GERD) in Adults. Health Information. National Institute of Diabetes and Digestive and Kidney Diseases. http://www.niddk.nih.gov/health-information/health-topics/digestive-diseases/ger-and-gerd-in-adults/Pages/over view.aspx. Accessed Winter 2015.
2. Gastroesophageal Reflux Disease. A.D.A.M. Medical Encyclopedia. U.S. National Library of Medicine; 2013. http://www.ncbi.nlm.nih.gov/pubmedhealth/PMH0001311/
3. Treatment of GERD. International Foundation for Functional Gastrointestinal Disorders; 2014. http://www.aboutgerd.org/site/treatment/
4. Lie DA. Can Complementary and Alternative Therapies Relieve GERD Symptoms? Medscape Family Medicine; 2014. http://www.medscape.com/viewarticle/827662
5. Neu M, Schmiege SJ, Pan Z, et al. Interactions during feeding with mothers and their infants with symptoms of gastroesophageal reflux. *Journal of Alternative and Complementary Medicine* 2014;20(6):493–499. http://www.ncbi.nlm.nih.gov/pubmed/24742255
6. O'Malley P. Gastric Ulcers and GERD: The New "Plagues" of the 21st Century Update for the Clinical Nurse Specialist. Medscape; 2003. http://www.medscape.com/viewarticle/465049
7. Simic PJ. Acid Reflux (GERD). eMedicineHealth; 2014. http://www.emedicinehealth.com/acid_reflux_disease_gerd/article_em.htm

Hepatitis

1. Living with Hepatitis. U.S. Department of Veterans Affairs. http://www.hepatitis.va.gov/patient/daily/daily-index.asp. Accessed Winter 2015.
2. Managing Side Effects of Hepatitis C Treatment. VA Hepatitis C Resource Centers; 2007. http://www.hepatitis.va.gov/pdf/treatment-side-effects.pdf
3. Hepatitis B Information for Health Professionals. Centers for Disease Control and Prevention; 2012. http://www.cdc.gov/hepatitis/HBV/index.htm
4. Hepatitis A FAQs for Health Professionals. Centers for Disease Control and Prevention; 2013. http://www.cdc.gov/hepatitis/HAV/HAVfaq.htm
5. Viral Hepatitis Surveillance—United States, 2010. Centers for Disease Control and Prevention; 2013. http://www.cdc.gov/hepatitis/statistics/2010surveillance/Commentary.htm
6. Hepatitis A. World Health Organization; 2014. http://www.who.int/mediacentre/factsheets/fs328/en/
7. Hepatitis B. World Health Organization; 2014. http://www.who.int/mediacentre/factsheets/fs204/en/
8. Hepatitis C. World Health Organization; 2014. http://www.who.int/mediacentre/factsheets/fs164/en/
9. Nonalcoholic Steatohepatitis. Health Information. National Institute of Diabetes and Digestive and Kidney Diseases; 2014. http://www.niddk.nih.gov/health-information/health-topics/liver-disease/nonalcoholic-steatohepatitis/Pages/facts.aspx
10. Hepatitis C: A Focus on Dietary Supplements. National Center for Complementary and Integrative Health; 2014. https://nccih.nih.gov/sites/nccam.nih.gov/files/Get_The_Facts_Hepatitis_C.pdf
11. Hepatitis C Information for Health Professionals. Centers for Disease Control and Prevention; 2015. http://www.cdc.gov/hepatitis/HCV/HCVfaq.htm
12. Jhaveri R. What's New in the Alphabet Soup of Viral Hepatitis. Medscape Infectious Diseases; 2011. http://www.medscape.com/viewarticle/743651
13. Mauss S, Berg T, Rockstroh J, et al. *Hepatology 2014: a clinical textbook*. Flying Publisher. http://emedicine.medscape.com/article/185856-overview

Irritable Bowel Syndrome

1. Irritable Bowel Syndrome and Complementary Health Practices: What the Science Says. NCCIH Clinical Digest. National Center for Complementary and Integrative Health; 2013. https://nccih.nih.gov/health/providers/digest/IBS-science

2. About Irritable Bowel Syndrome (IBS). International Foundation for Functional Gastrointestinal Disorders; 2014. http://www.aboutibs.org/
3. Cremon C, Stanghellini V, Pallotti F, et al. Salmonella gastroenteritis during childhood is a risk factor for irritable bowel syndrome in adulthood. *Gastroenterology* 2014;147(1):69–77. http://www.gastrojournal.org/article/S0016-5085(14)00362-X/fulltext
4. Lehrer JK. Irritable Bowel Syndrome. Medscape; 2015. http://emedicine.medscape.com/article/180389-overview
5. Martinez-Martinez LA, Mora T, et al. Sympathetic nervous system dysfunction in fibromyalgia, chronic fatigue syndrome, irritable bowel syndrome, and interstitial cystitis: a review of case-control studies. *Journal of Clinical Rheumatology* 2014;20(3):146–150. http://www.medscape.com/viewarticle/823084
6. McPartland JM, Guy GW, Di Marzo V. Care and feeding of the endocannabinoid system: a systematic review of potential clinical interventions that upregulate the endocannabinoid system. *PLoS One* 2014;9(3):e89566. http://www.ncbi.nlm.nih.gov/pmc/articles/PMC3951193/

Liver Cancer

1. Liver Cancer Overview. American Cancer Society. http://www.cancer.org/cancer/livercancer/overviewguide/index. Accessed Winter 2015.
2. What You Need To Know About Liver Cancer. National Cancer Institute; 2009. http://www.cancer.gov/publications/patient-education/liver.pdf
3. Adult Primary Liver Cancer Treatment. National Cancer Institute; 2014. http://www.cancer.gov/cancertopics/pdq/treatment/adult-primary-liver/Patient/AllPages
4. Cicalese L. Hepatocellular Carcinoma. Medscape; 2014. http://emedicine.medscape.com/article/197319-overview
5. Kulik LM, Fisher RA, Rodrigo DR, et al. Outcomes of living and deceased donor liver transplant recipients with hepatocellular carcinoma: results of the A2ALL cohort. *American Journal of Transplantation* 2012;12(11):2997–3007. http://www.ncbi.nlm.nih.gov/pmc/articles/PMC3523685/

Pancreatic Cancer

1. What is Pancreatic Cancer? Pancreatica. http://pancreatica.org/faq/pancreatic-cancer/, Accessed Winter 2015.
2. Pancreatic Cancer. National Cancer Institute. http://www.cancer.gov/cancertopics/types/pancreatic. Accessed Winter 2015.
3. What You Need To Know About Cancer of the Pancreas. National Cancer Institute; 2010. http://www.cancer.gov/publications/patient-education/wyntk-pancreas
4. How is pancreatic cancer staged? American Cancer Society; 2015. http://www.cancer.org/cancer/pancreaticcancer/detailedguide/pancreatic-cancer-staging
5. Abate-Daga D, Rosenberg SA, Morgan RA. Pancreatic cancer: hurdles in the engineering of CAR-based immunotherapies. *Oncoimmunology* 2014;3:e29194. http://www.ncbi.nlm.nih.gov/pmc/articles/PMC4108460/
6. Bittoni A, Santoni M, Lanese A, et al. Neoadjuvant therapy in pancreatic cancer: an emerging strategy. *Gastroenterology Research and Practice* 2014;2014:183852. http://www.hindawi.com/journals/grp/2014/183852/
7. Dragovich T. Pancreatic Cancer. Medscape; 2014. http://emedicine.medscape.com/article/280605-overview

Pancreatitis

1. Pancreatitis. Health Topics. National Institute of Diabetes and Digestive and Kidney Diseases; 2012. http://www.niddk.nih.gov/health-information/health-topics/digestive-diseases/pancreatitis/Pages/facts.aspx
2. Anand B. Peptic Ulcer Disease. Medscape; 2015. http://emedicine.medscape.com/article/181753-overview
3. Gardner TB. Acute Pancreatitis. Medscape; 2014. http://emedicine.medscape.com/article/181364-overview
4. Huffman JL. Chronic Pancreatitis. Medscape; 2014. http://emedicine.medscape.com/article/181554-overview
5. Lee P, Stevens T. Acute Pancreatitis. Disease Management Project. Cleveland Clinic. http://www.clevelandclinicmeded.com/medicalpubs/diseasemanagement/gastroenterology/acute-pancreatitis/. Accessed Winter 2015.
6. Lee P, Stevens T. Chronic Pancreatitis. Disease Management Progress. Cleveland Clinic. http://www.clevelandclinicmeded.com/medicalpubs/diseasemanagement/gastroenterology/chronic-pancreatitis/. Accessed Winter 2015.

Peptic Ulcers

1. What is *Helicobacter pylori*. The Helicobacter Foundation. http://www.helico.com/whatishelicobacterpylori.html. Accessed Winter 2015.
2. Peptic Ulcer Disease and *H. pylori*. National Digestive Diseases Information Clearinghouse. National Institute of Diabetes and Digestive and Kidney Diseases; 2014. http://www.niddk.nih.gov/health-information/health-topics/digestive-diseases/peptic-ulcer/Documents/hpylori_508.pdf
3. Peptic Ulcer Disease and NSAIDs. National Digestive Diseases Information Clearinghouse. National Institute of Diabetes and Digestive and Kidney Diseases; 2014. http://www.niddk.nih.gov/health-information/health-topics/digestive-diseases/peptic-ulcer/Documents/NSAIDS_PepticUlcers_508.pdf
4. What I Need to Know About Peptic Ulcer Disease. National Digestive Diseases Information Clearinghouse. National Institute of Diabetes and Digestive and Kidney Diseases; 2014. http://www.niddk.nih.gov/health-information/health-topics/digestive-diseases/peptic-ulcer/Documents/WINTKA-PepticUlcers_508.pdf
5. What is *H. pylori*? WebMD; 2014. http://www.webmd.com/digestive-disorders/h-pylori-helicobacter-pylori
6. Aksenova AM, Teslenko OI, Boganskaia OA. Changes in the immune status of peptic ulcer patients after combined treatment including deep massage. *Voprosy Kurortologii, Fizioterapii, i Lechebnoĭ Fizicheskoĭ Kultury* 1999;(2):19–20. http://www.ncbi.nlm.nih.gov/pubmed/24742255
7. Charpignon C, Lesgourgues B, Pariente A, et al. Peptic ulcer disease: one in five is related to neither *Helicobacter pylori* nor aspirin/NSAID intake. *Alimentary Pharmacology and Therapeutics* 2013;38(8):946–954. http://www.medscape.com/viewarticle/811649
8. Huang TC, Lee CL. Diagnosis, treatment, and outcome in patients with bleeding peptic ulcers and *Helicobacter pylori* infections. *BioMed Research International* 2014;2014:658108. http://www.hindawi.com/journals/bmri/2014/658108/

Stomach Cancer

1. Stomach Cancer. Conditions & Treatments. Cedars-Sinai. http://www.cedars-sinai.edu/Patients/Health-Conditions/Stomach-Cancer.aspx. Accessed Winter 2015.

2. What You Need To Know About Stomach Cancer. Patient Education Publications. National Cancer Institute; 2009. http://www.cancer.gov/publications/patient-education/wyntk-stomach-cancer/AllPages
3. *Helicobacter pylori* and Cancer. National Cancer Institute; 2013. http://www.cancer.gov/cancertopics/factsheet/Risk/h-pylori-cancer
4. Stomach Cancer. American Cancer Society; 2015. http://www.cancer.org/acs/groups/cid/documents/webcontent/003141-pdf.pdf
5. Bartol TG. *H. pylori* Eradication to Prevent Gastric Cancer: What Does the Evidence Really Mean? Medscape Nurses; 2014. http://www.medscape.com/viewarticle/828408
6. Cabebe EC. Gastric Cancer. Medscape; 2014. http://emedicine.medscape.com/article/278744-overview
7. Khorana AA. New Standard of Care in Gastric Cancer. Medscape Oncology; 2014. http://www.medscape.com/viewarticle/819830
8. Lin WL, Sun JL, Chang SC, et al. Factors predicting survival of patients with gastric cancer. *Asian Pacific Journal of Cancer Prevention* 2014;15(14):5835–5838. http://www.apocpcontrol.org/paper_file/issue_abs/Volume15_No14/5835-5838%205.22%20Wen-Li%20Lin.pdf

Chapter 9

Diabetes Mellitus

1. Diabetic Neuropathies: The Nerve Damage of Diabetes. National Diabetes Information Clearinghouse. National Institute of Diabetes and Digestive and Kidney Diseases; 2013. http://diabetes.niddk.nih.gov/dm/pubs/neuropathies/index.aspx
2. Kidney Disease of Diabetes. National Kidney and Urologic Diseases Information Clearinghouse. National Institute of diabetes and Digestive and Kidney Diseases; 2014. http://kidney.niddk.nih.gov/KUDiseases/pubs/kdd/index.aspx
3. National Diabetes Statistics Report, 2014. Centers for Disease Control and Prevention; 2014. http://www.cdc.gov/diabetes/pubs/statsreport14/national-diabetes-report-web.pdf
4. Canaway R, Manderson L, Oldenburg B. Perceptions of benefit of complementary therapy use among people with diabetes and cardiovascular disease. *Forschende Komplementarmedizin* 2014;21(1):25–33. http://www.ncbi.nlm.nih.gov/pubmed/24603627
5. Castro-Sanchez AM, Moreno-Lorenzo C, Mataran-Penarrocha GA, et al. Connective tissue reflex massage for type 2 diabetic patients with peripheral arterial disease: randomized controlled trial. *Evidence-Based Complementary and Alternative Medicine* 2011;2011:804321. http://www.hindawi.com/journals/ecam/2011/804321/
6. Hawk C, Ndetan H, Evans MW, Jr. Potential role of complementary and alternative health care providers in chronic disease prevention and health promotion: an analysis of National Health Interview Survey data. *Preventive Medicine* 2012;54(1):18–22. http://www.ncbi.nlm.nih.gov/pubmed/21777609
7. Hendrick B. CDC: 26 Million Americans Have Diabetes. Medscape; 2011. http://www.medscape.com/viewarticle/736400
8. Khardori R. Type 1 Diabetes Mellitus. Medscape; 2014. http://emedicine.medscape.com/article/117739-overview
9. Khardori R. Type 2 Diabetes Mellitus. Medscape; 2014. http://emedicine.medscape.com/article/117853-overview
10. Lazaro-Martinez JL, Aragon-Sanchez J, Garcia-Morales E. Response to comment on Lazaro-Martinez et al. Antibiotics versus conservative surgery for treating diabetic foot osteomyelitis: a randomized comparative trial. *Diabetes Care* 2014;37:789–795. *Diabetes Care* 2014;37(5):e116–e117. http://www.medscape.com/viewarticle/821788
11. Marsh K, Brand-Miller J. Vegetarian diets and diabetes. *American Journal of Lifestyle Medicine* 2011;5(2):135–143. http://www.medscape.com/viewarticle/739101
12. Sajedi F, Kashaninia Z, Hoseinzadeh S, et al. How effective is Swedish massage on blood glucose level in children with diabetes mellitus? *Acta Medica Iranica* 2011;49(9):592–597. http://acta.tums.ac.ir/index.php/acta/article/view/4400
13. Wandell PE, Arnlov J, Nixon Andreasson A, et al. Effects of tactile massage on metabolic biomarkers in patients with type 2 diabetes. *Diabetes and Metabolism* 2013;39(5):411–417. http://www.ncbi.nlm.nih.gov/pubmed/23642641

Hyperthyroidism

1. NINDS Thyrotoxic Myopathy Information Page. Disorders A-Z. National Institute of Neurological Disorders and Stroke; 2011. http://www.ninds.nih.gov/disorders/thyrotoxic_myopathy/thyrotoxic_myopathy.htm
2. Graves' Disease. National Endocrine and Metabolic Diseases Information Service. National Institute of Diabetes and Digestive and Kidney Diseases; 2012. http://www.endocrine.niddk.nih.gov/pubs/graves/
3. Hyperthyroidism. National Endocrine and Metabolic Diseases Information Service. National Institute of Diabetes and Digestive and Kidney Diseases; 2012. http://www.endocrine.niddk.nih.gov/pubs/Hyperthyroidism/
4. Pregnancy and Thyroid Disease. National Endocrine and Metabolic Diseases Information Service. National Institute of Diabetes and Digestive and Kidney Diseases; 2012. http://endocrine.niddk.nih.gov/pubs/pregnancy/Pregnancy_Thyroid_Disease_508.pdf
5. Hyperthyroidism. American Thyroid Association; 2014. http://www.thyroid.org/wp-content/uploads/patients/brochures/Hyper_brochure.pdf
6. Anderson P. Hyperthyroidism Increases Stroke Risk in Young Adults. Medscape; 2010. http://www.medscape.com/viewarticle/719675
7. Lee SL. Hyperthyroidism. Medscape; 2014. http://emedicine.medscape.com/article/121865-overview
8. Schraga ED. Hyperthyroidism, Thyroid Storm, and Graves Disease. Medscape; 2014. http://emedicine.medscape.com/article/767130-overview
9. Tachi J, Amino N, Miyai K. Massage therapy on neck: a contributing factor for destructive thyrotoxicosis? *Thyroidology* 1990;2(1):25–27. http://www.ncbi.nlm.nih.gov/pubmed/1715747

Hypothyroidism

1. Hypothyroidism. National Endocrine and Metabolic Diseases Information Service. National Institute of Diabetes and Digestive and Kidney Diseases; 2013. http://www.endocrine.niddk.nih.gov/pubs/Hypothyroidism/
2. Hypothyroidism. American Thyroid Association; 2013. http://www.thyroid.org/wp-content/uploads/patients/brochures/Hypothyroidism_web_booklet.pdf

3. Allen PJ, Fomenko SD. Congenital hypothyroidism. *Pediatric Nursing* 2011;37(6):324–326. http://www.medscape.com/viewarticle/756520
4. Almandoz JP, Gharib H. Hypothyroidism: etiology, diagnosis, and management. *Medical Clinics of North America* 2012;96(2):203–221. http://saludesa.org.ec/biblioteca/MEDICINA%20INTERNA/hipotiroidismo_manejo.pdf
5. Mayer O Jr, Simon J, Filipovsky J, et al. Hypothyroidism in coronary heart disease and its relation to selected risk factors. *Vascular Health Risk Management* 2006;2(4):499–506. http://www.ncbi.nlm.nih.gov/pubmed/17323605
6. Orlander PR. Hypothyroidism. Medscape; 2014. http://emedicine.medscape.com/article/122393-overview
7. Yamada M, Mori M. Mechanisms related to the pathophysiology and management of central hypothyroidism. *Nature Clinical Practice Endocrinology and Metabolism* 2008;4(12):683–694. http://www.medscape.com/viewarticle/584468

Thyroid Cancer

1. What You Need To Know About Thyroid Cancer. Patient Education Publications. National Cancer Institute; 2012. http://www.cancer.gov/publications/patient-education/wyntk-thyroid-cancer/AllPages
2. Thyroidectomy. MedlinePlus. U.S. National Library of Medicine; 2013. http://www.nlm.nih.gov/medlineplus/ency/presentations/100135_1.htm
3. Thyroid Cancer. American Cancer Society; 2014. http://www.cancer.org/acs/groups/cid/documents/webcontent/003144-pdf.pdf
4. Goodman AL. Thyroid Cancer Symptoms, Possible Causes, and Risk Factors. EndocrineWeb; 2014. http://www.endocrineweb.com/guides/thyroid-cancer/thyroid-cancer-symptoms-possible-causes-risk-factors
5. Ito Y, Miyauchi A, Kobayashi K, et al. Static and dynamic prognostic factors of papillary thyroid carcinoma [review]. *Endocrine Journal* 2014. https://www.jstage.jst.go.jp/article/endocrj/advpub/0/advpub_EJ14-0303/_pdf
6. Lentsch EJ. Thyroid Cancer Staging. Medscape; 2013. http://emedicine.medscape.com/article/2006643-overview
7. Lentsch EJ. Thyroid Cancer Treatment Protocols. Medscape; 2013. http://emedicine.medscape.com/article/2007769-overview
8. Sharma PK. Thyroid Cancer. Medscape; 2014. http://emedicine.medscape.com/article/851968-overview

Chapter 10

Bladder Cancer

1. Bladder Cancer. Cancer Care. Memorial Sloan Kettering Cancer Center. http://www.mskcc.org/cancer-care/adult/bladder. Accessed Winter 2015.
2. Bladder Cancer. Cancer Information. University of Texas MD Anderson Cancer Center. http://www.mdanderson.org/patient-and-cancer-information/cancer-information/cancer-types/bladder-cancer/index.html. Accessed Winter 2015.
3. What You Need To Know About Bladder Cancer. Patient Education Publications. National Cancer Institute; 2010. http://www.cancer.gov/publications/patient-education/wyntk-bladder-cancer/AllPages
4. Cigarette smoking implicated in half of bladder cancers in women; NIH study confirms bladder cancer risk from smoking is higher than previously estimated. News. National Cancer Institute; 2011. http://www.cancer.gov/newscenter/newsfromnci/2011/SmokingBladderRisk
5. Bladder Cancer. A.D.A.M. Medical Encyclopedia. U.S. National Library of Medicine; 2014. http://www.ncbi.nlm.nih.gov/pubmedhealth/PMH0001517/
6. Bladder Cancer. Urology Care Foundation; 2014. http://www.urologyhealth.org/urology/index.cfm?article=100
7. Bladder Cancer. Cancer Immunotherapy. Cancer Research Institute; 2014. http://www.cancerresearch.org/cancer-immunotherapy/impacting-all-cancers/bladder-cancer
8. Bladder Cancer. American Cancer Society; 2015. http://www.cancer.org/acs/groups/cid/documents/webcontent/003085-pdf.pdf
9. Steinberg GD. Bladder Cancer. Medscape; 2014. http://emedicine.medscape.com/article/438262-overview

Interstitial Cystitis

1. Interstitial Cystitis/Bladder Pain Syndrome. U.S. Department of Health and Human Services, Office on Women's Health; 2010. http://www.womenshealth.gov/publications/our-publications/fact-sheet/interstitial-cystitis.pdf
2. Interstitial Cystitis/Painful Bladder Syndrome. National Kidney and Urologic Diseases Information Clearinghouse. National Institute of Diabetes and Digestive and Kidney Diseases; 2013. http://kidney.niddk.nih.gov/kudiseases/pubs/interstitialcystitis/
3. IC Treatment Guideline. Interstitial Cystitis Association; 2014. http://www.ichelp.org/Page.aspx?pid=429
4. FitzGerald MP, Payne CK, Lukacz ES, et al. Randomized multicenter clinical trial of myofascial physical therapy in women with interstitial cystitis/painful bladder syndrome and pelvic floor tenderness. *Journal of Urology* 2012;187(6):2113–2118. http://www.ncbi.nlm.nih.gov/pmc/articles/PMC3351550/
5. Hanno PM, Erickson D, Moldwin R, et al. Diagnosis and treatment of interstitial cystitis/bladder pain syndrome: AUA guideline amendment. *Journal of Urology* 2015. http://www.auanet.org/education/guidelines/ic-bladder-pain-syndrome.cfm
6. Metts JF. Interstitial cystitis: urgency and frequency syndrome. *American Family Physician* 2001;64(7):1199–1206. http://www.aafp.org/afp/2001/1001/p1199.html
7. Oyama IA, Rejba A, Lukban JC, et al. Modified Thiele massage as therapeutic intervention for female patients with interstitial cystitis and high-tone pelvic floor dysfunction. *Urology* 2004;64(5):862–865. http://www.ncbi.nlm.nih.gov/pubmed/15533464
8. Persu C, Cauni V, Gutue S, et al. From interstitial cystitis to chronic pelvic pain. *Journal of Medicine and Life* 2010;3(2):167–174. http://www.ncbi.nlm.nih.gov/pmc/articles/PMC3019050/
9. Rovner ES. Interstitial Cystitis. Medscape; 2014. http://emedicine.medscape.com/article/2055505-overview
10. Webster DC, Brennan T. Self-care strategies used for acute attack of interstitial cystitis. *Urologic Nursing* 1995;15(3):86–93. http://www.ncbi.nlm.nih.gov/pubmed/7481892
11. Weiss JM. Pelvic floor myofascial trigger points: manual therapy for interstitial cystitis and the urgency-frequency syndrome. *Journal of Urology* 2001;166(6):2226–2231. http://www.ncbi.nlm.nih.gov/pubmed/11696740

Kidney Stones

1. Kidney Stones—Overview. Diseases & Conditions. Cleveland Clinic. http://my.clevelandclinic.org/services/urology-kidney/diseases-conditions/kidney-stones-overview. Accessed Winter 2015.
2. Kidney Stones. National Kidney Foundation. https://www.kidney.org/atoz/content/kidneystones. Accessed Winter 2015.
3. Kidney Stones in Adults. National Kidney and Urologic Diseases Information Clearinghouse. National Institute of Diabetes and Digestive and Kidney Diseases; 2013. http://kidney.niddk.nih.gov/kudiseases/pubs/stonesadults/
4. Alexander RT, Hemmelgarn BR, Wiebe N, et al. Kidney stones and kidney function loss: a cohort study. *BMJ* 2012;345:e5287. http://www.ncbi.nlm.nih.gov/pmc/articles/PMC3431443/
5. Smith JK. Urinary Calculi Imaging. Medscape; 2013. http://emedicine.medscape.com/article/381993-overview
6. Wedro B. Kidney Stones. eMedicineHealth; 2014. http://www.emedicinehealth.com/kidney_stones/article_em.htm
7. Wolf JS. Nephrolithiasis. Medscape; 2014. http://emedicine.medscape.com/article/437096-overview

Polycystic Kidney Disease

1. The Science of PKD. PKD Foundation. http://www.pkdcure.org/learn/science-of-pkd. Accessed Winter 2015.
2. Polycystic Kidney Disease. National Kidney Foundation. https://www.kidney.org/atoz/content/polycystic. Accessed Winter 2015.
3. Polycystic Kidney Disease. National Kidney and Urologic Diseases Information Clearinghouse. National Institute of Diabetes and Digestive and Kidney Diseases; 2010. http://kidney.niddk.nih.gov/kudiseases/pubs/polycystic/
4. Polycystic Kidney Disease. Diseases & Conditions. Mayo Clinic; 2014. http://www.mayoclinic.org/diseases-conditions/polycystic-kidney-disease/basics/definition/con-20028831
5. Balbo BE, Sapienza MT, Ono CR, et al. Cyst infection in hospital-admitted autosomal dominant polycystic kidney disease patients is predominantly multifocal and associated with kidney and liver volume. *Brazilian Journal of Medical and Biological Research* 2014;47(7):584–593. http://www.ncbi.nlm.nih.gov/pmc/articles/PMC4123838/pdf/1414-431X-bjmbr-47-07-00584.pdf
6. Mufarrij AJ, Hitti E. Acute cystic rupture and hemorrhagic shock after a vigorous massage chair session in a patient with polycystic kidney disease. *American Journal of the Medical Sciences* 2011;342(1):76–78. http://www.ncbi.nlm.nih.gov/pubmed/21642815
7. Torra R. Polycystic Kidney Disease. Medscape; 2014. http://emedicine.medscape.com/article/244907-overview
8. Verghese P. Pediatric Polycystic Kidney Disease. Medscape; 2014. http://emedicine.medscape.com/article/983281-overview

Pyelonephritis

1. Pyelonephritis: Kidney Infection. National Kidney and Urologic Diseases Information Clearinghouse. National Institute of Diabetes and Digestive and Kidney Diseases; 2012. http://kidney.niddk.nih.gov/kudiseases/pubs/pyelonephritis/
2. Fulop T. Acute Pyelonephritis. Medscape; 2014. http://emedicine.medscape.com/article/245559-overview
3. Hinfrey PB. Pediatric Pyelonephritis. Medscape; 2014. http://emedicine.medscape.com/article/968028-overview
4. Lohr JW. Chronic Pyelonephritis. Medscape; 2013. http://emedicine.medscape.com/article/245464-overview
5. Ramakrishnan K, Scheid DC. Diagnosis and management of acute pyelonephritis in adults. *American Family Physician* 2005;71(5):933–942. http://www.aafp.org/afp/2005/0301/p933.html
6. Shetty S. Emphysematous Pyelonephritis (EPN). Medscape; 2013. http://emedicine.medscape.com/article/2029011-overview

Renal Cancer

1. Wilms' Tumor. Diseases and Conditions. Mayo Clinic; 2014. http://www.mayoclinic.org/diseases-conditions/wilms-tumor/basics/definition/con-20043492
2. About Kidney Cancer. Kidney Cancer Association; 2014. http://www.kidneycancer.org/knowledge/learn/about-kidney-cancer/
3. Kidney Cancer (Adult)—Renal Cell Carcinoma. American Cancer Society; 2015. http://www.cancer.org/acs/groups/cid/documents/webcontent/003107-pdf.pdf
4. Drug Information Sheets. Kidney Cancer Association; 2015. http://www.kidneycancer.org/knowledge/learn/drug-information-sheets/
5. Sachdeva K. Renal Cell Carcinoma. Medscape; 2014. http://emedicine.medscape.com/article/281340-overview

Renal Failure

1. About Chronic Kidney Disease. National Kidney Foundation. https://www.kidney.org/kidneydisease/aboutckd. Accessed Winter 2015.
2. NSAIDs and Chronic Kidney Disease. Centers for Disease Control and Prevention. http://www.cdc.gov/diabetes/news/pdf/nsaid_transcript.pdf. Accessed Winter 2015.
3. Living Kidney Donors Network Mission. Living Kidney Donors Network. http://www.lkdn.org/mission.html. Accessed Winter 2015.
4. Kidney Disease Statistics for the United States. National Kidney and Urologic Diseases Information Clearinghouse. National Institute of Diabetes and Digestive and Kidney Diseases; 2012. http://kidney.niddk.nih.gov/KUDiseases/pubs/kustats/KU_Diseases_Stats_508.pdf
5. Kidney Failure: Choosing a Treatment That's Right for You. National Kidney and Urologic Diseases Information Clearinghouse. National Institute of Diabetes and Digestive and Kidney Diseases; 2013. http://kidney.niddk.nih.gov/kudiseases/pubs/choosingtreatment/index.aspx
6. Chronic Kidney Disease. eMedicineHealth; 2014. http://www.emedicinehealth.com/chronic_kidney_disease/article_em.htm
7. National Chronic Kidney Disease Fact Sheet, 2014. Centers for Disease Control and Prevention; 2014. http://www.cdc.gov/diabetes/pubs/pdf/kidney_factsheet.pdf
8. Organ Donation and Transplantation Statistics. National Kidney Foundation; 2014. https://www.kidney.org/news/newsroom/factsheets/Organ-Donation-and-Transplantation-Stats
9. Arora P. Chronic Kidney Disease. Medscape; 2014. http://emedicine.medscape.com/article/238798-overview
10. Cho YC, Tsay SL. The effect of acupressure with massage on fatigue and depression in patients with end-stage renal disease. *Journal of Nursing Research* 2004;12(1):51–59. http://www.ncbi.nlm.nih.gov/pubmed/15136963
11. Gulati S. Chronic Kidney Disease in Children. Medscape; 2015. http://emedicine.medscape.com/article/984358-overview

12. Shahgholian N, Dehghan M, Mortazavi M, et al. Effect of aromatherapy on pruritus relief in hemodialysis patients. *Iranian Journal of Nursing and Midwifery Research* 2010;15(4):240–244. http://www.ncbi.nlm.nih.gov/pmc/articles/PMC3203284/
13. Workeneh BT. Acute Kidney Injury. Medscape; 2014. http://emedicine.medscape.com/article/243492-overview

Urinary Tract Infection

1. Urinary Tract Infection (UTI). U.S. Department of Health and Human Services, Office on Women's Health; 2008. http://www.womenshealth.gov/publications/our-publications/fact-sheet/urinary-tract-infection.pdf
2. Urinary Tract Infections in Adults. National Kidney and Urologic Diseases Information Clearinghouse. National Institute of Diabetes and Digestive and Kidney Diseases; 2012. http://kidney.niddk.nih.gov/KUDiseases/pubs/uti adult/index.aspx
3. Cranberry. National Center for Complementary and Integrative Health; 2012. https://nccih.nih.gov/health/cranberry
4. Urinary Tract Infection. University of Maryland Medical Center; 2013. http://umm.edu/health/medical/reports/articles/urinary-tract-infection
5. Urinary Tract Infection in Women—Self-Care. MedlinePlus. U.S. National Library of Medicine; 2013. http://www.nlm.nih.gov/medlineplus/ency/patientinstructions/000391.htm
6. Brusch JL. Cystitis in Females. Medscape; 2014. http://emedicine.medscape.com/article/233101-overview

Chapter 11

Benign Prostatic Hyperplasia

1. Deters LA. Benign Prostatic Hypertrophy. Medscape; 2014. http://emedicine.medscape.com/article/437359-overview
2. Enlarged Prostate. MedlinePlus: U.S. National Library of Medicine; 2013. http://www.nlm.nih.gov/medlineplus/ency/article/000381.htm
3. Woods E. Laser ablation of the prostate: a safe effective treatment of obstructive benign prostatic disease. *Canadian Urological Association Journal* 2010;4(5):344–346. http://www.ncbi.nlm.nih.gov/pmc/articles/PMC2950757/
4. Prostate Changes That Are Not Cancer. Cancer Topics. National Cancer Institute; 2009. http://www.cancer.gov/cancertopics/screening/understanding-prostate-changes/changes
5. Prostate Enlargement: Benign Prostatic Hyperplasia. National Kidney and Urologic Diseases Information Clearinghouse: National Institute of Diabetes and Digestive and Kidney Diseases; 2014. http://kidney.niddk.nih.gov/KUDiseases/pubs/prostateenlargement/ProstateEnlargement_508.pdf
6. Muruve NA. Transurethral Needle Ablation of the Prostate (TUNA). Medscape; 2014. http://emedicine.medscape.com/article/449477-overview

Breast Cancer

1. Breast Cancer Treatment. Cancer Topics: National Cancer Institute; 2014. http://www.cancer.gov/cancertopics/pdq/treatment/breast/Patient/page1
2. Stages of Breast Cancer. Cancer Topics: National Cancer Institute; 2014. http://www.cancer.gov/cancertopics/pdq/treatment/breast/Patient/page2
3. What You Need To Know About Breast Cancer. Patient Education Publications: National Cancer Institute; 2014. http://www.cancer.gov/publications/patient-education/wyntk-breast-cancer
4. Medicines to Reduce Breast Cancer Risk. American Cancer Society; 2014. http://www.cancer.org/acs/groups/cid/documents/webcontent/002585-pdf.pdf
5. Mammograms and Other Breast Imaging Tests. American Cancer Society; 2014. http://www.cancer.org/acs/groups/cid/documents/webcontent/003178-pdf.pdf
6. Stage Information for Breast Cancer. Cancer Topics. National Cancer Institute; 2015. http://www.cancer.gov/cancertopics/pdq/treatment/breast/healthprofessional/page3
7. Fernandez-Lao C, Cantarero-Villanueva I, Diaz-Rodriguez L, et al. Attitudes towards massage modify effects of manual therapy in breast cancer survivors: a randomised clinical trial with crossover design. *European Journal of Cancer Care* 2012;21(2):233–241. http://www.ncbi.nlm.nih.gov/pubmed/22060159
8. Fernandez-Lao C, Cantarero-Villanueva I, Diaz-Rodriguez L, et al. The influence of patient attitude toward massage on pressure pain sensitivity and immune system after application of myofascial release in breast cancer survivors: a randomized, controlled crossover study. *Journal of Manipulative and Physiological Therapeutics* 2012;35(2):94–100. http://www.ncbi.nlm.nih.gov/pubmed/22018755
9. Kim JI, Lee MS, Kang JW, et al. Reflexology for the symptomatic treatment of breast cancer: a systematic review. *Integrative Cancer Therapies* 2010;9(4):326–330. http://www.ncbi.nlm.nih.gov/pubmed/21106613
10. Krohn M, Listing M, Tjahjono G, et al. Depression, mood, stress, and Th1/Th2 immune balance in primary breast cancer patients undergoing classical massage therapy. *Supportive Care in Cancer* 2011;19(9):1303–1311. http://www.ncbi.nlm.nih.gov/pubmed/20644965
11. Lee MS, Lee EN, Ernst E. Massage therapy for breast cancer patients: a systematic review. *Annals of Oncology* 2011;22(6):1459–1461. http://annonc.oxfordjournals.org/content/22/6/1459.long
12. Mayer M, Batur P. Breast Disorders and Breast Screening. Center for Continuing Education. Cleveland Clinic. http://www.clevelandclinicmeded.com/medicalpubs/disease-management/womens-health/breast-disorders-and-cancer-screening/. Accessed Winter 2015.
13. Mustian KM, Roscoe JA, Palesh OG, et al. Polarity therapy for cancer-related fatigue in patients with breast cancer receiving radiation therapy: a randomized controlled pilot study. *Integrative Cancer Therapies* 2011;10(1):27–37. http://www.ncbi.nlm.nih.gov/pmc/articles/PMC3085180/
14. Stopeck AT. Breast Cancer. Medscape; 2014. http://emedicine.medscape.com/article/1947145-overview
15. Swart R. Breast Cancer in Men Overview of Male Breast Cancer. Medscape; 2014. http://emedicine.medscape.com/article/1954174-overview

Cervical Cancer

1. Recurrent Cervical Cancer. Texas Oncology. http://www.texasoncology.com/types-of-cancer/cervical-cancer/recurrent-cervical-cancer/. Accessed Winter 2015.
2. HPV and Cancer. Cancer Topics. National Cancer Institute; 2012. http://www.cancer.gov/cancertopics/factsheet/Risk/HPV
3. What You Need To Know About Cervical Cancer. Cancer Topics. National Cancer Institute; 2012. http://www.cancer.gov/publications/patient-education/wyntk-cervical-cancer/AllPages

4. Get the Facts About Gynecologic Cancer. Centers for Disease Control and Prevention; 2012. http://www.cdc.gov/cancer/knowledge/pdf/CDC_GYN_Comprehensive_Brochure.pdf
5. Comprehensive cervical cancer prevention and control: a healthier future for girls and women. World Health Organization; 2013. http://www.who.int/immunization/hpv/learn/comprehensive_cervical_cancer_who_2013.pdf
6. Cervical Cancer Treatments. Cancer Topics. National Cancer Institute; 2014. http://www.cancer.gov/cancertopics/pdq/treatment/cervical/Patient/AllPages
7. Cervical Cancer. American Cancer Society; 2014. http://www.cancer.org/acs/groups/cid/documents/webcontent/003094-pdf.pdf
8. Preventing Cervical Cancer: The Development of HPV Vaccines. Cancer Research Progress. National Cancer Institute; 2014. http://www.cancer.gov/aboutnci/servingpeople/cancer-research-progress/discovery/hpvvaccines
9. Cervical Cancer. Gynecologic Cancers. Centers for Disease Control and Prevention; 2015. http://www.cdc.gov/cancer/cervical/
10. Boardman CH. Cervical Cancer Staging. Medscape; 2013. http://emedicine.medscape.com/article/2006486-overview
11. Nakano T, Ohno T, Ishikawa H, et al. Current advancement in radiation therapy for uterine cervical cancer. *Journal of Radiation Research* 2010;51(1):1–8. https://www.jstage.jst.go.jp/article/jrr/51/1/51_09132/_pdf

Dysmenorrhea

1. Dysmenorrhea. Diseases & Conditions. Cleveland Clinic; 2014. http://my.clevelandclinic.org/health/diseases_conditions/hic_Dysmenorrhea
2. Calis KA. Dysmenorrhea. Medscape; 2014. http://emedicine.medscape.com/article/253812-overview
3. Marzouk TM, El-Nemer AM, Baraka HN. The effect of aromatherapy abdominal massage on alleviating menstrual pain in nursing students: a prospective randomized cross-over study. *Evidence-Based Complementary and Alternative Medicine* 2013;2013:742421. http://www.hindawi.com/journals/ecam/2013/742421/
4. Apay SE, Arslan S, Akpinar RB, et al. Effect of aromatherapy massage on dysmenorrhea in Turkish students. *Pain Management Nursing* 2012;13(4):236–240. http://www.ncbi.nlm.nih.gov/pubmed/23158705
5. Chen HM, Wang HH, Chiu MH, et al. Effects of acupressure on menstrual distress and low back pain in dysmenorrheic young adult women: an experimental study. *Pain Management Nursing* 2014 (electronic publication ahead of print). http://www.ncbi.nlm.nih.gov/pubmed/25175554
6. Menstrual Cramps (Dysmenorrhea). University of Illinois at Urbana-Champaign McKinley Health Center. http://www.mckinley.illinois.edu/handouts/menstrual_cramps.html. Accessed Winter 2015.
7. Davis AR, Westhoff C, O'Connell K, et al. Oral contraceptives for dysmenorrhea in adolescent girls: a randomized trial. *Obstetrics and Gynecology* 2005;106(1):97–104. https://pedclerk.uchicago.edu/sites/pedclerk.uchicago.edu/files/uploads/OCP.RCT_.2005.pdf
8. Ou MC, Hsu TF, Lai AC, et al. Pain relief assessment by aromatic essential oil massage on outpatients with primary dysmenorrhea: a randomized, double-blind clinical trial. *Journal of Obstetrics and Gynaecology Research* 2012;38(5):817–822. http://www.ncbi.nlm.nih.gov/pubmed/22435409
9. Painful Menstrual Periods. MedlinePlus. U.S. National Library of Medicine; 2012. http://www.nlm.nih.gov/medlineplus/ency/article/003150.htm
10. Primary Dysmenorrhea Consensus Guideline. The Society of Obstetricians and Gynaecologists of Canada; 2005. http://sogc.org/guidelines/primary-dysmenorrhea-consensus-guideline/
11. Kannan P, Claydon LS. Some physiotherapy treatments may relieve menstrual pain in women with primary dysmenorrhea: a systematic review. *Journal of Physiotherapy* 2014;60(1):13–21. http://www.journalofphysiotherapy.com/article/S1836-9553(14)00004-6/abstract

Endometriosis

1. Johnson NP, Hummelshoj L. Consensus on current management of endometriosis. *Human Reproduction* 2013;28(6):1552–1568. http://humrep.oxfordjournals.org/content/28/6/1552.long
2. Deep Endometriosis. Pelvic Pain Support Network; 2015. http://www.pelvicpain.org.uk/index.php?page=deep-endometriosis
3. Valiani M, Ghasemi N, Bahadoran P, et al. The effects of massage therapy on dysmenorrhea caused by endometriosis. *Iranian Journal of Nursing and Midwifery Research* 2010;15(4):167–171. http://www.ncbi.nlm.nih.gov/pmc/articles/PMC3093183/
4. Stoppler MC. Endometriosis. eMedicineHealth; 2014. http://www.emedicinehealth.com/endometriosis/article_em.htm
5. Acien P, Velasco I. Endometriosis: a disease that remains enigmatic. *ISRN Obstetrics and Gynecology* 2013;2013:242149. http://www.ncbi.nlm.nih.gov/pmc/articles/PMC3730176/
6. Bernardi LA, Pavone ME. Endometriosis: an update on management. *Womens Health (Lond Engl)* 2013;9(3):233–250. http://www.medscape.com/viewarticle/803830
7. Missmer SA, Bove GM. A pilot study of the prevalence of leg pain among women with endometriosis. *Journal of Bodywork and Movement Therapies* 2011;15(3):304–308. http://www.ncbi.nlm.nih.gov/pmc/articles/PMC3115527/
8. Harding A. Severe Acne in Teen Years Linked to Increased Endometriosis Risk. Medscape; 2014. http://www.medscape.com/viewarticle/830653

Fibroid Tumors

1. Mara M, Kubinova K. Embolization of uterine fibroids from the point of view of the gynecologist: pros and cons. *International Journal of Womens Health* 2014;6:623–629. http://www.ncbi.nlm.nih.gov/pmc/articles/PMC4074023/
2. Leppert PC, Jayes FL, Segars JH. The extracellular matrix contributes to mechanotransduction in uterine fibroids. *Obstetrics and Gynecology International* 2014;2014:783289. http://www.ncbi.nlm.nih.gov/pmc/articles/PMC4106177/
3. Evans P, Brunsell S. Uterine fibroid tumors: diagnosis and treatment. *American Family Physician* 2007;75(10):1503–1508. http://www.aafp.org/afp/2007/0515/p1503.html
4. Uterine Fibroids. National Women's Health Information Center. U.S. Department of Health and Human Services, Office on Women's Health; 2008. http://www.womenshealth.gov/publications/our-publications/fact-sheet/uterine-fibroids.pdf
5. Uterine Fibroids. American Congress of Obstetricians and Gynecologists; 2011. http://www.acog.org/Patients/FAQs/Uterine-Fibroids
6. Stoppler MC. Uterine Fibroids. eMedicineHealth; 2014. http://www.emedicinehealth.com/uterine_fibroids/article_em.htm

Menopause

1. Darsareh F, Taavoni S, Joolaee S, et al. Effect of aromatherapy massage on menopausal symptoms: a randomized placebo-controlled clinical trial. *Menopause* 2012;19(9):995–999. http://www.ncbi.nlm.nih.gov/pubmed/22549173
2. Taavoni S, Darsareh F, Joolaee S, et al. The effect of aromatherapy massage on the psychological symptoms of postmenopausal Iranian women. *Complementary Therapies in Medicine* 2013;21(3):158–163. http://www.ncbi.nlm.nih.gov/pubmed/23642946
3. Oliveira DS, Hachul H, Goto V, et al. Effect of therapeutic massage on insomnia and climacteric symptoms in postmenopausal women. *Climacteric* 2012;15(1):21–29. http://www.ncbi.nlm.nih.gov/pubmed/22017318
4. Hormones and Menopause Tips from the National Institute on Aging. National Institute on Aging; 2012. http://www.nia.nih.gov/sites/default/files/hormones_and_menopause_0.pdf
5. Shoupe D. Individualizing hormone therapy to minimize risk: accurate assessment of risks and benefits. *Womens Health (London, England)* 2011;7(4):475–485. http://www.medscape.com/viewarticle/747269
6. Lewis R. Introducing 'Genitourinary Syndrome of Menopause'. Medscape; 2014. http://www.medscape.com/viewarticle/830398
7. Menopausal Symptoms and Complementary Health Practices. National Center for Complementary and Integrative Healthcare; 2013. https://nccih.nih.gov/sites/nccam.nih.gov/files/Get_The_Facts_Menopause_09-19-2013.pdf
8. Menopause. National Institute on Aging; 2015. http://www.nia.nih.gov/health/publication/menopause
9. Coney P. Menopause. Medscape; 2014. http://emedicine.medscape.com/article/264088-overview
10. Manson JE. Overview of Menopause. North American Menopause Society. http://www.menopause.org/docs/2012/cg_a.pdf?sfvrsn=2. Accessed Winter 2015.
11. Rossouw JE, Anderson GL, Prentice RL, et al. Risks and benefits of estrogen plus progestin in healthy postmenopausal women: principal results from the Women's Health Initiative randomized controlled trial. *JAMA* 2002;288(3):321–333. http://jama.jamanetwork.com/article.aspx?articleid=195120
12. Saetung S, Chailurkit LO, Ongphiphadhanakul B. Thai traditional massage increases biochemical markers of bone formation in postmenopausal women: a randomized crossover trial. *BMC Complementary and Alternative Medicine* 2013;13:69. http://www.ncbi.nlm.nih.gov/pmc/articles/PMC3770450/
13. WHI Study Data Confirm Short-Term Heart Disease Risks of Combination Hormone Therapy for Postmenopausal Women. NIH News. National Institutes of Health; 2010. http://www.nih.gov/news/health/feb2010/nhlbi-15.htm

Ovarian Cancer

1. Get the Facts About Gynecologic Cancer. Centers for Disease Control and Prevention; 2012. http://www.cdc.gov/cancer/knowledge/pdf/CDC_GYN_Comprehensive_Brochure.pdf
2. Gross AH, Cromwell J, Fonteyn M, et al. Hopelessness and complementary therapy use in patients with ovarian cancer. *Cancer Nursing* 2013;36(4):256–264. http://www.ncbi.nlm.nih.gov/pubmed/23086133
3. Ovarian Cancer. Johns Hopkins University, Department of Pathology. http://pathology2.jhu.edu/ovca/menu_understanding.cfm. Accessed Winter 2015.
4. Ovarian Cancer. American College of Obstetricians and Gynecologists; 2014. http://www.acog.org/~/media/For%20Patients/faq096.pdf
5. Green AE. Ovarian Cancer. Medscape; 2014. http://www.menopause.org/docs/2012/cg_a.pdf?sfvrsn=2
6. Ovarian Cancer Overview. American Cancer Society; 2015. http://www.cancer.org/acs/groups/cid/documents/webcontent/003070-pdf.pdf
7. Bodurka DC, Sun CC, Basen-Engquist K. Ovarian Cancer Quality of Life Issues. National Ovarian Cancer Coalition; 2006. http://www.ovarian.org/assets/pdf/NOCC_Quality_of_Life_Issues.pdf
8. Ovarian Cancer Staging System, FIGO System & TNM System. HealthCommunities.com; 2015. http://www.healthcommunities.com/ovarian-cancer/figo-system-tnm-system.shtml
9. Ward SM. Salpingo-Oophorectomy. Medscape; 2015. http://emedicine.medscape.com/article/1894587-overview
10. Helm CW. TNM and FIGO Classifications for Ovarian Cancer. Medscape; 2013. http://emedicine.medscape.com/article/2007140-overview
11. Treatment Side-Effects. National Ovarian Cancer Coalition. http://www.ovarian.org/treatment_side_effects.php. Accessed Winter 2015.

Ovarian Cysts

1. Gene linked to excess male hormones in female infertility disorder. News & Events. Eunice Kennedy Shriver National Institute of Child Health and Human Development; 2014. http://www.nih.gov/news/health/apr2014/nichd-15.htm
2. Gallenberg MM. Is there a link between ovarian cysts and fertility? Diseases and Conditions. Mayo Clinic; 2012. http://www.mayoclinic.org/diseases-conditions/ovarian-cysts/expert-answers/ovarian-cysts-and-infertility/FAQ-20057806?p=1
3. Ovarian Cysts. American College of Obstetricians and Gynecologists; 2014. http://www.acog.org/~/media/For%20Patients/faq075.pdf
4. Helm CW. Ovarian Cysts. Medscape; 2014. http://emedicine.medscape.com/article/255865-overview
5. Ovarian Cysts and Tumors. WebMD; 2014. http://www.webmd.com/women/guide/ovarian-cysts
6. Polycystic Ovary Syndrome. A.D.A.M. Medical Encyclopedia. U.S. National Library of Medicine; 2014. http://www.ncbi.nlm.nih.gov/pubmedhealth/PMH0001408/
7. Polycystic Ovary Syndrome (PCOS): Condition Information. Heath & Research. Eunice Kennedy Shriver National Institute of Child Health and Human Development; 2013. http://www.nichd.nih.gov/health/topics/PCOS/conditioninfo/Pages/default.aspx

Pregnancy

1. Rigby FB. Common Pregnancy Complaints and Questions. Medscape; 2014. http://emedicine.medscape.com/article/259724-overview
2. Deligiannidis KM, Freeman MP. Complementary and alternative medicine therapies for perinatal depression. *Best Practice and Research. Clinical Obstetrics and Gynaecology*

2014;28(1):85–95. http://www.ncbi.nlm.nih.gov/pmc/articles/PMC3992885/

3. Sepilian VP. Ectopic Pregnancy. Medscape; 2014. http://emedicine.medscape.com/article/2041923-overview
4. High Blood Pressure in Pregnancy. Health Information for the Public: National Heart, Lung, and Blood Institute. http://www.nhlbi.nih.gov/health/resources/heart/hbp-pregnancy. Accessed Winter 2015.
5. Hollenbach D, Broker R, Herlehy S, et al. Non-pharmacological interventions for sleep quality and insomnia during pregnancy: a systematic review. *Journal of the Canadian Chiropractic Association* 2013:57(3):260–270. http://www.ncbi.nlm.nih.gov/pmc/articles/PMC3743652/
6. Pregnancy Care. A.D.A.M. Medical Encyclopedia. U.S. National Library of Medicine; 2012. http://www.ncbi.nlm.nih.gov/pubmedhealth/PMH0004480/
7. Pregnancy Statistics. Statistic Brain; 2014. http://www.statisticbrain.com/pregnancy-statistics/
8. DeSisto CL, Kim SY, Sharma AJ. Prevalence estimates of gestational diabetes mellitus in the United States, Pregnancy Risk Assessment Monitoring System (PRAMS), 2007–2010. *Preventing Chronic Disease* 2014;11:E104. http://www.cdc.gov/pcd/issues/2014/13_0415.htm

Premenstrual Syndrome

1. Direkvand-Moghadam A, Sayehmiri K, Delpisheh A, et al. Epidemiology of premenstrual syndrome (PMS)-a systematic review and meta-analysis study. *Journal of Clinical and Diagnostic Research* 2014;8(2):106–109. http://www.ncbi.nlm.nih.gov/pmc/articles/PMC3972521/
2. Premenstrual Dysphoric Disorder. A.D.A.M. Medical Encyclopedia. U.S. National Library of Medicine; 2012. http://www.ncbi.nlm.nih.gov/pubmedhealth/PMH0004461/
3. Premenstrual Syndrome. U.S. Department of Health and Human Services, Office on Women's Health; 2010. http://www.womenshealth.gov/publications/our-publications/fact-sheet/premenstrual-syndrome.pdf
4. Moreno MA. Premenstrual Syndrome. Medscape; 2012. http://emedicine.medscape.com/article/953696-overview
5. Premenstrual Syndrome—Self-Care. MedlinePlus: U.S. National Library of Medicine; 2014. http://www.nlm.nih.gov/medlineplus/ency/patientinstructions/000556.htm
6. Tolossa FW, Bekele ML. Prevalence, impacts and medical managements of premenstrual syndrome among female students: cross-sectional study in College of Health Sciences, Mekelle University, Mekelle, northern Ethiopia. *BMC Womens Health* 2014;14:52. http://www.ncbi.nlm.nih.gov/pmc/articles/PMC3994244/
7. Gallenberg MM. What's the difference between premenstrual dysphoric disorder and premenstrual syndrome? Diseases and Conditions. Mayo Clinic; 2010. http://www.mayoclinic.org/diseases-conditions/premenstrual-syndrome/expert-answers/pmdd/FAQ-20058315?p=1

Prostate Cancer

1. Humphrey PA. Pathology of Hormonal Therapy on Prostate Cancer. Medscape; 2014. http://emedicine.medscape.com/article/1612087-overview
2. About the Prostate. Understanding Prostate Cancer. Prostate Cancer Foundation. http://www.pcf.org/site/c.leJRIROrEpH/b.5802023/k.B322/About_the_Prostate.htm. Accessed Winter 2015.
3. Ornish D, Magbanua MJ, Weidner G, et al. Changes in prostate gene expression in men undergoing an intensive nutrition and lifestyle intervention. *Proceedings of the National Academy of Sciences of the United States of America* 2008;105(24):8369–8374. http://www.ncbi.nlm.nih.gov/pmc/articles/PMC2430265/
4. Prostate Cancer. American Cancer Society; 2015. http://www.cancer.org/acs/groups/cid/documents/webcontent/003134-pdf.pdf
5. Ghavamian R. Prostate Cancer Treatment Protocols. Medscape; 2014. http://emedicine.medscape.com/article/2007095-overview
6. Prostate-Specific Antigen (PSA) Test. Cancer Topics. National Cancer Institute; 2012. http://www.cancer.gov/cancertopics/factsheet/detection/PSA
7. PSA: The Test. Lab Tests Online. American Association for Clinical Chemistry; 2012. http://labtestsonline.org/understanding/analytes/psa/tab/test
8. SEER Stat Fact Sheets. Prostate Cancer. Cancer Statistics. National Cancer Institute. http://seer.cancer.gov/statfacts/html/prost.html. Accessed Winter 2015.
9. Kim JH, Lee HJ, Song YS. Stem cell based gene therapy in prostate cancer. *BioMed Research International* 2014;2014:549136. http://www.ncbi.nlm.nih.gov/pmc/articles/PMC4120795/

Prostatitis

1. Ahuja SK. Chronic Bacterial Prostatitis. Medscape; 2014. http://emedicine.medscape.com/article/458391-overview
2. Watson RA. Chronic Pelvic Pain in Men. Medscape; 2015. http://emedicine.medscape.com/article/437745-overview
3. Yang CC. Neuromodulation in male chronic pelvic pain syndrome: rationale and practice. *World Journal of Urology* 2013;31(4):767–772. http://www.ncbi.nlm.nih.gov/pmc/articles/PMC3753408/
4. Strauss AC, Dimitrakov JD. New treatments for chronic prostatitis/chronic pelvic pain syndrome. *Nature Reviews. Urology* 2010;7(3):127–135. http://www.ncbi.nlm.nih.gov/pmc/articles/PMC2837110/
5. Van Alstyne LS, Harrington KL, Haskvitz EM. Physical therapist management of chronic prostatitis/chronic pelvic pain syndrome. *Physical Therapy* 2010;90(12):1795–1806. http://ptjournal.apta.org/content/90/12/1795.long
6. Prostate Changes That Are Not Cancer. Cancer Topics. National Cancer Institute; 2009. http://www.cancer.gov/cancertopics/screening/understanding-prostate-changes/changes
7. Turek PJ. Prostatitis. Medscape; 2014. http://emedicine.medscape.com/article/785418-overview
8. Fitzgerald MP, Anderson RU, Potts J, et al. Randomized multicenter feasibility trial of myofascial physical therapy for the treatment of urological chronic pelvic pain syndromes. *Journal of Urology* 2013;189(1 Suppl):S75–S85. http://www.ncbi.nlm.nih.gov/pubmed/23234638
9. Self-massage shows benefit in CP/CPPS patients with myofascial pain. Urology Times; 2011. http://urologytimes.modernmedicine.com/urology-times/news/modernmedicine/modern-medicine-news/self-massage-shows-benefit-cpcpps-patients-my?page=full

Sexually Transmitted Infections

1. Bacterial Vaginosis (BV)—CDC Fact Sheet. Centers for Disease Control and Prevention; 2014. http://www.cdc.gov/STD/bv/STDFact-Bacterial-Vaginosis.htm

2. Chlamydia—CDC Fact Sheet. Centers for Disease Control and Prevention; 2014. http://www.cdc.gov/std/chlamydia/STDFact-Chlamydia-detailed.htm
3. Chesson HW, Kirkcaldy RD, Gift TL, et al. Ciprofloxacin resistance and gonorrhea incidence rates in 17 cities, United States, 1991–2006. *Emerging Infectious Diseases* 2014;20(4):612–619. http://www.ncbi.nlm.nih.gov/pmc/articles/PMC3966369/
4. Jenkins WD, Nessa LL, Clark T. Cross-sectional study of pharyngeal and genital chlamydia and gonorrhoea infections in emergency department patients. *Sexually Transmitted Infections* 2014;90(3):246–249. http://www.medscape.com/viewarticle/824390
5. Hofstetter AM, Rosenthal SL, Stanberry LR. Current thinking on genital herpes. *Current Opinion in Infectious Diseases* 2014;27(1):75–83. http://www.medscape.com/viewarticle/820140
6. Wilbanks MD, Galbraith JW, Geisler WM. Dysuria in the emergency department: missed diagnosis of chlamydia trachomatis. *Western Journal of Emergency Medicine* 2014;15(2):227–230. http://www.ncbi.nlm.nih.gov/pmc/articles/PMC3966459/
7. Genital HPV Infection—Fact Sheet. Centers for Disease Control and Prevention; 2014. http://www.cdc.gov/std/HPV/STDFact-HPV.htm
8. Gonorrhea—CDC Fact Sheet (Detailed Version). Centers for Disease Control and Prevention; 2014. http://www.cdc.gov/std/Gonorrhea/STDFact-gonorrhea-detailed.htm
9. Molluscum Contagiosum. A.D.A.M. Medical Encyclopedia. U.S. National Library of Medicine; 2013. http://www.ncbi.nlm.nih.gov/pubmedhealth/PMH0001829/
10. Nongonococcal Urethritis (NGU) in Men. Diseases & Conditions. Cleveland Clinic; 2010. http://my.clevelandclinic.org/health/diseases_conditions/hic_Chlamydia/hic_NongonococcalUrethritis_NGU_in_Men
11. Patton ME, Su JR, Nelson R, et al. Primary and secondary syphilis—United States, 2005–2013. *Morbidity and Mortality Weekly Report* 2014;63(18):402–406. http://www.cdc.gov/mmwr/preview/mmwrhtml/mm6318a4.htm?s_cid=mm6318a4_w
12. Sexually Transmitted Infections: Overview. U.S. Department of Health and Human Services, Office on Women's Health; 2009. http://www.womenshealth.gov/publications/our-publications/fact-sheet/sexually-transmitted-infections.pdf
13. Syphilis—CDC Fact Sheet. Centers for Disease Control and Prevention; 2014. http://www.cdc.gov/std/syphilis/STDFact-Syphilis-detailed.htm
14. Trichomoniasis—CDC Fact Sheet. Centers for Disease Control and Prevention; 2012. http://www.cdc.gov/std/trichomonas/STDFact-Trichomoniasis.htm

Testicular Cancer

1. Nichols CR, Roth B, Albers P, et al. Active surveillance is the preferred approach to clinical stage I testicular cancer. *Journal of Clinical Oncology* 2013;31(28):3490–3493. http://jco.ascopubs.org/content/31/28/3490.full.pdf+html
2. How to Do a Testicular Self Examination. Testicular Cancer Resource Center; 2012. http://tcrc.acor.org/tcexam.html
3. Koerth-Baker M. Positive pregnancy test diagnoses man's cancer. BoingBoing.net; 2012. http://boingboing.net/2012/11/08/positive-pregnancy-test-diagno.html
4. SEER Stat Fact Sheets: Testis Cancer. Surveillance, Epidemiology, and End Results Program. National Cancer Institute. http://seer.cancer.gov/statfacts/html/testis.html. Accessed Winter 2015.
5. Testicular Cancer. American Cancer Society; 2014. http://www.cancer.org/acs/groups/cid/documents/webcontent/003142-pdf.pdf
6. Testicular Cancer. Cancer Topics. National Cancer Institute; 2014. http://www.cancer.gov/cancertopics/types/testicular
7. Testicular Cancer Info: Staging. Teticiular Cancer Resource Center; 2012. http://tcrc.acor.org/staging.html
8. Testicular Cancer Treatment. Cancer Topics. National Cancer Institute; 2014. http://www.cancer.gov/cancertopics/pdq/treatment/testicular/HealthProfessional
9. Brown CG. Testicular cancer: an overview. *Medsurg Nursing* 2003;12(1):37–43; quiz 44. http://www.medscape.com/viewarticle/473629

Uterine Cancer

1. Nelson R. BRCA1 Linked to Higher Risk for Aggressive Uterine Cancer. Medscape; 2014. http://www.medscape.com/viewarticle/822542
2. Rich WM. Cancer of the Uterus. Introduction to Gynecologic Oncology. http://www.gyncancer.com/uterus.html [Accessed Winter 2015.]
3. Endometrial Cancer Treatment. Cancer Topics. National Cancer Institute; 2014. http://www.cancer.gov/cancertopics/pdq/treatment/endometrial/Patient/AllPages
4. Get the Facts About Gynecologic Cancer. Centers for Disease Control and Prevention; 2012. http://www.cdc.gov/cancer/knowledge/pdf/CDC_GYN_Comprehensive_Brochure.pdf
5. Gor HB. Hysterectomy. Medscape; 2015. http://emedicine.medscape.com/article/267273-overview
6. Salani R, Preston MM, Hade EM, et al. Swelling among women who need education about leg lymphedema: a descriptive study of lymphedema in women undergoing surgery for endometrial cancer. *International Journal of Gynecological Cancer* 2014;24(8):1507–1512. http://www.ncbi.nlm.nih.gov/pubmed/25078342
7. Chiang JW. Uterine Cancer. Medscape; 2013. http://emedicine.medscape.com/article/258148-overview
8. What You Need To KNow About Cancer of the Uterus. Patient Education Publications: National Cancer Institute; 2010. http://www.cancer.gov/publications/patient-education/wyntk-uterus

Chapter 12

1. Screening for Various Cancers. Programmes. World Health Organization. http://www.who.int/cancer/detection/variouscancer/en/. Accessed Winter 2015.
2. SEER Stat Fact Sheets: All Cancer Sites. Surveillance, Epidemiology, and End Results Program. National Cancer Institute. http://seer.cancer.gov/statfacts/html/all.html. Accessed Winter 2015.
3. What Are Cancer Cell and Gene Therapies? Alliance for Cancer Gene Therapies. http://www.acgtfoundation.org/cell-and-gene-therapy/what-are-cancer-cell-and-gene-therapies/. Accessed Winter 2015.
4. The World Health Organization's Fight Against Cancer: Strategies That Prevent, Cure, and Care. World Health Organization; 2007. http://www.who.int/cancer/publicat/WHOCancerBrochure2007.FINALweb.pdf

5. Are the number of cancer cases increasing or decreasing in the world? World Health Organization; 2008. http://www.who.int/features/qa/15/en/
6. Cancer Vaccines. Cancer Topics. National Cancer Institute; 2011. http://www.cancer.gov/cancertopics/factsheet/Therapy/cancer-vaccines
7. Metastatic Cancer. Cancer Topics. National Cancer Institute; 2013. http://www.cancer.org/cancer/cancercauses/othercarcinogens/generalinformationaboutcarcinogens/known-and-probable-human-carcinogens
8. Chronological History of ACS Recommendations for the Early Detection of Cancer in People Without Cancer Symptoms. American Cancer Society; 2014. http://www.cancer.org/healthy/findcancerearly/cancerscreeningguidelines/chronological-history-of-acs-recommendations
9. Known and Probable Human Carcinogens. American Cancer Society; 2014. http://www.cancer.org/cancer/cancercauses/othercarcinogens/generalinformationaboutcarcinogens/known-and-probable-human-carcinogens
10. Cancer. Media Centre. World Health Organization; 2015. http://www.who.int/mediacentre/factsheets/fs297/en/
11. Cancer Prevention Overview. Cancer Topics. National Cancer Institute; 2015. http://www.cancer.gov/cancertopics/pdq/prevention/overview/HealthProfessional
12. Berrettoni BA, Carter JR. Mechanisms of cancer metastasis to bone. *Journal of Bone and Joint Surgery, American Volume* 1986;68(2):308–312. http://jbjs.org/content/68/2/308
13. Emanuel L. Combating Compassion Fatigue and Burnout in Cancer Care. Medscape Nurses; 2011. http://www.medscape.com/viewarticle/742941

Glossary

Ablate A medical procedure in which tissue is removed.

Abscess A deposit of purulent exudate appearing in an acute or chronic localized infection.

Acanthosis nigricans A condition characterized by the formation of velvety brown or black patches on the skin, usually around creases and folds.

Acetylcholine A common neurotransmitter that is necessary for the nervous system to stimulate muscle movement.

Acidosis The state of having abnormally acidic body fluids or tissues.

Acinar Describing a raspberry-shaped cluster of cells that produces a secretion.

Acropachy A condition characterized by clubbing and swelling of the ends of the fingers and toes.

Acute chest syndrome A complication of infection or a sickle cell blockage; can be life-threatening.

Adenocarcinoma A malignant tumor of glandular epithelial cells.

Adenoma A benign tumor of glandular epithelial cells.

Adipocyte A fat cell.

Adjunctive therapy A secondary treatment used to support the primary treatment method for a condition.

Adjuvant A substance added to a medication that affects the action of the drug in a predictable way.

Adult respiratory distress syndrome (ARDS) An acute condition characterized by widespread inflammation of the lungs.

Adventitia The outermost connective tissue layer that covers organs and vessels.

Aflatoxin B1 A toxin produced by some strains of *Aspergillus flavus* that causes cancer in some animals.

Agglutinate To stick together, as when red blood cells form clumps.

Albumin A protein found in blood.

Allergen A substance that elicits an allergic reaction.

Allodynia A condition in which a normally painless stimulus causes pain.

Allogeneic A graft transplanted between genetically different individuals of the same species.

Alopecia Baldness. Can refer to body and facial hair as well as hair on the head.

Alpha 1-antitrypsin A protein that protects alveoli.

Alpha fetoprotein A protein produced by a fetus. Levels can be measured to detect neural tube defects before birth.

Alveolus, Alveoli Small cavities or sockets. Specifically, the tiny air sacs in the lungs where the exchange of gases takes place.

Amenorrhea Absence of menses.

Amines A category of organic compounds found in the body.

Aminosalicylates A type of medicines used to treat inflammatory bowel disease.

Ampulla The dilated end of a duct.

Amyloidosis A disease characterized by extracellular accumulation of amyloid proteins in various organs and tissues.

Angina pectoris Severe chest pain.

Angiogenesis Development of new blood vessels.

Angioplasty A procedure for opening a blood vessel, usually by means of balloon dilation or the placement of a stent.

Angular cheilitis A condition characterized by inflammation and cracking at the corners of the mouth.

Anosmia Total or partial absence of the sense of smell.

Anoxia The absence of oxygen.

Anticholinergic Antagonistic to the action of parasympathetic or other cholinergic nerve fibers.

Antidiuretic hormone (ADH) A hormone that encourages water retention and increased blood pressure. Also called vasopressin.

Antigen Any substance that elicits an immune response on contact with sensitive cells.

Antinuclear antibodies Antibodies produced by the immune system that attack the body's own cells.

Aphasia A loss of language and communication skills due to brain damage.

Aphtha, Aphthae A small ulcer on a mucous membrane, especially the mouth.

Aplastic Referring to conditions characterized by defective regeneration, e.g., forms of cancer.

Apophysitis Inflammation of a bony process or outgrowth.

Apoptosis Programmed cell death.

Arbovirus A virus transmitted by arthropods, such as mosquitoes, ticks, and midges.

Arrhythmia Irregularity of the heartbeat.

Arterial embolization A surgical procedure in which an artery is deliberately blocked in order to reduce blood flow to a tumor or other affected area.

Arteriosclerosis Hardening of the arteries.

Arteriovenous malformation An abnormal connection between veins and arteries, usually found in the cranium.

Arthroplasty Joint replacement surgery.

Arthroscopy A minimally invasive surgery in which the inside of a joint is examined using an arthroscope.

Ascites The accumulation of fluid in the peritoneal cavity.

Asphyxia Impaired or absent exchange of carbon dioxide and oxygen in the respiratory system. Suffocation.

Astrocyte Star-shaped glial cell in the central nervous system.

Ataxic Unable to coordinate muscle activity for smooth movement.

Athetoid Slow, writhing, involuntary movements of the fingers and hands, sometime the toes and feet.

Atopic Referring to an allergic reaction.

Atrophy Wasting of tissues.

ATP energy crisis The cycle of involuntary muscle cell contraction that leads to an increased need for fuel and a decreased supply of blood.

Atrium, Atria The upper chambers of the heart.

Autodigestion A process in which cells are digested by enzymes produced within them.

Autogenic A transplant using a person's own tissues.

Autoimmune polyglandular syndrome A descriptor for a group of conditions that frequently appear together or within families, including Graves disease, type I diabetes, systemic lupus erythematosus, and others.

Autonomic dysreflexia A condition in which an ordinary stimulus results in an uncontrollable sympathetic reaction. Caused by a spinal cord injury above T6.

Autosomal recessive Describing a condition that requires two copies of the gene in question to be present in order for the disease to develop.

Axon The long process of a nerve cell that conducts impulses away from the cell body.

Babinski sign An abnormal reflexive extension of the great toe, indicating an injury to the central nervous system.

Balloon sinusotomy A procedure in which a balloon is inflated inside the sinuses in order to restructure them without extensive scarring.

Bariatric surgery Stomach surgery used to induce weight loss.

Barotraumas An injury to the inner ear resulting from rapid changes in pressure. Most often seen in scuba divers.

Barrett esophagus A condition in which normal esophageal tissue is replaced by tissue similar to intestinal lining.
Basal ganglia Large masses of gray matter at the base of the cerebral hemispheres.
Basophil A phagocytic leukocyte.
Beta amyloid A type of protein associated with formation of plaque in the brain.
Beta cell A type of cell, located in the islets of Langerhans of the pancreas, which produces insulin.
Bile salts Salts created from bile acid, which serve to assist in the digestion of fats.
Biliary colic Acute pain associated with the impaction of a gallstone in the cystic duct.
Bilirubin A dark bile pigment formed from the hemoglobin of dead red blood cells.
Biopsy The process of removing tissue from a patient for examination.
Bismuth A chemical element sometimes used in the treatment of ulcers.
Bisphosphonates A class of drug used to restrict bone loss by reducing the number of bone-clearing cells.
Blood–brain barrier A highly selective filter formed by endothelial cells and astrocytes to prevent the passage of material from the blood directly into the central nervous system.
Body mass index A scale calculated using the ratio between a person's height and weight.
Bony labyrinth The rigid outer wall of the inner ear.
Bouchard nodes Enlargement of the proximal interphalangeal joints due to bone spurs associated with osteoarthritis.
Bowman capsule The beginning segment of a nephron, which surrounds the glomerulus.
Brachytherapy A medical procedure in which radioactive materials are implanted directly into tissue.
Bradycardia Slow heart rate.
Brain-gut axis The ongoing process of biochemical interaction between the gastrointestinal tract and the nervous system.
Bruxism Habitual teeth grinding, especially while sleeping.
Buerger disease Inflammation of the intima of a blood vessel with thrombosis.
Bulbar Bulb-shaped. Referring to a problem involving the medulla oblongata.
Bulla, Bullae A lesion in the lungs where alveoli join in cavities of 1 cm or larger.
Bursa, Bursae Fluid-filled sacs that reduce the friction where a muscle or tendon slides across bone.
Bypass surgery A surgery in which a diseased blood vessel is bypassed by a grafted vessel in order to restore blood flow.
Cachexia Dramatic weight loss and muscle atrophy seen in people with chronic, often terminal diseases.
Calcinosis Accumulation of calcium deposits in the skin, especially in the fingers.
Capsaicin The compound that gives hot peppers their hotness. Also used topically in diluted form for pain relief.
Capsular ligament A thickened part of the capsule that surrounds synovial joints.
Carbidopa A drug used to treat symptoms of Parkinson disease.
Carcinoid tumors A rare kind of cancer found in the digestive tract.
Carcinoma Any kind of malignant tumor that arises in epithelial tissue.
Cardiac tamponade Pathological compression of the heart, related to increased fluid volume within the pericardium.
Cardiomegaly Abnormal enlargement of the heart.
Cardiomyopathy Disease of the myocardium.
Caries Severe decay of tooth or bone.
Cataplexy A transient attack of extreme generalized muscular weakness, often precipitated by an emotional reaction or surprise.
Catheter A tube inserted into the body in order to drain fluid.
Cauda equina Bundle of spinal nerve roots at the base of the spinal column. Literally "horse tail."
Cauda equina syndrome A condition in which the inferior part of the spinal cord is damaged,

resulting in loss of function.

Cavitation The formation of pits or holes.

Celiac sprue Chronic inflammation and atrophy of the mucosa of the small intestine, related to an allergy to gluten. Also called celiac disease.

Central sensitization A change in the central nervous system in response to repeated incidences of pain, leading the person to feel more pain in response to the same stimulus, or even to feel pain in response to a stimulus that would not normally be considered painful.

Cesarian section A surgical procedure in which a mother's abdomen is cut open in order to remove the infant directly.

Chancre The primary lesion of syphilis.

Chiari II formation A malformation of the brain in which part of the brain protrudes through the foramen magnum.

Cholangitis Inflammation of the bile ducts.

Cholecyst Another name for the gallbladder.

Cholecystectomy The surgical removal of the gallbladder.

Cholecystitis Inflammation of the gallbladder.

Choledocholithiasis The presence of a gallstone in the common bile duct.

Cholelithiasis The presence of a gallstone in the gallbladder or bile ducts.

Chondral Having to do with cartilage.

Chondroblasts A cell that produces cartilage cells.

Chondrocytes A cartilage cell.

Chondroitin sulfate An important component of cartilage, sometimes taken as a dietary supplement for joint health.

Chondromalacia A condition in which the cartilage behind the kneecap becomes irritated.

Choriocarcinoma A very invasive cancer, usually of the placenta, but which also occurs sometimes in the ovaries and testes.

Chronic obstructive pulmonary disease COPD. A progressive respiratory disease characterized by difficulty breathing.

Chronic traumatic encephalopathy A degenerative condition of the brain resulting from multiple head injuries.

Chronic venous insufficiency A condition in which the valves in the veins are weakened, resulting in edema as blood fails to return to the heart.

Chyme Partially digested food in the stomach or small intestine.

Circadian rhythm The biological 24-hour cycles that occur within the body.

Clasp-knife effect An abnormal reflex in which passive flexion of a joint is resisted at first, but gives way suddenly with continued pressure.

Clubbing A deformity of the fingers and fingernails that is associated with several lung and heart conditions.

Cochlea The coiled part of the inner ear where sound is converted into nerve impulses.

Coelomic metaplasia A theory about the cause of endometriosis based on the fact that coelomic epithelium is the common ancestor of endometrial and peritoneal cells, and may undergo a change in formation later in life.

Cognitive-behavioral therapy A technique in psychotherapy whereby negative patterns of thought are challenged in order to alter them.

Collagenase An enzyme that dissolves collagen.

Colostomy A procedure in which an artificial opening is created between the skin of the abdomen and the colon.

Comedome An acne lesion, a dilated hair follicle filled with bacteria and other material.

Complement A combination of many serum proteins that react with each other in various ways to disable antigens and assist immune system response.

Condylomata acuminata Genital warts.

Cone biopsy The removal of a cone-shaped section of tissue from the cervix in order to examine it for cancer.

Congenital hepatic fibrosis Liver damage present as a result of a recessive genetic trait.

Contractility The ability to contract.

Contracture An abnormal contraction or shortening of a muscle. Can become permanent.

Contusion A bruise, usually severe.

Cor pulmonale Enlargement of the right ventricle of the heart, often arising from lung disease.

Corpus luteum A temporary hormone-secreting structure in an ovary that exists where the a follicle containing an egg used to be.

Cortical bone The dense outer layer of bone. Also called compact bone.

Cortical spreading depression A wave of increased followed by decreased brain activity that usually begins in the occipital lobes and spreads anteriorly.

Coryza Inflammation of the mucous membrane of the nose.

Costoclavicular space The space between the clavicle and the first rib.

Counterirritant An agent that causes mild irritation or inflammation of the skin on order to relieve symptoms of inflammation in deeper tissues.

Coup-contrecoup A brain injury that occurs both directly beneath the impact and also on the opposite side of the head.

C-reactive protein A liver enzyme secreted in the presence of inflammation. A predictor of heart attack and stroke.

Crepitus A crackling sound, often created by joints.

CREST A mnemonic for the most common scleroderma symptoms: calcinosis, Raynaud phenomenon, esophageal motility disorders, sclerodactyly, and telangiectasia.

Creutzfeldt-Jakob disease A degenerative and fatal neurological disease caused by prions. Commonly known as mad cow disease.

Crural fascia The deep fascia (connective tissue) of the leg.

Cryotherapy A medical procedure that uses extremely cold temperatures to kill or slow the growth of cancerous tissue.

Cryptorchidism The failure of one or both of the testes to descend.

Cupula, Cupulae The gelatinous mass inside the ampulla that senses spatial orientation.

Cyanosis A bluish coloration of the skin and mucous membranes due to insufficient oxygenation.

Cyclooxygenase-1 pathway (COX-1 pathway) The sequence of events that leads to an inflammatory process.

Cystoscope A thin, lighted tube used to see inside the body with minimal damage.

Cytotoxic The quality of being detrimental or destructive to certain cells.

Debridement The removal of dead tissue and foreign matter from a wound.

Dendrite The process of a nerve cell that carries impulses towards the cell body.

Dengue fever A disease transmitted by mosquitos that is characterized by fever, aches, and a measles-like rash.

Dermatitis herpetiformis A chronic condition characterized by a rash of extremely itchy blisters.

Dermatophyte A fungus that causes superficial infections of the skin, hair, and nails.

Desensitization A therapy by which a person is introduced to gradually increasing amounts of an allergen in order to eliminate allergic reaction.

Diaphysis The shaft of a long bone.

Diastole The phase of the heartbeat during which heart muscles relax, allowing the chambers to fill with blood.

Diethylstilbestrol A synthetic estrogen. Formerly given to pregnant women in the mistaken belief that it would help prevent miscarriage.

Diffuse axonal injury Injury to white matter in the central nervous system, often associated with a persistent vegetative state.

Diffuse idiopathic skeletal hyperostosis A bony hardening of ligaments that attach to the spine.

Dihydrotestosterone A form of testosterone.

Dilatation and curettage Enlargement of the cervix and scraping of the endometrium to remove growths or other abnormal tissues.

Dioxin A toxic, carcinogenic compound that is the byproduct of some herbicides.

Discectomy The surgical removal of some or all of a vertebral disc.

Disease-modifying anti-rheumatic drugs (DMARDs) Agents that apparently alter the course and progression of rheumatoid arthritis, rather than simply suppressing inflammation and pain.

Diverticulum An abnormal bulging out of the intestine. (**Plural:** diverticula.)

Dopamine A neurotransmitter in the basal ganglia, associated with attention and pleasure.

Double crush syndrome Irritation of peripheral nerves at multiple sites, leading to confusing signs and symptoms. Also called "multiple crush syndrome."

Ductal ectasia A condition in which the milk ducts of the breast becomes clogged.

Dysarthria Difficulty articulating words.

Dyspepsia Indigestion.

Dysphagia Difficulty swallowing.

Dysplasia Abnormal tissue development.

Dyspnea Difficulty breathing.

Dyssomnias A category including sleep disorders that involve difficulty falling asleep or remaining asleep.

Dystrophic Wasting away.

Dystrophin A protein found in skeletal muscle tissue; it is missing in people with some forms of muscular dystrophy.

Eclampsia Convulsions caused by pregnancy-induced hypertension.

Electrocauterization A medical procedure in which electricity is used to remove unwanted tissue or seal a blood vessel.

Embryonic carcinoma A rare cancer of the ovaries and testes.

Empyema Pus in a body cavity.

Encephalopathy A disease affecting brain function.

Endarterectomy Excision of the diseased layers of an artery along with obstructing plaques.

Endemic Present in a given community or people.

Endocervical curettage A medical procedure in which the lining on the inside of the cervix is scraped with an instrument in order to obtain a tissue sample.

Endogenous Originating in the body.

Endolymph The fluid filling the membranous labyrinth of the ear.

Endometrioma A type of cyst that forms when endometrial tissue grows on the ovaries.

Endometrium The inner layers of the uterine wall.

Endomysium The connective tissue membrane surrounding individual muscle fibers.

Endoscopy Examination of the interior of a hollow area by means of an endoscope.

Endosteum The layer of cells lining the inner surface of bone in the central medullary cavity of long bones.

Enterovirus Any of a group of viruses that attack the intestines.

Enthesitis Inflammation of sites where ligaments or tendons meet bone.

Epididymis The winding duct that connects the testes to the vas deferens.

Epididymitis Inflammation of the epididymis

Epiglottis The flap of tissue that covers the windpipe during swallowing.

Epimysium The connective tissue membrane surrounding a skeletal muscle.

Epistaxis Nosebleed.

Erythema migrans A "bull's eye" rash, usually seen as an early symptom of Lyme disease.

Erythropoietin A hormone produced by the kidneys that stimulates the production of red blood cells.

Esophageal hiatus The opening in the diaphragm through which the esophagus passes.

Estradiol An estrogen produced in the ovaries.

Estriol An estrogen produced in the ovaries, primarily during pregnancy.

Estrogen dominance A condition in which the ratio of estrogen to progesterone in the body is abnormally high.

Estrone An estrogen produced in the ovaries that is less potent than estradiol.

Ethanol Ethyl alcohol.

Excitotoxicity A pathologic state in which nerve cells are damaged by excessive exposure to excitatory neurotransmitters.

Excretion Material that has been excreted (discharged) by the body because it serves no further use.

Exenteration A radical surgery in which all the organs from the pelvic cavity are removed.

Exogenous Originating outside the body.

Exophthalmos Abnormal bulging of the eyes. Also called eye proptosis.

Expiratory reserve volume The amount of air that can still be expelled from the lungs after a normal exhalation.

Extracellular matrix A collective term for connective tissue fibers and the liquid medium in which they are suspended.

Extracorporeal shockwave lithotripsy A medical procedure in which intense sound waves are used to break up stones in the body such as kidney stones and gallstones.

False negative A test result that mistakenly reports the absence of a condition when it is actually present.

False positive A test result that mistakenly reports the presence of a condition when it is actually absent.

Familial adenomatous polyposis Genetic condition characterized by the presence of numerous polyps, which can become cancerous.

Fascicle, fasciculi A band bundle of fibers.

Fasciculations An involuntary twitching contraction of fasciculi.

Fasciotomy A surgical procedure to cut fascia in order to relieve internal pressure.

Fat necrosis The death of fat cells, often in the breast.

Febrile seizures Seizures brought on by sudden increase in body temperature. Most common in infants and young children.

Fecalith A hard, rock-like mass of feces in the intestine.

Female athlete triad The combination of disordered eating, amenorrhea, and osteopenia or osteoporosis that is sometimes seen with women athletes, and is predictive of later serious health problems.

Festinating gait The small, shuffling steps characteristic of Parkinson disease.

Fetal alcohol syndrome A pattern of health problems that arises in children of mothers who consume excessive amounts of alcohol during pregnancy.

Fibrillation Rapid twitching of muscular fibrils.

Fibrin A protein that aids in blood clotting.

Fibroblast A cell capable of forming collagen fibers.

Fibromatosis A condition in which connective tissue cells multiply into tumors called fibromas. Usually not cancerous.

Fimbria, Fimbriae The fringe-like projections at the ends of the fallopian tubes.

Fistula, Fistulae An abnormal passage from one epithelialized surface to another.

Flagellum, Flagella The whiplike "tail" that enables a sperm cell to swim.

Fomite An object that can harbor and transmit infectious agents.

Fragile X syndrome A condition in which a pinch appears in the X chromosome, leading to mental disability.

Fulminant Sudden and severe.

Fundoplication Suture of the fundus of the stomach around the esophagus to prevent reflux with hiatal hernia.

GABA An inhibitory neurotransmitter in the central nervous system. Stands for gamma-amino-butyric acid.

Gastritis Inflammation of the stomach.

Gastrostomy Creation of an artificial external opening into the stomach for nutritional support.

Geniculate ganglion A cluster of sensory fibers of the facial nerve, running through the facial canal.

Gerota fascia The layer of connective tissue surrounding the kidneys and adrenal glands.

Geste antagoniste The habit of touching an area of the body to relieve symptoms of dystonia.

Gingivitis Inflammation of the gums.

Gliadin A class of proteins found in gluten.

Globus pallidus The inner and lighter gray portion of the lentiform nucleus in the brain. Literally "pale globe."

Glomerular filtrate The liquid pushed from the glomerulus into the Bowman capsule.
Glomerular filtration rate (GFR) The rate at which blood passes through the glomeruli of the kidneys.
Glomerulations A tiny hemorrhage of the bladder.
Glomerulonephritis Acute kidney inflammation.
Glottis The vocal cords and the slit between them. Part of the larynx.
Glucocorticoids A category of hormones with anti-inflammatory effects.
Glucosamine A compound found in connective tissue, sometimes taken as a dietary supplement for joint health.
Gluten-sensitive enteropathy Another name for celiac disease.
Glycogen The form in which the body stores carbohydrates.
Goiter An enlarged thyroid gland that can be seen as a swelling in the neck.
Gomerulus, Glomeruli The tiny knot of capillaries at the end of a kidney tubule.
Gonococcal arthritis A joint infection caused by gonorrhea.
Gram-negative Describing a class of bacteria that can be identified by the way in which they do not retain violet coloring when using a Gram stain.
Granuloma A mass of granulation tissue formed in response to infection or a foreign substance.
Graves ophthalmopathy Bulging of the eyes caused by increased water content in the eye tissues. Often associated with hyperthyroidism.
Ground substance The gel-like substance that surrounds connective tissue cells.
HAART Highly active antiretroviral therapy. A combination of at least three drugs used to suppress HIV.
Hand-foot syndrome A complication of chemotherapy in which the palms and soles become red, swollen, numb, and flaky. Also called palmar-plantar erythrodysesthesia.
Haustrum, Haustra The small pouches of the colon.
Heberden node A bulging at the distal interphalangeal joints caused by arthritis.
HELLP syndrome A mnemonic for Hemolysis, Elevated Liver enzymes, and Low Platelet count. Associated with pregnancy-induced hypertension.
Hemagglutinin A type of protein that causes agglutination of red blood cells. Found on the outer coating of influenza and other antigens.
Hematologic Having to do with blood.
Hematoma A mass of clotted blood within an organ or tissue.
Hematuria The presence of blood in the urine.
Heme The non-protein part of hemoglobin, which contains iron.
Hemiparesis Muscle weakness of one side of the body.
Hemiplegia Paralysis of one side of the body.
Hemochromatosis A genetic disorder characterized by the over-absorption of iron.
Hemodialysis A medical procedure in which blood is purified outside of the body, used when the kidneys cannot perform this function normally. Commonly called dialysis.
Hemoglobin The protein in red blood cells that binds to oxygen.
Hemolysis The destruction of red blood cells.
Hemolytic uremic syndrome An infection in which red blood cells are destroyed, which in turn damages the kidneys.
Hemophilic arthritis Joint damage and inflammation, associated with hemophilia-related bleeding into joint cavities.
Hemoptysis Coughing up blood.
Hepatocytes An active liver cell.
Hepatomegaly Abnormal enlargement of the liver.
Hepatorenal syndrome Renal failure in a person with liver disease.
Hereditary nonpolyposis colorectal cancer syndrome A genetic condition that causes a predisposition to colorectal cancer. Also called Lynch syndrome.
High-density lipoprotein (HDL) A compound made up of both lipids and proteins, which is associated with a reduced risk of cardiovascular disease.
Hippocampus A structure in the brain located within the temporal lobe. Part of the limbic system and involved in the consolidation of information from short- to long-term memory.

Hirsutism Abnormally strong presence of bodily and facial hair in a male pattern, especially in women.

Homeostasis The tendency to maintain a stable internal environment.

Homocysteine An amino acid in the blood

HPA axis The hypothalamic-pituitary-adrenal axis, consisting of the complex interactions between these three glands.

Hunner ulcer A star-shaped lesion in the wall of the bladder.

Hyaline Describing translucent articular cartilage.

Hydrocephalus A condition marked by the excessive accumulation of cerebrospinal fluid.

Hydrophilic Inclined to mix with water. Literally, "water-loving."

Hydrostatic pressure The pressure exerted by a fluid due to the effects of gravity.

Hyperacusis Abnormally acute hearing due to irritability of sensory nerves.

Hyperalgesia Extreme sensitivity to painful stimuli.

Hypercalcemia Abnormally high calcium levels.

Hypercoagulability An excessive tendency to form blood clots.

Hyperglycemia Abnormally high blood sugar levels.

Hyperlipidemia Abnormally high levels of fats in the blood.

Hypernephroma The most common form of cancer of the kidneys.

Hyperosmolality Increased concentration of a solution.

Hyperplasia An increase in the number of cells in a tissue or organ, outside of tumor formation.

Hyperpyrexia Dangerously high fever.

Hypersensitivity reactions Exaggerated responses to the stimulus of a foreign agent.

Hyperthermia Abnormally high body temperature.

Hyperuricemia An abnormally high concentration of uric acid in the blood.

Hypnagogic hallucinations Vivid hallucinations that occur while transitioning from wakefulness to sleep or vice versa.

Hypnic myoclonia A muscular jerk experienced at the onset of sleep that may replicate the feeling of falling.

Hypocretin A neurotransmitter produced by the hypothalamus that regulates wakefulness and appetite. Also called orexin.

Hypoglycemia insensitivity Loss of the ability to sense when one's blood sugar is low.

Hypothalamus-pituitary-thyroid The interrelationship between the hypothalamus, the pituitary gland, and the thyroid gland, and the hormones they each secrete, which serve to modify the activity of the others.

Hypoxia Abnormally low oxygen levels in the body.

Icterus Abnormal yellowing of the skin and eyes. Also called jaundice.

Idiopathic Relating to a condition or disease of unknown cause.

Idiopathic endolymphatic hydrops The accumulation of excess endolymph inside the membranous labyrinth. Meniere disease.

Ileocecal valve The passage from the small intestine to the large intestine.

Immunoglobulin A protein that helps the immune system recognize and attack foreign objects. Also called antibodies.

In situ In its own place. Carcinomas found in situ have not grown beyond where those cells would normally be found, and are sometimes categorized as precancerous.

Incarcerated Describing a hernia that is entrapped to the degree that it cannot be repaired without surgery.

Indurated Hardened.

Infarct An area of dead tissue resulting from lack of blood supply.

Infarction The obstruction of blood supply to a tissue.

Inflammatory bowel disease An umbrella term encompassing both Crohn disease and ulcerative colitis.

Infundibulum The hollow structure that connects the hypothalamus to the posterior pituitary gland.

Inguinal ring The entrance to the inguinal canal, through which the vas deferens passes into the abdomen.

Instillation A medical procedure in which medication is administered directly into the bladder with a catheter.

Interleukin-1 A protein that raises body temperature, among other things.

Intermittent claudication Exercise-induced leg cramping caused by blocked arteries.

Interosseous membrane A thin membrane of connective tissue extending from one bone to another. The interosseous membrane of the leg is also called the middle tibiofibular ligament.

Interpersonal therapy A type of psychotherapy focused on interpersonal relationships and skills.

Intertrigo Inflammation of the skin in and around folds.

Intervertebral foramina The openings between adjacent vertebrae. A single spinal nerve exits through each intervertebral foramen.

Intrathecal An injection directly into the central nervous system.

Involutional Describing something that is entangled or turned inward on itself.

Iritis Inflammation of the iris of the eye.

Ischemic penumbra The area surrounding an ischemic stroke.

Kerion A secondary bacterial infection of tinea capitis, leading to a raised, spongy lesion.

Ketoacidosis A dangerous metabolic state characterized by high blood acidity (acidosis), which occurs when the body, unable to break down sugars, instead uses fats, releasing an acidic byproduct called ketones.

Ketogenic Giving rise to ketones in the metabolism.

Ketone Potentially toxic byproduct of metabolism.

Kinin Any of a variety of chemicals with physiological effects on cell activity, including visceral muscle contraction along with vascular muscle relaxation, which leads to vasodilation.

Koebner phenomenon Heightened susceptibility to the effects of trauma and chemical exposure.

Kupffer cells Phagocytes (cell-eating cells) found in the liver.

Labile (Of cells) constantly multiplying.

Lacteals Lymphatic vessels of the small intestine, through which fats are absorbed.

Lacunar infarctions Tiny areas of damage caused by stroke occurring in a small vessel.

Laparoscopy Examination of the abdominal contents with a scope passed through the abdominal wall.

Laparotomy An incision into the abdominal wall.

Latent infection A condition in which a virus is present in a person but is dormant, causing no symptoms.

Lavage The washing out of a hollow cavity.

Laxity Looseness.

Leiomyoma A benign tumor that grows in smooth muscle tissue, such as in the uterus. Also called a fibroid tumor.

Lentigo A brown macule resembling a large freckle.

Leptomeninges The inner two meninges, the pia mater and arachnoid layers.

Levodopa The biologically active form of dopa; a precursor of dopamine.

Levulose A sugar found in many fruits. Also called fructose.

Lewy body disease A multisystem disease involving abnormal proteins in the brain that contribute to dementia and Parkinson disease symptoms.

Lichenification An area of thick and leathery skin or the process by which the epidermis becomes thick and leathery.

Ligamentum flavum One of the ligaments of the spinal column that connect the laminae of adjacent vertebrae.

Limbic system A group of brain structures that exert major influence on the endocrine and autonomic nervous systems.

Lipodystrophy The abnormal redistribution of fat in the body.

Lobectomy The surgical removal of a lobe of an organ.

Locked-in syndrome A condition in which the body and most of the face are paralyzed, but consciousness remains.

Loop electrosurgical excision procedure (LEEP) A medical procedure in which a wire loop heated by electricity is used to remove abnormal cells from the cervix or vagina.

Loop of Henle The U-shaped loop of tubule in the nephron of a kidney.

Low-density lipoprotein (LDL) A compound made up of both lipids and proteins, which is associated with an increased risk of cardiovascular disease.

Lower esophageal sphincter The bundle of muscles surrounding the passage from the esophagus to the stomach.

Lower motor neurons Motor neurons that link upper motor neurons and skeletal muscles.

Lumen The space inside a tube, such as an artery or intestine.

Lymphadenitis Inflammation of one or more lymph nodes.

Lymphangion A lymphatic vessel.

Lymphedema Swelling caused by the build-up of proteins in the body's interstitial spaces.

Lymphoid Producing or related to lymphocytes and antibodies.

Macrophage A type of phagocytic white blood cell.

Macrosomia A condition in which a fetus grows abnormally large as a result of gestational diabetes.

Malabsorption Impaired absorption of nutrients by the small intestine.

Malar A rash of the cheeks, often associated with lupus or erysipelas. Also known as a "butterfly rash."

MAOIs Monoamine oxidase inhibitors, group of chemicals used in the treatment of depression.

Mast cell A white blood cell found in connective tissue that contains heparin and histamine.

Mastitis Inflammation of the mammary gland of the breast.

Mediastinal Relating to the mediastinum, the space in the chest containing all of the thoracic organs except the lungs.

Melatonin A hormone secreted by the pineal gland that is associated with cycles of sleeping and waking.

Membranous labyrinth An organ of the ear lying within the bony labyrinth. Filled with endolymph.

Menarche The first occurrence of menstruation.

Meniscus A crescent-shaped fibrocartilaginous structure; found in the knee, TMJ, and other joints.

Menses The periodic discharge of blood and tissue from the uterus, usually as a result of ovulation not followed by pregnancy.

Meralgia paresthetica Paresthesia of the lateral thigh.

Mesentery A fold of tissue that anchors the intestines and other abdominal organs to the posterior abdominal wall.

Mesothelioma Cancer of the mesothelium.

Metabolite Any product of metabolism.

Microaerophilic Describing a type of bacteria that requires very little oxygen to live.

Microglia Glial cells that act as on-site macrophages in the central nervous system.

Micrographia Handwriting that grows progressively more cramped.

Microstomia Literally, "small mouth." A possible sequela of scleroderma.

Mineralocorticoid One of the steroids from the adrenal cortex that influence salt metabolism.

Mittelschmerz Pain upon ovulating.

Monoclonal gammopathy of undetermined significance A condition in which there are abnormal antibodies present in the blood.

Monoclonal immunoglobulins Nonfunctioning antibodies produced by myeloma cells. Also called M-proteins.

Monocyte A relatively large leukocyte; normally comprises 3% to 7% of the leukocytes in circulating blood.

Mononeuropathy A disorder of a single nerve.

Morphea A localized form of scleroderma.

Motility The ability to move.

Motor unit A motor neuron and the skeletal muscle fibers it innervates.

Mucopolysaccharide Long chain of sugars, commonly found in mucus. Often called glycosaminoglycan.

Mucormycosis A fungal infection of the sinuses.

Mucus blanket The mucus covering of the respiratory epithelium.

Multiple crush syndrome Irritation of peripheral nerves at multiple sites, leading to confusing signs and symptoms. Also called "double crush syndrome"

Myalgic encephalomyelitis Another name for chronic fatigue syndrome.

Mycosis Any disease caused by a fungus.

Myelin The insulating cover surrounding the axons of nerve cells.

Myelodysplastic anemia A form of anemia in which bone marrow manufactures abnormal cells. May be a precursor to myeloma or leukemia.

Myeloid Relating to bone marrow.

Myelopathy Disease or injury of the spinal cord.

Myofiber A muscle fiber

Myofibroblast An atypical type of fibroblast with some qualities of smooth muscle cells.

Myotonia Delayed relaxation of a muscle after a strong contraction.

Myxedema coma A profound loss of consciousness resulting from low levels of thyroid hormone in the body.

Needle aponeurotomy A minimally invasive treatment for Dupuytren contracture, in which the offending band is weakened using microscopic punctures.

Negative feedback loop A process in which a response reduces the stimulus causing it.

Neoadjuvant A treatment administered prior to the primary therapy.

Nephroblastoma A type of kidney cancer that occurs primarily in children. Also called Wilms tumor.

Nephrolithiases A crystalline mass found in the kidneys or ureters. Also called a kidney stone.

Nephron A functional unit of the kidney

Neti pots A container used to administer nasal flushing in order to clear the sinuses.

Neural tube An embryonic structure from which the brain and spinal cord eventually develop.

Neuraminidase A protein found on the outer surface of influenza viruses.

Neuraminidase inhibitors A class of antiviral drugs that targets influenza.

Neurilemma The outermost sheath surrounding nerve cells.

Neuroendocrine tumors Tumors of tissues of the endocrine and neurological systems, which can be either benign or malignant.

Neurofibrillary tangles Intraneural accumulations of filaments with twisted, contorted patterns. Associated with Alzheimer disease.

Neurogenic bladder A condition in which there is a lack of motor control over the process of urination.

Neuroplasticity The ability of the central nervous system to change functionally and structurally as a result of injury or damage

Neutropenia A condition in which the body lacks sufficient neutrophils, leaving it susceptible to infection.

Neutrophil A type of mature white blood cell formed in the bone marrow.

Nidus, Nidi A tiny crystal around which a larger stone can form.

Nitrate A common preservative in meats. Contains one more oxygen than nitrites.

Nitrite A salt or ester of nitrous acid, commonly used as a preservative

Nocturia The need to wake and urinate during the night.

Nonalcoholic fatty liver disease A condition, often asymptomatic, characterized by fatty deposits in the liver of a person who consumes little to no alcohol.

Nonalcoholic steatohepatitis (NASH) Inflammation of fatty tissue in the liver.

Nonseminoma A type of testicular cancer.

Nosocomial A hospital-acquired infection.

Nystagmus Abnormal involuntary eye movements.

Oligodendrocyte A type of glial cell found in the central nervous system. They provide protection and insulation to CNS neurons.

Omentum An apron-like layer of fatty tissue that hangs down over the abdominal organs.

Oncogene Any of a family of genes that normally code for proteins related to cell growth, but which can encourage the development of cancer if mutated or abnormally activated.

Onycholysis Loosening of the nails.

Oophorectomy Surgical removal of the ovaries.

Opioid peptides Chemicals that bind to opioid receptors in the brain.

Orchitis Inflammation of the testes.

Osteocyte A bone cell.

Osteomalacia A condition characterized by the progressive softening of bones.

Osteonecrosis Death of bone tissue on a macroscopic scale.

Osteopenia The condition of low bone density, but not low enough to be considered osteoporosis.

Osteophyte A bony outgrowth.

Osteotomy The surgical cutting of bone.

Otolith A tiny ear stone of hardened material found in the vestibule of the inner ear.

Pain-spasm-ischemia A cycle traditionally thought to create trigger points: sensations of pain cause spasm, which limits blood flow, resulting in more pain, and so on.

Palliative Describing any treatment aimed at relieving symptoms rather than treating the underlying condition.

Pancolitis Inflammation of the entire colon.

Papain An enzyme derived from papayas that is used to dissolve connective tissue. Also used as a meat tenderizer.

Papanicolaou test A screening procedure for cervical cancer in which a few cells are removed from the cervix for examination under a microscope. Commonly called a Pap test.

Papule A small, raised bump in the skin, similar to a pimple but without producing pus.

Paraplegia Paralysis of both lower extremities and (usually) the lower trunk.

Parasomnia Disruption of the sleep cycle.

Parenchyma The functional tissue of an organ.

Paresthesia An abnormal sensation, such as burning, prickling, tickling, or tingling.

Pars interarticularis The part of the vertebra between the superior and inferior articular process.

Patent foramen ovale A condition in which the valve in the atrial septum of the heart does not fully close after birth.

Pauciarticular JRA Juvenile rheumatoid arthritis affecting fewer than five joints.

PCBs Polychlorinated biphenyls, chemicals that were banned in the US when their harmful impact on human health and the environment was discovered.

Pedunculate Having a peduncle; suspended from a stalk.

Pepsin The main digestive enzyme in the stomach.

Peptide A compound made up of two or more amino acids.

Percutaneous nephrolithotomy A medical procedure in which an incision is made through the skin of the back directly to the kidney in order to remove a stone.

Percutaneous transluminal coronary angioplasty (PTCA) A procedure in which a balloon is used to enlarge an artery.

Perforator veins Veins that perforate the superficial fascia, connecting superficial veins to the deep ones into which they drain.

Perfusion pressure The gradient between arterial and venous pressure in a comparable location.

Perilymph The fluid surrounding the membranous labyrinth of the ear.

Perimysium The connective tissue membrane surrounding a bundle of muscle fibers.

Perineurium The connective tissue wrapping around bundles of nerve fibers.

Periodic limb movement disorder A disorder characterized by problematic episodes of limb movements during sleep.

Periosteum The connective tissue membrane covering the outside surface of a bone.

Peristalsis The wave-like contractions of the intestines that move their contents forward.

Peritoneum The membrane that lines the abdominal cavity.

Periurethral Related to the tissues that surround the urethra.

Pernicious anemia A condition in which the body does not produce enough red blood cells due to insufficient amounts of vitamin B_{12} (either due to inadequate consumption or because it is not properly absorbed).

Persistent vegetative state A state characterized by normal levels of arousal (including sleep-wake cycles), but complete lack of awareness.

Phalen's test A common test for carpal tunnel syndrome in which the wrists are held in flexion for 60 seconds or longer.

Philadelphia chromosome A dysfunctional chromosome associated with the development of leukemia.

Phlebectomy The surgical removal of a part of a vein.

Photosensitivity Abnormal sensitivity to light.

Placenta abruption A condition in which the placenta prematurely separates from the uterus.

Plasma cell A B-cell that produces a single type of antibody.

Plastocytoma A tumor made of mutated immature B-cells.

Platelets An irregularly shaped fragment of a megakaryocyte that aids in blood clotting.

Pleural effusion The accumulation of fluid in the pleural cavity.

Plexus, Plexi A network of nerves, blood vessels, or lymphatic vessels.

Pneumatic compression A technique in which venous circulation in a limb is manually increased through the use of intermittently inflated sleeves.

Pneumonectomy The surgical removal of a lung.

Pneumothorax The presence of air or gas in the pleural cavity.

Podagra A painful condition of the foot (usually the great toe) caused by gout.

Polyarticular JRA Juvenile rheumatoid arthritis affecting five or more joints.

Polycythemia An abnormally high number of red cells in the blood.

Polydipsia Excessive thirst.

Polyneuropathy A condition affecting multiple peripheral nerves.

Polyphagia Excessive eating.

Polyp An abnormal growth that projects from a mucous membrane.

Polysomnography Continuous monitoring of physiological functioning during sleep.

Polyuria Excessive urination.

Pons A part of the brainstem, located between the medulla oblongata and the thalamus.

Portal hypertension Elevated pressure in the hepatic portal due to damaged liver tissue.

Positive feedback loop A process in which a stimulus prompts a response, which in turn amplifies the stimulus, heightening the response.

Post concussion syndrome A condition in which concussion symptoms last for weeks or months after the concussion itself.

Post-mastectomy pain syndrome A condition characterized by chronic pain in the axilla, shoulder, arm, or chest wall following breast surgery.

Postthrombotic syndrome A combination of swelling, pain, and skin damage that sometimes follows deep vein thrombosis.

Post-treatment Lyme disease syndrome (PTLDS) Chronic symptoms of pain and fatigue that may continue for months in some people after contracting Lyme disease.

Preeclampsia A condition occurring in pregnant women characterized by hypertension along with elevated proteins in the urine and sometimes systemic swelling

Pretibial myxedema A rash that occurs in the tibial region, specifically associated with hyperthyroidism.

Proctitis Ulcerative colitis that is present only in the rectum or anus.

Proctosigmoiditis Ulcerative colitis that is present in both the rectum and the sigmoid colon.

Prodrome An early symptom or warning of the onset of a disease.

Proliferant A substance that stimulates the growth of cells.

Proliferative inflammatory atrophy A condition of the prostate and other tissues involving chronic inflammation, which leads to cellular proliferation and an increased risk of cancer.

Prophylaxis Prevention of a disease or of a process that can lead to a disease.

Proprioceptor A sensory neuron that conveys information about muscle tension and joint position.

Proptosis Abnormal bulging of the eyes or other body part.

Prostatic intrathelial neoplasia (PIN) The presence of abnormal cells in the epithelium of the prostate.

Prostadynia, Prostatodynia Chronic pelvic pain in men that is not the result of an infection or other obvious cause. Also called chronic pelvic pain syndrome (CPPS).

Prosthesis, prostheses Artificial body part.

Proteoglycan Large, negatively charged molecule that attracts water.

Pruritis Itchiness.

Pseudogout A painful joint disease with symptoms similar to gout, but which does not involve uric acid.

Psychodynamic therapy A form of psychotherapy that focuses on how unresolved inner conflicts affect one's decision-making.

Psychosis A mental and behavioral disorder affecting a person's ability to recognize reality.

Pulmonary hypertension Abnormally high blood pressure in the arteries of the lungs.

Punch biopsy The surgical removal of a cylindrical portion of tissue for examination.

Pustule A small bump in the skin containing pus. A pimple.

Pyloric valve The ring of muscle at the passage from the stomach to the small intestine. Also called the pyloric sphincter.

Pyrexia Fever.

Pyrogen A fever-inducing agent.

Q-angle The angle formed by the line from the ASIS to the middle of the patella, and the line from the middle of the patella to the tibial tubercle.

Quadriplegia Paralysis of all four limbs. Also called tetraplegia.

Radiculopathy Any disorder of the spinal nerve roots.

Radon A radioactive gas.

Rales An abnormal rattling sound when breathing.

RANK ligand inhibitors A class of drugs used to treat osteoporosis by interfering with bone resorption.

Recombinant factors Manufactured blood clotting proteins.

Reducible Able to be reduced, or put back in proper position.

Reed Sternberg cells Large transformed lymphocytes, indicative of Hodgkin disease.

Reflex arc A neural pathway for an action reflex, which bypasses the brain.

Refractory Relapsed or recurring.

Renal colic Severe pain caused by the impaction or passage of a kidney stone.

Renin An enzyme produced by the kidneys that is involved in vasoconstriction and hypertension.

Respiratory syncytial virus (RSV) A common virus that causes colds in healthy adults, but can be serious in infants and the immunocompromised.

Restenosis Recurring stenosis after corrective surgery.

Reticulocyte Immature red blood cell.

Retinopathy Noninflammatory degenerative disease of the retina of the eye.

Rh sensitization A complication that occurs when a person with Rh-negative blood becomes pregnant with an Rh-positive child for the second time, in which the mother's antibodies attack the fetus' red blood cells.

Rheumatic nodules Lumps under the skin that occur near joints affected with rheumatoid arthritis.

Rhinitis Inflammation of the nasal mucous membrane.

Rhinophyma A large, bulbous, and red nose, often caused by rosacea.

Rhupus Term for the common combination of rheumatoid arthritis and lupus.

Sarcolemma The plasma membrane of a muscle fiber.

Sarcoma Any kind of malignant tumor that arises in muscle or connective tissue.

Sarcomere The contracting part of a myofibril.

Savant A condition in which a person with developmental disorders shows one or more areas of unusually strong ability or skill.

Schistosoma haematobium A parasitic flatworm that can infect the urinary system of humans.

Sciatica Irritation of the sciatic nerve. Often causes pain that radiates down the leg through the buttocks.

Sclera The white, outer layer of the eye.

Sclerodactyly Stiffness of the skin of the fingers.

Sclerosing agent A medicine injected into blood vessels in order to shrink them.

Selective estrogen receptor modulators A group of medications developed to reduce the risk of estrogen-dependent cancers and conditions (SERMs).

Seminiferous tubules The location in the testes where sperm cells develop.

Seminoma The most common type of testicular cancer.

Sentinel lymph node The first lymph node to receive lymph drainage from a malignant tumor.

Sentinel node biopsy A biopsy of the first lymph node to receive lymph drainage from a malignant tumor; used to determine whether cancer has spread.

Sepsis An inflammation of the whole body in response to an infection. Can be fatal.

Septicemia Systemic disease caused by the spread of microorganisms and their toxins in the circulating blood. Also known as blood poisoning.

Septum A wall between two chambers.

SERMs See selective estrogen receptor modulators.

Seronegative spondyloarthropathy An autoimmune disease of the vertebral column that does not result in antinuclear antibodies in the blood.

Serotonin A chemical found in many tissues, functioning as a neurotransmitter in the brain, and a vasoconstrictor, stimulator of smooth muscle contractions, and gastric secretion inhibitor in other parts of the body.

Severe acute respiratory syndrome SARS. A highly contagious respiratory illness caused by a type of coronavirus.

Sine An unusual form of systemic scleroderma with significant organ involvement and minimal affect on the skin

Sinus A channel for the passage of material without the layers of an ordinary vessel.

Sitz baths A bath in which only the hips and buttocks are immersed, leaving the legs outside the tub.

SNRIs Serotonin and norepinephrine reuptake inhibitors, classes of drugs used to relieve depression.

Somatotropin Another term for growth hormone.

Spasticity A state of increased muscle tone with exaggerated muscle tendon reflexes.

Sphygmomanometer An instrument for measuring blood pressure.

Spinal cord shock The period immediately following a spinal cord injury, characterized by swelling of the spinal cord and impairment of various bodily functions.

Splenomegaly Enlargement of the spleen.

Sputum Mucus and other material that is coughed up from the respiratory tract.

SSRI Selective serotonin reuptake inhibitor, a type of drug used to relieve depression.

Stapedius A muscle in the ear that stabilizes the stapes bone. The smallest skeletal muscle.

Starling equilibrium The principle that the amount of fluid squeezed out of circulatory capillaries should be almost equal to the amount being drawn into lymphatic capillaries.

Steatorrhea Abnormal amounts of fat in the feces resulting from poor absorption of fats in the intestines.

Stenosis An abnormal narrowing of a canal.

Stereotactic radiotherapy A targeted form of radiotherapy in which beams of radiation from various positions are all aimed at one place.

Steroids A group of chemical compounds that includes some types of hormones.

Strabismus A lack of parallel alignment of the eyes.

Stricture Narrowing of a tube, duct, or hollow structure.

Stroma The connective tissue, fat, and blood cells that support an epithelial organ.

Stromal tumors A tumor that arises from the connective tissue stroma rather than epithelium.

Subacute cutaneous lupus A type of cutaneous lupus that is between chronic and acute in nature.

Subglottis The lower portion of the larynx, which connects it to the trachea.

Subluxation An incomplete dislocation.

Substantia nigra A large mass in the brainstem, composed of pigmented cells. Synthesizes dopamine.

Sulcus, Sulci The grooves or furrows on the surface of the brain.

Superior vena cava syndrome A condition caused by compression of the superior vena cava, usually by a tumor.

Supraglottis The upper part of the larynx.

Symbiosis A mutually beneficial relationship between two organisms.

Sympathectomy The surgical removal of a section of sympathetic nerve or one or more of the sympathetic ganglia.

Synapse The junction between two nerve cells.

Syndesmophytes A bone spur attached to a ligament.

Synkinesis An involuntary movement that follows a voluntary one.

Synovium The soft tissue found between the joint capsule and the joint cavity of synovial joints.

Systemic JRA/Still's disease The most serious type of juvenile rheumatoid arthritis, affecting at least one joint as well as causing inflammation in various internal organs.

Systole The phase of the heartbeat during which heart muscles contract, pushing blood out of the chambers.

Tachycardia Rapid heartbeat.

Tamoxifen An antiestrogen agent used in the treatment of breast cancer.

Tarsal coalition An abnormal fusion of tarsal bones.

Tau A protein that helps to maintain the structure of the cytoskeleton. Found in the plaques of people with Alzheimer disease.

Telangiectasias Small dilated blood vessels, usually in the skin. Also called as "Spider veins."

Tenesmus A constant or recurring feeling of needing to have a bowel movement, regardless of the actual contents of the colon.

Tenocyte A tendon cell.

TENS unit A transcutaneous electrical nerve stimulation device, used to control pain.

Teratoma A tumor that contains tissues not normally found in the tissue in which it arises. Usually found in the ovaries and testes.

Testis, Testes The male reproductive organ that produces sperm cells.

Tethered cord A group of malformations that all involve the restriction of the movement of the spinal cord within the spinal canal.

Tetraplegia Quadriplegia.

Thrombocytopenia Decreased number of thrombocytes.

Thrombolytics Related to the therapeutic dissolving of blood clots.

Thrush Candida infection of the mouth.

Thyroidectomy Surgical removal of the thyroid gland.

Thyrotoxic myopathy A neuromuscular disorder connected to hyperthyroidism that involves weakness, the breakdown of muscle tissue, and intolerance to heat.

Thyrotoxicosis Excessive levels of thyroid hormone.

Tinea A fungal infection of the skin, hair, or nails.

Tinel's sign A test used to detect an irritated nerve (such as in carpal tunnel syndrome) by tapping directly over the nerve.

Tinnitus Ringing in the ears.

Tissue pressure The pressure of interstitial tissue fluid in an enclosed space.

Titers A measurement of concentration (as in the concentration of a virus in the blood).

Tonometer An instrument for measuring pressure or tension.

Torsion Twisting. In the case of ovarian torsion, the ovary is rotated in such a way that the artery to the ovary becomes blocked.

Toxic megacolon Acute nonobstructive dilation of the colon.

Trabecular bone The softer bone tissue generally found at the ends of long bones and in the interior of vertebrae. Also called spongy bone.

Transcranial magnetic stimulation A treatment using magnetic fields to stimulate nerves in the brain in order to relieve depression.

Transcriptase An enzyme that converts RNA to DNA

Transitional The transitional portion of the prostate surrounds part of the urethra. It continues to grow throughout life and is responsible for benign prostatic hyperplasia (BPH).

Transmembrane conductance regulator gene A gene that is responsible for proteins that conduct chloride in and out of cells. Mutation is associated with cystic fibrosis.

Tricyclic antidepressants A class of drugs used to relieve depression.

Triglyceride A major component of natural fats and oils, containing glycerol and three fatty acids.

Tuberous sclerosis A rare genetic disease that causes nonmalignant tumors to grow in the brain and other vital organs.

Tumor suppressor genes A gene that suppresses or protects against cancer. Also called an antioncogene.

Tunica externa The tough outermost layer of blood vessel walls.

Tunica intima The endothelial, innermost layer of blood vessel walls.

Tunica media The smooth muscle middle layer of blood vessel walls.

Type I collagen The most common form of collagen in the body, found in places including tendons, skin, artery walls, and scar tissue.

Type III collagen A form of collagen that is thinner and weaker than Type I.

Upper motor neurons Motor neurons that originate in the brain, and carry signals to lower motor neurons.

Ureterolithiasis A kidney stone that is lodged in a ureter.

Urothelial carcinoma A cancer of the kidneys, ureters, bladder, and urethra.

Urushiol An oil that causes an allergic skin reaction in most people.

Uterine artery embolization A medical procedure in which blood supply is cut off to a uterine body such as a fibroid tumor.

Uterine hyperplasia The excessive growth of cells of the lining of the uterus.

Uveitis Inflammation of the uvea of the eye.

Vagus nerve stimulation A treatment for relieving depression.

Valgus Laterally deviated

Vapocoolant spray A topical anesthetic aerosol spray.

Varix, varices Dilated, distended vein.

Varus Medially deviated

Vas deferens The secretory duct of the testicle, along which sperm travel from the testes.

Vasculitis Inflammation of a blood or lymphatic vessel

Vasoconstriction Tightening of blood vessels, including capillaries.

Vasodilation Loosening of blood vessels, including capillaries.

Vasospasm The sudden constriction of a blood vessel.

Venous thromboembolism (VTE) The combination of deep vein thrombosis and pulmonary embolism.

Ventricles A cavity, in this case, the inferior chambers of the heart.

Verruca A wart.

Vertigo A sensation of being spun around.

Vesicle A blister.

Vesicouretal reflux The flow of urine from the bladder backwards into the kidneys.

Vesicouretal valve A valve in the ureters that prevents urine from passing from the bladder back up into the ureters.

Vestibular rehabilitation A program of exercises designed to improve balance and decrease dizziness.

Vestibule The central part of the bony labyrinth of the ear.

Villus, Villi Fingerlike projections that increase the surface area of the small intestine, which in turn increases nutrient absorption.

Viscosity The degree to which a fluid resists flowing. Stickiness.

von Hippel-Lindau syndrome A genetic condition that increases the risk of several different kinds of cancer.

Wernicke-Korsakoff syndrome A combination of conditions related to prolonged alcohol abuse and thiamin deficiency, including tremor, psychosis, confusion, memory loss, and delirium tremens.

Yolk sac tumors A rare form of cancer, usually found in the ovaries or testes of children under the age of 2.

Illustration Credits

Chapter 1

1.2 Harvey RA, Cornelissen CN. *Microbiology*. 3rd ed. Philadelphia, PA: Lippincott Williams & Wilkins; 2012.
1.3 Asset provided by Anatomical Chart Co.
1.4 Porth CM. *Pathophysiology*. 7th ed. Philadelphia, PA: Lippincott Williams & Wilkins; 2004.
1.5 Harvey RA, Cornelissen CN. *Microbiology*. 3rd ed. Philadelphia, PA: Lippincott Williams & Wilkins; 2012.
1.6 Harvey RA, Cornelissen CN. *Microbiology*. 3rd ed. Philadelphia, PA: Lippincott Williams & Wilkins; 2012.
1.7 Harvey RA, Cornelissen CN. *Microbiology*. 3rd ed. Philadelphia, PA: Lippincott Williams & Wilkins; 2012.
1.8 Stoller JK. *The Cleveland Clinic Foundation intensive review of internal medicine*. 6th ed. Philadelphia, PA: Lippincott Williams & Wilkins; 2014.
1.9 Dr. Stan Erlandsen; Dr. Dennis Feely. Public Health Images Library, Centers for Disease Control and Prevention, 1982. http://phil.cdc.gov
1.10 James Gathany. Public Health Images Library, Centers for Disease Control and Prevention, 2014. http://phil.cdc.gov
1.11 Koneman EW, Allen SD, Janda WM, et al. *Color atlas and textbook of diagnostic microbiology*. 5th ed. Philadelphia, PA: Lippincott Williams & Wilkins; 1997.
1.12 Williams A. *Massage mastery*. Philadelphia, PA: Lippincott Williams & Wilkins; 2012.

Chapter 2

2.2 Goodheart HP. *Goodheart's photoguide of common skin disorders*. 2nd ed. Philadelphia, PA: Lippincott Williams & Wilkins; 2003.
2.3 Goodheart HP. *Goodheart's photoguide of common skin disorders*. 2nd ed. Philadelphia, PA: Lippincott Williams & Wilkins; 2003.
2.4 Koneman EW, Allen SD, Janda WM, et al. *Color atlas and textbook of diagnostic microbiology*. 5th ed. Philadelphia, PA: Lippincott Williams & Wilkins; 1997.
2.5 Dr. Dennis D. Juranek. Public Health Images Library, Centers for Disease Control and Prevention. http://phil.cdc.gov
2.6 Koneman EW, Allen SD, Janda WM, et al. *Color atlas and textbook of diagnostic microbiology*. 5th ed. Philadelphia, PA: Lippincott Williams & Wilkins; 1997.
2.7 Goodheart HP. *Goodheart's photoguide of common skin disorders*. 2nd ed. Philadelphia, PA: Lippincott Williams & Wilkins; 2003.
2.8 Public Health Images Library, Centers for Disease Control and Prevention. http://phil.cdc.gov
2.9 Goodheart HP. *Goodheart's photoguide of common skin disorders*. 2nd ed. Philadelphia, PA: Lippincott Williams & Wilkins; 2003.
2.10 Goodheart HP. *Goodheart's photoguide of common skin disorders*. 2nd ed. Philadelphia, PA: Lippincott Williams & Wilkins; 2003.
2.11 Sutton DA, Fothergill AW, Rinaldi MG. *Guide to clinically significant fungi*. Baltimore, MD: Lippincott Williams & Wilkins; 1998.
2.12 Goodheart HP. *Goodheart's photoguide of common skin disorders*. 2nd ed. Philadelphia, PA: Lippincott Williams & Wilkins; 2003.
2.13 Goodheart HP. *Goodheart's photoguide of common skin disorders*. 2nd ed. Philadelphia, PA: Lippincott Williams & Wilkins; 2003.
2.14 Image provided by Stedmans. (Dr. Barankin Dermatology Collection 2)
2.15 Fleisher GR, Ludwig S, Baskin MN. *Atlas of pediatric emergency medicine*. Philadelphia, PA: Lippincott Williams & Wilkins; 2004.
2.16 Public Images Library, Centers for Disease Control and Prevention.
2.17 Goodheart HP. *Goodheart's photoguide of common skin disorders*. 2nd ed. Philadelphia, PA: Lippincott Williams & Wilkins; 2003.
2.18 Goodheart HP. *Goodheart's photoguide of common skin disorders*. 2nd ed. Philadelphia, PA: Lippincott Williams & Wilkins; 2003.
2.19 McDonagh DO, Lereim I, Micheli LJ, et al. *FIMS sports medicine manual*. Philadelphia, PA: Lippincott Williams & Wilkins; 2011.
2.20 Image provided by Stedmans. (Dr. Barankin Dermatology Collection.)
2.22 Bruno Coignard, M.D.; Jeff Hageman, M.H.S. Public Health Images Library, Centers for Disease Control and Prevention. http://phil.cdc.gov
2.23 Anderson MK. *Foundations of athletic training*. 5th ed. Philadelphia, PA: Lippincott Williams & Wilkins; 2012.
2.24 Goodheart HP. *Goodheart's photoguide of common skin disorders*. 2nd ed. Philadelphia, PA: Lippincott Williams & Wilkins; 2003.
2.25 Goodheart HP. *Goodheart's photoguide of common skin disorders*. 2nd ed. Philadelphia, PA: Lippincott Williams & Wilkins; 2003.
2.26 Image provided by Stedmans. (Dr. Barankin Dermatology Collection.)
2.27 Rassner G. *Atlas of dermatology*. 3rd ed. Philadelphia, PA: Lea & Febiger; 1994.
2.28 Goodheart HP. *Goodheart's photoguide of common skin disorders*. 2nd ed. Philadelphia, PA: Lippincott Williams & Wilkins; 2003.
2.29 Burkhart C, Morrell D, Goldsmith LA, et al. *VisualDx: essential pediatric dermatology*. Philadelphia, PA: Lippincott Williams & Wilkins; 2009.

2.30 Lugo-Somolinos A, McKinley-Grant L, Goldsmith LA, et al. *VisualDx: essential dermatology in pigmented skin*. Philadelphia, PA: Lippincott Williams & Wilkins; 2011.
2.31 Goodheart HP. *Goodheart's photoguide of common skin disorders*. 2nd ed. Philadelphia, PA: Lippincott Williams & Wilkins; 2003.
2.32 Goodheart HP. *Goodheart's photoguide of common skin disorders*. 2nd ed. Philadelphia, PA: Lippincott Williams & Wilkins; 2003.
2.33 Sauer GC, Hall JC. *Manual of skin diseases*. 10th ed. Philadelphia, PA: Lippincott Williams & Wilkins; 2010.
2.34 Craft N, Taylor E, Tumeh PC, et al. *VisualDx: essential adult dermatology*. Philadelphia, PA: Lippincott Williams & Wilkins; 2010.
2.36 Goodheart HP. *Goodheart's photoguide of common skin disorders*. 2nd ed. Philadelphia, PA: Lippincott Williams & Wilkins; 2003.
2.37 Lugo-Somolinos A, McKinley-Grant L, Goldsmith LA, et al. *VisualDx: essential dermatology in pigmented skin*. Philadelphia, PA: Lippincott Williams & Wilkins; 2011.
2.38 Image provided by Stedmans. (Dr. Barankin Dermatology Collection.)
2.39 Goodheart HP. *Goodheart's photoguide of common skin disorders*. 2nd ed. Philadelphia, PA: Lippincott Williams & Wilkins; 2003.
2.40 Craft N, Taylor E, Tumeh PC, et al. *VisualDx: essential adult dermatology*. Philadelphia, PA: Lippincott Williams & Wilkins; 2010.
2.41 Goodheart HP. *Goodheart's photoguide of common skin disorders*. 2nd ed. Philadelphia, PA: Lippincott Williams & Wilkins; 2003.
2.42 Goodheart HP. *Goodheart's photoguide of common skin disorders*. 2nd ed. Philadelphia, PA: Lippincott Williams & Wilkins; 2003.
2.43 Lugo-Somolinos A, McKinley-Grant L, Goldsmith LA, et al. *VisualDx: essential dermatology in pigmented skin*. Philadelphia, PA: Lippincott Williams & Wilkins; 2011.
2.44 Craft N, Taylor E, Tumeh PC, et al. *VisualDx: essential adult dermatology*. Philadelphia, PA: Lippincott Williams & Wilkins; 2010.
2.45 Stedman's Medical Dictionary.
2.46 Lippincott's Nursing Advisor 2011.
2.47 Edwards L, Lynch PJ. *Genital dermatology atlas*. 2nd ed. Philadelphia, PA: Lippincott Williams & Wilkins; 2010.
2.48 Craft N, Taylor E, Tumeh PC, et al. *VisualDx: essential adult dermatology*. Philadelphia, PA: Lippincott Williams & Wilkins; 2010.
2.49 Goodheart HP. *Goodheart's photoguide of common skin disorders*. 2nd ed. Philadelphia, PA: Lippincott Williams & Wilkins; 2003.
2.50 Goodheart HP. *Goodheart's photoguide of common skin disorders*. 2nd ed. Philadelphia, PA: Lippincott Williams & Wilkins; 2003.
2.51 Image provided by Stedmans. (Dr. Barankin Dermatology Collection.)
2.52 Rubin E, Farber JL. *Pathology*. 3rd ed. Philadelphia, PA: Lippincott Williams & Wilkins; 1999.
2.53 Goodheart HP. *Goodheart's photoguide of common skin disorders*. 2nd ed. Philadelphia, PA: Lippincott Williams & Wilkins; 2003.
2.54 The Podiatry Institute; Southerland J, Alder D, Boberg J, et al. *McGlamry's comprehensive textbook of foot and ankle surgery*. 4th ed. Philadelphia, PA: Lippincott Williams & Wilkins; 2012.
2.55 Lawrence PF, Bell RM, Dayton MT, et al. *Essentials of general surgery*. 5th ed. Philadelphia, PA: Lippincott Williams & Wilkins; 2012.
2.56 Goodheart HP. *Goodheart's photoguide of common skin disorders*. 2nd ed. Philadelphia, PA: Lippincott Williams & Wilkins; 2003.
2.57 Asset provided by Anatomical Chart Co.
2.58 Miller M, Berry D. *Emergency response management for athletic trainers* (Photo courtesy of George A. Datto III, MD). Philadelphia, PA: Lippincott Williams & Wilkins; 2010.
2.59 Image provided by Stedmans. (Dr. Barankin Dermatology Collection.)
2.60 McGreer MA, Carter PJ. *Workbook for Lippincott's textbook for personal support workers*. (Photo © John Radcliffe Hospital/ Photo Researchers, Inc.). Philadelphia, PA: Lippincott Williams & Wilkins; 2010.
2.61 Lugo-Somolinos A, McKinley-Grant L, Goldsmith LA, et al. *VisualDx: essential dermatology in pigmented skin*. Philadelphia, PA: Lippincott Williams & Wilkins; 2011.
2.62 Creason C. *Stedman's medical terminology*. Philadelphia, PA: Lippincott Williams & Wilkins; 2010.
2.63 Assets provided by Anatomical Chart Company.
2.64 Rubin E, Gorstein F, Schwarting R, et al. *Rubin's pathology: clinicopathologic foundations of medicine*. 4th ed. Philadelphia, PA: Lippincott Williams & Wilkins; 2005.

Chapter 3

3.2 Asset modified from Anatomical Chart Co.
3.3 Escott-Stump S. *Nutrition and diagnosis-related care*. 7th ed. Philadelphia, PA: Lippincott Williams & Wilkins; 2011.
3.6 From Wikimedia. http://commons.wikimedia.org/wiki/File:Osteosarcoma_of_the_thigh_bone,_Egyptian,_5th_Dynasty_Wellcome_M0018166.jpg
3.7 Berg D, Worzala K. *Atlas of adult physical diagnosis*. Philadelphia, PA: Lippincott Williams & Wilkins; 2006.
3.8 Roentgen EJ. *Diagnosis of diseases of bone*. 3rd ed. Baltimore, MD: Lippincott Williams & Wilkins; 1981.
3.10 Rubin E, Gorstein F, Schwarting R, et al. *Rubin's pathology: clinicopathologic foundations of medicine*. 4th ed. Philadelphia, PA: Lippincott Williams & Wilkins; 2005.
3.13 Waldman S. *Comprehensive atlas of ultrasound-guided pain management injection techniques* (Photo courtesy of Mary L. Brandt, MD). Philadelphia, PA: Lippincott Williams & Wilkins; 2013.
3.14 Rubin E, Gorstein F, Schwarting R, et al. *Rubin's pathology: clinicopathologic foundations of medicine*. 4th ed. Philadelphia, PA: Lippincott Williams & Wilkins; 2005.
3.15 Berg D, Worzala K. *Atlas of adult physical diagnosis*. Philadelphia, PA: Lippincott Williams & Wilkins; 2006.
3.16 Lugo-Somolinos A, McKinley-Grant L, Goldsmith LA, et al. *VisualDx: essential dermatology in pigmented skin*. Philadelphia, PA: Lippincott Williams & Wilkins; 2011.
3.17 Anderson MK. *Foundations of athletic training*. 5th ed. Philadelphia, PA: Lippincott Williams & Wilkins; 2012.
3.18 Smith WL. *Radiology 101*. 4th ed. Philadelphia, PA: Lippincott Williams & Wilkins; 2013.
3.19 Asset provided by Anatomical Chart Co.
3.20 Asset provided by Anatomical Chart Co.
3.21 Centers for Disease Control and Prevention, Public Health Images Library. http://phil.cdc.gov
3.22 James Gathany, Centers for Disease Control and Prevention, Public Health Images Library. http://phil.cdc.gov

3.23 Asset provided by Anatomical Chart Co.
3.24 Asset provided by Anatomical Chart Co.
3.26 MacNab I, McCulloch J. *Neck ache and shoulder Pain*. Baltimore, MD: Williams & Wilkins; 1994.
3.27 MacNab I, McCulloch J. *Neck ache and shoulder Pain*. Baltimore, MD: Williams & Wilkins; 1994.
3.31 Asset modified from Anatomical Chart Co.
3.33 Moore KL, Dalley AF. *Clinically oriented anatomy*. 4th ed. Baltimore, MD: Lippincott Williams & Wilkins; 1999.
3.34 Weber J, Kelley J. *Health assessment in nursing*. 2nd ed. Philadelphia, PA: Lippincott Williams & Wilkins; 2003.
3.35 Elder DE, Elenitsas R, Rubin AI, et al. *Atlas and synopsis of lever's histopathology of the skin*. 3rd ed. Philadelphia, PA: Lippincott Williams & Wilkins; 2012.
3.36 The Podiatry Institute; Southerland J, Alder D, Boberg J, et al. *McGlamry's comprehensive textbook of foot and ankle surgery*. 4th ed. Philadelphia, PA: Lippincott Williams & Wilkins; 2012.
3.37 Asset provided by Anatomical Chart Co.
3.38 Asset provided by Anatomical Chart Co.
3.39 Smeltzer SC, Bare BG. *Textbook of medical-surgical nursing*. 9th ed. Philadelphia, PA: Lippincott Williams & Wilkins; 2000.
3.41 Anderson MK. *Foundations of athletic training*. 5th ed. Philadelphia, PA: Lippincott Williams & Wilkins; 2012.
3.42 Berg D, Worzala K. *Atlas of adult physical diagnosis*. Philadelphia, PA: Lippincott Williams & Wilkins; 2006.
3.43 Schaaf CP, Zschocke J, Potocki L. *Human genetics*. Philadelphia, PA: Lippincott Williams & Wilkins; 2011.
3.44 Asset provided by Anatomical Chart Co.
3.47 Creason C. *Stedman's medical terminology*. Philadelphia, PA: Lippincott Williams & Wilkins; 2010.
3.48 Castillo M. *Neuroradiology companion: methods, guidelines, and imaging fundamentals*. 4th ed. Philadelphia, PA: Lippincott Williams & Wilkins; 2012.
3.49 Premkumar K. *The massage connection, anatomy and physiology*. 2nd ed. Baltimore, MD: Lippincott Williams & Wilkins; 2004.
3.50 Bucci C. *Condition-specific massage therapy*. Philadelphia, PA: Lippincott Williams & Wilkins; 2011.
3.54 Image provided by Stedmans. (Dr. Barankin Dermatology Collection.)
3.58 Wiesel SW. *Operative techniques in orthopaedic surgery. Four volume set*. Philadelphia, PA: Lippincott Williams & Wilkins; 2010.
3.60 Bickley LS, Szilagyi P. *Bates' guide to physical examination and history taking*. 8th ed. Philadelphia, PA: Lippincott Williams & Wilkins; 2003.
3.61 Asset provided by Anatomical Chart Co.

Chapter 4

4.3 Rubin E, Strayer DS. *Rubin's pathology: clinicopathologic foundations of medicine*. 5th ed. Philadelphia, PA: Lippincott Williams & Wilkins; 2008.
4.4 Asset provided by Anatomical Chart Co.
4.5 Rowland LP. *Merritt's neurology*. 11th ed. Philadelphia, PA: Lippincott Williams & Wilkins; 2005.
4.6 Onofrey BE, Skorin L, Holdeman NR. *Ocular therapeutics handbook*. 3rd ed. Philadelphia, PA: Lippincott Williams & Wilkins; 2011.
4.8 Schalock PC, Hsu JT, Arndt KA. *Lippincott's primary care dermatology*. Philadelphia, PA: Lippincott Williams & Wilkins; 2010.
4.9 Nelson LB. *Wills eye institute: pediatric ophthalmology*. Philadelphia, PA: Lippincott Williams & Wilkins; 2011.
4.10 Image provided by Stedmans. (Dr. Barankin Dermatology Collection.)
4.13 Asset provided by Anatomical Chart Co.
4.14 *Lippincott Williams & Wilkins' comprehensive dental assisting*. Philadelphia, PA: Lippincott Williams & Wilkins; 2011.
4.18 The Podiatry Institute; Southerland J, Alder D, Boberg J, et al. *McGlamry's comprehensive textbook of foot and ankle surgery*. 4th ed. Philadelphia, PA: Lippincott Williams & Wilkins; 2012.
4.19 Yochum TR, Rowe LJ. *Essentials of skeletal radiology*. 2nd ed. Baltimore, MD: Williams & Wilkins; 1996.
4.21 Asset provided by Anatomical Chart Co.
4.24 American College of Sports Medicine. *ACSM's introduction to exercise science*. 2nd ed. Philadelphia, PA: Lippincott Williams & Wilkins; 2013.
4.30 Modified from Moore KL, Agur AM, Dalley AF. *Essential clinical anatomy*. 4th ed. Philadelphia, PA: Lippincott Williams & Wilkins; 2010.
4.31 Wiesel SW. *Operative techniques in orthopaedic surgery*. Philadelphia, PA: Lippincott Williams & Wilkins; 2010.
4.32 McConnell TH, Hull KL. *Human form, human function*. Philadelphia, PA: Lippincott Williams & Wilkins; 2010.
4.34 Asset modified from Anatomical Chart Co.
4.35 Asset modified from Anatomical Chart Co.

Chapter 5

5.1 Archer P, Nelson LA. *Applied anatomy & physiology for manual therapists*. Philadelphia, PA: Lippincott Williams & Wilkins; 2012.
5.2 Anatomical Chart Co.
5.3 Modified from Anatomical Chart Co.
5.4 Anatomical Chart Co.
5.7 Anatomical Chart Co.
5.9 Salter RB. *Textbook of disorders and injuries of the musculoskeletal system*. 3rd ed. Philadelphia, PA: Lippincott Williams & Wilkins; 1998.
5.10 Pereira I, George TI, Arber DA. *Atlas of peripheral blood*. Philadelphia, PA: Lippincott Williams & Wilkins; 2011.
5.11 Anatomical Chart Co.
5.13 Anatomical Chart Co.
5.14 Rubin E, Farber J. *Pathology*. 3rd ed. Philadelphia, PA: Lippincott Williams & Wilkins; 1999.
5.16 Anatomical Chart Co.
5.17 Harwood-Nuss A, Wolfson AB, et al. *The clinical practice of emergency medicine*. 3rd ed. Philadelphia, PA: Lippincott Williams & Wilkins; 2001.
5.19 Courtesy of International Scleroderma Network, www.sclero.org
5.21 Craft N, Taylor E, Tumeh PC, et al. *VisualDx: essential adult dermatology*. Philadelphia, PA: Lippincott Williams & Wilkins; 2010.
5.22 Moore KL, Dalley AF. *Clinically oriented anatomy*. 4th ed. Baltimore, MD: Lippincott Williams & Wilkins; 1999.

Chapter 6

6.1 Adapted from Moore KL, Dalley AF. *Clinically oriented anatomy*. 5th ed. Philadelphia, PA: Lippincott Williams & Wilkins; 2005.
6.2 Sussman C, Bates-Jensen B. *Wound care*. 4th ed. (Photo copyright © Evonne Fowler, RN, CNS, CWOCN.). Philadelphia, PA: Lippincott Williams & Wilkins; 2011.

6.3 Reprinted with permission from Fitzpatrick J, Aeling J. *Dermatology secrets in color*. 2nd ed. Philadelphia, PA: Hanley & Belfus; 2000.
6.4 Bickley LS. *Bates' guide to physical examination and history taking*. 7th ed. Philadelphia, PA: Lippincott Williams & Wilkins; 1999.
6.5 Miller MD, Chhabra AB, Konin J, et al. *Sports medicine conditions: return to play: recognition, treatment, planning*. Philadelphia, PA: Lippincott Williams & Wilkins; 2013.
6.6 Neville B, et al. *Color atlas of clinical oral pathology*. Philadelphia, PA: Lea & Febiger; 1991.
6.7 Anatomical Chart Co.
6.8 DeVita VT, Hellamen S, Rosenberg S, et al. *AIDS: etiology, diagnosis, treatment, and prevention*. 4th ed. Philadelphia, PA: Lippincott Williams & Wilkins; 1997.
6.9 Modified from Porth CM. *Pathophysiology*. 7th ed. Philadelphia, PA: Lippincott Williams & Wilkins; 2004.
6.11 Goodheart HP. *Goodheart's photoguide of common skin disorders*. 2nd ed. Philadelphia, PA: Lippincott Williams & Wilkins; 2003.
6.12 Porth CM. *Essentials of pathophysiology: concepts of altered health states*. 2nd ed. Philadelphia, PA: Lippincott Williams & Wilkins; 2007.
6.14 Anatomical Chart Co.
6.16 Rubin E, Gorstein F, Schwarting R, et al. *Rubin's pathology: clinicopathologic foundations of medicine*. 4th ed. Philadelphia, PA: Lippincott Williams & Wilkins; 2005.
6.17 Goodheart HP. *Goodheart's photoguide of common skin disorders*. 2nd ed. Philadelphia, PA: Lippincott Williams & Wilkins; 2003.
6.18 Lugo-Somolinos A, McKinley-Grant L, Goldsmith LA, et al. *VisualDx: essential dermatology in pigmented skin*. Philadelphia, PA: Lippincott Williams & Wilkins; 2011.
6.19 Goodheart HP. *Goodheart's photoguide of common skin disorders*. 2nd ed. Philadelphia, PA: Lippincott Williams & Wilkins; 2003.
6.20 Rubin E, Farber JL. *Pathology*. 3rd ed. Philadelphia, PA: Lippincott Williams & Wilkins; 1999.
6.21 Kroumpouzos G. *Text atlas of obstetric dermatology*. Philadelphia, PA: Lippincott Williams & Wilkins; 2013.
6.22 Goodheart HP. *Goodheart's photoguide of common skin disorders*. 2nd ed. Philadelphia, PA: Lippincott Williams & Wilkins; 2003.
6.23 Goodheart HP. *Goodheart's photoguide of common skin disorders*. 2nd ed. Philadelphia, PA: Lippincott Williams & Wilkins; 2003.
6.24 Adapted from Anatomical Chart Co.

Chapter 7

7.1 Anatomical Chart Co.
7.2 Anatomical Chart Co.
7.4 Anatomical Chart Co.
7.6 Harvey RA, Cornelissen CN. *Microbiology*. 3rd ed. Philadelphia, PA: Lippincott Williams & Wilkins; 2012.
7.7 Fleisher GR, Ludwig W, Baskin MN. *Atlas of pediatric emergency medicine*. Philadelphia, PA: Lippincott Williams & Wilkins; 2004.
7.8 Rubin E, Farber JL. *Pathology*. 3rd ed. Philadelphia, PA: Lippincott Williams & Wilkins; 1999.
7.9 Anatomical Chart Co.
7.10 Anatomical Chart Co.
7.11 Anatomical Chart Co.
7.12 Anatomical Chart Co.
7.13 Anatomical Chart Co.
7.14 Moore KL, Dalley AF. *Clinically oriented anatomy*. 4th ed. Baltimore, MD: Lippincott Williams & Wilkins; 1999.

Chapter 8

8.2 A: Stocker JT, Dehner LP, Husain AN. *Stocker and Dehner's pediatric pathology*. 3rd ed. Philadelphia, PA: Lippincott Williams & Wilkins; 2010. B: Rubin R, Strayer DS. *Rubin's pathology: clinicopathologic foundations of medicine*. 5th ed. Philadelphia, PA: Lippincott Williams & Wilkins; 2008.
8.3 Moore KL, Agur AMR, Dalley AF. *Clinically oriented anatomy*. 7th ed. Philadelphia, PA: Lippincott Williams & Wilkins; 2013.
8.4 Anatomical Chart Co.
8.6 Anatomical Chart Co.
8.7 Anatomical Chart Co.
8.8 Anatomical Chart Co.
8.9 Rubin E, Farber JL. *Pathology*. 3rd ed. Philadelphia, PA: Lippincott Williams & Wilkins; 1999.
8.10 Anatomical Chart Co.
8.11 Anatomical Chart Co.
8.12 LifeART.
8.13 Anatomical Chart Co.
8.14 Sun T. *Parasitic disorders: pathology, diagnosis, and management*. 2nd ed. Philadelphia, PA: Lippincott Williams & Wilkins; 1999.
8.15 Rubin E, Farber JL. *Pathology*. 3rd ed. Philadelphia, PA: Lippincott Williams & Wilkins; 1999.
8.17 Rubin E, Farber JL. *Pathology*. 3rd ed. Philadelphia, PA: Lippincott Williams & Wilkins; 1999.
8.18 Anatomical Chart Co.
8.19 LWW's Organism Central.

Chapter 9

9.1 Anatomical Chart Co.
9.2 Adapted from Rosdahl CB, Kowalski MT. *Textbook of basic nursing*. 10th ed. Philadelphia, PA: Lippincott Williams & Wilkins; 2011.
9.3 Smeltzer SC, Bare BG. *Brunner & Suddarth's textbook of medical-surgical nursing*. 9th ed. Philadelphia, PA: Lippincott Williams & Wilkins; 2000.
9.5 Weber J, Kelley J. *Health assessment in nursing*. 2nd ed. Philadelphia, PA: Lippincott Williams & Wilkins; 2003.
9.7 Anatomical Chart Co.

Chapter 10

10.1 Adapted from LifeART.
10.3 Rubin E, Gorstein F, Schwarting R, et al. *Rubin's pathology: clinicopathologic foundations of medicine*. 4th ed. Philadelphia, PA: Lippincott Williams & Wilkins; 2005.
10.4 Anatomical Chart Co.
10.5 Anatomical Chart Co.
10.6 Creason C. *Stedman's medical terminology*. Philadelphia, PA: Lippincott Williams & Wilkins; 2010.
10.7 Anatomical Chart Co.
10.8 Porth CM. *Essentials of pathophysiology*. 3rd ed. Philadelphia, PA: Lippincott Williams & Wilkins; 2010.

10.9 Jenkins B. *Step-up to USMLE Step 1*. 6th ed. Philadelphia, PA: Lippincott Williams & Wilkins; 2013.
10.10 Anatomical Chart Co.
10.11 Anatomical Chart Co.

Chapter 11

11.1 Modified from Anatomical Chart Co.
11.2 Modified from Anatomical Chart Co.
11.3 Anatomical Chart Co.
11.4 Anatomical Chart Co.
11.5 Anatomical Chart Co.
11.6 Adapted from Anatomical Chart Co.
11.7 Anatomical Chart Co.
11.8 Adapted from Anatomical Chart Co.
11.9 Mitchell GW. *The female breast and its disorders*. Baltimore, MD: Lippincott Williams & Wilkins; 1990.
11.10 Anatomical Chart Co.
11.11 Anatomical Chart Co.
11.12 Rubin E, Gorstein F, Schwarting R, et al. *Rubin's pathology: clinicopathologic foundations of medicine*. 4th ed. Philadelphia, PA: Lippincott Williams & Wilkins; 2005.
11.14 Anatomical Chart Co.
11.16 A, B, D: Anatomical Chart Co. C: McClatchey KD. *Clinical laboratory medicine*. 2nd ed. Philadelphia, PA: Lippincott Williams & Wilkins; 2002.
11.17 Anatomical Chart Co.

Chapter 12

12.1 Anatomical Chart Co.
12.2 A: Lippincott's Nursing Advisor 2012. B: *Wound care made incredibly visual!* 2nd ed. Philadelphia, PA: Lippincott Williams & Wilkins; 2011. C: Adapted from Stein SM. *Boh's pharmacy practice manual: a guide to the clinical experience*. 4th ed. (From the patient information Web site of Cancer Research UK: http://www.cancerresearchuk.org/cancer-help.) Philadelphia, PA: Lippincott Williams & Wilkins; 2014.
12.3 Gold DH, Weingeist TA. *Color atlas of the eye in systemic disease*. Philadelphia, PA: Lippincott Williams & Wilkins; 2001.
12.4 Rubin E, Gorstein F, Schwarting R, et al. *Rubin's pathology: clinicopathologic foundations of medicine*. 4th ed. Philadelphia, PA: Lippincott Williams & Wilkins; 2005.
12.5 Photo by Stephen Fischer. Courtesy Tracy Walton & Associates, LLC, www.tracywalton.com

Index

A

B

C

D

E

H

J

K

L

M

P

Q

R

S

T